KRUGMAN'S

INFECTIOUS DISEASES OF CHILDREN

ELEVENTH EDITION

ANNE A. GERSHON, MD
PROFESSOR OF PEDIATRICS;
DIRECTOR, DIVISION OF INFECTIOUS DISEASES,
COLLEGE OF PHYSICIANS AND SURGEONS,
COLUMBIA UNIVERSITY,
NEW YORK, NEW YORK

PETER J. HOTEZ, MD, PhD
PROFESSOR AND CHAIR,
DEPARTMENT OF MICROBIOLOGY AND TROPICAL MEDICINE;
PROFESSOR OF GLOBAL HEALTH, EPIDEMIOLOGY,
INTERNATIONAL AFFAIRS AND HUMAN SCIENCES,
THE GEORGE WASHINGTON UNIVERSITY,
WASHINGTON, DC

SAMUEL L. KATZ, MD
WILBURT C. DAVISON PROFESSOR AND CHAIRMAN EMERITUS,
DEPARTMENT OF PEDIATRICS,
DUKE UNIVERSITY MEDICAL CENTER,
DURHAM, NORTH CAROLINA

WITH *186* ILLUSTRATIONS AND *54* COLOR PLATES

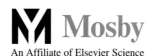
Mosby
An Affiliate of Elsevier Science

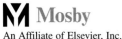 Mosby

An Affiliate of Elsevier, Inc.

The Curtis Center
Independence Square West
Philadelphia, Pennsylvania 19106

Krugman's Infectious Diseases of Children, 11th edition   ISBN 0-323-01756-8
Copyright © 2004, Mosby, Inc. All rights reserved.

Notice

Pediatrics is an ever-changing field. Standard safety precautions must be followed, but as new research and clinical experience broaden our knowledge, changes in treatment and drug therapy may become necessary or appropriate. Readers are advised to check the most current product information provided by the manufacturer of each drug to be administered to verify the recommended dose, the method and duration of administration, and contraindications. It is the responsibility of the licensed prescriber, relying on experience and knowledge of the patient, to determine dosages and the best treatment for each individual patient. Neither the publisher nor the author assumes any liability for any injury and/or damage to persons or property arising from this publication.

Previous editions copyrighted 1958, 1960, 1964, 1968, 1973, 1977, 1981, 1985, 1992, 1998

Library of Congress Cataloging-in-Publication Data

Krugman's infectious diseases of children—11th ed. / [edited by] Anne A. Gershon, Peter J. Hotez, Samuel L. Katz.
    p.; cm.
   Includes bibliographical references and index.
   ISBN 0-323-01756-8
    1. Communicable diseases in children. I. Title: Infectious diseases of children. II.
  Krugman, Saul, 1911-III. Gershon, Anne A. IV. Hotez, Peter J. V. Katz, Samuel L.,
  1927-
   [DNLM: 1. Communicable Diseases—Child. 2. Communicable Diseases—Infant. WC
  100 K931 2004]
  RJ401.K7 2004
  618.92′9—dc22
                                  2003059984

Acquisitions Editor: Judith Fletcher
Developmental Editor: Andrew C. Hall
Publishing Services Manager: Pat Joiner
Project Manager: Karen M. Rehwinkel
Senior Designer: Mark A. Oberkrom

Printed in the United States of America

Last digit is the print number: 9 8 7 6 5 4 3 2 1

CONTRIBUTORS

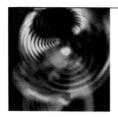

Stuart P. Adler, MD
Professor and Chair,
Division of Pediatric Infectious Diseases,
Virginia Commonwealth University,
Medical College of Virginia Campus,
Richmond, Virginia

Paula W. Annunziato, MD
Director, Biologics Clinical Research,
Merck & Co., Inc.
West Point, Pennsylvania

Carol J. Baker, MD
Professor of Pediatrics,
Molecular Virology and Immunology;
Head, Section of Infectious Diseases,
Department of Pediatrics,
Baylor College of Medicine,
Houston, Texas

William Borkowsky, MD
Department of Pediatrics,
New York University School of Medicine,
New York, New York

Kenneth Boyer, MD
Chairman, Department of Pediatrics;
Chief, Division of Pediatric Infectious Diseases,
Rush Presbyterian St. Luke's Medical Center
and Rush University School of Medicine,
Chicago, Illinois

Kenneth Bromberg, MD
Vice Chairman, Community Pediatrics;
Attending Physician, Pediatric Infectious
Diseases,
The Children's Hospital at Downstate;
Professor of Clinical Pediatrics,
Associate Professor, Microbiology,
Immunology, and Medicine,
Downstate Medical Center,
Brooklyn, New York

Margaret Burroughs, MD
Clinical Project Director,
Hepatology/Gastroenterology,
Schering-Plough Research Institute,
Kenilworth, New Jersey

Stephen J. Chanock, MD
Senior Investigator, Pediatric Oncology
Branch,
National Cancer Institute,
National Institutes of Health,
Bethesda, Maryland

James D. Cherry, MD, MSc
Professor of Pediatrics,
David Geffen School of Medicine at UCLA,
University of California at Los Angeles;
Attending Physician,
Mattel Children's Hospital at UCLA,
Los Angeles, California

Thomas G. Cleary, MD
Director, Division of Infectious Diseases,
Department of Pediatrics,
The University of Texas Medical School,
Houston, Texas

Dennis A. Clements, MD, PhD
Professor, Primary Care and Infectious
Diseases,
Department of Pediatrics,
Duke University Medical Center,
Durham, North Carolina

Johanna P. Daily, MD
Instructor in Medicine,
Harvard Medical School;
Associate Physician, Brigham and Women's
    Hospital;
Instructor in Immunology in Infectious
    Disease,
Harvard School of Public Health,
Boston, Massachusetts

Gail J. Demmler, MD
Professor of Pediatrics,
Baylor College of Medicine;
Attending Physician, Infectious Diseases
    Service;
Director, Diagnostic Virology Laboratory,
Texas Children's Hospital,
Houston, Texas

Emily DiMango, MD
Department of Medicine,
College of Physicians and Surgeons,
Columbia University,
New York, New York

Morven S. Edwards, MD
Professor, Department of Pediatrics,
Baylor College of Medicine,
Houston, Texas

Anne A. Gershon, MD
Professor of Pediatrics;
Director, Division of Infectious Diseases,
College of Physicians and Surgeons,
Columbia University,
New York, New York

Laura Gutman, MD
Infectious Diseases Division, Department of
    Pediatrics,
Duke University Medical Center,
Durham, North Carolina

Caroline Breese Hall, MD
Professor of Pediatrics and Medicine in
    Infectious Diseases,
Departments of Pediatrics and Medicine,
University of Rochester School of Medicine
    and Dentistry,
Rochester, New York

Margaret R. Hammerschlag, MD
Professor of Pediatrics and Medicine;
Director, Division of Pediatric Infectious
    Diseases,
SUNY Downstate Medical Center,
Brooklyn, New York

Maria-Arantxa Horga, MD
Assistant Professor of Pediatrics,
Mount Sinai School of Medicine,
New York, New York

Margaret K. Hostetter, MD
Professor of Pediatrics and Microbial
    Pathogenesis;
Chair, Department of Pediatrics,
Yale University School of Medicine,
New Haven, Connecticut

Peter J. Hotez, MD, PhD
Professor and Chair,
Department of Microbiology and Tropical
    Medicine;
Professor of Global Health, Epidemiology,
    International Affairs and Human Sciences,
The George Washington University,
Washington, DC

Shirley Jankelevich, MD
Division of AIDS,
National Institute of Allergy and Infectious
    Diseases,
National Institute of Health,
Department of Health and Human Services,
Besthesda, Maryland

Niranjan Kanesa-Thasan, MD, MTMH
Chief, Clinical Studies Department, Medical
    Division,
US Army Medical Research Institute of
    Infectious Diseases,
Fort Detrick, Maryland;
Attending Staff, Walter Reed Army Medical
    Center,
Washington, DC;
Adjunct Assistant Professor, Preventive
    Medicine and Biometrics,
Uniformed Services University of the Health
    Sciences,
Bethesda, Maryland

Barrett Katz, MD, MBA
Professor and Chair,
Department of Ophthalmology,
The George Washington University Medical
    Center,
Washington, DC

Ben Z. Katz, MD
Associate Professor,
Department of Pediatrics,
Northwestern University Medical School;
Attending Physician,
Children's Memorial Hospital,
Chicago, Illinois

Samuel L. Katz, MD
Wilburt C. Davison Professor and Chairman
    Emeritus,
Department of Pediatrics,
Duke University Medical Center,
Durham, North Carolina

Jerome O. Klein, MD
Department of Pediatrics,
Boston University School of Medicine;
Maxwell Finland Laboratory for Infectious
    Diseases,
Boston Medical Center,
Boston, Massachusetts

William C. Koch, MD
Associate Professor of Pediatrics,
Division of Pediatric Infectious Diseases,
Virginia Commonwealth University,
Medical College of Virginia Campus,
Richmond, Virginia

Keith M. Krasinski, MD
Professor of Pediatrics and Environmental
    Medicine,
New York University School of Medicine,
New York, New York

Saul Krugman, MD†
Professor and Chairman Emeritus,
Department of Pediatrics,
New York University Medical Center,
New York, New York

Philip LaRussa, MD
Professor of Clinical Pediatrics,
College of Physicians and Surgeons,
Columbia University,
New York, New York

Sarah S. Long, MD
Professor of Pediatrics,
Drexel University College of Medicine;
Chief, Section of Infectious Diseases,
St. Christopher's Hospital for Children,
Philadelphia, Pennsylvania

George H. McCracken, Jr., MD
Professor of Pediatrics,
GlaxoSmithKline Distinguished Professor of
    Pediatric Infectious Disease,
The Sarah M. and Charles E. Seay Chair in
    Pediatric Infectious Disease,
University of Texas Southwestern Medical
    Center at Dallas,
Dallas, Texas

Rima McLeod, MD
Jules and Doris Stein RPB Professor,
The University of Chicago,
Chicago, Illinois

George Miller, MD
John F. Enders Professor of Pediatric
    Infectious Diseases;
Professor of Epidemiology and Molecular
    Biophysics and Biochemistry,
Department of Pediatrics,
Yale University School of Medicine,
New Haven, Connecticut

John F. Modlin, MD
Professor of Pediatrics and Medicine;
Chair, Department of Pediatrics,
Dartmouth Medical School;
Medical Director, Children's Hospital at
    Dartmouth,
Dartmouth-Hitchcock Medical Center,
Lebanon, New Hampshire

Edward A. Mortimer, Jr., MD†
Professor Emeritus,
Department of Epidemiology and Biostatistics,
Case Western Reserve University,
Cleveland, Ohio

Anne Moscona, MD
Professor of Pediatrics,
Vice Chair for Research,
Department of Pediatrics,
Mount Sinai School of Medicine,
New York, New York

Matthew T. Murrell, BA, MD
PhD Candidate,
Department of Pediatrics,
Mount Sinai School of Medicine,
New York, New York

Larry K. Pickering, MD, FAAP
Senior Advisor to the Director,
National Immunization Program,
Centers for Disease Control and Prevention,
Atlanta, Georgia

Stanley A. Plotkin, MD
Emeritus Professor of Pediatrics,
University of Pennsylvania;
Philadelphia, Pennsylvania;
Medical and Scientific Consultant,
   Aventis Pasteur,
Doylestown, Pennsylvania

Alice S. Prince, MD
Professor of Pediatrics,
College of Physicians and Surgeons,
Columbia University,
New York, New York

Sarah A. Rawstron, MB, BS
Attending Physician, Pediatric Infectious
   Diseases,
The Children's Hospital at Downstate;
Assistant Professor, Pediatrics,
Downstate Medical Center,
Brooklyn, New York

Fiona Roberts, BSc, MD, MRC
Path Consultant and Honorary Clinical Senior
   Lecturer in Ophthalmic Pathologist,
University Department of Pathology,
Western Infirmary,
Glasgow, Scotland, United Kingdom

Anne H. Rowley, MD
Professor of Pediatrics and
   Microbiology/Immunology,
Northwestern University Feinberg School of
   Medicine;
Attending Physician, Division of Infectious
   Diseases,
The Children's Memorial Hospital,
Chicago, Illinois

Edward T. Ryan, MD, DTM&H
Director, Tropical and Geographic Medicine
   Center,
Division of Infectious Diseases,
Massachusetts General Hospital and
   Massachusetts General Hospital for
   Children;
Assistant Professor of Medicine,
Harvard Medical School;
Assistant Professor of Public Health,
Department of Immunology and Infectious
   Diseases,
Harvard School of Public Health,
Boston, Massachusetts

Xavier Sáez-Llorens, MD
Professor of Pediatrics,
University of Panama School of Medicine;
Vice-Chairman and Head,
Division of Pediatric Infectious Diseases,
Hospital del Niño,
Panama City, Republic of Panama

Lisa Saiman, MD, MPH
Columbia University,
Department of Pediatrics,
Division of Pediatric Infectious Diseases,
The Children's Hospital of New York,
New York, New York

Mohammed Abdus Salam, MBBS
Chief Physician,
Clinical Research and Service Centre Scientist,
Head, Clinical Sciences Division,
International Centre for Diarrheal Disease
   Research, Bangladesh (ICDDR, B),
Dhaka, Bangladesh

Eugene D. Shapiro, MD
Professor of Pediatrics, Epidemiology and
   Investigative Medicine,
Yale University School of Medicine,
New Haven, Connecticut

Robert E. Shope, MD
Professor of Pathology,
Center for Tropical Diseases,
University of Texas Medical Branch,
Galveston, Texas

Jeffrey R. Starke, MD
Professor of Pediatrics,
Department of Pediatrics,
Baylor College of Medicine,
Houston, Texas

James K. Todd, MD
Professor of Pediatrics, Microbiology, and
    Preventative Medicine/Biometrics,
University of Colorado School of Medicine;
Director of Epidemiology, Clinical
    Microbiology, and Clinical Outcomes,
Denver, Colorado

David W. Vaughn, MD
Director, Military Infectious Diseases Research
    Program,
US Army Medical Research and Materiel
    Command,
Fort Detrick, Maryland

Gonzalo Vicente, MD
Assistant Clinical Professor of Ophthalmology,
Department of Ophthalmology,
The George Washington University,
Washington, DC;
Attending Physician,
Department of Ophthalmology,
Boston Children's Hospital,
Boston, Massachusetts;
University Ophthalmic Consultants,
Chevy Chase, Maryland

Kathleen McKenna Vozzelli, MD
Staff Physician,
Department of Pediatrics,
Division of Infectious Diseases,
The Barbara Bush Children's Hospital,
Maine Medical Center,
Portland, Maine

Melinda Wharton, MD, MPH
Director, Epidemiology and Surveillance
    Division,
National Immunization Program,
Centers for Disease Control and Prevention,
Atlanta, Georgia

Richard J. Whitley, MD
Leob Professor of Pediatrics;
Professor of Pediatrics, Microbiology,
    Medicine and Neurosurgery,
The University of Alabama at Birmingham,
Birmingham, Alabama

Catherine Wilfert, MD
Professor Emerita,
Pediatrics and Virology,
Duke University Medical Center,
Durham, North Carolina;
Scientific Director,
Elizabeth Glaser Pediatric AIDS Foundation,
Santa Monica, California

To Sylvia Stern Krugman
(1912-2002)

For nine editions she was the critical editor (behind the scene) who improved much of the syntax, vocabulary, and grammar of many chapters. For 55 years she enriched the life of her partner, our mentor Saul, whose leadership and knowledge guided this book for 37 years through its continuing evolution.

To my husband, Dr. Michael Gershon, and our children and grandchildren.
AAG

To my wife, Ann Hotez, and our children.
PJH

To my wife, Dr. Catherine Wilfert, and all our children and grandchildren.
SLK

PREFACE

Each year the World Health Organization prepares a new edition of *The World Health Report*, a document that distills and analyzes vast amounts of data in order to provide an annual summary of the state of global health. *The World Health Report 2002* provides a chilling reminder of the devastating toll of infectious diseases on child health. This year we learned that infections are still the leading killers of children. It was reported that more than 1 million children died from falciparum malaria, and almost 750,000 children died from measles. Together, pertussis and tetanus killed more than 500,000 children. Children also comprised the majority of the estimated 2 million people who died from infectious diarrheas and the more than 3 million who perished from lower respiratory infections.

To better assess the disease burden caused by different conditions, *The World Health Report 2002* measured not only the numbers of deaths caused by disease, but also the impact of non-fatal illnesses that cause disability and, ultimately, shorten lifespan. The Disability-Adjusted Life Year, or "DALY," is a health gap measure that combines this information in order to compare more than 100 different conditions. One DALY is considered equivalent to 1 lost year of healthy life. Based on DALY estimates, we learned that a list of non-fatal infectious diseases, such as helminth infections, dengue, and trachoma, further adds to the misery of children growing up in developing countries.

For this eleventh edition of *Krugman's Infectious Diseases of Children,* we believed it was important to expand our commitment to the health of all children by adding new chapters on major childhood and emerging infectious disease problems in the developing world. For the first time we have included chapters on cholera, dengue fever, helminth infections, and malaria. In addition, the chapter on smallpox and vaccinia provides the latest recommendations on use of the vaccine in our post 9-11 era. Finally, we have both extensively revised and updated all of the chapters from the previous edition. Many of these chapters have new authors. We believe that the final product is a highly readable and balanced single-volume textbook that will be used by pediatric practitioners, house officers in training, and students in all of the health sciences.

The days and weeks following September 11, 2001 were a wake-up call to the medical community that all health issues are global in scope. This edition of *Krugman's Infectious Diseases of Children* provides concise yet detailed information on the natural history, management, and treatment of the major infections affecting children worldwide. We hope it is a fitting tribute to the legacy of Dr. Saul Krugman, a pioneer of medical science, whose thoughts, discoveries, and writings had direct relevance to the health of children worldwide.

Anne A. Gershon
Peter J. Hotez
Samuel L. Katz

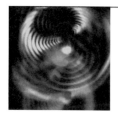

CONTENTS

†Deceased

[†]Deceased.

KRUGMAN'S

INFECTIOUS DISEASES OF CHILDREN

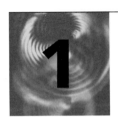

ACQUIRED IMMUNODEFICIENCY SYNDROME AND HUMAN IMMUNODEFICIENCY VIRUS

WILLIAM BORKOWSKY

In 1980 an outbreak of community-acquired *Pneumocystis carinii* pneumonia (PCP) was recognized in California and New York, and, simultaneously, Kaposi's sarcoma was recognized to be occurring at 50 times the expected rate in male homosexuals. These events combined to define an immunodeficiency syndrome never before described. This syndrome was soon observed in intravenous drug users, recipients (both male and female) of standard blood products, and non–drug-using female sex partners of individuals with the disease.

In 1982 an *acquired immunodeficiency syndrome* (AIDS) was recognized in children (Centers for Disease Control and Prevention [CDC], 1982); occurrences in New Jersey (Oleske et al., 1983), New York (Rubinstein et al., 1983), San Francisco (Ammann et al., 1983), and Miami (Scott et al., 1984), were described. In less than a decade a previously unknown disease became the single most important communicable disease in the United States and many other nations, a position it still holds today. Although pediatric human immunodeficiency virus (HIV) infection makes up only 2% of the total number of reported cases of AIDS in the United States, the rapid increase in reported cases in children and the emergence of the virus as a cause of death in young infants and children are clear.

ETIOLOGY

The causative agents of AIDS were isolated from the blood of patients and were described by researchers in both France (Barre-Sinoussi et al., 1983) and the United States (Gallo et al., 1984; Levy et al., 1984). These researchers referred to the viruses as the *lymphadenopathy-associated viruses* (LAV), the *human T-cell lymphotropic viruses* (HTLV-III), and the *AIDS-related retroviruses* (ARV), respectively.

By consensus these agents now are termed the HIVs. These enveloped RNA viruses are in the lentivirus subfamily of retroviruses and are 80 to 120 nm in diameter. Characteristics of HIV that resemble those of lentiviruses include (1) the long incubation period; (2) the ability to establish latent or persistent infection; (3) the ability to produce immunosuppression; (4) a tropism to lymphoid cells, particularly macrophages; (5) the ability to affect the hematopoietic system; (6) a tropism to the central nervous system (CNS); and (7) the ability to produce cytopathic effects observed in appropriate cell types (Bryant and Ratner, 1991). The major targets of HIV are CD4-antigen–bearing cells such as helper T cells, monocytes and macrophages, Langerhans cells, and glial cells of the CNS. HIV has also been reported to be capable of infecting non–CD4-bearing cells such as enterocytes and certain neuronal cells. Virtually all individuals with primary HIV infection have viruses, isolated from peripheral blood mononuclear cells, which are monocytotropic and do not multiply in T-cell leukemia cell lines. As the infection progresses over the years and immune function fails, viruses capable of multiplying in T-cell lines such as HUT-76 and CEM emerge. Those viruses that grow very rapidly in tissue culture and to high titer have been described as *syncytium-inducing* viruses or *rapid-high isolates*. The monocytotropic isolates are said to be *non–syncytium inducing*.

In vivo, virus production from infected lymphocytes continues for a relatively short time (i.e., a viral half life of 1.6 days) (Ho et al., 1995), with 99% of virus production coming from recently infected cells (30% to 50% of virions in the plasma have come from a CD4 T cell infected the previous day).

HIV has a cylindrical eccentric core, or nucleoid, that contains the diploid RNA genome (Figure 1-1). A nucleic acid–binding protein and reverse transcriptase are associated with the genome. Nucleocapsid structure is completed by the capsid antigen (p24), which encloses the nucleoid components. Surrounding the core of the virus is p17, the matrix antigen, which lines the inner surface of the envelope. Knoblike projections formed by the envelope glycoprotein, gp120, are on the surface of the virus. An associated intermembranous portion of the envelope, gp41, anchors the gp120 component.

A portion of the gp120 domain of the envelope binds to the CD4 molecule of human cells with high affinity, and a segment of the gp41 plays a crucial role in the fusion of the viral envelope with the host cell (Figure 1-2). Several non-CD4 antigens also play an important role in viral entry. These include the fusin molecule (CXCR4) in T cells (Feng et al., 1996) and a chemokine receptor (CCR-5) on monocyte-macrophage lineage cells (Deng et al., 1996) and activated T cells. After viral entry and uncoating, the reverse transcriptase characteristic of all retroviruses produces double-stranded virally encoded DNA that enters the nucleus and integrates randomly in the host genome by using the long–terminal repeat (LTR) segments

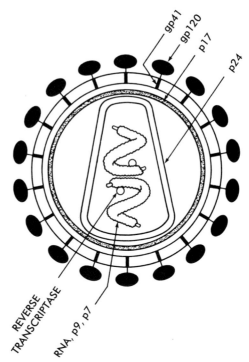

Fig. 1-1 Schematic representation of the morphologic structure of HIV-1. ENV gene products, gp120 and gp41; gag gene products, p24, p17, p9, and p7; pol gene product, RT.

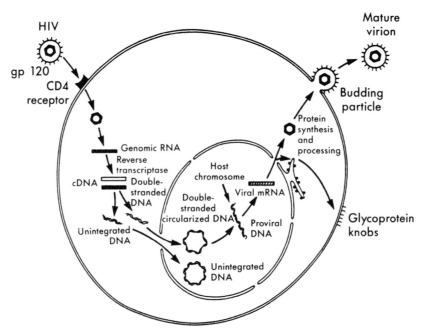

Fig. 1-2 The life cycle of the human immunodeficiency virus. (From Pizzo P, Wilfert CM [eds]: Pediatric AIDS. Baltimore, Williams & Wilkins, 1991.)

that flank the other genes of the virus. The virus is then in a latent state, in which it may remain indefinitely. A variety of stimuli—including antigens, mitogens, ultraviolet light, heat shock, hypoxia, and proteins derived from other viruses—are capable of initiating the transcription of HIV messenger RNA, which is first translated into complex spliced messages. These encode a group of regulatory molecules that ultimately govern the production of HIV messenger RNA capable of producing full-length transcripts and the associated structural proteins. The ribonucleoprotein core buds from the cellular membrane and acquires a coat of viral envelope glycoprotein and the lipid bilayer from the host cell. A viral enzyme (protease) completes the maturation of the virion by cleaving specific internal core components.

The individual isolates of HIV-1 from different persons vary a great deal. There is also considerable variation between sequential isolates obtained from the same infected person. HIV can spread from cell to cell independent of release of virus from the cell. This spread may occur through syncytial formation or fusion of an infected cell and uninfected cell(s).

PATHOGENESIS

HIV infection in children is characterized by an incubation period or asymptomatic interval that may be much shorter than it is in adults, but is not always so. The inevitable consequence of infection with HIV is profound immunosuppression, which leaves the host susceptible to the development of infections and neoplasms.

T4 Cells

The depletion of helper T cells (CD4) in symptomatic patients has been noted since 1981. HIV is capable of causing a profound cytopathic effect in T4 cells in vitro. However, only a small proportion of cells are infected with the virus, and not all are killed. Uninfected cells also die by a process of programmed cell death, such as apoptosis, or are dysfunctional; this may be mediated by the binding of gp120 to CD4, which interferes with its essential association with major histocompatibility complex (MHC) class II molecules. The virus is capable of establishing latency or a low level of replication in some cells.

T4-cell depletion is due in part to direct virus-induced damage, and there is some indication that "memory" helper T cells are more selectively depleted than "virgin" cells as a result of selective replication in the former cell type. The budding of large numbers of virus particles disrupting the external cell membrane contributes to destruction of the cell by creating osmotic disequilibrium. HIV replication results in the accumulation of a number of foreign products, including viral DNA, RNA, and core proteins, which may interfere with normal cellular function and contribute to the death of the cell. Syncytia, or multinucleated giant cells, are observed in vitro with HIV replication. Such syncytia can form when CD4 molecules of uninfected T4 cells bind to the gp120 expressed on the surface of HIV-infected T4 cells. It is unknown whether syncytial formation contributes to cell death. The functional abnormalities of T4 cells from HIV-infected individuals are numerous despite the fact that the virus is present in only a small percentage of circulating T4 cells. These abnormalities include (1) defective helper interaction with B cells for immunoglobulin production; (2) defective proliferative responses to antigenic stimuli; (3) diminished expression of interleukin (IL-2) receptors; and (4) defective lymphokine production in response to antigenic stimuli, particularly of IL-2 and gamma interferon. These defects would be expected to predispose infected persons to infections with intracellular pathogens.

In the course of a normal immune response the CD4 molecule binds to the class II MHC molecules on the surface of an antigen-presenting immune cell. However, the CD4 molecule binds to gp120 of HIV with a greater affinity than for its normal ligand (class II MHC molecules). This high-affinity binding of gp120 to CD4 may contribute to the impaired T-cell responses and may also be the basis of autoimmune reactions that destroy T4 cells. The gp41 of the virus possesses a region of homology with the class II MHC molecule. Anti-gp41 HIV antibodies from AIDS patients can react with class II MHC antigens and may therefore be involved in cytotoxicity or complement-mediated cell killing of uninfected target cells carrying only the class II MHC molecule. Antibody-dependent cellular cytotoxicity (ADCC) may contribute to cell death of both infected cells and uninfected cells. If an uninfected T4 cell binds free gp120 to its surface, the cell can be mistakenly identified as infected and subsequently be destroyed by ADCC or by gp120-specific, CD4-positive cytotoxic T cells. It has also been noted that HIV-infected T4 cells can kill adjacent uninfected T4 cells in vitro. It is estimated that as many as 2 billion cells (i.e., 5% of the total CD4 T-cell population) are destroyed daily. To maintain constant CD4 T-cell numbers, comparable numbers of cells must be produced daily. The thymus is the major source of new T cells, and its productive capacity in children and young adolescents is superior to that seen in the adult thymus gland (Zhang et al., 1999).

T8 Cells

Soon after HIV infection, CD8+ T cells increase in frequency and number. In addition, these cells appear to be activated (Plaeger-Marshall S et al., 1993), most likely by HIV (Landay et al., 1993), but perhaps also by herpes viruses. Some of these cells may perform as cytotoxic T cells (Koup et al., 1994); others may inhibit viral replication in the absence of cytotoxicity (Walker et al., 1986).

Monocyte, Macrophage, and Dendritic Cells

HIV also infects cells of the CD4-expressing monocyte-macrophage lineage. The virus is not cytopathic to these cells but may interfere in their ability to present antigens to helper T cells. Intact virus particles may replicate to high numbers in these cells and may also be disseminated to tissues such as the brain, spinal cord, lung, bone marrow, liver, heart, and gut, where soluble virus products may produce organ dysfunction. Alternatively, virus particles may be borne to tissues wherein they replicate directly, thereby producing cell damage. These infected cells may also produce increased quantities of IL-1, IL-6, prostaglandins, and other molecules that may affect adjacent cell functions.

HIV has been shown to adhere to antigen-processing dendritic cells at high concentration but not to replicate in them. The virus binds to a specific antigen, called DC-SIGN, allowing it to be protected from the environment and allowing for prolonged infectivity (Geijtenbeek et al., 2000). This probably serves as an important source of infection to T4 cells that come in contact with them.

B Cells

No spontaneously infected B cells have been observed in vivo, although some B lymphocytes bear CD4 on their surfaces and can be infected in vitro. Nevertheless, HIV infection results in profound effects on B-cell function. In vitro the HIV envelope can induce polyclonal B-cell activation (Pahwa et al., 1985). It may also produce increased IL-6 production by other cells, with resulting hypergammaglobulinemia. In spite of the observed hypergammaglobulinemia that is commonly seen, both primary and secondary antibody responses to some antigens may be impaired (Bernstein et al., 1985b), contributing to the high incidence of infection with common bacterial pathogens. The B-cell impairment often is observed in association with impaired T-cell responses to the same antigens (Borkowsky et al., 1987), and these findings are correlated with a poorer clinical outcome (Blanche et al., 1986).

Neutrophils

Although neutrophils are not directly infected by HIV, autoimmune neutropenias have been observed and neutrophil dysfunction has been described (Roilides et al., 1990). This defect may contribute to the immunodeficiency-related infections that occur.

PATHOLOGY

The primary pathologic effects of HIV infection are seen in the lymphoreticular system, in which marked cell depletion is the end-stage pathology. HIV probably infects the epithelial cells of the thymus, and thymitis has been described. This initial inflammatory response is characterized by multinucleated giant cells in the medulla of the thymus or by diffuse lymphoplasmocytic or lymphomononuclear infiltrates of the cortex and medulla. These changes precede the involution noted in end-stage disease. The involution is characterized by depletion of lymphocytes, loss of corticomedullary differentiation, and microcystic dilation of Hassall's corpuscles (Joshi, 1991). In a few instances a reduction of Hassall's corpuscles has also been described, and this constellation is termed *dysinvolution*. The severe effects of the virus on the thymus of the young infant or fetus may contribute to the more rapid progression of the immunologic compromise. It is likely that thymic dysfunction continues to contribute to illness in adult life.

Lymphoproliferation in lymph nodes, the gastrointestinal tract, and lungs has been observed. It is now known that the concentration of HIV in these nodes vastly exceeds that seen in peripheral blood lymphocytes. Multinucleated giant cells are present. Late in the disease, lymph nodes are depleted of lymphocytes in the paracortex, ultimately progressing to marked lymphocyte depletion of the entire lymph node. Atrophic changes of the spleen, appendix, and Peyer's patches are also described in late stages. The pathologic features in the brain include atrophy; sclerosis; microglial nodules; and necrosis, with or without an inflammatory cell infiltrate, loss of myelin, vasculitis, and calcification of vessels and basal ganglia (Sharer, et al., 1985; Sharer et al., 1986). The virus has been localized by in situ hybridization in macrophages, microglia, and giant cells and less frequently in glial cells and neurons (Shaw et al., 1985; Stoler et al., 1986). Brain atrophy with compensatory ventricular dilatation is a common finding in children with clinically evident encephalopathy.

Opportunistic infections and malignancies of the CNS are infrequently seen in children. Pathologic findings associated with a broad spectrum of infectious agents—including *P. carinii* in the lungs, *Candida* infection of the mucous membranes, *Mycobacterium avium-intracellulare* in almost all tissues, and cryptosporidiosis of the gastrointestinal tract—are seen in biopsy and autopsy specimens. Viruses that are common causes of infection include herpes simplex virus (HSV), cytomegalovirus (CMV), Epstein-Barr virus (EBV), and varicella-zoster virus (VZV). In contrast to adults, infections with human herpes virus 8 (HHV8), the probable agent causative of Kaposi's sarcoma, rarely is found in HIV-infected children in the USA but can be seen in children from Africa.

Other findings of undetermined pathogenesis appear frequently on tissue examinations. Dilated cardiomyopathy is observed with microscopic hypertrophy of myocardial fibers, focal vacuolation, interstitial edema, small foci of fibrosis, and endocardial thickening. Unusually sparse inflammatory infiltrates are seen.

Clinically important renal disease is accompanied by microscopic findings of focal segmental glomerulosclerosis and mesangial proliferative glomerulonephritis (Connor et al., 1988). Immunoglobulin and complement deposits are evident under immunofluorescence. It is speculated that circulating immune complexes may contribute to the pathogenesis of the renal disease. By in situ hybridization p24 antigen has been demonstrated in tubular and glomerular epithelial cells in renal biopsy specimens of adults.

Hepatobiliary disease is not uncommon. Unfortunately, a variety of causes (i.e., HIV, EBV, CMV, hepatitis C virus [HCV], drug toxicity) have been implicated, and it is rare that the liver histologic findings can clarify the process. Fatty infiltration, portal inflammation, lymphoplasmacytic inflammation, and cholestasis can be seen. Infection with CMV or *Cryptosporidium* has also been associated with cholecystitis and sclerosing cholangitis-like conditions.

A variety of neoplastic disorders of the gastrointestinal tract—including lymphoma, leiomyosarcoma, and Kaposi's sarcoma (rarely)—have been described. The first two appear to have EBV genome in the tumor cells. Longer survival of children may result in more frequent occurrence of malignancies.

LABORATORY DIAGNOSIS

Antibody to HIV can be measured accurately and is the mainstay of laboratory diagnosis of HIV infection in adults, in children perinatally infected who are more than 15 months old, and in children of any age who have acquired HIV infection through transfusion or blood products. The enzyme-linked immunosorbent assay (ELISA) and Western blot assay measure antibodies to the major structural proteins or antigens of the virus and are commercially available. A positive ELISA must be confirmed by a second assay plus a positive Western blot assay on the same specimen to reduce the rate of false positive results to approximately 1 in 100,000. Because all newborns receive maternal antibodies during the latter part of pregnancy through the placenta, any infant born to a mother with antibodies to HIV will also test positive, regardless of whether actually infected with HIV. The titer of maternal antibodies is usually high and may be detected in a dilution of 1 to several million. Because the half-life of IgG1, the predominant maternally transmitted immunoglobulin, is approximately 3 to 4 weeks, maternally derived anti-HIV antibody may persist for 15 or more months. Consequently, standard antibody assays for HIV may be misleading for the diagnosis of HIV infection in infants less than 18 months of age. Assays that measure IgA subclass HIV-specific antibodies may facilitate the serologic diagnosis of HIV infection in young infants between 2 months and 1 year of age.

HIV can be grown in tissue culture from the majority of HIV-infected adults and children. HIV is detected in peripheral blood mononuclear cells and as cell-free virus in plasma and cerebrospinal fluid. These cultures may prove positive as soon as 3 days after initiation but may require as long as 4 to 6 weeks for the diagnosis of low levels of virus. Early experience with attempts to isolate HIV from newborn or cord-blood lymphocytes suggests that no more than half of infected children are culture positive for HIV in the neonatal period. The HIV recovery rate increases substantially during the ensuing months, and almost all infected infants can be diagnosed by culture within the first 2 to 3 months of life. HIV core (p24) antigen can be detected in body fluids by ELISA. This antigen appears soon after HIV infection and then often becomes undetectable, associated with the appearance of anti-p24 antibody in most infected adults. The antigen reappears as the HIV infection progresses and can be found with increasing frequency in more symptomatic individuals. This antigen can be found in more than half of HIV-infected infants during the first year of life but in substantially fewer babies during the first months of life and in only 10% of infected newborns (Borkowsky et al., 1989). The measurement of p24 antigen may also help identify the 10% of HIV-infected hypogammaglobulinemic children who test negative for anti-HIV on ELISA (Borkowsky et al., 1987). Dissociation of anti-p24 antibodies from p24 antigen may increase the sensitivity of the assay during the first month of life (Miles et al., 1993; Chandwani et al., 1993).

One of the most sensitive diagnostic techniques is the polymerase chain reaction (PCR), a method by which the viral DNA can be amplified a million times. Viral culture and detection of viral DNA by PCR in infant blood appear to be equally sensitive as tests to diagnose infection in an infant. The sensitivity of PCR in early diagnosis of infection of infants born to HIV-infected mothers was first shown in a study conducted by the CDC in collaboration with the New York City Department of Health and several hospitals in New York (Rogers et al., 1989). Many subsequent studies have verified the sensitivity of PCR and have shown that it is comparable to HIV culture for early diagnosis. The technical problems with PCR relate to the extreme sensitivity of the test. Even very small amounts of contaminating DNA in the material tested can be amplified and result in either ambiguous or false-positive results. Modifications of the assay have made these inaccuracies less likely to occur. The test can be completed in <2 days. A licensed test to measure HIV RNA copy numbers also can be completed within this period and may prove even more sensitive than DNA PCR for early diagnosis.

Other nonspecific laboratory parameters that may be helpful in the diagnosis of infection include immunologic measurements. The classic hallmarks of infection are a low CD4 cell count and an altered CD4:CD8 ratio. Age-appropriate normal values must be used for comparison. Elevated serum immunoglobulin levels are characteristic of infection. A minority (approximately 10%) of untreated children may have hypogammaglobulinemia. These children usually have severe T-cell depletion.

Other assays for early detection of HIV infection in babies use measurement of antibody production by the infant. Several approaches have been used. Peripheral blood lymphocytes have been harvested and stimulated with pokeweed mitogen or EBV and the supernatant fluids tested for the production of specific HIV antibody (Amadori et al., 1988; Pahwa et al., 1989; Pollack et al., 1993). Alternatively, peripheral blood mononuclear cells have been placed into cell-culture wells containing HIV antigens. When labeled antihuman globulin is used, the cells producing antibody are identified by "spots" in the wells (Lee et al., 1989). Maternal IgA antibody does not cross the placenta, so the presence of HIV-specific antibody of this subclass indicates that an infant is infected. The presence of specific IgA antibody is being evaluated as a means of making an early diagnosis of HIV infection in young infants, and it has been detected in cohorts of infected infants by 6 months of age (Mann et al., 1994). The ability to make HIV-specific antibody does not become fully developed until a few months of age, well after HIV antigen or nucleic acid can be detected.

EPIDEMIOLOGY AND NATURAL HISTORY

The World Health Organization (WHO) estimates that as of 2000, 40 million adults and adolescents and 3 million children had been infected with HIV. Sub-Saharan Africa is home to 90% of those who are infected, but the disease is spreading rapidly in Eastern Europe and South and Southeast Asia. Sexual transmission is the major mode of spread of HIV-1 infection in most developing countries. In some African and Caribbean cities 15% to 50% of pregnant women are HIV seropositive. Bidirectional heterosexual transmission has been well documented. The incidence of heterosexual transmission is steadily increasing in the United States. Perinatal transmission parallels heterosexual transmission, because a substantial proportion of infected people are women of reproductive age. The male-female ratio of reported AIDS cases approaches 1 when heterosexual transmission of infection predominates, and the percentage of pediatric AIDS cases increases dramatically with this ratio (Centers for Disease Control and Prevention, 1995).

The risk factors associated with the development of AIDS among women are also risk factors for the transmission of HIV to infants and children. They include (1) intravenous drug use, which was an admitted risk behavior in almost 50% of HIV-infected women in the United States a decade ago but is now half that percentage; (2) heterosexual contact with a person who is HIV infected, which is the risk behavior of 40% of infected women in the United States (two thirds of the partners are admitted intravenous drug users; sexual exposure in prepubertal children may occur in the context of childhood sexual abuse [Gutman et al., 1991]); and (3) receiving infected blood products (whole blood and its components, including clotting factor concentrates). Although the screening of blood products for HIV antibody as of May 1984 has largely eliminated any transmission of HIV through blood products in the United States, such transmission continues to plague developing countries.

Perinatal Infection

In the United States the major risk factor for pediatric HIV infection is an infected mother. Black and Hispanic populations are disproportionately infected. In 1995, 84% of children reported to have AIDS were in these categories. In the U.S. population, lower socioeconomic status is also disproportionately represented (Centers for Disease Control and Prevention, 1995). HIV transmission probably can occur by more than one mechanism. There is evidence that in utero infection occurs, based on the recovery of HIV in cell culture from fetuses that have been aborted between weeks 9 and 20 of gestation (Sprecher et al., 1986; Kashkin et al., 1988; Jovais et al., 1985; Di Maria et al., 1986). Evidence of severe thymic depletion has been seen in such abortuses. These and other observations suggest that a portion of the cohort found to be infected perinatally is infected in utero. In Africa, studies of placentas demonstrated chorioamnionitis in placentas of women who delivered infected babies. These women had advanced HIV disease, and it is not possible to determine whether this inflammatory response was a result of secondary infection or a direct consequence of the severity of the HIV infection. Recovering HIV from placental tissue has been difficult, but HIV has been found in placentas by in situ hybridization (Chandwani, 1991) and by PCR (Andiman and Modlin, 1991). HIV has been demonstrated in placental macrophages (Hofbauer cells) in fetal villi. These cells could serve either as a barrier to or as a means of fetal HIV infection. The detection of HIV in the placenta does not predict whether an infant has acquired infection.

In spite of the timing of perinatal infection, virtually all newborns of HIV-infected mothers are born without obvious signs of clinical or immunologic abnormalities. Studies performed worldwide have found that 15% to 30% of children born to infected women will prove to be infected with HIV, even in the absence of breast-feeding. Yet half of this group cannot be shown to have evidence of HIV infection at birth using current virologic, immunologic, and molecular biologic techniques.

A variety of factors have been found to correlate with increased HIV transmission to the fetus or young infant. These include (1) maternal blood viral burden (Weiser et al., 1994; Borkowsky et al., 1994); (2) exposure to high levels of vaginal HIV burden (Minkoff et al., 1995); (3) low maternal CD4 level (Blanche et al., 1989); (4) high maternal CD8 level (St. Louis et al., 1993); and (5) vaginal delivery (Tovo et al., 1995).

The increase in HIV transmission to the first (twin A) of multiple births with discordant HIV infection has been used to suggest that exposure to vaginal HIV is an important risk factor (Duliege et al., 1995). However, this pattern was also seen in those delivered by cesarean section. In addition, a perinatal intervention trial in Malawi that studied the effect of vaginal cleansing on HIV transmission failed to show an effect. Nevertheless, prolonged (>4 hours) ruptured membranes (Landesman et al., 1996) appears to be a risk factor for HIV transmission since it increases the duration of potential exposure.

Combined treatment of an HIV-infected mother during the last trimester of pregnancy and her offspring for 6 weeks with a nucleoside analog, zidovudine (ZDV), was found to result in a reduction of transmission from 26% to 8% (Connor et al., 1994); consequently, this regimen with ZDV has become the standard of care.

It remains likely that some HIV transmission occurs at the time of parturition, as in the model of hepatitis B transmission. Although some studies have suggested that children infected at this time are more likely to have a better clinical outcome than children infected in utero (Dickover et al., 1994; Mayaux et al., 1996), the effect of the timing of infection on outcome as an isolated high-risk factor has been disputed, and it has been suggested that the extent of viral replication in the first months of life may be a better correlate (Arlievsky et al., 1995; Papaevangelou et al., 1996). This has been borne out by findings of an improved clinical outcome when effective antiretroviral intervention begins early in life (Luzuriaga et al., 2000).

Data suggest that maternal HIV infection results in lower birth weights for infants. Many of the studies have been complicated by the high rate of illegal drug use in HIV-1 seropositive women, and infants born to cocaine- or heroin-using women have significantly lower birth weights and higher mortality rates than non–drug-using women (Selwyn et al., 1989). Studies in developing nations have been free of the confounding effects of illegal drug use, but women having babies in these nations have more advanced HIV disease. In both Africa and Haiti the birth weights of infants born to HIV-1–seropositive women are significantly lower than the birth weights of infants born to seronegative women (Ryder et al., 1989; Halsey et al., 1990). In addition, the mortality rates in both Africa and Haiti are higher for infants born to seropositive women. This rate has been reported to be 89% by 3 years of age in a cohort from Malawi (Taha et al., 2000). This may be due to increased exposure to other infectious agents or to decreased accessibility of medical care. Mortality rates in infants born to HIV-negative women are substantially higher in these areas than in developed nations, and it is apparent that HIV and AIDS are increasing the overall perinatal mortality rate. A prospective natural history study in the United States showed that HIV-infected infants were 0.28 kg lighter and 1.64 cm shorter at birth than uninfected infants (Moye et al., 1996). The children maintained their decrease in height and weight and had a sustained decrement in head circumference by 18 months of age relative to noninfected infants. In this study, ZDV therapy was not associated with improved growth. Results have also shown diminished stature in HIV-infected newborns (Pollack et al., 1996), with catch-up growth seen in those who demonstrate limited HIV viral burden as measured by RNA copy number but sustained short stature and diminished weight seen in those with high viral burden.

The majority of infected children become symptomatic during the first 6 months of life (median of 5.2 months, range of 0.03 to 56 months), with the development of lymphadenopathy as the initial finding (Galli et al., 1995). The most common signs in the first year of life are lymphadenopathy (70%), splenomegaly (58%), and hepatomegaly (58%), with only 19% of infected children remaining asymptomatic for a year. Some HIV-infected children develop a severe failure to thrive or encephalopathy during the first year of life. These children appear to have exceptionally high levels of HIV in their blood during the first few months of life (Arlievsky et al., 1995). Survival in such children, as well as in those who develop symptoms before 5 months of age, is significantly lower than in those with a later onset of symptoms as determined through assessments at both 1 year and 5 years of age.

Transfusion and Coagulation Factor Acquired Disease

Of all cases of pediatric and adolescent AIDS, those acquired through exposure to blood products used to treat coagulation factor deficiency now represents fewer than 10%. The use of recombinant factors and methods that effectively eliminate the possibility of survival of HIV in today's products should make this cause of pediatric HIV infection extraordinarily rare.

Screening of blood products for HIV, initiated in 1984, has made the use of such products a rare cause of HIV infection in children, adolescents, and adults. One study estimates the risk of infection as 1 in 493,000 (95% confidence interval of 202,000 to 2,778,000; Schreiber et al., 1996). Antibody screening alone will not reveal acute HIV infection in donors of blood products. The use of assays that detect actual virus should prevent the likelihood that such blood will be used for transfusion.

Adolescents

The absolute number of cases of AIDS among adolescents 13 to 19 years of age is now greater than that reported in children less than 13 years of age. Approximately 2400 males and 1700 females in this adolescent age group had been diagnosed with AIDS as of December 2000. About 1500 of these adolescents are still living with AIDS, and almost as many are living with HIV infection in the absence of AIDS. About a third of the male patients cite homosexuality or exposure to blood products as risk factors, and half of the female patients cite heterosexual exposure. The incubation period is sufficiently long that adolescents who have acquired infection may not become ill until they are older (i.e., in their twenties or thirties). The number of cases of AIDS in the 20-to-24–year age group is almost 20,000 in males and 8,000 in females.

CLINICAL MANIFESTATIONS

Children with untreated or poorly treated HIV infection have a broad spectrum of clinical manifestations. With the advent of highly active antiretroviral therapies (HAART, discussed later in this chapter), most of these conditions can be prevented or resolved. The existence of such therapies has completely changed the nature of HIV infection in developed countries, where they are accessible. Since the initiation of these therapies, the mortality rate of HIV infection has plummeted. Nevertheless, for the rest of the world, the facts regarding HIV infection in the pre-HAART era still apply.

The original classification was a useful way to categorize illness, and it demonstrated the array of infectious agents and organ systems that may be involved. With the original classification system, however, only clinical problems were used to stage HIV infection with regard to natural history and prognosis. Table 1-1 presents the new modified classification system for HIV in children developed by the CDC in 1994 (MMWR Sept. 30). This new classification system incorporates both clinical (Boxes 1-1 and 1-2) and immunologic variables (Table 1-2) to stage infection in children. A comparison of the old classification system and the new one is shown in Table 1-3. In addition to characterizing clinical syndromes, the classification system has proved useful for determining who should receive prophylaxis against PCP.

TABLE 1-1	Pediatric Human Immunodeficiency Virus (HIV) Classification*			
	CLINICAL CATEGORIES			
Immunologic categories	*N: No signs/symptoms*	*A: Mild signs/symptoms*	*B:[†] Moderate signs/symptoms*	*C:[†] Severe signs/symptoms*
1: No evidence of suppression	N1	A1	B1	C1
2: Evidence of moderate suppression	N2	A2	B2	C2
3: Evidence of severe suppression	N3	A3	B3	C3

From Centers for Disease Control and Prevention: MMWR 1994;43:1-10
*Children whose HIV infection status is not confirmed are classified by using the above grid with a letter E (for perinatally exposed) placed before the appropriate classification code (e.g., EN2).
[†]Both Category C and lymphoid interstitial pneumonitis in Category B are reportable to state and local health departments as AIDS.

TABLE 1-2   Immunologic Categories Based on Age-Specific CD4+ T-lymphocyte Counts and Percentage of Total Lymphocytes

| Immunologic category | AGE OF CHILD | | | | | |
| | <12 MO | | 1-5 YR | | 6-12 YR | |
	μl	(%)	μl	(%)	μl	(%)
1: No evidence of suppression	≥1,500	(≥25)	≥1,000	(≥25)	≥500	(≥25)
2: Evidence of moderate suppression	750-1,499	(15-24)	500-999	(15-24)	200-499	(15-24)
3: Evidence of severe suppression	<750	(<15)	<500	(<15)	<200	(<15)

From Centers for Disease Control and Prevention: MMWR 1994;43:1-10

TABLE 1-3   Comparison of the 1987 and 1994 Pediatric HIV Classification Systems

1987 Classification	1994 Classification
P-0	Prefix "E"
P-1	N
P-2A	A, B, and C
P-2B	C
P-2C	B
P-2D1	C
P-2D2	C
P-2D3	B
P-2E1	C
P-2E2	B
P-2F	B

From Centers for Disease Control and Prevention: MMWR 1994;43:1-10

PCP is the most commonly reported AIDS-indicating disease in children. Infants presenting with PCP are usually less than 1 year of age. In adults with AIDS there is a correlation between the CD4 count and the subsequent occurrence of PCP. Seven percent of adults with a CD4 count of <200/mm³ will develop PCP within 6 months, 15% within 12 months, and 30% within 36 months (Phair et al., 1990). Infection correlates with the degree of immuno-compromise, and CD4 counts are predictive of risk of PCP. Correlations with CD4 counts in children can also be made, although infants normally have much higher CD4 levels than adults. CD4 counts of <1500/mm³ have been observed in 90% of reported cases of PCP in patients younger than 12 months (Centers for Disease Control and Prevention, 1991).

PCP may occur in children 1 to 2 years old when CD4 counts are <750/mm³ and in children 2 to 6 years old when CD4 counts are <500/mm³. These values reflect the higher numbers of CD4 cells normally present in young children. Thus prophylaxis for PCP can be empirically based on the CD4 values and be offered to all children with "severe suppression" (category 3).

In the original classification of HIV disease in children, multiple or recurrent serious bacterial infections were included as a prominent manifestation of AIDS. Two or more serious infections in a 2-year period met the case definition of AIDS in an HIV-seropositive infant. When AIDS was first identified in children, bacteremia appeared to occur in almost half of the children who were diagnosed. More recent estimates of the frequency of bacteremia suggest that it occurs less often, particularly if only community-acquired infections are evaluated. The relative risk for invasive bacteremia with community-acquired organisms is about three-fold to twelvefold higher (with about 1 infection per 100 person-months) than that seen in HIV-uninfected children born to infected mothers (Andiman et al., 1994; Felowyn et al., 1994). This decrease in cases of bacteremia may in part be attributable to the ability to diagnose HIV infection before such severe complications cause a child to be brought for medical attention. Children less than 2 years old have an evolving immunologic ability to identify polysaccharide antigens. Thus even normal infants are susceptible to pathogens such as pneumococcus. Children with HIV infection not only are susceptible, but, with their compromised immune systems their susceptibility is

---

BOX 1-1

CLINICAL CATEGORIES FOR CHILDREN WITH HIV INFECTION

Category N: Not Symptomatic

Children who have no signs or symptoms considered to be the result of HIV infection or who have only one of the conditions listed in Category A.

Category A: Mildly Symptomatic

Children with two or more of the conditions listed below but none of the conditions listed in Categories B and C.
- Lymphadenopathy ($\geq$0.5 cm at more than two sites; bilateral = one site)
- Hepatomegaly
- Splenomegaly
- Dermatitis
- Parotitis
- Recurrent or persistent upper respiratory infection, sinusitis, or otitis media

Category B: Moderately Symptomatic

Children who have symptomatic conditions other than those listed for Category A or C that are attributed to HIV infection. Examples of conditions in clinical Category B include but are not limited to the following:
- Anemia (<8 gm/dl), neutropenia (<1,000/mm^3), or thrombocytopenia (<100,000/mm^3) persisting $\geq$30 days
- Bacterial meningitis, pneumonia, or sepsis (single episode)
- Candidiasis, oropharyngeal (thrush), persisting (>2 months) in children >6 months of age
- Cardiomyopathy
- CMV infection, with onset before 1 month of age
- Diarrhea, recurrent or chronic
- Hepatitis
- HSV stomatitis, recurrent (more than two episodes within 1 year)
- HSV bronchitis, pneumonitis, or esophagitis with onset before 1 month of age
- Herpes zoster (shingles) involving at least two distinct episodes or more than one dermatome
- Leiomyosarcoma
- Lymphoid interstitial pneumonia (LIP) or pulmonary lymphoid hyperplasia complex
- Nephropathy
- Nocardiosis
- Persistent fever (lasting >1 month)
- Toxoplasmosis, onset before 1 month of age
- Varicella, disseminated (complicated chickenpox)

Category C: Severely Symptomatic

Children who have any condition listed in the 1987 surveillance case definition for AIDS (10), with the exception of LIP (Box 1-2).

From Centers for Disease Control and Prevention: MMWR 1994;43:1-10

---

prolonged. Hypergammaglobulinemia is a common development in children with HIV infection because of polyclonal activation of B cells. These antibodies are largely nonspecific, and children do not recognize antigens or respond well as their disease progresses. Thus, elevated IgG levels in these children indicate an abnormal host response and one that is functionally antibody deficient. The major bacterial diseases in HIV-infected children are bacteremia and sepsis, but meningitis, cellulitis, wound infection, gastroenteritis, and pneumonia also occur frequently. A primary focus of infection is not uniformly identified in bacteremic children; more than half may have no known focus. Several reports (Krasinski et al., 1988; Bernstein

---

BOX 1-2

CONDITIONS INCLUDED IN CLINICAL CATEGORY C FOR CHILDREN INFECTED WITH HIV

Category C: Severely Symptomatic*

- Serious bacterial infections, multiple or recurrent (i.e., any combination of at least two culture-confirmed infections within a 2-year period), of the following types: septicemia, pneumonia, meningitis, bone or joint infection, or abscess of an internal organ or body cavity (excluding otitis media, superficial skin or mucosal abscesses, and indwelling catheter-related infections)
- Candidiasis, esophageal or pulmonary (bronchi, trachea, lungs)
- Coccidioidomycosis, disseminated (at site other than or in addition to lungs or cervical or hilar lymph nodes)
- Cryptococcosis, extrapulmonary
- Cryptosporidiosis or isosporiasis with diarrhea persisting >1 month
- Cytomegalovirus disease with onset of symptoms at age >1 month (at a site other than liver, spleen, or lymph nodes)
- Encephalopathy (at least one of the following progressive findings present for at least 2 months in the absence of a concurrent illness other than HIV infection that could explain the findings): (a) failure to attain or loss of developmental milestones or loss of intellectual ability, verified by standard developmental scale or neuropsychological tests; (b) impaired brain growth or acquired microcephaly demonstrated by head circumference measurements or brain atrophy demonstrated by computerized tomography or magnetic resonance imaging (serial imaging is required for children <2 years of age); (c) acquired symmetric motor deficit manifested by two or more of the following: paresis, pathologic reflexes, ataxia, or gait disturbance
- Herpes simplex virus infection causing a mucocutaneous ulcer that persists for >1 month; or bronchitis, pneumonitis, or esophagitis for any duration affecting a child >1 month of age
- Histoplasmosis, disseminated (at a site other than or in addition to lungs or cervical or hilar lymph nodes)
- Kaposi's sarcoma
- Lymphoma, primary, in brain
- Lymphoma, small, noncleaved cell (Burkitt's), or immunoblastic or large-cell lymphoma of B-cell or unknown immunologic phenotype
- *Mycobacterium tuberculosis*, disseminated or extrapulmonary
- *Mycobacterium*, other species or unidentified species, disseminated (at a site other than or in addition to lungs, skin, or cervical or hilar lymph nodes)
- *Mycobacterium avium* complex or *Mycobacterium kansasii*, disseminated (at site other than or in addition to lungs, skin, or cervical or hilar lymph nodes)
- *Pneumocystis carinii pneumonia*
- Progressive multifocal leukoencephalopathy
- Salmonella (nontyphoid) septicemia, recurrent
- Toxoplasmosis of the brain with onset at >1 month of age
- Wasting syndrome in the absence of a concurrent illness other than HIV infection that could explain the following findings: (a) persistent weight loss >10% of baseline OR (b) downward crossing of at least two of the following percentile lines on the weight-for-age chart (e.g., 95th, 75th, 50th, 25th, 5th) in a child ≥1 year of age OR (c) <5th percentile on weight-for-height chart on two consecutive measurements, ≥30 days apart PLUS (a) chronic diarrhea (i.e., at least two loose stools per day for ≥30 days) OR (b) documented fever (for ≥30 days, intermittent or constant)

From Centers for Disease Control and Prevention: MMWR 1994;43:1-10
*See the 1987 AIDS surveillance case definition (10) for diagnosis criteria.

---

et al., 1985a) have indicated that *Streptococcus pneumoniae* is the most common pathogen in bacteremic disease and is reported in approximately 30% of infections. A National Institute of Child Health and Human Development (NICHD) study has estimated that pneumococcal bacteremia in untreated symptomatic patients occurs at a rate of 37 per 1,000 patients per year. Infections with *Haemophilus influenzae*, *Salmonellae* species, staphylococci, and a variety of other encapsulated organisms have been reported. Unfortunately, many of these children have had community- and hospital-acquired gram-negative bacteremias. Upper-respiratory infections, including sinusitis and otitis media, are very common. Recurrent episodes of these infections are frequent sources of chronic fever and require vigorous antibiotic therapy. Chronic sinusitis may require prolonged intravenous antibiotic therapy or aggressive surgical drainage.

Chronic Pneumonitis

Lymphoid interstitial pneumonitis (LIP), or pulmonary lymphoid hyperplasia, is a common occurrence and was reported in 28% of children with AIDS in 1988 and 1989. The etiology of this syndrome is unknown, with both EBV and HIV being implicated in the disease process (Andiman et al., 1985; Chayt et al., 1986). However, EBV is not always found, and HIV may be isolated from bronchoalveolar fluid and lung tissue even in the absence of LIP.

LIP usually is diagnosed in children with perinatally acquired HIV infection who are more than 1 year of age. It often begins as an asymptomatic pulmonary infiltrate but can progress to severe pulmonary compromise with superimposed complications of disease such as pneumonia or congestive heart failure. The chronic illness and hypoxemia can be similar to that with chronic bronchiectasis. Children with LIP tend to have a longer survival time than children with encephalopathy or a history of PCP. The entity frequently is associated with chronic parotitis, hypergammaglobulinemia, and lymphadenopathy. A possible adult equivalent of LIP has been described and appears to occur exclusively in individuals with a particular HLA class II haplotype (Itescu et al., 1989). As children with LIP develop progressive T4 lymphopenia with advanced age, the LIP syndrome appears to improve, although their overall HIV disease actually worsens.

Encephalopathy and Myelopathy

CNS involvement is frequent in children with HIV infection. Studies reporting children with advanced HIV disease suggest that up to 60% will have neurologic manifestations (Belman et al., 1988; Epstein et al., 1986). Reported neurologic findings include impaired brain growth, generalized weakness with pyramidal signs, pseudobulbar palsy, ataxia, seizures, myoclonus, and extrapyramidal rigidity. Approximately 40% of HIV-infected children may develop progressive encephalopathy, resulting in the loss of developmental

milestones or subcortical dementia. However, some preliminary natural history studies suggest that progressive encephalopathy may be present in a smaller proportion (i.e., 9% to 20%) of children (European Collaborative Study, 1988; Blanche et al., 1989; Mok et al., 1987). These children were observed to a mean age of 18 months and included those with mild and asymptomatic disease. It has also been reported that approximately 25% of children have an encephalopathy that does not progress (Epstein et al., 1988). A study of children who were evaluated at a mean age of 9.5 years revealed that two thirds had normal IQs. However, 54% had abnormal results on visual-spatial and time orientation tests. Children with normal school achievement had higher CD4+ cells during the first years of life (Tardieu et al., 1995). Although the manifestations of CNS involvement with HIV may vary considerably, it is agreed that the virus does infect the CNS and that the young infant with an immature CNS is uniquely susceptible to damage, resulting in an array of developmental deficits and neurologic abnormalities such as spastic paraparesis. In addition to the harmful effects of HIV infection per se on the CNS, HIV-infected children can develop additional CNS complications, including neoplasm, stroke, and infections with other pathogenic organisms.

Wasting Syndrome and Diarrhea

The gastrointestinal tract is also a source of invasive pathogens, and children with HIV infection sustain symptomatic infections with the common bacterial organisms such as *Salmonella, Shigella, Campylobacter,* and *Clostridium difficile. Salmonella* species occur more commonly than in normal children and cause invasive disease. Relapse of symptomatic illness has been reported. Adult studies have suggested that ceftriaxone may be more successful in eradicating *Salmonella* species than more commonly used forms of therapy such as ampicillin or trimethoprim-sulfamethoxazole (Rolston et al., 1989). In children with exceptionally low T4 counts ($<50/mm^3$ absolute), disseminated *M. avium-intercellulare* may produce a profound wasting disease. Anemia, daily fever, and leukopenia are also commonly seen in such cases. Treatment with multiple drugs—including ethambutol, long-acting macrolides, rifabutin, quinolones, and aminoglycosides—may result in transient improvement.

Gastrointestinal tract infections with protozoal organisms are usually of short duration in normal persons. However, in persons with a compromised immune system, such as children with AIDS, the clinical course often is protracted. *Cryptosporidium, Isospora belli, Giardia lamblia,* and *Microsporida* infection have been reported in AIDS patients. *Cryptosporidium* species are probably the most common parasitic causes of diarrhea in adult AIDS patients and have produced similar chronic disease, although less frequently, in children. Failure to thrive, or the HIV wasting syndrome, may be due to a complex array of infectious agents, including HIV. HIV-infected adult patients may have malabsorption even when no opportunistic infections are present. HIV infection can be associated with abnormal small bowel mucosa, and the histologic conditions vary from normal to villous atrophy with crypt hypoplasia. HIV RNA has been demonstrated in macrophages and lymphocytes in the lamina propria of intestinal biopsies (Fox et al., 1989; Nelson et al., 1988). A child may have acute diarrhea, chronic nonspecific diarrhea, or failure to thrive. In addition to these problems, HIV-infected individuals apparently are in a hypermetabolic state, which probably increases normal caloric and fluid requirements.

Opportunistic Infections

Opportunistic infections are a common complication in HIV-infected children but are somewhat different from those in adults. Oral *Candida* infection is extremely common in immunocompetent infants because they may acquire the organism as early as parturition. It is thought that 80% of infants are colonized by 4 weeks of age (Russell and Lay, 1973). It is estimated that 15% to 40% of children with HIV infection have oral candidiasis. In the normal child, oral *Candida* infection is often mild and readily treated. *Candida* infection in children with HIV infection appears as oral mucosal candidiasis, gingivostomatitis, and periodontitis. Although it may respond initially to simple therapy such as oral nystatin solution, the hallmark of HIV infection is the persistence of *Candida* species.

Children who develop severe *Candida* infection are likely to have diminished numbers of CD4 cells. Candidiasis may extend to the esophagus and the larynx. Esophageal candidiasis is an indicator disease of AIDS, and it can occur without obvious oral pharyngeal candidiasis. Disseminated candidiasis is an unusual occurrence in HIV-infected children. Infections with agents of the herpesvirus group—including HSV, CMV, and VZV—are among the reported manifestations of HIV infection in children. These are ubiquitous pathogens of children, and their ability to establish latency and the potential to induce severe infections in immunocompromised hosts are manifest as both severe and chronic infection in children with HIV infection. Coinfection with perinatal CMV and HIV has been associated with more profound T-cell depletion and decreased survival (Doyle et al., 1996).

Hematologic Syndromes

Although cervical lymphadenopathy is a very nonspecific sign, the presence of axillary and inguinal nodes in a young infant should arouse suspicion of HIV infection. Hepatosplenomegaly may accompany the lymphadenopathy. CD4+ cell numbers may remain normal at this time. The most common abnormality is microcytic or normocytic anemia, which occurs even with elevated erythropoietin levels. Thrombocytopenia resulting from the clearance of immune-complex–coated platelets by the reticuloendothelial system occurs in approximately 10% of patients. This syndrome can be differentiated from idiopathic thrombocytopenic purpura (ITP) by the presence of complement on the platelet surface, but it may respond to standard therapies effective in treating ITP. Treatment with antiviral medications that inhibit HIV replication may be the treatment of choice for this disorder. Alternate therapies include high dose monthly infusions of IVIG, intermittent treatment with anti-D immunoglobulin (Rhogam), and splenectomy. Lupus anticoagulants are seen in HIV-infected adults and are probably also found in HIV-infected children.

Anemia and leukopenia are common manifestations of advanced HIV disease. In some cases these have been associated with infections (e.g., disseminated *M. avium-intercellulare,* CMV, parvovirus), whereas in others toxicity from multidrug therapy has been implicated (e.g., ZDV, trimethoprim-sulfa). HIV may also directly interfere with hematopoietic stem cell maturation.

Hepatitis Syndrome

Liver transaminase and alkaline phosphatase levels are often elevated in HIV-infected children. Hyperbilirubinemia occurs infrequently, but obstructive jaundicelike conditions have been seen in young infants (Persaud et al., 1993). Although this hepatitis may be due to infection with secondary pathogens or may be a reaction to drugs such as trimethoprim-sulfamethoxazole and fluconazole, it is often intrinsic to HIV infection alone. HIV can replicate in hepatoma cell lines and can be found in liver macrophages. Chronic hepatitis B infection is usually milder in HIV-infected immunocompromised individuals than in those not infected, reaffirming the theory that chronic active hepatitis is immunologically mediated. HCV infection is often present in HIV-infected women and may be transmitted to their offspring at increased frequency (15% to 50%), often in the absence of anti-HCV antibody in coinfected children (Papaevangelou et al., 1998). The contribution of HCV to the hepatitis syndrome remains to be elucidated in children.

Renal Syndrome

Some children (particularly of African descent) with HIV infection may present with a rapidly progressive glomerulopathy. Light microscopy demonstrates focal segmental glomerulosclerosis and mesangial glomerulonephritis (Connor et al., 1988). Immunoglobulin and complement deposits are evident by immunofluorescence. It is speculated that circulating immune complexes may contribute to the disease. HIV p24 antigen has been demonstrated by in situ hybridization in tubular and glomerular epithelial cells in renal biopsy specimens of adults. Increased production of IL-6, a lymphokine associated with other glomerulopathies, may also play a role in pathogenesis.

Cardiac Syndrome

Abnormalities, including progressive left ventricular dilatation and poor myocardial contractility with compensatory hypertrophy, may occur early in children with HIV disease without obvious clinical consequences (Lipshultz et al., 1992). The progression of this disease and the occurrence of myocarditis, pericardial effusion, and the effects of LIP on function of the right side of the heart may ultimately produce congestive heart failure. EBV coinfection is strongly correlated with chronic congestive

failure (Luginbuhl et al., 1993). As children progress to a diagnosis of AIDS, significant cardiac dysfunction is seen with tachycardia, bradycardia, hypertension, hypotension, and dysrhythmias. Secondary agents such as CMV, enteroviruses, and M. *avium-intracellulare* may contribute to this syndrome. HIV RNA has been found in macrophages infiltrating myocardial tissue in children with this disorder.

Malignancies

Although Kaposi's sarcoma, recently associated with HHV8 infection, is the most common neoplasm in adults with AIDS, it occurs very rarely in children, possibly because of relative infrequent infection of young children with HHV8. Lymphoreticular malignancies are being reported with increasing frequency in both HIV-infected adults and children. These tumors can appear as both Hodgkin's and non-Hodgkin's lymphomas. The latter is most often a B-cell malignancy (e.g., Burkitt's lymphoma) but may also be a T-cell lymphoma. The lymphomas may be discrete or disseminated and commonly present in the CNS. The risk is increased in individuals who have lived with fewer than 50 CD4+ cells/mm^3 for more than 2 years. Rarely, leiomyosarcomas and progressive giant papillomas may also occur.

DIFFERENTIAL DIAGNOSIS

HIV infection can both mimic a host of other disorders and predispose a patient to certain of them. These disorders include the following:

- Maturational immunodeficiency of newborns, resulting in neonatal sepsis and severe infection with herpesviruses (especially CMV)
- Congenital infections, with associated lymphadenopathy and hepatosplenomegaly
- Congenital immunodeficiency states
  - Severe combined immunodeficiency
  - DiGeorge's syndrome
  - Wiskott-Aldrich syndrome
  - Agammaglobulinemia or hypogammaglobulinemia
  - Ataxia telangiectasia
  - Neutrophil defects in mobility or killing
  - Chronic mucocutaneous candidiasis
- Inflammatory bowel diseases
- Hereditary encephalopathies and neuropathies
- ITP
- Chronic allergies with sinusitis, otitis, and dermatitis

- Cystic fibrosis or α_1-antitrypsin deficiency
- Primary lymphoreticular malignancy

TREATMENT
Specific Retroviral Therapy

Primary infection with HIV results in HIV copy numbers in excess of a million/ml of plasma. Eventually this level of viremia decreases to a "set point" that is unique to each individual, ranging from 100 to several million copies/ml, remaining stable for months and occasionally years. There appears to be an inverse correlation between the set point HIV copy number and survival.

The ideal goal of treatment would be to eradicate all virus-infected cells and cure the infection. This is currently becoming feasible as more potent antiretroviral agents become available, in spite of the fact that 1 to 10 billion viral particles are produced daily. Available therapeutic agents (Table 1-4) suppress viral multiplication by 0.5 log to 3 log titers and improve or reverse some of the symptoms, improving the quality and duration of life. Newer viral load monitoring assays allow for the detection of as little as 50 copies of RNA/ml. Although suppression of plasma viremia below these levels is now possible for extended periods of time, the presence of virus in other sanctuaries (e.g., CNS, lymph nodes, mucosal sites) does not hold promise for total eradication in the near future. Moreover, the presence of latent virus in resting T cells has resulted in a prediction that virus may persist in an infected adult or child for over 50 years (Finzi et al., 1999; Persaud et al., 2000). Nevertheless, the historic evolution of antiretroviral agents is discussed below.

Azidothymidine (AZT), or ZDV, was the first antiretroviral agent approved for use in children. ZDV was shown to increase the rate of the patient's growth, decrease p24 antigen levels in the serum and cerebrospinal fluid, and decrease serum immunoglobulin levels (McKinney et al., 1991). ZDV, at higher doses and given intravenously, also improved the neurobehavioral status of children with HIV infection (Brouwers et al., 1994). The survival of ZDV-treated children with AIDS appears longer than that of historical controls. Prolonged use of ZDV is limited by bone marrow toxicity to erythroid and myeloid elements. Some of the toxicity can be modified by dose reduction. ZDV-resistant HIV isolates emerge after 6 to 12 months of therapy and limit its usefulness as a single agent.

Other nucleoside derivatives, including didanosine (DDI), zalcitabine (DDC), stavudine (D4T), and abacavir (ABC) have also proven effective in adults and children. Initial treatment with DDI was found to be superior to that of ZDV alone and equivalent to that of DDI and ZDV in children (Englund et al., 1997). However, more prolonged follow-up suggests that single drug therapy is unwise. Mutations in single bases in the reverse transcriptase molecule are sufficient to produce resistant virus. A given mutation (e.g., codon 184) may also result in cross-resistance to other nucleoside RT inhibitors. The use of drug combinations will likely result in a decrease in the emergence of resistant viruses. Nonnucleoside reverse transcriptase inhibitors (NNRTI) such as nevirapine, delavirdine, and efavirenz appear to be more potent (resulting in a 2- to 3-log reduction of viral RNA levels) than the nucleosides but also fraught with the likelihood of the appearance of highly resistant HIV isolates emerging within weeks of treatment initiation. In contrast to the nucleoside analogs, which are incorporated into nascent viral DNA and cause chain termination, the NNRTI drugs bind to the viral reverse transcriptase and inhibit its function. The combination of these drugs with several other anti-HIV drugs, including the nucleoside reverse transcriptase inhibitors, may result in a delay in the appearance of resistant virus.

The introduction of HIV protease inhibitors such as saquinavir, ritonavir, indinavir, nelfinavir, amprenavir, and lopinavir to the therapeutic armamentarium has resulted in far more dramatic reductions (1 log to 3 log) of HIV burden than any of the isolated nucleosides (0.5 log to 1.5 log) (Carpenter et al., 1996). Unfortunately, HIV resistance often develops rapidly in an environment of insufficient drug concentration. Although several mutations appear to be necessary to produce resistant virus, cross-resistance to other protease inhibitors (e.g., indinavir resistance may render a virus resistant to ritonavir) although not always (e.g., indinavir/ritonavir resistant virus remains sensitive to saquinavir). The combination of a protease inhibitor with two other nucleosides has resulted in even more dramatic reductions in HIV load and more delayed emergence of resistant virus (Nachman et al., 2000). Other combinations include the simultaneous administration of nucleosides, nonnucleosides, and protease inhibitors.

TABLE 1-4   Available Therapeutic Agents to Suppress Viral Multiplication

Generic name	Trade name	Dose	Preparation	Administration	Side effects	Drug interaction
Individual Nucleoside Agents						
abacavir (ABC)	Ziagen	8 mg/kg (300 max) bid	Tablet: 300 mg Liquid: 20 mg/ml		Severe hypersensitivity reaction	
didanosine (DDI)	Videx	90-150 mg/m² bid	Liquid: 10 mg/ml Powder: 100, 167, 250 mg Chewable: 25, 50, 100, 150, 200 mg	Empty stomach or 30 min before meal	Diarrhea, gastrointestinal disturbance Uncommon: pancreatitis, peripheral neuropathy	dapsone, ketoconazole, itraconazole, ethambutol, zalcitabine, metronidazole, fluoroquinolone
	Videx EC	<60 kg: 250 od >60 kg: 400 od	Delayed-release capsule: 125, 200, 250, 400 mg			
lamivudine (3TC)	Epivir	4 mg/kg bid >50 kg: 150 bid	Liquid: 10 mg/ml Tablets: 150 mg		Pancreatitis (8%-14%), peripheral neuropathy, rash (9%)	Trimethoprim/sulfa
stavudine (D4T)	Zerit	1 mg/kg bid <60 kg: 30 bid >60 kg: 40 bid	Liquid: 1 mg/ml Capsule: 15, 20, 30, 40 mg		Headache, gastrointestinal disturbance, skin rash Rare: lactic acidosis	ZDV
zalcitabine (DDC)	HIVID	0.01 mg/kg q8h Adolescent: 0.75 mg tid	Solution: 0.1 mg/ml Tablet: 0.375, 0.75 mg		Headache, gastrointestinal disturbances, peripheral neuropathy, pancreatitis, esophageal ulcers	cimetidine, amphotericin, aminoglycosides, pentamidine
zidovudine (ZDV, AZT)	Retrovir	PO *Full term:* <90 days: 2 mg/kg q6h *Premature:* <2 weeks: 1.5 mg/kg q12h >2 weeks 2 mg/kg q8h IV 1.5 mg/kg q6h *Pediatric:* 90-180 mg per m² q6-8h	Liquid: 10 mg/ml Capsule: 100 mg Tablet: 30 mg IV solution: 10 mg/ml		Anemia, neutropenia, headache Uncommon: myopathy, liver toxicity Rare: lactic acidosis	ganciclovir, fluconazole, rifampin, atovaquone, pentamidine, probenecid, valproic acid

Continued

Generic name	Trade name	Dose	Preparation	Administration	Side effects	Drug interaction
zidovudine (cont'd)		*Adolescent:* 200 mg tid, 300 mg bid				
Combination Nucleosides						
(ZDV+3TC) (300)+(150)	Combivir	Adolescent: 1 tab bid				
(ABC+3TC+ZDV) (300)+(150)+(300)	Trizivir	Adolescent: 1 tab bid				
Nucleotides						
tenofovir	Viread	Adolescent: 300 od			Gastrointestinal intolerance	
Non-Nucleosides						
delaviridine (DLV)	Rescriptor	Adolescent: 400 mg tid	Tablet: 100, 200 mg		Headache, fatigue, gastrointestinal disturbance, rash	*Induces p450 3A* antihistamines, sedative-hypnotics, calcium channel blockers, ergots, cisapride, warfarin, amphetamines, rifampin, anticonvulsants
efavirenz (EFV)	Sustiva	10-15 kg: 200 mg od 15-20 kg: 250 mg od 20-25 kg: 300 mg od 25-32.5 kg: 350 mg 32.5-40 kg: 400 mg od >40 kg: 600 mg od	Capsule: 50, 100, 200 mg	Bedtime dose recommended	Rash, CNS disturbances (somnolence, insomnia, abnormal dreams)	*Induces p450 3A4* antihistamines, sedative-hypnotics, calcium channel blockers, ergots, cisapride, warfarin, amphetamines, rifampin, anticonvulsants
nevirapine (NVP)	Viramune	Neonate: 120-200 mg/m² od for 14 days then bid <8 years: 7 mg/kg od for 14 days then bid	Liquid: 10 mg/ml Tablet: 200 mg		Rash (Stevens-Johnson), hepatitis (rarely fatal), hypersensitivity reactions	*Induces p450 3A* ketoconazole, rifampin/rifabutin, methadone, anticonvulsants, oral contraceptives

Protease Inhibitors

			Dose	Formulation	Administration	Side Effects	Interactions
			>8 years: 4 mg/kg od for 14 days then bid Adolescent: 200 mg od for 14 days then bid				
amprenavir (APV)	Agenerase		<50 kg: 22.5 mg/kg bid or 17 mg/kg tid Adolescent: 1200 mg bid	Liquid: 15 mg/ml Capsule: 50, 150 mg	Not to be taken with high-fat meal; take 1 hr before antacids or DDI Not recommended for <3 years of age	Gastrointestinal disturbances, perioral paresthesia, rash, taste alteration Rare: Stevens-Johnson	*CYP3A4 inhibitor* rifampin, sedative-hypnotics, calcium channel blockers, ergots, cisapride
indinavir (IDV)	Crixivan		500 mg per m² q8h, or for small individuals 300-400 mg per m² q8h Adolescent: 800 mg q8h	Capsule: 200, 400 mg	Empty stomach or light meal, not to be taken with high-fat meal, take 1 hr before antacids or DDI, drink 8 glasses of water daily	Nausea, headache, hyperbilirubinemia, nephrolithiasis	*CYP3A4 inhibitor* rifampin, sedative-hypnotics, calcium channel blockers, ergots, cisapride, ketoconazole, itraconazole, clarithromycin
lopionavir/ritonavir	Kaletra		7-15 kg: 12/3 mg/kg bid 15-40 kg: 10/2,5 mg/kg bid >40 kg: 400/100 mg bid	Liquid: 80 mg lopinvir/ 20 mg ritonavir per ml Capsule: 133.3 mg/lopinavir 33.3 mg/ritonavir	Take with food If taken with EFV, increase Kaletra dose by 10%-20% Liquid contains 42% alcohol	Diarrhea, headache, weakness, nausea, vomiting, increased triglycerides and cholesterol	*Induces p450 3A* antihistamines, sedative-hypnotics, calcium channel blockers, antiarrhythmics, ergots, cisapride, warfarin, amphetamines, rifampin, anticonvulsants, neuroleptics, clarithromycin, HMG-CoA redeuctase inhibitors, ethanyl estradiol

Continued

TABLE 1-4 Available Therapeutic Agents to Suppress Viral Multiplication—cont'd

Generic name	Trade name	Dose	Preparation	Administration	Side effects	Drug interaction
nelfinavir (NFV)	Viracept	20-30 mg/kg tid, but 30-45 mg/kg tid used often Adolescent: 1250 bid or 750 tid	Powder/Suspension: 50 mg/scoop 200 mg/tspn Tablet: 250 mg	Light meal increases SQV, increases IDV, increased NFV when taken with RTV 1-2 hrs before/after DDI	Diarrhea, asthenia, abdominal pain, rash, increased triglycerides and cholesterol	*CYP3A4 inhibitor* rifampin, sedative-hypnotics, calcium channel blockers, ergots, cisapride
ritnoavir (RTV)	Norvir	Pediatric: 350-400 mg per m² bid Adolescent: 600 mg bid Used as PI enhancer: 100-400 mg bid	Liquid: 80 mg/ml Capsule: 100 mg	With food, taken 1-2 hrs before/after DDI To neutralize poor taste and nausea, give with milk, ice cream, peanut butter, maple syrup, or frozen juices	Nausea, vomiting, diarrhea, anorexia, circumoral paresthesias, increased LFTs, increased triglycerides and cholesterol	*Induces p450 3A* antihistamines, sedative-hypnotics, calcium channel blockers, antiarrhythmics, ergots, cisapride, warfarin, amphetamines, rifampin, anticonvulsants, neuroleptics, clarithromycin, HMG-CoA redeuctase inhibitors, ethanyl estradiol
saquinavir (SQV)	Invirase (hard gel cap) Fortovase (soft gel cap)	Pediatric: 50 mg/kg q8h If taken with NFV: 33 mg/kg q8h If taken with RTV: 50 mg/kg bid Adolescent: 1200 mg tid 1600 mg bid Fortovase	Capsule: 200 mg	With food Grapefruit juice increases SQV concentration	Diarrhea, gastrointestinal disturbance, headache, paresthesia, rash, photosensitivity, hyperglycemia	*CYP3A4 inhibitor* rifampin, sedative-hypnotics, calcium channel blockers, ergots, cisapride

Despite all attempts to prevent resistance from developing, poor absorption, inadequate dosing, and lack of adherence to prescribed regimens all play a role in the development of resistance. Knowledge of resistance patterns may allow for a more effective selection of therapeutic agents in those in whom therapy has failed. One problem with using DNA sequencing to identify resistance mutations is the requirement that 20% or more of the circulating virus have this mutation. Archived virus with resistance to a given drug is not detectable in the absence of drug selection pressure. However, such resistant viruses are likely to emerge as the dominant strain when selective pressure is applied to competing quasispecies in the individual. Knowledge of treatment history is obviously critical in treatment decision-making, as well. The most common mutation selected by the various classes of antiretroviral agent can be seen on the Internet (http://hiv-web.lanl.gov).

The introduction of protease inhibitor therapy has resulted in the appearance of complications rarely described prior to the entrance of these drugs into large populations. These complications include insulin resistance, dyslipidemias, and lipodystrophy syndromes. The first of these has produced type II diabetes mellitus, and the latter has resulted in fat remodeling, which results in the disappearance of fat from the face and extremities while it is deposited in the waist, the upper back (buffalo hump), and the breasts. Although this syndrome appears to be less common in pediatric patients than in adults, this may prove, as therapy continues, not to be the case.

Newer classes of therapeutic agents have been developed. Tenofovir is a novel nucleotide analog with activity against human immunodeficiency virus types 1 and 2 (HIV-1 and HIV-2) and hepatitis B virus (HBV). Tenofovir diphosphate (PMPApp), the active intracellular moeity, is a potent inhibitor of retroviral reverse transcriptase and acts as a DNA chain terminator. An orally available prodrug of tenofovir, tenofovir disoproxil fumarate, was selected for clinical development because of its advantageous pharmacokinetic profile, oral bioavailability, potent antiviral activity, and unique in vitro resistance profile. This drug was recently approved by the Food and Drug Administration (FDA) for use in adults, although its antivirologic potency is similar to monotherapy with nucleoside drugs. Studies with children are ongoing. T-20 and T-1249 are peptides derived from the transmembrane portion of HIV and are unique among current antiretroviral agents in that they can prevent viral entry. The drugs are currently only bioavailable by parenteral injection. Short-term viral suppression in the order of 1 to 2 log has been achieved with monotherapy. T-20 was approved for use in adults in 2003. Additional experience will be needed for FDA approval in children.

When to begin antiretroviral therapy remains controversial. Initial studies in adults showed clear clinical benefit when initiation with monotherapy was begun late in the disease course. When monotherapy was begun with minimal clinical disease (i.e., CD4 counts >500 and CD4% >25), no benefit was observed. Subsequent studies have shown that early initiation of HAART and its maintenance in young infants can prevent immune attrition from occurring and can prevent the development of serologic evidence of HIV infection, despite the fact that HIV remains latent in such individuals (Luzuriaga et al., 2000).

Therapy is recommended for (1) all symptomatic individuals (clinical categories A, B, or C); (2) all asymptomatic individuals with moderate immunosuppression (i.e., categories 2 or 3) (3) asymptomatic children under 12 months of age; and (4) all asymptomatic individuals with >100,000 HIV RNA copies/ml plasma or rapidly declining CD4 cell counts. Therapy should be considered for patients with >15,000 HIV RNA copies/ml or those with HIV RNA increases in excess of 0.7 log (fivefold change) for those under 2 years of age or 0.5 log (threefold change) in those older. Updated recommendations by the Working Group on Antiretroviral Therapy and Medical Management of HIV-Infected Children for therapy initiation or therapy changes in adolescents or in children are available at the following World Wide Web sites:
- http://www.hivatis.org/trtgdlns.html#Pediatric
- http://www.hivatis.org/guidelines/adult/Aug 13_01/text/index.html

Substantial immunologic reconstitution has been described in children treated with HAART (Melvin et al., 1997; Essajee et al., 1999; Vigano et al., 1999). Recent studies suggest that this effect is long lasting and often dissociated from the degree of virologic suppression

(Nikolic-Djokic et al., 2002). Moreover, children who started therapy at immunologic stage 3 did as well as those who started at better immunologic strata.

Antiparasitic therapy. Recommendations recently have been made for prophylaxis of HIV-seropositive infants against *P. carinii* infection (MMWR, 1991). These guidelines are summarized in Figure 1-3 and Table 1-5 and depend on normal CD4 numbers in infants, the safety of available therapy, and problems of the early diagnosis of HIV infection in young infants. PCP prophylaxis may be discontinued in infants aged 4 months or older when HIV infection has been excluded (two or more negative viral diagnostic tests performed after 1 month of age, with the last performed at or after 4 months of age). Suitable viral diagnostic tests are HIV culture or PCR (Centers for Disease Control and Prevention, 1995).

Children with acute PCP should be treated with parenteral trimethoprim-sulfamethoxazole or parenteral pentamidine. Alternative therapies include dapsone, atovaquone, and a long-acting macrolide-sulfa combination. Recent evidence suggests that the introduction of corticosteroid therapy early in this infection in adults helps preserve residual pulmonary function in those who recover.

Immunomodulators. A controlled trial of intravenous immunoglobulin (IVIG) versus placebo conducted by the NICHD reported no difference in survival time but did report a decrease in the number of bacterial infections in children with CD4 counts >200/mm^3 who received IVIG (Mofenson et al, 1992). Most of these children did not receive retroviral therapy, and trimethoprim-sulfamethoxazole for prevention of PCP was progressively administered over the duration of the trial. The single most common pathogen was *S. pneumoniae*, which caused 19 bacteremias in 16 children. A study comparing the effect of IVIG to placebo in AZT-treated HIV-infected children also showed some benefit in reducing infections with common pathogens (Spector et al., 1995). However, IVIG was probably equivalent in efficacy with trimethroprim-sulfamethoxazole in this study.

Antifungal agents. Effective therapy for mucocutaneous candidal disease requires the use of ketoconazole or clotrimazole troches. Oral fluconazole is even more potent. Disseminated candidal disease can occur in the absence of neutropenia and requires treatment with parenteral amphotericin B. Cryptococcal pneumonia and meningitis require parenteral treatment with amphotericin, followed by life-

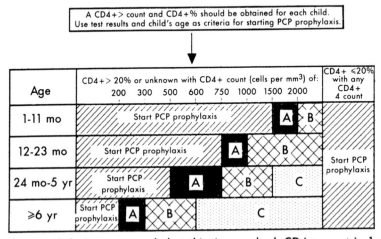

A: No prophylaxis recommended at this time; recheck CD4+ count in 1 month.

B: No prophylaxis recommended at this time; recheck CD4+ count at least every 3-4 months.

C: No prophylaxis recommended at this time; recheck CD4+ count at least every 6 months.

Fig. 1-3 Recommendations for initiation of PCP prophylaxis for children 1 month of age or older who are (1) HIV infected, (2) HIV seropositive, or (3) less than 12 months old and born to an HIV-infected mother. (From Centers for Disease Control and Prevention: MMWR 1991;40:1-14 [March 15].)

TABLE 1-5 Recommendations for Prophylaxis and Treatment of Specific Diseases Seen in HIV-infected Individuals

Disease state	Common organism	Prophylaxis regimen	Treatment regimen
Thrush	Candida	Nystatin Clotrimazole troche Ketoconazole Fluconazole	Fluconazole Amphotericin
Recurrent bacteremia	Pneumococcus/other organisms	Intravenous gammaglobulin Prophylactic antibiotics	Organism/sensitivity specific drug(s)
Wasting syndrome Fever Weight loss Anemia Diarrhea	M. avium/ M. intercellulare	Clarithromycin or azithromycin or rifabutin	Multidrug regimen: 1. Clarithromycin, or azithromycin and 2. Ethambutol and 3. Rifabutin ± aminoglycoside ± fluoroquinolone
Interstitial pneumonitis	P. carinii	Trimethoprim-sulfa or pentamidine or aerosolized pentamidine or dapsone	Trimethoprim/sulfa or pentamidine or atovaquone or clindamycin/primaquine
Retinitis, colitis, esophagitis,	CMV	Ganciclovir	Ganciclovir or foscarnet or cidofovir
Oral ulcers	Herpes simplex virus or	Acyclovir or valacyclovir	Acyclovir or valacyclovir or famciclovir
	Sterile		Topical steroid or thalidomide
Chronic diarrhea	CMV or M. avium M. intracellulare or Cryptosporidium or I. belli	Boil all water	Ganciclovir see MAI regimen above Paramomycin trimethoprim/sulfa
Chickenpox/ shingles	Varicella zoster virus	Immune globulin	Acyclovir or famciclovir

long suppressive maintenance therapy with fluconazole.

Antimycobacterial agents. Advanced immunosuppression, particularly when the CD4 percentage falls below 5, is often associated with disseminated infection with *M. avium-intercellulare* and an associated failure to thrive. Children in this risk group may reduce the risk for acquiring this infection by prophylactic treatment with weekly azithromycin, or daily clarithromycin or rifabutin. In studies of HIV-infected adults the use of weekly azithromycin was optimal, and the addition of rifabutin was additive in its effects.

Antiviral agents. HIV-infected children may develop overwhelming or chronic secondary viral infections. VZV may produce disseminated dis-

ease and death, or it may result in a necrotizing ulcerating zoster skin lesion. Varicella-zoster immune globulin should be used prophylactically to prevent or modify VZV infection when a known exposure occurs in a child susceptible to varicella. Acyclovir, valacyclovir, or famciclovir therapy may be used to modify VZV infection. Prolonged high-dose oral acyclovir therapy is often used to heal and prevent exacerbations of the skin ulcers (Jura et al., 1989). Measles may produce a fulminating and fatal disease in HIV-infected children (Krasinski et al., 1988). Gamma globulin may modify the clinical appearance of the disease but has not prevented measles. All HIV-infected children, even if vaccinated, should receive gamma globulin if a known exposure to measles occurs. Some limited experience with ribavirin, given parenterally, has suggested that it may be an effective antimeasles agent.

Respiratory syncytial virus infection in the HIV-infected infant results in delayed eradication of this respiratory pathogen. It also produces a modified clinical picture, with only the rare occurrence of wheezing and the more common appearance of pneumonia (Chandwani et al., 1990). Aerosolized ribavirin has not been systematically studied in this situation.

Immunizations. HIV-seropositive and HIV-infected children should receive all of their recommended childhood immunizations. Inactivated poliovirus vaccine should be substituted for oral poliovirus vaccine in both the children and their household contacts who are receiving vaccine, although this may not be possible in developing nations. In particular, HIV-seropositive infants should receive measles, mumps, and rubella vaccines unless the CD4 T-cell count is markedly reduced. Studies done in Africa have shown that protection attributable to vaccine in these children is substantial but less than that achieved in healthy children (Oxtoby et al., 1988). Varicella vaccine has been shown to be safe and somewhat (60% to 80%) immunogenic in children with >25% CD4 T cells (Levin et al., 2001). Studies are underway to evaluate the vaccine in those with CD4 T cells >15%. Although pneumococcal polysaccharide vaccine is relatively poor at eliciting immune responses in HIV-infected children, the conjugate vaccine has performed better in this population, although still less well than in HIV-uninfected children (King et al., 1996). It is likely that all vaccine responses will improve after the effects of HAART are seen.

There has been some concern raised about the potentially adverse effects of immune stimulation by vaccines, resulting in increased HIV RNA levels. Thus far, these increases appear to be limited to the immediate postvaccination period, with a return to baseline levels by 4 weeks (Rosok et al., 1996). The clinical consequences of such transient elevation in viremia appears to be minimal.

General nutrition. Many children with HIV infection are unable to sustain a positive nutritional balance. Some drugs, such as the steroid megestrol acetate (Megace), may improve appetite and increase patient weight. It should be noted that such increases are largely a result of fat and not protein. Protein and caloric support can be provided with tube feedings and/or total parenteral nutrition. It has, however, been shown that the risk of catheter infections is considerably higher in HIV-infected children than in other children requiring such intravenous support (e.g., those with malignancies), necessitating an individualized approach to choosing this option for any patient.

MEDICAL MANAGEMENT

Infants born to HIV-seropositive women should be identified so they can receive optimal medical care. Access to care is of critical importance. Ideally, identification of infected women would occur before or during pregnancy so that they too could receive optimal medical care. The recommendation by the U.S. Public Health Service is for seropositive women not to breast-feed because of the undefined risk of viral transmission in the postpartum period. However, in developing nations the benefits of breast-feeding may be more important than the small risk of transmission of the virus, and those women should breast-feed their infants when this is the case. The care of HIV-seropositive infants in the first year of life is very much the same as that for healthy infants. However, these infants should have a CD4 count and HIV culture done every 1 to 3 months if possible. Depending on the resources available, a PCR should be performed along with viral culture for diagnosis. Supportive care provided to children known to be seropositive is of critical importance. The response to an unknown febrile illness or the suspicion that pulmonary disease may be PCP can be lifesaving for these infants. Finally, the institution of PCP prophylaxis is probably the single most important lifesaving part of their medical management at the present time. It is possible that early administration of retroviral therapy may provide even greater benefit than its administration to symptomatic children; thus infected infants must be identified as early as possible.

Older children at risk for HIV infection or with suspicious symptoms suggesting HIV infection should be tested by HIV ELISA and, if positive, confirmed with Western blot assay. The current ELISA tests will detect both HIV-1 and HIV-2, which is found largely in Western Africa. Even if the result of the Western blot assay is positive, an additional serologic test at a different date is necessary to rule out lab error.

When HIV infection has been proved, measurements of both CD4 T cells and HIV RNA in the plasma are used to determine staging to evaluate risk for opportunistic infection, to determine prognostic implications, and to facilitate antiretroviral management. The presence of genotypically different HIV-1 in different geographic regions of the world has resulted in the division of these viruses into "clades." Clade B is found in North America and Europe. Other clades (A, C, E, recombinant forms, and so on) represent the predominant viruses in Africa, Asia, and South America. Some PCR assays, which measure HIV RNA copy numbers, may be restricted in their accurate detection of certain clades (e.g., Clade A). When these clades are believed to be present, the use of a branch chain DNA test to measure viral load will serve as a better assay.

PROGNOSIS

The epidemiologic and circumstantial data suggest that there are two groups of children who have different responses to HIV infection. The first group, who present with illness during the first year of life, has a more rapid progression of disease and death. These children may have been infected in utero (Dickover et al., 1994), although this remains controversial (Papaevengalou et al., 1996). Other infants may be infected in the first year but present with symptoms later; they appear to have a more sustained course of illness.

The diagnosis of PCP in an HIV-infected child carries a poor prognosis. The survival rate after diagnosis of PCP is shown in Figure 1-4 (Borkowsky, unpublished data based on 294 perinatally infected children seen at Bellevue Hospital). The 50% survival for this group is less than 2 years. This is in marked contrast to those perinatally infected children without PCP, with a 50% survival in excess of 12 years. Improved methods for early HIV diagnosis—coupled with earlier implementation of primary and adjunctive therapies, including prophylactic measures against PCP—should dramatically improve future survival.

The introduction of HAART has dramatically changed the outcome of pediatric HIV infection. Shown in Figure 1-5 is the effect of this therapy on mortality at NYU School of Medicine since its introduction in 1996. Since that time, deaths have virtually ceased. It remains to be seen whether this trend continues as antiretroviral resistance increases.

PROPHYLAXIS
Vertical Transmission

The institution of antiretroviral therapy during the late stages of pregnancy of an HIV-infected

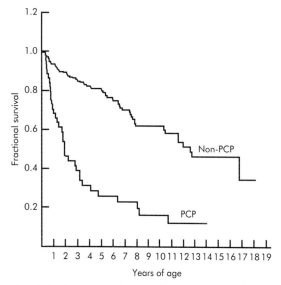

Fig. 1-4 The survival rate after diagnosis of PCP. (Borkowsky, unpublished data based on 294 perinatally infected children seen at Bellevue Hospital.)

woman and the continuation for the first weeks of infancy have resulted in a dramatic reduction of HIV transmission, from over 20% to under 10% (Connor et al., 1994). Although it appears reasonable that this effect was due to a reduction in maternal viral load, this was not the case in the original study (ACTG 076) (Sperling et al., 1996).

The regimen employed in ACTG 076 was maternal AZT 500 mg/day after 14 weeks of gestation. During labor a loading dose of AZT was intravenously given (2 mg/kg over 1 hour) followed by a continuous infusion of 1.5 mg/kg. Infants were begun on AZT within 8 to 12 hours of birth, either orally (2 mg/kg q6h) or intravenously (1.5 mg/kg q6h) and treated orally for 6 weeks, with close follow-up of hemoglobin levels for the presence of anemia, the major adverse event encountered. Abbreviated forms of this regimen also have demonstrated an almost 50% decrease in transmission (Wade et al., 1998).

Newer strategies have employed the more potent antiretroviral agent, nevirapine [NVP], as prophylaxis. A Ugandan trial demonstrated that the use of abbreviated regimens started intrapartum and followed with a single dose to the child at 48 to 72 hours of life resulted in a 50% decrease in perinatal transmission (Musoke et al., 1999; Guay et al., 1999). In pregnant women in the United States and Europe, successful antiretroviral regimens employing HAART as well as the previously mentioned therapies have decreased transmission to 2% to 3%. This change is reflected in the reduced number of infants

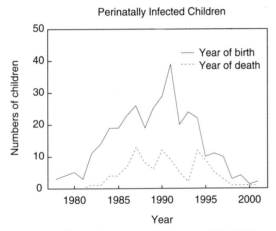

Fig. 1-5 Effects of HIV prophylaxis and HAART on perinatal births and deaths.

infected at birth seen at NYU (Figure 1-5). Guidelines for therapy of HIV-1–infected pregnant women have been recently updated. The most recent information is available on the HIV/AIDS Treatment Information Service Web site (http://www.hivatis.org). The decision as to what therapy should be offered is dependent on a number of considerations, including the potential for dose alteration due to changes in physiology that accompany pregnancy; the potential for short- and long-term effects on the fetus and newborn; and the effectiveness of a regimen in reducing transmission. When HIV RNA is decreased to <1000 copies of RNA per ml, transmission is reduced to <1%. Therefore, all regimens attempt to achieve this goal. The Antiretroviral Pregnancy Registry (www.apregistry.com/contact.htm; [800]-258-4263) anonymously monitors the effects of therapy on mothers and children. Obstetricians and pediatricians are urged to update the registry with their experiences.

Other strategies to decrease HIV perinatal transmission include the use of nonemergent cesarian section (International Perinatal HIV Group, 1999). Recent studies suggest that this strategy is best applied to those who have inadequate antiretroviral suppression of their HIV.

Because of some similarity between perinatal transmission of HIV and HBV, perinatal vaccination with recombinant HIV vaccines (Borkowsky et al., 2000; Cunningham et al., 2001) and with canarypox-based vectors for HIV antigens have been evaluated for safety and immunogenicity. Some combination of these vaccines, possibly with passively administered antiretroviral bio-

logic agents, may have a significant role to play in the future with regard to prevention.

Breast-feeding remains a significant risk for post-partum HIV transmission (Van de Perre et al., 1991) and should be discouraged wherever bottled formula is readily available and safe. Both mother and child may suffer adversely from continued breast-feeding (Nduati et al., 2001).

Postexposure Prophylaxis

Exposure to HIV by needle stick in a nosocomial setting or in the community unfortunately occurs all too often. Fortunately, the average risk for HIV infection from all types of percutaneous exposure is estimated to be only 0.3%. Guidelines have been drafted by the Centers for Disease Control and Prevention Task Force (Centers for Disease Control and Prevention, 1996;45:468-72) and were updated in June 2001 (MMWR June 29, 2001;50[RR11];1-42). These guidelines, based on a case-control study demonstrating a 79% reduction in HIV transmission in treated individuals and presumptions of relative antiviral efficacy, suggest that therapy with multiple antiretroviral drugs be initiated as soon as possible (within 48 to 72 hours) and continued for 4 weeks (or 3 or more drugs, given simultaneously, if the exposure represents an increased risk for transmission) if percutaneous exposure to blood from high- or increased-risk source material occurs. The definition of high risk would include a large volume of inoculum with a high titer of HIV in the inoculum (e.g., blood from a symptomatic individual). Increased risk would be a large volume of inoculum *or* a high-titer inoculum. Special circumstances (e.g., delayed exposure report, donor of blood products unknown, pregnancy, or suspected antiretroviral resistance in the source virus) should be approached by consulting with a local infectious disease expert or by calling the National Clinicians' Post-Exposure Prophylaxis Hotline (PEPline; 1-888-448-4911).

Combinations of nucleoside for postexposure prophylaxis (PEP) include ZDV/3TC, 3TC/d4T, and DDI/d4T. The increased prevalence of HIV resistance to ZDV/3TC may influence this choice. Reports of fatal lactic acidosis associated with the DDI/d4T combination in pregnant women have prompted warnings regarding this choice. The risk of hyperbilirubinemia in newborns has limited the use of IDV shortly before delivery. Initially, IDV and NFV were selected as drugs of first choice for high-risk exposures.

Subsequently, EFV, ABC, and lopinavir (Kaletra) have been added as potential drugs for use in situations where antiretroviral resistance to protease inhibitors is suspected. The National Surveillance System for Health Care Workers (NaSH) and the HIV Postexposure Registry report that 50% of health-care workers experience drug-related adverse symptoms during PEP and that 33% stop PEP because of them. Rapid HIV tests are likely to reduce the potential overuse of these drugs.

Mucous Membrane and Skin Exposure

The risk following exposure to HIV-containing fluids is estimated to be <0.1% and probably depends on the titer of HIV in the fluid. The risk increases if the duration of exposure is long or if there is a loss of integrity in the skin or mucous membrane barrier. An antiretroviral agent may be offered if the risk is believed to be increased. Urine and saliva are not likely to transmit HIV.

Sexual Exposure

In the absence of data, physicians should discuss the potential risk and unknown benefits of prophylactic antiretroviral intervention with those exposed to semen from an HIV-infected individual.

BIBLIOGRAPHY

Amadori A, De Rossi A, Giacquinto C, et al. In vitro production of HIV-specific antibody in children at risk for HIV infection. Lancet 1988;1:852-854.

Ammann AJ, Cowan MJ, Wara DW, et al. Acquired immunodeficiency in an infant: possible transmission by means of blood products. Lancet 1983;1:956-958.

Andiman W, Eastman RN, Martin K, et al. Opportunistic lymphoproliferations associated with EBV DNA in infants and children with AIDS. Lancet 1985;2:1390-1393.

Andiman WA, Mezger J, Shapiro E. Invasive bacterial infections in children born to women infected with human immunodeficiency virus type 1. J Pediatr 1994;124:846-852.

Andiman WA, Modlin JF. Vertical transmission. In Pizzo P, Wilfert CM (eds). Pediatric AIDS. Baltimore: Williams & Wilkins, 1991.

Arlievsky NZ, Pollack H, Rigaud M, et al. Shortened survival in infants with human immunodeficiency virus with elevated p24 antigenemia. J Pediatr 1995;127:538-543.

Barre-Sinoussi F, Cherman JC, Rey F, et al. Isolation of a T-lymphotropic retrovirus from a patient at risk for acquired immunodeficiency syndrome (AIDS). Science 1983;220:868-871.

Belman AL, Diamond G, Dixon D, et al. Pediatric acquired immunodeficiency syndrome: neurologic syndromes. Am J Dis Child 1988;149:29-35.

Bernstein LJ, Krieger BZ, Novick B, et al. Bacterial infection in the acquired immunodeficiency syndrome of children. Pediatr Infect Dis 1985a;4:472-475.

Bernstein LJ, Ochs HD, Wedgwood RJ, Rubinstein A. Defective humoral immunity in pediatric acquired immunodeficiency syndrome. J Pediatr 1985b;107:352-357.

Biggar RJ, Miotti PG, Taha TE, et al. Perinatal intervention trial in Africa: effect of a birth canal cleansing intervention to prevent HIV transmission. Lancet 1996;347:1647-1650.

Blanche S, Le Deist F, Fischer A, et al. Longitudinal study of 18 children with perinatal LAV/HTLV III infection: attempt at prognostic evaluation. J Pediatr 1986;109:965-970.

Blanche S, Rouziouz C, Moscato ML, et al. A prospective study of infants born to mothers seropositive for human immunodeficiency virus type 1. N Engl J Med 1989;320:1643-1648.

Blanche S, Rouzioux C, Moscato ML, et al. A prospective study of infants born to women seropositive for human immunodeficiency virus type 1. HIV Infection in Newborns French Collaborative Study Group.

Borkowsky W, Kaul A. Cholestatic hepatitis in children with HIV infection. Ped Infect Dis 1993;12:492-497.

Borkowsky W, Krasinski K, Cao Y, et al. Correlation of perinatal transmission of human immunodeficiency virus-1 with maternal viremia and lymphocyte phenotypes. J Pediatr 1994;125:345-351.

Borkowsky W, Krasinski K, Paul D, et al. Human immunodeficiency virus infections in infants negative for anti-HIV by enzyme linked immunoassay. Lancet 1987;1:1168-1171.

Borkowsky W, Krasinski K, Paul D, et al. Human immunodeficiency virus core protein antigenemia in children with HIV infection. J Pediatr 1989;114:940-945.

Borkowsky W, Wara D, Fenton T, et al. Lymphoproliferative responses to recombinant HIV-1 envelope antigens in neonates and infants receiving gp120 vaccines. J Infect Dis 2000;181(3):890-896.

Brouwers P, Decarli C, Tudor-Williams G, et al. Interrelations among patterns of change in neurocognitive, CT brain imaging, and CD4 measures associated with antiretroviral therapy in children with symptomatic HIV infection. Adv Neuroimmunol 1994;4:223-231.

Bryant ML, Ratner L. Biology and molecular biology of HIV. In Pizzo P, Wilfert CM (eds). Pediatric AIDS. Baltimore: Williams & Wilkins, 1991.

Carpenter C, Fischl MA, Hammer S, et al. Antiretroviral therapy for HIV infection in 1996. JAMA 1996;276:146-154.

Centers for Disease Control and Prevention. Unexplained immunodeficiency and opportunistic infections in infants: New York, New Jersey, California. MMWR 1982;31:665-667.

Centers for Disease Control and Prevention. Update: acquired immunodeficiency syndrome—United States, 1989. MMWR 1990;39:81-86.

Centers for Disease Control and Prevention. Pneumocystis carinii pneumonia prophylaxis in children. MMWR 1991;40:1-14.

Centers for Disease Control and Prevention. 1994 Recommendations of the U.S. Public Health Service Task Force on the use of zidovudine to reduce perinatal transmission of human immunodeficiency virus. MMWR 1994;43:1-20.

Centers for Disease Control and Prevention. 1994 Revised classification system for human immunodeficiency virus infection in children less than 13 years of age. MMWR 1994;43:1-10.

Centers for Disease Control and Prevention. 1995 Revised guidelines for Prophylaxis against Pneumocystis Carinii pneumonia for children infected with or perinatally exposed to human immunodeficiency virus. MMWR 1995;44:1-11.

Centers for Disease Control and Prevention. HIV/AIDS Surveillance Report. MMWR 1995;7:1-38.

Chandwani S, Borkowsky W, Krasinski K, et al. Respiratory syncytial virus infections in human immunodeficiency virus infected children. J Pediatr 1990;117:251-254.

Chandwani S, Greico A, Mittal K, et al. Pathology and human immunodeficiency virus expression in placentas of seropositive women. J Infect Dis 1991;163:1134-1138.

Chandwani S, Moore T, Krasinski K, Borkowsky W. Early diagnosis of HIV-1 infected infants by plasma p24 antigen assay after immune complex dissociation. Pediatr Infect Dis J 1993;12:96-97.

Chayt K, Harper M, Marselle L, et al. Detection of HTLV-III RNA in lungs of patients with AIDS and pulmonary involvement. JAMA 1986;256:2356-2359.

Connor E, Gupta S, Joshi V, et al. Acquired immunodeficiency syndrome: associated renal disease in children. J Pediatr 1988;113:38-44.

Connor EM, Sperling RS, Gelber R, et al. Reduction of maternal-infant transmission of human immunodeficiency virus type 1 with zidovudine treatment. N Engl J Med 1994;331:1173-1180.

Cunningham CK, Wara DW, Kang M, et al. Safety of two recombinant HIV-1 envelope vaccines in neonates born to HIV-1 infected mothers. Clin Infect Dis 2001;32:801-807.

Deng HK, Liu R, Ellmeier W, et al. Identification of a major co-receptor for primary isolates of HIV-1. Nature 1996;381:661-666.

Dickover RE, Dillon M, Gillette SG, et al. Rapid increases in load of human immunodeficiency virus correlate with early disease progression and loss of CD4 cells in vertically infected infants. J Infect Dis 1994;170:1279-1284.

Di Maria H, Courpotin C, Rouzioux C, et al. Transplacental transmission of human immunodeficiency virus. Lancet 1986;2:215-216.

Doyle M, Atkins JT, Rivera-Matos IR. Congenital cytomegalovirus infection in infants infected with human immunodeficiency virus type 1. Pediatr Infect Dis J 1996;15(12):1102-1106.

Duliege AM, Amos CI, Felton S, et al. Birth order, delivery route, and concordance in the transmission of human immunodeficiency virus type 1 from mothers to twins. J Pediatr 1995;126:625-632.

Englund JA, Baker CJ, Raskino C, et al. Didanosine and combination zidovudine/didanosine are superior to zidovudine monotherapy for the initial treatment of symptomatic children infected with human immunodeficiency virus. N Engl J Med 1997;326:1704-1712.

Epstein LG, Sharer LR, Goudsmit J. Neurologic and neuropathological features of HIV infection in children. Ann Neurol 1988;23:S19-S23.

Epstein LG, Sharer LR, Oleski JM, et al. Neurologic manifestations of human immunodeficiency virus infection in children. Pediatrics 1986;78:678-687.

Essajee SM, Kim M, Gonzalez C, et al. Immunologic and virologic responses to HAART in severely immunocompromised HIV-1 infected children. AIDS 1999;13:2523-2532.

European Collaborative Study. Mother to child transmission of HIV infection. Lancet 1988;2:1039-1042.

European Collaborative Study. Children born to women with HIV-1 infection: natural history and risk of transmission. Lancet 1991;337:253-260.

Eyster ME. Transfusion and coagulation factor acquired disease. In Pizzo P, Wilfert CM (eds). Pediatric AIDS. Baltimore: Williams & Wilkins, 1991.

Felowyn PA, Farley JJ, King JC, et al. Invasive pneumococcal disease among infected and uninfected children of mothers with human immunodeficiency virus infection. J Pediatr 1994;124:853-858.

Feng Y, Broder CC, Kennedy PE, Berger E. HIV-1 entry cofactor: functional cDNA cloning of a seven-transmembrane, G protein-coupled receptor. Science 1996;272:872-877.

Finzi D, Blankson J, Siliciano JD, et al. Latent infection of CD4+ T cells provides a mechanism for lifelong persistence of HIV-1, even in patients on effective combination therapy. Nat Med 1999;5(5):512-517.

Fox CH, Kotler D, Tierney A, et al. Detection of HIV-1 RNA in the lamina propria of patients with AIDS in GI disease. J Infect Dis 1989;159:467-471.

Galli L, de Martino M, Tovo PA, et al. Onset of clinical signs in children with HIV-1 perinatal infection. AIDS 1995;9:455-461.

Gallo RC, Salahuddin SZ, Popovic M, et al. Frequent detection and isolation of cytopathic retroviruses (HTLV-3) from patients with AIDS and at high risk for AIDS. Science 1984;224:500-503.

Geijtenbeek TB, Kwon DS, Torensma R, et al. DC-SIGN, a dendritic cell-specific HIV-1-binding protein that enhances trans-infection of T cells. Cell 2000;100(5):587-597.

Guay LA, Musoke P, Fleming T, et al. Intrapartum and neonatal single-dose nevirapine compared with zidovudine for prevention of mother-to-child transmission of HIV-1 in Kampala, Uganda: HIVNET 012 randomised trial. Lancet 1999;354:795-802.

Gutman LT, St.-Claire K, Weedy C, et al. Human immunodeficiency virus transmission by sexual abuse. Am J Dis Child 1991;145:137-141.

Halsey NA, Boulos R, Holt E, et al. Transmission of HIV-1 infections from mothers to infants and babies. Impact on childhood mortality and malnutrition. JAMA 1990;264:2088-2092.

Ho DD, Neumann AU, Perelson AU, et al. Rapid turnover of plasma virions and CD4 lymphocytes in HIV-1 infection. Nature 1995;373:123-126.

Hutto C, Parks WP, Lai S, et al. A hospital-based prospective study of perinatal infection with human immunodeficiency virus type 1. J Pediatr 1991;118:347-353.

The International Perinatal HIV Group. The mode of delivery and the risk of vertical transmission of human immunodeficiency virus type 1—a meta-analysis of 15 prospective cohort studies. N Engl J Med 1999;340(13):977-987.

Itescu S, Brancato LJ, Winchester R. A sicca syndrome in HIV infection: association with HLA-DR5 and CD8 lymphocytosis. Lancet 1989;2:466-468.

Joshi VV. Pathologic findings association with HIV infection in children. In Pizzo P, Wilfert CM (eds). Pediatric AIDS. Baltimore: Williams & Wilkins, 1991.

Jovais E, Koch MA, Schafer A, et al. LAV/HTLV-III in a 20-week fetus. Lancet 1985;2:1129 (letter).

Jura E, Chadwick E, Joseph S, et al. Varicella-zoster virus infections in children infected with human immunodeficiency virus. Pediatr Infect Dis 1989;8:586-590.

Kashkin JM, Shliozberg J, Lyman WD, et al. Detection of human immunodeficiency virus (HIV) in human fetal tissues. Pediatr Res 1988;23(2):355A.

King JC Jr, Vink PE, Farley JJ, et al. Comparison of the safety and immunogenicity of a pneumococcal conjugate with a licensed polysaccharide vaccine in human immunodeficiency virus and non-human immunodeficiency virus-infected children. Pediatr Infect Dis J 1996;15(3):192-196.

Koup RA, Safrit JT, Cao Y, et al. The initial control of viremia during primary HIV-1 syndrome is temporally associated with the presence of cellular immune responses. J Virol 1994;68:4650-4655.

Krasinski K, Borkowsky W, Bonk S, et al. Bacterial infections in human immunodeficiency virus infected children. Pediatr Infect Dis 1988;7:323-328.

Landay AL, Mackewicz CE, Levy JA. An activated CD8+T cell phenotype correlates with anti-HIV activity and asymptomatic clinical status. Clin Immunol Immunopath 1993;69:106-116.

Landesman SH, Kalish LA, Burns DN, et al. Obstetrical factors and the transmission of human immunodeficiency virus type 1 from mother to child. N Engl J Med 1996;334:1617-1623.

Lee FK, Nahmias AJ, Lowery S, et al. ELISPOT: a new approach to studying the dynamics of virus-immune system interaction for diagnosis and monitoring of HIV infection. AIDS Res Hum Retrovir 1989;5:517-523.

Levin MJ, Gershon AA, Weinberg A, et al. Immunization of HIV-infected children with varicella vaccine. J Pediatr 2001;139(2):305-310.

Levy JA, Hoffman AD, Kramer SM, et al. Retroviruses from San Francisco patients with AIDS. Science 1984;225:840-842.

Lipshultz SE, Orav EJ, Sanders SP, et al. Cardiac structure and function in children with human immunodeficiency virus infection treated with zidovudine. N Engl J Med 1992;327:1260-1265.

Luginbuhl LM, Orav J, McIntosh K, Lipshultz SE. Cardiac morbidity and related mortality in children with HIV infection. JAMA 1993;269:2869-2675.

Luzuriaga K, McManus M, Catalina M, et al. Early therapy of vertical human immunodeficiency virus type 1 (HIV-1) infection; control of viral replication and absence of persistent HIV-1 specific immune responses. J Virol 2000;74:6984-6991.

Mann DL, Hamlin-Green G, Willoughby A, et al. Immunoglobulin class and subclass antibodies to HIV proteins in maternal serum: association with perinatal transmission. J AIDS 1994;7:617-622.

Mayaux MJ, Burgard M, Teglas JP, et al. Neonatal characteristics in rapidly progressive perinatally acquired HIV-1 disease: the French Pediatric HIV Infection Study Group. JAMA 1996;275:606-610.

McKinney RE Jr, Maha MA, Connor EM et al. A multicenter trial of oral zidovudine in children with advanced human immunodeficiency virus disease. The Protocol 043 Study Group. N Engl J Med 1991;324(15):1018-1025.

Melvin AJ, Mohan KM, Arcuino LA, et al. Clinical, virologic and immunologic responses of children with advanced human immunodeficiency virus type 1 disease treated with protease inhibitors. Pediatr Infect Dis J 1997;16:968-974.

Miles SA, Balden E, Magpantay L et al. Rapid serologic testing with immune-complex-dissociated HIV p24 antigen for early detection of HIV infection in neonates. Southern California Pediatric AIDS Consortium. N Engl J Med 1993;328(5):297-302.

Minkoff H, Burns DN, Landesman S, et al. The relationship of the duration of ruptured membranes to vertical transmission of human immunodeficiency virus. Am J Obstet Gynecol 1995;173:585-589.

Mofenson LM, Moye J Jr, Bethel J et al. Prophylactic intravenous immunoglobulin in HIV-infected children with CD4+ counts of 0.20 × 10(9)/L or more. Effect on viral, opportunistic, and bacterial infections. The National Institute of Child Health and Human Development Intravenous Immunoglobulin Clinical Trial Study Group. JAMA 1992;268(4):483-488.

Mok JG, Gianquinto C, Derossi A, et al. Infants born to mothers seropositive for human immunodeficiency virus: preliminary findings from the multicenter European study. Lancet 1987;1:1164-1168.

Moye J, Rich KC, Kalish LA, et al. Natural history of somatic growth in infants born to women infected by human immunodeficiency virus. J Pediatr 1996;128:58-69.

Musoke P, Guay LA, Bagenda D, et al. A phase I/II study of the safety and pharmacokinetics of nevirapine in HIV-1 infected pregnant Ugandan women and their neonates (HIVNET 006). AIDS 1999;13:479-486.

Nachman S, Stanley K, Yogev R, et al. Nucleoside analogues plus ritonavir in stable antiretroviral therapy-experienced HIV-infected children: a randomized trial. JAMA 2000;283:492-498.

Nduati R, Richardson BA, John G, et al. Effect of breast-feeding on mortality among HIV-1 infected women: a randomised trial. Lancet 2001;357(9269):1651-1655.

Nelson JA, Wiley CA, Reynolds-Kohler C, et al. Human immunodeficiency virus detected in bowel epithelium from patients with gastrointestinal symptoms. Lancet 1988;1:259-262.

Nikolic-Djokic D, Essajee S, Rigaud M, et al. Immunoreconstitution in children on highly active antiretroviral therapy depends on the Cd4 % at baseline. J Infect Dis 2002 (in press).

Oleske J, Minnefor A, Cooper R, et al. Immune deficiency in children. JAMA 1983;249:2345-2349.

Oxtoby MS, Mvula M, Ryder R, et al. Measles and measles immunity in African children with HIV (abstract 1353). Interscience Conference on Antimicrobial Agents and Chemotherapy, Los Angeles, 1988.

Pahwa S, Chirmule N, Leombruno C, et al. In vitro synthesis of human immunodeficiency virus–specific antibodies in peripheral blood lymphocytes of infants. Proc Natl Acad Sci 1989;86:7532-7536.

Pahwa S, Pahwa R, Saxinger C, et al. Influence of the human T-lymphotropic virus/lymphadenopathy virus on functions of human lymphocytes: evidence for immunosuppressive effects and polyclonal B-cell activation by banded viral preparations. Proc Natl Acad Sci USA 1985;82:8198-8202.

Papaevangelou V, Pollack H, Rigaud M, et al. The amount of early p24 antigenemia and not the time of first detection of virus predicts the clinical outcome of vertically HIV-1 infected infants. J Infect Dis 1998;173:574-578.

Papaevangelou V, Pollack H, Rochford G et al. Enhanced transmission of vertical HCV infection to HIV-infected infants of HIV and HCV co-infected women. J Infect Dis 1998;178:1047-1052.

Persaud D, Bangaru B, Greco MA, et al. Cholestatic hepatitis in children with HIV infection. Ped Infect Dis 1993;12:492-499.

Persaud D, Pierson T, Ruff C, et al. A stable latent reservoir for HIV-1 in resting CD4(+) T lymphocytes in infected children. J Clin Invest 2000;105(7):995-1003.

Phair J, Munoz A, Detels R, et al. The risk of *Pneumocystis carinii* pneumonia among men infected with human immunodeficiency virus type 1. Multicenter AIDS Cohort Study Group. N Engl J Med 1990;322(3):161-165.

Plaeger-Marshall S, Hultin P, Bertolli J, et al. Activation and differentiation antigens on T cells of healthy, at-risk, and HIV-infected children. J AIDS 1993;6:984-990.

Pollack H, Zhan MX, Moore T et al. Ontogeny of Anti-HIV Antibody Production in HIV-infected infants. Proc Natl Acad Sci (USA) 1993;90:2340-2344.

Pollack H, Glasberg H, Lee E, et al. Neurodevelopment, growth, and viral load in HIV-infected infants. Brain Behav Immun 1996;10:298-312.

Quinn TC, Ruff A, Halsey N. Special considerations for developing nations. In Pizzo P, Wilfert CM (eds). Pediatric AIDS. Baltimore: Williams & Wilkins, 1991.

Rogers MF, Ou CY, Rayfield M et al. Use of the polymerase chain reaction for early detection of the proviral sequences of human immunodeficiency virus in infants born to seropositive mothers. New York City Collaborative Study of Maternal HIV Transmission and Montefiore Medical Center HIV Perinatal Transmission Study Group. N Engl J Med 1989;320(25):1649-1654.

Roilides E, Mertins S, Eddy J, et al. Impairment of neutrophil chemotactic and bactericidal function in children infected with HIV-1 and partial reversal after in vitro exposure to granulocyte-macrophage colony stimulating factor. J Pediatr 1990;117:531-540.

Rolston K, Rodriquez S, Mansell P. Therapy of salmonella infection in AIDS patients (abstract). Fifth international conference on AIDS, Montreal, June 1989.

Rosok B, Voltersvik P, Bjerknes R, et al. Dynamics of HIV-1 replication following influenza vaccination of HIV+ individuals. Clin Exp Immunol 1996;104:203-207.

Rubinstein A, Sicklick M, Gupta A, et al. Acquired immunodeficiency with reversed T4/T8 ratios in infants born to promiscuous and drug-addicted mothers. JAMA 1983;249:2350-2356.

Russell C, Lay K. Natural history of *Candida* species of the yeast in the oral cavities of infants. Arch Oral Biol 1973;18:957-962.

Ryder RW, Nsaw W, Hassigs E, et al. Perinatal transmission of the human immunodeficiency virus type 1 to infants of seropositive women in Zaire. N Engl J Med 1989;320:1637-1642.

Schreiber GB, Busch MP, Kleinman SH, et al. The risk of transfusion-transmitted viral infections. N Engl J Med 1996;334:1685-1690.

Scott GB, Buck BE, Leterman JG, et al. Acquired immunodeficiency syndrome in infants. N Engl J Med 1984;310:76-81.

Selwyn PA, Schoenbaum EE, Davenny K, et al. Prospective study of human immunodeficiency virus infection and pregnancy outcomes in intravenous drug users. JAMA 1989;261:1289-1294.

Sharer LR, Cho ES, Epstein LG. Multinucleated giant cells and HTLV/III in AIDS encephalopathy. Hum Pathol 1985;16:760.

Sharer LR, Epstein LG, Cho ES, et al. Pathologic features of AIDS encephalopathy in children: evidence for LAV/-HTLV-III infection of brain. Hum Pathol 1986;17:271-284.

Shaw GM, Harper ME, Hahn BH, et al. HTLV/III infection of brains of children and adults with AIDS encephalopathy. Science 1985;227:117-182.

Spector SA, Gelber RD, McGrath N et al. A controlled trial of intravenous immune globulin for the prevention of serious bacterial infections in children receiving zidovudine for advanced human immunodeficiency virus infection. Pediatric AIDS Clinical Trials Group. N Engl J Med 1994;331(18):1181-1187.

Sperling RS, Shapiro DE, Coombs RW, et al. Maternal viral load, zidovudine treatments, and the risk of transmission of human immunodeficiency virus type 1 from mother to infant. N Engl J Med 1996;335:1621-1629.

Sprecher S, Soumenkoff G, Puissant F, and Degueldre M. Vertical transmission of HIV in 15-week fetus. Lancet 1986;2:288-289.

St. Louis ME, Kamega M, Brown C, et al. Risk for perinatal HIV-1 transmission according to maternal immunologic, virologic, and placental factors. JAMA 1993;269:2853-2859.

Stoler MH, Eskins TA, Benn S, et al. Human T-cell lymphotropic virus type 3 infection of the central nervous system. A preliminary in situ analysis. JAMA 1986;256:2360-2364.

Taha TE, Graham SM, Kumwenda NI, et al. Morbidity among human immunodeficiency virus-1-infected and -uninfected African children. Pediatrics 2000;106(6):E77.

Tardieu M, Mayaux MJ, Seibel N, et al. Cognitive assessment of school-age children infected with maternally transmitted human immunodeficiency virus type 1. J Pediatr 1995;126:375-379.

Tovo PA, de Martino M, Gabiano C, et al. Mode of delivery and gestational age influence perinatal HIV-1 transmission: Italian register for HIV infection in children. J AIDS Hum Retrovirol 1995;Jan 11:88-94.

Uetmann MH, Belman WL, Ruff HA, et al. Developmental abnormalities in infants and children with acquired immune deficiency syndrome (AIDS) and AIDS-related complex. Dev Med Child Neurol 1985;27:563-571.

Van de Perre P, Simonon A, Msellati P, et al. Postnatal transmission of human immunodeficiency virus type 1 from mother to infant. A prospective cohort study in Kigali, Rwanda. N Engl J Med 1991;325(9):593-598.

Vigano A, Dally L, Bricalli D, et al. Clinical and immunovirologic characterization of the efficacy of stavudine, lamivudine, and indinavir in human immunodeficiency virus infection. J Pediatr 1999;135:675-682.

Wade NA, Birkhead GS, Warren BL, et al. Abbreviated regimens of zidovudine prophylaxis and perinatal transmission of the human immunodeficiency virus. N Engl J Med 1998;339(20):1409-1414.

Walker CM, Moody DJ, Stites DO, Levy JA. CD8+lymphocytes can control HIV infection in vitro by suppressing viral replication. Science 1986;234:1563-1566.

Weiser B, Nachman S, Tropper P, et al. Quantitation of human immunodeficiency virus type 1 during pregnancy: relationship of viral titer to mother-to-child transmission and stability of viral load. PNAS (USA) 1994;91:8037-8041.

Zhang L, Lewin S, Markowitz M, et al. Measuring recent thymic emigrants in blood of normal persons and HIV-1 infected patients before and after effective therapy. J Exper Med 1999;190:725-732.

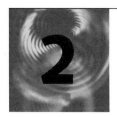

BOTULISM

SARAH S. LONG

Botulism is a neuroparalytic disease caused by the action of a heat-labile neurotoxin produced almost exclusively by *Clostridium botulinum*. The disease occurs under three circumstances: (1) botulism food poisoning, which results from consuming food that contains preformed toxin; (2) wound botulism, which occurs when toxin is produced by *C. botulinum* organisms contaminating traumatic wounds; and (3) infant botulism, which is due to toxin production by *C. botulinum* within the gastrointestinal tract. Infant botulism occurs occasionally in adults, usually in the setting of abdominal surgery, gastrointestinal tract abnormalities, or antibiotic use. Arnon and others have discussed aerosolization of toxin as a potential mode of bioterrorism. More than 1,500 cases of infant botulism have been confirmed in the United States since Pickett and associates reported the first case in 1976. Shapiro and associates report that since 1979 infant botulism has been the most frequent form of botulism, accounting for >60% of all cases, with a median of 71 cases identified annually by the Centers for Disease Control and Prevention (CDC). It is the exclusive form of botulism in infants.

ETIOLOGY AND PATHOPHYSIOLOGY

C. botulinum represents a heterogeneous group of gram-positive, anaerobic, spore-forming bacilli, individual strains of which can produce one of seven serologically distinct neurotoxins (types A to G). More than 90% of cases of infant botulism in the United States are due to type A or B. *C. baratii* and *C. butyricum* are responsible rarely for cases caused by botulinal neurotoxins type E and F.

Botulinal neurotoxin, produced with outgrowth of spores, is the most potent poison known. After systemic absorption, toxin binds irreversibly to receptors on presynaptic nerve endings of cranial and peripheral nerves where a portion is internalized and prevents release of acetylcholine at motorneuron terminals. Neutralizing antitoxin is effective only before internalization of the toxin molecule. Recovery depends on ultrasprouting of nerve endings.

Infant botulism results from ingestion of botulinal spores. In approximately 85% of cases the source is unknown and probably is unavoidable; less frequently, spores in honey are the source. Vulnerability of healthy infants is unique, with cases occurring from 6 days to 12 months of age but not later. The results of experiments performed on mice by Wells and Sugiyami in the 1980s, and observations in cases of infant botulism, suggest that transient lack of competitive microbial intestinal flora (and possibly alteration in motility or pH) permits outgrowth of vegetative forms following ingestion of spores.

The intestinal flora of breast-fed and formula-fed infants, as well as adults, would be expected to inhibit vegetative outgrowth of *C. botulinum* spores. Long has postulated that there are brief periods of permissiveness before flora are well established in infants fed formula and during the perturbation of flora at the time of weaning of infants fed human milk. The mean age of diagnosis of botulism is 7.6 weeks in formula-fed infants and 13.7 weeks in breast-fed infants.

EPIDEMIOLOGY

Risk factors for infant botulism are multifactorial and involve both the environment and the infant. The environment and naturally contaminated foodstuffs, such as honey and corn syrup, are potential sources of *C. botulinum*. *C. botulinum* spores are ubiquitous worldwide and are found in virgin and cultivated soils. In the United States, almost all type A spores are found west of the Mississippi River. Type B spores have a more general distribution but usually are present between 35 and 55 degrees north latitude, especially in soil with high organic content. Incidence of infant botulism and botulinum toxin types mirror the geographic presence and density of spores in the environment. Cases of infant botulism have been reported in 45 states in the United States and on all continents except Africa. The highest reported incidences of disease in the United States are in California (where toxin types are evenly distributed between A and B) and in a narrow arc from Delaware, across Southeastern Pennsylvania, to New Jersey (where toxin type B accounts for more than 90% of cases). When environmental investigation was performed in Pennsylvania and California, one or more samples from an affected infant's environment, such as yard soil, vacuum cleaner dust, crib, father's work shoes, or consumed honey, usually yielded spores of C. botulinum, always of matching toxin type.

Arnon, Spika, and Long have studied host susceptibility factors for infant botulism in addition to the well-recognized ones of age, feeding of human milk, and use of honey. Many, such as higher socioeconomic standard and race, may be markers for likelihood of breast-feeding, and others, such as suburban or rural residence and father's occupation, may be markers for heightened opportunity for exposure to soil. First introduction of foodstuffs to breast-fed infants marks a period of heightened risk. Constipation may be a risk factor (odds ratio of 2.9 in Spika study), but it also is an early manifestation of intoxication. When botulism occurs in infants fed formula, or is caused by toxin type A, the course is more rapidly paralytic. There is no apparent natural acquisition of immunity of the population to C. botulinum or its toxin. Infants recovering from botulism have demonstrable specific antibody to toxin, despite continued presence of toxin in stool for several weeks. There are no cases of distant recurrences, although occurrence after 12 months of age is rare in all individuals.

CLINICAL MANIFESTATIONS

Clinical manifestations (Table 2-1) are entirely due to progressive, symmetrical, *descending* neuromuscular blockade. Presynaptic autonomic nerves also are affected. The spectrum of infant botulism is broad, with sudden infant death syndrome (SIDS) an occasional presentation at one extreme and transient mild weakness and hypotonia, slow feeding, or constipation alone at the other.

Constipation (no spontaneous stools for 3 or more days) is the initial manifestation in most cases. Descending symmetric paralysis progresses over hours to 20 days (median 4.2 days) before medical recognition or hospitalization. Function of cranial nerves is affected before that of others that control muscles of trunk, extremities, and diaphragm. Subtly flat expression, a quiet voice, and less avid suck are

TABLE 2-1	Clinical Features of Infant Botulism		
Symptoms	Signs	Autonomic signs
Decreased frequency of stools	Quiet, stillness	Decreased tearing and salivation
Lack of expression	Poor head control	Fluctuating blood pressure and heart rate
Weak voice or cry	Diminished gag and suck	Flushed skin (sometimes harlequin)
Weak suck, prolonged feeding	Diminished range of eye movement	Constipation
Floppiness		Decreased anal sphincter tone
Gurgling, drooling	Sluggishly reactive or non-reactive pupils	Atony of the bladder
	Diminished movement against gravity	
	Hypotonia, hyporeflexia	

noted, usually only by parents. Floppiness, poor feeding, gurgling, and drooling are noted almost universally by the time of hospitalization.

The most notable immediate impression on physical examination is the infant's quiet, still demeanor. Although frequently the infant's condition is misinterpreted as "lethargic" or "septic," the infant is afebrile, alert, and interested in the environment (but unable to smile, vocalize, or move), and skin color is normal or robust rather than mottled. All cranial nerves are eventually involved. Hyporeflexia, which is relatively mild early in the course despite profound hypotonia, progresses over time. Autonomic dysfunction is common (see Table 2-1) but is underrecognized.

Except for complications directly related to hypotonia, secondary infections are most common. These predominantly are acute otitis media, aspiration pneumonia, urinary tract infection, and infections associated with hospitalization. Schechter and co-workers reported five cases of C. *difficile* colitis in infants during or after hospitalization for botulism. Toxic megacolon and necrotizing enterocolitis distinguished two cases.

DIAGNOSIS

The diagnosis is a clinical one. Results of standard laboratory tests, including cerebrospinal fluid examination, are normal. Although electromyographic findings in infant botulism are unique, the procedure is painful and generally unnecessary. Confirmation of the diagnosis requires isolation of the organism or, preferably, detection of toxin in stool. C. *botulinum* organisms and toxin can be identified in stool of affected infants for as long as 4 months after onset of symptoms, well into recovery. Electroencephalogram and findings from neuroimaging studies usually are normal, barring a hypoxic event.

Toxin neutralization bioassay in mice performed on stool filtrate at a state laboratory or at the CDC is the only reliable confirmatory test. Passed stool is the preferred specimen, but effluent from a small volume enema, using sterile nonbacteriostatic water, is acceptable. The specimen must be maintained at 4° C through all stages of transport. Fluorescent antibody or enzyme immunoassay for detection of toxin or organism is inferior, and use of poly-

merase chain reaction is confounded by extensive sharing of unexpressed toxin genes across species.

DIFFERENTIAL DIAGNOSIS

Several disorders can mimic infant botulism superficially. These include infectious disorders (septicemia, meningitis, poliomyelitis, encephalitis); biochemical or metabolic disorders (dehydration, electrolyte imbalance, genetic metabolic disorder, Leigh disease); endocrinologic disorders (hypothyroidism); neurologic conditions (myasthenia gravis, infantile polyneuropathy, Guillain-Barré syndrome, Werdnig-Hoffmann disease, congenital myopathy, tick paralysis); and drug or chemical poisoning. Felz and associates point out that tick paralysis typically affects children (but rarely infants), and early manifestations are paresthesias and leg weakness followed by *ascending* paralysis. In infant botulism, paralysis is descending and there are no sensory abnormalities. The constellation of findings of infant botulism in the setting of age, feeding history, and exposures is usually classic, and the possibility of another diagnosis is remote. Cerebrospinal fluid and peripheral blood studies are normal.

TREATMENT

A 5-year placebo (intravenous immunoglobulin)-controlled randomized clinical trial of efficacy of a single intravenous dose of human botulinum immunoglobulin (BIG) derived from pooled plasma of immunized adult volunteers was concluded in California under the sponsorship of the Office of Orphan Products Development of the U.S. Food and Drug Administration and the California Department of Health Services. As reported by Arnon, BIG recipients had a significant reduction in hospitalization, from 5.5 weeks to 2.5 weeks, and a two-thirds reduction in the rate of intubation. The Food and Drug Administration has approved human BIG for use as a Treatment Investigational New Drug only for infant botulism; it can be obtained from the California Department of Health Services 24 hours a day by calling 510-540-2646. BIG should be administered as early as possible to infants with suspected botulism to interrupt neuromuscular blockade. Equine botulinal antitoxin should not be used for infant botulism, and human BIG is not available for use in any form of botulism other than infant botulism.

The prognosis for patients with infant botulism usually is excellent. The challenge of management, after timely recognition and administration of antitoxin, is to prevent complications while awaiting neuromuscular recovery. Sudden catastrophic hypoxia is the most frequent, highly morbid, and preventable event. Observation in an intensive care unit with continuous monitoring for at least 48 hours is essential to determine progression. In infants older than 2 months of age, the tempo of progression becomes apparent; preemptive intubation can be performed as the infant's ability to protect the airway diminishes. In infants younger than 2 months of age, weakness, obstruction, and aspiration can occur concurrently, making intubation a prudent approach for most.

Enteral feedings should be provided immediately by continuous small volumes through a nasoenteric tube; such feedings are usually tolerated even by infants lacking bowel sounds. Use of an indwelling intravenous catheter, a urinary catheter, or antibiotics is not warranted generally, and each carries risk. Extubation and resumption of oral feeding depend on return of adequate ability to protect airway, suck, swallow, and sustain movement against gravity.

OUTCOME AND PREVENTION

Patients in whom supportive care is begun before a hypoxic episode occurs have an excellent prognosis, with <1% mortality rate even before the availability of human BIG. Full recovery without neurologic or neuromuscular sequelae depends on maintaining vigilance and meticulous supportive care while minimizing interventions that increase complications.

Botulism is uncommon, and environmental exposure to spores is unavoidable. Honey is an avoidable source of spores. The American Academy of Pediatrics and the CDC recommend not offering honey to children younger than 12 months. Considering that sterility of corn syrup cannot be guaranteed, the AAP also recommends against its use in infants. No case of infant botulism has been ascribed to spores contaminating corn syrup.

SUGGESTED READINGS

Arnon SS, Schechter R, Inglesby TV, et al. Botulinum toxin as a biological weapon: Medical and public health management. JAMA 2001;285:1059–1069.

Arnon SS. Infant botulism. In Feigin RD, Cherry JD (eds). Textbook of pediatric infectious diseases, ed 4. Philadelphia: WB Saunders, 1998.

Arnon SS, Midura TF, Clay SA, et al. Infant botulism: epidemiologic, clinical, and laboratory aspects. JAMA 1977;237:1946-1951.

Centers for Disease Control and Prevention. Summary of notifiable diseases, United States, 1999. MMWR 2001;48(R-53):1-81.

Committee on Infectious Diseases. Clostridial infections. Appendix VI. Potentially contaminated food products. In Pickering LK (ed). 2000 Red Book: Report of the Committee on Infectious Diseases, ed 25. Elk Grove Village, Ill.: American Academy of Pediatrics, 2000.

Felz MW, Smith CD, Swift TR. A six-year-old girl with tick paralysis. N Engl J Med 2000;342:90-94.

Long SS. Epidemiologic study of infant botulism in Pennsylvania: report of the infant botulism study group. Pediatrics 1985;75:928-934.

Long SS, Gajewski JL, Brown LW, et al. Clinical, laboratory, and environmental features of infant botulism in Southeastern Pennsylvania. Pediatrics 1985;75:935-941.

Pickett J. Syndrome of botulism in infancy: clinical and electrophysiologic study. N Engl J Med 1976;295:770.

Schechter R, Peterson B, McGee J, et al. *Clostridium difficile* colitis associated with infant botulism: near-fatal case analogous to Hirschsprung's enterocolitis. Clin Infect Dis 1999;29:367-374.

Shapiro RL, Hatheway C, Swerdlow DL. Botulism in the United States: a clinical and epidemiologic review. Ann Int Med 1998;129:221-228.

Spika JS, Shafer N, Hargrett-Bean N, et al. Risk factors for infant botulism in the United States. Am J Dis Child 1989;143:828-832.

Wells CL, Sugiyama H, Bland SE. Resistance of mice with limited intestinal flora to enteric colonization by *Clostridium botulinum*. J Infect Dis 1982;146:791-796.

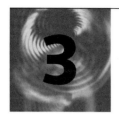

3 CHOLERA

EDWARD T. RYAN AND MOHAMMED ABDUS SALAM

Cholera is a watery diarrhea caused by infection with *Vibrio cholerae* O1 or O139. It is an infection of global importance, resulting in seven documented global pandemics in the last 200 years. The seventh pandemic began in the 1960s in Asia, has spread around the world, and is still ongoing.

Despite its often-catastrophic clinical manifestations, cholera remains an immensely preventable and treatable disease. The majority of cholera cases occur in areas of the world endemic for infection with *V. cholerae*, where the burden of disease is highest among children.

MICROBIOLOGY

V. cholerae is a facultatively anaerobic, curved gram-negative bacillus in the family Vibrionaceae. It is motile, possessing a unipolar flagellum, and has a characteristic darting or "shooting star" appearance on microscopic examination of freshly passed cholera stools. *V. cholerae* is oxidase positive, sucrose positive, and usually lactose negative. If infection with *V. cholerae* is suspected, stool or vomitus should be plated on selective media such as thiosulfate-citrate-bile salts-sucrose (TCBS) agar or taurocholate-tellurite-gelatin agar (TTGA).

Agglutinating antibody that reacts with surface lipopolysaccharide can be used to differentiate *V. cholerae* organisms into over 150 serogroups, of which *V. cholerae* O1 and O139 are capable of causing epidemic cholera (Chakraborty et al., 2000). Non-O1 and non-O139 *V. cholerae* organisms have been associated with occasional cases of diarrhea but do not express cholera toxin and have not been associated with epidemic outbreaks of cholera (Morris, 1994). *V. cholerae* O1 exists in two biotypes: classical and El Tor. These biotypes differ by biochemical profile and phage infectivity. Based on additional differences in the O antigen of the lipopolysaccharide, *V. cholerae* O1 can be further subdivided into serotypes Ogawa, Hikojima, and Inaba. During epidemics, *V. cholerae* O1 can switch among serotypes. Hikojima is thought to be an unstable variant, and Inaba and Ogawa strains cause the majority of disease worldwide (Stroeher et al., 1992). *V. cholerae* O139 is thought to have arisen from a *V. cholerae* O1 El Tor strain. It is not further subdivided into biotypes or serotypes and, in contrast to *V. cholerae* O1, has a different surface lipopolysaccharide and a capsule (*V. cholerae* O1 is not encapsulated).

PATHOGENESIS

V. cholerae O1 El Tor strain N16961 has recently been sequenced (Heidelberg et al., 2000). The genome is composed of two circular chromosomes: chromosome 1 (consisting of 2.96 Mbp) and chromosome 2 (consisting of 1.07 Mbp), in total encoding 3,885 open reading frames. The majority of potential proteins encoded by the open reading frames are currently of unknown function. A number of genes known to be involved in pathogenesis localize in a 45.3 kbp *Vibrio* chromosomal pathogenicity island (VPI) located on the large chromosome (Heidelberg et al., 2000; Karaolis et al., 1998).

Cholera toxin is the major virulence factor for all toxigenic strains of *V. cholerae*. Cholera toxin is a heterodimeric protein exotoxin consisting of a single, enzymatically active A subunit that is noncovalently attached to five identically sized B subunits (Gill, 1976). Cholera toxin is secreted by *V. cholerae* organisms via a dedicated type II secretion system encoded by extracellular protein secretion (*eps*) genes (Sandkvist et al., 1993). The B subunits of cholera holotoxin bind to ganglioside GM_1 molecules on the surface of eukaryotic cells.

After internalization, the enzymatically active A subunit is nicked, reduced, and translocated intracellularly, where it transfers ADP-ribose to the $G_s\alpha$ subunit of adenylate cyclase, elevating cAMP within intestinal epithelial cells. This increase in cAMP causes chloride secretion through the apical transmembrane cystic fibrosis transmembrane regulator (CFTR) channel, and sodium and water molecules follow, resulting in secretory diarrhea (Mekalanos et al., 1979; Cassel and Pfeuffer, 1978). Cholera toxin's effect on intestinal prostaglandin levels may also contribute to diarrhea (Speelman et al., 1985). Cholera toxin is expressed by both V. cholerae O1 (El Tor and classical strains) and V. cholerae O139. The genes encoding cholera toxin (ctxAB) are arranged in an operon and are encoded by a filamentous bacteriophage (designated CTXφ) (Waldor and Mekalanos, 1996).

A second major virulence factor involved in intestinal colonization by V. cholerae is the toxin coregulated pilus (TCP) (Herrington et al, 1988). The TCP operon contains a number of genes, including tcpA, which encodes the main structural gene involved in formation of the pilus (Kaufman et al., 1993). TCP not only is involved in the ability of V. cholerae to colonize the human intestine, but also acts as the receptor for CTXφ. Following infection of the bacterial cell, CTXφ integrates at a specific 18 base pair (bp) sequence on the V. cholerae chromosome termed attRS1 (Waldor and Mekalanos, 1996; Pearson et al., 1993). In vivo expression of both TCP and cholera toxin in V. cholerae is coregulated by a number of genes including toxR, tcpH, tcpP, and toxT, which together form the V. Cholerae virulence gene regulatory cascade (Hase, 1998; Caroll, 1997; Lee, 2001). Evaluation of V. cholerae gene expression during infection has shown up-regulation of genes involved in motility, chemotaxis, intestinal colonization, and toxin production (Lee, 2001; Xu, 2003), whereas V. cholerae recovered from stool have a distinct transcriptional profile that may reflect a hyper-infectious phenotype (Merrell, 2002). Another pilus antigen identified in V. cholerae is the mannose-sensitive hemagglutinin (MSHA) (Mukhopadhyay et al., 1996). The role of MSHA in colonization in humans is currently unclear (Finn et al., 1987). A third pilus identified in V. cholerae is encoded by a four-gene cluster pilABCD (Fullner, 1999). The role of this in human infection is still being defined.

A number of other proteins involved in pathogenesis have also been identified. These include a protease that degrades mucosal mucus (possibly facilitating colonization or motility) (Schneider and Parker, 1978); an accessory colonization factor (Trucksis et al., 1993); a zona occludens toxin (Fasano et al., 1991); an RTX toxin involved in rounding of epithethial cells (Fullner and Mekalanos, 2000); the iron-regulated proteins IrgA and IrgB (Goldberg et al., 1990); a hemolysin (Alm et al., 1991); and a neuraminidase that catalyzes conversion of ganglioside to GM_1 (Holmgren et al., 1975). The sequencing of the V. cholerae genome is facilitating identification of additional genes important in regulation and pathogenesis.

EPIDEMIOLOGY AND TRANSMISSION

V. cholerae exists in the environment in brackish water along coastal areas and in river estuaries. In these environments, V. cholerae is associated with zooplankton and other marine fauna with chitinous exoskeletons (Colwell, 1996). In this ecologic niche, V. cholerae may also exist in a viable but nonculturable state (Huq et al., 1990). Responding to poorly understood environmental signals, possibly including changes in water temperature and zooplankton levels, V. cholerae organisms multiply. Ingestion of water or food contaminated with V. cholerae then leads to incidental infection of humans. Although all V. cholerae organisms can cause mild diarrhea, only V. cholerae O1 and O139 contain the cholera toxin genetic element (CTXφ) and are capable of causing epidemic and secondary transmission of cholera. Animals are poorly colonized or infected with V. cholerae, and animal reservoirs are not thought to be important in transmission.

Cholera is predominantly a disease of impoverished and developing areas of the world. Secondary transmission among humans occurs most frequently in areas lacking potable water and adequate sanitary conditions. Social disruptions such as those that occur during or following war, famine, and natural disasters create fertile environments for secondary transmission among humans. Although cholera is a disease reportable to the World Health Organization (WHO), it is estimated that only a small minority of cases of cholera are either identified or reported to health authorities. Despite this, in the 1990s, over 100 countries reported cholera to the

WHO (World Health Organization, 2001), and it is estimated that approximately 5 to 7 million cases of cholera occur worldwide each year, resulting in over 100,000 to 150,000 deaths (Institute of Medicine, 1986; World Health Organization, 2001b).

Approximately one third of the deaths are thought to occur in children younger than 5 years of age, one quarter in children 5 to 14 years of age, and the remainder in adults (Anonymous, 2001). In Bangladesh alone, a country in which the disease is endemic, the annual incidence rate for cholera is estimated to be 3 to 5 cases per 1,000 individuals (Clemens et al., 1995).

Cholera may be characterized as endemic, epidemic, or pandemic. Recorded history has documented seven cholera pandemics since the early 1800s. The first six were caused by *V. cholerae* O1 classical biotype organisms. The seventh pandemic began in Indonesia in the 1960s and continues to the current day. The current pandemic, caused by *V. cholerae* O1 biotype El Tor, has spread throughout Asia, being introduced to the African continent in 1970s and to the Latin American mainland in the 1990s. Although slightly different from the strain responsible for the seventh pandemic, *V. cholerae* O1 biotype El Tor is also endemic in the southern United States along the Gulf of Mexico (Blake, 1993). A new virulent serogroup of *V. cholerae* capable of causing epidemic cholera (*V. cholerae* O139) was first recognized in Asia in the 1990s and is now reported in 11 Asian countries (Cholera Working Group, 1993). For unknown reasons, *V. cholerae* O139 has not replaced *V. cholerae* O1 as the predominant strain.

Cholera is transmitted by ingestion of contaminated food or water (Mintz et al., 1994) and usually results from ingestion of a relatively large inoculum (10^8 to 10^{11} organisms in individuals with normal gastric acidity) (Cash et al., 1974). Ingestion of antacids or the buffering of gastric juices through ingestion of food or liquid lowers the required inoculum (10^4 to 10^6 organisms in hypochlorhydric individuals) (Gitelson, 1971). Infected individuals excrete up to 10^{13} *V. cholerae* organisms per day in stool (10^6 to 10^8 organisms per ml) (Feachem, 1982; Gorbach, 1970), and contamination of food and water supplies can lead to rapid dissemi-

nation of infection in a population. When cholera first occurs in an immunologically naïve population, it usually affects children and adults equally since all are equally susceptible, and large epidemics may ensue. Such an epidemic occurred in 1994 in a refugee camp in Goma, Zaire, when 50,000 of approximately 500,000 to 800,000 refugees died within a 21-day period owing to explosive epidemics of cholera and shigellosis (Goma Epidemiology Group, 1995; Siddique et al., 1995).

In endemic situations, individuals are repetitively exposed to *V. cholerae* established in the local water supply. In areas of the world endemic for cholera, surviving adults are usually completely or partially immune, and clinical cholera is usually a pediatric disease having its highest incidence among children between 2 and 9 years of age (Glass et al., 1982). Maternal antibody may provide some protection to children younger than 2 years of age, and breast-feeding may protect against clinical disease, although breast-feeding does not protect against colonization by *V. cholerae* organisms themselves (Clemens et al., 1990; Glass et al., 1983). Chronic malnutrition does not appear to increase the risk of infection or disease due to *V. cholerae* (Glass et al., 1989).

Emergence of a new serogroup of toxigenic *V. cholerae* in any area of the world (including areas of the world endemic for cholera) can lead to massive epidemics. Such epidemics occurred when *V. cholerae* O139 was introduced in areas of the world endemic for *V. cholerae* O1, since immune responses against *V. cholerae* O1 do not protect against infection with *V. cholerae* O139 (Albert et al., 1993).

Cholera is predominantly a disease of impoverishment, but it can affect travelers. The incidence rate of development of cholera per month spent in a developing country has been estimated to be 0.01% to 0.001% (Ryan and Calderwood, 2001).

CLINICAL MANIFESTATIONS

The incubation period of cholera is usually 1 to 3 days, although it may be as short as a few hours or as long as 5 days, depending on the size of the inoculum and the gastric pH (Cash et al., 1974a). The hallmark of cholera is a profuse secretory diarrhea. Individuals with severe disease may lose more than 250 ml/kg of body weight in a 24-hour period (Molla et al.,

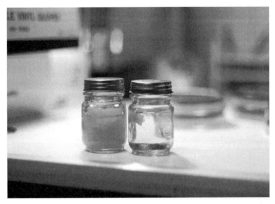

Fig. 3-1 Representative samples of diarrheal stools. On the left is a sample of a diarrheal stool from a patient with cholera. The cholera stool is voluminous and watery with flecks of mucus, resembling "rice water." On the right is a stool sample from a patient with bacillary dysentery due to shigellosis. The dysenteric sample is small volume, bloody and mucoid.

1981). As intestinal contents are evacuated, stool becomes progressively clearer, although it continues to contain flecks of mucus, resulting in a classic "rice water" appearance (Figure 3-1). Cholera stool has a fishy odor, and the darting or shooting star movement of *V. cholerae* organisms is readily apparent when a wet preparation of stool is examined under dark field microscopy. Because *V. cholerae* is a noninvasive organism, stool should contain neither blood nor fecal leukocytes, and fever is typically absent. In fact, individuals with cholera are usually hypothermic because of severe dehydration. Bowel movements may be frequent and voluminous. Nausea, vomiting, and abdominal cramping are common. In severe disease, as diarrhea and vomiting continue, isotonic dehydration occurs and can lead to vascular collapse, shock, and death within 6 to 12 hours of onset of disease (Bennish, 1994).

Although the above scenario describes the classic clinical presentation of severe cholera (cholera gravis), *V. cholerae* can actually cause a spectrum of disease. In endemic areas, asymptomatic stool passage or mild disease is most common in individuals with complete or partial preexisting immunity. Nonimmune individuals can develop disease ranging from moderate gastroenteritis to voluminous diarrhea. The severity of cholera relates to many factors including inoculum size; the presence or absence of preexisting immunity; blood group (individuals with blood group O are at the highest risk of cholera gravis); and the biotype of the infecting strain (Barua and Paguio, 1977; Sircar et al., 1981). Individuals who ingest classical *V. cholerae* organisms are more likely to have symptomatic and severe disease than those who ingest El Tor organisms.

Individuals with cholera should be classified as having severe, moderate (some), or mild (none) dehydration (Institute of Medicine, 1986). Individuals with severe dehydration will have lost greater than 10% of their total body weight in water (approximately 15% of their total body water) and have a fluid deficit of greater than 100 ml per kg. Individuals with severe dehydration have sunken eyes, minimal or absent urine production, dry mucous membranes, and a nonpalpable or rapid and feeble pulse. They are often tachypneic with labored respirations, and they may be comatose, lethargic, or markedly apprehensive. Infants and young children are most likely to be comatose when severely dehydrated. Individuals who are severely dehydrated have skin that retracts extremely slowly when pinched. The tachypnea may be related to a compensatory respiratory response to the severe metabolic acidosis accompanying the bicarbonate loss in diarrheal stool. It may also be due to primary respiratory compromise relating to aspiration of vomitus or concomitant pneumonia (Ryan, 2000b).

Individuals with moderate (some) dehydration will have lost approximately 6% to 10% of their body weight (approximately 7% to 12% of their body water) and have a fluid deficit of approximately 60 to 100 ml per kg World Health Organisation, 2001b). These individuals are usually arousable with increased thirst, and they may be irritable or restless. The individual may be tachypneic, and blood pressure is usually preserved although the pulse rate is rapid. Mucous membranes are dry. Skin retracts slowly when pinched. Eyes are moderately shrunken, and urine production continues, although the amount may be markedly decreased.

Individuals with mild or no dehydration may report thirst without other obvious signs of clinical dehydration and have a fluid deficit of less than 50 ml per kg. Mild cholera may be indistinguishable from other forms of infectious diarrhea.

Diarrhea associated with cholera is usually most severe during the first 1 to 2 days of illness, persisting for 4 to 6 days in most individuals (Hirschhorn et al., 1968). Cholera stools contain high concentrations of sodium, potassium, chloride, and bicarbonate (Table 3-1). Children with cholera may be predisposed to hypoglycemia, possibly relating to diminished food intake during the acute illness, depletion of hepatic glycogen stores, and general malnutrition. Acidosis may be prominent because of bicarbonate losses in diarrheal stools. Although total body potassium levels are often markedly depleted, coexisting acidosis may result in apparently normal serum potassium concentrations at initial presentation (Rapoport et al., 1947). Upon correction of fluid status, however, hypokalemia may become quite pronounced and often contributes to paralytic ileus. Administration of rehydration therapy containing bicarbonate may result in a rapid pH change and subsequent calcium shift, precipitating tetany (Ryan, 2000b). Muscle cramps and myalgia due to the many metabolic and electrolyte disturbances are common.

Severe hemodynamic compromise may precipitate cerebral vascular accidents or myocardial ischemia, particularly among elderly individuals (Ryan, 2000b). Renal blood flow is often compromised in all age groups, resulting in prerenal azotemia, acute tubular necrosis, and oliguria. Complete renal failure requiring dialysis is rare. Renal function usually improves with restitution of intravascular volume. Intravascular depletion may result in hemoconcentration and hyperproteinemia (Wang et al., 1986). Mild to moderate leukocytosis, probably related to stress responses and demargination, is not uncommon.

The death rate for individuals with untreated or poorly treated cholera is often 20% to 50% during epidemic disease (with death rates of 70% to 100% for individuals with cholera gravis) (Ryan, 2000a). Although death may occur within a few hours of onset of diarrhea, more commonly, untreated patients progress to shock in 12 to 24 hours and die within the first 1 to 3 days. Worldwide, many individuals, especially children, die of cholera before they can reach a medical facility. Individuals who do reach medical facilities capable of providing fluid replacement therapy are unlikely to die of dehydration, with death rates in such facilities falling to less than 1% (Ryan, 2000b). Death in individuals with cholera at medical facilities capable of providing adequate fluid replacement is usually due not to dehydration, but to

TABLE 3-1	Composition of Cholera Stool and Replacement Fluids					
	ELECTROLYTE CONCENTRATION (MMOL/L)					
	Na	*Cl⁻*	*K⁺*	*HCO₃⁻*	*Glucose*	*Osmolality (mosm/L)*
Cholera Stool						
Infants and young children	100-105	90	25-35	30		300
Older children and adults	130-135	100	15-20	35-45		300
Hydration Solutions						
Oral						
World Health Organization oral rehydration*	90	80	20	30⁺	111	331
Intravenous						
Ringer's lactate	130	109	4	28†	0‡	271
Normal saline	154	154	0	0	0‡	308

*Per sachet, to be added to 1 L of clean water: sodium chloride, 3.5 g; trisodium citrate, 2.9 g (longer shelf life than sodium bicarbonate, 2.5 g); potassium chloride, 1.5 g; and glucose, 20 g. A homemade alternative can be made by adding the following to 1 L of clean water: 1 level tsp of sodium chloride (approximately 5 g) and 50 g of precooked rice cereal or 40 g of sucrose (table sugar). If a homemade preparation is used, it should be supplemented with potassium, such as that in orange juice or coconut milk.

⁺As citrate: 10 mmol/L of citrate supplies 30 mmol HCO_3^-/L.

†Ringer's lactate does not contain bicarbonate, but does contain lactate.

‡Because of the risk of hypoglycemia, Ringer's lactate and normal saline should contain 50 g of dextrose per liter (5%, 277 mmol/L).

concomitant infection, especially pneumonia (Ryan, 2000b). Severe cholera during pregnancy carries a high mortality rate, with a 50% risk of fetal death during the third trimester (Hirschhorn, 1969).

DIAGNOSIS

Definitive diagnosis of cholera rests on identification of V. cholerae O1 or O139 in the stool or vomitus of an infected individual. If microscopy is performed by an experienced individual, rapid presumptive identification of V. cholerae can be made by noting the shooting star movement of the organism on dark field microscopy of a wet prep stool specimen, and inhibition of that movement after addition of specific agglutinating antibody (Benenson et al., 1964). In most areas of the world, however, standard microbiologic culturing techniques are usually required, often using selective media such as TCBS or TTGA. Enzyme-linked immunoabsorbent assays that detect cholera toxin and genetic probes and rapid DNA amplification assays that detect V. cholerae O1 and O139 have also been developed (although these are not commercially available). Suspected V. cholerae organisms should be sent to reference laboratories for further identification and confirmation, and suspected cholera cases should be immediately reported to the local Department of Public Health. Retrospectively, a suspected case can be confirmed by measuring an increase in the serum vibriocidal antibody response (see section on Immunity).

TREATMENT

The cornerstone of treatment of individuals with cholera is appropriate, rapid, and adequate fluid replacement (Table 3-2). Fluid may be administered either orally or intravenously depending on the severity of dehydration and the ability of the patient to drink. Individuals with diarrhea and dehydration should be rapidly assessed to ascertain their approximate level of dehydration (described above). The fluid deficit should then be calculated, and fluid replaced as quickly as possible. Individuals with severe dehydration initially require over 100 ml per kg body weight of fluid replacement, and patients with moderate or some dehydration require 60 to 100 ml per kg of body weight. Individuals with severe dehydration and those with heavy purging and frequent vomiting should initially receive intravenous fluids.

Fluid replacement therapy should also account for ongoing losses (losses through diarrhea and urine and insensible losses). The use of a cholera cot may help in correctly ascertaining ongoing fluid loss and replacing lost fluids. A cholera cot consists of a rubber sheet with a central hole leading to a bucket for collection of diarrheal stools (Figure 3-2). The collected stool

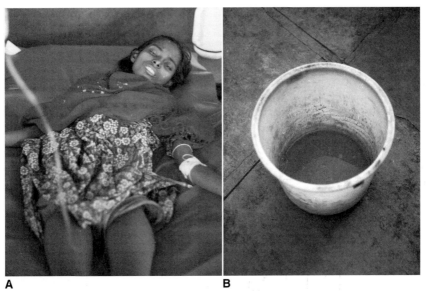

A   **B**

Fig. 3-2 A, Adolescent girl with cholera in Bangladesh. There is a central hole in her cholera cot leading to a bucket. **B,** The volume of diarrhea collected in the bucket can be frequently measured so that the rate of fluid replacement therapy may be accordingly adjusted.

TABLE 3-2	Fluid Replacement Therapy for Patients With Suspected Cholera

For Severe Dehydration
- Give intravenous fluid immediately. Use Ringer's lactate (or, if not available, normal saline) supplemented-with glucose and potassium. If the patient can drink, also begin ORT (see below).
- Age ≥1 year, give 100 ml/kg intravenously in 3 hours:
  30 ml/kg (rapidly) within 30 minutes, then
  70 ml/kg in the next 2 -2½ hours
- Age <1 year, give 100 ml/kg intravenously in 6 hours:
  30 ml/kg (rapidly) in the first hour, then
  70 ml/kg in the next 5 hours
- If after the initial 30 ml/kg the radial pulse is not strong, continue to administer intravenous fluid rapidly.
- Begin ORT, 5 ml/kg/hour, as soon as the patient can drink (in addition to intravenous fluid)
- *Reassess after 3 hours (infants after 6 hours)*
  - If *severe* dehydration still exists, repeat the above.
  - If *some* dehydration exists, continue as listed below.
  - If *no* dehydration exists, continue as listed below.

For Some (Moderate) Dehydration
Approximate amount of ORS to administer in the first 4 hours:

Age	Less than 4 months	4-11 months	12-23 months	2-4 years	5-14 years	15 years or older
Weight	Less than 5 kg	5-7.9 kg	8-10.9 kg	11-15.9 kg	16-29.9 kg	30 kg or more
ORS solution in ml	200-400	400-600	600-800	800-1200	1200-2200	2200-4000

- Use the patient's age when weight not known. The approximate amount of oral rehydration salt-solution (ORS) required (in ml) can also be estimated by multiplying the patient's weight (in kg) by 75.
- If the patient passes watery stools or desires more ORS than listed, administer more.
  Monitor closely.
- *Reassess after 4 hours*
  - If *severe* dehydration, administer intravenous fluids (see above).
  - If *some* dehydration, repeat ORS as listed.
  - If *no* dehydration, continue as listed below.

For No (Mild) Dehydration
Maintenance fluid

Age	Amount of ORS after each loose stool
Less than 24 months	50-100 ml
2-9 years	100-200 ml
10 years or more	As much as wanted

Monitor and assess frequently
If a patient is unable to maintain hydration orally, is vomiting frequently, or develops abdominal distension, stop ORS and administer intravenous fluid, 50 ml/kg in 3 hours, then attempt to resume ORS.
If an antibiotic is to be administered (see text), it should be administered orally after the patient has been rehydrated (usually within 4-6 hours), and after vomiting has stopped.

Modified from World Health Organization. Management of the patient with cholera, World Health Organization Emergency and Other Communicable Diseases, Surveillance and Control, WHO/CDD/SER/91.15 Rev.1 Surveillance and Response Web site]. Available at: www.who.int/csr/resources/publications/cholera/who_cdd_ser_91_15/ent, accessed 4/28/03.

may then be measured, and fluid replacement therapy accordingly adjusted.

As is shown in Table 3-1, cholera stools are isotonic, containing sodium, potassium, chloride, and bicarbonate. Intravenous fluid replacement therapy should, therefore, replace these electrolytes, and should also contain glucose to prevent concomitant hypoglycemia. Ringer's lactate is the most commonly available crystalline fluid that approximates required fluid. Because of the large total body potassium deficit, supplemental potassium should also be administered with Ringer's lactate. Inadequate or inappropriate rehydration is extremely common in treatment of individuals with cholera, especially in areas of the world with limited experience. Although much discussed, over-rehydration during administration of intravenous fluids is an infrequent occurrence in individuals with severe cholera. When it does occur, it is most common in young children, usually first manifests as puffiness around the eyes, and can lead to pulmonary edema, even in children with normal cardiovascular reserve.

All individuals with cholera who can drink should receive oral rehydration therapy (ORT). For individuals with mild or moderate disease, only oral therapy is usually required. Individuals with severe dehydration should begin oral replacement therapy when they awaken, and intravenous fluid replacement should continue until they are no longer severely dehydrated and are able to maintain adequate oral fluid intake. ORT is based upon use of a glucose-coupled sodium chloride cotransport mechanism (Field et al, 1989a, 1989b). This transport mechanism permits uptake of sodium chloride with glucose through a different pump than that involved in the extracellular intraluminal secretion of sodium chloride and water caused by cholera toxin. ORT has reduced mortality from cholera from over 50% to less than 1% in many areas of the world (Ryan, 2000b). The World Health Organization (WHO) recommends oral rehydration salt (ORS) solution contain 3.5 g of sodium chloride, 2.9 g of trisodium citrate (or 2.5 g of sodium bicarbonate), 1.5 g of potassium chloride, and 20 g of glucose (or 40 g of sucrose) per liter of water. ORT based on rice- or cereal-based carbohydrate sources may also be used and may more effectively reduce diarrhea in children with cholera than do glucose-containing solutions (Gore et al., 1992). Oral rehydration solutions available in many industrialized countries contain a lower concentration of sodium (60 mmol/L) than that lost in cholera stool (100 to 130 mmol/L). This lower concentration more closely approximates the losses that occur during infection with organisms more commonly diagnosed in the industrialized world, such as rotavirus. Use of such industrialized-world oral rehydration solutions in individuals with cholera, especially children, may lead to severe hyponatremia. Administration of ORT in children often requires the constant presence of a dedicated attendant or care-giver to encourage frequent ingestion of small volumes of liquid. Intermittent vomiting is not a contraindication to the administration of ORT.

Although commonly used, antimicrobial agents play a purely secondary role in the treatment of individuals with cholera. The primary risk of death during cholera is from dehydration, not from overwhelming infection or sepsis. Administration of antibiotics is, however, associated with reduction in the duration of diarrhea and volume of stool by approximately 50%, increased clearance of *V. cholerae* from the intestine, and decreased incidence of secondary transmission. These are important considerations in areas of the world in which resources are limited and the risk of secondary transmission is high. Oral tetracycline (50 mg/kg per day, maximum 2 g per day in 4 divided doses for 3 days) or doxycycline (6 mg/kg, maximum 300 mg, as a single dose) are usually considered the drugs of choice for individuals with cholera. Use of tetracyclines is contraindicated in children younger than 8 years old, and although trimethoprim-sulfamethoxazole (8 to 10 mg/kg per day of trimethoprim and 40 to 50 mg/kg per day of sulfamethoxazole in 2 divided doses for 3 days) or furazolidone (5 to 8 mg/kg per day, maximum 400 mg, in four divided doses for 3 days) is often recommended for use in young children, increasing resistance to these agents has greatly limited their usefulness (Yamamoto et al., 1995). Currently, erythromycin (40 mg/kg per day, maximum 1000 mg, in four divided doses for 3 days) has become the antibiotic of choice for treating young children and pregnant women with cholera in many areas of the world. Fluoroquinolones such as ciprofloxacin, ofloxacin, and levofloxacin and newer macrolides such as azithromycin may also be effective in treating individuals with cholera, although their use is rarely indicated.

IMMUNITY

Infection with *V. cholerae* induces protective immunity against subsequent cholera infection that lasts for at least a few years (Cash, 1974a, 1974b). Volunteer studies in nonendemic settings have demonstrated that infection with classical biotype *V. cholerae* O1 provides 100% protection from subsequent disease due to classical biotype organisms for at least 3 years (the time period last examined), while an El Tor infection provides 90% protection from subsequent disease due to El Tor strains (Levine et al.,

1981). In the field, cholera (severe enough to require medical attention at a health-care facility) caused by *V. cholerae* O1 classical organisms also decreases the risk of subsequent clinical cholera by approximately 90%, with a lower level of protection associated with El Tor strains (Glass et al., 1985; Clemens et al., 1991). In endemic areas, recurrent ingestion of *V. cholerae* organisms is probably common, resulting in repetitive stimulation of immune responses.

Antibacterial immune responses appear to be more important than antitoxin immune responses following cholera, because (1) protection from clinical disease is associated with inability to culture *V. cholerae* organisms from the stool of immune volunteers after rechallenge; (2) previous disease due to cholera toxin–producing *V. cholerae* O1 does not protect from subsequent disease caused by cholera toxin–producing *V. cholerae* O139; and (3) nontoxigenic recombinant vaccine strains of *V. cholerae* induce protective immunity in volunteers equivalent to that conferred by toxigenic parent strains.

The best characterized of the antibacterial immune responses following cholera is the vibriocidal antibody response. Vibriocidal antibodies are measured in a bactericidal assay requiring the presence of complement-fixing antibody bound specifically to vibrios (Losonsky et al., 1996). Vibriocidal antibodies are thought to be directed against *V. cholerae* lipopolysaccharide and other surface-expressed molecules. In nonendemic settings and in volunteer studies, marked increases in both vibriocidal and antitoxin antibody titers occur in infected individuals after infection with clinical cholera (Snyder et al., 1981, Clements et al., 1982). Vibriocidal antibody levels return to baseline within 6 months of primary disease, and antitoxin levels decline over 1 to 2 years (Snyder et al., 1981). In Bangladesh, vibriocidal antibody levels increase with age and are detectable in approximately 40% to 80% of individuals by the age of 10 to 15 years (Glass et al., 1985; Mosley et al., 1968). In endemic areas, an inverse relationship exists between the vibriocidal antibody titer and susceptibility to intestinal colonization with *V. cholerae* and symptomatic cholera (Glass et al., 1985; Mosley et al., 1968). Every twofold rise in the vibriocidal geometric mean titer is associated with an approximately 50% decrease in the attack rate of cholera (Glass et al, 1985; Mosley et al., 1968). No such association is found for any other immune response examined.

It is currently unclear why the vibriocidal antibody response is the only recognized predictor of protection from clinical cholera and why no such association exists for serum antitoxin responses (Benenson et al., 1968). Because *V. cholerae* is a noninvasive organism and because there is no disruption of the intestinal epithelium during cholera, a serum complement-fixing antibody response would be predicted to have minimal, if any, activity during mucosal infection with *V. cholerae*. Noncomplement binding secretory IgA (sIgA) is the primary antibody in the intestinal lumen. It is possible that the vibriocidal antibody response is a surrogate marker for an as-yet-unidentified intestinal sIgA response. Immunologic analysis is ongoing.

PREVENTION

V. cholerae in water may be eliminated by filtration or killed by boiling or addition of chlorine or iodine. Food, especially shellfish, should be well cooked and eaten hot. Hands and utensils should be appropriately washed. Although cholera may be avoided if water and food are kept uncontaminated, potable water and appropriate waste disposal are not possible in many areas of the developing world. Secondary transmission in households in the developing world may be as high as 20% to 50% (McCormack et al., 1969). In such situations, prophylactic administration of tetracycline antibiotics to household members markedly decreases the risk of secondary transmission. Whether prophylactic use of other antibiotics would be similarly effective is unclear. Prophylactic use of antibiotics is not, however, recommended for household contacts of individuals with cholera in the industrialized world, because adequate water and sewage facilities in these countries make secondary transmission unlikely.

A number of cholera vaccines are currently available, although none is commercially available in the United States (Ryan, 2000b; Ryan and Calderwood, 2001). A phenol-killed *V. cholerae* O1 parenteral vaccine has been approved by the Food and Drug Administration in the United States but is no longer commercially available. The vaccine is only approximately 50% effective for approximately 3 to 6 months against cholera caused by *V. cholerae* O1, and it does not protect against cholera caused by *V. cholerae* O139. The vaccine was evaluated only in areas of the world endemic for cholera and had its lowest efficacy among young children. This suggests that the parenteral vaccine may boost immunologic responses that are already present and that it would be a poor vaccine for control of epidemics in immunologically naïve populations. The parenteral vaccine has a high adverse event profile including local pain, erythema, induration, fever, malaise, and headache in most individuals. The vaccine should not be administered to infants less than 6 months of age, and its adverse event profile precludes its use in pregnant women. The vaccine requires two or three parenteral administrations, does not interrupt transmission of *V. cholerae* organisms in the community, and has been associated with impedance of other, more useful sanitary and therapeutic interventions, especially during outbreaks. For these and other reasons, the World Health Assembly removed the requirement for cholera vaccination for international travel in 1973. No country currently requires documentation of cholera vaccination for entry.

Two oral cholera vaccines are also currently available. One is a killed whole-cell vaccine supplemented with recombinant B subunit (WC-rBS). The vaccine is administered in 2 to 3 doses, each separated by 7 to 42 days. In a field trial in Bangladesh (in which 3 doses of the vaccine were administered at 6-week intervals), a WC-BS vaccine induced approximately 85% protection during the initial 6 months of the study (Clemens et al., 1986). At 12 months the vaccine was approximately 62% effective, and at 36 months (the end of follow up in the study) the vaccine was approximately 50% protective. During the first 6 months of evaluation, the vaccine provided protection in both young and older children as well as in adults; however, the protective effect in young children rapidly decreased, and at 36 months the vaccine had its lowest efficacy—approximately 26%—among children aged 2 to 5 years, compared with 63% among individuals older than 5 years (Clemens et al., 1990b). These findings once again suggest that this vaccine is most efficacious when administered to individuals with preexisting immunity. WC-rBS vaccine is currently available in Europe; it does not provide any protection against *V. cholerae* O139 infection.

A live, attenuated *V. cholerae* classical biotype vaccine strain, CVD 103-HgR, is also available in Europe, Canada, and Latin America. After a single oral administration, this vaccine provided 63% to 100% (depending on the challenge strain of *V. cholerae* O1) short-term (1- to

6-month) protection against cholera in immunologically naïve North American volunteers (Tacket, 1992; Tacket, 1999). Unfortunately, in a large field trial in an area of the world endemic for cholera (Indonesia), the vaccine showed no protective efficacy (Richie et al., 2000).

None of the three commercially available cholera vaccines provide any protection against cholera caused by *V. cholerae* O139. A number of additional cholera vaccines are currently under development (Ryan, 2000a; Ryan and Calderwood, 2001).

ACKNOWLEDGMENTS

This work was supported in part by grants from the National Institute of Allergy and Infectious Diseases, AI/K08-01332 and AI-40725 (E.T.R), and an International Collaborations in Infectious Disease Research Award, HD39165, from the National Institute of Allergy and Infectious Diseases and the National Institute of Child Health and Human Development (E.T.R.). The International Centre for Diarrheal Disease Research, Bangaladesh (ICDDR, B) is supported by many donors, including the United Nations Children's Fund (UNICEF), the Bill and Melinda Gates Foundation, and the governments of Australia, Bangladesh, Belgium, Canada, Saudi Arabia, Sweden, Switzerland, the United Kingdom, and the United States.

BIBLIOGRAPHY

Albert MJ, Siddique AK, Islam MS, et al. Large outbreak of clinical cholera due to *Vibrio cholerae* non-O1 in Bangladesh. Lancet 1993;341:704.

Alm RA, Mayrhofer G, Kotlarski I, et al. Amino-terminal domain of the El Tor haemolysin of *Vibrio cholerae* O1 is expressed in classical strains and is cytotoxic. Vaccine 1991;9:588-594.

Barua D, Paguio AS. ABO blood groups and cholera. Ann Hum Biol 1977;4:489-492.

Benenson AS, Islam MR, Greenough WB III. Rapid identification of *Vibrio cholerae* by darkfield microscopy. Bull World Health Organ 1964;30:827-831.

Benenson AS, Saad A, Mosley WH, et al. Serological studies in cholera. 3. Serum toxin neutralization—rise in titre in response to infection with *Vibrio cholerae*, and the level in the "normal" population of East Pakistan. Bull World Health Organ 1968;38:287-295.

Bennish ML. Cholera: pathophysiology, clinical features, and treatment. In Wachsmuth IK, Blake PA, Olsvik O (eds). *Vibrio cholerae* and cholera: molecular to global perspectives. Washington, D.C.: ASM Press, 1994.

Blake PA. Epidemiology of cholera in the Americas. Gastroenterol Clin North Am 1993;22:639-660.

Carroll PA, Tashima KT, Rogers MB, et al. Phase variation in tcpH modulates expression of the ToxR regulation in *Vibrio cholerae*. Mol Microbiol 1997;25(6):1099-1111.

Cash RA, Music SI, Libonati JP, et al. Response of man to infection with *Vibrio cholerae*. I. Clinical, serologic, and bacteriologic responses to a known inoculum. J Infect Dis 1974a;129:45-52.

Cash RA, Music SI, Libonati JP, et al. Response of man to infection with *Vibrio cholerae*. II. Protection from illness afforded by previous disease and vaccine. J Infect Dis 1974b;130:325-333.

Cassel D, Pfeuffer T. Mechanism of cholera toxin action: covalent modification of the guanyl nucleotide-binding protein of the adenylate cyclase system. Proc Natl Acad Sci USA 1978;75:2669-2673.

Chakraborty S, Mukhopadhyay AK, Bhadra RK, et al. Virulence genes in environmental strains of *Vibrio cholerae*. Appl Environ Microbiol 2000;66:4022-4028.

Cholera Working Group, International Centre for Diarrhoeal Diseases Research, Bangladesh. Large epidemic of cholera-like disease in Bangladesh caused by *Vibrio cholerae* O139 synonym Bengal. Lancet 1993;342:387-390.

Clemens J, Albert MJ, Rao M, et al. Impact of infection by *Helicobacter pylori* on the risk and severity of endemic cholera. J Infect Dis 1995;171:1653-1656.

Clemens JD, Sack DA, Harris JR, et al. Field trial of oral cholera vaccines in Bangladesh. Lancet 1986;2:124-127.

Clemens JD, Sack DA, Harris JR, et al. Breast feeding and the risk of severe cholera in rural Bangladeshi children. Am J Epidemiol 1990a;131:400-411.

Clemens JD, Sack DA, Harris JR, et al. Field trial of oral cholera vaccines in Bangladesh: results from three-year follow-up [see comments]. Lancet 1990b;335:270-273.

Clemens JD, Van LF, Sack DA, et al. Biotype as determinant of natural immunising effect of cholera. Lancet 1991;337:883-884.

Clements ML, Levine MM, Young CR, et al. Magnitude, kinetics, and duration of vibriocidal antibody responses in North Americans after ingestion of *Vibrio cholerae*. J Infect Dis 1982;145:465-473.

Colwell RR. Global climate and infectious disease: the cholera paradigm. Science 1996;274:2025-2031.

DiRita VJ, Mekalanos JJ. Periplasmic interaction between two membrane regulatory proteins, ToxR and ToxS, results in signal transduction and transcriptional activation. Cell 1991;64:29-37.

Fasano A, Baudry B, Pumplin DW, et al. *Vibrio cholerae* produces a second enterotoxin, which affects intestinal tight junctions. Proc Natl Acad Sci USA 1991;88:5242-5246.

Feachem RG. Environmental aspects of cholera epidemiology. III. Transmission and control. Trop Dis Bull 1982;79:1-47.

Field M, Rao MC, Chang EB. Intestinal electrolyte transport and diarrheal disease (1). N Engl J Med 1989a;321:800-806.

Field M, Rao MC, Chang EB. Intestinal electrolyte transport and diarrheal disease (2). N Engl J Med 1989b;321:879-883.

Finn TM, Reiser J, Germanier R, et al. Cell-associated hemagglutinin-deficient mutant of *Vibrio cholerae*. Infect Immun 1987;55:942-946.

Fullner KJ, Mekalanos JJ. Genetic characterization of a new type IV-A pilus gene cluster found in both classical and E1 Tor biotypes of *Vibrio cholerae*. Infect Immun 1999;67(3):1393-1404.

Fullner KJ, Mekalanos JJ. In vivo covalent cross-linking of cellular actin by the *Vibrio cholerae* RTX toxin. EMBO J 2000;19:5315-5323.

Gill DM. The arrangement of subunits in cholera toxin. Biochemistry 1976;15:1242-1248.

Gitelson S. Gastrectomy, achlorhydria and cholera. Isr J Med Sci 1971;7:663-667.

Glass RI, Becker S, Huq MI, et al. Endemic cholera in rural Bangladesh, 1966-1980. Am J Epidemiol 1982;116:959-970.

Glass RI, Svennerholm AM, Khan MR, et al. Seroepidemiological studies of El Tor cholera in Bangladesh: association of serum antibody levels with protection. J Infect Dis 1985;151:236-242.

Glass RI, Svennerholm AM, Stoll BJ, et al. Protection against cholera in breast-fed children by antibodies in breast milk. N Engl J Med 1983;308:1389-1392.

Glass RI, Svennerholm AM, Stoll BJ, et al. Effects of under-nutrition on infection with *Vibrio cholerae* O1 and on response to oral cholera vaccine. Pediatr Infect Dis J 1989;8:105-109.

Goldberg MB, Boyko SA, Calderwood SB. Transcriptional regulation by iron of a *Vibrio cholerae* virulence gene and homology of the gene to the *Escherichia coli* Fur system. J Bacteriol 1990;172:6863-6870.

Goma Epidemiology Group. Public health impact of Rwandan refugee crisis: what happened in Goma, Zaire, in July, 1994? Lancet 1995;345:339-344.

Gorbach SL, Banwell JG, Jacobs B, et al. Intestinal microflora in Asiatic cholera. II. The small bowel. J Infect Dis 1970;121:38-45.

Gore SM, Fontaine O, Pierce NF. Impact of rice based oral rehydration solution on stool output and duration of diarrhoea: meta-analysis of 13 clinical trials. BMJ 1992;304:287-291.

Hase CC, Mekalanos JJ. TcpP protein is a positive regulator of virulence gene expression in *Vibrio cholerae*. Proc Natl Acad Sci USA 1998;95(2):730-734.

Heidelberg JF, Eisen JA, Nelson WC, et al. DNA sequence of both chromosomes of the cholera pathogen *Vibrio cholerae*. Nature 2000;406:477-483.

Herrington DA, Hall RH, Losonsky G, et al. Toxin, toxin-coregulated pili, and the *toxR* regulon are essential for *Vibrio cholerae* pathogenesis in humans. J Exp Med 1988;168:1487-1492.

Hirschhorn N, Chaudhury AKMA, Ledenbaum J. Cholera in pregnant women. Lancet 1969:1230-1232.

Hirschhorn N, Kinzie JL, Sachar DB, et al. Decrease in net stool output in cholera during intestinal perfusion with glucose-containing solutions. N Engl J Med 1968;279:176-181.

Holmgren J, Lonnroth I, Mansson J, et al. Interaction of cholera toxin and membrane GM_1 ganglioside of small intestine. Proc Natl Acad Sci USA 1975;72:2520-2524.

Huq A, Colwell RR, Rahman R, et al. Detection of *Vibrio cholerae* O1 in the aquatic environment by fluorescent-monoclonal antibody and culture methods. Appl Environ Microbiol 1990;56:2370-2373.

Institute of Medicine. New vaccine development: establishing priorities. Vol II. Diseases of importance in developing countries. Washington, D.C.: National Academy Press, 1986.

Karaolis DK, Johnson JA, Bailey CC, et al. A *Vibrio cholerae* pathogenicity island associated with epidemic and pandemic strains. Proc Natl Acad Sci USA 1998;95:3134-3139.

Kaufman MR, Shaw CE, Jones ID, et al. Biogenesis and regulation of the *Vibrio cholerae* toxin-coregulated pilus:

analogies to other virulence factor secretory systems. Gene 1993;126:43-49.

Lee SH, Butler SM, Camilli A. Selection for in vivo regulators of bacterial virulence. Proc Natl Acad Sci USA 2001:98(12):6889-6894.

Levine MM, Black RE, Clements ML, et al. Duration of infection-derived immunity to cholera. J Infect Dis 1981;143:818-820.

Losonsky GA, Yunyongying J, Lim V, et al. Factors influencing secondary vibriocidal immune responses: relevance for understanding immunity to cholera. Infect Immun 1996;64:10-15.

McCormack WM, Islam MS, Fahimuddin M, et al. A community study of inapparent cholera infections. Am J Epidemiol 1969;89:658-664.

Mekalanos JJ, Collier RJ, Romig WR. Enzymic activity of cholera toxin. II. Relationships to proteolytic processing, disulfide bond reduction, and subunit composition. J Biol Chem 1979;254:5855-5861.

Merrell DS, Butler SM, Qadri F, et al. Host-induced epidemic spread of the cholera bacterium. Nature 2002:417 (6889):642-645.

Mintz ED, Popovic T, Blake PA. Transmission of *Vibrio cholerae* O1. In Wachsmuth IK, Blake PA, Olsvik O (eds). *Vibrio cholerae* and cholera: molecular to global perspectives. Washington D.C.: ASM Press, 1994.

Molla, AM, Rahman M, Sarker SA, et al. Stool electrolyte content and purging rates in diarrhea caused by rotavirus, enterotoxigenic *E. coli*, and *V. cholerae* in children. J Pediatr. 1981;98:835-838.

Morris JGJ. Non-O group 1 *Vibrio cholerae* strains not associated with epidemic disease. In Wachsmuth IK, Blake PA, Olsvik O (eds). *Vibrio cholerae* and cholera: molecular to global perspectives. Washington, D.C.: American Society for Microbiology, 1994.

Mosley WH, Ahmad S, Benenson AS, et al. The relationship of vibriocidal antibody titre to susceptibility to cholera in family contacts of cholera patients. Bull World Health Organ 1968;38:777-785.

Mosley WH, Benenson AS, Barui R. A serological survey for cholera antibodies in rural East Pakistan. 1. The distribution of antibody in the control population of a cholera-vaccine field-trial area and the relation of antibody titre to the pattern of endemic cholera. Bull World Health Organ 1968;38:327-334.

Mukhopadhyay S, Ghosh C, Ghose AC. Phenotypic expression of a mannose-sensitive hemagglutinin by a *Vibrio cholerae* O1 El Tor strain and evaluation of its role in intestinal adherence and colonization. FEMS Microbiol Lett 1996;138:227-232.

Pearson GD, Woods A, Chiang SL, et al. CTX genetic element encodes a site-specific recombination system and an intestinal colonization factor. Proc Natl Acad Sci USA 1993;90:3750-3754.

Rapoport SM, Dodd M, Clark M, et al. Postacidotic state of infantile diarrhea: symptoms and chemical data: postacidotic hypocalcemia and associated decreases in levels of potassium, phosphorous, and phosphatase in the plasma. Am J Dis Child 1947;73:391-441.

Richie EE, Punjabi NH, Sidharta YY, et al. Efficacy trial of single-dose live oral cholera vaccine CVD 103-HgR in North Jakarta, Indonesia, a cholera-endemic area. Vaccine 2000;18:2399-2410.

Ryan ET, Calderwood SB. Cholera vaccines. Clin Infect Dis 2000a;31:561-565.

Ryan ET, Calderwood SB. Cholera vaccines. J Travel Med 2001;8:82-91.

Ryan ET, Dhar U, Khan WA, et al. Mortality, morbidity, and microbiology of endemic cholera among hospitalized patients in Dhaka, Bangladesh. Am J Trop Med Hyg 2000b;63:12-20.

Sandkvist M, Morales V, Bagdasarian M. A protein required for secretion of cholera toxin through the outer membrane of *Vibrio cholerae*. Gene 1993;123:81-86.

Schneider DR, Parker CD. Isolation and characterization of protease-deficient mutants of *Vibrio cholerae*. J Infect Dis 1978;138:143-151.

Sircar BK, Dutta P, De SP, Sikdar SN, et al. ABO blood group distributions in diarrhoea cases including cholera in Calcutta. Ann Hum Biol 1981;8:289-291.

Siddique, AK, Salam A, Islam MS, et al. Why treatment centres failed to prevent cholera deaths among Rwandan refugees in Goma, Zaire [see comments]. Lancet 1995;345:359-361.

Snyder JD, Allegra DT, Levine MM, et al. Serologic studies of naturally acquired infection with *Vibrio cholerae* serogroup O1 in the United States. J Infect Dis 1981;143:182-187.

Speelman P, Rabbani GH, Bukhave K, et al. Increased jejunal prostaglandin E_2 concentrations in patients with acute cholera. Gut 1985;26:188-193.

Stroeher UH, Karageorgos LE, Morona R, et al. Serotype conversion in *Vibrio cholerae* O1. Proc Natl Acad Sci USA 1992;89:2566-2570.

Tacket CO, Losonsky G, Nataro JP, et al. Onset and duration of protective immunity in challenged volunteers after vaccination with live oral cholera vaccine CVD 103-HgR. J Infect Dis 1992;166(4):837-841.

Tacket CO, Cohen MB, Wasserman SS, et al. Randomized, double-blind, placebo-controlled, multicentered trial of the efficacy of a single dose of live oral cholera vaccine CVD 103-HgR in preventing cholera following challenge with *Vibrio cholerae* O1 E1 inaba three months after vaccination. Infect Immun 1999;67(12):6341-6345.

Trucksis M, Galen JE, Michalski J, et al. Accessory cholera enterotoxin (Ace), the third toxin of a *Vibrio cholerae* virulence cassette. Proc Natl Acad Sci USA 1993;90:5267-5271.

Waldor MK, Mekalanos JJ. Lysogenic conversion by a filamentous phage encoding cholera toxin. Science 1996;272:1910-1914.

Wang F, Butler T, Rabbani GH, et al. The acidosis of cholera. Contributions of hyperproteinemia, lactic acidemia, and hyperphosphatemia to an increased serum anion gap. N Engl J Med 1986;315:1591-1595.

World Health Organization. Cholera in 1994. Part 1. Wkly Epidemiol Rec 2001a;70:201-208.

World Health Organization. Management of the patient with cholera, World Health Organization Emergency and Other Communicable Diseases, Surveillance and Control, WHO/ CDD/SER/91.15 Rev.1 Surveillance and Response Web site]. Available at: www.who.int/csr/ resources/publications /cholera/who_cdd_ser_91_15/ent, accessed 4/28/03.

Xu Q, Dziejman M, Mekalanos JJ. Determination of the transcriptome of *Vibrio cholerae* during intraintestinal growth and midexponential phase in vitro. Proc Natl Acad Sci USA. 2003:100(3):1286-1291.

Yamamoto T, Nair GB, Albert MJ, et al. Survey of in vitro susceptibilities of *Vibrio cholerae* O1 and O139 to antimicrobial agents. Antimicrob Agents Chemother 1995;39:241-244.

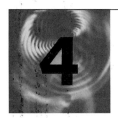

CYTOMEGALOVIRUS

GAIL J. DEMMLER

ytomegalovirus (CMV) is a ubiquitous agent that commonly infects people from all backgrounds, races, ethnicities, ages, and geographic locations. Most infections with this virus are asymptomatic, but CMV can cause serious, even life-threatening and permanently disabling disease in the fetus and newborn and in immunocompromised hosts.

HISTORY

Infections in newborns caused by CMV were first recognized in the latter part of the nineteenth century. It was believed at that time that these infections were caused by a protozoan or represented a form of syphilis, and the salivary glands were believed to be the major pathologic site. By the 1950s, the virus was isolated in cell culture and called "salivary gland virus" or "cytomegalovirus" (Rowe, 1956; Smith, 1956; Weller et al., 1957). A constellation of clinical signs and symptoms associated with this virus was then recognized, and included hepatosplenomegaly, thrombocytopenia, jaundice, intracerebral calcifications, chorioretinitis, and poor growth, with eventual development of microcephaly and mental retardation. The syndrome was called "cytomegalic inclusion disease" (Weller and Hanshaw, 1962). In 1960, Weller, Hanshaw, and Scott proposed "cytomegalovirus infection" for the illness, because it better reflected the nature of the disease, and this term remains in common use today. Although the infection was once thought to be rare, it is now known that congenital CMV infection is relatively common and that the infants with obvious "cytomegalic inclusion disease" represented only the proverbial "tip of the iceberg."

CMV also has been shown to cause infection and disease in older infants, children, and adults. It was discovered in 1966 to be a cause of "posttransfusion syndrome," with subsequent studies leading eventually to screening of blood-product donors and processing of blood products to reduce the risk of transfusion-acquired disease due to the virus (Kaariainen et al.,1966; Adler, 1983; Demmler et al., 1986a; Lambertson et al., 1988). In the 1970s and 1980s, CMV emerged as an important pathogen in immunocompromised hosts, especially in those patients undergoing cancer chemotherapy, those receiving an organ or marrow transplant, or those with AIDS. In 1976 the results of the first clinical trial of a live attenuated CMV vaccine were published, and research continues today for a safe and effective vaccine candidate (Plotkin et al., 1976). In 1989, ganciclovir was the first antiviral licensed specifically for the treatment of CMV disease, and now several therapeutic options are available to clinicians to manage CMV infections.

ETIOLOGY

Despite initial confusion concerning the cause of cytomegalic inclusion disease, some investigators suspected this illness was caused by a virus long before the agent itself was identified. Similarities seen on pathologic examination between cytomegalic inclusion cells (Goodpasture and Talbot, 1921) and cells in herpetic lesions were noted by early investigators (von Glahn and Pappenheimer, 1925); these similarities were remarkable in light of the modern classification of CMV as a member of the Herpesviridae family of viruses. In 1954, Smith was the first to propagate murine CMV in mouse cell cultures (Smith, 1954), and shortly thereafter, human CMV was isolated by three independent investigators (Rowe, 1956; Smith, 1956; Weller et al., 1957). CMV is now routinely cultured in a variety of human fibroblast cells and produces a characteristic focal cytopathic effect with cytomegaly and intranuclear and cytoplasmic inclusions that contain viral antigenic structures.

In the cell, CMV causes both permissive infections, in which viral progeny are produced, and abortive infections, in which there are no progeny produced, but messenger RNA (mRNA) expression, DNA replication, and formation of early viral antigens occur. Virus also may remain latent and reactivate into a productive infection if host cell factors allow. The site of latency of CMV probably is cells of lymphoid origin, including granulocytes and mononuclear cells (Merigan and Resta, 1990; Taylor-Wiedeman et al., 1994; Schrier et al., 1985; Spector and Spector, 1985). The virus also resides in the kidney and salivary glands. Oncogenic transformation also has been observed in cell culture systems (Heggie et al., 1986), but to date no specific malignancies in humans have been convincingly linked to CMV.

The virus is a member of the Herpesviridae family and contains a genome composed of double-stranded DNA, approximately 240 kilobases (kb) in length. Viral particles consist of an inner core with a diameter of 65 nm, a capsid composed of 162 capsomeres arranged in icosahedral symmetry that measures 110 nm in diameter, a surrounding amorphous tegument, and an envelope; the complete viral particle measures 200 nm in diameter (Figure 4-1). The CMV genome consists of over 208 open reading frames, and replication occurs in a regulated sequence, with immediate early gene products controlling subsequent transcription and translation of early and late gene products (Merigan and Resta, 1990; Baldick and Shenk, 1996). The genome encodes for at least 30 structural and nonstructural proteins. The envelope glycoproteins are antigenic and at least two, gB and gH, are believed to play an important role in viral infectivity and in generating immune responses from the infected host. The tegument proteins, especially pp65, also may play important roles in host response to CMV (Kozinowski et al., 1987; Plotkin, 1999; Boppana et al., 2001).

CMV is not differentiated into traditional serotypes, as many other viruses are, but there appear to be many genotypes or "molecular strains" of CMV (Wilfert et al., 1982; Griller et al., 1988; Bale et al, 2000). Traditional molecular methods using restriction-enzyme analysis of whole viral DNA have shown simi-

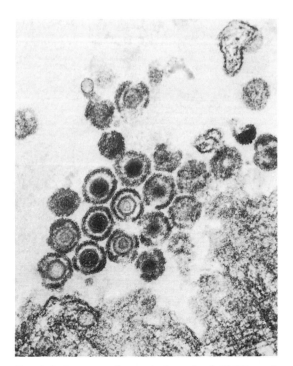

Fig. 4-1 A group of negatively stained CMV particles propagated in human lung fibroblast cell culture. The nucleocapsid core exhibits typical herpesvirus icosahedral symmetry and is surrounded by a tegument and a double-layered envelope. (Magnification × 155,000.) (Courtesy Janet D. Smith, PhD.)

lar DNA fragment mapping patterns in CMV strains isolated serially from the same person, mother-infant pairs, and family members, and differences in CMV strains isolated from individuals who are not epidemiologically linked (Huang et al., 1980; Spector and Spector, 1982; Sokol et al., 1992). More recent studies using polymerase chain reaction (PCR)–based methods show that nucleotide polymorphisms occur in a variety of CMV genes, including the *a* sequence, the major immediate early gene, and the glycoprotein B (gB or UL55) and the UL144 regions (Bale et al., 2000). The variability of at least four gB genotypes has been characterized and, although definite effects of these polymorphisms on the biology and disease expression of CMV infections are not known, some studies suggest adverse outcomes after CMV infection may be linked to infection with a specific gB genotype. For example, infection with CMV gB3 genotype may be a risk factor for fatality in bone marrow transplant recipients, whereas gB2 and gB4 genotypes appear more often to be fatal in patients with AIDS (Fries et al., 1994;

Rasmussen et al., 1997). One study of gB geno-type and congenital CMV disease showed that all four major gB genotypes could be vertically transmitted from mother to infant, but it did not find a relationship between gB genotype and neonatal disease expression or neurodevelopmental outcome (Bale et al., 2000).

PATHOLOGY, PATHOGENESIS, AND IMMUNE RESPONSE

The histologic lesion of CMV infection is characterized by enlarged cells that contain intranuclear and cytoplasmic inclusion bodies. The intranuclear inclusion body appears reddish purple after being stained with hematoxylin and eosin and is surrounded by a halo, resulting in an "owl's eye" appearance. The paranuclear inclusion or dense body is more granular and more basophilic in appearance. In disseminated disease, inclusion-bearing cytomegalic cells may be seen in every tissue and organ system in the body. Infiltration of mononuclear cells and necrosis may occur. In the brain, necrotizing lesions with extensive calcifications, usually in the periventricular area, may occur in congenital infections involving the central nervous system (Figure 4-2). The inner ear of congenitally infected newborns also may show classic cytomegalic inclusion cells. The liver and spleen may display extramedullary hematopoiesis. The virus also may cause vasculitis, with inclusion bodies and thrombi in endothelial cells in the submucosa and muscle wall of blood vessels (Tatum et al., 1989). Furthermore, some controversial studies suggest CMV may be associated with atherosclerosis (Melnick et al., 1983).

The natural history of CMV infection in the human is complicated. First of all, infection with the virus may be primary or recurrent. Primary infections are infections for the first time with CMV, whereas recurrent infections may be reactivation of a latent infection or reinfection with a new "strain" of CMV (Figure 4-3). Furthermore, infections with CMV also may be latent and nonproductive, where the host is well and does not shed the virus in body secretions; productive yet asymptomatic, where the host remains well but is actively shedding the virus in body secretions; or productive and symptomatic, where the host is ill and virus replication is present and detectable in a variety of body fluids. Infections may be acquired prenatally (producing congenital infection); perinatally (producing infection in young infants); or postnatally (producing infection in older infants, children, adolescents, and adults). Once a host acquires CMV,

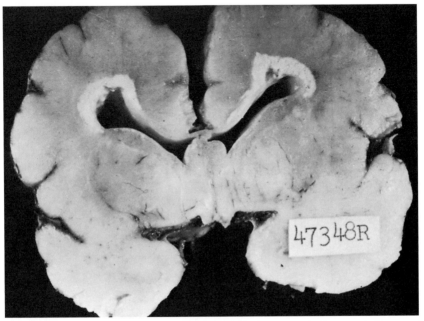

Fig. 4-2 Brain of an infant with congenital CMV disease with characteristic central nervous system involvement that produces periventricular necrosis and calcification.

infection is lifelong. Multiple strains of CMV may infect a person at one time, or reinfection with different strains may occur sequentially over time (Spector et al., 1984; Chou, 1986; Chou, 1989a; McFarlane and Koment, 1986; Chandler et al., 1987; Adler, 1991b).

The immune response of the host to an infection with CMV is very important in limiting the infection and in determining the amount of disease expression. The cell-mediated immune response—both early and nonspecific with natural killer cells and interferon production, and later with CMV-specific cytotoxic T cells—appears to be very important in the host defense of CMV (Rola-Pleszczynski et al., 1977; Starr et al., 1979; Reynolds et al., 1979; Schrier et al. 1986). In addition, gB-specific lymphocyte responses and CD8+ and CD4+ cytolytic responses are produced after CMV infection and appear important in limiting the infection (Navarro et al., 1997). Individuals with an immature or deficient cellular immune response therefore will be more vulnerable to CMV-associated disease than individuals with mature, normal immune systems. Humoral immunity does not appear to prevent infection with CMV, but it does appear to lessen the severity of symptoms associated with disease, and the important factors associated with protective humoral immunity are beginning to be elucidated. For example, antibodies to the envelope glycoproteins gB and gH appear to represent most of the neutralizing activity in sera from CMV-infected individuals. Studies of the antigenic and functional structure of gB suggest that certain regions of the molecule are immunodominant and that in vitro these antibodies block virus entry into cells, as well as cell-to-cell transmission of the virus. The abundance of these antibodies in convalescent sera in normal hosts further suggests they may be important in limiting dissemination of the virus. Strain-specific neutralizing epitopes within regions of the envelope glycoprotein gH also occur, and a study of serial serum samples from transplant recipients and women of childbearing age shed light on why CMV-specific humoral immunity may be only partially pro-

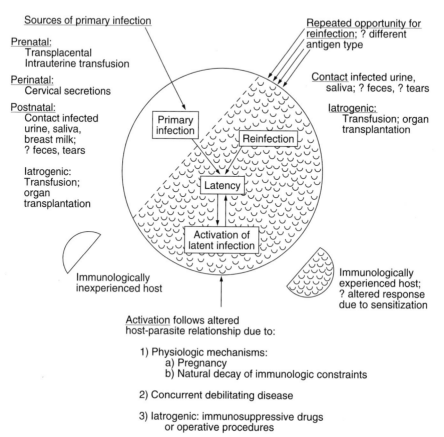

Fig. 4-3 Natural history of human CMV infection. (From Weller TH: N Engl M Med 1970;285:203).

tective and may allow recurrent infection with a new strain of CMV to occur (Chou, 1989b; Boppana et al., 2001). To further complicate our understanding of the immune response to CMV, the virus has been shown to express gene products that allow it to evade the immune system (Gilbert et al., 1993). Also, homology between CMV proteins and host histocompatibility antigens allows "molecular mimicry" to trigger end organ tissue destruction. Finally, CMV itself may be an immunosuppressive agent, suppressing the proliferative responses to T cells in individuals with mononucleosis and patients who are immunocompromised (Rinaldo et al., 1980; Paya, 2001).

EPIDEMIOLOGY

Infection with CMV is common worldwide, and most infections are without symptoms. There is no apparent seasonal occurrence. However, there do appear to be several important periods of acquisition during the lifetime of an individual, including the newborn period, early childhood, adolescence, and the child-bearing years.

Approximately 1% of all newborns are congenitally infected with CMV, with ranges of 0.2% to 2.5% reported (Stagno et al., 1986; Demmler, 1991). Given current birth rates in the United States, this means CMV infection is the most common congenital infection in the United States, affecting 30,000 to 40,000 newborns annually. Both primary and recurrent infections (reinfection and reactivation) in the mother can result in transmission of CMV to the fetus (Yow et al., 1988). However, transmission rates are much higher after primary maternal infections (up to 40% in primary versus 1% or less in recurrent infections), and primary maternal infections are more likely to be associated with disease in the fetus and newborn (Stagno et al., 1977b; Stagno et al., 1982; Fowler et al., 1992). Symptomatic congenital CMV infection can occur, however, even after a nonprimary or recurrent maternal infection with CMV (Ahlfors et al., 1981; Ahlfors et al., 1999; Rutter et al., 1985; Boppana et al., 1999). CMV also may be transmitted from mother to infant during the perinatal period through exposure to CMV-infected maternal cervicovaginal secretions or through ingestion of human milk after delivery (Stagno et al., 1980). This type of infection usually is benign in normal-term infants but can be serious in

extremely low–birth weight, premature infants (Dworsky et al., 1983b, Vochem et al., 1998; Maschmann et al., 2001).

Infants not infected with CMV during the neonatal period may be infected during the toddler or preschool years, usually through contact with other children who may be shedding the virus (Yow et al., 1987). It is common for children who attend group day care to be infected with CMV, with both primary infections and reinfections with new strains. These children also shed the virus for prolonged periods of time and transmit the virus horizontally, sometimes in genotype clusters, to one another (Pass et al., 1982; Murph et al., 1986; Adler, 1985; Adler, 1991b; Lasry et al., 1996). They also may transmit the virus to day-care–center workers, as well as to parents and siblings at home (Pass et al., 1986; Pass et al., 1987; Adler, 1988a; Adler, 1988b). Furthermore, CMV strains from day-care settings, when transmitted from toddlers to their pregnant mothers at home, may be the source of congenital CMV infection (Murph et al., 1998). Once CMV enters the family setting, transmission occurs quite readily, with annual attack rates between 47% and 53%, and may take one of three patterns: between siblings, between parents, and between children and parents (Dworsky et al., 1984; Taber et al., 1985). Although direct contact with an infected person's secretions is the most likely route of transmission in these settings, inanimate objects, such as toys, also may be contaminated with CMV (Hutto et al., 1986).

Sexual activity appears to be a risk factor for acquisition of CMV by adolescents and adults (Rosenthal et al., 1997). The virus is shed in saliva, cervical secretions, and semen and may be acquired and transmitted between partners during primary or reactivation infections or through reinfection with a new strain of CMV (Lang and Kummer, 1975; Handsfield et al., 1985; Demmler et al., 1986b; Sohn et al., 1991). Vertical transmission of CMV acquired by sexually active adolescents may result in congenital infection of their offspring (Kumar et al., 1984c), and some studies suggest that adolescents are at higher risk for having a baby with congenital CMV disease than mothers who are older than 20 years of age at the time of giving birth (Istas et al., 1995).

CMV also may be transmitted within the hospital setting through blood-product transfusion, organ and marrow transplantation and, very rarely, through person-to-person transmission. Apparent infant-to-infant transmission of CMV has been documented in two busy units with a high prevalence of CMV excretion (Spector, 1983; Demmler et al., 1987), but transmission from patient to health-care worker has not been documented, despite numerous attempts to do so (Yow et al., 1982; Dworsky et al., 1983a; Adler et al., 1986; Demmler et al., 1987). In addition, seroepidemiologic studies have shown that, despite their daily exposure to CMV in the hospital setting, health-care workers do not appear to be at greater risk than the general population for acquiring CMV infection (Friedman et al., 1984; Balfour et al., 1986). Blood-product transfusion is a well-recognized source of CMV infection (Adler, 1983). Posttransfusion CMV hepatitis and mononucleosis can occur in older children and adults, especially if they receive large volumes of whole, fresh blood from CMV-seropositive donors (Lang et al., 1969), and newborns, especially those who are premature, may experience a viral sepsis–like syndrome with shock, pneumonitis, lymphocytosis, and thrombocytopenia (Yeager, 1974). Screening donors for CMV antibody, as well as administering leukocyte-depleted blood products, can reduce the risk of posttransfusion CMV infection and disease in both adults and neonates (Yeager et al., 1981; Demmler et al., 1986a; Gilbert et al., 1989; Bowden et al., 1995).

Primary and reactivation infections and reinfection with CMV commonly occur in organ- and marrow-transplant recipients and most commonly manifest clinically and virologically 30 to 90 days after transplantation (Pollard, 1988; Singh et al., 1988). Earlier and later infections also occur and may be influenced by donor or recipient CMV serostatus, degree of immunosuppression, graft-versus-host disease, molecular strain or gB genotype of CMV causing infection, and administration of prophylactic antiviral agents or immune globulin. Immunosuppression associated with AIDS, severe burns, cancer chemotherapy, and immunosuppressive therapy for connective-tissue diseases also may be associated with severe disease caused by CMV. Infants infected perinatally with human immunodeficiency virus (HIV) who also acquire CMV infection congenitally or in the first 18 months of life appear at significant risk for rapid disease progression and debilitating central nervous system disease (Scott et al, 1984; Doyle et al., 1996; Kovacs et al., 1999).

CLINICAL MANIFESTATIONS

Most infections with CMV are asymptomatic; clinical manifestations can occur, however, and cover a broad spectrum of signs and symptoms (Figure 4-4).

Symptomatic Congenital Infection

The clinical manifestations seen at birth that are associated with symptomatic congenital CMV infection most commonly include small size for gestational age, hepatosplenomegaly, skin lesions such as petechiae or purpura, and jaundice (Figure 4-5 and Table 4-1). Severely ill infants also may have pneumonitis, lethargy, and a viral sepsis–like syndrome. Central nervous system involvement is present in approximately two thirds of affected infants and may produce microcephaly, neurologic abnormalities, and seizures. Almost half of the infants may have deafness, and 10% to 20% will have chorioretinitis that may produce visual impairment. Death in the newborn period may occur in approximately 8% to 9% of severely affected newborns (Boppana et al., 1992; Istas et al., 1995; CMV Updates, 2002). In infants who survive, jaundice usually subsides in a few weeks but may persist for several months. Hepatosplenomegaly may persist for several months, as well. The skin lesions often resolve within days to a week after birth. Urinary excretion of CMV, on the other hand, persists for many years in most infants (Figure 4-6) (Stagno et al., 1983; Noyola et al., 2000). Laboratory findings in these infants include anemia, lymphopenia or neutropenia, and thrombocytopenia. Liver transaminase levels may be elevated, but rarely more than 10 times normal. Urine and saliva cultures will grow CMV, and the virus also may be detectable in the blood and plasma through viral culture, CMV antigenemia assay, or PCR. The cerebrospinal fluid (CSF) in affected infants often is normal and rarely grows the virus; however, the presence of CMV DNA detected through PCR is associated with adverse neurodevelopmental outcome (Jamison and Hathorn, 1978; Atkins et al., 1994). Imaging by traditional skull radiographs rarely shows abnormalities, except in extreme cases (Figure 4-7). However, cranial

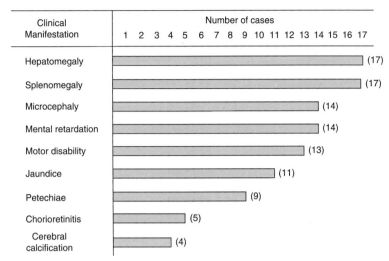

Fig. 4-4 Clinical features in 17 infants with congenital CMV disease. (From Weller TH, Hanshaw JB: N Engl J Med 1962; 266:1233).

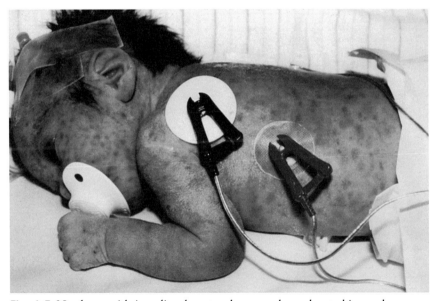

Fig. 4-5 Newborn with jaundice, hepatosplenomegaly, and petechiae and purpura due to congenital CMV disease. Infant also had intracranial calcifications, chorioretinitis, and bilateral sensorineural deafness.

imaging with modern ultrasound or computed tomography (CT) often shows intracranial calcifications, usually in a periventricular distribution (Figure 4-8) (Bale et al., 1990; Boppana et al., 1997; Noyola et al., 2001). Associated abnormalities include ventriculomegaly, periventricular leukomalacia, cortical atrophy, and neuronal migration abnormalities. Ophthalmologic findings occur in over 20% of infants with symptomatic congenital CMV infection, and include chorioretinitis, optic atrophy, cortical blindness, and strabismus (Stagno et al., 1977a; Coats et al., 2000). Long-term sequelae associated with symptomatic congenital CMV infection include sensorineural deafness, which is usually bilateral and progresses to a severe-to-profound loss over time, and visual impairment (Peckham et al., 1987).

| TABLE 4-1 | Signs and Symptoms in Newborn Infants With Congenital CMV Disease, as Reported to the National Congenital CMV Registry (N = 786, as of January, 2002) |

Sign or Symptom	N (%)*
Petechiae or purpura	417 (54)
Small for gestational age	362 (47)
Thrombocytopenia[†]	392 (54)
Hepatomegaly	360 (47)
Splenomegaly	336 (44)
Intracranial calcifications	288 (43)
Jaundice at birth	272 (36)
Microcephaly	301 (40)
Hearing impairment	213 (41)
Hemolytic anemia	83 (13)
Chorioretinitis	67 (11)
Seizures	59 (8)
Pneumonia	77 (11)
Abnormal neurologic exam	197 (28)
Hyperbilirubinemia[‡]	274 (40)
Elevated transaminase level (ALT)[§]	175 (30)
Death	49 (8)
Congenital coinfection	19 (7)
Treated with antiviral agent	62 (22)

*Percentage was calculated based on denominator of case reporting forms that had denoted a response for that particular sign or symptom.
[†]Thrombocytopenia defined as platelet count <75,000/mm3
[‡]Hyperbilirubinemia defined as total bilirubin >3.0 mg/dL
[§]ALT = alanine aminotransferase; elevated >100 U/L

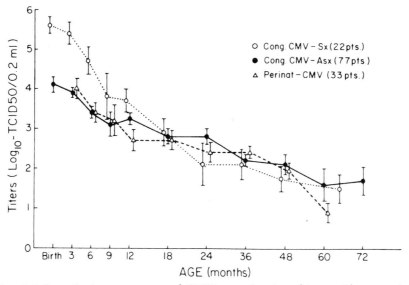

Fig. 4-6 Quantitative assessment of CMV excretion in subjects with congenital symptomatic *(open circles)*, congenital asymptomatic *(closed circles)*, and perinatal *(triangles)* infections. (From Stagno S et al: Semin Perinatol 1983;7:24-42).

Developmental and motor disabilities also may occur and may be predicted by head size and CT findings at birth (Pass et al., 1980; Williamson et al., 1982; Conboy et al., 1987; Noyola et al., 2001). In contrast to rubella virus, CMV appears to have only weak teratogenic capabilities. Structural abnormalities associated with congenital CMV infection

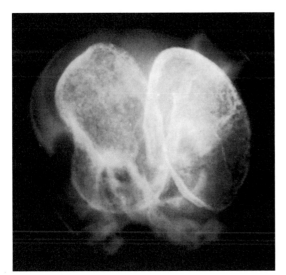

Fig. 4-7 Skull radiograph demonstrating massive intracranial calcifications in a 1-week-old infant born with severe neurologic involvement from congenital CMV disease.

include inguinal hernias, abnormalities of the first brachial arch, hypoplasia or agenesis of central nervous system structures, and defects of enamel of primary dentition (Fig. 4-9) (Reynolds et al., 1986). These malformations associated with CMV infection may result from tissue necrosis rather than interference with organogenesis; others may be just coincidental findings.

Asymptomatic Congenital Infection

Most (85% to 90%) of infants born congenitally infected with CMV are asymptomatic at birth or "silently" infected (Demmler, 1991). Asymptomatic congenital infection may result from a maternal infection during pregnancy that is primary or recurrent in nature and is identified in the well-appearing newborn by isolation of CMV from the urine or saliva obtained in the first 2 to 3 weeks of life. Urinary excretion of the virus then persists for many years (Noyola et al., 2000). Up to 15% of children born with asymptomatic congenital CMV infection will develop hearing loss, more often unilateral than bilateral, and usually progressive in nature (Williamson et al., 1992; Fowler et al., 1997). Late-onset hearing loss, detected for the first time after the first 3 months of life, also may occur, making it likely that universal newborn screening programs will miss many of these children (Fowler et al., 1999). Rarely, retinal lesions

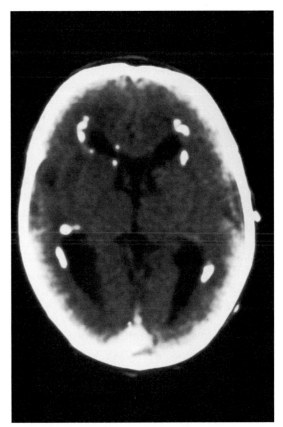

Fig. 4-8 Unenhanced CT scan of the brain demonstrating linear, periventricular calcifications in a newborn with congenital CMV disease.

may occur in these children (Coats et al., 2000). Earlier studies suggested "school failure" or developmental disabilities were likely in children born with "silent" congenital CMV infection, but more recent studies suggest overall cognitive development in these children appears to be normal when compared with that in uninfected children (Kumar et al., 1973; Reynolds et al., 1974; Hanshaw et al., 1975; Conboy et al., 1986; Williamson et al., 1990; Kashden et al., 1998).

Perinatal Infection

Despite the presence of maternal antibody to CMV, normal-term infants may be infected with CMV at the time of birth, during passage through the cervix, where secretions harbor infectious CMV. These perinatal infections are common and result in viral shedding of CMV for a month or longer; they usually are of little clinical significance in affected infants. Pneumonitis, hepatosplenomegaly, and bronchopulmonary dysplasia, however, have been associated with perinatally acquired CMV infection (Stagno et al., 1981; Kumar et al., 1984b; Sawyer et al., 1987; Whitley et al, 1976). Furthermore, developmental sequelae may occur in preterm infants who acquire CMV during the first 2 months of life (Paryani et al., 1985). Healthy, full-term infants also may acquire CMV from maternal milk; again, infection acquired in this manner is usually not associated with symptoms or sequelae in the infant (Dworsky et al., 1983b; Kumar et al., 1984a). However, CMV acquired by preterm infants from blood-product transfusion or from human milk from CMV-seropositive donors may produce not only infection, but also serious, potentially fatal, multisystem disease, with thrombocytopenia, hepatosplenomegaly, pneumonitis, and viral sepsis–like syndrome (Yeager, 1974; Maschmann et al., 2001).

Postnatal Infection—Normal Hosts

Postnatal infections with CMV in both children and adults are usually not apparent. However, clinical manifestations occur with about 10% of these infections and include fever; severe, intense, and persistent malaise and fatigue; or a heterophil-negative mononucleosis-like syndrome with hepatosplenomegaly, hepatitis, and nonexudative pharyngitis with cervical or generalized adenopathy (Horwitz et al., 1986). Occasionally a rash may accompany the illness. Upper-respiratory illness and mild gastrointestinal symptoms also have been temporally associated with CMV infections. The virus also has been isolated from the middle-ear fluid from normal hosts with otitis media; however, in contrast to congenital infection, hearing loss has rarely, if ever, been associated with postnatal CMV infection (Chonmaitree et al., 1992). Postnatal CMV infection also has been associated with development of autoimmune disorders and type I diabetes mellitus in children (Pak et al., 1988). Other complications of postnatal CMV infection are rare but include pneumonitis, myocarditis, pericarditis, hemolytic anemia, thrombocytopenia, hemophagocytic syndrome, arthralgias or arthritis, Guillain-Barré syndrome, and meningoencephalitis. Severe, icteric hepatitis and granulomatous hepatitis also can occur during an infection with CMV, but cirrhosis or hepatic necrosis with liver failure has not been convincingly documented to occur in the normal host.

Postnatal Infection—Immunocompromised Hosts

Systemic and overt end organ disease, as well as mortality, due to CMV are more likely to occur in immunocompromised hosts than in those who have normal immune systems. Furthermore, the type of CMV disease can often be predicted by the underlying immune disorder of the host. For example, bone marrow–transplant recipients are likely to experience fever and leukopenia syndromes or interstitial pneumonitis. They are at greatest risk if they are CMV-seronegative recipients who have received marrow from a CMV-seropositive donor, and the presence of acute or chronic graft-versus-host disease also is a significant risk factor for CMV-associated disease in these patients. Solid organ–transplant recipients, on the other hand, are likely to experience CMV disease in the transplanted organ (Paya, 2001). Recipients of transplanted livers are likely to experience post-transplantation CMV hepatitis, usually occurring 1 month after transplantation, with a range of 2 weeks to 4 months (Kanj et al., 1996). It is associated with fever, leukopenia, thrombocytopenia, elevated liver transaminase levels, hyperbilirubinemia, and rarely, liver graft failure. Unusual complications include pneumonia, gastritis, and colitis. CMV infection in these patients may coexist with acute or chronic rejection, and antirejection therapy with OKT3 carries considerable risk (Portela et al., 1995). CMV myocarditis has been seen most commonly in heart- and kidney-transplant recipients, usually as part of a disseminated CMV disease and associated with graft rejection that requires treatment with immunosuppressive agents (Egan et al., 2002). Presenting symptoms may include unexplained fever, heart failure, cardiomegaly, electrocardiographic abnormalities, and poor ventricular function on echocardiogram. The virus also may cause coronary artery vasculitis, with thrombosis and infarction in heart-transplant recipients. Recipients of heart-lung and lung transplants also may experience CMV pneumonitis, and children who receive intestinal transplants may experience colitis, gastritis, and pneumonitis due to CMV (Bueno et al., 1997).

In patients with AIDS, CMV causes colitis, encephalitis, pneumonia, or progressive retinitis that often leads to blindness (Drew, 1988). HIV-infected infants who are congenitally infected with CMV or who acquire CMV infection early in life also are at risk for progression of HIV disease, for central nervous system disease, and for decreased survival when compared with HIV-infected infants who are not infected with CMV (Doyle et al., 1996; Kovacs et al., 1999). Patients who are immunocompromised because of cancer chemotherapy or treatment for autoimmune disorders and those who have been burned extensively also may have serious disease associated with CMV infection (Cox and Hughes, 1975; Mera et al., 1996).

Another consequence of CMV infection in the immunocompromised host is an increased risk for opportunistic infections and graft rejection, not only because CMV infection is a marker for severe immunosuppression, but also because CMV itself appears to be an immunomodulator (Grundy et al., 1988; Grundy, 1990; Paya, 2001). In several studies of solid organ– and bone marrow–transplant recipients and of patients with AIDS, CMV infection has appeared to be an independent risk factor for the development of other systemic infections, such as gram-negative enteric bacterial infections, invasive aspergillosis, *Pneumocystis carinii* pneumonia, and Epstein-Barr virus (EBV)–associated lymphoproliferative disease (Chandwani et al., 1996; Husni et al., 1998). Also, infants with HIV infection who have *P. carinii* pneumonia commonly are coinfected with CMV, and those with dual infection have more severe disease (Williams et al., 2001).

Differential Diagnosis

The differential diagnosis of congenital CMV disease includes congenital toxoplasmosis, congenital rubella syndrome, congenital HIV infection, neonatal infection with herpes simplex virus or enterovirus, neonatal early onset bacterial sepsis, congenital syphilis, and congenital infection with lymphocytic choriomeningitis virus (Wright et al., 1997). These infectious diseases can be differentiated from congenital CMV disease by paying careful attention to important clinical clues and by obtaining appropriate viral and bacterial cultures, using DNA and RNA detection methods; and conducting serologic tests. Noninfectious conditions may mimic congenital infections and should be considered if microbiologic, virologic, and serologic tests are negative. These conditions include genetic syndromes, metabolic disorders, hematologic diseases such as erythroblastosis fetalis and

neonatal thrombocytopenia syndromes, and maternal toxin or drug exposure (Bale, 1994).

The differential diagnosis of CMV-associated mononucleosis includes infections with other viruses, such as EBV, hepatitis A and B virus, and HIV. Also, acquired toxoplasmosis can produce a mononucleosis syndrome. CMV syndromes in immunocompromised hosts may take many forms that mimic infection with other viral pathogens, bacteria, and fungi, and often are accompanied by coinfection with other opportunistic pathogens.

LABORATORY DIAGNOSIS

Congenital infection with CMV should be considered in a fetus or newborn with growth retardation, enlarged liver and spleen, jaundice, or a petechial rash present at birth, especially if thrombocytopenia, microcephaly, or intracranial calcifications also are present. Microcephaly, developmental and motor disabilities, deafness, and visual impairment or strabismus may be the presenting signs and symptoms in older infants and children whose congenital infection with CMV went unrecognized. Acquired infections with CMV should be considered in immunocompromised hosts with unexplained fever, hepatitis, or pneumonia and in healthy individuals with heterophil-negative mononucleosis, unexplained hepatitis, or persistent fatigue. Laboratory tests will be able to determine if a CMV infection is present, but careful clinical correlation is required to determine which role, if any, the virus is playing in the patient's presenting illness.

Serology

The host serologic response to CMV infection can be detected by CMV-IgG and CMV-IgM antibody tests. Historically, a variety of methods have been used to detect antibody responses to CMV, and currently enzyme immune assay and the latex agglutination test are widely used commercial assays that are available to clinicians (Hursh et al., 1989; Demmler et al., 1986c). Results may vary among methodologies and even among laboratories using similar methodologies, so the clinician should be familiar with the performance of the test used in each laboratory (Demmler et al., 2000). Also, even though detection of CMV antibody is available and relatively easy to perform, interpretation of the meaning of the results, especially if they are positive, requires careful thought. Up to 80% of the general population may have IgG antibody to CMV. A positive result merely reflects a past or present infection with the virus and the potential for recurrence. A negative result excludes the infection in most cases; severely immunocompromised patients, however, may lose their humoral immune response to the virus. Seroconversion from CMV-IgG–antibody negative to CMV-IgG–antibody positive occurs during primary CMV infections. Detection of CMV-IgM antibody suggests a recent primary infection has occurred, but it is difficult to pinpoint exactly when the infection has occurred, because IgM antibody usually persists for 8 to 12 weeks in normal hosts, with a broad range of 2 weeks to over a year (Griffiths et al., 1982a; Schaeffer et al., 1988; Demmler et al., 1986c). CMV-IgM antibody also may be elevated during recurrent infections, and false-positive and false-negative results also can occur (McEvoy and Adler, 1989). Western blot assays using viral structural proteins separated from purified viral particles or from recombinant viral proteins appear sensitive and specific for CMV-IgM detection. Currently these tests are available only in research or reference laboratories, but may soon be offered commercially (Lazzarotto et al., 1997). The CMV-IgG avidity index may be useful in providing information on the timing of a CMV infection. A low avidity index (less than 30%) suggests a recent primary infection (i.e., within 3 months), while a high avidity index (greater than 60%) suggests a past or recurrent infection (Grangeot-Keros et al., 1997).

Virus Isolation

CMV is routinely and reliably isolated in diagnostic virology laboratories using cell cultures of human fibroblasts or by a popular adaptation of traditional cell culture, called the *shell vial assay* (Demmler et al., 2000). Both methods detect live, infectious virus and can be performed in a variety of body fluids and tissue. Detection of live virus in a peripheral body fluid, such as saliva, nasal wash, urine, cervical secretions, or semen suggests an active infection but does not differentiate between a primary or recurrent infection. The presence of CMV in the blood is a condition called *viremia*, and suggests a recent primary infection or a clinically significant recurrent infection in an immocompromised host.

Detection of Viral Antigen and DNA

Surrogates for viral replication, and viremia in particular, using antigen and DNA detection methods are now available to clinicians. CMV-antigenemia tests, using commercially available immunofluorescence assay kits that detect the pp65 tegument protein in circulating white blood cells, are being performed in many diagnostic virology laboratories, especially those that serve clinicians caring for immunocompromised hosts (Schafer et al., 1997). Results of this test—which are positive during serious CMV disease—can be obtained within 24 hours in most cases. Because surveillance studies have shown CMV antigenemia results occur 1 to 2 weeks before onset of CMV-associated disease, this test also may be used to predict which patients may be at risk for CMV disease and may allow clinicians to institute preemptive therapy. The results of this test also can be quantified, and it can be used to assess antiviral response to therapy. Traditional DNA-DNA hybridization methods and, more recently, PCR-based methods for detection of CMV DNA are available in many reference laboratories, as well. These very sensitive tests may be used to detect CMV DNA in a variety of samples, including blood, CSF, tissue, and peripheral body fluids. Detection of CMV DNA in CSF supports the diagnosis of central nervous system infection in congenitally infected infants and immunocompromised hosts (Atkins et al., 1994; Arribas et al., 1995). Detection of CMV DNA in white blood cells and plasma also is used for early detection of CMV infection, especially in immunocompromised hosts. However, although the detection method is extremely sensitive, the presence of CMV DNA in blood is not always specific for predicting serious disease. Many patients in whose white blood cells CMV DNA can be detected do not develop disease. Therefore, some experts believe that PCR tests that quantify the amount of CMV DNA in the sample or detect CMV DNA only in plasma more accurately predict which patients ultimately develop CMV-associated disease (Wolf and Spector, 1993; Gallez-Hawkins et al., 1997; Zipeto et al., 1995). The presence of mRNA signals may also be a marker for early CMV infection, but this test remains a research tool at present time. False-negative results of PCR tests also may occur if the samples are inhibitory to the reaction or contain inadequate nucleic acid for analysis.

Histopathology

The effects of the virus on cells can also be assessed histopathologically in tissue, lavage samples, and even in urine. Cells that are productively infected with CMV will be enlarged and exhibit type A Cowdry intranuclear inclusions with a central area of clearing. Immunohistochemical staining may be used to enhance the detection of these "cytomegalic inclusion cells." The presence of these cells suggests active infection and end organ disease due to CMV. Virus particles, if present in abundant amounts, also may be detected by electron microscopy in tissue and in the urine of congenitally infected newborns.

Prenatal Diagnosis

The prenatal diagnosis of in utero CMV infection often is sought if a woman seroconverts from CMV-IgG–antibody negative to CMV-IgG–antibody positive during pregnancy or if CMV-IgM antibody is detected in a single sample. Since IgM antibody may persist for weeks or months after a primary infection and also may be present during a recurrent infection, other methods are under investigation to specifically diagnose primary maternal infections that produce a risk to the fetus. For example, some centers have shown low IgG antibody avidity assay results (less than 30%) appear to correlate with a higher likelihood of a recent primary infection and higher risk for transmission of CMV to the fetus (Ruellan-Eugene et al., 1996; Boppana and Britt, 1995; Grangeot-Keros et al., 1997). Infection of the fetus may be documented by isolation of CMV or detection of CMV DNA by PCR assay in amniotic fluid obtained at least 2 weeks after the suspected time of the primary maternal infection. Fetal condition may be assessed by serial fetal ultrasound examinations and, on some occasions, by fetal blood sampling for blood counts, transaminase levels, CMV-IgM antibody, and CMV DNA determination (Donner et al., 1993; Revello et al., 1995; Hohlfeld et al., 1991). The prenatal screening of pregnant women and the prenatal diagnosis of congenital CMV infection are offered routinely in many European countries but remain controversial in the United States. Negative results can be reassuring, but positive results can offer more questions than answers and should be accompanied by careful prenatal counseling by personnel knowledgeable about all the possible outcomes that can occur in congenital CMV infection and disease and all the options that are available to the parents (Enders et al., 2001).

Congenital Infection

Congenital infection with CMV in the newborn is best diagnosed by isolation of the virus from urine or saliva obtained in the first 3 weeks of life (Demmler, 1991). Urinary excretion of the virus may persist for years in congenitally infected children (Figure 4-9) (Stagno et al., 1983; Noyola et al., 2000). The presence of CMV DNA detected on PCR or histopathologic evidence of classic "cytomegalic inclusion cells" in body fluids or tissue samples obtained during this period also provide supporting evidence for the diagnosis (Demmler et al., 1991). Standard serologic tests also can be applied to diagnose congenital CMV infection but are not the recommended approach. Presence of CMV-IgG antibody in the newborn merely reflects passive maternal transfer, but the presence of CMV-IgM antibody in the newborn usually indicates symptomatic congenital infection (Griffiths et al., 1982b; Stagno et al., 1985). However, a congenitally infected newborn may have a negative CMV-IgM antibody test (Nelson et al., 1995), so the results of this serologic test should not be the sole means of establishing the diagnosis. The absence of CMV-IgG specific antibody in the newborn or older infant or child suggests congenital CMV infection was not present. Serial serologic tests at 1, 3, and 6 months of age may also be obtained. If CMV-IgG antibody level declines and the antibodies disappear over the first few months of life, then congenital infection also is ruled out. However, if the CMV-IgG antibody level persists during infancy, congenital infection is possible, as is perinatal or early postnatal infection with the virus (Demmler, 1991).

Perinatal and Postnatal Infections

The diagnosis of perinatal infection is difficult but is best documented by a negative CMV urine or saliva culture at birth and a positive culture with persistence of CMV-IgG antibody at 2 to 4 months of age.

Postnatal primary infections in both immunocompromised and normal hosts are best documented by CMV-IgG antibody conversion, but the presence of CMV-IgM

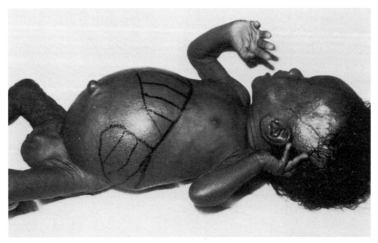

Fig. 4-9 Four-month-old child with congenital CMV disease manifesting severe failure to thrive, hepatitis with hepatosplenomegaly, bilateral inguinal hernias, and micropenis. (From Stagno S: Curr Prob Pediatr 1986;16:646).

antibody in significant titers or levels in a single serum sample also supports the diagnosis. Primary infections, especially if symptomatic, also may be accompanied by positive viral cultures of blood, urine, saliva, and other body fluids for several weeks or more. Postnatal recurrent infections are difficult to document but are suggested by an increase in CMV-IgG antibody levels, fluctuating CMV-IgM antibody levels, and intermittent viral shedding in peripheral body fluids. In the immunocompromised host, especially organ- and marrow-transplant recipients, shedding of CMV from peripheral sites such as in saliva and urine is common and nonspecific, but prospective monitoring of the blood for CMV-viremia or surrogates of viremia such as CMV-antigenemia and CMV-DNA-emia appear helpful in detecting both primary and clinically significant recurrent infections that may cause disease in these special hosts. Also, presence of CMV detected through histopathology, culture, antigen, or DNA-detection methods in bronchoalveolar lavage samples may be significant in immunocompromised hosts with or at risk for interstitial pneumonitis (Stover et al., 1984; Springmeyer et al., 1986). Early preemptive therapy with specific antiviral agents then can be administered and continued during the period of risk, with the goal of preventing a silent infection from evolving into end organ involvement or disseminated disease (van der Bij and Speich, 2001).

MANAGEMENT, TREATMENT, AND PREVENTION

Specific antiviral therapy for CMV infection and disease is available (Collaborative DHPG Treatment Study Group, 1986). Antiviral agents with activity against CMV include ganciclovir, valganciclovir, cidofovir, and foscarnet. Acyclovir and valacyclovir also may have limited activity against the virus under certain conditions (Balfour et al., 1989). In addition, biological agents, such as immune globulin and CMV-hyperimmune globulin, may be of benefit in certain clinical conditions, and novel approaches to therapy are under investigation, as well. Treatment of asymptomatic CMV infection and mild-to-moderate disease in the normal host is not indicated; antiviral therapy, however, may be beneficial for immunocompromised hosts and newborns with serious CMV disease (Fan-Hovard et al., 1989). Prevention of CMV infection and disease remains a challenging target for clinical research.

Congenital Infections

Treatment of newborns or infants with asymptomatic or "silent" congenital CMV infection is not currently indicated. However, since up to 15% of these children experience a progressive form of sensorineural deafness, clinical trials are needed to identify affected children and assess the efficacy of early or preemptive treatment in this selected group at risk for deafness.

Treatment of infants with symptomatic congenital CMV infection remains controversial. Clinicians as early as 1990 reported their experience treating newborns with serious disease associated with congenital infection. Two infants critically ill with severe, life-threatening pneumonitis, with evidence of active viral replication in urine, endotracheal secretions, lung tissue, and blood, received intravenous ganciclovir, and virologic and clinical improvement was observed during treatment. Both infants developed chronic lung disease. One of them died at 3 months of age from hypoxia associated with complications of chronic lung disease (Hocker et al., 1990; Vallejo et al., 1994). Another infant who suffered severe, and ultimately fatal, CMV disease that was presumably acquired from an in utero transfusion also showed virologic and clinical improvement while receiving intravenous ganciclovir therapy (Evans and Lyon, 1991). However, two additional anecdotal reports that focused on infants with symptoms traditionally associated with congenital CMV disease showed a virologic response during treatment, but not a definite clinical response after limited follow-up (Nigro et al., 1994; Reigstad et al., 1992). The first effort to systematically and scientifically address the issue in clinical trials began in 1989. A multicenter phase I and II study of the pharmacokinetics, safety, and antiviral effect of intravenous ganciclovir was conducted in 47 newborn infants with symptomatic congenital CMV infection who also had evidence of neurologic involvement (Trang et al., 1993; Zhou et al., 1996; Whitley et al., 1997). This initial study showed that an intravenous regimen of 6 mg per kilogram administered every 12 hours for 6 weeks produced a significant reduction in urine virus quantity during antiviral treatment; viral shedding, however, recurred at near pretreatment levels once ganciclovir treatment was terminated. Neutropenia (≤ 500 mm^3) was commonly observed during treatment. Thrombocytopenia and elevated liver transaminase levels also were observed, but the relationship to ganciclovir treatment was difficult to determine in this study. Limited clinical follow-up in 30 of the infants showed hearing improved or stabilized in 16%. Based on these findings, a phase III, multicenter, randomized clinical trial began in 1991. One hundred infants were enrolled; the infants had virologically confirmed congenital CMV disease with evidence of neurologic disease, such as microcephaly, intracranial calcifications, abnormal spinal fluid, retinitis, or hearing loss. The study was completed in 1999. It showed that 6 mg per kilogram of ganciclovir administered intravenously every 12 hours for 6 weeks to these severely affected neonates appeared to slightly improve hearing, maintain normal hearing, or prevent hearing deterioration at 6 months of age, with some effect even measurable at 12 months of age. Furthermore, those infants randomized to receive ganciclovir treatment had a more rapid resolution of their transaminase elevations and a greater degree of short-term increase in weight and head circumference. Surprisingly, no significant difference in resolution of thrombocytopenia was observed. The effect of treatment on neurodevelopmental outcome was not able to be evaluated in this trial. Treatment was also significantly associated with absolute neutropenia, which necessitated dosage adjustment or cessation but which was reversible in all infants (Kimberlin et al., 2000). Some experts administered granulocyte-stimulating factors to those infants who experienced significant neutropenia, with favorable response. However, since only 44% of enrolled subjects had careful follow-up that could be evaluated, the enduring effect on growth, development, or hearing loss is being evaluated in a long-term study of these infants.

Currently, the decision to administer antiviral therapy to a newborn with congenital CMV disease remains at the discretion of the clinician. Short-term antiviral therapy is likely to be beneficial to infants with evidence of a viral sepsis–like syndrome or multisystem disease with viremia, pneumonitis, or active retinitis, where an acute reduction in viral replication is likely to improve the overall clinical condition or resolve end organ disease. However, the role of short-term treatment in the newborn period with the goal of improving long-term audiologic or neurodevelopmental outcome is unclear at this time. The active infection associated with congenital CMV disease is chronic, lasting several years in most infants. Furthermore, although a significant portion of the neurologic disease is evident at birth, some of the sequelae observed, especially progressive or late-onset deafness, may be due to continued viral replication or a host response to the chronic infection. Therefore, it is possible that a longer period of therapy with an orally administered antiviral agent could improve outcome. Oral ganciclovir is not easily administered to newborns and small infants, but clinical trials of valganciclovir, a new, orally available prodrug of ganciclovir, may soon be conducted in newborns and small infants (Martin et al., 2002).

In addition to the consideration of antiviral therapy, the management of infants with congenital CMV disease includes vigorous supportive care of severely ill infants, including ventilatory and pressor support, seizure control, and platelet transfusions. Some infants also may have feeding difficulties, both in the immediate newborn period and also during the first few years of life, especially if they are developmentally challenged. Long-term care involves frequent assessments of growth and development, periodic ophthalmologic evaluations if retinitis was present at birth or if strabismus or optic nerve atrophy develop, and annual audiologic evaluations, even if hearing was normal at birth. Full diagnostic auditory brain stem evoked responses, with otoaucoustic emission studies, are recommended in children less than 3 years of age, and behavioral audiometry may be performed in older children. Routine annual assessments should be performed, with more frequent evaluations if a hearing loss progression is discovered or suspected. It is unclear at this time how long the annual hearing assessments should be continued, since progression of hearing loss has been documented in longitudinal studies of these children to occur up to almost 10 years of age.

Infections in the Pregnant Woman and Fetus

Prenatal diagnosis may be offered to pregnant women with serologic evidence of primary CMV infection; its use, however, remains controversial, and there does not appear to be a consensus regarding how to best manage this difficult situation. Therefore, the decision-making process must be shared with both the parents and a knowledgeable perinatologist. Most perinatologists agree that if a woman is diagnosed serologically with a primary CMV infection during pregnancy or shortly before conception, serial fetal ultrasound examinations and counseling of the parents are indicated. Most obstetricians also offer amniotic fluid samples for CMV culture and/or DNA

detection by PCR. Collection of amniotic fluid as early as 20 to 22 weeks gestation may be used to diagnose fetal infection, and serial ultrasound examinations even at as early as 19 weeks gestation can help asses fetal well-being (Hohlfeld et al., 1991; Donner et al., 1993; Revello et al., 1993; Enders et al., 2001). Fetal infection may be excluded in most cases if amniotic fluid studies performed at least 2 weeks and preferably 6 to 8 weeks after diagnosis of a maternal primary infection are negative. However, a negative result on assessment of an amniotic fluid sample does not exclude congenital infection in all cases, and some experts stress the importance of repeat amniotic fluid sampling (Donner et al., 1993; Revello et al., 1995). A positive result on amniotic fluid study, on the other hand, indicates fetal infection, but does not predict outcome. If an ultrasound examination reveals abnormalities, sampling of amniotic fluid and fetal blood for diagnosis, including detection of CMV by culture or PCR and fetal CMV-IgM antibody may be recommended (Enders et al., 2001). Some experts, on the other hand, prefer a strategy of noninvasive management, counseling the parents about all possible outcomes and following the fetus with serial ultrasounds while awaiting the natural course of the pregnancy. Still others consider termination of the pregnancy, especially if severe fetal disease with central nervous system involvement is diagnosed early in the pregnancy. Antiviral therapy for the pregnant woman or the fetus cannot be recommended at this time, since no clinical trials have been conducted to determine optimal dosing, safety, and efficacy. However, the prenatal treatment of an in utero CMV infection at 29 weeks gestation by fetal intravascular administration of ganciclovir has been reported (Revello et al., 1993). In this case report, reduction of virus titer in amniotic fluid and fetal urine was observed, with disappearance of viral DNA in fetal blood and normalization of fetal platelet count and results of liver function tests. However, fetal bradycardia and decreased fetal movements were noted following administration of ganciclovir, and the fetus died in utero at 32 weeks gestation; histopathologic evidence of CMV was seen in multiple organs.

Prevention of CMV infection in the pregnant woman and her fetus is not yet possible through routine vaccination, as has been possible, for example, with congenital rubella syndrome. However, because congenital CMV infection and disease remain a major public health problem, prevention by some means, while awaiting the formulation of a successful vaccine, seems reasonable. Controversy, therefore, looms in this arena, as well. One approach is to recommend routine screening of women of childbearing age for CMV infection or selective screening of women who have contact with young children at home or at child-care centers, both of which are environments proven to be at high risk for CMV transmission. By screening pregnant women prenatally or early in the first trimester, CMV-seronegative women can be provided with basic information about common sources of CMV and offered behavioral strategies that may reduce their risk of acquiring the virus during pregnancy (Demmler and Yow, 1992; Grose et al., 1992; Enders et al., 2001). They also should avoid intimate contact with anyone who is experiencing an active CMV infection, such as a spouse with CMV mononucleosis (Demmler et al., 1986b). The use of hygienic precautions has been shown in at least one controlled trial to reduce the risk of transmission of CMV in the family setting to women of childbearing age (Adler et al., 1996). Other experts feel more information is needed before this strategy can be recommended, preferring to wait until a more definitive preventive strategy, such as a vaccine, becomes available.

Infections in the Immunocompromised Host

Treatment of CMV-associated disease, such as retinitis, pneumonitis, colitis, esophagitis, encephalitis, or hepatitis, in the immunocompromised host usually involves a period of induction therapy with an intravenous antiviral medication, usually ganciclovir (Laskin et al., 1987; Reed et al., 1988). In special circumstances, foscarnet or cidofovir may be indicated. Since most published information on the antiviral treatment of CMV infections is on adult patients, the doses, indications, and monitoring for pediatric patients must be extrapolated from available published information on adult patients and complemented with anecdotal clinical experience (Lim et al., 1988). The usual duration of induction therapy is 2 to 3 weeks and should result in clinical and virologic response. If the host is expected to continue to be immunocompromised, then maintenance therapy at a reduced dosage

schedule, administered intravenously or orally, through the expected period of immunosuppression is indicated; in patients with AIDS, maintenance therapy is continued indefinitely. In adult patients with AIDS who have CMV retinitis, local treatment with a ganciclovir implant may augment systemic therapy with ganciclovir, but published experience evaluating this approach in children is not available. In one study, valganciclovir, the oral prodrug of ganciclovir, was as effective as intravenous ganciclovir for induction therapy for CMV retinitis (Martin et al., 2002). Valganciclovir also may be considered for long-term maintenance therapy. Clinical trials evaluating valganciclovir to treat CMV disease in children who are immunocompromised are underway, as well.

In immunocompromised hosts, CMV disease may persist or progress, despite antiviral therapy, and both host and viral factors may be responsible. The patient's immunosuppression should be assessed, coinfections and other comorbid conditions should be treated, and resistance to antiviral medications should be considered. Drug resistance is especially likely to occur in patients who receive long-term maintenance or suppression therapy with one or more antiviral agents. Resistance to ganciclvoir has been documented most often in patients with AIDS but also has been seen in patients with hematologic malignancy and in transplant recipients (Chou et al., 1995; Jacobs et al., 1998). Most ganciclovir CMV strains have a mutation in the UL97 phosphotransferase gene, but some specific mutations in the UL54 DNA polymerase gene also may occur alone or in combination with UL97 mutations. Most ganciclovir-resistant CMV strains exhibit cross-resistance to cidofovir. Multidrug resistance to ganciclovir, cidofovir, and foscarnet also may rarely occur (Chou et al., 1997). In general, if ganciclovir resistance is suspected clinically, the CMV isolate, if available, should be sent to a reference laboratory for antiviral resistance testing, and another antiviral medication, usually foscarnet, should be added to the patient's antiviral treatment, if the patient's medical condition allows.

Prevention of CMV disease is important because CMV disease continues to cause significant morbidity and mortality in immunocompromised hosts; is associated with the development of other posttransplantation complications, such as opportunistic coinfections and graft rejection; and also appears to increase resource use in transplant program. Current strategies to prevent CMV disease in transplant recipients include prophylaxis and preemptive therapy.

Prophylaxis entails administration of an antiviral agent or biologic compound prior to and at the time of engraftment, and for a period thereafter (usually 3 months), to all or to a predefined at-risk group of individuals. Its major disadvantage, however, is exposure of many low-risk patients to a potentially toxic drug and development of antiviral resistance. Numerous clinical trials have evaluated a variety of agents in many different groups of transplant recipients, and these studies have used different definitions of CMV disease, have administered antiviral therapy for different durations or by different routes of administration, and have used different follow-up periods to assess efficacy (Meyers et al., 1983; Meyers et al., 1986; Merigan et al., 1992; Paya, 2001). Therefore, successful results with one particular agent in, for example, renal-transplant recipients, does not necessarily mean the same agent will be effective in another transplant population. Furthermore, late-onset CMV disease may occur in patients who received successful prophylaxis during the immediate 3 months after transplantation. In general, prophylaxis usually is favored in patients at high risk for CMV disease, such as CMV-seronegative recipients of CMV-seropositive transplants or those CMV-seropositive recipients in whom antibodies to T-cell receptors are used in the immediate posttransplant period (Snydman et al., 1987). CMV hyperimmune globulin appears more effective than unselected immune globulin preparations, especially in renal-transplant recipients (Meyers et al., 1983; Adler, 1991a). Acyclovir and valacyclovir appear to be mildly to moderately effective in some transplant recipients compared with no treatment or placebo, but these agents clearly appear suboptimal when compared with ganciclovir, which is the antiviral compound of choice for most centers.

Preemptive therapy involves treatment with an antiviral compound, usually ganciclovir, administered to transplant recipients who develop virologic markers that suggest active viral replication and that appear predictive of CMV disease (Paya, 2001). This strategy exposes fewer patients to potentially toxic antiviral agents, but it does require an available, sensitive, and predictive test that identifies all patients at risk for posttransplantation CMV disease. A variety of diagnostic tests have been evaluated for their ability to predict the development of CMV disease in transplant recipients. Surveillance cultures of urine or saliva for CMV are nonspecific and generally not helpful. Detection of CMV viremia by viral blood culture is insensitive, often developing at or very close to the time of disease and often taking a week or longer to provide positive results. Currently, tests of choice include CMV antigenemia tests, which can provide results within 24 hours and also can quantify the antiviral effect of treatment. Tests to detect CMV DNA in blood or plasma also are commonly used and appear more sensitive and less selective or specific in predicting which patients will develop disease. Quantitative PCR assays may provide more information on viral load thresholds, which may be used to predict CMV disease. If a positive marker is detected, then preemptive therapy is initiated and continued for a defined period of time. This approach has been shown effective in randomized trials and appears to be effective in many transplant centers. The optimal duration of preemptive therapy varies, depending on the patient's immunosuppression and viral load, and recurrences of CMV infection can occur after apparently successful preemptive therapy.

Prevention of CMV infection and disease in immunocompromised patients can also be accomplished by reducing the host's exposure to CMV in potentially infected organs, marrow, and blood products. The use of CMV-seronegative and filtered leukocyte-reduced blood products can prevent transfusion-associated CMV infection in transplant recipients (Bowden et al., 1986; Bowden et al., 1995). This strategy also is effective in preventing CMV infection and disease in neonates (Gilbert et al., 1989). The optimal mode of preventing transmission of CMV from human milk to preterm and extremely low–birth weight neonates—one that inactivates CMV while preserving the nutritional and immunologic components of the milk—is currently not known, but clinical trials are being conducted (Dworsky et al., 1982; Maschmann et al., 2001). The use of universal hygienic precautions in the hospital setting appears effective in preventing the person-to-person transmission of CMV in that environment.

Prevention Through Active Immunization

Prevention of CMV disease through active immunization recently was recommended to be a priority for the twenty-first century (Stratton et al, 1999). Prevention of congenital and acquired CMV disease not only would reduce mortality and morbidity and therefore improve the quality of life for many individuals, but also has been shown to be financially beneficial (Porath et al., 1990). However, although most experts agree that the rationale for the development of a CMV vaccine is sound, a safe and effective CMV vaccine remains elusive. Since the original studies in 1975 with the first potential CMV vaccine, strain Towne 125, many different vaccines and vaccine strategies have been investigated (Plotkin et al., 1975; Plotkin et al., 1976; Plotkin et al., 1984). These strategies have included live virus vaccines that are improved versions of the original Towne strain and appear to be more immunogenic, as well as unique mutant hybrid strains in which the safety of the Towne strain is combined with enhanced immunogenicity and possibly, also, enhanced virulence, from another CMV strain, the Toledo (Adler et al., 1998; Plotkin, 1999). Other investigators are evaluating subunit vaccines that include purified gB, a glycoprotein of CMV that appears to induce abundant neutralizing antibodies in naturally infected, healthy individuals. To be immunogenic, however, this viral glycoprotein must be complexed with powerful adjuvants or inserted into vaccine vectors such as live adenovirus or canarypox virus (Marshall et al., 1990; Pass et al., 1999). Most recently, "DNA vaccines" that encode glycoprotein pp65 or gB are being evaluated as immunogens that may induce protective cellular immunity against CMV (Pande et al., 1998; Endresz et al., 1999). Finally, adoptive immunotherapy using T cells sensitized and active against CMV may some day be evaluated in bone marrow–transplant recipients as a way to reduce morbidity and mortality resulting from CMV infection.

BIBLIOGRAPHY

Adler SP. Transfusion-associated cytomegalovirus infections. Rev Infect Dis 1983;5:977-993.

Adler SP. The molecular epidemiology of cytomegalovirus transmission among children attending a day care center. J Infect Dis 1985;52:760-768.

Adler SP. Cytomegalovirus transmission among children in day care, their mothers, and caretakers. Pediatr Infect Dis J 1988a;7:279-285.

Adler SP. Molecular epidemiology of cytomegalovirus: viral transmission among children attending a day care center, their parents, and caretakers. J Pediatrics 1988b;112:366-372.

Adler SP. Cytomegalovirus hyperimmune globulin: who needs it? Pediatr Infect Dis J 1991a;11:266-269.

Adler SP. Molecular epidemiology of cytomegalovirus: a study of factors affecting transmission among children at three day-care centers. Pediatr Infect Dis J 1991b;10:584-590.

Adler SP, Baggett J, Wilson M, et al. Molecular epidemiology of cytomegalovirus in a nursery: lack of evidence for nosocomial transmission. J Pediatr 1986;117-123.

Adler SP, Finney JW, Manganello AM, et al. Prevention of child-to-mother transmission of cytomegalovirus by changing behaviors: a randomized controlled trial. Pediatr Infect Dis J 1996;15:240-246.

Adler SP, Hempfling SH, Starr SE, et al. Safety and immunogenicity of the Towne strain cytomegalovirus vaccine. Pediatr Infect Dis J 1998;17:200-206.

Ahlfors K, Harris S, Ivarsson S, et al. Secondary maternal cytomegalovirus infection causing symptomatic congenital infection. N Engl J Med 1981;305:284.

Ahlfors K, Ivarsson S, Harris S. Report on a long-term study of maternal and congenital cytomegalovirus infection in Sweden: review of prospective studies in the literature. Scand J Infect Dis 1999;31:443-457.

Arribas JR, Clifford DB, Fichtenbaum CJ, et al. Level of cytomegalovirus (CMV) DNA in cerebrospinal fluid of subjects with AIDS and CMV infection of the central nervous system. J Infect Dis 1995;172:527-531.

Atkins JT, Demmler GJ, Williamson WD, et al. Polymerase chain reaction to detect cytomegalovirus DNA in the cerebrospinal fluid of neonates with congenital infection. J Infect Dis 1994;169:1334-1337.

Baldick CJ, Shenk T. Proteins associated with purified human cytomegalovirus. J Virol 1996;6097-6105.

Bale J. Conditions mimicking congenital infections. In Bordenstein JB (ed). Seminars in pediatric neurology, vol 1, Philadelphia: WB Saunders, 1994.

Bale JF, Blackman JA, Sato, Y. Outcome in children with symptomatic congenital cytomegalovirus infection. J Child Neurol 1990;5:131-136.

Bale JF, Murph JR, Demmler GJ, et al: Intrauterine cytomegalovirus infection and glycoprotein B genotypes. J Infect Dis 2000;182:933-936.

Balfour CL, Balfour HH Jr. Cytomegalovirus is not an occupational risk for nurses in renal transplant and neonatal units: results of a prospective surveillance study. JAMA 1986;256:1909-1914.

Balfour HH, Chace BA, Stapleton JT, et al. A randomized placebo-controlled trial of oral acyclovir for the prevention of cytomegalovirus disease in recipients of renal allografts. N Engl J Med 1989;320:1381-1387.

Boppana S, Pass RF, Britt WJ, et al. Symptomatic congenital cytomegalovirus infection: neonatal morbidity and mortality. Pediatr Infect Dis J 1992;11:93-99.

Boppana SB, Britt WJ. Antiviral antibody responses and intrauterine transmission after primary maternal cytomegalovirus infection. J Infect Dis 1995;171:1115-1121.

Boppana SB, Fowler KB, Britt WJ, et al. Symptomatic congenital cytomegalovirus infection in infants born to mothers with preexisting immunity to cytomegalovirus. Pediatrics 1999;104:55-60.

Boppana SB, Fowler KB, Vaid Y, et al. Neuroradiographic findings in the newborn period and long-term outcome in children with symptomatic congenital cytomegalovirus infection. Pediatrics 1997;99:409-414.

Boppana SB, Rivera L, Fowler KB, et al. Intrauterine transmission of cytomegalovirus to infants of women with preconceptional immunity. N Engl J Med 2001;18:1360-1371.

Bowden RA, Sayers M, Fluornoy N, et al. Cytomegalovirus immune globulin and seronegative blood products to prevent primary cytomegalovirus infection after bone marrow transplantation. N Engl J Med 1986;314:1006-1010.

Bowden RA, Slichter SJ, Sayers M, et al. A comparison of filtered leukocyte-reduced and cytomegalovirus (CMV) seronegative blood products for the prevention of transfusion-associated CMV infection after marrow transplantation. Blood 1995;86:3598-3607.

Bueno J, Green M, Kocochis S, et al. Cytomegalovirus infection after intestinal transplantation in children. Clin Infect Dis1997;25:1078-1083.

Chandler SH, Handsfield HH, McDougall JK. Isolation of multiple strains of cytomegalovirus from women attending a clinic for sexually transmitted diseases. J Infect Dis 1987;155:655-660.

Chandwani S, Kaul A, Bebenroth D, et al. Cytomegalovirus infection in human immunodeficiency virus type 1-infected children. Pediatr Infect Dis J 1996;15:310-314.

Chonmaitree T, Owen MJ, Patel J, et al. Presence of cytomegalovirus and herpes simplex virus in middle ear fluids from children with acute otitis media. Clin Infect Dis 1992;15:650-653.

Chou S. Acquisition of donor strains of cytomegalovirus by renal transplant recipients. N Engl J Med 1986;314:1418-1423.

Chou S. Reactivation and recombination of multiple cytomegalovirus strains from individual organ donors. J Infect Dis 1989a;160:11-15.

Chou S. Neutralizing antibody responses to reinfecting strains of cytomegalovirus in transplant recipients. J Infect Dis 1989b;160:16-21.

Chou S, Guentzel S, Michels KR, et al. Frequency of UL97 phosphotransferase mutations related to ganciclovir resistance in clinical cytomegalovirus isolates. J Infect Dis 1995;172:238-242.

Chou S, Marousek G, Guentzel S, et al. Evolution of mutations conferring multidrug resistance during prophylaxis and therapy for cytomegalovirus disease. J Infect Dis 1997;172:786-789.

Coats DK, Demmler GJ, Paysse EA, et al. Ophthalmologic findings in children with congenital cytomegalovirus infection. J AAPOS 2000;4:110-116.

Collaborative DHPG Treatment Study Group. Treatment of serious cytomegalovirus infections with 9-(1,3-dihydroxy-2-propoxymethyl) guanine in patients with AIDS and other immunodeficiencies. N Engl J Med 1986;314:801-805.

Conboy TJ, Pass RF, Stagno S, et al. Intellectual development in school-aged children with asymptomatic congenital cytomegalovirus infection. Pediatrics 1986;77:801-805.

Conboy TJ, Pass RF, Stagno S, et al. Early clinical manifestations and intellectual outcome in children with symp-tomatic congenital cytomegalovirus infection. J Pediatr 1987;111:343-348.

Cox F, Hughes WT. Cytomegalovirus in children with acute lymphatic leukemia. J Pediatr 1975;87:190.

Demmler GJ. Summary of a workshop on surveillance for congenital cytomegalovirus disease. Rev Infect Dis 1991;13:315-329.

Demmler GJ, Brady M, Bijou H, et al. Posttransfusion cytomegalovirus infection in neonates: role of saline-washed red blood cells. J Pediatr 1986a;108:762-765.

Demmler GJ, Istas A, Easley K, et al. Results of a quality assurance program for detection of cytomegalovirus infection in the pediatric pulmonary and cardiovascular complications of vertically transmitted human immunodeficiency virus infection study. J Clin Microbiol 2000;38: 3942-3945.

Demmler GJ, O'Neil GW, O'Neil JH, et al. Transmission of cytomegalovirus from husband to wife. J Infect Dis 1986b;154:545-546.

Demmler GJ, Six HR, Hurst M, et al. Enzyme-linked immunosorbent assay for the detection of IgM class antibodies to cytomegalovirus. J Infect Dis 1986c;153:1152-1155.

Demmler GJ, Yow MD. Congenital cytomegalovirus disease—20 years is long enough. N Engl J Med 1992;326:702-703.

Demmler GJ, Yow MD, Spector S, et al. Nosocomial cytomegalovirus infections within two hospitals caring for infants and children. J Infect Dis 1987;156:9-16.

Donner C, Liesnard C, Congent J, et al. Prenatal diagnosis of 52 pregnancies at risk for congenital cytomegalovirus infection. Obstet Gynecol 1993;82:481-486.

Doyle M, Atkins JT, Rivera-Matos IR. Congenital cytomegalovirus infection in infants infected with human immunodeficiency virus type 1. Pediatr Infect Dis J 1996;15:1102-1106.

Drew LW. Cytomegalovirus infection in patients with AIDS. J Infect Dis 1988;158:449-456.

Dworsky M, Lakeman A, Stagno S. Cytomegalovirus transmission within a family. Pediatric Infect Dis J 1984;3:236-238.

Dworsky M, Stagno S, Pass RF, et al. Persistence of cytomegalovirus in human milk after storage. J Pediatr 1982;101:440-443.

Dworsky M, Stagno S, Pass RF, et al. Occupational risk for primary cytomegalovirus infection among pediatric health-care workers. N Engl J Med 1983a; 309:950-953.

Dworsky M, Yow M, Stagno S, et al. Cytomegalovirus infection of breast milk and transmission in infancy. Pediatrics 1983b;72:295-299.

Egan JJ, Carroll KB, Yonan N, et al. Valacyclovir prevention of cytomegalovirus reactivation after heart transplantation: a randomized trial. J Heart Lung Transplant 2002;4:460-466.

Enders G, Bader V, Lindemann, et al. Prenatal diagnosis of congenital cytomegalovirus infection in 189 pregnancies with known outcome. Prenat Diagn 2001;21:326-377.

Endresz V, Kari L, Berensci K, et al. Induction of human cytomegalovirus (HCMV)-glycoprotein B (gB)-specific neutralizing antibody and phosphoprotein 65 (pp65)-specific cytotoxic T-lymphocyte responses by naked DNA immunization. Vaccine 1999;17:50-58.

Evans DGR, Lyon AJ. Fatal congenital cytomegalovirus infection acquired by an intra-uterine transfusion. Eur J Pediatr 1991;150:780-781.

Fan-Hovard P, Nahata MC, Brady MT. Ganciclovir-a review of pharmacology, therapeutic efficacy and potential use for the treatment of congenital cytomegalovirus infections. J Clin Pharm Therapeut 1989;14:329-340.

Fowler KB, Dahle AJ, Boppana SB, et al. Newborn hearing screening: will children with hearing loss caused by congenital cytomegalovirus infection be missed? J Pediatr 1999;135:60-64.

Fowler KB, McCollister FP, Dahle AJ, et al. Progressive or fluctuating sensorineural hearing loss in children with asymptomatic congenital cytomegalovirus infection. J Pediatr 1997;130:626-630.

Fowler KB, Stagno S, Pass R, et al. The outcome of congenital cytomegalovirus infection in relation to maternal antibody status. N Engl J Med 1992;326:663-667.

Friedman HM, Lewis MR, Nemerofsky DM, et al. Acquisition of cytomegalovirus infection among female employees at a pediatric hospital. Pediatr Infect Dis J 1984;3:233-235.

Fries BC, Chou S, Boeckh M, et al. Frequency distribution of cytomegalovirus envelope glycoprotein genotypes in bone marrow transplant recipients. J Infect Dis 1994;169:759-764.

Gallez-Hawkins GM, Tegtmeier BR, terVeer A, et al. Evaluation of a quantitative plasma PCR plate assay detection with cytomegalovirus infection in marrow transplant recipients. J Clin Microbiol 1997;35:788-790.

Gilbert GL, Hayes K, Hudson I, et al. Prevention of transfusion-acquired cytomegalovirus infection in infants by blood filtration to remove leucocytes. Lancet 1989;1:1228-1231.

Gilbert MJ, Riddell SR, Li CR, et al. Selective interference with class I major histocompatibility complex presentation of the major immediate-early protein following infection with human cytomegalovirus. J Virol 1993;67:3461-3469.

Goodpasture EW, Talbot FB. Concerning the nature of "protozoan-like" cells in certain lesions of infancy. Am J Dis Child 1921;21:415.

Grangeot-Keros L, Mayaux MJ, Lebon P, et al. Value of cytomegalovirus (CMV) IgG avidity index for the diagnosis of primary CMV infection in pregnant women. J Infect Dis 1997;175:944-950.

Griffiths PD, Stagno S, Pass RF, et al. Infection with cytomegalovirus during pregnancy: specific IgM antibodies as a marker of recent primary infection. J Infect Dis 1982a;145:647-653.

Griffiths PD, Stagno S, Pass RF, et al. Congenital cytomegalovirus infection: diagnostic and prognostic significance of the detection of specific immunoglobulin M antibodies in cord serum. Pediatrics 1982b;69:544-549.

Griller L, Ahlfors K, Ivarsson S, et al. Endonuclease cleavage pattern of cytomegalovirus DNA of strains isolated form congenitally infected infants with neurologic sequelae. Pediatrics 1988;81:27-30.

Grose C, Meehan T, Weinder C. Prenatal diagnosis of congenital cytomegalovirus infection by virus isolation after amniocentesis. Pediatr Infect Dis J 1992;11:605-607.

Grundy JE. Virologic and pathologic aspects of cytomegalovirus infection. Rev Infect Dis 1990;12 (suppl):S711-S719.

Grundy JE, Ayles HM, McKeating JA, et al. Enhancement of class I HLA antigen expression by cytomegalovirus: role in amplification of virus infection. J Med Virol 1988;25:483-495.

Handsfield HH, Chandler SH, Caine VA, et al. Cytomegalovirus infections in sex partner: evidence for sexual transmission. J Infect Dis 1985;151:344-348.

Hanshaw JB, Scheiner AP, Moxley AW, et al. School failure and deafness after "silent" congenital cytomegalovirus infection. N Engl J Med 1975;295:468-470.

Heggie AD, Wentz WB, Reagan JW, et al. Roles of cytomegalovirus and *Chlamydia trachomatis* in the induction of cervical neoplasia in the mouse. Cancer Res 1986;46:5211-5214.

Hocker JR, Cook LN, Adams G, et al. Ganciclovir therapy of congenital cytomegalovirus pneumonia. Pediatr Infect Dis J 1990;9:743-745.

Hohlfeld P, Vial Y, Maillard-Grignon C, et al. Cytomegalovirus fetal infections. Prenatal Diag 1991;78:615-618.

Horwitz CA, Henle W, Henle G, et al. Clinical and laboratory evaluation of cytomegalovirus-induced mononucleosis in previously healthy individuals: report of 82 cases. Medicine 1986;65:124-134.

Huang ES, Alford C, Reynolds DW, et al. Molecular epidemiology of cytomegalovirus infections in women and their infants. N Engl J Med 1980;303:958-962.

Hursh DA, Abbot AD, Sun R, et al. Evaluation of a latex particle agglutination assay for the detection of cytomegalovirus antibody in patient serum. J Clin Microbiol 1989;27:2878-2879.

Husni RN, Gordon SM, Longworth DL, et al. Cytomegalovirus infection is a risk factor for invasive Aspergillosis in lung transplant recipients. Clin Infect Dis 1998;26:753-755.

Hutto C, Little A, Ricks R, et al. Isolation of CMV from toys and hands in a day-care center. J Infect Dis 1986;154:527-530.

Istas AS, Demmler GJ, Dobbin JG, et al. Surveillance for congenital cytomegalovirus disease: a report from the national congenital cytomegalovirus disease registry. Clin Infect Dis 1995;20:665-670.

Jacobs DA, Enger C, Dunn JP, et al. cytomegalovirus retinitis and viral resistance: ganciclovir resistance. J Infect Dis 1998;177:770-773.

Jamison RM, Hathorn AW. Isolation of cytomegalovirus from cerebrospinal fluid of a congenitally infected infant. Am J Dis Child 1978;132:63-64.

Kaariainen L, Klemola E, Paloheimo J. Rise of cytomegalovirus antibodies in an infectious mononucleosis-like syndrome after transfusion. Br Med J 1966;2:1270-1272.

Kanj SS, Sharar AI, Clavien PA, et al. Cytomegalovirus infection following liver transplantation: Review of the literature. Clin Infect Dis 1996;22:537-549.

Kashden J, Frison S, Fowler KB, et al. Intellectual assessment of children with asymptomatic congenital cytomegalovirus infection. Develop Behav Pediatr 1998;19:254-259.

Kimberlin DW, Lin C-Y, Sanchez P, et al. Antiviral treatment of symptomatic congenital cytomegalovirus (CMV) infection. Results of a Phase III randomized trial. Program and Abstracts of the 40th Interscience Conference on Antimicrobial Agents and Chemotherapy, 2000.

Kovacs A, Schluchter M, Easley K, et al. Cytomegalovirus infection and HIV-1 disease progression in infants born to HIV-1 infected women. N Engl J Med 1999;341: 77-84.

Kozinowski UH, Reddehase MJ, Keil GM, et al. Host immune response to cytomegalovirus: products of transfected viral immediate-early genes are recognized by cloned cytolytic T lymphocytes. J Virol 1987;61:2054-2058.

Kumar ML, Nankervis GA, Cooper AR, et al. Postnatally acquired cytomegalovirus infected infants of CMV-excreting mothers. J Pediatr 1984a;104:674-679.

Kumar ML, Nankervis GA, Gold E, et al. Inapparent congenital cytomegalovirus infection: a followup study. N Engl J Med 1973;288:1370-1372.

Kumar ML, Nankervis GA, Jacobs IB, et al. Congenital and postnatally acquired cytomegalovirus infections: long-term follow up. J Pediatr 1984b;104:669-673.

Kumar ML, Gold E, Jacobs I, et al. Primary cytomegalovirus infection in adolescent pregnancy. Pediatrics 1984c;74: 493-500.

Lambertson HV, McMillan JA, Weiner LB, et al. Prevention of transfusion-associated cytomegalovirus (CMV) infection in neonates by screening blood donors for IgM to CMV. J Infect Dis 1988;157:820-823.

Lang DJ, Hanshaw JB. Cytomegalovirus infection and the postperfusion syndrome: recognition of primary infections in four patients. N Engl J Med 1969;280:1145-1150.

Lang DJ, Kummer JF. Cytomegalovirus in semen: observations in selected populations. J Infect Dis 1975;132:472-475.

Laskin O, Cederberf D, Mills J, et al. Ganciclovir for the treatment and suppression of serious infections caused by cytomegalovirus. Am J Med 1987;83:201-207.

Lasry S, Deny P, Asselot C, et al. Interstrain variation in the cytomegalovirus (CMV) glycoprotein B gene sequence among CMV-infected children attending six day care centers. J Infect Dis 1996;174:606-609.

Lazzarotto T, Maine GT, Dalmonte P, et al. A novel western blot test containing both viral and recombinant proteins for anticytomegalovirus immunoglobulin M detection. J Clin Microbiol 1997;35:393-397.

Lim W, Kahn E, Gupta A, et al. Treatment of cytomegalovirus enterocolitis with ganciclovir in an infant with acquired immunodeficiency syndrome. Pediatr Infect Dis J 1988;7:354-357.

Marshall GS, Ricciardi RP, Rando RF, et al. An adenovirus recombinant that expresses the human cytomegalovirus major envelope glycoprotein and induces neutralizing antibodies. J Infect Dis 1990;162:1177-1181.

Martin DF, Sierra-Madero J, Walmsley S, et al. A controlled trial of valganciclovir as induction therapy for cytomegalovirus retinitis. N Engl J Med 2002;346:1119-1126.

Maschmann J, Hamprecht K, Dietz K, et al. Cytomegalovirus infection of extremely low-birth weight infants via breast milk. Clin Infect Dis 2001;33:1998-2002.

McEvoy MA, Adler S. Immunologic evidence for frequent age-related cytomegalovirus reactivation in seropositive immunocompetent individuals. J Infect Dis 1989;160: 1-10.

McFarlane ES, Koment RW. Use of restriction endonuclease digestion to analyze strains of human cytomegalovirus isolated concurrently from an immunocompetent heterosexual man. J Infect Dis 1986;154:167-168.

Melnick JL, Petrie BL, Dreesman GR, et al. Cytomegalovirus antigen within human arterial smooth muscle cells. Lancet 1983;2:644-647.

Mera JR, Whimbey E, Elting L, et al. Cytomegalovirus pneumonia in adult nontransplantation patients with cancer: review of 20 cases occurring from 1964 through 1990. Clin Infect Dis 1996;22:1046-1050.

Merigan T, Renlund D, Keay S, et al. A controlled trial of ganciclovir to prevent CMV disease after transplantation. N Engl J Med 1992;326:1182-1186.

Merigan T, Resta S. Cytomegalovirus: where have we been and where are we going? Rev Infect Dis 1990;12(suppl);S693-S700.

Meyers JD, Flournoy N, Thomas ED. Risk factors for cytomegalovirus infection after human marrow transplantation. J Infect Dis 1986;153:478-488.

Meyers JD, Leszczynski J, Zaia JA, et al. Prevention of cytomegalovirus infection by cytomegalovirus immune globulin after marrow transplantation. Ann Intern Med 1983;98:442-446.

Murph JR, Bale JF, Murran JC, et al. Cytomegalovirus transmission in a Midwest day-care center: possible relationship to child care practices. J Pediatr 1986;109: 35-39.

Murph JR, Souza IE, Dawson JD, et al. Epidemiology of congenital cytomegalovirus infection: maternal risk factors and molecular analysis of cytomegalovirus strains. Am J Epidemiol 1998;147:940-947.

National Congenital CMV Disease Registry. CMV Updates [serial online] 2002;7(1). Available at: www.bcm.tmc.edu/pedi/infect/cmv.

Navarro D, Lennette E, Tugizov S, et al. Humoral immune response to functional regions of cytomegalovirus glycoprotein b. J Med Virol 1997;52:451-459.

Nelson CT, Istas AS, Wilkerson MK, et al. PCR detection of cytomegalovirus DNA in serum as a diagnostic test for congenital cytomegalovirus infection. J Clin Microbiol 1995;33:3317-3318.

Nigro G, Scholz H, Bartmann U. Ganciclovir therapy for symptomatic congenital cytomegalovirus infection in infants: a two regimen experience. J Pediatr 1994;124:318-322.

Noyola DF, Demmler GJ, Nelson CT, et al. Early predictors of neurodevelopmental outcome in symptomatic congenital cytomegalovirus infection. J Pediatr 2001;138:325-331.

Noyola DF, Demmler GJ, Williamson WD, et al. Cytomegalovirus urinary infection and long term outcome in children with congenital cytomegalovirus infection. Pediatr Infect Dis J 2000;19:505-510.

Pak CY, Eun HM, McArthur RG, et al. Association of cytomegalovirus infection with autoimmune type I diabetes. Lancet 1988;2:1-4.

Pande H, Campo K, Tanamachi B, et al. Direct DNA immunization of mice with plasmid DNA encoding the tegument protein pp65 (ppUL83) of human cytomegalovirus induces high levels of circulating antibody to the encoded protein. Scand J Infect Dis Suppl 1998;99:117-120.

Paryani SG, Yeager AS, Hosford-Dunn H, et al. Sequelae of acquired cytomegalovirus infection in premature and sick term infants. J Pediatr 1985;107:451-456.

Pass RF, August AN, Dworsky M, et al. Cytomegalovirus infection in a day care center. N Engl J Med 1982;307:477-479.

Pass RF, Duliege A-M, Boppana S, et al. A subunit cytomegalovirus vaccine based on recombinant envelope glycoprotein B and a new adjuvant. J Infect Dis 1999; 180:990-995.

Pass RF, Hutto C, Ricks R, et al. Increased rate of cytomegalovirus infection among parents of children attending day-care centers. N Engl J Med 1986;314: 1414-1416.

Pass RF, Little EA, Stagno S, et al. Young children as a probable source of maternal and congenital cytomegalovirus infection. N Engl J Med 1987;316:1366-1370.

Pass RF, Stagno S, Myers G, et al. Outcome of symptomatic congenital cytomegalovirus infection: results of long-term longitudinal follow-up. Pediatr 1980;66:758-762.

Paya C. Prevention of cytomegalovirus disease in recipients of solid-organ transplants. Clin Infect Dis 2001;32:596-603.

Peckham CS, Stark O, Dudgeon JA, et al. Congenital cytomegalovirus infection: a cause of sensorineural hearing loss. Arch Dis Child 1987;62:1233-1237.

Plotkin SA. Vaccination against cytomegalovirus, the challenging demon. Pediatr Infect Dis J 1999;313-326.

Plotkin SA, Farquhar J, Hornberger E. Clinical trials of immunization with the Towne 125 strain of human cytomegalovirus. J Infect Dis 1976;134:470-475.

Plotkin SA, Friedman HM, Fleisher GR, et al. Towne-vaccine-induced prevention of cytomegalovirus disease after renal transplants. Lancet 1984;1:528-530.

Plotkin SA, Furukawa T, Zygraich N, et al. Candidate cytomegalovirus strain for human vaccination. Infect Immun 1975;12:521-527.

Pollard RB. Cytomegalovirus infections in renal, heart, heart-lung, and liver transplantation. Pediatr Infect Dis J 1988;7:S97-S102.

Porath A, McNutt RA, Smiley LM, Weigle KA. Effectiveness and cost benefit of a proposed live cytomegalovirus vaccine in the prevention of congenital disease. Rev Infect Dis 1990;12:31-40.

Portela D, Patel R, Larson-Keller JJ, et al. OKT3 treatment for allograft rejection is a risk factor for cytomegalovirus disease in liver transplantation. J Infect Dis 1995;171: 1014-1019.

Rand KH, Pollard RB, Merigan TC. Increased pulmonary superinfections in cardiac transplant patients undergoing primary cytomegalovirus infection. N Engl J Med 1988;298:951-957.

Rasmussen L, Hong C, Zipeto D, et al. Cytomegalovirus gB genotype distribution differs in human immunodeficiency virus-infected patients and immunocompromised allograft recipients. J Infect Dis 1997;175:179-184.

Reed EC, Bowden RA, Dandliker PS, et al. Treatment of cytomegalovirus pneumonia with ganciclovir and intravenous cytomegalovirus immunoglobulin in patients with bone marrow transplants. Ann Intern Med 1988;109:783-788.

Reigstad H, Bjerknes R, Markestad T, et al. Ganciclovir therapy of congenital cytomegalovirus disease. Acta Pediatr 1992;81:707-708.

Revello MG, Baldanti F, Furione M, et al. Polymerase chain reaction for prenatal diagnosis of congenital human cytomegalovirus infection. J Med Virol 1995;47:462-466.

Revello MG, Percivalle E, Baldanti F, et al. Prenatal treatment of congenital human cytomegalovirus infection by fetal intravascular administration of ganciclovir. Clin Diag Virol 1993;1:61-67.

Reynolds DW, Dean PH, Pass RF, Alford CA. Specific cell-mediated immunity in children with congenital and neonatal cytomegalovirus infection and their mothers. J Infect Dis 1979;140:493-499.

Reynolds DW, Stagno S, Alford C. Congenital cytomegalovirus infection. In. Reynolds DW, Stagno S, Alford C (eds). Teratogen update: environmentally induced birth defect risks. New York: Alan R. Liss, 1986.

Reynolds DW, Stagno S, Stubbs G, et al. Inapparent congenital cytomegalovirus infection with elevated cord IgM levels: causal relation with auditory and mental deficiency. N Engl J Med 1974;290:291-296.

Rinaldo CR, Carney WP, Richter BS, et al. Mechanisms of immunosuppression of cytomegalovirus mononucleosis. J Infect Dis 1980;141:488-495.

Rola-Pleszczynski M, Frenkel L, Fuceillo DA, et al. Specific impairment of cell-mediated immunity in mothers of infants with congenital infection due to cytomegalovirus. J Infect Dis 1977;135:386-391.

Rosenthal SL, Stanberry LR, Biro FM, et al. Seroprevalence of herpes simplex virus types 1 and 2 and cytomegalovirus in adolescents. Clin Infect Dis 1997;24: 135-139.

Rowe WP. Cytopathogenic agent resembling human salivary gland virus recovered from tissue cultures of human adenoids. Proc Soc Exp Biol Med 1956;92:4181.

Ruellan-Eugene G, Barjot P, Campet M, et al. Evaluation of virological procedures to detect fetal human cytomegalovirus infection: avidity of IgG antibodies, virus detection in amniotic fluid, and maternal serum. J Med Virol 1996;50:9-15.

Rutter D, Griffiths P, Trompeter RS. Cytomegalic inclusion disease after recurrent maternal infection. Lancet 1985;2:1182.

Sawyer MH, Edwards DK, Spector SA. Cytomegalovirus infection and bronchopulmonary dysplasia in premature infants. Am J Dis Child 1987;141:303-305.

Schaeffer L, Cesario A, Demmler G, et al. Evaluation of Abbot CMV-M enzyme immunoassay for detection of cytomegalovirus immunoglobulin M antibody. J Clin Microbiol 1988;26:2041-2043.

Schafer P, Tenschat W, Gutensohn, K, et al. Minimal effects of delayed sample processing on results of quantitative PCR for cytomegalovirus DNA in leucocytes compared to results of an antigenemia assay. J Clin Microbiol 1997;35:741-744.

Schrier RD, Nelson JA, Oldstone MBA. Detection of human cytomegalovirus in peripheral blood leucocytes in a natural infection. Science 1985;230:1048-1051.

Schrier RD, Rice GPA, Oldstone MBA. Suppression of natural killer cell activity and T cell proliferation by fresh isolates of human cytomegalovirus. J Infect Dis 1986;153:1084-1091.

Scott GB, Buck BE, Leterman JG, et al. Acquired immunodeficiency syndrome in infants. N Engl J Med 1984;310:76-81.

Singh N, Dummer JS, Kusne S, et al. Infections with cytomegalovirus and other herpesviruses in 121 liver transplant recipients: transplantation by donated organ and the effect of OKT3 antibodies. J Infect Dis 1988;158:124-131.

Smith MG. Propagation of salivary gland virus of the mouse in tissue cultures. Proc Soc Exp Biol Med 1954;86:435.

Smith MG. Propagation in tissue cultures of a cytopathogenic virus from human salivary gland virus (SGV) disease. Proc Soc Exp Biol Med 1956;92:424.

Snydman DR, Werner BG, Heize-Lacey B, et al. Use of cytomegalovirus immune globulin to prevent cytomegalovirus disease in renal transplant recipients. N Engl J Med 1987;317:1049-1054.

Sokol DM, Demmler GJ, Buffone GJ. Rapid epidemiologic analysis of cytomegalovirus by using polymerase chain reaction assays of the L-S junction. J Clin Microbiol 1992;30:839-844.

Sohn N, Ohm Y, Balcarek K, et al. Cytomegalovirus infection in sexually active adolescents. J Infect Dis 1991;163:460-463.

Spector SA. Transmission of cytomegalovirus among infants in hospital documented by restriction-endonuclease-digestion analyses. Lancet 1983;1:378-381.

Spector SA, Hirata KK, Neuman TR. Identification of multiple cytomegalovirus strains in homosexual men with acquired immunodeficiency syndrome. J Infect Dis 1984;150:953-956.

Spector SA, Spector DH. Molecular epidemiology of cytomegalovirus infections in premature twin infants and their mother. Pediatr Infect Dis J 1982;1:405-409.

Spector SA, Spector DH. The use of DNA probes in studies of human cytomegalovirus. Clin Chem 1985;31:1514-1520.

Springmeyer SC, Hackman RC, Holle R, et al. Use of bronchoalveolar lavage to diagnose acute diffuse pneumonia in the immunocompromised host. J Infect Dis 1986;154:604-610.

Stagno S, Brasfield DM, Brown MB, et al. Infant pneumonitis associated with cytomegalovirus, chlamydia, pneumocystis, and ureaplasma: a prospective study. Pediatrics 1981;68:322-329.

Stagno S, Pass RF, Dworsky ME, et al. Congenital cytomegalovirus infection: the relative importance of primary and recurrent maternal infection. N Engl J Med 1982;306:945-949.

Stagno S, Pass R, Dworsky M, et al. Congenital and perinatal cytomegalovirus infections. Semin Perinatol 1983;7:31-43.

Stagno S, Pass RF, Dworsky ME, et al. Primary cytomegalovirus infection in pregnancy. Incidence, transmission to fetus, and clinical outcome. JAMA 1986;256:1904-1908.

Stagno S, Reynolds D, Amos CS, et al. Auditory and visual defects resulting from symptomatic and subclinical congenital cytomegaloviral and toxoplasma infections. Pediatrics 1977a;59:669-678.

Stagno S, Reynolds DW, Huang ES, et al. Congenital cytomegalovirus infection. Occurrence in an immune population. N Engl J Med 1977b;296:1254-1258.

Stagno S, Reynolds DW, Pass RF, Alford CA. Breast milk and the risk of cytomegalovirus infection. N Engl J Med 1980;302:1073-1076.

Stagno S, Tinker M, Elrod C, et al. Immunoglobulin M antibodies detected by enzyme-linked immunosorbent assay and radioimmunoassay in the diagnosis of cytomegalovirus infections in pregnant women and newborn infants. J Clin Microbiol 1985;31:930-935.

Starr SE, Tolpin MD, Friedman HM, et al. Impaired cellular immunity to cytomegalovirus in congenitally infected children and their mothers. J Infect Dis 1979;140:500-505.

Stover DE, Zaman MB, Hajdu SI, et al. Bronchoalveolar lavage in the diagnosis of diffuse pulmonary infiltrates in the immunosuppressed host. Ann Intern Med 1984;101:1-7.

Stratton KR, Durch JS, Lawrence RS. Vaccines for the 21st century: a tool for decision making. Report of the Committee to Study Priorities for Vaccine Development; Division of Health Promotion and Disease Prevention; Institute of Medicine; National Academy of Sciences. Washington , D.C.: National Academy Press, 1999.

Taber LH, Frank AI, Yow MD, et al. Acquisition of cytomegaloviral infections in families with young children: a serologic study. J Infect Dis 1985;151:948-952.

Tatum ET, Sun PC, Cohn DJ. Cytomegalovirus vasculitis and colon perforation in a patient with the acquired immunodeficiency syndrome. Pathology 1989;21:235-238.

Taylor-Wiedeman J, Sissons P, Sinclair J. Induction of endogenous human cytomegalovirus gene expression after differentiation of monocytes from healthy carriers. J Virol 1994;1597-1604.

Trang JM, Kidd L, Gruber W, et al. Linear single-dose pharmacokinetics of ganciclovir in newborns with congenital cytomegalovirus infections. Clin Pharmacol Ther 1993;53:15-21.

Vallejo JG, Englund JA, Garcia-Prats JA, et al. Ganciclovir treatment of steroid-associated cytomegalovirus disease in a congenitally infected neonate. Pediatr Infect Dis J 1994;13:239-241.

Van der Bij W, Speich R. Management of cytomegalovirus infection and disease after solid-organ transplantation. Clin Infect Dis 2001;33(suppl 1):533-537.

Vochem M, Hamprecht K, Jahn G, et al. Transmission of cytomegalovirus to preterm infants through breast milk. Pediatr Infect Dis J 1998;17:53-58.

von Glahn WC, Pappenheimer AM. Intranuclear inclusions in visceral disease. Am J Pathol 1925;1:445.

Walmus BF, Yow MD, Lester JW, et al. Factors predictive of cytomegalovirus immune status in pregnant women. J Infect Dis 1988;157:172-177.

Weller TH, Hanshaw JB. Virologic and clinical observations on cytomegalic inclusion disease. N Engl J Med 1962;26:1233-1240.

Weller TH, Macaulay JC, Craig JM, et al. Isolation of intranuclear inclusion agents from infants and illnesses resembling cytomegalic inclusion disease. Proc Soc Exp Biol Med 1957;94:4.

Whitley RJ, Brasfield D, Reynolds DW, et al. Protracted pneumonitis in young infants associated with perinatally acquired cytomegaloviral infection. J Pediatr 1976;89:16-22.

Whitley RJ, Cloud G, Gruber W, et al. Ganciclovir treatment of symptomatic congenital cytomegalovirus infection: results of a Phase II study. J Infect Dis 1997;175:1080-1086.

Wilfert CM, Huang ES, Stagno S. Restriction endonuclease analysis of cytomegalovirus deoxyribonucleic acid as an epidemiologic tool. Pediatrics 1982;70:717-721.

Williamson WD, Demmler GJ, Percy AK, et al. Progressive hearing loss in infants with asymptomatic congenital cytomegalovirus infection. Pediatrics 1992;90:862-866.

Williamson WD, Desmond MM, LaFevers N, et al. Symptomatic congenital cytomegalovirus: disorders of language, learning and hearing. Am J Dis Child 1982;136:902-905.

Williamson WD, Percy AK, Yow MD, et al. Asymptomatic congenital cytomegalovirus infection: audiologic, neuro-radiologic and neurodevelopmental abnormalities during the first year. Am J Dis Child 1990;144:1365-1368.

Williams AJ, Duong T, McNally LM, et al. *Pneumocystis carinii* pneumonia and cytomegalovirus infection in children with vertically acquired HIV infection. AIDS 2001;15:335-339.

Wolf DC, Spector SA. Early diagnosis of human cytomegalovirus disease in transplant recipients by DNA amplification in plasma. Transplantation 1993;56:330-334.

Wright R, Johnson D, Neumann M, et al. Congenital lymphocytic choriomeningitis syndrome: a disease that mimics congenital toxoplasmosis or cytomegalovirus infections. Pediatrics 1997;100:1-6.

Yeager AS. Transfusion-acquired cytomegalovirus infection in newborn infants. Am J Dis Child 1974;128:478-483.

Yeager AS, Grumet FC, Hafleigh EB, et al. Prevention of transfusion-acquired cytomegalovirus infections in newborn infants. J Pediatr 1981;98:281-287.

Yow MD, Lakeman AD, Stagno S, et al. Use of restriction enzymes to investigate the source of a primary cytomegalovirus infection in a pediatric nurse. Pediatrics 1982;70:713-716.

Yow MD, White N, Taber L, et al. Acquisition of cytomegalovirus infection from birth to 10 years: a longitudinal serologic study. J Pediatr 1987;110:37-42.

Yow MD, Williamson DW, Leeds LJ, et al. Epidemiologic characteristics of cytomegalovirus infection in mothers and their infants. Am J Obstet Gynecol 1988;158:1189-1195.

Zhou X-S, Gruber W, Demmler G, et al. Population pharmacokinetics of ganciclovir in newborns with congenital cytomegalovirus infections. Antimicrob Agents Chemother 1996;40:2202-2205.

Zipeto D, Morris S, Hong C, et al. Human cytomegalovirus (CMV) DNA in plasma reflects quantity of CMV DNA present in leukocytes. J Clin Microbiol 1995;33:2607-2612.

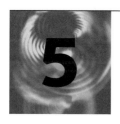

5 DENGUE AND DENGUE HEMORRHAGIC FEVER

Niranjan Kanesa-thasan, David W. Vaughn, and Robert E. Shope

Dengue is the leading disease of humans caused by an insect-borne virus. With over 100 million cases occurring annually, dengue takes a higher toll than do other major flaviviral pathogens, such as yellow fever, Japanese encephalitis, tick-borne encephalitis, and the West Nile virus (Innis, 1995). In the tropics and subtropics, dengue is a major public-health burden in terms of disability-adjusted life-years and hospitalization costs (Gubler and Meltzer, 1999). In the United States, cases of dengue contracted elsewhere occur sporadically, with occasional small foci of indigenous transmission in Hawaii and on the borders (Centers for Disease Control and Prevention, 2001).

HISTORY

The first English description of dengue was provided in 1789 by Benjamin Rush, who described the clinical characteristics of the acute illness (Rush, 1789). However, the role of *Aedes aegypti* mosquitoes in transmission of the virus was not understood until 1906 (Siler et al., 1926). The cause of dengue was attributed to a virus in 1907, making it the second viral infection of humans identified after the discovery of the etiologic agent of yellow fever by Walter Reed (Ashburn and Craig, 1907). Experimental studies of dengue that established many features of the disease were conducted by the U.S. military in the Philippines from 1924 to 1931 (Siler, Hall, and Hitchens, 1926; Simmons et al., 1931).

World War II resulted in the epidemic spread of dengue because of mass movements of infected men and mosquito-contaminated materiel, particularly throughout the Pacific. This epidemic raised sufficient concern to accelerate scientific studies of the virus by both Japanese and U.S. researchers (Hotta, 1969).

Albert Sabin successfully identified and propagated dengue-1 and dengue-2 virus serotypes during the 1940s from virus strains obtained in Hawaii, New Guinea, and India (Sabin, 1952). This led to the rapid development of diagnostic tests and, in the next decade, the first experimental attenuated vaccines (Sabin, 1955; Sabin and Schlesinger, 1945).

The next major events in the history of dengue were the description of dengue hemorrhagic fever (DHF) in Southeast Asia in 1953 and 1954 (Hammon et al., 1960) and the recognition in the 1960s that the syndrome was caused by the dengue virus (Halstead, 1966). The reported number of cases has expanded exponentially in the decades since the 1970s; this expansion has been accelerated in part by the decline of mosquito-control campaigns (Monath, 1994). A large outbreak in Cuba in 1981 resulted in 160,000 hospitalizations and heralded the arrival of DHF in the Americas (Kouri et al., 1987). Since then, dengue and DHF have become endemic throughout the tropics and subtropics (Rigau-Perez et al., 1998).

ETIOLOGY

The dengue virus is a flavivirus of the family Flaviviridae, related to the prototype yellow fever virus (Kuno et al., 1998). Within the flavivirus group, four serotypes exist in the dengue virus complex, named dengue virus types 1, 2, 3, and 4 (Calisher et al., 1989). These four dengue viruses share 78% amino acid homology (Tsarev et al., 2000), yet several genotypic variants have been identified within each serotype (Rico-Hesse, 1990). Many genotypes cluster in geographic regions, but substantial genetic heterogeneity within genotypes has also been demonstrated (Worobey et al., 1999). Genotypic diversity may have implications for disease (see the discussion on pathogenesis, later in this chapter).

The dengue virion is a 40- to 50-nm enveloped spherical particle, composed of three structures: the core, the membrane, and the envelope (Henchal and Putnak, 1990). These assemble into an outer protein shell, a lipid membrane, and a nucleocapsid enclosing a single-stranded, plus-sense RNA genome of approximately 10.7 kilobases (kb) (Kuhn et al., 2002). The virion attaches to host cells, typically cells of reticuloendothelial lineage such as monocyte/macrophages and dendritic cells (Wu et al., 2000), through receptors that include heparin-containing glycosaminoglycans (Putnak et al., 1997). Once attached, the coat fuses with the cellular membrane, enters the cytoplasm, and begins translation from the viral RNA. Eventually, transcription results in viral replication within the cytoplasm of infected cells and subsequent extracellular shedding of infectious virions (Burke and Monath, 2001). The infection may induce apoptosis in vitro (Marianneau et al., 1998; Duarte dos Santos et al., 2000).

Transmission of dengue viruses occurs directly from humans to mosquitoes to humans without an intermediate vector or amplifying host. The principal insect vectors are *Aedes* species, especially *A. aegypti*, which are widely dispersed and anthropophilic (preferentially feed on humans) and primarily feed at dusk and dawn (Rodhain and Rosen, 1997). These vectors are extremely well adapted to humans and infest small freshwater-collection areas in homes and adjacent places. While nonhuman primate-mosquito transmission cycles have been demonstrated in rural areas, they are of minor importance compared with the urban epidemic and endemic transmission of dengue (de Silva et al., 1999).

EPIDEMIOLOGY

Dengue is a threat in mosquito-infested areas throughout the tropics and subtropics and at present affects more than 2.5 billion persons. Travelers to these areas are also affected (Jelinek, 2000). Epidemic dengue may enter a susceptible population and subside rapidly, with many years between outbreaks in more remote populations. Dengue affects all age groups when the virus is first introduced into an area. Endemic dengue transmission follows after one or more circulating dengue viruses are established, with periodic cycles of increased disease. As multiple serotypes circulate (hyperendemicity), the adult population becomes immune and disease is seen primarily among children (Hay et al., 2000). However, the numbers of cases in endemic areas may be underestimated because infections often result in minor or undifferentiated febrile illnesses (see discussion of clinical manifestations later in this chapter).

The risk for DHF increases if a new dengue serotype is introduced into an area previously endemic for another serotype. DHF occurs more frequently, but not exclusively, in individuals with secondary infections with dengue virus (Innis, 1997). In Thailand, the risk of DHF as a secondary infection is estimated to be more than 100 times greater than that of DHF as a primary infection (Sangkawibha et al., 1984). DHF primarily affects school-age children (age less than 15 years) in areas where three or more dengue serotype viruses circulate simultaneously or sequentially. Infants with circulating maternal antibodies to dengue virus are also susceptible to severe primary infection (Kliks et al., 1988).

Prior exposure to dengue virus provides only a partial explanation for DHF, as DHF occurs only 1 in every 200 secondarily infected children (Halstead, 1988). No single clinical or epidemiologic factor discriminates between those predisposed to severe dengue and those who experience uncomplicated secondary dengue virus infections (Bravo et al., 1987). Clinical and epidemiologic features of DHF are not altered significantly in different ecologic locations, such as Latin America and Asia. In other areas, for example, India, the reasons for emergence of DHF are less certain, because both viruses and vectors had been present for several decades prior to emergence (Pushpa et al., 1998).

PATHOGENESIS

Dengue virus infection begins with inoculation of virus into skin and blood vessels by an infected *Aedes* mosquito. Viral entry and infection of resident dendritic cells in the skin—Langerhans cells—may occur at the site (Taweechaisupapong et al., 1996). These phagocytic cells may then relay the virus to draining lymphoid tissues, where further viral replication occurs. Secondary viremia results in onset of symptoms and seeding of secondary organs (McBride and Bielefeldt-Ohmann, 2000). This phase of viremia may be detectable for 4 to 5 days then ceases with the appearance of adaptive immune responses (Vaughn et al., 1997). No persistence of dengue virus has been defined in humans.

Host Factors in DHF

In secondary dengue, particularly in DHF, a major hypothesis has been the possibility of enhanced viral replication with waning neutralizing antibody titer (Cardosa, 2000). In vitro, the rate and intensity of infection with dengue virus may be enhanced by cross-reactive, nonneutralizing antibody (antibody-dependent enhancement) (Halstead et al., 1973). The virus binds available group-specific antibody from a previous dengue virus infection and enters the cell through Fc receptors displayed on the cell surface (Morens, 1994). This route facilitates replication of virus, particularly if the number of Fc receptors is increased by other precedent stimuli, such as gamma interferon (Kontny et al., 1988). Apparent replicative advantages may be influenced by specificities of antisera, other virus receptors, or cell maturation and differentiation state (O'Sullivan and Killen, 1994). Other host factors such as race and human leukocyte antigen (HLA) status may also affect susceptibility to DHF (Bravoet al., 1987; Chiewsilp et al., 1981). Moreover, female gender, good nutritional status (well nourished), and coexistent chronic disease such as asthma or diabetes are epidemiologic risk factors associated with increased incidence and severity of DHF (Guzman and Kouri, 2002).

Viral Factors in DHF

Primary infections may rarely lead to DHF, suggesting that a single virulent virus genotype may be sufficient to induce DHF. Presumably, this viral virulence factor would only be augmented in the presence of enhancing dengue-specific antibody in secondary infections. Dengue viruses of Southeast Asian origin, particularly dengue-2 viruses, have been associated with all DHF and dengue shock syndrome (DSS) epidemics to date (Rico-Hesse et al., 1997; Leitmeyer et al., 1999). Conversely, dengue-2 viruses originating from the Americas have not induced DHF, despite the occurrence of a dengue-1 epidemic in Peru (Watts et al., 1999).

Immune Activation in DHF

Early activation of cells of the immune system is apparent in dengue (Green et al., 1999a). This activation reflects direct and indirect (bystander) effects of the virus following infection of monocyte/macrophages, dendritic cells, lymphocytes, and other cells. Elevated levels of potent cytokines, including tumor necrosis factor-a (TNF-a), interleukin-1ß (IL-1ß), and γ-interferon, are found in individuals with dengue (Kurane and Ennis, 1994) and are generally associated with increasing severity of disease (Bethell et al., 1998). TNF-a and IL-1ß and their receptors are mediators produced by altered virus-monocyte interactions, reflecting their sustained stimulation in DHF (Hober et al., 1998; Green et al., 1999b). Furthermore, other inflammatory molecules, such as the chemokine interleukin-8 and α- and β-interferons, are also elevated in the acute phase of the disease (Raghupathy et al., 1998; Kurane et al., 1993).

The endothelium is the target of the immunopathologic mechanisms in DHF and where the hallmark vascular permeability and coagulation disorders originate. Various inflammatory molecules such as histamine, C3a, or leukotrienes have been sought as inducers of vascular permeability in DHF, yet the final common mediators of endothelial leakage are largely unknown. Final integration of pathogenetic mechanisms in DHF will involve multiple cell and tissue interactions with dengue virus, based on better understanding of differences in kinetics of replication of virus, immunologic response of cell to virus entry, or both.

PATHOLOGY

The pathology of dengue fever is limited by the benign nature of the acute disease. Evaluation of skin rash in dengue reveals no specific inflammation or dengue viral antigens around vessels (de Andino et al., 1985), but activated dendritic cells have been demonstrated (Wu et al., 2000). In DHF and DSS, the liver, the reticuloendothelial system, and the vascular system are affected, with focal hyaline necrosis of hepatocytes and Kupffer's cells, expansion of lymphocyte mass with increased circulating atypical forms, and vasculopathy as evidenced by increased capillary fragility and coagulopathy (Bhamarapravati et al., 1967). The presence of hemorrhage with an absence of overt inflammation or tissue injury is most striking and suggests the action of biologic mediators in the pathogenesis of DHF (Rothman and Ennis, 1999). Active proliferation and lymphocytolysis of germinal centers in lymph nodes and spleen are also seen (Aung-Khin et al., 1975). Dengue antigen has been detected by use of immunofluorescence within tissue macrophages in affected target organs (liver, spleen, kidney, and skin). Skin biopsies have shown infiltration of capillary vessel walls with mononuclear cells, and deposits of IgM, complement, and fibrinogen. Perivascular edema and endothelial cell swelling accompany these peripheral vascular changes (Bhamarapravati, 1997).

CLINICAL MANIFESTATIONS

The spectrum of dengue disease ranges from subclinical infection to shock (Figure 5-1). Most infections are asymptomatic or result in minor febrile illnesses (Burke et al., 1988). This may be particularly true for dengue virus serotypes 2 and 4 (Vaughn, 2000). Symptomatic infections commonly produce an acute febrile syndrome, termed *dengue fever*, which may be incapacitating but is rarely fatal. However, in uncommon severe DHF infections, presenting symptoms may include vascular leakage and hemorrhage; such infections rarely progresses to DSS.

Symptoms of dengue fever typically develop after an incubation period of 7 days, with a range of 3 to 15 days following the bite from an infected mosquito. The illness may have a mild prodrome but classically begins with sudden onset of high fevers to 39° to 41° C (102° to 105° F), headache, myalgia, and prostration. Children with dengue are more likely than children with other febrile illnesses to report gastrointestinal symptoms of anorexia, nausea, and vomiting (Kalayanarooj et al., 1997). When present, retroorbital pain, arthralgias, and myalgia may prove helpful in the differential diagnosis but are not pathognomonic features for arboviral illness. Facial flushing with conjunctival injection, generalized macular or maculopapular rash, and lymphadenopathy are present in 20% to 50% of patients after onset of fever (Figure 5-2) (Teeraratkul et al., 1990; Trofa et al., 1997). Symptoms and signs, with the exception of rash, may be more frequent in children with secondary dengue (Cobra et al., 1995). A tourniquet test (inflate blood pressure cuff to a point midway between systolic and diastolic blood pressures, maintain for 5 minutes, then count the number of petechiae that appear in a 2.5-cm diameter area on the skin distal to the cuff) may be helpful; more than 20 petechiae indicate vascular injury. Results of the tourniquet test are posi-

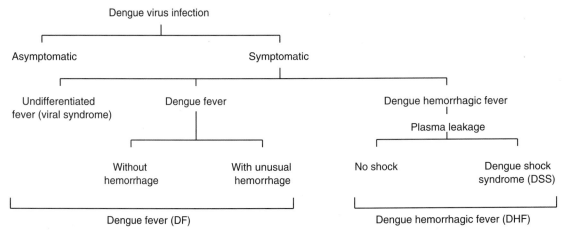

Fig. 5-1 The spectrum of dengue illness. Dengue may occur as an asymptomatic infection, an undifferentiated febrile illness, classical dengue fever, or dengue hemorrhagic fever (DHF). The latter two conditions may have hemorrhagic manifestations as presenting symptoms; however, only DHF has clinical evidence of plasma leakage including hemoconcentration (rise in hematocrit >20%) accompanied by thrombocytopenia (platelet count <100,000/mm³). (Modified from World Health Organization: Dengue Haemorrhagic Fever: Diagnosis, Treatment, Prevention and Control, ed 2. Geneva: World Health Organization, 1997.)

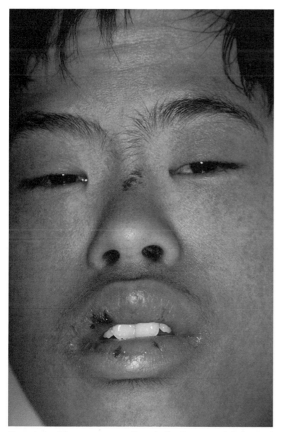

Fig. 5-2 Characteristic facial flushing and bilateral bulbar conjunctivitis are present in this child with dengue fever. Malaise and redness and cracking of lips are also apparent. Note ecchymoses over bridge of nose and on upper lip, which may accompany uncomplicated dengue infection. (Photograph courtesy Dr. Siripen Kalayanarooj, Queen Sirikit Institute for Child Health, Bangkok, Thailand.)

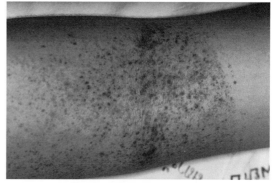

Fig. 5-3 Marked petechial reaction over dorsal surface of forearm after tourniquet test. While indicative of capillary fragility, this finding is not specific for dengue virus infection and can not be used to differentiate between dengue fever and DHF. Positive test results in a child with fever and other signs of bleeding should prompt further evaluation for dengue. (Photograph courtesy Dr. Siripen Kalayanarooj, Queen Sirikit Institute for Child Health, Bangkok, Thailand.)

tive in 83% of children with dengue, but this is a nonspecific finding (Kalayanarooj et al., 1997) (Figure 5-3). Depression of total white blood cell counts, with neutropenia (<1.5 × 106/mm³) and monocytopenia, is a characteristic finding in dengue, with a rapid rebound to normal levels after cessation of fever (Simmons et al., 1931). Plasma alanine and aspartate (AST) aminotransferase levels are higher in children with dengue than in children with other febrile illnesses, and plasma AST levels are higher still in children who develop DHF than in those with DF (Kalayanarooj et al., 1997). Typically, there is a rapid resolution of symptoms after defervescence, which occurs on approximately the third to fifth day of illness. In adults, malaise and fatigue may persist for many weeks after recovery.

The clinical presentation of DHF is indistinguishable from dengue fever during the acute febrile phase (Monath, 1997). DHF is a reversible systemic capillary leakage syndrome that typically develops upon defervescence; paradoxically, the presence of hemorrhagic manifestations is not essential to the disease. Prodromal symptoms are often vague and may consist of nausea and abdominal pain accompanied by pallor and clammy skin. Clinical diagnosis of DHF requires the presence of a rising hematocrit and thrombocytopenia, reflecting the interstitial leakage of plasma and consumption of platelets that are characteristic of the disease (Figure 5-4). The World Health Organization has published the diagnostic criteria for DHF, based on hemoconcentration (change in hematocrit >20%) or other evidence of plasma leakage (pleural effusion or ascites) and platelet count <100,000/mm³ (WHO criteria, 1997) (Figure 5-5). Gallbladder-wall thickening is commonly found by radiographic studies in children with evidence of vascular leakage (Setiawan et al., 1998). Increasing severity of plasma leakage in DHF may result in relative bradycardia, narrowing of pulse pressure (grade III DHF), hypotension (blood pressure below 90/60), and rarely progression to severe shock (grade IV DHF) if decreased plasma volume is not adequately replenished. Hepatomegaly and diffuse abdominal

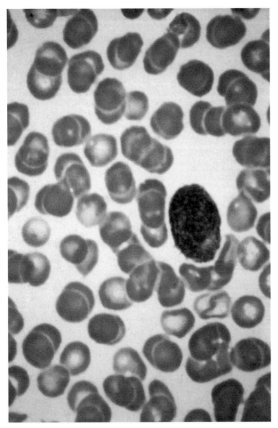

Fig. 5-4 Hematologic picture consistent with DHF reveals marked absence of platelets and paucity of white blood cells, with an atypical lymphocyte present in the field. The red blood cells are normal and there are no intracellular malarial parasites. (Photograph courtesy Dr. Siripen Kalayanarooj, Queen Sirikit Institute for Child Health, Bangkok, Thailand.)

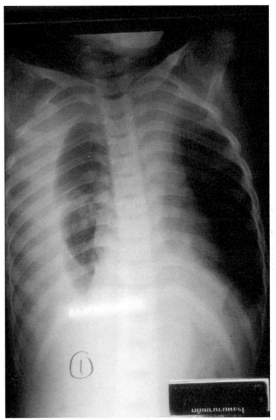

Fig. 5-5 This radiograph shows a significant right pleural effusion in a child with dengue hemorrhagic fever. The presence and volume of pleural fluid are positively correlated with increasing severity of disease. Mild hepatomegaly is also present. (Photograph courtesy Dr. Siripen Kalayanarooj, Queen Sirikit Institute for Child Health, Bangkok, Thailand.)

tenderness without guarding may be found in children with DHF (Nimmannitya, 1987). Increased vascular permeability in DHF is apparent in detectable petechiae or purpura, and through the results of the tourniquet test (Cao et al., 2002) (see Figure 5-3).

Bleeding may be present in children with dengue fever and DHF. Studies have consistently revealed a marked reduction of complement, particularly C3, in individuals with DHF; levels decrease progressively with increasing severity of infection (Bokisch et al., 1973). Other hematologic phenomena have been correlated with the decline in C3, including fibrinogen and platelet levels (World Health Organization, 1973). Complement is activated by both the classical (antigen-antibody) and alternate pathways. There is a mixed picture of concurrent fibrinolysis and coagulation in patients with DHF (Krishnamurti et al., 2001). Disseminated intravascular coagulation has been reported but is an uncommon event. The coagulation and fibrinolytic pathways may be disrupted by immune mechanisms that affect endothelial and platelet function or may be modified by activities expressed by infected cells. The actual mechanism(s) are not known.

Unusual manifestations of dengue include neurologic and hepatitis syndromes. Encephalitis due to dengue has been increasingly reported as an uncommon outcome of infection (Kankirawatana et al., 2000; Solomon et al., 2000). Prognosis for recovery is generally good except in children with concomitant DHF, where direct central nervous system invasion may occur (Cam et al., 2001). Febrile convulsions are sometimes associated with dengue (Familusi et al., 1972). Mild hepatic dysfunction has been recognized in up to 80% of individuals with dengue and is more frequent in children with DHF (Kalayanarooj et al., 1997; Mohan et al., 2000). The disease is uncommonly fulminant (Innis et al., 1990; Lum et al., 1993) and may be associated with encephalopathy or a Reye's-like syndrome (Sinniah et al., 1990). Although rare vertical transmission of dengue virus has been documented (Thaithumyanon et al., 1994), there is no evidence of fetal malformation.

DIAGNOSIS
Differential Diagnosis

Dengue should be suspected in an individual with fever after entry into an endemic area or after return from the tropics. The diagnosis of malaria should be ruled out with a minimum of three blood smears. Other causes of fever with typical exanthem (prominent maculopapular, blanching rash over trunk and extremities, sparing palms and soles) may be considered in the pediatric population, such as measles (Dietz et al., 1992); rubella (Bustos et al., 1990); Kawasaki disease, leptospirosis (Ko et al., 1999); and Mayaro virus disease and chikungunya (alphavirus illnesses found in the Americas and Asia, respectively) (Pinheiro et al., 1981; Halstead et al., 1969). Measles may be differentiated by the presence of coryza, respiratory symptoms, Koplik's spots, and discrete rash from face to trunk; rubella may include postauricular lymph nodes. For suspected DHF in children and adolescents, the diagnosis of meningococcal fever, with abrupt onset of painful, palpable purpura and shock, should be excluded. Other hemorrhagic fever viruses, such as yellow fever, must be kept in mind (Monath, 1999). In semirural environments, rickettsial or other bacterial fevers whose presenting symptoms include vesicular or petechial rashes including the palms and soles should be considered when appropriate.

Laboratory Diagnosis

Confirmation of dengue virus infection is achieved through isolation of virus from blood or sera, demonstration of dengue-specific IgM antibody in serum, or a fourfold rise in dengue-specific antibody titers. Recently, reverse transcriptase polymerase chain reaction has been used to identify dengue RNA in clinical specimens (Harris et al., 1998; Houng et al., 2001). Cross-reactive antibodies may complicate serologic diagnosis using the hemagglutination-inhibiting or enzyme linked immunosorbent antibody assays, particularly in areas where two or more flaviviruses may circulate (Cuzzubbo et al., 1999; Groen et al., 2000; Innis et al., 1989; Vaughn et al., 1999). Infectious virus is best isolated from sera collected from febrile individuals, whereas antibodies are typically detected in specimens obtained after defervescence.

IMMUNITY

In uncomplicated primary dengue virus infection, viremia ceases as IgM antibody appears, with cessation of fever by the fifth day of illness (Vaughn et al., 1997). In general, the most severe symptoms occur as the immune response clears extracellular and intracellular virus from the blood and tissues. The virus envelope glycoprotein is the major target of humoral immunity, resulting in development of hemagglutinin-inhibiting, neutralizing and other antibodies that protect in vivo (Chang, 1997). Maternal transfer of these antibodies is believed to protect infants against dengue disease in the first 6 months of life; DHF appears in some infants with waning of titers (Kliks et al., 1988). Circulating viral antigens (envelope protein and nonstructural 1 protein), antibodies, and their immune complexes are increased in the sera of individuals with dengue (Young et al., 2000). As with other viral infections, cell-mediated immunity may have a role in clearance of infection. Both CD4+ and CD8+ T cells are activated during dengue illness and stimulated to proliferate to virus antigens (Kurane et al., 1991). More refined analysis of T-cell clones reveals that CD4 and CD8 populations are stimulated to specific dengue viral epitopes, but CD8 cells may possess cytotoxic activity correlated with more broadly cross-reactive responses (Bukowski, 1989).

Protection against infection correlates with the appearance of type-specific neutralizing antibody. Infection with one dengue virus serotype protects against reinfection with the same serotype (homotypic immunity) but does not confer long-lasting protection against infection with other serotypes (heterotypic immunity) (Sabin, 1952). Hence, infection with two or more serotypes is possible, even simultaneously (Kanesa-thasan et al., 1994). Secondary infection with dengue virus occasionally provokes a strong anamnestic immune response to the infecting virus, and prospective studies identify truncated duration of viremia in the presence of these antibody responses (Vaughn et al., 2000). In DHF, the equation may be more complex, with maximal peak viremia titers along with dysregulated immune responses responsible for much of the pathophysiology of severe dengue (Rothman and Ennis, 1999). These disrupted responses are apparent in differential patterns of antibody, T-cell, and cytokine responses (Koraka et al., 2001; Loke et al., 2001; Chaturvedi et al., 2000).

TREATMENT

Dengue is usually a self-limited, nonfatal illness. There is no specific treatment, and only supportive treatment with bed rest, fluids, and administration of analgesic and antiinflammatory agents is required until symptoms resolve. Use of aspirin or other compounds that may interfere with coagulation is discouraged. The key to management is recognition of the syndrome of dengue fever with fever, headache, and myalgias, since diagnostic confirmation is usually unavailable at time of treatment. Patients with suspected dengue should be shielded from mosquitoes, and precautions should be used with body fluids. Outpatient management is adequate for most dengue patients (Chin, 1993). All cases of dengue should be reported.

Consider DHF or other hemorrhagic fevers in the dengue patient who does not improve or has clinical deterioration (decreasing blood pressure, bleeding) with symptomatic treatment (Chin, 1993). Patients with suspected DHF require aggressive monitoring of vital signs and fluid support (Figure 5-6). Either colloids or crystalline fluids may be used for resuscitation (Ngo et al., 2001); this simple treatment used judiciously and without fluid overload decreases mortality with DHF. There is no indication for the use of steroids in dengue (Sumarmo et al., 1982; Tassniyom et al., 1993). Consult intensive care experts for all DHF patients, as they may require substantial medical monitoring and support.

PREVENTION AND CONTROL

Avoidance of exposure to infectious mosquitoes is achieved by screening windows and doors, using bed nets, and wearing protective clothing such as long-sleeved shirts. The use of insect repellents is strongly recommended as a measure of personal protection against insect bites. Containers that hold small freshwater pools, such as plant pots or cisterns, are potential breeding sites for *Aedes* mosquitoes and should be removed from households if possible. *Aedes* vectors are difficult to eradicate using volume spraying with insecticides because of their propensity to dwell indoors.

Most effective strategies for dengue control incorporate community education and participation to identify and eliminate common breeding sites in conjunction with vector control plans (Gubler and Clark, 1994).

Dengue vaccines have been pursued for many decades but have proved difficult to achieve (Kanesa-thasan, 1998). Although humans are the principal mammalian host for dengue viruses and infection induces apparently lifelong monotypic immunity, the presence of four dengue serotypes and antibody-dependent enhancement complicates the development of vaccines (Cardosa, 1998). The objectives for dengue vaccines have been the prevention of infection and protection against disease, with the goal of a tetravalent vaccine to decrease the possibility of immune potentiation of disease (Chambers et al., 1997). Selection of vaccine candidates has been hindered by the lack of an animal model of disease, which has prevented a full understanding of molecular pathogenic or attenuating properties of the virus and correlates of long-term natural immunity. Most vaccine strategies have focused on the envelope protein as the target of protective antibody response. Development of dengue vaccines is in its infancy, yet three major classes of dengue vaccines show promise: replicating vaccines, including live-attenuated viruses and infectious complementary DNA (cDNA); vectored replicating vaccines using yellow fever virus or other viral vectors; and nonreplicating vaccines, such as inactivated viruses, recombinant or subunit vaccines, and nucleic acid vaccines (Bhamarapravati and Yoksan, 1997). In the future, dengue vaccines may be administered in childhood in regions with early and intense exposure to dengue and other flaviviruses. Future issues include the possibility of viral interference and blocking of replicating vaccines by maternal antibodies.

Dengue Treatment Algorithm

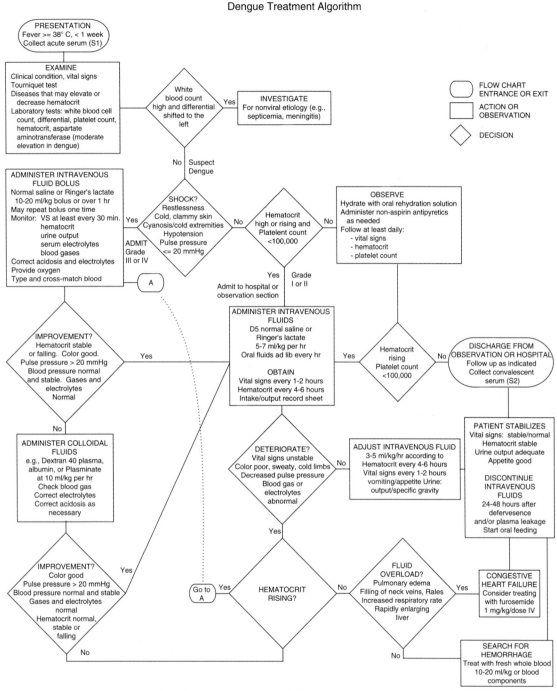

Fig. 5-6 Algorithm for the treatment of dengue. Patients suspected of having dengue should have their blood pressure and pulse monitored carefully during the later febrile phase (third or fourth day of fever). In clinically suspected DHF, serial hematocrits during the period of defervescence may show a >10% rise as a result of vascular leakage. In case of dropping blood pressure, narrowing pulse pressure, or rising hematocrit, a bolus of fluid should restore vital signs to normal. Fluids should be used to restore volume deficits only, as extravascular fluid resolves spontaneously within 1 to 2 days. (Modified from Vaughn DW, Green S (eds). Dengue and dengue hemorrhagic fever. In Strickland, GT (ed): Hunter's Textbook of Tropical Medicine and Emerging Infectious Diseases, ed 8. Philadelphia: WB Saunders, 2000.)

BIBLIOGRAPHY

Ashburn PM, Craig CF. Experimental investigations regarding the etiology of dengue fever. J Infect Dis 1907;4:440-475.

Aung-Khin M, Ma-Ma K, Thant Z. Changes in the tissues of the immune system in dengue haemorrhagic fever. J Trop Med Hyg 1975;78:256-261.

Bethell DB, Flobbe K, Cao XT, et al. Pathophysiologic and prognostic role of cytokines in dengue hemorrhagic fever. J Infect Dis 1998;177:778-782.

Bhamarapravati N. Pathology of dengue infections. In Gubler DA, Kuno G (eds). Dengue and Dengue Hemorrhagic Fever. New York: CAB International, 1997.

Bhamarapravati N, Tuchinda P, Boonyapaknavik V. Pathology of Thailand haemorrhagic fever: a study of 100 autopsy cases. Ann Trop Med Parasitol 1967;61:500-510.

Bhamarapravati N, Yoksan S. Live attenuated tetravalent dengue vaccine. In Gubler DA, Kuno G (eds). Dengue and Dengue Hemorrhagic Fever. New York: CAB International, 1997.

Bokisch VA, Top FH Jr, Russell PK, et al. The potential pathogenic role of complement in dengue hemorrhagic shock syndrome. N Engl J Med 1973;289:996-1000.

Bravo JR, Guzman MG, Kouri GP. Why dengue haemorrhagic fever in Cuba? 1. Individual risk factors for dengue haemorrhagic fever/dengue shock syndrome (DHF/DSS). Trans R Soc Trop Med Hyg;81:816-820.

Bukowski JF, Kurane I, Lai CJ, et al. Dengue virus-specific cross reactive CD8+ human cytotoxic T lymphocytes. J Virol 1989;13:5086-5091.

Burke DS, Monath TP. Flaviviruses. In Knipe DM, Mowley PM (eds). Fields Virology, ed 4. Philadelphia: Lippincott Williams & Wilkins, 2001.

Burke DS, Nisalak A, Johnson DE, Scott RM. A prospective study of dengue infections in Bangkok. Am J Trop Med Hyg 1988;38:172-180.

Bustos J, Hamdan A, Lorono MA, et al. Serologically proven acute rubella infection in patients with clinical diagnosis of dengue. Epidemiol Infect 1990;104:297-302.

Calisher CH, Karabatsos N, Dalrymple JM, et al. Antigenic relationships between flaviviruses as determined by cross-neutralization tests with polyclonal antisera. J Gen Virol 1989;70:37-43.

Cam BV, Fonsmark L, Hue NB, et al. Prospective case-control study of encephalopathy in children with dengue hemorrhagic fever. Am J Trop Med Hyg 2001;65:848-851.

Cao XT, Ngo TN, Wills B, et al. Evaluation of the World Health Organization standard tourniquet test and a modified tourniquet test in the diagnosis of dengue infection in Viet Nam. Trop Med Int Health 2002;7:125-132.

Cardosa MJ. Dengue vaccine design: issues and challenges. Br Med Bull 1998;54:395-405.

Cardosa MJ. Dengue haemorrhagic fever: questions of pathogenesis. Curr Opin Infect Dis 2000;13:471-475.

Centers for Disease Control and Prevention. Underdiagnosis of dengue—Laredo, Texas, 1999. JAMA 2001;285:877.

Chambers TJ, Tsai TF, Pervikov Y, Monath TP. Vaccine development against dengue and Japanese encephalitis: report of a World Health Organization meeting. Vaccine 1997;15:1494-1502.

Chang GJ. Molecular biology of dengue viruses. In Gubler DJ, Kuno G (eds). Dengue and Dengue Hemorrhagic Fever. New York: CAB International, 1997.

Chaturvedi UC, Agarwal R, Elbishbishi EA, Mustafa AS. Cytokine cascade in dengue hemorrhagic fever: implications for pathogenesis. FEMS Immunol Med Microbiol 2000;28:183-188.

Chiewsilp P, Scott RM, Bhamarapravati N. Histocompatibility antigens and dengue hemorrhagic fever. Am J Trop Med Hyg 1981;30:1100-1105.

Chin CK. Outpatient management of dengue infection in the University Hospital, Kuala Lumpur. Malays J Pathol 1993;15: 21-23.

Cobra C, Rigau-Perez JG, Kuno G, Vorndam V. Symptoms of dengue fever in relation to host immunologic response and virus serotype, Puerto Rico, 1990-1991. Am J Epidemiol 1995;142:1204-1211.

Cuzzubbo AJ, Vaughn DW, Nisalak A, et al. Comparison of PanBio dengue duo enzyme-linked immunosorbent assay (ELISA) and MRL dengue fever virus immunoglobulin M capture ELISA for diagnosis of dengue virus infections in southeast Asia. Clin Diagn Lab Immunol 1999;6:705-712.

de Andino RM, Botet MV, Gubler DJ, et al. The absence of dengue virus in the skin lesions of dengue fever. Int J Dermatol 1985;24:48-51.

de Silva AM, Dittus WP, Amerasinghe PH, Amerasinghe FP. Serologic evidence for an epizootic dengue virus infecting toque macaques (Macaca sinica) at Polonnaruwa, Sri Lanka. Am J Trop Med Hyg 1999;60:300-306.

Dietz VJ, Nieburg P, Gubler DJ, Gomez I. Diagnosis of measles by clinical case definition in dengue-endemic areas: implications for measles surveillance and control. Bull World Health Organ 1992:70;745-750.

Duarte dos Santos CN, Frenkiel MP, Courageot MP, et al. Determinants in the envelope E protein and viral RNA helicase NS3 that influence the induction of apoptosis in response to infection with dengue type 1 virus. Virology 2000;274:292-308.

Familusi JB, Moore DL, Fomufod AK, Causey OR. Virus isolates from children with febrile convulsions in Nigeria. A correlation study of clinical and laboratory observations. Clin Pediatr (Phila) 1972;11:272-276.

Green S, Pichyangkul S, Vaughn DW, et al. Early CD69 expression on peripheral blood lymphocytes from children with dengue hemorrhagic fever. J Infect Dis 1999a;180:1429-1435.

Green S, Vaughn DW, Kalayanarooj S, et al. Early immune activation in acute dengue illness is related to development of plasma leakage and disease severity. J Infect Dis 1999b;179:755-762.

Groen J, Koraka P, Velzing J, et al. Evaluation of six immunoassays for detection of dengue virus-specific immunoglobulin M and G antibodies. Clin Diagn Lab Immunol 2000;7:867-871.

Gubler DJ, Clark GG. Community-based integrated control of Aedes aegypti: a brief overview of current programs. Am J Trop Med Hyg 1994;50:50-60.

Gubler DJ, Meltzer M. Impact of dengue/dengue hemorrhagic fever on the developing world. Adv Virus Res 1999;53:35-70.

Guzman MG, Kouri G. Dengue: an update. Lancet Infect Dis 2002;2:33-42.

Halstead SB. Mosquito-borne haemorrhagic fevers of South and South-East Asia. Bull World Health Org 1966;35:3-15.

Halstead SB. Pathogenesis of dengue: challenges to molecular biology. Science 1988;239:476-481.

Halstead SB, Chow J, Marchette NJ. Immunologic enhancement of dengue virus replication. Nature New Biology 1973;243:24-26.

Halstead SB, Udomsakdi S, Singharaj P, Nisalak A. Dengue and chikungunya virus infection in man in Thailand, 1962-1964. III. Clinical, epidemiologic, and virologic observations on disease in non-indigenous white persons. Am J Trop Med Hyg 1969;18:984-996.

Hammon WM, Rudnick A, Sather GE. Viruses associated with epidemic hemorrhagic fevers of the Philippines and Thailand. Science 1960;131:1102-1103.

Harris E, Roberts TG, Smith L, et al. Typing of dengue viruses in clinical specimens and mosquitoes by single-tube multiplex reverse transcriptase PCR. J Clin Microbiol 1998;36:2634-2639.

Hay SI, Myers MF, Burke DS, et al. Etiology of interepidemic periods of mosquito-borne disease. Proc Natl Acad Sci USA 2000;97:9335-9339.

Henchal EA, Putnak JR. The dengue viruses. Clin Microbiol Rev 1990;3:376-396.

Hober D, Nguyen TL, Shen L, et al. Tumor necrosis factor alpha levels in plasma and whole-blood culture in dengue-infected patients: relationship between virus detection and pre-existing specific antibodies. J Med Virol 1998;54:210-218.

Hotta S. In Sanders M (ed). Dengue and Related Hemorrhagic Diseases. St Louis, Mo: Warren H. Green, 1969.

Houng HH, Chung-Ming Chen R, Vaughn DW, Kanesa-thasan N. Development of a fluorogenic RT-PCR system for quantitative identification of dengue virus serotypes 1-4 using conserved and serotype-specific 3' noncoding sequences. J Virol Methods 2001;95:19-32.

Innis BL. Dengue and dengue hemorrhagic fever. In Porterfield JS (ed). Kass Handbook of Infectious Diseases: Exotic Virus Infections, ed 1. London: Chapman & Hall Medical, 1995.

Innis BL. Antibody responses to dengue virus infection. In Gubler DJ, Kuno G (eds). Dengue and Dengue Hemorrhagic Fever. New York: CAB International, 1997.

Innis BL, Myint KSA, Nisalak A, et al. Acute liver failure is one important cause of fetal dengue infection. Southeast Asian J Trop Med Public Health. 1990;31:695-696.

Innis BL, Nisalak A, Nimmannitya S, et al. An enzyme-linked immunosorbent assay to characterize dengue infections where dengue and Japanese encephalitis co-circulate. Am J Trop Med Hyg 1989;40:418-427.

Jelinek T. Dengue fever in international travelers. Clin Infect Dis 2000;31:144-147.

Kalayanarooj S, Vaughn DW, Nimmannitya S, et al. Early clinical and laboratory indicators of acute dengue illness. J Infect Dis 1997;176:313-321.

Kanesa-thasan N. Development of dengue vaccines: an overview. Indian Pediatr 1998;35:97-100.

Kanesa-thasan N, Iacono Connors L, Magill A, et al. Dengue serotypes 2 and 3 in U.S. forces in Somalia. Lancet 1994;343:678.

Kankirawatana P, Chokephaibulkit K, Puthavathana P, et al. Dengue infection presenting with central nervous system manifestation. J Child Neurol 2000;15:544-547.

Kliks SC, Nimmannitya S, Nisalak A, Burke DS. Evidence that maternal dengue antibodies are important in the development of dengue hemorrhagic fever in infants. Am J Trop Med Hyg 1988;38:411-419.

Ko AI, Galvao Reis M, Ribeiro Dourado CM, et al. Urban epidemic of severe leptospirosis in Brazil. Salvador Leptospirosis Study Group. Lancet 1999;354:820-825.

Kontny U, Kurane I, Ennis FA. Gamma interferon augments Fc gamma receptor-mediated dengue virus infection of human monocytic cells. J Virol 1988;62:3928-3933.

Koraka P, Suharti C, Setiati TE, et al. Kinetics of dengue virus-specific serum immunoglobulin classes and subclasses correlate with clinical outcome of infection. J Clin Microbiol 2001;39:4332-4338.

Kouri GP, Guzman MG, Bravo JR. Why dengue haemorrhagic fever in Cuba? 2. An integral analysis. Trans R Soc Trop Med Hyg 1987;81:821-823.

Krishnamurti C, Kalayanarooj S, Cutting MA, et al. Mechanisms of hemorrhage in dengue without circulatory collapse. Am J Trop Med Hyg 2001;65:840-847.

Kuhn RJ, Zhang W, Rossmann MG, et al. Structure of dengue virus. Implications for flavivirus organization, maturation, and fusion. Cell 2002;108:717-725.

Kuno G, Chang GJ, Tsuchiya KR, et al. Phylogeny of the genus Flavivirus. J Virol 1998;72:73-83.

Kurane I, Ennis FA. Cytokines in dengue virus infections: role of cytokines in the pathogenesis of dengue hemorrhagic fever. Semin Virol 1994;5:443-448.

Kurane I., Innis BL, Nimmannitya S, et al. Activation of T lymphocytes in dengue virus infections. High levels of soluble interleukin 2 receptor, soluble CD4, soluble CD8, interleukin 2, and interferon-gamma in sera of children with dengue. J Clin Invest 1991;88:1473-1480.

Kurane I, Innis BL, Nimmannitya S, et al. High levels of interferon-alpha in the sera of children with dengue virus infection. Am J Trop Med Hyg 1993;48:222-229.

Leitmeyer KC, Vaughn DW, Watts DM, et al. Dengue virus structural differences that correlate with pathogenesis. J Virol 1999;73: 4738-4747.

Loke H, Bethell DB, Phuong CX, et al. Strong HLA class I–restricted T cell responses in dengue hemorrhagic fever: a double-edged sword? J Infect Dis 2001;184:1369-1373.

Lum LC, Lam SK, George R, Devi S. Fulminant hepatitis in dengue infection. Southeast Asian J Trop Med Public Health 1993;24:467-471.

Marianneau P, Flamand M, Deubel V, Despres P. Apoptotic cell death in response to dengue virus infection: the pathogenesis of dengue haemorrhagic fever revisited. Clin Diagn Virol 1998;10:113-119.

McBride WJ, Bielefeldt-Ohmann H. Dengue viral infections; pathogenesis and epidemiology. Microbes Infect 2000;2:1041-1050.

Mohan B, Patwari AK, Anand VK. Hepatic dysfunction in childhood dengue infection. J Trop Pediatr 2000;46:40-43.

Monath TP. Dengue: the risk to developed and developing countries. Proc Natl Acad Sci USA 1994;91:2395-2400.

Monath TP. Early indicators in acute dengue infection. Lancet 1997;350:1719-1720.

Monath TP. Facing up to re-emergence of urban yellow fever. Lancet 1999;353:1541.

Morens DM. Antibody-dependent enhancement of infection and the pathogenesis of viral disease. Clin Infect Dis 1994;19:500-512.

Ngo NT, Cao XT, Kneen R, et al. Acute management of dengue shock syndrome: a randomized double-blind comparison of 4 intravenous fluid regimens in the first hour. Clin Infect Dis 2001;32:204-213.

Nimmannitya S. Clinical spectrum and management of dengue haemorrhagic fever. Southeast Asian J Trop Med Public Health 1987;18:392-397.

O'Sullivan MA, Killen HM. The differentiation state of monocytic cells affects their susceptibility to infection and the effects of infection by dengue virus. J Gen Virol 1994;75:2387-2392.

Pinheiro FP, Freitas RB, Travassos da Rosa JF, et al. An outbreak of Mayaro virus disease in Belterra, Brazil. I. Clinical and virological findings. Am J Trop Med Hyg 1981;30:674-681.

Pushpa V, Venkatadesikalu M, Mohan S, et al. An epidemic of dengue haemorrhagic fever/dengue shock syndrome in tropical India. Ann Trop Paediatr 1998;18:289-293.

Putnak JR, Kanesa-Thasan N, Innis BL. A putative cellular receptor for dengue viruses. Nat Med 1997;3:828-829.

Raghupathy R, Chaturvedi UC, Al-Sayer H, et al. Elevated levels of IL-8 in dengue hemorrhagic fever. J Med Virol 1998;56:280-285.

Rico-Hesse R. Molecular evolution and distribution of dengue viruses type 1 and 2 in nature. Virology 1990;174:479-493.

Rico-Hesse R, Harrison LM, Salas RA, et al. Origins of dengue type 2 viruses associated with increased pathogenicity in the Americas. Virology 1997;230:244-251.

Rigau-Perez JG, Clark GG, Gubler DJ, et al. Dengue and dengue haemorrhagic fever. Lancet 1998;352:971-977.

Rodhain F, Rosen L. Mosquito vectors and dengue virus-vector relationships. In Gubler DJ, Kuno G (eds). Dengue and Dengue Hemorrhagic Fever. New York: CAB International, 1997.

Rothman AL, Ennis FA. Immunopathogenesis of dengue hemorrhagic fever. Virology 1999;257:1-6.

Rush B. An account of the bilious remitting fever, as it appeared in Philadelphia, in the summer and autumn of the year 1780. Philadelphia: Prichard and Hall, 1789.

Sabin AB. Research on dengue during World War II. Am J Trop Med Hyg 1952;1:30-50.

Sabin AB. Recent advances in our knowledge of dengue and sandfly fever. Am J Trop Med Hyg 1955;4:198-207.

Sabin AB, Schlesinge, RW. Production of immunity to dengue with virus modified by propagation in mice. Science 1945;101:640-642.

Sangkawibha N, Rojanasuphot S, Ahandrik S, et al. Risk factors in dengue shock syndrome: a prospective epidemiologic study in Rayong, Thailand. I. The 1980 outbreak. Am J Epidemiol 1984;120:653-669.

Setiawan MW, Samsi TK, Wulur H. et al. Dengue haemorrhagic fever: ultrasound as an aid to predict the severity of the disease. Pediatr Radiol 1998;28:1-4.

Siler JF, Hall MW, Hitchens AP. Dengue: its history, epidemiology, mechanism of transmission, etiology, clinical manifestations, immunity, and prevention. Philippine J Sci 1926;29:1-304.

Simmons JS, St John JH, Holt JR, Reynolds FHK. The possible transfer of dengue virus from infected to normal mosquitoes during copulation. Am J Trop Med 1931;11:199-216.

Simmons JS, St John JH, Reynolds FHK. Experimental studies of dengue. Philippine J Sci 1931;44:1-252.

Sinniah D, Sinniah R, Yap YF, et al. Reye and Reye-like syndromes: results of a pilot study in Peninsular Malaya, 1986. Acta Paediatr Jpn 1990;32:385-390.

Solomon T, Dung NM, Vaughn DW, et al. Neurological manifestations of dengue infection. Lancet 2000;355:1053-1059.

Sumarmo, Talogo W, Asrin A, et al. Failure of hydrocortisone to affect outcome in dengue shock syndrome. Pediatrics 1982;89:48-49.

Tassniyom S, Vasanawathana S, Chirawatkul A, Rojanasuphot S. Failure of high-dose methylprednisolone in established dengue shock syndrome: a placebo-controlled, double-blind study. Pediatrics 1993;92:111-115.

Taweechaisupapong S, Sriurairatana S, Angsubhakorn S, et al. Langerhans cell density and serological changes following intradermal immunisation of mice with dengue 2 virus. J Med Microbiol 1996;45:138-145.

Teeraratkul A, Limpakarnjanaral K, Nisalek A, Nimmannitya S. Predictive value of clinical and laboratory findings for early diagnosis of dengue and dengue hemorrhagic fever. Southeast Asian J Trop Public Health 1990;21:696-697.

Thaithumyanon P, Thisyakorn U, Deerojnawong J, Innis BL Dengue infection complicated by severe hemorrhage and vertical transmission in a parturient woman. Clin Infect Dis; 1994;18:248-249.

Trofa AF, DeFraites RF, Smoak BL, et al. Dengue fever in U.S. military personnel in Haiti. JAMA 1997; 277:1546-1548.

Tsarev SA, Sanders ML, Vaughn DW, Innis BL. Phylogenetic analysis suggests only one serotype of Japanese encephalitis virus. Vaccine 2000;18(suppl 2):36-43.

Vaughn DW. Invited commentary: dengue lessons from Cuba. Am J Epidemiol 2000;152:800-803.

Vaughn DW, Green S. Dengue and dengue hemorrhagic fever. In Strickland GT (ed). Hunter's Textbook of Tropical Medicine and Emerging Infectious Diseases, ed 8. Philadelphia: W.B. Saunders, 2000.

Vaughn DW, Green S, Kalayanarooj S, et al. Dengue in the early febrile phase: viremia and antibody responses. J Infect Dis 1997;176:322-330.

Vaughn DW, Green S, Kalayanarooj S, et al. Dengue viremia titer, antibody response pattern, and virus serotype correlate with disease severity. J Infect Dis 2000;181:2-9.

Vaughn DW, Nisalak A, Solomon T, et al. Rapid serologic diagnosis of dengue virus infection using a commercial capture ELISA that distinguishes primary and secondary infections. Am J Trop Med Hyg 1999;60:693-698.

Watts DM, Porter KR, Putvatana P, et al. Failure of secondary infection with American genotype dengue 2 to cause dengue haemorrhagic fever. Lancet 1999;354:1431-1434.

World Health Organization. Pathogenetic mechanisms in dengue haemorrhagic fever: report of an international collaborative study. Bull World Health Organ 1973;48:117-133.

World Health Organization. Dengue Haemorrhagic Fever: Diagnosis, Treatment, Prevention and Control, ed 2. Geneva: World Health. Organization, 1997.

Worobey M, Rambaut A, Holmes EC. Widespread intra-serotype recombination in natural populations of dengue virus. Proc Natl Acad Sci USA 1999;96:7352-7357.

Wu SJ, Grouard-Vogel G, Sun W, et al. Human skin Langerhans cells are targets of dengue virus infection. Nat Med 2000;6:816-820.

Young PR, Hilditch PA, Bletchly C, Halloran W. An antigen capture enzyme-linked immunosorbent assay reveals high levels of the dengue virus protein NS1 in the sera of infected patients. J Clin Microbiol 2000;38:1053-1057.

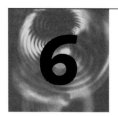

6

DIPHTHERIA

MELINDA WHARTON

Diphtheria is a preventable acute disease caused by *Corynebacterium diphtheriae*. The microorganism produces an exotoxin that is responsible for many of the severe manifestations of diphtheria. The disease is characterized clinically by a sore throat and a membrane that may cover the tonsils, pharynx, and larynx. Diphtheria is rare today in developed areas of the world and is seldom considered in differential diagnosis. Nevertheless, sporadic cases still occur, and epidemic diphtheria reemerged in the Soviet Union in the early 1990s. In addition, it is prevalent in many developing countries, and importation of cases into the United States and other developed countries may occur.

HISTORY

The recognition of diphtheria as a disease probably dates back to the second century. It was in 1826, however, that Bretonneau named the illness *la diphthérite* and accurately described the clinical manifestations. He distinguished scarlet fever from diphtheria and identified membranous croup as a form of diphtheria.

Corynebacterium diphtheriae was discovered by Klebs in 1883 and was isolated in pure culture by Löffler. It was called the *Klebs-Löffler bacillus*, and its etiologic relationship to the disease was demonstrated in 1884. In 1888 Roux and Yersin showed that the bacillus produced an exotoxin that was responsible for the various clinical manifestations of the disease such as myocarditis and neuritis. In 1890 von Behring showed that the toxin stimulated the production of antitoxin. Subsequently, in 1894 Roux and Martin used equine antitoxin for treatment of diphtheria in children at one hospital, with a reduction in mortality from 51% to 24%. In the same year, von Behring used toxin neutralized by antitoxin to induce immu-nity in animals and man. A large-scale immunization program to protect children was initiated by Park in 1922. Finally, in 1923 Ramon showed that formalin-treated toxin, currently known as *toxoid*, was superior to toxin-antitoxin as an immunizing agent. A century of progress culminated in 1923 in the development of a safe and effective vaccine capable of preventing the disease.

EPIDEMIOLOGY

Diphtheria is worldwide in distribution. The extensive use of diphtheria toxoid in industrialized countries in the 1940s and 1950s has led to a marked decrease in diphtheria incidence. Since 1980 no more than five cases of respiratory diphtheria have been reported each year in the United States (Figure 6-1). Although some cases may be unrecognized, the low level of reported disease likely reflects the near absence of respiratory diphtheria in this country.

In developing countries with effective childhood immunization programs, diphtheria incidence has decreased dramatically, but the proportion of cases among older adolescents and adults has increased. Because immunity induced by diphtheria toxoid is not lifelong, additional doses of diphtheria toxoid are needed to extend protection into adolescence and adulthood. In some developing countries that have achieved high levels of vaccination among children, diphtheria epidemics have occurred among older children, adolescents, and adults, highlighting the importance of vaccination of these age groups (Galazka and Robertson, 1995).

In 1990 a diphtheria epidemic began in Russia that by 1994 had spread to all the New Independent States (NIS) of the former Soviet Union. From 1990 to 1995 approximately 125,000 cases and 4,000 deaths resulting from

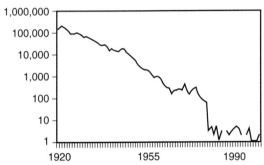

Fig. 6-1 Reported cases of diphtheria, United States, 1920-2001. Since 1980, only respiratory diphtheria has been reportable. No cases were reported in 1986, 1993, and 1995; two cases were reported in 1994. Data for 2001 are provisional. From Centers for Disease Control and Prevention. National Notifiable Diseases Surveillance System. Atlanta, Ga: Centers for Disease Control and Prevention.

diphtheria were reported in the NIS. Lack of routine vaccination of adults and delayed vaccination of children may have lead to increased susceptibility of the population; socioeconomic instability and population movement may have been contributing factors (Dittmann et al., 2000). Adults who never received a full primary series of diphtheria toxoid in childhood were at increased risk of severe disease and death. Outbreak control strategies included achieving and maintaining high immunization coverage among children and administering a single dose of diphtheria toxoid to adults; additional doses were recommended for age cohorts that had not necessarily received a full primary series in childhood. With implementation of these strategies, the outbreak came under control.

Diphtheria is acquired by contact with an ill person with the disease or with an asymptomatic carrier of the organism. Persons with cutaneous diphtheria serve as a reservoir of C. diphtheriae. In tropical countries, cutaneous infection is common among children and results in naturally acquired immunity. Milkborne epidemics have been reported. The organism can also be spread by fomites.

In temperate climates the highest seasonal incidence occurs during the autumn and winter months, and epidemics of respiratory diphtheria occur in susceptible populations. Increased disease incidence among school-age children during the first few months of the school year has been reported (Naiditch and Bower, 1954).

In the prevaccine era, achieving high vaccination coverage among school-age children, combined with moderate coverage among preschool-age children, was associated with control of epidemics, suggesting that children of school age may play an important role in spread of diphtheria. In tropical climates, seasonality is less distinct, and cutaneous infections are more common.

ETIOLOGY

C. diphtheriae is the only major human pathogen of the corynebacterial group. These organisms are taxonomically related to the mycobacteria and *Nocardia* species.

Morphology

C. diphtheriae organisms are slender gram-positive rods that measure 2 to 4 μm in length. When grown on suboptimal media, the bacteria are pleomorphic. The cells vary in diameter, and the ends are broader than the center, producing a typical club-shaped appearance. A beaded or bandlike appearance is produced by the metachromatic granules, which are accumulations of polymerized polyphosphates. As a result of cell division the bacteria appear in palisades or as individual cells at sharp angles to each other.

Cultural Characteristics

C. diphtheriae is an aerobe easily grown on standard microbiologic media, such as sheep blood agar, and complex media are not required for its isolation. However, because clinical specimens from which it is isolated (nose and throat swabs) are obtained from sites characterized by abundant normal flora, tellurite-containing media (e.g., cystine-tellurite or Tinsdale medium) that selectively inhibit a number of these organisms are helpful for isolation of C. diphtheriae. There are four biotypes of C. diphtheriae—gravis, mitis, intermedius, and belfanti—which can be distinguished biochemically and by their colonial morphology. No constant relationship exists between biotype and disease severity.

Other *Corynebacterium* Species Associated With Respiratory Disease

Pseudomembranous pharyngitis clinically indistinguishable from respiratory diphtheria has been reported in association with infection with both *C. pseudodiphtheriticum* and *C. ulcerans*. Although uncommon causes of human infection, strains of *C. ulcerans* and *C. pseudotuberculosis* can produce diphtheria toxin. Susceptible patients with disease associated with toxigenic *C. ulcerans* can develop severe disease.

PATHOGENESIS AND PATHOLOGY

Diphtheria toxin is responsible for many for the serious clinical manifestations of the disease. It is extremely unstable and is easily destroyed by heat (75° C for 10 minutes), light, and aging. Toxin is produced by strains of *C. diphtheriae* that are lysogenic for bacteriophage carrying the *tox* gene (Freeman and Morse, 1953). Thus, a person may harbor *C. diphtheriae*, and the organism may acquire beta corynebacteriophage, converting the bacterium to a toxin producer. Toxin production does not require lytic growth of the phage. The *tox* gene is thought to confer an advantage in survival both to the phage and to *C. diphtheriae* in the human host. In vitro, diphtheria toxin is maximally produced when there is a limited amount of iron present. When adequate iron is present, a repressor-iron complex binds to the *tox* gene and prevents toxin formation. When the iron concentration is lowered, dissociation of the repressor complex from the *tox* gene occurs, and toxin is produced.

The toxin is synthesized on membrane-bound polysomes and is released extracellularly as a single inactive precursor polypeptide chain. Cleavage exposes the active enzymatic site of toxin, and the biologically active toxin consists of two functionally distinct polypeptides, A and B, linked by a disulfide bond. Fragment A is extremely stable, enzymatically active, and responsible for the toxic effects, which are due to inhibition of cellular protein synthesis. Fragment A inactivates elongation factor 2, which is a protein common to all eukaryotic cells. This protein is essential for translocation of peptidyl transfer RNA on ribosomes. Fragment B is unstable, is not enzymatically active, and is required for attachment of the activated toxin molecule to receptors of sensitive host cells. All human cells have receptor sites for fragment B, and the binding is rapid and irreversible. The attachment of B is necessary for penetration of fragment A into the cell. Both A and B are necessary for cytotoxicity.

Following attachment of the diphtheria organism to the nasopharyngeal mucosa of a susceptible person, the toxin is elaborated and absorbed locally. The toxic effect on the cells causes tissue necrosis, which provides the environment for growth of the organism and production of more toxin. In addition to the necrosis, an inflammatory and exudative reaction is induced by the toxin. The necrotic epithelial cells, leukocytes, red blood cells, fibrinous material, diphtheria bacilli, and other bacterial inhabitants of the nasopharynx combine to form the typical membrane. The superficial epithelial cells of the mucosa form an integral part of this membrane and cause it to adhere; attempts to separate it are followed by bleeding and the formation of a new membrane, which sloughs off during the recovery period.

The toxin produced at the site of the membrane is distributed through the bloodstream to tissues all over the body. The size of the membrane usually reflects the amount of toxin produced. The toxin reaches the circulation more readily from the pharynx and tonsils than from the larynx and trachea. Consequently, laryngotracheal diphtheria produces less toxemia than pharyngotonsillar involvement, but the obstruction of the airway by the laryngotracheal membrane may be life threatening.

Differential effects on various tissues are not well understood. The most striking clinical manifestations are seen in the heart and the nervous system, but other organs may also be affected. Pathologic changes associated with diphtheria myocarditis include hyaline degeneration and necrosis, associated with inflammation in the interstitial spaces. The maximal pathologic effects of fatty degeneration and fibrosis occur after the first week of illness, consistent with the observation that myocarditis usually develops 10 to 14 days after onset of illness.

In the nervous system, segmental demyelination of nerve fibers within the sensory ganglia is found, along with demyelination of adjacent parts of peripheral nerves and anterior and posterior roots. Degeneration is limited to short segments of the myelin sheath (Fisher and Adams, 1956). Macrophages ingest myelin; otherwise, there is little inflammation. It has been suggested that Schwann's cells are sensitive to toxin, with resulting inhibition of synthesis of myelin basic protein, leading to development of segmental lesions. When myelinization is resumed, recovery occurs.

Although diphtheria toxin is the most important virulence factor of C. *diphtheriae*, colonization of mucous membranes can be accomplished by both toxigenic and nontoxigenic strains. The well-documented occurrence of pseudomembranous pharyngitis in persons infected with nontoxigenic strains suggests that there are important virulence factors other than diphtheria toxin. The organisms have a toxic glycolipid and a cord factor, which is considered necessary for virulence; in addition, other virulence factors may exist.

CLINICAL MANIFESTATIONS

Diphtheria usually develops after a short incubation period of 2 to 4 days, with a range of 1 to 5 days. For clinical purposes, the disease may be classified by the anatomic location of infection. More than one anatomic site may be involved at the same time.

Nasal Diphtheria

The onset of nasal diphtheria is indistinguishable from that of the common cold. It is characterized by a nasal discharge and a lack of constitutional symptoms. Fever, if present, is usually low grade. The nasal discharge, which at first is serous, subsequently becomes serosanguineous. In some cases there may be frank epistaxis. The discharge, which may be unilateral or bilateral, becomes mucopurulent, and the anterior nares and upper lip usually have an impetiginous appearance. The discharge may obscure the presence of a white membrane on the nasal septum. The poor absorption of toxin from this site accounts for the mildness of the disease and the paucity of constitutional symptoms. In the untreated patient the nasal discharge may persist for many days or weeks. This rich source of diphtheria bacilli becomes a menace to all susceptible contacts.

Tonsillar and Pharyngeal Diphtheria

Tonsillar diphtheria usually begins insidiously with malaise, anorexia, sore throat, and low-grade fever. Within 24 hours a patch of exudate or membrane appears in the faucial area. In vaccinated persons the membrane may be limited, resembling tonsillitis, but in susceptible persons it may spread rapidly and within 12 to 24 hours involve the anterior and posterior fau-

cial pillars, the soft palate, and the uvula. It is smooth, adherent, and white or gray (Plate 1); in the presence of bleeding it may be black. Forcible attempts to remove it are followed by bleeding. Pharyngotonsillar involvement is characterized by a variable amount of cervical adenitis, and in severe cases the marked swelling produces a "bull-neck" appearance.

The course of the illness is variable, but disease is usually mild in previously vaccinated persons. The temperature remains either normal or slightly elevated, but the pulse is disproportionately rapid. In mild cases the membrane sloughs off between the seventh and the tenth day and the patient has an uneventful recovery. In moderately severe cases, convalescence is slow, with the course frequently complicated by myocarditis and neuritis. Severe cases are characterized by increasing toxemia manifested by severe prostration, striking pallor, rapid thready pulse, stupor, coma, and death within 6 to 10 days.

Laryngeal Diphtheria

Laryngeal diphtheria most often develops as an extension of pharyngeal involvement. Occasionally, however, it may be the only manifestation of the disease. The illness is ushered in by fever, hoarseness, and cough, which develop a barking quality. Increasing obstruction of the airway by the membrane is manifested by inspiratory stridor followed by suprasternal, supraclavicular, and subcostal retractions. The membrane may extend downward to involve the entire tracheobronchial tree.

The clinical picture of laryngeal diphtheria is dominated by the consequences of the mechanical obstruction to the air passages caused by the membrane, congestion, and edema. In mild cases or in those modified by antitoxin therapy the airway remains patent and the membrane is coughed up between the sixth and tenth day. A sudden acute and fatal obstruction may occur in a mild case in which a partially detached piece of membrane blocks the airway. In very severe cases there is increasing obstruction followed by progressive hypoxia, which is manifested by restlessness, cyanosis, severe prostration, coma, and death.

Signs of toxemia are minimal in primary laryngeal involvement because toxin is poorly absorbed from the mucous membrane of the larynx. In most instances, however, the laryngeal involvement is associated with tonsillar and pharyngeal diphtheria. Consequently, the clinical manifestations are those of both obstruction and severe toxemia.

Cutaneous Diphtheria

Cutaneous diphtheria classically has been described as a deep, rounded, "punched out" ulcer with sharply demarcated edges and a membranous base; the ulcer does not extend into the subcutaneous tissue. However, other clinical presentations occur; because *C. diphtheriae* can colonize preexisting skin lesions (wounds, dermatitis, and insect bites, for example), the clinical presentation may be highly variable (Höfler, 1991). Cutaneous diphtheria may be important epidemiologically; chronic skin infection may serve as a reservoir of the organism. Because toxin is absorbed slowly from cutaneous sites, complications are relatively uncommon following cutaneous infection.

Unusual Types of Diphtheria

Diphtheritic infections occasionally develop in sites other than the respiratory tract or the skin. Conjunctival, aural, and vulvovaginal infections may occur. The conjunctival lesion primarily involves the palpebral surface, which is reddened, edematous, and membranous. Involvement of the external auditory canal is usually manifest by a persistent purulent discharge. Vulvovaginal lesions are usually ulcerative and confluent.

DIAGNOSIS

An early diagnosis of diphtheria is essential because delay of administration of antitoxin may impose a serious and preventable risk to the patient. Accurate bacteriologic confirmation by means of culture requires special media, a proficient laboratory, and a minimum of 15 to 20 hours; smears are not reliable. Consequently, the initial diagnosis, as a basis for therapy, must be made on clinical grounds alone.

The diagnosis of diphtheria is confirmed by the demonstration of diphtheria bacilli cultured from material obtained from the site of infection. Care should be exercised in obtaining the culture. The swab should be rubbed firmly over the lesion or, if possible, should be inserted beneath the membrane; if it can be obtained, a fragment of the membrane should be submitted

for culture. Swabs should be taken from the nasopharynx and from any wounds or other skin lesions in patients with suspected diphtheria. Lesions should be cleaned with sterile normal saline, crusted material removed, and the swab applied firmly to the base of the lesion. The physician must notify the laboratory that diphtheria is suspected to have correct media used. If swabs must be shipped to a reference laboratory, a transport medium such as that containing silica gel should be used. A blood agar plate and a tellurite plate should be streaked with the swab. The plates should be placed in the incubator at 37° C without delay. After incubation for 24 to 48 hours, the organisms on the plates should be identified by an experienced laboratorian.

Diphtheria bacilli that are isolated on culture should be classified by biotype (mitis, gravis, intermedius, or belfanti) and tested for toxigenicity. Although the original assays for toxigenicity were performed in vivo, the method now most commonly used for determining toxigenicity is the Elek immunoprecipitation test. Because diphtheria has become a rare diagnosis in most developed countries, many laboratories are not proficient in performing the test, and specimens will need to be forwarded to a reference laboratory for toxigenicity testing. A polymerase chain reaction (PCR) assay detecting the A and B subunit of the *tox* gene, which correlates well with the Elek test, has also been developed. The PCR assay may be performed directly on clinical specimens, allowing rapid confirmation of the presence of toxigenic *Corynebacterium* organisms.

DIFFERENTIAL DIAGNOSIS

The differential diagnosis of diphtheria varies with the particular anatomic site of involvement. The presentation of nasal diphtheria may be clinically indistinguishable from that of a foreign body in the nose. Tonsillar and pharyngeal diphtheria may resemble streptococcal infection; coinfection with both toxigenic *C. diphtheriae* and group A streptococcus is well documented. Other diagnoses that may be considered in patients with diphtheria of these sites are infectious mononucleosis, nonbacterial membranous tonsillitis, primary herpetic tonsillitis, and thrush. Laryngeal diphtheria may present with signs and symptoms resembling laryngotracheitis or epiglottitis.

COMPLICATIONS

The most common and most serious complications are those caused by the effect of the toxin on the heart and central nervous system.

Myocarditis

Myocarditis occurs frequently as a complication of severe diphtheria, but it may also follow milder forms of the disease. The more extensive the local lesion is and the more delayed the institution of antitoxin therapy is, the more frequently myocarditis occurs. In most instances the cardiac manifestations appear during the second week of the disease. Occasionally, myocarditis may be noted as early as the first week and as late as the sixth week of the disease. Abnormal electrocardiographic findings include flattening and inversion of T waves; elevation of the ST segment; and conduction abnormalities, including complete heart block. Myocarditis may be followed by cardiac failure.

Neuritis

Neuritis also is generally a complication of severe diphtheria. The manifestations of neuritis appear after a variable latent period, are predominantly bilateral, and usually resolve completely. Neuropathy affecting cranial nerves typically occurs early in the course of illness, during the first 4 weeks after the onset of disease; peripheral neuropathy occurs later, 5 to 8 weeks after onset of disease. Cranial nerve involvement rarely if ever occurs as a complication of cutaneous diphtheria without respiratory involvement. Paralysis of the limbs has been reported following cutaneous infection, and the latent period may be quite prolonged.

Paralysis of the soft palate. Soft palate paralysis is the most common manifestation of diphtheritic neuritis. It may occur as early as the first week after onset of illness. It is characterized by a nasal quality to the voice and nasal regurgitation. The paralysis usually subsides completely within 1 to 2 weeks.

Ocular palsy. This palsy usually occurs between the third and fifth week and is characterized by paralysis of the muscles of accommodation, causing blurring of vision. Less commonly there may be involvement of the extraocular muscles, causing strabismus. Involvement of the lateral rectus muscle, causing an internal squint, may also occur.

Paralysis of diaphragm. Paralysis of the diaphragm may occur between the fifth and seventh week as a result of neuritis of the phrenic nerve. Death occurs if mechanical respiratory support is not provided.

Paralysis of limbs. Limb paralysis may occur between the fifth and tenth week. Both sensory and motor nerves are involved. Paresthesias are followed by weakness of the extremities and loss of deep tendon reflexes. Nerve conduction studies show slowing of conduction; prolongation of distal motor latency; and, in severe cases, conduction block. The absence of deep tendon reflexes, bilateral symmetric involvement, and the presence of an elevated level of spinal fluid protein make this complication clinically indistinguishable from the Guillain-Barré syndrome.

Other Complications

In severe diphtheria, thrombocytopenia and coagulation abnormalities are not uncommon. The peripheral blood smear may show evidence of microangiopathic hemolytic anemia, and frank disseminated intravascular coagulation may occur. These abnormalities are thought to be a result of the effects of diphtheria toxin on the vascular endothelium. Likewise, proteinuria is commonly found in severe disease, and renal failure may occur.

PROGNOSIS

Before the turn of the century the mortality rate of diphtheria was 30% to 50%. The advent of diphtheria antitoxin in 1894 and the beginning of large-scale active immunization programs in 1922 led to a dramatic reduction in the mortality rate to approximately 10%. In spite of subsequent improvements in the care of critically ill patients, case-fatality ratios of 5% to 10% have been reported in most series. Extensive disease and delays in seeking medical care, diagnosis, and receipt of diphtheria antitoxin are risk factors for death resulting from diphtheria. Mortality rates are consistently lower for cases receiving antitoxin within the first 2 days of illness. The susceptibility of the patient is also critical; illness is usually mild in vaccinated persons.

The prognosis in the individual case of diphtheria must be guarded. Sudden death may be caused by a variety of unpredictable events, including the sudden complete obstruction of the airway by a detached piece of membrane, the development of myocarditis and heart failure, or the late occurrence of respiratory paralysis caused by phrenic nerve involvement. Patients who survive myocarditis or neuritis generally recover completely. Occasionally, however, diphtheritic myocarditis may be followed by permanent damage to the heart.

IMMUNITY

Antibody to diphtheria toxin (antitoxin) confers protection from severe clinical manifestations of diphtheria. Antitoxin levels of 0.01 to 0.09 IU (international unit)/ml are thought to confer some protection, and with levels of ≥0.1 IU/ml, protection is considered reliable. However, persons with "protective" levels of antitoxin have developed diphtheria (Ipsen, 1946). Antibodies to other components of C. diphtheriae may also play a role in immunity.

Antitoxin levels are most commonly measured by in vitro neutralization in tissue culture. Both enzyme-linked immunosorbent assays (ELISA) and passive hemagglutination have been used, but both are unreliable at low concentrations of antitoxin (<0.1 IU/ml). The poor correlation between results of ELISA and in vitro neutralization at low antitoxin concentrations is thought to be caused by the binding of nonneutralizing antibodies.

Passive Immunity

Passive immunity may be acquired either by transplacental transfer of antibody from an immune mother or by parenteral administration of diphtheria antitoxin. Congenitally acquired passive immunity persists for approximately 6 months. Protection after injection of diphtheria antitoxin disappears after 2 to 3 weeks.

Active Immunity

Active immunity may be induced either by previous infection with C. diphtheriae or, more commonly today, by vaccination with diphtheria toxoid. The toxin is more toxic than immunogenic; thus, reliable immunity is produced only by vaccination. Persons with diphtheria should therefore be immunized. Recurrent attacks of the disease frequently occurred in the prevaccine era, but by late adolescence most of those persons were immune.

Immunization with diphtheria toxoid can be relied on to prevent serious or fatal disease. The widespread and routine immmunization of infants and children has had a profound effect on the immune status of the population at large. Fully immunized individuals have antibody to toxin but do not have antibody to the organism and may become nasopharyngeal carriers or, uncommonly, may develop mild disease.

TREATMENT
Antitoxin Therapy

Diphtheria antitoxin must be given promptly and in adequate dosage (Table 6-1). Any delay increases the possibility that myocarditis, neuritis, or death may occur. During an infection, diphtheria toxin may be present in three forms: (1) circulating or unbound; (2) bound to the cells; or (3) internalized in cytoplasm. Antitoxin will neutralize circulating toxin and may affect bound toxin but will not affect internalized toxin. Because bacteriologic confirmation of the diagnosis cannot be obtained immediately, the decision to administer diphtheria antitoxin must be made on clinical and epidemiologic grounds.

Currently available diphtheria antitoxin is of equine origin, and, like any heterologous serum, its administration may be followed by an immediate reaction, such as acute anaphylactic shock, or a delayed type of reaction, such as serum sickness. Any history regarding previous horse serum injections or possible allergy should be obtained before administering the product, and the patient must be tested for hypersensitivity by skin or eye tests. When testing for hypersensitivity or administering diphtheria antitoxin, health-care workers should always have a syringe loaded with a

TABLE 6-1	Dosage of Antitoxin Recommended for Treatment of Diphtheria
Type of diphtheria	*Dosage (units)*
Anterior nasal	10,000-20,000
Tonsillar	15,000-25,000
Pharyngeal ≤48 hr duration	20,000-40,000
Laryngeal ≤48 hr duration	20,000-40,000
Nasopharyngeal	40,000-60,000
Extensive disease of ≥3 days duration or any patientwith brawny swelling of the neck	80,000-120,000

1:1,000 solution of epinephrine ready and available for emergency use.

Skin test. An injection of 0.1 ml of a 1:100 dilution of diphtheria antitoxin in physiologic saline solution is given intracutaneously. The test is read in 20 minutes and is positive if a wheal 1 cm or more in diameter is present. In persons with a history of allergy to equine serum the dose should be reduced to 0.05 ml of a 1:1,000 dilution intracutaneously. The use of undiluted antitoxin will invariably cause a false-positive reaction; dilution is therefore mandatory. A negative skin test does not preclude the occurrence of serum reactions.

Conjunctival test. One drop of a 1:10 dilution of the serum in physiologic saline solution is instilled inside the lower lid of one eye; 1 drop of physiologic saline solution is used as a control for the other eye. The test is read in 20 minutes and is positive if conjunctivitis and lacrimation are present. If a positive reaction occurs, the eye should be treated with 1 drop of a 1:100 solution of epinephrine.

If the history and sensitivity tests are negative, the total recommended dose of antitoxin should be given without delay. The precise dose and route of administration of antitoxin is determined by the location and extent of the membrane, the degree of toxemia, and the duration of the illness. Dosage does not vary by the patient's age and weight. The dosages shown in Table 6-1 are recommended for the various types of diphtheria.

To neutralize toxin as rapidly as possible, the preferred route of administration is intravenous; antitoxin may also be administered by intramuscular injection, but peak antitoxin levels may not be reached for several days. If intravenous therapy is indicated, antitoxin should be diluted in 500 ml of saline and administered by intravenous drip. The rate should be very slow over the first half hour to allow for desensitization; the entire dose should be administered within 90 minutes. The patient must be carefully monitored, and the infusion must be stopped if signs of shock appear. The addition of 0.1 to 0.3 ml of 1:1,000 dilution of epinephrine to the solution is a useful precaution. If administered by intramuscular injection, antitoxin is injected undiluted into the buttocks.

If a patient is sensitive to horse serum, the indications for the diphtheria antitoxin should be reevaluated because of this potential risk. If the antitoxin is indicated, it can be given following desensitization by the intravenous, intradermal, subcutaneous, or intramuscular regimen, as described in Tables 6-2 and 6-3. Signs of acute anaphylaxis call for the immediate intravenous injection of 0.2 to 0.5 ml of 1:1,000 epinephrine solution.

In the United States, diphtheria antitoxin is no longer commercially available, but it is available from the Centers for Disease Control and Prevention as an investigational agent. Physicians caring for patients with suspected diphtheria should contact their state health department for assistance in obtaining diphtheria antitoxin.

Antibacterial Therapy

Penicillin and erythromycin are effective against most strains of diphtheria bacilli. Penicillin is the preferred drug and may be given as aqueous procaine penicillin (25,000 to 50,000 units per kilogram of body weight per day for children, with a maximum dosage of 1.2 million units per day, in two divided doses). Patients who are sensitive to penicillin should be given parenteral erythromycin in a daily dosage of 40 to 50 mg per kilogram, with a maximum dosage of 2 g per day. When the

| TABLE 6-2 | Desensitization to Serum: Intravenous Route |

Dose number*	Dilution of serum in isotonic sodium chloride	Amount of injection (mL)
1	1:1,000	0.1
2	1:1,000	0.3
3	1:1,000	0.6
4	1:100	0.1
5	1:100	0.3
6	1:100	0.6
7	1:10	0.1
8	1:10	0.3
9	1:10	0.6
10	Undiluted	0.1
11	Undiluted	0.3
12	Undiluted	0.6
13	Undiluted	1.0

From American Academy of Pediatrics. Passive immunization. In Pickering LK (ed). 2000 Red Book: Report of the Committee on Infectious Diseases, ed 25. Elk Grove Village, Ill: American Academy of Pediatrics, 2000.

*Administer consistently at 15-minute intervals.

TABLE 6-3 Desensitization to Serum: Intradermal (ID), Subcutaneous (SC), and Intramuscular (IM) Routes

Dose number*	Route of administration	Dilution of serum in isotonic sodium chloride	Amount of injection (mL)
1	ID	1:1,000	0.1
2	ID	1:1,000	0.3
3	SC	1:1,000	0.6
4	SC	1:100	0.1
5	SC	1:100	0.3
6	SC	1:100	0.6
7	SC	1:10	0.1
8	SC	1:10	0.3
9	SC	1:10	0.6
10	SC	Undiluted	0.1
11	SC	Undiluted	0.3
12	IM	Undiluted	0.6
13	IM	Undiluted	1.0

From American Academy of Pediatrics. Passive immunization. In Pickering LK (ed). 2000 Red Book: Report of the Committee on Infectious Diseases, ed 25. Elk Grove Village, Ill: American Academy of Pediatrics, 2000.
ID, Intradermal; *SC*, subcutaneous; *IM*, intramuscular.
*Administer consistently at 15-minute intervals

patient can swallow comfortably, oral erythromycin in four divided doses or oral penicillin V (125 to 250 mg four times daily) may be substituted for a recommended total treatment period of 14 days. Antimicrobial therapy is not a substitute for antitoxin treatment.

Eradication of the organism should be documented by culture. Persons who continue to harbor the organism after treatment with either penicillin or erythromycin should receive an additional 10-day course of erythromycin, and follow-up cultures should be obtained.

Supportive Treatment

Bed rest is more important in the management of diphtheria than in most other infectious diseases. It should be enforced for at least 12 days because of the possibility of complicating myocarditis. The patient's activity subsequently is guided by the results of the daily physical examinations, the serial electrocardiograms, and the presence or absence of complications. In addition to requiring antitoxin, penicillin, and other supportive measures, patients with laryngeal diphtheria may require treatment for the relief of airway obstruction. Intubation and/or tracheostomy may be necessary. Steroid therapy did not prevent myocarditis or neuritis in one controlled trial (Thisyakorn et al., 1984).

Treatment of Complications

Myocarditis and neuritis are the most important complications requiring therapy. In general the management of diphtheritic myocarditis and its sequelae is the same as that used for any other type of acute myocardial damage. Bed rest and inactivity may be beneficial. Sudden death caused by myocardial failure may be precipitated by excessive activity. The administration of digoxin is controversial; however, it should not be withheld if there is evidence of cardiac decompensation. Conduction abnormalities may require use of a temporary pacemaker.

Palatal and pharyngeal paralysis may be complicated by aspiration because of the tendency for regurgitation and difficulty in swallowing. Under these circumstances, gastric or duodenal intubation is indicated. Mechanical ventilation may be required in patients with paralysis of the diaphragm resulting from phrenic nerve involvement.

Treatment of Diphtheria Carriers

A carrier is an individual who has no symptoms and harbors virulent diphtheria bacilli in the nasopharynx. The eradication of these microorganisms may be extremely difficult. A single dose of intramuscular benzathine penicillin G (600,000 units for children <6 years of age) or a 7- to 10-day course of oral ery-thromycin (40 mg/kg/day for children, 1 g/day for adults) is recommended. Although there is some evidence that erythromycin may be more effective in eradicating the carrier state, intra-muscular penicillin is preferred if compliance is in doubt. Because neither regimen is 100% effective and bacteriologic relapse may occur, specimens should be obtained for repeated cul-ture a minimum of 14 days after completion of therapy. Persons who continue to harbor the organism after treatment with either penicillin or erythromycin should receive an additional 10-day course of oral erythromycin, and fol-low-up cultures should be obtained (Farizo et al., 1993). Occasionally an undetected foreign body in the nose may be responsible for persis-tence of a carrier state.

ISOLATION AND QUARANTINE

The patient is infective until diphtheria bacilli can be no longer cultured from the site of the infection. Isolation should be maintained until elimination of the organism is demonstrated by negative cultures of two samples obtained at least 24 hours after completion of antimicro-bial therapy.

Care of Exposed Persons

Close contacts of the patient should be identi-fied, evaluated, and maintained under surveil-lance for 7 days. Close contacts include household members and other persons with a history of direct contact with a case (e.g., care-takers, relatives, or friends who regularly visit the home), as well as medical staff exposed to oral or respiratory secretions of the case. Both nasal and pharyngeal swabs should be obtained for culture from close contacts, regardless of vaccination status. As soon as specimens are obtained, antimicrobial prophylaxis is recom-mended, using either a single dose of intramus-cular penicillin (600,000 units for children <6 years of age and 1.2 million units for those ≥6 years of age) or a 7- to 10-day course of oral erythromycin (40 mg/kg/day for children, 1 g/day for adults). If compliance is in question, intramuscular penicillin is preferred.

The diphtheria vaccination status of contacts should be reviewed, and persons who have not been vaccinated should receive an immediate dose of diphtheria toxoid and complete the series in accordance with the recommended schedule for vaccination. In addition, contacts who have not received a booster dose within the last 5 years should receive a booster. If the contact has received diphtheria toxoid within 5 years, no additional vaccine is needed (Farizo et al., 1993).

Notification of Public Health Authorities

If the diagnosis of diphtheria is suspected, local or state public health authorities should be notified immediately. Measures to prevent additional cases should be undertaken promptly. In the United States, diphtheria anti-toxin is available through state health depart-ments. Notification is mandatory in all states and in most countries.

PREVENTIVE MEASURES

The dramatic decline in the incidence of diph-theria since 1922 can be attributed for the most part to mass immunization programs and routine immunization of infants and children. Diphtheria toxoid is prepared by formalde-hyde treatment of diphtheria toxin. The limit of flocculation (Lf) content of each toxoid (quantity of toxoid as assessed by flocculation) varies among products. The concentration of diphtheria toxoid used in preparations intended for adult use is reduced because adverse reactions to diphtheria toxoid are directly related to the quantity of antigen and to the age or previous vaccination history of the recipient, and because a smaller dosage of diphtheria toxoid produces an adequate immune response in adults. In the United States, diphtheria toxoid is administered in combination with acellular pertussis vaccine and tetanus toxoids (DTaP) or with tetanus toxoid (DT or Td). Pediatric formulations of diphtheria toxoid (DTaP and DT) are for use among infants and children <7 years of age. Each 0.5-ml dose is formulated to contain 6.7 to 25 Lf units of diphtheria toxoid. Adult for-mulation diphtheria and tetanus toxoids (Td) is for use among persons ≥7 years of age; each 0.5-ml dose is formulated to contain ≤2 Lf units of diphtheria toxoid. The vaccine is administered by intramuscular injection. In infants the anterolateral aspect of the thigh provides the largest muscle mass and is the rec-ommended site for intramuscular injection. In toddlers and older children the deltoid may be used if the muscle mass is adequate.

In the United States the routine diphtheria, tetanus, and pertussis vaccination schedule for children <7 years of age is composed of 5 doses of vaccine containing diphtheria, tetanus, and pertussis antigens. Three doses should be administered during the first year of life, generally at 2, 4, and 6 months of age. The fourth dose is recommended for children 15 to 18 months old to maintain adequate immunity during the preschool years. The fourth dose should be administered at least 6 months after the third. The fifth dose is recommended for children 4 to 6 years of age to confer continued protection against disease during the early elementary school years. A fifth dose is not necessary if the fourth dose in the series is administered on or after the fourth birthday.

For children <7 years of age in whom pertussis vaccine is contraindicated, DT should be used instead of DTaP. To ensure that there is no interference with the response to DT antigens from maternal antibodies, previously unvaccinated children who receive their first DT dose when <1 year of age should receive a total of 4 doses of DT as the primary series—the first three doses at 4- to 8-week intervals and the fourth dose 6 to 12 months later. If additional doses of pertussis vaccine become contraindicated after the series is begun in the first year of life, DT should be substituted for each of the remaining scheduled DTaP doses. If a child develops acute anaphylaxis following a dose of DTaP, further doses of the vaccine or any of its components should be deferred. Because of the importance of tetanus vaccination, referral to an allergist for evaluation and possible desensitization should be strongly considered.

Unvaccinated children 1 to 6 years of age for whom pertussis vaccine is contraindicated should receive 2 doses of DT 4 to 8 weeks apart, followed by a third dose 6 to 12 months later to complete the primary series. Children who have already received 1 or 2 doses of DT or DTaP after their first birthday and for whom further pertussis vaccine is contraindicated should receive a total of 3 doses of DT (if <7 years of age) or Td (≥7 years of age), with the third dose administered 6 to 12 months after the second dose. Children who complete a primary series of DT before their fourth birthday should receive a fifth dose of DT before entering kindergarten or elementary school. This dose is not necessary if the fourth dose was given after the fourth birthday.

Diphtheria infection may not confer immunity; therefore vaccination should be initiated

at the time of recovery from the illness, and arrangements should be made to ensure that all doses of a primary series are administered on schedule.

Because immunity induced by both diphtheria and tetanus toxoids wanes with time, booster vaccination with Td is recommended at 10-year intervals throughout life, following administration of a primary series. Administering the first Td booster vaccination at an adolescent immunization visit at 11 to 12 years of age is recommended to increase compliance and thereby reduce the susceptibility of adolescents to tetanus and diphtheria.

BIBLIOGRAPHY

American Academy of Pediatrics. 2000 Red Book: Report of the Committee on Infectious Diseases, ed 25. Elk Grove Village, Ill: American Academy of Pediatrics, 2000.

Belsey MA. Skin infections and the epidemiology of diphtheria: acquisition and persistence of C. diphtheriae infections. Am J Epidemiol 1975;102:179-184.

Centers for Disease Control and Prevention. Immunization of adolescents: recommendations of the Advisory Committee on Immunization Practices, the American Academy of Pediatrics, the American Academy of Family Physicians, and the American Medical Association. MMWR 1996;45(No. RR-13):1-16.

Centers for Disease Control and Prevention. Pertussis vaccination: use of acellular pertussis vaccines among infants and young children. Recommendations of the Advisory Committee on Immunization Practices (ACIP). MMWR 1997;46(No. RR-7):1-25.

Collier RJ. Understanding the mode of action of diphtheria toxin: a perspective on progress during the 20th century. Toxicon 2001;39:1793-1803.

Dittmann S, Wharton M, Vitek C, et al. Successful control of epidemic diphtheria in the states of the former Union of Soviet Socialist Republics: lessons learned. J Infect Dis 2000;181(suppl 1):S10-S22.

Dobie RA, Tobey DN. Clinical features of diphtheria in the respiratory tract. JAMA 1979;242:2197-2201.

Dolman CE. Landmarks and pioneers in the control of diphtheria. Can J Public Health 1973;64:317-336.

Efstratiou A, Maple PAC. Manual for the Laboratory Diagnosis of Diphtheria. WHO Regional Office for Europe, Copenhagen, 1994.

English PC. Diphtheria and theories of infectious diseases: centennial appreciation of the critical role of diphtheria in the history of medicine. Pediatrics 1985;76:1-9.

Farizo KM, Strebel PM, Chen RT, et al. Fatal respiratory disease due to Corynebacterium diphtheriae: case report and review of guidelines for management, investigation, and control. Clin Infect Dis 1993;16:59-68.

Fisher CM, Adams RD. Diphtheritic polyneuritis: a pathological study. J Neuropathol Exp Neurol 1956;15:243-268.

Freeman VJ, Morse U. Further observations on the change of virulence of bacteriophage-infected avirulent strains of

Corynebacterium diphtheriae. J Bacteriol 1953;63:407-414.

Funke GT, Bernard KA. Coryneform gram-positive rods. In Murray PR, Baron EJ, Pfaller MA, et al. (eds). Manual of Clinical Microbiology, ed 7. Washington, D.C.: American Society for Microbiology, 2000.

Funke G, von Graevenitz A, Clarridge JE, Bernard KA. Clinical microbiology of coryneform bacteria. Clin Micro Rev 1997;10:125-159.

Galazka AM, Robertson SE. Diphtheria: changing patterns in the developing world and the industrialized world. European J Epidemiol 1995;11:107-117.

Godfrey ES. Study in the epidemiology of diphtheria in relation to the active immunization of certain age groups. Am J Public Health 1932;22:237-256.

Hardy IRB, Dittmann S, Sutter RW. Current situation and control strategies for resurgence of diphtheria in newly independent states of the former Soviet Union. Lancet 1996;347:1739-1744.

Höfler W. Cutaneous diphtheria. Int J Dermatol 1991;30:845-847.

Holmes, RK. Biology and molecular biology of diphtheria toxin and the *tox* gene. J Infect Dis 2000;181(suppl 1): S156-S167.

Ipsen J. Circulating antitoxin at the onset of diphtheria in 425 patients. J Immunol 1946;54:325-347.

Liebow AA, MacLean PD, Bumstead JH, Welt LG. Tropical ulcers and cutaneous diphtheria. Arch Intern Med 1946;78:255-295.

Mikhailovich VM, Melnikov VG, Mazurova IK, et al. Application of PCR for detection of toxigenic *Corynebacterium diphtheriae* strains isolated during the Russian diphtheria epidemic, 1990 through 1994. J Clin Microbiol 1995;33:3061-3063.

Morgan BC. Cardiac complications of diphtheria. Pediatrics 1963;32:549-557.

Naiditch MJ, Bower AG. Diphtheria: a study of 1,433 cases observed during a ten-year period at the Los Angeles County Hospital. Am J Med 1954;17:229-245.

Neubauer C. Clinical signs of diphtheria in inoculated children. Lancet 1943;2:192-194.

Soldiers G, Nennesmo I, Persson A. Diphtheritic neuropathy, an analysis based on muscle and nerve biopsy and repeated neurophysiological and autonomic function tests. J Neurol Neurosurg Psychiatry 1989;52:876-880.

Piradov MA, Pirogov VN, Popova LM, Avdunina IA. Diphtheritic polyneuropathy: clinical analysis of severe forms. Arch Neurol 2001;58:1438-1442.

Tao X, Schiering N, Zeng H, et al. Iron, DtxR, and the regulation of diphtheria toxin expression. Mol Microbiol 1994;14:191-197.

Thisyakorn U, Wongvanich J, Kampeng V. Failure of corticosteroid therapy to prevent diphtheritic myocarditis or neuritis. Pediatr Infect Dis J 1984;3:126.

Wesley AG, Pather M, Chrystal V. The hemorrhagic diathesis in diphtheria with special reference to disseminated intravascular coagulation. Ann Trop Paediatr 1981;1:51-56.

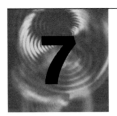

7 ENDOCARDITIS

Lisa Saiman

Endocarditis is an infection of the endothelium of the heart and most typically involves the heart valves, although infectious lesions can occur on the myocardial wall, at the site of a septal defect, or within an extracardiac shunt. The characteristic lesion of endocarditis is vegetation that consists of fibrin, platelets, host inflammatory cells, and the infecting microorganisms. Despite this relatively straightforward pathologic description, the diagnosis and management of endocarditis presents considerable challenges. Recent reviews have been written about endocarditis, but these have focused on adult patients (Mylonakis and Calderwoood, 2001; Wilson et al., 1995). Adult patients may have prosthetic valves or degenerative valvular disease, which are not generally seen in children; adults are also more likely to have risk factors such as intravenous drug abuse, poor dental hygiene, long-term hemodialysis, and diabetes. Historically, endocarditis has been divided into two categories: (1) acute, fulminant infection of normal hearts, and (2) subacute, chronic infection of valves damaged by rheumatic fever. However, numerous changes in medical and surgical practices during the past three decades have created new risk factors that make these historic categories less applicable. Rheumatic fever has been decreasing in the developed world. Children with complex cyanotic heart disease are having palliative and corrective surgery, often with placement of shunts and prosthetic valves. Premature infants and critically ill children in intensive care units with central venous catheters are at risk for hospital-acquired (nosocomial) endocarditis secondary to bloodstream infections. Mitral valve prolapse (MVP) is a relatively common lesion in the general population and can be a risk factor for endocarditis. In addition, whereas endocarditis is often caused by predictable pathogens, the widespread problem of antibiotic resistance has had a substantial impacted on the management of endocarditis, and less common pathogens including fungi and molds are causing endocarditis with increasing frequency.

EPIDEMIOLOGY

It is difficult to ascertain precise rates at which endocarditis occurs in children. Endocarditis is not a reportable disease and most data regarding occurrence rates have been derived from case series from tertiary care pediatric referral centers. Thus, referral patterns can have a dramatic impact on occurrence-rate data. Despite this limitation, there appears to be an increase in the incidence of endocarditis, particularly due to the increase in occurrence of hospital-acquired endocarditis. From 1930 to 1972, endocarditis accounted for 1 in 2,000 to 5,000 hospital admissions in children; from 1960 to 1980, this proportion increased to 1 in 500 to 1,000 admissions (Stull and LiPuma, 1992; Kaplan, 1977; Caldwell et al., 1971; Zakrewski and Keith, 1965). No recent reviews have calculated the rate of endocarditis in children in the developed world, although in the developing world, where rheumatic heart disease is still common, the incidence of endocarditis from 1997 to 2000 was 32 per 1,000 pediatric admissions (Sadiq et al., 2001).

Additional changes in epidemiology have been noted. Rheumatic valvulitis is no longer the most important risk factor for endocarditis in the developing world. Since the 1970s, congenital heart disease is the most common risk factor for endocarditis. Thus, staphylococci, including coagulase-negative staphylococci and *Staphylococcus aureus*, and not viridans streptococci, are the most common etiologic agents in some series of cases of pediatric endocarditis; fungal species, particularly *Candida albicans*, are causing endocarditis with increasing frequency (Saiman et al., 1993; Aspesberro et al., 1999). With the increasing use of indwelling central venous catheters, intralipids, and hyperalimentation in critically ill children and neonates with normal and abnormal hearts, nosocomial endocarditis is being diagnosed with increased frequency.

RISK FACTORS
Rheumatic Carditis

The relationship between rheumatic carditis and endocarditis has been understood for decades (Feinstein et al., 1964a). Approximately one third of patients with rheumatic fever develop carditis, and most recover uneventfully. In contrast, some patients have recurrent episodes of rheumatic fever with progressive cardiac damage (Feinstein et al., 1964b). Approximately 5% of patients with rheumatic carditis develop endocarditis (Griffiths and Gersony, 1990). In series of cases of pediatric endocarditis from the 1940s to the 1960s, rheumatic carditis was the underlying lesion in one third of the children (Blumenthal et al., 1960; Johnson et al., 1975). In case series from the 1970s to the 1990s, as the incidence of rheumatic fever declined, rheumatic carditis was the underlying lesion in only 12% of children with endocarditis (Normand et al., 1995; Saiman et al., 1993). In contrast, rheumatic fever is the underlying lesion in 40% to 50% of children from the developing world who have endocarditis (Sadiq et al., 2001; Dhawan et al., 1993; Bitar et al., 2000).

Congenital Heart Disease

The link between the pathophysiology of endocarditis and the anatomic defects of congenital heart disease was first noted in autopsy studies (Johnson et al., 1975; Cutler et al., 1958; Gelfman and Levine, 1942). In an autopsy series describing 181 children with unrepaired congenital heart disease, 16.5% had endocarditis (Cutler et al., 1958). In these early series, ventricular septal defect (VSD), patent ductus arteriosus, and tetralogy of Fallot were the most common lesions associated with endocarditis. Patients with these lesions had a relatively prolonged life expectancy before the advent of cardiac surgery, and these lesions caused turbulent blood flow that increased the risk of endocarditis. In one series, previously undiagnosed VSD and MVP were detected as the *result* of endocarditis (Saiman et al., 1993).

Cardiac Surgery

The link between surgical palliation or correction of congenital heart disease and endocarditis was noted in initial surgical reports of patent ductus arteriosus ligation and construction of a palliative shunt for tetralogy of Fallot (Johnson et al., 1975; Linde and Heins, 1960; Geva and Frand, 1988). Equipment, the operating field, and the operative site became contaminated, but with improvements in surgical technique and standards for sterilization, intraoperative contamination decreased. Furthermore, as surgical techniques for complex congenital cyanotic heart disease improved, such lesions became increasingly reported as the underlying lesion in children with endocarditis. From 1930 to 1951, only 5% of children with endocarditis had tetralogy of Fallot, but from 1952 to 1972, 33% had this lesion (Johnson et al., 1975). Cardiac surgery has been shown to *protect* patients from endocarditis. The Natural History Study prospectively followed patients with VSDs, aortic stenosis, and pulmonic stenosis until they were 30 years of age and demonstrated that the risk of endocarditis in unrepaired VSDs was 9.7%, compared with 2% after surgical repair (Gersony and Hayes, 1977).

Despite improvements in surgical techniques for treatment of heart disease, patients can develop endocarditis postoperatively. Postoperative endocarditis is divided into two categories: early postoperative endocarditis, and late postoperative endocarditis (Table 7-1). In adult patients, the use of mechanical prosthetic valves poses an increased risk for development of early postoperative endocarditis when compared with bioprosthetic valves (Mylonakis and Calderwood, 2001), but this conclusion cannot be drawn for children because of the relative rarity of valve replacement. However, children do have extracardiac shunts, valves, stents, and patches placed to repair complex congenital heart disease, and the presence of these foreign materials is a risk factor for endocarditis. There has been an increasing trend to repair the mitral valve rather than to replace it and to use homografts and bioprostheses rather than mechanical valves for aortic valve replacement. Both of

TABLE 7-1	Timing of Early Versus Late Postoperative Endocarditis	
Postoperative category	*Time after surgery*	*Types of pathogens*
Early	<2 months	Hospital-acquired (e.g., coagulase negative staphylococci or *Candida* spp.)
Mixed	2-12 months	Hospital and community acquired
Late	>12 months	Community-acquired (e.g., viridans streptococci)

these trends are associated with a reduced rate of early postoperative endocarditis in adults (Gordon et al., 2000).

More recently, technologic advances in treatment of heart disease have introduced new foreign bodies that put patients at risk for endocarditis. These include left ventricular assist devices, cardioverter-defibrillators, and pacemaker wires and the pacemaker pouch (Arber et al., 1994; Laguno et al., 1998; Klug et al., 1997; Giamarellou, 2002).

Hospital-Acquired (Nosocomial) Endocarditis

Nosocomial endocarditis can occur in seriously ill patients with and without structural heart disease or prosthetic valves as a complication of bloodstream infection from another source such as a central venous catheter, an infection in the genitourinary or gastrointestinal tract, or a wound (Giamarellou, 2002; Gilleece and Fenelon, 2000; Terpenning et al., 1988; Gouello et al., 2000). Several different definitions of nosocomial endocarditis have been used in the literature (Table 7-2). However, the definition of nosocomial endocarditis is complicated by

the often-prolonged incubation period of some pathogens, particularly fungi and molds. Morbidity and mortality are high in patients with nosocomial endocarditis as a result of the presence of comorbid conditions and the subsequent difficulties and delay in diagnosing endocarditis. Endocarditis may not be diagnosed until autopsy (Saiman et al., 1993; Terpenning et al., 1988). The incidence of nosocomial endocarditis appears to be increasing because of an increasing number of patients at risk, as well as the increased survival of such patients (Table 7-3).

Premature Infants

Neonatal endocarditis appears to be increasing in frequency (Saiman et al., 1993; Aspesberro et al., 1999; Pearlman et al., 1998; Zafar et al., 2001; Freeman et al., 1990; Gaynes et al., 1991). In this age group, endocarditis is more often a complication of extreme prematurity, major surgery, and/or the prolonged use of central venous catheters, rather than the result of congenital heart disease. Congenital heart disease is the underlying risk factor in only 30%

TABLE 7-2	Proposed Definitions of Nosocomial Endocarditis	
Timing relative to hospitalization		*Definition*
≥72 hr after admission		Endocarditis occurs 72 hours or more after admission for unrelated condition*
Previous hospitalization within 4-8 weeks		Hospital intervention including cardiac surgery performed 4-8 weeks prior to diagnosis of endocarditis
Prosthetic device placed within 12 months		Endocarditis that develops within 12 months of placement of an implanted prosthetic device‡

*Data from Terpenning MS, Buggy BP, Kauffman CA: Arch Intern Med 1988;148:1601-1603; Friedland G, von Reyn CF, Levy B, et al: Infect Control 1984;5:284-288; and Chen SC, Dwyer DE, Sorrell TC: Am J Cardiol 1992;70:1449-1452.
†Data from Chen SC, Dwyer DE, Sorrell TC: Am J Cardiol 1992;70:1449-1452; and Fernandez-Guerrero ML, Verdejo C, Azofra J, et al: Clin Infect Dis 1995; 20:16-23; and Sobel JD: In Kaye D (ed). Infective endocarditis, ed 2, New York: Raven Press, 1992; 361-373.
‡Data from Emori TG, Culver DH, Horan TC, et al: National nosocomial infections surveillance system (NNIS): description of surveillance methods. Am J Infect Control 1991;19:19-35.

TABLE 7-3	Factors That May Contribute to the Increased Incidence of Nosocomial Endocarditis
Factor	*Etiology of increased incidence*
Nosocomial bloodstream infection	Increased rate of nosocomial bacteremia and fungemia; bloodstream infection is the most frequently occurring hospital-acquired infection in children
Immunocompromised hosts	Increased number of immunocompromised children (e.g., transplant recipients and oncology patients); increased survival rate of such children
Intensive Care Units	Increased number of ICU beds, prolonged hospitalizations, and invasive procedures
Central venous catheters	Increased use of indwelling (e.g., Broviac catheters) and nonindwelling central venous catheters
Preterm infants	Increased number of preterm births and increasing survival of low–birth-weight infants (<1,500 g) and extremely low–birth-weight infants (<1,000 g)

Modified from Giamarellou H: Nosocomial cardiac infections. J Hosp Infect 2002; 50:91-105.

of infants with endocarditis, compared with 70% to 90% of older children (Gaynes et al., 1991). In infants with normal cardiac anatomy, following injury to the endothelium of the right atrium by central venous catheters, endocarditis develops on the right and then promotes thrombus formation. In addition, turbulent blood flow from a patent ductus arteriosus and persistent fetal circulation can cause endovascular damage and thrombus formation (Edwards et al., 1977; Morrow et al., 1982; Symchych et al., 1977; Oelberg et al., 1983). Prolonged hospitalization, use of central venous catheters with frequent manipulations of the catheter and administration set, potentially contaminated infusions, and invasive procedures are risk factors for bacteremia or fungemia. Endocarditis can develop when the sterile thrombus becomes infected during bacteremia or fungemia.

Mitral Valve Prolapse

MVP is a relatively common lesion and a well-known risk factor for endocarditis (Clemens et al., 1982). MVP occurs in about 5% of children (Greenwood, 1984), but not all patients with MVP are at equal risk for endocarditis. Risk factors for endocarditis associated with MVP include the presence of valve thickening and mitral regurgitation (Zuppiroli et al., 1995). It is estimated that the risk of endocarditis occurring in persons with mitral valve insufficiency due to prolapse is 0.1 per 100 subject years (Zuppiroli et al., 1995) or 1.5% to

3% over 20 years (McNamara, 1982). In adult patients with MVP, increased age is associated with increased risk (Zuppiroli et al., 1995).

PATHOGENESIS
Subacute Endocarditis

The pathogenesis of subacute endocarditis has been gleaned from both animal models (Durack et al., 1973) and from human studies of rheumatic carditis (Weinstein and Schlesinger, 1974a; Weinstein and Schlesinger, 1974b; Scheld et al., 1983). During an episode of rheumatic fever, a generalized pancarditis can occur, but valvulitis leads to the most serious sequelae. Valvulitis is the result of an incompletely understood immunopathogenic process that causes valvular thickening with fibrin and inflammatory cells. This initial inflammation organizes to fibrosis, stenosis, and calcification that usually affect the mitral and aortic valve; the tricuspid and pulmonary valves are rarely involved. The resultant valvular stenosis causes turbulent blood flow that damages the endothelium and exposes the collagen beneath the damaged endothelium of the heart wall and valves. Fibrin and platelets are deposited on this collagen, and a sterile thrombus is created. Transient bacteremia with endogenous oral flora (e.g., viridans streptococci) leads to infection of the thrombus, and more platelets and fibrin are deposited over the microbes. Thus, an early and critical event in the pathogenesis of endocarditis is adherence by the infecting microorganisms to the thrombus. Adherence is mediated by several virulence factors including dextran, the platelet aggregating ability of *Streptococcus* and *Staphylococcus* species, and teichoic acid of staphylococci (Scheld et al., 1983).

Acute Endocarditis

The pathogenesis of acute endocarditis has been explained by correlating clinical findings with autopsy findings (Weinstein and Schlesinger, 1974a; Weinstein and Schlesinger, 1974b; Arnett and Roberts; 1976). Unlike subacute endocarditis, which generally occurs in patients with heart disease, 50% to 60% of cases of acute endocarditis occur in patients with normal cardiac anatomy. Initially, an extracardiac site becomes infected, bacteremia occurs, and the heart is then infected. Alternatively, intravenous drug abuse can be associated with bacteremia and right-sided endocarditis. *S. aureus* is a common cause of acute endocarditis, and this pathogen can bind to collagen, fibronectin, laminin, vitronectin, and fibrinogen. However, the bacterial adhesins involved in binding are less well understood. *S. aureus* is a virulent pathogen and can cause extensive valvular destruction and intracardiac extension, including abscesses.

Postoperative Endocarditis

As described previously, cardiac surgery is a risk factor for endocarditis. Early postoperative endocarditis can be caused by intraoperative contamination of the surgical site, the prosthetic valve, conduit, or patch, the bypass pump, and indwelling catheters or it can spread from extracardiac infections. A bacterial capsular polysaccharide adhesin has been implicated in the pathogenesis of prosthetic valve endocarditis caused by *Staphylococcus epidermidis* (Shiro et al., 1995).

The pathogenesis of late postoperative endocarditis is different than that of early postoperative endocarditis, as operative sites are almost completely endothelialized by 6 months (Arnett and Roberts, 1976). Late postoperative infections are similar to those of subacute endocarditis in that endogenous flora, such as streptococci, can infect prosthetic material such as valves, patches, and shunts during transient bacteremia. Patients with prosthetic mechanical valves are at particular risk of developing endocarditis; 1% to 4% of adult patients with mechanical valves develop endocarditis within

the year after valve replacement, and 1% of patients develop endocarditis thereafter (Bayer, 1993).

MICROBIOLOGY

Understanding the different risk factors that are associated with different pathogens can be helpful both diagnostically and therapeutically. Gram-positive cocci such as streptococci, staphylococci, and enterococci are the most common pathogens causing endocarditis. However, there have been changes in the epidemiology of infecting microorganisms resulting from changes in risk factors (Table 7-4). Staphylococci, including *S. aureus* and coagulase-negative staphylococci, have become increasingly common; in some series staphylococcal species have replaced streptococci as the most frequent causes of endocarditis (Saiman et al., 1993; del Pont et al., 1995). Fungal pathogens, particularly *Candida* species, are increasingly common and cause endocarditis more frequently in children than in adults (Mylonakis and Calderwoood, 2001).

Viridans streptococci are the alpha-hemolytic and nonhemolytic endogenous flora of the oral cavity and the gastrointestinal tract. Viridans streptococci are the most common cause of subacute, community-acquired endocarditis in children with congenital or rheumatic heart disease or late postoperative endocarditis. Viridans streptococci include *Streptococcus sanguis*, *Streptococcus bovis*, *Streptococcus mutans*, and *Streptococcus mitis*, and less commonly *Streptococcus salivarius*, *Streptococcus oralis* and others.

S. aureus organisms are normal skin and mucosal flora. Infection with *S. aureus* is a common cause of acute bacterial endocarditis and associated with a high rate of morbidity and mortality. However, *S. aureus* can cause a surprisingly indolent course in children with congenital heart disease (Saiman et al., 1993). *S. aureus* endocarditis is a well-known complication of intravenous drug abuse, and more than one episode of endocarditis may occur in the same patient. It may be difficult to distinguish *S. aureus* bacteremia from endocarditis, as patients with *S. aureus* endocarditis may not always have classic signs and symptoms. In a study of 103 adults with one or more positive blood cultures for *S. aureus*, 26 (25%) had endocarditis (Fowler et al., 1997). However, only 7 of 26 patients had vegetations

TABLE 7-4	Risk Factors and Diagnostics Tests Used to Identify Pathogens Causing Endocarditis	
Pathogen	Risk factors	Diagnostic tests
Viridans streptococci	Rheumatic heart disease Late postoperative endocarditis	Routine blood cultures as media are now supplemented for nutritionally deficient streptococci
S. aureus	Acute endocarditis Neonatal endocarditis Intravenous drug abuse Long-term indwelling catheters	Routine blood cultures
Coagulase-negative staphylococci	Early postoperative endocarditis Hospital-acquired, often in patient with prosthetic valve Rarely infects native valve	Routine blood cultures
Enterococci	Hospital-acquired endocarditis Often secondary to bacteremia from the genitourinary tract	Routine blood cultures
Gram-negative pathogens	Rare, early postoperative endocarditis Rare, hospital-acquired endocarditis *Pseudomonas* in dialysis patients	Routine blood cultures
HACEK organisms: *Haemophilus parainfluenzae,* *Actinobacillus actinomycetemcomitans,* *Cardiobacterium hominis,* *Eikenella corrodens, Kingella kingae*	Native valve Late postoperative endocarditis, particularly of valves	Blood cultures may require prolonged incubation (7-28 days)
Coxiella burnettii (Q fever)	Native valve Postoperative endocarditis	Serologic tests Polymerase chain reaction, Giemsa staining, immunohistology for operative specimens
Bartonella henselae or *B. quintana*		Polymerase chain reaction Prolonged incubation (4 weeks) of cultures processed by lysis-centrifugation
Fungi: *Candida* spp., *Cryptococcus neoformans,* *Histoplasma capsulatum,* *Trichosporon* spp.	Neonatal endocarditis Infected homografts Early postoperative endocarditis Hospital-acquired secondary to central venous catheters, noncardiac surgery, immunosuppression	Routine blood cultures for *Candida*, Lysis-centrifugation for endemic fungi Antigen testing for *Cryptococcus* or *Histoplasma*, serology for *Aspergillus* remains investigational
Molds: *Aspergillus* spp.	Transplant recipients Homografts	Blood cultures rarely positive Cultures of skin lesions and emboli

demonstrated by transthoracic echocardiography (TTE), whereas transesophageal echocardiography (TEE) detected vegetations in an additional 19 patients (Fowler et al., 1997). The distinction between bacteremia and endocarditis is important, as an inadequate duration of therapy for undiagnosed endocarditis may be associated with relapse and increased morbidity and mortality. However, similar studies to distinguish bacteremia from endocarditis due to *S. aureus* have not been performed in children.

Early postoperative endocarditis is usually caused by *S. epidermidis*, other coagulase-negative staphylococci, *S. aureus*, enterococci, fungi, and more rarely, Enterobacteriaceae (Gordon et al., 2000).

Most episodes of nosocomial endocarditis are caused by staphylococcal species including coagulase-negative staphylococci, particularly *S. epidermidis*, and *S. aureus*. Enterococci, particularly *Enterococcus faecalis*, are frequent causes of nosocomial endocarditis, in part as a result of the relatively high incidence of nosocomial bacteremia caused by enterococcal species. Despite the frequency of bacteremia caused by gram-negative pathogens, these organisms are rarely associated with hospital-acquired endocarditis, as they do not adhere well to the endothelium and heart valves. In contrast, fungi, particularly *C. albicans*, are increasingly frequent causes of nosocomial endocarditis, most likely because of the marked increase in candidemia (Saiman et al., 2000; Blumberg et al., 2001). Similarly, molds including *Aspergillus* species are increasingly described causes of nosocomial endocarditis (Giamarellou, 2002; Barst et al., 1981). There have been several case reports of endocarditis caused by *Candida* or *Aspergillus* species due to homografts (Kuehnert et al., 1998; Fedalen et al., 1999). Homografts may become infected because of contaminated preservative fluid, or they may be contaminated intraoperatively. Endocarditis caused by *Aspergillus* species has also been described in transplant recipients secondary to extension from pulmonary or gastrointestinal tract disease (Gilbey et al., 2000; Demaria et al., 2000; Viertel et al., 1999).

There has been an increase in the diagnosis of more unusual pathogens causing endocarditis (Table 7-4). These include the so-called HACEK organisms (*Haemophilus parainfluenzae*, *Actinobacillus actinomycetemcomitans*, *Cardiobacterium hominis*, *Eikenella corrodens*, *Kingella kingae*); *Coxiella burnettii*, the causative agent of Q fever; and *Bartonella* species (Normand et al., 1995). These pathogens are relatively rare in children and often require serologic or molecular diagnosis.

CLINICAL MANIFESTATIONS AND COMPLICATIONS

The clinical manifestations of endocarditis are varied and depend on the infecting organism as well as the site of cardiac involvement. Early complications of endocarditis are unfortunately frequent and include emboli, cardiac, and immunologic phenomenon (Table 7-5). In subacute endocarditis, extracardiac disease is immune mediated, whereas in acute endocarditis extracardiac disease is caused by embolic phenomenon from bulky, friable vegetations. The prognosis of endocarditis is related to the extent of complications.

Subacute Endocarditis

The clinical presentation of subacute endocarditis has been well described and classically includes fever (including fever of unknown origin), malaise, splenomegaly, regurgitant murmur, weight loss, night sweats, and fatigue that may be present for weeks to months. Other prominent features of subacute endocarditis are the immunologic phenomena caused by continuous antigenic stimulation by microorganisms within the vegetation. This antigenic stimulation leads to the formation of circulating immune complexes (Weinstein and Schlesinger, 1974a; Weinstein and Schlesinger, 1974b) that can deposit in the skin, kidney, and retina, and cause the classic clinical manifestations of subacute endocarditis. These include: (1) Roth's spots located on the optic disk, (2) Janeway lesions, which are nontender nodules noted at the pulp of the fingers or thenar eminence, (3) Osler's nodes, which are tender, erythematous, hemorrhagic, or pustular lesions, (4) conjunctival or mucosal petechiae, (5) splinter hemorrhages located beneath the fingernails or toenails, and (6) glomerulonephritis (Mylonakis and Calderwood, 2001; Weinstein and Schlesinger, 1974a; Weinstein and Schlesinger, 1974b; Scheld et al., 1983). Thus, meticulous examination of the skin, extremities, and retina should always be performed in patients with suspected endocarditis.

TABLE 7-5	Early Phase Complications of Endocarditis	
Type of complication	Site	Description
Embolic	Central nervous system	Stroke, hemiparesis, intraventricular hemorrhage
	Extremities	Cool, painful, pulseless limb or digit
	Coronary arteries	Myocardial ischemia, congestive heart failure
	Spleen	Prolonged fever, pleuritic pain, shoulder pain
	Kidneys	Hematuria, sterile pyuria
	Lungs	Shortness of breath, chest pain, hemoptysis
Cardiac	Valvular insufficiency	Papillary muscle or chordae tendineae rupture
	Myocardial abscess	Prolonged fever
	Dehiscence of annular ring	Congestive heart failure
	Conduction abnormalities	Arrhythmias
Immunologic	Skin or mucous membranes	Petechiae, splinter hemorrhages,
	Digits	Janeway lesions, Osler's nodes
	Ocular	Roth's spots, conjunctival hemorrhages
	Glomerulonephritis	Low complement (C3,C4), proteinuria, hematuria

Acute Endocarditis

Acute endocarditis is a fulminant process marked by a new murmur, congestive heart failure caused by valvular destruction, sepsis, and systemic emboli. Left-sided endocarditis may cause emboli in the central nervous system, the extremities, the liver and spleen, the kidneys, and occasionally the coronary arteries. Embolic phenomenon may be the presenting sign or symptom of endocarditis. Of 260 adults with endocarditis caused by S. aureus, 61 (23%) presented with neurologic symptoms (Røder et al., 1997a; Røder et al., 1997b). Right-sided endocarditis may cause emboli in the lungs unless a right-to-left intracardiac shunt exists.

Nosocomial Endocarditis

The clinical presentations of nosocomial endocarditis in the neonate, in surgical patients in the early postoperative period, or in critically ill patients are not generally suggestive of endocarditis. Patients rarely have the immunologic or embolic phenomena that are noted in patients with subacute and acute endocarditis. Furthermore, the comorbid conditions of such patients are often complicated by symptoms (such as fever, hypotension, tachycardia, drug rashes, and edema) that make the clinical diagnosis of endocarditis even less straightforward. Although patients with nosocomial endocarditis almost always have positive blood cultures, it can be difficult to distinguish endocarditis from more common clinical entities such as

bacteremia or sepsis. Persistently positive blood cultures, particularly after removal of a central venous catheter, a new murmur, embolic phenomenon, or cardiac failure are clues that point to endocarditis.

EMBOLIC PHENOMENON

Emboli may occur before, during or after antibiotic treatment, although as reported in adults, emboli are more common before effective antimicrobial therapy has been started and during the first week of treatment (Bayer, 1993). Emboli are rare after 2 weeks of treatment (Steckelberg et al., 1991) and more common with endocarditis caused by S. aureus (Røder et al., 1997a; Røder et al., 1997b; Tornos et al., 1999) and fungi (Ellis et al., 2001). Emboli present in different ways, depending on the site involved (Table 7-5). Septic emboli can cause mycotic aneurysms in the artery intima and vessel wall. The clinical manifestations of a mycotic aneurysm range from headache and meningeal irritation to an intracranial hemorrhage. Thus, daily physical examinations, including the evaluation of neurologic status, must be performed.

DIAGNOSIS

Endocarditis is a syndrome, and therefore its diagnosis depends on a constellation of signs and symptoms. The diagnosis of endocarditis is not always straightforward and may require a high index of clinical suspicion. Two sets of criteria have been developed to diagnose endocarditis in adults: von Reyn's criteria (von Reyn et al., 1981) and Duke University's criteria (Durack et al., 1994). In each set of criteria, the diagnosis of endocarditis is based on a combination of diagnostic evaluations such as histopathology, autopsy findings, or echocardiography; blood cultures; and supportive laboratory data such as elevated sedimentation rate, anemia, or abnormal urine analysis. Each set of criteria grades the likelihood of endocarditis (e.g., definite, probable, possible, or unlikely) depending on the signs and symptoms present.

The earlier (von Reyn's) criteria required intraoperative histopathology or autopsy findings to make a definitive diagnosis of endocarditis. To remedy the omission of echocardiographic findings used to assist in the diagnosis of endocarditis, the Duke criteria included the results of echocardiograms. The Duke criteria have been independently validated by other investigators and found to have a high degree of predictive value (Bayer, 1993; Bayer et al., 1998; Bayer et al., 1994; Hoen et al., 1995). The Duke diagnostic criteria have also been validated in children with suspected endocarditis and proved superior to the von Reyn criteria (del Pont et al., 1995). Suggestions to modify the Duke criteria have recently been made which incorporate the use of TEE to distinguish *S. aureus* bacteremia from endocarditis and the use of serology to diagnose Q fever caused by *C. burnettii* (Li et al., 2000). The criteria proposed by Li et al. use a combination of major and minor criteria to diagnose definite or possible endocarditis (Table 7-6). In this proposed modification,

TABLE 7-6	Modified Duke Criteria for the Diagnosis of Endocarditis	
Criteria	*Comments*
Major Criteria	
Microbiologic	Typical microorganisms isolated from ≥2 blood cultures: Viridans streptococci HACEK organisms *Staphylococcus aureus* Community-acquired enterococci *or* Persistently positive blood cultures *or* *Coxiella burnettii* detected in ≥1 blood culture or antiphase titer IgG > 1:800
Endocardial involvement	New regurgitant murmur *or* Findings on echocardiogram including: Echogenic, oscillating intracardiac mass Periannular abscess New dehiscence of prosthetic valve
Minor Criteria	
Predisposing risk factors for endocarditis	*High risk:* previous endocarditis, aortic valve disease, rheumatic heart disease, prosthetic valve, coarctation, complex cyanotic heart disease *Moderate risk:* mitral valve prolapse (regurgitation or valve thickening), mitral stenosis, tricuspid disease, pulmonary stenosis, cardiomyopathy *Low/no risk:* atrial septal defect, ischemic heart disease, coronary artery bypass surgery, mitral valve prolapse without regurgitation or thickening
Clinical manifestations	Fever Vascular phenomenon (e.g., emboli, intracranial hemorrhage, Janeway lesions) Immunologic phenomenon (e.g., glomerulonephritis, rheumatoid factor)
Microbiologic manifestations	Single positive blood culture (except coagulase-negative staphylococci or gram-negative bacilli) or serologic evidence of active infection with organism associated with endocarditis

Modified from Li JS, Sexton DJ, Mick N, et al: Clin Infect Diseases 2000;30:633-638.

"definite endocarditis" is diagnosed if two major criteria, one major plus three minor criteria, or five minor criteria are present; "possible endocarditis" is diagnosed if one major and one minor criteria or three minor criteria are present.

Blood Cultures

Blood cultures are the most important diagnostic test for endocarditis (Washington, 1982). Ninety percent of patients with endocarditis have positive blood cultures. At least two sets of blood cultures should be obtained within 2 hours from clinically stable patients using different venipuncture sites, and three sets of blood cultures should be obtained within minutes from patients who are clinically unstable (e.g., hypotensive). Microorganisms are not more likely to be recovered from arterial blood cultures than from venous blood cultures.

Approximately 5% to 15% of patients are diagnosed with culture-negative endocarditis (Walterspiel and Kaplan, 1986). The most common reasons for culture-negative endocarditis are antecedent antibiotics or endocarditis caused by less common, fastidious organisms that are difficult to culture and whose identification requires special diagnostic techniques such as polymerase chain reaction (PCR), serology, special media or growth conditions, or prolonged incubation (Table 7-4). It is imperative to inform the clinical microbiology laboratory that endocarditis is being considered to ensure appropriate handling and testing of the diagnostic specimens. The use of broad-range PCR amplification using the 16S rRNA gene from bacteria and 18S and 28S rRNA from fungi has been studied recently (Millar et al., 2001; Goldenberger et al., 1997). Unfortunately, these molecular tools are still investigational.

Echocardiography

TTE revolutionized the diagnosis of endocarditis almost three decades ago by visualizing vegetations and diagnosing valvular abnormalities. However, only 70% to 80% of children diagnosed with endocarditis have visible vegetations (Geva and Frand, 1988; del Pont et al., 1995; Bricker et al., 1985). Results of TTE may be negative, as vegetations smaller than 2 mm cannot be visualized. Preexisting valvular abnormalities or palliative shunts may obscure vegetations. Obesity and chest wall deformities can lead to false-negative TTE results.

TEE has been used with increased frequency to diagnose endocarditis in adult populations. TEE can improve the visualization of vegetations <5 mm, valvular abnormalities, intracardiac abscesses, periannular complications, and intracardiac anatomy in patients with chest wall abnormalities, obesity, recent cardiothoracic surgery, or prosthetic valves (Bayer, 1993; Bayer et al., 1994; Bayer et al., 1998; Rohmann et al., 1995; Lindner et al., 1996). Although there are numerous reports describing the use of TEE to assess intraoperative cardiac repairs in children, TEE has rarely been used to diagnosis endocarditis in children because of technical limitations of the probe size and the relative invasiveness of the procedure.

Ancillary Tests

Several ancillary tests may be used to assist in the diagnosis of endocarditis. Children with suspected endocarditis should have a complete blood count, a sedimentation rate, a urine analysis, liver function tests, and an electrocardiogram. Complement levels and rheumatoid factor may be diagnostically useful in subacute cases of endocarditis, and the latter test may serve as minor criterion in the diagnosis.

TREATMENT OF ENDOCARDITIS
General Principles

Treatment of endocarditis with prolonged courses of parenteral antimicrobial agents remains the cornerstone of therapy (Wilson et al., 1995; Fleming, 1987; Besnier and Choutet, 1995). Daily monitoring of hemodynamic status, careful observation for embolic complications, and, when indicated, timely surgical intervention are critical to ensure the best possible outcome. Optimal management often depends on collaboration among several subspecialists, including infectious disease physicians, cardiologists, cardiothoracic surgeons, neurologists, and the clinical microbiology laboratory staff. Bactericidal, not bacteriostatic, antibiotics are used because the organisms within the infected thrombus grow slowly; antibiotics do not diffuse well into the thrombus; and complement, antibodies, and inflammatory cells are often excluded from the avascular thrombus. Adequate therapy requires higher, more sustained blood levels, usually with more than one agent. Duration of therapy is guided by duration of symptoms before diagnosis, the presence of prosthetic material, and complications.

Initial antimicrobial management may be empiric until a causative agent is identified. The initial choice of antimicrobial agents is guided by (1) the risk factors of the infected patient, (2) the clinical presentation, (3) the presence of prosthetic material, and (4) the epidemiology of antibiotic resistance in specific settings (e.g., intensive care units). Antibiotic therapy is modified when the pathogen is identified and antibiotic susceptibilities are determined.

Serum cidal levels are no longer recommended when treating a patient with endocarditis. Standardized laboratory methods have not been developed for this assay and, in general, results are not correlated with clinical outcome. However, vancomycin and/or gentamicin levels need to be determined and monitored if the patient has renal insufficiency, if renal function changes, or if concomitant nephrotoxic drugs are used.

Empiric Antibiotic Therapy

As described previously, two or more blood cultures must be obtained prior to starting empiric antimicrobial treatment. Subacute endocarditis in a child with rheumatic heart disease can be treated initially with penicillin and gentamicin. Empiric antimicrobial therapy for community-acquired endocarditis should include three agents; penicillin; a semisynthetic β-lactam agent, such as oxacillin (or nafcillin); and low-dose gentamicin. Community-acquired methicillin-resistant *S. aureus* (MRSA) is increasingly common, even in patients without traditional risk factors including previous hospitalizations (Gorak et al., 1999; Centers for Disease Control and Prevention, 1999). Thus, vancomycin can be used in place of penicillin and oxacillin in patients with type I hypersensitivity reactions to penicillin or if community-acquired MRSA is of concern. However, vancomycin should be used with caution. Vancomycin has been shown to be a less effective agent against *S. aureus* than semisynthetic penicillins (Wilson et al., 1995) Overuse has also been strongly associated with the growing problem of vancomycin-resistant enterococci, and most recently vancomycin-resistant *S. aureus* has been described (Centers for Disease Control and Prevention, 2002).

DRUG REGIMENS FOR SPECIFIC PATHOGENS

Following identification and susceptibility testing of the pathogen, antibiotic therapy can be

modified, when appropriate. Treatment recommendations for endocarditis in children are largely derived from treatment recommendations for adults with endocarditis, although adults may have different risk factors such as calcified or artificial valves, intravenous drug abuse, or higher rates of rheumatic fever (Wilson et al., 1995). However, these recommendations have been supported by case series and anecdotal experience treating endocarditis in children. An overview of treatment regimens for the most frequent causes of endocarditis is shown in Table 7-7.

Streptococci

Viridans streptococci are often highly susceptible to penicillin with minimum inhibitory concentration (MIC) values ≤0.1 µg/ml. Treatment regimens for uncomplicated endocarditis without foreign bodies are as follows: 4 weeks of penicillin G or 4 weeks of ceftriaxone alone. Once treatment has been initiated in the hospital and the patient is stable, antibiotics can be successfully completed in the outpatient setting (Francioli et al., 1992). A 2-week course of penicillin G and gentamicin has proven successful for treatment of endocarditis of a native valve without complications (i.e., no intracardiac extension or abscesses). Cure rates of 98% have been obtained with all three medical regimens. These recommendations also apply to *S. bovis*, but this is a very infrequent cause of pediatric endocarditis. Vancomycin can replace penicillin in patients with documented type I hypersensitivity allergy to β-lactam agents.

Streptococci are considered relatively resistant to penicillin if the MIC is >0.1 µg/ml and ≤0.5 µg/ml. Patients infected with these organisms should be treated with 4 weeks of penicillin G and 2 weeks of gentamicin. There are not adequate data to support the use of single daily dosing of aminoglycosides for treatment of endocarditis. Resistant streptococci, including nutritionally variant streptococci, defined by MIC of >0.5 µg/ml, should be treated using regimens similar to those for enterococcal endocarditis (Besneir and Choutet, 1995).

Enterococci

Treatment of enterococcal endocarditis has become increasingly complex as multidrug-resistant strains of enterococci with high levels of resistance to penicillin, gentamicin,

TABLE 7-7	Antimicrobial Treatment Regimens for Endocarditis in Children	
Pathogen	Native valves—no foreign material	Prosthetic valves—foreign material
Viridans streptococci or other *Streptococcus* spp. that are penicillin susceptible (penicillin MIC ≤ 0.1 μg/ml)	Penicillin G for 4 weeks *or* Ceftriaxone for 4 weeks *Alternative regimen:* Penicillin or ceftriaxone and gentamicin for 2 weeks if uncomplicated course	Penicillin G for 6 weeks and Gentamicin for 2 weeks
Streptococci that are relatively resistant to penicillin (penicillin MIC >0.1 to ≤0.5 μg/ml)	Penicillin G for 4 weeks and Gentamicin for 2 weeks	Penicillin G for 6 weeks and Gentamicin for 4 weeks
Streptococci that are resistant to penicillin (MIC >0.5 μg/ml) Enterococci that are susceptible to penicillin	Penicillin G (or ampillicin) and Gentamicin for 4-6 weeks *6 weeks if longer duration of symptoms (>3 months) or complications*	Penicillin G (or ampillicin) and gentamicin for 6 weeks
Methicillin–susceptible*; *S. aureus* or coagulase-negative staphylococci	Oxacillin (or nafcillin) for 4-6 weeks and gentamicin for 3-5 days	Oxacillin (or nafcillin) for 6 weeks and rifampin for 6 weeks and gentamicin for 2 weeks
Methicillin-resistant *S. aureus* or coagulase-negative staphylococci	Vanocomycin for 4-6 weeks and gentamicin for 3-5 days	Vancomycin for 6 weeks and rifampin for 6 weeks and gentamicin for 2 weeks *If resistant to gentamicin, select another ant-staphylococcal agent on the basis of in vitro susceptibilities*

Modified from Mylonakis E, Calderwood SB: N Engl J Med 2001;345:1318-1330.
*Applies to enterococci that are susceptible to penicillin.

vancomycin, and/or linezolid have been documented (Murray, 2000; Gonzales et al., 2001). Enterococcal endocarditis caused by strains susceptible to penicillin should be treated for 6 weeks with penicillin (or ampicillin) and low-dose gentamicin. If the strain exhibits high-level resistance to gentamicin, susceptibility to streptomycin should be determined, as resistance is encoded by different aminoglycoside-modifying enzymes. Strains resistant to penicillin are generally susceptible to vancomycin, but vancomycin resistance is well documented, particularly in *E. faecium*. Management of vancomycin-resistant endocarditis is limited to case reports and animal models, which suggest that multidrug regimens (Francioli et al., 1992; Landman et al., 1995; Landman et al., 1996) may be successful (Patel et al., 2001).

Streptococcus Pneumoniae, Streptococcus pyogenes, *and Other F streptococci.* Other streptococcal species such as *S. pneumoniae, S. pyogenes*, and group B streptococci are rela-

tively rare causes of endocarditis. Management is guided by antimicrobial susceptibilities as streptococci, including the pneumococci, have become increasingly resistant to penicillin. Treatment of endocarditis caused by pneumococci with intermediate or high resistance to penicillin is derived from treatment of other infections caused by *S. pneumoniae*. Pneumococci with an MIC to penicillin ≤0.1 μg/ml can be treated with penicillin alone. Intermediately resistant strains (those with MIC between 0.1 and 1.0 μg/ml), can be managed with a third-generation cephalosporin (e.g., ceftriaxone or cefotaxime). Resistant strains with an MIC ≥2 μg/ml that cause central nervous system involvement should be managed with vancomycin and a third-generation cephalosporin (McCracken, 1995). Some experts recommend the addition of an aminoglycoside for treatment of group B, C, and G streptococci.

S. Aureus *and Coagulase-Negative* Staphylococci. Treatment of *S. aureus* endocarditis is also complex and is guided by several considerations, including antibiotic susceptibility, location (i.e., right-sided versus left-sided disease), the presence of prosthetic valves or material, and/or the occurrence of embolic events or intracardiac extension. Antimicrobial therapy should be continued for 6 weeks or occasionally longer in patients with a slow clinical response or complications such as persistently positive blood culture, intracardiac extension, valve replacement, or embolic phenomena. Rifampin should be added if prosthetic material is present or a myocardial abscess is diagnosed. Data suggest that intravenous drug addicts with right-sided endocarditis of native valves caused by methicillin-susceptible *S. aureus* can be successfully treated with oxacillin and gentamicin for 2 weeks provided there are no complications and the vegetation is smaller than 1 to 2 cm (Chambers et al., 1988; Hecht and Berger, 1992). Treatment recommendations for coagulase-negative staphylococci are similar to those used for treatment of *S. aureus* (Wilson et al., 1995). The majority of cases of coagulase negative staphylococci occur in the postoperative setting associated with infection of prosthetic materials.

Fungal Endocarditis

Management of fungal endocarditis requires both medical and surgical treatment (Ellis et al., 2001). Amphotericin B is used to treat endocarditis arising from either *Candida* or *Aspergillus* species. The toxicities of amphotericin are considerable, and the patient's renal function, electrolytes, and blood counts must be carefully monitored during the prolonged antimicrobial course. However, it is unknown if lipid-associated amphotericin products are more effective than conventional amphotericin for the treatment of endocarditis. Lipid-associated amphotericin (e.g., Abelcet or Ambisome), although costly, is associated with less toxicity, and higher dosages may be tolerated (Melamed et al., 2000). Surgical excision of the vegetation and removal of the prosthetic valve have been widely recommended. Recurrence among survivors is unfortunately common; 30% may have another episode of fungal endocarditis. Some experts recommend the use of fluconazole for at least 2 years after apparent cure of endocarditis caused by *Candida* and the use of itraconazole for fungi and molds resistant to fluconazole (Ellis et al., 2001) to prevent

relapse by presumed residual foci of fungi (Muehrcke et al., 1995). However, there are several case reports of children, including premature infants, with inoperable fungal endocarditis who survived with medical management alone (Sanchez et al., 1991; Aspesberro et al., 1999; Mayayo et al., 1996). In adult patients, surgery improves survival. Even when managed both surgically and medically, fungal endocarditis carries a mortality rate of 50% to 90% (Ellis et al., 2001). Newer agents such as caspofungin and voriconazole may prove more effective in treating endocarditis Caused by Candida or Aspergillus spp., respectively.

Culture-Negative Endocarditis

Therapy of community-acquired, culture-negative endocarditis should include ampicillin, oxacillin, and low-dose gentamicin. If there has been recent cardiac surgery, vancomycin should be used instead of oxacillin. As described in Table 7-4, all efforts should be made to identify the etiologic agent, as it is very difficult to design effective empiric regimens given the wide variety of potential pathogens. Continual surveillance of the clinical course is imperative to demonstrate response to the initial choice of antimicrobial agents (Kupferwasser and Bayer, 2000). In a clinically stable patient with culture-negative endocarditis, antibiotics can be discontinued for 4 to 5 days, and repeat diagnostic studies, including blood cultures, can be obtained (Bayer, 1993; Bayer et al., 1998; Bayer et al., 1994).

Anticoagulant Therapy

Anticoagulant therapy has not been shown to reduce the incidence of embolic complications and may *increase* the risk of intracranial hemorrhage. In a review of 56 adult patients with left-sided endocarditis, 21 had prosthetic valves; of the 21, 19 were being managed with oral anticoagulant therapy when they were diagnosed with endocarditis (Tornos et al., 1999). Central nervous system and embolic complications were comparable in patients with native versus prosthetic valve endocarditis. However, mortality was higher in patients with prosthetic valves because of central nervous system complications, particularly stroke. Thus, anticoagulant therapy should be used with great caution in patients being anticoagulated prior to the diagnosis of endocarditis of a prosthetic valve. Anticoagulation should be stopped in patients with endocarditis caused by *S. aureus* during the initial phase of illness or if central nervous system complications occur (Mylonakis and Calderwoood, 2001). In an experimental model of catheter-induced *S. aureus* endocarditis in rabbits, acetylsalicylic acid reduced the size of vegetations and the rate of embolization, presumably because of antiplatelet effects and the reduction of bacterial binding to exposed collages (Kupferwasser et al., 1999). Clinical studies with aspirin have not been performed.

SURGICAL MANAGEMENT

Surgical intervention is often necessary to effectively manage endocarditis. Surgery may be performed during the acute episode of endocarditis; this is termed *early-phase surgery* by some authors. Alternatively, surgery may be performed within 3 months of antibiotic treatment (termed *recent surgery*) or after 3 months of treatment (termed *late-phase surgery*) (Acar et al., 1995). Surgery may be performed to correct valvular dysfunction, to excise tissue that cannot be sterilized, to remove intracardiac abscesses, to close interventricular fistulas, or to remove vegetations that are sources of emboli (Acar et al., 1995).

The indications for early phase surgical treatment of endocarditis are often categorized as absolute indications or relative indications. Absolute indications include (1) intractable heart failure secondary to valvular obstruction, (2) prosthetic valve dehiscence, (3) fungal endocarditis, (4) persistently positive blood cultures for more than 1 week despite appropriate antibiotics accompanied by signs of heart failure due to valvular dysfunction, and (5) intracardiac extension causing myocardial abscess, or rupture of the papillary muscles, chorda tendineae, or ventricular septum. Early postoperative prosthetic valve endocarditis is usually an indication for valve replacement. In adults with early postoperative endocarditis, patients who underwent both surgical and medical management had improved survival, but unstable patients may not have been considered surgical candidates (Gordon et al., 2000).

One of the most difficult management decisions is whether or not to surgically remove the vegetation. The presence of large vegetation, even when present on the left side of the heart, is *not* an absolute indication for surgery. Size alone is not predictive of embolic complications, and, except in the case of fungal endocarditis, the type of infecting organism does not dictate surgery. However, left-sided embolic events, particularly those to the central nervous system, do represent a relative indication for surgery. Because of the surgical risks associated with endocarditis, many experts wait until a second embolic event occurs before recommending surgery.

Many patients who have been successfully treated for endocarditis will require valve replacement (Cabell and Peterson, 2001). As many as 47% of adults with endocarditis will require late-phase surgery despite microbiologic cure of endocarditis, and most will undergo valve replacement within the first 2 years after treatment. Although these are data from adult studies, children with endocarditis may also require late-phase valve replacement (Saiman et al., 1993).

PROGNOSIS

The outcome for children with endocarditis appears to be improving but depends largely on the pathogen. Mortality rates in the 1950s and 1960s were as high as 38% (Zakrewski and Keith, 1965). In the late 1970s and 1980s, the mortality rates in published series of endocarditis in pediatrics patients ranged from 14% to 22%, and more recent studies have shown mortality rates ranging from 5% to 11% (Saiman et al., 1993; Normand et al., 1995). Streptococcal endocarditis is associated with excellent outcomes and minimal mortality. Increased morbidity and mortality are associated with endocarditis caused by *S. aureus*, gram-negative bacilli, fungi, or molds. Younger infants also have a higher risk of morbidity and mortality. In a small study of long-term follow-up of children after endocarditis, the majority of patients were hemodynamically stable up to 27 years after their episode of endocarditis (Fisher et al., 1985).

Relapse and recurrences do occur (Table 7-8). Relapse with the same pathogen occurs in approximately 2% to 3% of adult patients (Mansur et al., 2001) and most often occurs in patients with complex congenital, cyanotic heart disease with prosthetic valves and shunts. Recurrences with different pathogens or >6 months after treatment for the initial episode occurs in approximately 10% of adults and 5% to 10% of children.

PREVENTION

Prophylactic administration of antibiotics to prevent endocarditis is recommended for

TABLE 7-8	Late Complications of Endocarditis in Adults	
Complication	Adult patients (%)	Comment
Valve replacement	20-47	Earlier valve replacement may reduce late valve replacement and mortality*
Relapse	1-3	Defined as episode of endocarditis with same organism ≤6 months after initial episode Increased risk among older adults
Recurrence	10	Defined as episode of endocarditis with different organism or >6 months after initial episode Increased risk among older adults
10-year mortality	23-80	Higher mortality found in studies conducted before 1980s.[†] Older age and recurrent endocarditis are risk factors for death.

*Data from Castillo JC, Anguita MP, Ramirez A, et al: Heart 2000;83:525-530; and Peric M, Vuk F, Huskic R, et al: Cardiovasc Surg 2000;8:208-213.
[†]Data from Cabell CH, Peterson GE: Am Heart J 2001;141:6-8; and Cabell CH, Jollis JG, Peterson GE, et al: Changing patient characteristics and the effect on mortality in endocarditis. Arch Intern Med 2002;162:90-94.

patients with cardiac lesions that are risk factors for endocarditis who are undergoing procedures that are potentially associated with transient bacteremia with gram-positive cocci such as streptococcal, enterococcal, or staphylococcal organisms. Thus, host factors, ability of organisms to adhere to sterile thrombi, and risk of transient bacteremia have been considered when developing prophylactic regimes (Moreillon, 2000; Dajani et al., 1997). The most recent recommendations for prophylaxis by the American Heart Association have simplified the regimens, clarified the lesions that represent the highest risk (Table 7-9), and shortened the list of procedures for which prophylaxis is indicated (Table 7-10). Prophylaxis

TABLE 7-9	Conditions That Put Patients at Risk for Endocarditis
Condition	Comments
Highest Risk	
Prosthetic valves	Includes bioprosthetic and homograft valves
Previous endocarditis	Bacterial or fungal
Complex congenital cyanotic heart disease	VSD, transposition of the great vessels, tetralogy of Fallot
Systemic pulmonary shunts or conduits	Surgically constructed
Moderate Risk	
Other congenital heart disease	Uncorrected VSD, PDA, ASD, coarctation, bicuspid aortic valve
Acquired valvular dysfunction	Rheumatic heart or collagen vascular disease with residual valvular dysfunction
Hypertrophic cardiomyopathy	
Mitral valve prolapse	With valvular regurgitation or thickened leaflets
Low or No Risk	
ASD	
Surgical repair of ASD, VSD, PDA	>6 months after surgery
Cardiac pacemakers	Intravascular or epicardial
Previous Kawasaki disease	Without valvular dysfunction

Modified from Dajani AS, Taubert KA, Wilson W, et al: Circulation 1997;96:358-366.
VSD, Ventricular septal defect; *PDA,* patent ductus arteriosus; *ASD,* atrial septal defect.

TABLE 7-10	Procedures Requiring Prophylaxis and Prophylactic Regimens for Endocarditis		
Type of procedure	Description of procedure	Recommended regimen	Alternative regimen if patient is allergic to penicillin
Dental or oral	Associated with bleeding, e.g., cleaning by dental hygienist, extractions, initial placement of orthodontic bands	Amoxicillin 50 mg/kg po 1 h before procedure Maximum 2 g	Clindamycin Cephalexin Azithromycin Clarithromycin
Esophageal	Stricture dilatation Sclerotherapy of esophageal varices	Same as for dental and oral procedures	
Respiratory	Rigid bronchoscopy, tonsillectomy, adenoidectomy, Surgery involving respiratory mucosa	Same as for dental and oral procedures	
Gastrointestinal	Biliary tract surgery Surgery that involves the intestinal mucosa	Ampicillin 50 mg/kg, maximum 2 g within 30 min Ampicillin 25 mg/kg 6 h later *Add gentamicin 1.5 mg/kg (maximum 120 mg) within 30 min of procedure for patients at high risk; no second dose recommended*	Vancomycin 20 mg/kg IV, maximum 2 g within 30 min *(No second dose recommended)*
Genitourinary	Cystoscopy Urethral dilatation	Same as for gastrointestinal procedures	

does not appear to reduce bacteremia, but rather antimicrobial prophylaxis appears to kill the microbes that adhere to the damaged endothelium. Thus, effective prophylaxis requires a prolonged concentration of antibiotics at concentrations above the MIC. Recommendations are continually being updated, and physicians should review the literature periodically (http://www.americanheart.org/Scientific/Statme nts/1997/07970L.html). However, most of the studies of prophylaxis have been performed in animal models, and their conclusions have not been supported by clinical trials. It is unlikely, because of ethical concerns, that such a trial will ever be performed. Furthermore, most of the episodes of endocarditis are not preceded by an antecedent event for which prophylaxis would be prescribed and are attributed to transient bacteremia caused by chewing, teeth brushing, defecating or other everyday events. Thus, good dental hygiene and the prevention of gingivitis may be an important preventive strategy. Despite these limitations, antimicrobial prophy-

laxis to prevent endocarditis has been established as routine medical practice.

BIBLIOGRAPHY

Acar J, Michel PL, Varenne O, et al. Surgical treatment of infective endocarditis. Eur Heart J 1995;16(suppl B): 94-98.

Arber N, Pras E, Copperman Y, et al. Pacemaker endocarditis. Report of 44 cases and review of the literature. Medicine (Baltimore) 1994;73:299-305.

Arnett EN, Roberts WC. Prosthetic valve endocarditis: clinicopathologic analysis of 22 necropsy patients with comparison observations in 74 necropsy patients with active infective endocarditis involving natural left-sided cardiac valves. Am J Cardiol 1976;38:281-292.

Aspesberro F, Beghetti M, Oberhansli I, et al. Fungal endocarditis in critically ill children. Eur J Pediatr 1999;158:275-280.

Barst RJ, Prince AS, Neu HC. *Aspergillus* endocarditis in children: case report and review of the literature. Pediatrics 1981;68:73-78.

Bayer AS. Infective endocarditis. Clin Infect Dis 1993;17:313-322.

Bayer AS, Bolger AF, Taubert KA, et al. Diagnosis and management of infective endocarditis and its complications. Circulation 1998;98:2936-2948.

Bayer AS, Ward JI, Ginzton LE, et al. Evaluation of new clinical criteria for the diagnosis of infective endocarditis. Am J Med 1994;96:211-219.

Besnier JM, Choutet P. Medical treatment of infective endocarditis: general principles. Eur Heart J 1995;16(suppl B):72-74.

Bitar FF, Jawdi RA, Dbaibo GS, et al. Paediatric infective endocarditis: 19-year experience at a tertiary care hospital in a developing country. Acta Paediatr 2000;89:427-430.

Blumberg HM, Jarvis WR, Soucie JM, et al. Risk factors for candidal bloodstream infections in surgical intensive care unit patients: the NEMIS prospective multicenter study. The National Epidemiology of Mycosis Survey. Clin Infect Dis 2001;33:177-186.

Blumenthal S, Griffiths SP, Morgan SP. Bacterial endocarditis in children with heart disease: a review based on the literature and experience with 58 cases. Pediatrics 1960;26:993.

Bricker JT, Latson LA, Huhta JC, et al. Echocardiographic evaluation of infective endocarditis in children. Clin Pediatr (Phila) 1985;24:312-317.

Cabell CH, Jollis JG, Peterson GE, et al. Changing patient characteristics and the effect on mortality in endocarditis. Arch Internal Med 2002;162:90-94.

Cabell CH, Peterson GE. Factors affecting long-term mortality in endocarditis: the bugs, the drugs, the knife or the patients? Am Heart J 2001;141:6-8.

Caldwell RL, Hurwitz RA, Girod DA. Subacute bacterial endocarditis in children. Current status. Am J Dis Child 1971;122:312-315.

Castillo JC, Anguita MP, Ramirez A, et al. Long term outcome of infective endocarditis in patients who were not drug addicts: a 10 year study. Heart 2000;83:525-530.

Centers for Disease Control and Prevention. Four pediatric deaths from community-acquired methicillin-resistant Staphylococcus aureus—Minnesota and North Dakota, 1997-1999. JAMA 1999;282:1123-1125.

Centers for Disease Control and Prevention. Staphylococcus aureus resistant to vancomycin—United States, 2002. MMWR 2002;51:565-566.

Chambers HF, Miller RT, Newman MD. Right-sided Staphylococcus aureus endocarditis in intravenous drug abusers: two-week combination therapy. Ann Intern Med 1988;109:619-624.

Chen SC, Dwyer DE, Sorrell TC. A comparison of hospital and community-acquired infective endocarditis. Am J Cardiol 1992;70:1449-1452.

Clemens JD, Horwitz RI, Jaffe CC, et al. A controlled evaluation of the risk of bacterial endocarditis in persons with mitral-valve prolapse. N Engl J Med 1982;307:776-781.

Cutler JG, Ongley PA, Shwachman H, et al. Bacterial endocarditis in children with heart disease. Pediatrics 1958;22:706-713.

Dajani AS, Taubert KA, Wilson W, et al. Prevention of bacterial endocarditis. Recommendations by the American Heart Association. Circulation 1997;96:358-366.

del Pont JM, de Cicco LT, Vartalitis C, et al. Infective endocarditis in children: clinical analyses and evaluation of two diagnostic criteria. Pediatr Infect Dis J 1995;14:1079-1086.

Demaria RG, Durrleman N, Rispail P, et al. Aspergillus flavus mitral valve endocarditis after lung abscess. J Heart Valve Dis 2000;9:786-790.

Dhawan A, Grover A, Marwaha RK, et al. Infective endocarditis in children: profile in a developing country. Ann Trop Paediatr 1993;13:189-194.

Durack DT, Beeson PB, Petersdorf RG: Experimental bacterial endocarditis. 3. Production and progress of the disease in rabbits. Br J Exp Pathol 1973;54:142-151.

Durack DT, Lukes AS, Bright DK. New criteria for diagnosis of infective endocarditis: utilization of specific echocardiographic findings. Duke Endocarditis Service. Am J Med 1994;96:200-209.

Edwards K, Ingall D, Czapek E, et al. Bacterial endocarditis in 4 young infants. Is this complication on the increase? Clin Pediatr (Phila) 1977;16:607-609.

Ellis ME, Al-Abdely H, Sandridge A, et al. Fungal endocarditis: evidence in world literature, 1965-1995. Clin Infect Dis 2001;32:50-62.

Emori TG, Culver DH, Horan TC, et al. National nosocomial infections surveillance system (NNIS): description of surveillance methods. Am J Infect Control 1991;19:19-35.

Fedalen PA, Fisher CA, Todd BA, et al. Early fungal endocarditis in homograft recipients. Ann Thorac Surg 1999;68:1410-1411.

Feinstein AR, Harrison HF, Spagnuolo M, et al. Rheumatic fever in children and adolescents: a long term epidemiologic study of subsequent prophylaxis, streptococcal infections and clinical sequelae. VII. Cardiac change and sequelae. Ann Intern Med 1964a;60:87-122.

Feinstein AR, Spagnuolo M, Wood HF, et al. Rheumatic fever in children and adolescents: a long term epidemiologic study of a subsequent prophylaxis, streptococcal infections and clinical sequelae. VI. Clinical features of streptococcal infections and rheumatic recurrences. Ann Intern Med 1964b;60:68-86.

Fernandez-Guerrero ML, Verdejo C, Azofra J, et al. Hospital-acquired infectious endocarditis not associated with cardiac surgery: an emerging problem. Clin Infect Dis 1995;20:16-23.

Fisher RG, Moodie DS, Rice R. Pediatric bacterial endocarditis. Long-term follow-up. Cleve Clin Q 1985;52:41-45.

Fleming HA. General principles of the treatment of infective endocarditis. J Antimicrob Chemother 1987;20 (suppl):143-145.

Fowler VG, Li J, Corey GR, et al. Role of echocardiography in evaluation of patients with Staphylococcus aureus bacteremia: experience in 103 patients. J Am Coll Cardiol 1997;30:1072-1078.

Francioli P, Etienne J, Hoigne R, et al. Treatment of streptococcal endocarditis with a single daily dose of ceftriaxone sodium for 4 weeks. Efficacy and outpatient treatment feasibility. JAMA 1992;267:264-267.

Freeman J, Platt R, Epstein MF, et al. Birth weight and length of stay as determinants of nosocomial coagulase-negative staphylococcal bacteremia in neonatal intensive care unit populations: potential for confounding. Am J Epidemiol 1990;132:1130-1140.

Friedland G, von Reyn CF, Levy B, et al. Nosocomial endocarditis. Infect Control 1984;5:284-288.

Gaynes RP, Culver DH, Emori TG, et al. The National Nosocomial Infections Surveillance System: plans for the 1990s and beyond. Am J Med 1991;91:116S-120S.

Gelfman R, Levine SA. The incidence of acute and subacute bacterial endocarditis in congenital heart disease. Am J Med Sci 1942;204:324-333.

Gersony WM, Hayes CJ. Bacterial endocarditis in patients with pulmonary stenosis, aortic stenosis, or ventricular septal defect. Circulation 1977;56:84-87.

Geva T, Frand M. Infective endocarditis in children with congenital heart disease: the changing spectrum, 1965-85. Eur Heart J 1988;9:1244-1249.

Giamarellou H. Nosocomial cardiac infections. J Hosp Infect 2002;50:91-105.

Gilbey JG, Chalermskulrat W, Aris RM. *Aspergillus* endocarditis in a lung transplant recipient. A case report and review of the transplant literature. Ann Transplant 2000;5:48-53.

Gilleece A, Fenelon L. Nosocomial infective endocarditis. J Hosp Infect 2000;46:83-88.

Goldenberger D, Kunzli A, Vogt P, et al. Molecular diagnosis of bacterial endocarditis by broad-range PCR amplification and direct sequencing. J Clin Microbiol 1997;35:2733-2739.

Gonzales RD, Schreckenberger PC, Graham MB, et al. Infections due to vancomycin-resistant Enterococcus faecium resistant to linezolid. Lancet 2001;357:1179.

Gorak EJ, Yamada SM, Brown JD. Community-acquired methicillin-resistant *Staphylococcus aureus* in hospitalized adults and children without known risk factors. Clin Infect Dis 1999;29:797-800.

Gordon SM, Serkey JM, Longworth DL, et al. Early onset prosthetic valve endocarditis: the Cleveland Clinic experience 1992-1997. Ann Thoracic Surg 2000;69:1388-1392.

Gouello JP, Asfar P, Brenet O, et al. Nosocomial endocarditis in the intensive care unit: an analysis of 22 cases. Crit Care Med 2000;28:377-382.

Greenwood RD. Mitral valve prolapse. Incidence and clinical course in a pediatric population. Clin Pediatr (Phila) 1984;23:318-320.

Griffiths SP, Gersony WM. Acute rheumatic fever in New York City (1969 to 1988): a comparative study of two decades. J Pediatr 1990;116:882-887.

Hecht SR, Berger M. Right-sided endocarditis in intravenous drug users. Prognostic features in 102 episodes. Ann Intern Med 1992;117:560-566.

Hoen B, Selton-Suty C, Danchin N, et al. Evaluation of the Duke criteria versus the Beth Israel criteria for the diagnosis of infective endocarditis. Clin Infect Dis 1995;21:905-.

Johnson DH, Rosenthal A, Nadas AS. A forty-year review of bacterial endocarditis in infancy and childhood. Circulation 1975;51:581-588.

Kaplan EL. Infective endocarditis in the pediatric age group: an overview. Infective Endocarditis: an American Heart Association Symposium, Dallas, 1977.

Klug D, Lacroix D, Savoye C, et al. Systemic infection related to endocarditis on pacemaker leads: clinical presentation and management. Circulation 1997;95:2098-2107.

Kuehnert MJ, Clark E, Lockhart SR, et al. *Candida albicans* endocarditis associated with a contaminated aortic valve allograft: implications for regulation of allograft processing. Clin Infect Dis 1998;27:688-691.

Kupferwasser LI, Bayer AS. Update on culture-negative endocarditis. Curr Clin Top Infect Dis 2000;20:113-133.

Kupferwasser LI, Yeaman MR, Shapiro SM, et al. Acetylsalicylic acid reduces vegetation bacterial density, hematogenous bacterial dissemination, and frequency of embolic events in experimental *Staphylococcus aureus* endocarditis through antiplatelet and antibacterial effects. Circulation 1999;99:2791-2797.

Laguno M, Miro O, Font C, et al. Pacemaker-related endocarditis. Report of 7 cases and review of the literature. Cardiology 1998;90:244-248.

Landman D, Quale JM, Mobarakai N, et al. Ampicillin plus ciprofloxacin therapy of experimental endocarditis caused by multidrug-resistant *Enterococcus faecium.* J Antimicrob Chemother 1995;36:253-258.

Landman D, Quale JM, Burney S, et al. Treatment of experimental endocarditis caused by multidrug resistant *Enterococcus faecium* with ramoplanin and penicillin. J Antimicrob Chemother 1996;37:323-329.

Li JS, Sexton DJ, Mick N, et al. Proposed modifications to the Duke criteria for the diagnosis of infective endocarditis. Clin Infect Dis 2000;30:633-638.

Linde LM, Heins HL. Bacterial endocarditis following surgery for congenital heart disease. N Engl J Med 1960;263:65-69.

Lindner JR, Case RA, Dent JM, et al. Diagnostic value of echocardiography in suspected endocarditis. An evaluation based on the pretest probability of disease. Circulation 1996;93:730-736.

Mansur AJ, Dal Bo CM, Fukushima JT, et al. Relapses, recurrences, valve replacements, and mortality during the long-term follow-up after infective endocarditis. Am Heart J 2001;141:6-8, 78-86.

Mayayo E, Moralejo J, Camps J, et al. Fungal endocarditis in premature infants: case report and review. Clin Infect Dis 1996;22:366-368.

McCracken GH. Emergence of resistant *Streptococcus pneumoniae*: a problem in pediatrics. Pediatr Infect Dis J 1995;14:424-428.

McNamara DG. Idiopathic benign mitral leaflet prolapse. The pediatrician's view. Am J Dis Child (1960) 1982;136:152-156.

Melamed R, Leibovitz E, Abramson O, et al. Successful non-surgical treatment of *Candida tropicalis* endocarditis with liposomal amphotericin-B (Ambisome). Scand J Infect Dis 2000;32:86-89.

Millar B, Moore J, Mallon P, et al. Molecular diagnosis of infective endocarditis—a new Duke's criterion. Scand J Infect Dis 2001;33:673-680.

Moreillon P. Endocarditis prophylaxis revisited: experimental evidence of efficacy and new Swiss recommendations. Swiss Working Group for Endocarditis Prophylaxis. Schweizerische Medizinische Wochenschrift. J Suisse Med 2000;130:1013-1026.

Morrow WR, Haas JE, Benjamin DR. Nonbacterial endocardial thrombosis in neonates: relationship to persistent fetal circulation. J Pediatr 1982;100:117-122.

Muehrcke DD, Lytle BW, Cosgrove DM. Surgical and long-term antifungal therapy for fungal prosthetic valve endocarditis. Ann Thoracic Surg 1995;60:538-543.

Murray BE. Vancomycin-resistant enterococcal infections. N Engl J Med 2000;342:710-721.

Mylonakis E, Calderwood SB. Infective endocarditis in adults. N Engl J Med 2001;345:1318-1330.

Normand J, Bozio A, Etienne J, et al. Changing patterns and prognosis of infective endocarditis in childhood. Euro Heart J 1995;16(suppl B):28-31.

Oelberg DG, Fisher DJ, Gross DM, et al. Endocarditis in high-risk neonates. Pediatrics 1983;71:392-397.

Patel R, Rouse MS, Piper KE, et al. Linezolid therapy of vancomycin-resistant *Enterococcus faecium* experimental endocarditis. Antimicrob Agents Chemother 2001;45:621-623.

Pearlman SA, Higgins S, Eppes S, et al. Infective endocarditis in the premature neonate. Clin Pediatr (Phila) 1998;37:741-746.

Peric M, Vuk F, Huskic R, et al. Active infective endocarditis: low mortality associated with early surgical treatment. Cardiovasc Surg 2000;8:208-213.

Røder BL, Wandall DA, Espersen F, et al. Neurologic manifestations in *Staphylococcus aureus* endocarditis: a review of 260 bacteremic cases in nondrug addicts. Am J Med 1997a;102:379-386.

Røder BL, Wandall DA, Espersen F, et al. A study of 47 bacteremic *Staphylococcus aureus* endocarditis cases: 23 with native valves treated surgically and 24 with prosthetic valves. *Scand Cardiovasc J* 1997b;31: 305-309.

Rohmann S, Erbel R, Mohr-Kahaly S, et al. Use of transesophageal echocardiography in the diagnosis of abscess in infective endocarditis. Euro Heart J 1995;16(suppl B):54-62.

Sadiq M, Nazir M, Sheikh SA. Infective endocarditis in children—incidence, pattern, diagnosis and management in a developing country. Int J Cardiol 2001;78: 175-182.

Saiman L, Ludington E, Pfaller M, et al. Risk factors for candidemia in Neonatal Intensive Care Unit patients. The National Epidemiology of Mycosis Survey study group. Ped Infect Dis J 2000;19:319-324.

Saiman L, Prince A, Gersony WM. Pediatric infective endocarditis in the modern era. J Pediatr 1993;122: 847-853.

Sanchez PJ, Siegel JD, Fishbein J. Candida endocarditis: successful medical management in three preterm infants and review of the literature. Pediatr Infect Dis J 1991;10:239-243.

Scheld WM, Strunk RW, Balian G, Calderone RA. Microbial adhesion to fibronectin in vitro correlates with production of endocarditis in rabbits. Proc Soc Exp Biol Med 1985;180:474-482.

Shiro H, Meluleni G, Groll A, et al. The pathogenic role of *Staphylococcus epidermidis* capsular polysaccharide/adhesin in a low-inoculum rabbit model of prosthetic valve endocarditis. Circulation 1995;92:2715-2722.

Sobel JD. Nosocomial infective endocarditis. In Kaye D (ed): Infective Endocarditis, ed 2. New York, NY: Raven Press, 1992.

Steckelberg JM, Murphy JG, Ballard D, et al. Emboli in infective endocarditis: the prognostic value of echocardiography. Ann Intern Med 1991;114:635-640.

Stull TL, LiPuma. Endocarditis in children. In Kaye D (ed). Infective Endocarditis, ed 2. New York: Raven Press, 1992.

Symchych PS, Krauss AN, Winchester P. Endocarditis following intracardiac placement of umbilical venous catheters in neonates. J Pediatr 1977;90:287-289.

Terpenning MS, Buggy BP, Kauffman CA. Hospital-acquired infective endocarditis. Arch Intern Med 1988; 148:1601-1603.

Tornos P, Almirante B, Mirabet S, et al. Infective endocarditis due to *Staphylococcus aureus*: deleterious effect of anticoagulant therapy. Arch Intern Med 1999;159: 473-475.

Viertel A, Ditting T, Pistorius K, et al. An unusual case of *Aspergillus* endocarditis in a kidney transplant recipient. Transplantation 1999;68:1812-1813.

von Reyn CF, Levy BS, Arbeit RD, et al. Infective endocarditis: an analysis based on strict case definitions. Ann Intern Med 1981;94:505-518.

Walterspiel JN, Kaplan SL. Incidence and clinical characteristics of "culture-negative" infective endocarditis in a pediatric population. Pediatr Infect Dis 1986;5:328-332.

Washington JA. The role of the microbiology laboratory in the diagnosis and antimicrobial treatment of infective endocarditis. Mayo Clinic Proc 1982;57:22-32.

Weinstein L, Schlesinger JJ. Pathoanatomic, pathophysiologic and clinical correlations in endocarditis (first of two parts). N Engl J Med 1974a;291:832-837.

Weinstein L, Schlesinger JJ. Pathoanatomic, pathophysiologic and clinical correlations in endocarditis (second of two parts). N Engl J Med 1974b;291:1122-1126.

Wilson WR, Karchmer AW, Dajani AS, et al. Antibiotic treatment of adults with infective endocarditis due to streptococci, enterococci, staphylococci, and HACEK microorganisms. American Heart Association. JAMA 1995;274:1706-1713.

Zafar N, Wallace CM, Kieffer P, et al. Improving survival of vulnerable infants increases neonatal intensive care unit nosocomial infection rate. Arch Pediatr Adolesc Med 2001;155:1098-1104.

Zakrewski T, Keith JD. Bacterial endocarditis in infants and children. J Pediatr 1965;67:1179.

Zuppiroli A, Rinaldi M, Kramer-Fox R, et al. Natural history of mitral valve prolapse. Am J Cardiol 1995;75: 1028-1032.

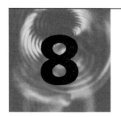

ENTEROVIRUSES

JOHN F. MODLIN

The human enteroviruses are small, positive-strand RNA viruses that cause ubiquitous infection, most commonly in infants and young children, and most frequently in the summer and fall at temperate latitudes. The 64 known enterovirus serotypes are traditionally divided among five subgenera: polioviruses, group A coxsackieviruses, group B coxsackieviruses, echoviruses, and enteroviruses (King et al., 2000). Poliovirus infections have been eliminated by immunization programs in most parts of the world and are targeted for global eradication. The other enterovirus subgenera cause diverse clinical manifestations with outcomes ranging from trivial, self-limited illness to serious disability and death.

HISTORY

The prototypical enteroviral disease, poliomyelitis became a major public health problem with the emergence of epidemic disease in northern Europe and the United States in the late nineteenth century (Paul, 1971; Vermont State Department of Public Health, 1924; Wickman, 1907). Landsteiner and Popper demonstrated that the etiologic agent of poliomyelitis was a filterable virus in 1908 by transmitting disease to monkeys by intraperitoneal injection of human neural tissue (Landsteiner and Popper, 1908). The next decades brought significant advances in understanding the virology and the pathophysiology of poliovirus infection but prevention was not possible until polioviruses were isolated in primate cell culture by Enders, Weller, and Robbins in 1949 (Enders et al., 1949). This landmark achievement led to development of both inactivated and live vaccines (Salk, 1953; Francis et al., 1957; Sabin, 1985) and to rapid control of poliomyelitis where these vaccines were universally administered.

The first nonpolio enteroviruses were isolated in newborn mice in the late 1940s by Dalldorf and Sickles, who were seeking an alternative animal host for poliomyelitis studies (Dalldorf and Sickles, 1948). These agents were termed *coxsackieviruses* because of their origin in patients living in the town of Coxsackie, New York. Shortly thereafter, Melnick and colleagues noted that the coxsackieviruses could be divided into two separate groups, designated A and B, according to the distribution of inflammatory lesions they produced in newborn mice (Curnen et al., 1949; Melnick, 1993). The nearly simultaneous development of cell culture led to the discovery of another group of enteroviruses that did not replicate in either mice or monkeys (Ramos-Alvarez and Sabin, 1954). These viruses were initially termed *enteric cytopathic human orphan (ECHO) viruses* because of their uncertain relationship to human disease (Committee on the ECHO Viruses, National Foundation for Infantile Paralysis, 1955). Within a short period of time, the coxsackieviruses and echoviruses were found to cause aseptic meningitis (also called *nonparalytic poliomyelitis*) and other acute diseases.

By the 1960s, it became apparent that not all enterovirus serotypes could be unambiguously characterized on the basis of host susceptibility. Subsequently, newly discovered agents were simply termed *enterovirus* rather than coxsackievirus or echovirus (Rosen et al., 1970). Four new serotypes (enteroviruses 68 through 71) were subsequently characterized. The last unique enterovirus to be described, enterovirus 71, was isolated in 1969 (Mirkovic et al., 1974).

VIROLOGY
Classification

The genus *Enterovirus* belongs to the family Picornaviridae, a large family of morphologically identical single-strand RNA viruses that share a common genomic and structural organization. Variations in the capsid proteins are responsible for the antigenic diversity among the 64 recognized human enterovirus serotypes (King et al., 2000), and each serotype is defined and distinguished from other serotypes by in vitro neutralization. Additional isolates considered "nontypable" by reference laboratories may represent previously undescribed serotypes (Oberste et al., 2000). By convention, each serotype is assigned to one of five subgenera on the basis of host range and, for the coxsackieviruses, the distribution of pathologic lesions in newborn mice (Table 8-1) (King et al., 2000; Melnick, 1993).

The biologic relationships among different subgenera and serotypes are sometimes indistinct. Some enterovirus isolates defy classification strictly on the basis of host range (see footnotes, Table 8-1), and cross-neutralization occurs between some serotypes (Box 8-1). In addition, mutation in the capsid coding region of the genome during sustained human transmission leads to variable neutralization among epidemiologically unrelated isolates of the same serotype (Melnick, 1996) and to difficulties in determination of serotype with reference sera raised against prototypic strains isolated decades before (Oberste et al., 2000; Melnick and Wimberly, 1985; Centers for Disease Control and Prevention, 2002b).

A new classification scheme based on genetic relatedness will circumvent some of these prob-

---

BOX 8-1

ANTIGENICALLY RELATED ENTEROVIRUS SEROTYPES

Coxsackieviruses A3 and A8
Coxsackieviruses A11 and A15
Coxsackieviruses A13 and A18
Echoviruses 1 and 8
Echoviruses 6 and 30
Echoviruses 12 and 29

---

lems associated with the traditional classification. Accordingly, four groups of enteroviruses are designated A through D based on homology within RNA regions coding for capsid proteins (Figure 8-1) (Oberste et al., 1999; Norder et al., 2001). Sequencing of regions coding for both VP1, VP2, and VP4 produces similar results, but classification based on VP1 homology is theoretically more useful as this protein contains the major epitopes associated with neutralization (Oberste et al., 1999; Caro et al., 2001; Ishiko et al., 2002). Isolates of the same serotype characteristically diverge in the VP1 region by less than 25% and 12%, respectively, within corresponding nucleotide and amino acid sequences (Oberste et al., 1999).

Physical Properties and Viral Replication

The enteroviruses are composed of a 27- to 30-nm protein capsid surrounding a positive-strand

---

| TABLE 8-1 | Conventional Classification and Host Range of Human Enterovirus |

		HOST RANGE		
Species	Serotypes	Primates	Newborn mice	Cell culture
Polioviruses	1-3	++	0[a]	++
Coxsackieviruses A	1-24[b]	0[c]	+++	±[d]
Coxsackieviruses B	1-6	0	+++	++
Echoviruses	1-34[e]	0	0[f]	++
Enteroviruses	68-72[g]	Variable	Variable	+

[a]Some strains have been adapted to mice.
[b]Coxsackievirus A23 has been reclassified as echovirus 9, which leaves 23 coxsackievirus serotypes in group A.
[c]Coxsackievirus A7 is pathogenic for the primate central nervous system.
[d]Most coxsackievirus serotypes of group A are not readily isolated in cell cultures, but exceptions exist (e.g., serotypes A9 and A16); additional serotypes have been adapted to cell cultures.
[e]Echovirus 10 has been reclassified as reovirus 1, and echovirus 28 as rhinovirus 1. Echovirus 34 is a variant of coxsackievirus A24. Echoviruses 22 and 23 have been assigned to the genus *Parechovirus* as parechovirus serotypes 1 and 2, respectively. Therefore, a total of 29 of the original 34 serotypes of echovirus remain.
[f]Except echovirus 21.
[g]Hepatitis A virus was briefly classified as enterovirus 72 but is now assigned to the genus *Heparnavirus*.

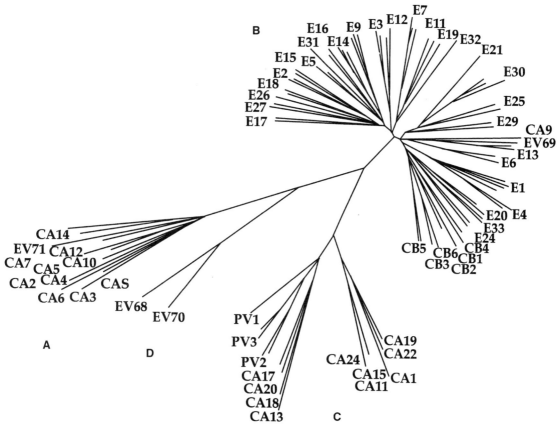

Fig. 8-1 Dendrogram representing genetic relationships among human enterovirus serotypes. (Modified from Norder H, Bjerregaard L, Magnius LO: J Med Virol 2001;63:35.)

RNA genome of approximately 7.4 kilobases (kb) in length and are distinguished from other picornaviruses by their resistance to inactivation over a broad pH range (Rueckert, 1990). Infection of the cell is initiated by attachment of the virion to one or more specific cell membrane protein receptors. The receptors for many of the human enteroviruses have been identified and characterized (Table 8-2). Penetration, uncoat-ing, and release of the positive-strand RNA genome into the cytoplasm occurs within min-utes at 37° C. The RNA genome serves as a monocistronic messenger whose product is a large polyprotein that is cleaved via a series of steps into both virion proteins and nonstruc-tural, regulatory proteins. Noncoding sequences at the 5′ and 3′ ends of the genome are critical for both translation and transcription. The four

TABLE 8-2	Enterovirus Cell Membrane Receptors
Enterovirus serotypes	*Receptor protein*
Polioviruses 1-3	PVR
Coxsackieviruses A13, A18, A21	ICAM-1
Coxsackieviruses B1-B6	CAR
Coxsackieviruses B1, B3, B5	DAF
Echoviruses 1, 8	VLA-2 ($\alpha 2\beta 1$)
Echoviruses 6, 7, 11-13, 20, 21, 29, 33	DAF
Enterovirus 70	DAF

CAR, Coxsackie adenovirus receptor; *DAF*, decay accelerating factor; *ICAM*, intracellular adhesion molecule 1; *PVR*, Poliovirus receptor; *VLA*, very late antigen.

virion proteins (VP1, VP2, VP3, and VP4) are assembled into the capsid in equimolar amounts of 60 copies each. Progeny RNA are copied from the genome via a negative-strand RNA intermediary and encapsidated to complete the replication cycle. In vitro infection produces about 10^4 to 10^5 viral particles per cell, but the number of infectious virions is 10- to 1,000-fold lower. Host cell protein and RNA synthesis are compromised within 3 hours of cell infection, and cell lysis occurs within 8 hours with virion release (Rueckert, 1990).

EPIDEMIOLOGY

Enterovirus infections are ubiquitous, occurring in all regions of the world and throughout the calendar year (Gelfand, 1961). A marked seasonal periodicity is observed in temperate climates, where infection peaks during summer and autumn months and diminishes to basal levels in late winter and early spring (Gelfand, 1961; Moore, 1982; Berlin et al., 1993). Enterovirus activity at higher latitudes is characterized by lower year-round excretion rates among healthy children and concentrated seasonal epidemic disease in all age groups (Moore, 1982), whereas in children living in warmer climates higher excretion rates are observed and disease occurs in an endemic pattern (Gelfand, 1961; Gelfand et al., 1963; Parks et al., 1967).

Surveillance

Poliomyelitis remains a reportable disease throughout the world. As of January 2002, wild-type poliovirus infections were confined to countries in sub-Saharan Africa, the Middle East, and the Indian subcontinent (Centers for Disease Control and Prevention, 2002c). Fewer than 1,000 cases were reported by the World Health Organization (WHO) for calendar year 2001 despite improved surveillance, and disease caused by type 2 poliovirus was last observed in northern India in October 1999 (Centers for Disease Control and Prevention, 1999).

Information on activity of other enteroviruses, which relies on passive reporting to national and international reference centers such as the Centers for Disease Control and Prevention (CDC) and WHO, shows marked variation in secular trends of disease activity among different serotypes. Table 8-3 lists the 15 most common enterovirus isolates submitted from state and local public health laboratories to the Enterovirus Surveillance Program of the CDC during the 2-year period or 2000 and 2001 (Centers for Disease Control and Prevention, 2000b). These serotypes accounted for 93.5% of all identifiable isolates submitted during this period. In the United States, typically one to three serotypes predominate each season, and these serotypes may vary in incidence from one

TABLE 8-3	Most Common Enterovirus Serotypes Submitted by State and Local Public Health Laboratories to CDC, 2000 and 2001
Enterovirus serotype	**Percent**
Echovirus 18	22.0
Echovirus 13	20.8
Coxsackievirus B5	11.9
Coxsackievirus B2	6.3
Echovirus 6	6.1
Echovirus 11	4.5
Coxsackievirus A9	4.0
Echovirus 9	3.3
Coxsackievirus B4	3.2
Echovirus 4	3.1
Coxsackievirus B3	2.4
Coxsackievirus B1	2.0
Echovirus 30	1.8
Echovirus 25	1.2
Enterovirus 71	1.1
Total	93.5

From Centers for Disease Control and Prevention: Enterovirus surveillance–United States, 2000-2001. MMWR 2002; 51:1047.

region to another. Overall, the prevalent serotypes change little from year to year (Moore, 1982; Centers for Disease Control and Prevention, 1997; Strikas et al., 1986). However, some serotypes may emerge, or reemerge after years of relative inactivity, such as occurred with echovirus serotypes 18 and 13 in 2001 (Centers for Disease Control and Prevention, 2000; Centers for Disease Control and Prevention, 1990; Rice et al., 1995). This periodic activity may depend on the accumulation of a sufficient number of susceptible persons since the previous appearance of the serotype (Gondo et al., 1995). Infection caused by many coxsackie A virus serotypes is probably underreported because of the difficulty of isolating these viruses in cell culture.

Transmission

Humans are the only reservoir for the enteroviruses in nature, and multiple routes of person-to-person transmission are known or inferred. Indirect transmission from contamination of the environment and self-inoculation via contaminated hands is the principal mode of spread, which is enhanced by the stability of enteroviruses at ambient conditions (Melnick, 1996) and the low inoculum required to cause infection (Minor et al., 1981). Most enteroviruses are spread via fecal contamination. Poor sanitation, low socioeconomic status, large family size, and crowding encourage transmission via this route. Transmission via contaminated food or water is theoretically possible but rarely documented (Melnick, 1996).

Respiratory secretions are known to transmit coxsackie A21 infections (Couch et al., 1970) and are probably an important source for other enterovirus infections, especially where fecal contamination is limited by adequate sanitation (Gelfand et al., 1959). Virus present in tears and conjunctival secretions may contribute to the explosive spread of acute hemorrhagic conjunctivitis due to coxsackie A24 and enterovirus 70 (Kono, 1975; Christopher et al., 1982; Onorato et al., 1985). Nosocomial transmission, which occurs via the hands of care-givers, is another indirect route (Kinney et al., 1986).

Vertical transmission from mother to infant occurs during parturition or in the immediate postpartum period, but rarely in utero (Modlin, 1994).

Descriptive Epidemiology

Enteroviruses spread rapidly in households and other closed settings. Infection is more likely to be introduced into households containing larger numbers of children and where school-age children are present (Hall et al., 1970). Nonimmune family members experience high rates of infection, whereas infection rates among those with preexisting serotype specific antibody are lower but still substantial (Kogon et al., 1969). Polioviruses and group B coxsackieviruses are associated with secondary attack rates of >75% within families. The lower rates for echoviruses have been attributed to their shorter duration of excretion (Kogon et al., 1969).

There is a strong inverse relationship between age and risk of enteroviral disease, with the highest risk of disease occurring in the first months of life (Berlin et al., 1993; Grist et al., 1978; Wilfert et al., 1975; Marier et al., 1975). Jenista et al. (1984), found that 13% of all healthy infants born between June and October in Rochester acquired a nonpolio enterovirus infection during the first month of life, and 21% of infected infants were admitted to the hospital with fever. Overall rates of enteroviral disease are several fold higher for infants under 12 months of age than older children, and they decline progressively after the first decade of life (Moore, 1982). Infants and young children are particularly susceptible to neurologic infection. Prospective studies demonstrate that most cases of enterovirus meningitis occur before 4 months of age (Berlin et al., 1993) and more serious infections, such as enterovirus 71 brainstem encephalitis, most commonly occur during the first 2 years of life (Chumakov et al., 1979; Alexander et al., 1994; Ho et al., 1999). For unknown reasons, boys have higher rates of enteroviral disease than girls throughout infancy and childhood by a factor of approximately 2:1 (Morens and Pallansch, 1995).

The higher prevalence of enterovirus infections among children of lower socioeconomic status in the United States (Honig et al., 1956) and living in poverty in developing countries (Parks et al., 1967; Otatume and Addy, 1975) is probably due to crowding and poor sanitation. Paradoxically, the early acquisition of infection among infants living in poor hygienic conditions may be associated with a lower risk of serious enteroviral disease because of partial protection conferred by passively acquired maternal antibody (Fox, 1964). In fact, the appearance of epidemic paralytic poliomyelitis in Europe and North America in the last half of the nineteenth century has been attributed to improved sanitation (Nathanson and Martin, 1979), and the recent epidemics of enterovirus 71 encephalitis in mid-developing countries in Eastern Europe and Southeast Asia may also be due to this phenomenon.

Molecular Epidemiology

Regular mutation in the RNA genome permits the study of the epidemiologic relationships among enteroviruses of the same serotype. The most informative method, RNA sequencing, has been used to trace the spread of polioviruses (Kew et al., 1990; Poyry et al., 1990) and to characterize the evolution of coxsackievirus A24 and enterovirus 70, viruses that cause acute hemorrhagic conjunctivitis (Ishiko et al., 1992; Lin et al., 2001; Miyamura et al., 1986).

PATHOPHYSIOLOGY

Challenge studies with attenuated polioviruses and with coxsackievirus A12 indicate that less than 100 $TCID_{50}$ of virus is sufficient to initiate infection of susceptible human volunteers (Minor et al., 1981; Koprowski, 1956; Schiff and Sherwoood, 2000). The incubation period for most enteroviral diseases has not been carefully studied. The time from exposure to onset of symptoms probably varies from relatively short periods (3 to 5 days) for acute localized illness such as upper respiratory tract disease to as long as 9 to 12 days for poliomyelitis (Horstmann and Paul, 1947).

The pathophysiologic events that lead to clinical disease can be inferred from studies in experimental animals. Bodian demonstrated replication of poliovirus in ileal lymphoid tissue of chimpanzees within 1 to 3 days after oral challenge (Bodian, 1952). Although inflammatory changes are not seen in gastrointestinal mucosa and lymphoreticular tissues (Bodian, 1949) and virus cannot be recovered from mucosal tissue (Bodian, 1955), viral replication in submucosal lymphoid tissue gives rise to a sustained viremia that distributes virus to distant lymph nodes, muscle, and susceptible target organs. Poliomyelitis follows spread of virus from peripheral sites to the central nervous system (CNS) via neural pathways (Sabin, 1956; Kaufman et al., 1992).

Mice infected with coxsackievirus B3 either orally or parenterally develop myocarditis. Virus titers in the heart peak 3 to 4 days after parenteral or oral challenge and diminish to undetectable levels by 7 to 10 days (Woodruff, 1980; Modlin and Crumpacker, 1982). In these animals, myocardial infection is enhanced by immature age (Kaplan and Melnick, 1951; Khatib et al., 1980), advanced age (Rytel and Kilbourne, 1971), late pregnancy (Modlin and Crumpacker, 1982; Knox, 1950; Dalldorf and Gifford, 1954), combined T- and B-cell immunodeficiency (Chow et al., 1992), corticosteroid treatment (Woodruff, 1979), irradiation (Cheever, 1953), starvation (Woodruff and Kilbourne, 1970), cold stress (Boring et al., 1956), and forced exercise (Gatmaitan et al., 1970).

Immune Response and Immunopathogenesis

Antibodies that recognize specific epitopes on capsid proteins, especially VP1, neutralize enteroviruses both in vitro and in vivo, probably by interfering with viral attachment to the cell membrane (Chow and Baltimore, 1985). The detection of serum neutralizing antibodies 5 to 7 days after infection in animals is temporally associated with clearance of viremia and reduction in virus titers in solid organs (Rabin et al., 1964). In the murine myocarditis model, expression of proinflammatory cytokines and an acute inflammatory infiltration follows peak viral replication (Woodruff, 1980; Woodruff and Kilbourne, 1970; Rabin et al., 1964; Kawai, 1999; Schmidtke et al., 2000). Macrophages predominate in the early stages and probably play a significant role in viral clearance (Rager-Zisman and Allison, 1973; Woodruff and Woodruff, 1974), whereas natural killer and T lymphocyte immune responses contribute to necrosis of infected cardiac myocytes (Woodruff and Woodruff, 1974; Huber et al., 1984; Godeny and Gauntt, 1987). An inflammatory response may persist long after viral replication has ceased, and ongoing cardiac damage may be mediated by virus-induced antibodies against cardiac antigens (Gauntt, 1997) or by cytotoxic T lymphocyte–mediated myocyte lysis (Kawai, 1999; Huber et al., 1984; Liao et al., 1995; Schwimmbeck et al., 1997).

Persistence of Infection

In both experimental primate and human infection, enteroviruses are generally recovered in higher titer and for longer periods from the gastrointestinal tract than from the upper respiratory tract. Normal children with primary poliovirus infection excrete virus in feces usually for 3 to 4 weeks, but for as long as 6 to 8 weeks (Alexander et al., 1997). In marked contrast, patients with B-cell immunodeficiency disorders may remain infected with the same enterovirus serotype for many years (McKinney et al., 1987; Kew et al., 1998). Some investigators, but not all, have detected enterovirus RNA in biopsied or explanted myocardium from patients with dilated cardiomyopathy (Andreoletti et al., 1996; Giacca et al., 1994; de Leeuw et al., 1998; Grasso et al., 1992; Griffin et al., 1995). In virtually all such cases, however, virus has not been recovered in cell culture, and the significance of the presence of genomic viral RNA is unknown.

Reinfection

Reinfections with the same serotype may occur, but they are not associated with illness, and the duration of excretion of virus is considerably shorter than in the primary infection (Kogon, 1969).

CLINICAL DISEASE
Coxsackie A Virus, Coxsackie B Virus, Echovirus, and Enterovirus 68-71 Infections

Nonspecific febrile illness. Acute febrile illness without an apparent source is the most common manifestation of enteroviral infection in infants and young children. Infants <3 months of age with nonspecific fever often come to medical attention and undergo evaluation and treatment for serious bacterial infection in the hospital. However, more than 90% of these febrile illnesses are caused by viruses, and during the summer and fall months, enteroviruses account for the majority of these cases (Sanders and Cramblett, 1968; Linnemann et al., 1974; Dagan et al., 1989; Dagan, 1996; Byington et al., 1999). One prospective study during the 1981 enterovirus season in Rochester, NY found that 13% of all newborn infants developed enterovirus infection in the first month of life, and 21% of infected infants were readmitted to the hospital (Jenista et al., 1984). The risk of enterovirus infection in this age group is higher for infants from lower socioeconomic status households and infants who do not breast-feed (Jenista et al., 1984), and symptoms occur only in

infants without passively acquired maternal antibody to the enterovirus serotype causing infection (Dagan, 1996).

Abrupt onset of fever may occur in association with irritability, lethargy, poor feeding, vomiting, diarrhea, exanthems, or signs of upper respiratory tract infection (Dagan, 1996; Rorabaugh et al., 1993). Peak fever, which coincides with the presence of viremia, exceeds 39° C in about two thirds of infected infants (Dagan, 1996). Approximately one half of enterovirus-infected febrile infants have aseptic meningitis in the absence of meningeal signs (Krober et al., 1985; Dagan et al., 1988). Virtually all infants recover within 7 days without sequelae (Dagan, 1996). However, new infections with other enterovirus serotypes during the same season are not uncommon.

Exanthems and enanthems. The enteroviruses cause a spectrum of common cutaneous and mucosal eruptions including many that present as nonspecific maculopapular rashes and some that mimic exanthems associated with other viruses including measles, rubella, parvovirus, herpes simplex, human herpesvirus 6, and varicella.

Maculopapular eruptions are often observed during echovirus outbreaks and are less commonly associated with other enteroviruses (Neva, 1956; Neva et al., 1954; Hall et al., 1977; Moritsugu et al., 1968). Enterovirus exanthems typically occur in children less than 10 years of age (Sabin et al., 1958). Fever, pharyngitis, and malaise may be present at onset; however, illness is invariably mild and resolves within a few days (Neva, 1956; Neva et al., 1954; Bell et al., 1975; Lerner et al., 1960). Petechial and purpuric rashes have been described with infections with echovirus 9 (Sabin et al., 1958; Frothingham, 1958) and coxsackievirus A9 (Cherry and Jahn, 1966), which have been confused with meningococcal disease. Other cutaneous manifestations reported in association with enterovirus infections include localized vesicular lesions, urticaria, and papular acrodermatitis (Dechamps et al., 1988; Cherry et al., 1963; James et al., 1982).

Hand-foot-and-mouth (HMF) disease is a distinctive illness characterized by fever, vesicular stomatitis, and, in about 75% of affected persons, peripherally distributed papular and/or vesicular lesions (Hughes and Roberts, 1972; Lindenbaum et al., 1975; Robinson et al., 1958; Adler et al., 1970). Children are most often affected, but spread to other household members commonly occurs. Patients complain of a sore throat or a sore mouth. Infants and young children may refuse to eat. Scattered 1- to 3-mm vesicles are found in the oral cavity, chiefly on the buccal mucosa and tongue, and these lesions may ulcerate by the time the patient is examined. The skin lesions of HFM disease occur on the distal extremities, especially on the hands and feet, and sometimes on the buttocks or genitalia. They consist of papules or clear vesicles with a surrounding rim of erythema and are tender to touch. These lesions consist of a subepidermal mixed lymphocytic and polymorphonuclear infiltrate with acantholysis of the overlying epidermis (Miller, 1968). The most common virus isolated is coxsackievirus A16, but other group A coxsackieviruses, group B coxsackieviruses, and enterovirus 71 have been recovered from skin lesions, the oropharynx, or feces. Most patients recover within a few days although HFM disease may accompany more serious neurologic disease when caused by enterovirus 71 (Wang et al., 1999).

Generalized vesicular eruptions with lesions similar to those of HFM disease have been reported in association with infections with coxsackievirus A9 and echovirus 11 in both immunocompetent and immunocompromised patients (Cherry et al., 1963; Deseda-Tous et al., 1977) They may be differentiated from varicella by the absence of pustular lesions.

Herpangina is a vesicular enanthem of the fauces and soft palate that occurs in seasonal outbreaks among children, adolescents, and young adults (Parrott et al., 1951; Howlett et al., 1957). Fever and other systemic symptoms such as headache, myalgias, and vomiting are present at onset. Sore throat and pain on swallowing are prominent symptoms that herald the appearance of the characteristic oral lesions. Examination of the oral cavity reveals pharyngeal erythema, a mild tonsillar exudate, and punctate macules, which evolve rapidly to 2- to 4-mm erythematous papules that progress to small vesicles and then ulcerate. These lesions are located on the soft palate and uvula and less commonly on the tonsils, posterior pharyngeal wall, or buccal mucosa. They number less than a dozen and are moderately tender. The systemic symptoms are generally brief, and the entire illness, including the enanthem, subsides within 7 days. Herpangina may be mistaken for bacterial or viral pharyngitis,

herpes simplex stomatitis, and aphthous stomatitis, although the clinical features are sufficiently distinctive to permit a diagnosis on clinical grounds alone. The group A coxsackieviruses are the most common viruses recovered from patients with herpangina, although many group B coxsackievirus and echovirus serotypes have also been implicated (Cherry and Jahn, 1965).

CNS infections. Enteroviruses are the most commonly recognized cause of viral CNS disease, and all enterovirus subgenera and most enterovirus serotypes are neurotropic. Meningitis and meningoencephalitis are relatively common, generalized infections that are caused by many enterovirus serotypes. Focal cerebritis, brainstem encephalitis, and transverse myelitis are less common, but often more serious diseases associated with a limited group of serotypes. Motor neuron disease, which is the hallmark of poliovirus CNS infection (see discussion of poliovirus infections elsewhere in this chapter), is an unusual, but well-documented manifestation of infection by other enteroviruses. In most cases, clinical illness is marked by abrupt onset during acute enterovirus infection and ability to recover infectious virus from CNS tissue or cerebrospinal fluid (CSF), the oropharynx, and the gastrointestinal tract.

The echoviruses and group B coxsackieviruses cause more than 90% of cases of all cases of *viral meningitis*, whereas meningitis caused by the group A coxsackieviruses is less common (Berlin et al., 1993). Infection with some serotypes, particularly the group B coxsackieviruses and echovirus 30, is more likely to result in meningitis than infection with other common enterovirus serotypes (Dagan et al., 1988). All age groups are susceptible, but the majority of cases are recognized among infants less than 12 months of age (Rorabaugh et al., 1993). Fever, irritability, and anorexia are often the only symptoms in infants and toddlers (Rorabaugh et al., 1993; Dagan et al., 1988). Older children and adults may develop illness in a biphasic manner in which a brief prodrome of fever and sore throat is followed by sudden onset of headache and meningeal irritation, or these symptoms may occur simultaneously. The headache is often severe. Complaints of neck stiffness, and the presence of meningeal irritation on examination are variable findings with enteroviral meningitis. Complications such as febrile seizures, complex seizures, lethargy, coma, and movement disorders occur early in the course in 5% to –10% of patients (Rorabaugh et al., 1993; Lepow et al., 1962b). Acute disease in adults appears to be more severe and to persist longer than in infants and young children (Helfand et al., 1994; Rotbart et al., 1998).

The diagnosis of viral meningitis can be inferred, and bacterial meningitis excluded, by laboratory examination of CSF. Enteroviral meningitis produces CSF which may appear clear or slightly turbid, may contain from 0 to >1,000 WBC/µl (Berlin et al., 1993; Wilfert et al., 1975; Haynes et al., 1969; Lake et al., 1976; Wenner et al., 1981; Amir et al., 1991) and will often demonstrate a predominance of neutrophils during the first 1 to 2 days of illness, with an invariable shift to a lymphocyte predominance later (Amir et al., 1991; Feigin and Shackelford, 1973). In most cases, the CSF glucose concentration is normal, but values slightly lower than normal are reported in 18% to –33% of cases (Avner et al., 1975; Singer et al., 1980; Sumaya and Corman, 1982), and the CSF protein concentration is normal or slightly elevated. Confirmation of the diagnosis depends on detection of an enterovirus in the CSF by isolation in cell culture or by polymerase chain reaction (PCR).

Patients with viral meningitis may be given analgesics for headache and often receive antibiotics until bacterial disease can be ruled out with confidence. Pleconaril, an experimental, orally administered antipicornavirus agent, significantly reduces the duration of headache and other symptoms in older children and adults (Weiner et al., 1997). Subtle disturbances of motor function such as limitation of passive motion, muscle spasm, and poor coordination may persist for weeks after resolution of the acute illness, but slowly resolve (Lepow et al., 1962a). Despite concern raised by early studies (Farmer et al., 1975; Sells et al., 1975), viral meningitis does not lead to long-term neurologic or cognitive sequelae (Bergman et al., 1987).

Nonpolio enterovirus infection is reported to cause up to 23% of cases of *viral encephalitis* in several series dating to the early 1960s (Lennette et al., 1962; Meyer et al., 1960), but more recent studies, including those using PCR methods, suggest that enterovirus infections contribute to less than 5% of cases

(Rantakallio et al., 1986; Read and Kurtz, 1999; Rantala and Uhari, 1989). Many enterovirus serotypes have been implicated, including serotypes representing group A coxsackieviruses, group B coxsackieviruses, echoviruses, and enterovirus 71. Enteroviral encephalitis is characterized by abrupt onset of fever, headache, personality changes, and alterations in consciousness that may range from lethargy to coma. Muscle weakness and seizures accompany more serious cases. Symptoms and signs of focal encephalitis such as partial motor seizures, hemichorea, and acute cerebellar ataxia are known to occur in infants and toddlers, particularly during infection with some group A coxsackieviruses (Modlin et al., 1991; Chalhub et al., 1977; Peters et al., 1979; Roden et al., 1975). These cases may closely mimic herpes simplex encephalitis (Modlin et al., 1991; Whitley et al., 1989). Cases of severe focal brainstem encephalitis associated with peripheral vasoconstriction and pulmonary edema have been observed in young children infected during recent epidemics of enterovirus 71 infection in Malaysia and Taiwan (Miller, 1968; Whitley et al., 1989).

The CSF findings in enteroviral encephalitis are similar to those found with viral meningitis. Electroencephalogram (EEG) and neuroimaging abnormalities usually reflect the extent and severity of brain involvement. Although many patients with coxsackievirus and echovirus encephalitis beyond the neonatal period recover fully, neurologic sequelae and rare deaths occur (Lennette et al., 1962; Chalhub et al., 1977; Klapper et al., 1984; Price RA et al., 1970).

Enterovirus 71 and coxsackievirus A7 have been associated with outbreaks of acute motor neuron disease clinically indistinguishable from poliomyelitis (Voroshilova and Chumakov, 1959; Grist and Bell, 1970; Gilbert et al., 1988; Shindarov et al., 1979). Sporadic cases are reported to have occurred with these two serotypes, as well as many other group A coxsackieviruses, group B coxsackieviruses, and echoviruses (Assaad and Cockburn, 1972; Godtfredsen and Hansen, 1961; Grist and Bell, 1975; Kibrick, 1964). Motor neuron disease caused by the nonpolio enteroviruses generally has a better outcome than poliomyelitis. Transient muscle weakness is more common than flaccid paralysis, and the paresis is usually not permanent. Cranial nerve involvement has occasionally resulted in complete unilateral oculomotor palsy (Hertenstein et al., 1976). Rare cases of fatal bulbar involvement have been reported (Steigman and Lipton, 1960).

Enterovirus infection has also been reported in association with other CNS syndromes including Guillain-Barré syndrome (Lepow et al., 1962a; Dery et al., 1974; Geer, 1961), transverse myelitis (Dery et al., 1974; Barak and Schwartz, 1988), and the opsoclonus-myoclonus syndrome (Kuban et al., 1983).

Myocarditis, pericarditis, and dilated cardiomyopathy. Enteroviruses are the most common cause of viral myocarditis, a disease characterized by acute inflammation of the heart and myocyte necrosis. The group B coxsackieviruses account for at least one half of etiologically diagnosed myocarditis cases (Grist and Bell, 1974; Ayuthya et al., 1974; Martino et al., 1995). Strong evidence supports a role for many group A coxsackievirus and echovirus serotypes (Kibrick, 1964; Johnson et al., 1961; Berkovich et al., 1968; Grist and Bell, 1969; Russell and Bell, 1970; Meehan and Bertrand, 1970; Bendig et al., 2001), as well as adenoviruses (Martin et al., 1994; Shimizu et al., 1995; Grumbach et al., 1999), influenza A viruses (Hildebrandt et al., 1962), mumps virus (Centers for Disease Control and Prevention, 1980), vaccinia virus (Caldera et al., 1961), and human immunodeficiency virus (HIV) (Lipschultz et al., 1998). A diagnosis of acute pericarditis is appropriate for occasional patients with clinical findings limited to fever, chest pain, and a pericardial friction rub. However, myocarditis and pericarditis share a common etiology, and both may be present in biopsied or postmortem heart tissue (Smith, 1966).

Enterovirus myocarditis is observed in all age groups but has a special predilection for physically active adolescents and young adults (Feldman and McNamara, 2000). Pharyngitis often occurs 7 to 14 days before the onset of cardiac symptoms, which may include dyspnea, precordial pain, fever, and malaise (Helin et al., 1968; Smith, 1970; Koontz and Ray, 1971). The chest pain may be dull, sharp, or pleuretic and is sometimes aggravated by lying in a recumbent position. Examination reveals a pericardial friction rub, often transient, in 35% to −80% of cases, and a gallop rhythm and other signs of frank congestive heart failure are

observed in roughly 20% (Smith, 1970; Koontz and Ray, 1971). Some patients have clinical evidence of viral meningitis or pleurodynia. Sudden death may be the presenting manifestation (Noren et al., 1977).

Enlargement of the cardiac silhouette on chest radiograph films represents either pericardial effusion or cardiac dilatation. Electrocardiographic abnormalities range from S-T segment elevation and nonspecific S-T segment and T wave changes with pericarditis or mild myocarditis to Q waves, ventricular tachyarrhythmias, and all degrees of heart block in more severe myocardial involvement (Wiles et al., 1992; Lee et al., 1999). Echocardiography may demonstrate left ventricular wall abnormalities and a diminished cardiac ejection fraction (Lee et al., 1999; Chan et al., 1991; Camargo et al., 1995), and other noninvasive methods such as antimyosin scintigraphy and magnetic resonance imaging may be useful in localizing and assessing the extent of cardiac inflammation (Kuhl et al., 1998; Friedrich et al., 1998). Serum levels of creatine kinase and cardiac troponin enzymes are inconsistently elevated (Feldman and McNamara, 2000; Smith et al., 1997; Lauer et al., 1997). It is possible to isolate virus in cell culture or to detect viral RNA by PCR in pericardial fluid or biopsied myocardial tissue, although, in practice, these techniques are most often nondiagnostic (Sutton et al., 1967; Sutton et al., 1963; Weiss et al., 1991b; Jin et al., 1990; Fujioka et al., 1996). In many cases, the diagnosis rests on circumstantial evidence provided by recovery of the agent from the oropharynx or feces and/or serologic evidence of recent infection by a group B coxsackievirus.

Supportive treatment consists of bed rest, pain relief, and medical management of arrhythmias and heart failure (Feldman and McNamara, 2000). Although one study reported improved cardiac function and a trend toward increased survival for children with acute myocarditis who received intravenous immune globulin (IVIG) when compared with historical controls (Drucker et al., 1994), randomized trials of immunosuppressive therapy, including IVIG, prednisone, and other drugs have failed to show any consistent treatment effect (Latham et al., 1989; Mason et al., 1995; Garg et al., 1998). Compassionate release of the experimental antiviral agent pleconaril has been associated with favorable outcomes in a small number of patients (Rotbart, 1998), but controlled studies have not been done.

The prognosis for children with acute myocarditis is better than for adults. Fewer than 15% die during the acute illness from intractable heart failure or uncontrolled arrhythmias, and fewer than 10% develop persistent or recurrent compromise from dilated cardiomyopathy requiring cardiac transplantation (Lee et al., 1999). The remaining patients recover uneventfully with little or no cardiac disability. The risk of developing long-term cardiac sequelae may be higher for children with less severe acute myocarditis (McCarthy et al., 2000).

Dilated cardiomyopathy is an important cause of chronic congestive heart failure that is the final result of multiple infectious and non-infectious cardiac insults (Codd et al., 1989), including both clinically apparent and unrecognized past enterovirus infections (Kawai, 1999; Smith, 1970; Koontz and Ray, 1971; Sainani et al., 1968). Some investigators have detected enterovirus RNA in cardiac tissue months to years after onset of dilated cardiomyopathy, but others who have searched with similar methods have not (Andreoletti et al., 1996; Giacca et al., 1994; de Leeuw et al., 1998; Grasso et al., 1992; Griffin et al., 1995; Weiss et al., 1991a; Muir et al., 1996).

Pleurodynia and myositis. Pleurodynia is an acute illness characterized by fever and localized myositis of the intercostal and abdominal muscles, leading to local sharp, spasmodic thoracic and abdominal pain (Sylvest, 1934). The group B coxsackieviruses cause pleurodynia more commonly than other enteroviruses (Curnen et al., 1949; Weller et al., 1950). Focal outbreaks with high attack rates within affected households are typical, and major epidemics occur as infrequently as every 10 to 20 years. Disease is observed more frequently in adolescents and older children than in infants.

Sore throat and headache may accompany muscle pain, but cough and other symptoms of respiratory infection are absent. The dominant complaint is chest wall or abdominal wall pain that is enhanced by respiration and that may result in splinting of the chest and rapid, shallow breathing. Muscle tenderness can be detected by direct palpation; less commonly, localized swelling is observed (Sylvest, 1934). The chest pain may mimic pneumonia or the preeruptive phase of herpes zoster. Although pleurodynia is often misdiagnosed clinically as pneumonia, the chest x-ray film inevitably reveals clear lung fields. Abdominal pain brought on by pleurodynia may suggest a variety of causes of acute abdomen. In fact, during a 1951 outbreak in Birmingham, England, 9 of 49 children who were hospitalized with pleurodynia underwent laparotomy (Disney et al., 1953). Analgesics and limitation of physical activity are helpful in reducing pain, which is generally most severe on presentation and then progressively diminishes during the course of illness (which is typically 4 to 6 days but which may last as long as 3 weeks) (Warin et al., 1953).

Acute enterovirus myositis may be localized to other muscles (De Renck et al., 1977; Jehn and Fink, 1980), especially those of the thigh, or generalized muscle involvement may be present (Fukuyama et al., 1977; Schiraldi and Iandolo, 1978; Gyorkey et al., 1978). These patients present with fever, chills, and generalized weakness, and examination may reveal hypotonia, tenderness, and edema of the involved muscle groups. Laboratory studies may demonstrate myoglobinemia, myoglobinuria, and an elevated creatine-phosphokinase level. Most patients have been reported to have recovered rapidly, but at least one fatal case of systemic echovirus 11 myositis has been reported in a 3-month-old infant (Halfon and Spector, 1981).

Diabetes mellitus. The evidence supporting a role for group B coxsackieviruses in the pathogenesis of type 1 insulin-dependent diabetes mellitus includes a number of clinical, epidemiologic, and experimental studies (Craighead, 1975; Barrett-Connor, 1985; Banatvala, 1987; Rewers and Atkinson, 1995; Yoon, 1990; Craighead et al., 1990). New onset juvenile diabetes cases sometimes occur in clusters (Huff et al., 1974; Rewers et al., 1987) or according to a seasonal pattern that peaks 1 to 3 months after enterovirus activity (Gamble et al., 1969; Gleason et al., 1982). Group B coxsackievirus infection of pancreatic islets has been demonstrated both in a murine model (Craighead, 1975; Hartig et al., 1983) and in the pancreases of two children dying of new onset ketoacidosis (Gladish et al., 1976; Yoon et al., 1979). Both enterovirus RNA (Clements et al., 1995; Andreoletti et al., 1997) and group B coxsackievirus–specific IgM antibody (Banatvala et al., 1985; Frisk et al., 1992; Dahlquist et al., 1995;

Helfand et al., 1995) have been found in sera from children experiencing new onset diabetes. Other evidence suggests that viral infection may initiate an immune response mediated by anti–islet cell antibodies (Kaufman et al., 1992; Solimena and De Camilli, 1995; Hiltunen et al., 1997; Lonnrot et al., 2000).

Other diseases. A preponderance of case reports suggest that group B coxsackieviruses and echoviruses cause some cases of pancreatitis (Craighead, 1975; Ursing, 1973; Arnesjo et al., 1976; Imrle et al., 1977) and orchitis in adolescent boys (Craighead et al., 1962; Welliver and Cherry, 1978; Ager et al., 1964; Murphy and Simmul, 1964). Enteroviruses have also been associated with many other acute diseases, including acute gastroenteritis (Kilbrick, 1964; Yow et al., 1963; Ramos-Alverez and Olarte, 1964; Steinhoff, 1978), hepatitis (Lansky et al., 1979; Leggiadro et al., 1982), arthritis (Kujala and Newman, 1985; Blotzer and Myers, 1978), acute infectious lymphocytosis (Van der Sar, 1979; Norwitz and Moore, 1968), and the hemolytic-uremic syndrome (Glasgow and Balduzzi, 1965; Ray et al., 1970; Oregan et al., 1980), although quality of the evidence supporting an etiologic relationship is variable.

Poliovirus Infections

Paralytic poliomyelitis. Acute neuroparalytic disease caused by naturally occurring poliovirus infection is now limited to certain regions in sub-Saharan Africa and the Indian subcontinent and is targeted for global eradication before 2005. However sporadic cases of motor neuron disease are caused by other enteroviruses, especially enterovirus 71, which also caused outbreaks in Eastern Europe in the late 1970s (Voroshilova and Chumakov, 1959; Grist and Bell, 1970; Shindarov et al., 1979).

The majority of persons infected with naturally occurring polioviruses experience few or no symptoms. Fewer than 10% of infections result in a "minor" illness consisting of fever, headache, and sore throat; and fewer than 1% of patients experience a "major" illness that is characterized by abrupt onset of viral meningitis and myalgias. Although the major illness is limited to viral meningitis, which resolves within 5 to 10 days (i.e., "nonparalytic poliomyelitis") in about one third of cases the majority of patients develop progressive asymmetric paresis of one or more extremities over a period of hours to days (Nathanson and Martin, 1979; Melnick and Ledinko, 1951).

The severity of disease ranges from mild weakness of a single extremity to complete flaccid quadriplegia. Proximal limb muscles are more involved than distal, and legs are more commonly involved than arms. "Bulbar poliomyelitis" complicates 5% to 35% of paralytic cases, most commonly affecting function of the ninth and tenth cranial nerves, causing dysphagia, dyspnea, difficulty with secretions, anxiety, and respiratory compromise. There is probably little correlation between age and severity of disease after the decline of maternal antibody (Nathanson and Martin, 1979; Melnick and Ledinko, 1951). However, the risk of neuroparalytic disease is enhanced by pregnancy (Weinstein et al., 1951; Anderson et al., 1952; Paffenbarger and Wilson, 1955), B-cell immunodeficiency (Wyatt, 1973; Davis et al., 1977), strenuous exercise during the incubation period (Horstmann, 1950), recent trauma or intramuscular injection (Hill and Knowelden, 1950; Greenberg et al., 1952; Sutter et al., 1992), and tonsillectomy (Paffenbarger and Wilson, 1955).

The disease most often confused with acute poliomyelitis is the Guillain-Barré syndrome, which, unlike poliomyelitis, causes paralysis that is classically ascending in nature, symmetric, and accompanied by sensory abnormalities. In addition, the CSF pleocytosis noted during the major illness of poliomyelitis is uncharacteristic of the Guillain-Barré syndrome, which is associated with a normal CSF leukocyte count and an elevated CSF protein concentration.

A period of recovery of muscle function follows that may extend up to 6 to 9 months; however, some motor deficit, ranging from minor debility to permanent, flaccid paralysis, persists in two thirds of cases. Of patients with acute paralytic poliomyelitis, 4% to 6% died of respiratory paralysis in the era predating modern intensive care. A postpoliomyelitis syndrome occurs 20 to 40 years later in approximately 25% of persons who survived acute paralytic poliomyelitis. Typically there is development of chronic pain and atrophy of the same muscle groups affected during the original acute infection (Dalakas and Illa, 1991). The etiology of this debilitating relapse is not known.

Enterovirus Infections in Special Hosts

Neonates. The high mortality rates observed during newborn nursery outbreaks of group B coxsackievirus myocarditis in southern Africa in the 1950s (Montgomery et al., 1955; Javett et al., 1956) provided the first evidence of serious disease from enterovirus infection acquired in the perinatal period. Since then, many cases of overwhelming neonatal disease caused by group B coxsackieviruses and echoviruses have been reported. The group A coxsackieviruses cause very rare cases of neonatal disease (Wright et al., 1963; Baker and Phillips, 1980; Talsma et al., 1984). An effective placental barrier prevents intrauterine enterovirus transmission (Selzer, 1969; Modlin and Bowman, 1987). Consequently, most neonatal infections are acquired in the perinatal period from their infected mothers, as many as 3% of whom may excrete enteroviruses at term during periods of high enterovirus activity (Modlin et al., 1981). Nosocomial infections also occur (Gear and Measroch, 1973; Modlin, 1986), and infection can be spread within nurseries via the hands of personnel engaged in mouth care, gavage feeding, and other activities requiring close direct contact (Kinney et al., 1986).

The pathophysiologic basis for the unique susceptibility of newborns, which extends to about 7 to 10 days of age, is not fully understood. Experimental data suggest that macrophage function, which does not sufficiently mature until several weeks of age in the human infant, is necessary to limit initial enteroviral replication (Rager-Zisman and Allison, 1973; Mills, 1983). In addition, the outcome of neonatal infection is strongly influenced by the presence or absence of passively acquired maternal type-specific neutralizing antibody (Modlin et al., 1981; Modlin, 1980; Berry and Nagington, 1982; Nagington, et al., 1978). Thus the timing of maternal infection in relation to development of maternal IgG antibody, and delivery of the infant, may be the most critical factor in determining the outcome of neonatal enterovirus infection.

The majority of infants with serious coxsackievirus and echovirus disease develop nonspecific symptoms of lethargy and poor feeding between 3 and 7 days of life before progression to one of two clinical syndromes: either myocarditis or severe, often fulminate hepatitis (Modlin, 1986, Kaplan et al., 1983). In addition, neonatal enterovirus pneumonia has been reported in a small number of cases, all of them fatal (Boyd et al., 1987; Cheeseman et al., 1977; Toce and Keenan, 1988).

Neonatal myocarditis, which is often accompanied by encephalitis and sometimes by hepatitis, is usually caused by one of the group B coxsackievirus serotype 1 to 5 viruses (Kibrick, 1964; Gear and Measroch, 1973) and less commonly by echovirus 11 infection (Berkovich et al., 1968; Drew, 1973). After a brief prodrome, infected infants rapidly develop clinical signs of heart failure, systolic murmurs, and arrhythmias. Infants with encephalitis may develop seizures, a bulging fontanel, and a CSF pleocytosis. Cyanosis and hypotension are poor prognostic signs. Surviving infants generally experience improvement of cardiac function within 7 days of onset. Reported mortality rates are 30% to 50%. Infants dying of myocarditis have enlarged, dilated hearts, extensive myonecrosis, and a variable degree of inflammation of the heart and less commonly the brain, meninges, lungs, liver, pancreas, or adrenal glands.

Echovirus 11 is prominent among the multiple echovirus serotypes reported to cause neonatal enterovirus hepatitis, which is often erroneously referred to as *enterovirus sepsis or sepsis syndrome* because of progressive hypotension, profuse bleeding, jaundice, and secondary multiple organ dysfunction due to fulminate liver failure (Modlin, 1986; Georgieff et al., 1987; Spector and Straube, 1983; Speer and Yawn, 1984; Wreghitt et al., 1984; Chambon et al., 1997). Hepatic transaminase levels rise rapidly to extremely high levels. Thrombocytopenia generally is profound, and markedly prolonged prothrombin times and partial thromboplastin times are indicative of profound hepatic failure. Despite therapy with blood products and intensive supportive care, more than half of infants with severe neonatal echovirus hepatitis die within days after onset of symptoms. Postmortem findings include hepatic necrosis and extensive hemorrhage into the cerebral ventricles, pericardial sac, renal medullae, and interstitial spaces of many solid organs (Mostoufizadeh et al., 1983). Inflammation is commonly limited to the liver and adrenal glands.

Supportive management of neonatal enteroviral disease includes medical therapy for heart failure and judicious use of packed red blood cells, platelets, and fresh-frozen plasma for infants with bleeding and coagulopathy caused by acute hepatic failure. Vitamin K should be administered intravenously in pharmacologic doses. Large doses of IVIG are sometimes given (Johnston and Overall, 1989) and pleconaril is available on a compassionate-use basis from the manufacturer (see the discussion of treatment, later in this chapter) (Rotbart, 1998). Neither agent has been evaluated in a controlled manner in infants with serious enterovirus infections.

Congenital B-cell immunodeficiency. Enterovirus infections in persons with hereditary and acquired B-cell immunodeficiency disorders may persist for months to years and cause a variety of serious complications including chronic meningoencephalitis, motor neuron disease, chronic hepatitis, and a dermatomyositis-like syndrome. Most affected patients have X-linked agammaglobulinemia or other conditions associated with hypogammaglobulinemia, including common variable immunodeficiency (McKinney et al., 1987). The risk of developing chronic enterovirus infections has diminished with the introduction of IVIG as standard antibody replacement therapy (Webster et al., 1993).

The increased susceptibility of patients with these disorders was first reported in young children infected with naturally occurring and attenuated polioviruses. Since then, about 30% of reported cases of vaccine-associated paralytic poliomyelitis (VAPP) have been immunodeficient (Sutter and Prevots, 1994). These patients may develop acute paralysis or, alternatively, follow an atypical course with an incubation period of months to years following administration of or exposure to oral polio vaccine (OPV) viruses, with development of prolonged febrile illness, chronic meningitis, and progressive motor weakness (Wyatt, 1973; Davis et al., 1977; Sutter and Prevots, 1994). Fecal excretion of virus in surviving cases has been estimated to occur for as long as 9 years (Kew et al., 1998). Immunodeficient VAPP patients have a higher mortality than patients who are immunocompetent (Sutter and Prevots, 1994).

Persistent CNS infection with other enteroviruses causes prolonged or recurrent nuchal rigidity, headache, lethargy, papilledema, seizures, motor weakness, tremors, and ataxia (McKinney et al., 1987). Most cases have been caused by echoviruses, with individual cases reported with group A coxsackievirus serotypes 4, 11, and 15, and group B coxsackievirus serotypes 2 and 3 (McKinney et al., 1987; O'Neil et al., 1988). Symptoms and signs of CNS infection may fluctuate, disappear, or steadily progress. Routine examination of the CSF demonstrates a lymphocytic pleocytosis and high protein concentration, and enteroviruses are readily identified by cell culture or PCR (Webster et al., 1993; Rotbart et al., 1990). Concomitant skeletal muscle infection is associated with a dermatomyositis-like syndrome in more than half of these patients (McKinney et al., 1987; Mease et al., 1981). Some patients develop chronic hepatitis.

Historically, most enterovirus infections in patients with agammaglobulinemia have ended in death. Some patients have experienced improvement when IVIG has been injected directly into the ventricles, but relapse of infection may occur even after long-term therapy (McKinney et al., 1987; Mease et al., 1981). The use of the antiviral drug pleconaril holds more promise, but the reported experience with it is uncontrolled and limited to a small number of patients (Rotbart and Webster, 2001).

Other immunodeficiency disorders. Hematopoietic stem cell allograft recipients have profoundly suppressed immunologic responses during the immediate posttransplant period, including the ability to mount a humoral immune response. A small number have developed enterovirus infections in the posttransplant period that were disseminated and prolonged and contributed to fatal outcomes (Biggs et al., 1990; Aquino et al., 1996; Galama et al., 1996). In contrast, persons with HIV infection appear to have little or no increased risk from enterovirus infection. VAPP has been reported in only two children with HIV infection (Ion-Neldescu et al., 1994; Chitsike and van Furth, 1999) despite the administration of many thousands of doses of OPV to HIV-infected infants (von Reyn et al., 1987; Onorato et al., 1988).

DIAGNOSIS

The laboratory diagnosis of enterovirus infection is accomplished by isolation and identification of virus in cell culture, by detection of enterovirus RNA by polymerase chain reaction (PCR), or by serologic methods. Each method has unique advantages and disadvantages.

Cell Culture

Enteroviruses produce characteristic cytopathic effect (CPE) in susceptible cultured cells, permitting their isolation and identification (Melnick et al., 1949; Gordon et al., 1959). In practice, clinical laboratories use three or four different cell lines to optimize recovery of a virus (Dagan and Menegus, 1986) Development of visible CPE usually requires 2 to 6 days in primary cultures (Dagan and Menegus, 1986). Some laboratories use a broadly specific monoclonal antibody to confirm that CPE is due to enteroviral replication (Trabelsi et al., 1995). Cell culture is labor intensive and expensive. However, recovery of an isolate in cell culture is necessary if serotype identification is important for clinical, epidemiologic, or research purposes. Regardless of the type of illness, the submission of clinical specimens from multiple sites enhances the likelihood of isolation of an enterovirus in cell culture. Stool and rectal swabs are most likely to produce an isolate. Often, CSF (in cases of CNS disease), orapharyngeal secretions, urine, and serum are sampled. "False-positive" results may occur when an untyped enterovirus is isolated from stool in locations where OPV viruses are widely prevalent, and because children excrete enteroviruses for up to 8 weeks in stool from a previous infection.

Polymerase Chain Reaction

PCR using an initial reverse transcriptase step and primers derived from the highly conserved 5′-noncoding region of the genome has superior sensitivity compared with cell culture for enterovirus detection. PCR detects enterovirus RNA in 66% to 86% of patients with acute viral meningitis, compared with cell culture isolation rates of approximately 30% (Rotbart et al., 1994; Sawyer et al., 1994; Yerly et al., 1996; Pozo et al., 1998). Experience with specimens other than CSF is limited. PCR compares favorably with culture for throat and serum specimens but may be less sensitive for urine specimens (Rotbart et al., 1997). Enterovirus PCR is not generally available in hospital laboratories but is offered by many reference and commercial laboratories.

Serology

Serologic assays are mainly used for determination of prior immunity for epidemiologic or research purposes. They are not very useful for diagnosis of acute disease except when infection with a specific serotype or one of a small number of serotypes is suspected. The microneutralization test is the standard method for determination of antibodies to enteroviruses, and the one to which other serologic methods are compared. Because microneutralization is serotype specific, it has limited usefulness in the routine diagnosis of nonpolio enterovirus infections because of the low feasibility of testing multiple live viral antigens, and because methods based on neutralization are relatively insensitive, poorly standardized, and labor intensive. Immunoassays (e.g., enzyme immunoassay [EIA] and indirect fluorescent antibody [IFA] test) offered in commercial laboratories to test antibodies against group B coxsackie virus serotypes 1 to 6, a few echoviruses, and one or two group A coxsackie virus serotypes are easier to perform but show some degree of cross-reactivity among different serotypes and may be difficult to interpret. These assays require both acute and convalescent sera.

Serum IgM antibody to the group B coxsackieviruses can often be detected in a single serum specimen early in the course of illness, but positive test results are not serotype specific (Pozetto et al., 1989; Bell et al., 1986).

TREATMENT

The great majority of enterovirus infections are self-limited and do not require specific therapy. Exceptions may include acute myocarditis and infections in neonates and B-cell deficient hosts, which may be life-threatening, and acute viral meningitis, which can cause short-term morbidity, especially in older children, adolescents, and adults. The therapeutic options for these more serious infections are quite limited. Serum immune globulin and IVIG have been given to individual, persistently infected B-cell deficient patients with mixed results (McKinney et al., 1987; Mease et al., 1981) and have been used in nonrandomized trials in children with myocarditis with uncertain effect (Drucker et al., 1994).

Although an effective antiviral drug to treat serious enterovirus infections has not been licensed, a variety of agents have shown activity against enteroviruses in animal models and in early clinical trials (Schiff and Sherwood, 2000). The most promising of these are antipicornavirus compounds that bind avidly to a pocket in the viral capsid, altering virus attachment and uncoating (Zhang et al., 1992). The best studied of the capsid-binding drugs is pleconaril, which inhibits replication of most enterovirus serotypes at concentrations of <0.1 μg/ml in vitro (Pevear et al., 1989) and which has favorable pharmacologic and safety profiles (Rotbart, 2002). Placebo-controlled trials of pleconaril in patients with enterovirus meningitis (age range 8 to 65 years) have shown significant reductions in the duration and severity of headache and other symptoms and a shorter period of viral shedding when the drug was administered within 24 hours of symptom onset (Weiner et al., 1997; Rotbart, 2000; Sawyer et al., 1999; Shafran et al., 1999). In addition, uncontrolled experience with pleconaril for B-cell deficient patients with persistent enterovirus infections and patients with potentially fatal infections, including neonates and persons of all ages with acute myocarditis, suggests substantial clinical benefit (Rotbart, 1998). Pleconaril can be obtained for compassionate use for patients with life-threatening enterovirus infections from ViroPharma, Inc. (Exton, Penn, 610-458-7300).

PREVENTION
Infection Control

Simple hygienic measures, such as hand washing and careful disposal or autoclaving of potentially infected feces and secretions, may prevent the spread of enteroviruses during community epidemics or when patients are hospitalized with enteroviral diseases. Use of gowns or masks or isolation of patients is unwarranted, except in the newborn nursery. Pregnant women near term should be advised to avoid contact with patients suspected of having enterovirus illness.

Passive Immunoprophylaxis

The preexposure administration of immunoglobulin is known to reduce the risk of paralytic poliomyelitis (Stevens, 1959). Immunoglobulin may also prevent nonpolio enteroviral disease, but this strategy is rarely applicable to clinical practice.

Active Immunization

Vaccines for poliovirus infections have been used worldwide in universal immunization programs to prevent paralytic poliomyelitis, and within the past two decades to eradicate

poliovirus infections. Vaccines are not available to prevent other enterovirus infections, although an inactivated vaccine was developed to control outbreaks of serious enterovirus 71 infections in Eastern Europe in the 1970s; this vaccine was never used on a widespread basis (Melnick, 1984).

Poliovirus Vaccines

Both inactivated poliovirus vaccine (IPV) and live, attenuated OPV were developed in the 1950s (Salk, 1953; Francis et al., 1957; Sabin, 1985), and both have been widely used throughout the world, albeit under different circumstances in different locations. Although both IPV and OPV have contributed to the successful control of poliomyelitis, these two vaccines possess different risks and benefits for individuals and for whole populations. IPV is now the only vaccine currently recommended for routine infant and childhood immunization in the United States and many other countries that have eradicated polio. Because OPV maintains certain advantages for children in developing countries, it is the vaccine recommended by the WHO Expanded Program on Immunization (EPI).

IPV is prepared by inactivation of naturally occurring polioviruses with dilute formalin. The "enhanced potency" IPV currently available in the United States (IPOL) is produced in monkey kidney (Vero) cells and contains 40, 8, and 32 D antigen units of poliovirus types 1, 2, and 3, respectively. IPV stimulates neutralizing antibodies to all three poliovirus types in 99% of recipients after two doses, and in 100% following the third dose (Simoes and John, 1986; McBean et al., 1988). Detectable antibody persists at protective levels for at least 5 years, although geometric mean antibody titers decline considerably (Swartz et al., 1986). Under conditions of natural exposure, efficacy rates of 36% and 89% have been demonstrated against poliovirus type 1 for one and two IPV doses, respectively (Robertson et al., 1988). Because most IPV recipients experience a substantial boost in antibody titer following a third dose, it is likely that efficacy after three IPV doses would be quite high. The incidence of local reactions following Vero cell derived IPV is the same as placebo, and there is no evidence that IPV is associated with more serious reactions. In the United States, IPV is routinely administered in four doses at 2 months, 4 months, 6 to 18 months, and 4 to 6 years of age (Centers for Disease Control and Prevention, 2000a).

The OPV vaccine strains were attenuated by passage in monkeys and in monkey kidney cell culture (Sabin, 1957). The trivalent OPV formulation distributed for many years in the United States (Orimune) contained $10^{6.5}$ $TCID_{50}$, $10^{5.4}$ $TCID_{50}$, and $10^{6.3}$ $TCID_{50}$, respectively, of poliovirus types 1, 2, and 3 (Patriarca et al., 1991). OPV vaccines produced in other countries are now similarly formulated. The unequal contribution of each type to the trivalent preparation represents a "balanced" formulation designed to account for the more efficient replication of type 2 OPV virus in the gastrointestinal tract, that is, if the three types are administered in equal concentrations, type 2 virus would interfere with the replication of types 1 and 3 (Robertson et al., 1962).

Multiple OPV doses are required to assure protection against all three poliovirus serotypes. In developed countries, three doses given at least 2 months apart are sufficient, with antibody prevalence to all three types ≥96% after the third dose (McBean et al., 1988). Detectable serum antibody to all three types persists in 84% to 98% of vaccinees 5 years after primary immunization (Krugman et al., 1977). Use of OPV for more than three decades—from 1961 to 1999—in the United States provides overwhelming evidence of effectiveness in developed countries. OPV vaccine efficacy was estimated to be 82%, 96%, and 98% for one, two, and three or more doses, respectively, during a type 1 poliovirus outbreak in Taiwan (Kim-Farley et al., 1984).

However, in tropical countries the EPI-recommended series of OPV at 6, 10, and 14 weeks of age may fail to produce active immunity in a significant proportion of infants. Low seroconversion rates to three OPV doses have been documented in many locations (de Brito et al., 1974; Domok et al., 1974; Hanlon et al., 1987; John and Jayabal, 1972; John and Christopher, 1975; Lasch et al., 1984), averaging 73%, 90%, and 70% for types 1, 2, and 3, respectively (Patriarca et al., 1991). The reason for the less-than-optimal responses to OPV is not fully understood, but interference by concurrent diarrheal disease appears to be an important factor (World Health Organization, 1992; Myaux et al., 1996).

The most important adverse outcome associated with OPV administration is the rare occurrence of vaccine-associated paralytic poliomyelitis (VAPP) affecting approximately 1 in 750,000 primary vaccinees, mostly infants receiving their first OPV dose, and also nonimmune household contacts of vaccinees (Strebel et al., 1992). Approximately 30% of reported VAPP cases occur among persons with B-cell immunodeficiency syndromes (Sutter and Prevots, 1994; Strebel et al., 1992). The risks of VAPP in the presence of immunodeficiency due to other causes, such as hematologic malignancy, cancer chemotherapy, radiation, organ transplantation, and HIV infection, have not been quantified, but are likely to be much lower than with B-cell disorders. However, because IPV is available as a safe alternative, OPV should not be given to these individuals (Centers for Disease Control and Prevention, 2000). OPV does not increase the risk of fetal malformation or other adverse pregnancy outcome (Harjulehto et al., 1989).

Recently among underimmunized children living in certain economically deprived regions, outbreaks of paralytic poliomyelitis have occurred that have been caused by OPV vaccine-derived polioviruses that circulate for long periods because of low immunization rates. These viruses have acquired virulent biologic properties that are indistinguishable from naturally occurring wild polioviruses (Centers for Disease Control and Prevention, 2000c; Kew et al., 2002; Centers for Disease Control and Prevention, 2001a; Centers for Disease Control and Prevention, 2001b; Centers for Disease Control and Prevention, 2002a). The discovery of these OPV vaccine–derived polioviruses has influenced plans for the eventual cessation of poliovirus immunization following eradication of poliomyelitis, which may include a strategy to simultaneously discontinue OPV use worldwide, development of an OPV vaccine stockpile, and a plan for containment of laboratory stocks of naturally occurring and attenuated polioviruses (Technical Consultative Group, 2002).

BIBLIOGRAPHY

Adler JL, Mostow SR, Mellin II, et al. Epidemiologic investigation of hand, foot, and mouth disease: infection caused by coxsackievirus A16 in Baltimore, June through September 1968. Am J Dis Child 1970;120:309.

Ager EA, Felsenstein WC, Alexander ER, et al. An epidemic of illness due to coxsackievirus group B, type 2. JAMA 1964;187:251.

Alexander JP, Baden L, Pallansch MA, et al. Enterovirus 71 infections and neurologic disease—United States, 1977-1991. J Infect Dis 1994;169:905.

Alexander JP, Gary HE Jr, Pallansch M. Duration of poliovirus excretion and its implications for acute flaccid paralysis surveillance: a review of the literature. J Infect Dis 1997;175:S176.

Amir J, Harel L, Frydman M, et al. Shift in cerebrospinal polymorphonuclear cell percentage in the early stage of aseptic meningitis. J Pediatr 1991;119:938.

Anderson GW, Anderson G, Skaar A, et al. Poliomyelitis in pregnancy. Am J Hyg 1952;55:127.

Andreoletti L, Hober D, Decoene C, et al. Detection of enteroviral RNA by polymerase chain reaction in endomyocardial tissue of patients with chronic cardiac diseases. J Med Virol 1996;48:53.

Andreoletti L, Hober D, Hober-Vandenberghe C, et al. Detection of coxsackie B virus RNA sequences in whole blood samples from adult patients at the onset of type I diabetes mellitus. J Med Virol 1997;52:121.

Aquino VM, Farah RA, Lee ME, et al. Disseminated cox-sackie A9 infection complicating bone marrow trans-plantation. Pediatr Infect Dis J 1996;15:1053.

Arnesjo B, Eden T, Ihse I, et al. Enterovirus infections in acute pancreatitis—a possible etiologic connection. Scand J Gastroenterol 1976;11:645.

Assaad F, Cockburn WC. Four year study of WHO virus reports on enteroviruses other than poliovirus. Bull World Health Org 1972;46:329.

Avner E, Satz J, Plotkin SA. Hypoglycorrhachia in young infants with viral meningitis. J Pediatr 1975;87: 883.

Ayuthya PSN, Jayavasu JJ, Pongpanich B. Coxsackie group B virus and primary myocardial disease in infants and children. Am Heart J 1974;88:311.

Baker DA, Phillips CA. Maternal and neonatal infection with coxsackievirus. Obstet Gynecol 1980;55:12.

Banatvala JE. Insulin-dependent (juvenile-onset, type 1) diabetes mellitus coxsackie B viruses revisited. Prog Med Virol 1987;34:33.

Banatvala JE, Bryant J, Schernthaner G, et al. Coxsackie B, mumps, rubella, and cytomegalovirus specific IgM responses in patients with juvenile-onset insulin-dependent diabetes mellitus in Britain, Austria, and Australia. Lancet 1985;2:1279.

Barak Y, Schwartz JF. Acute transverse myelitis associated with ECHO type 5 infection (letter). Am J Dis Child 1988;142:128.

Barrett-Connor E. Is insulin-dependent diabetes mellitus caused by coxsackievirus B infection? A review of the epidemiologic evidence. Rev Infect Dis 1985;7:207.

Bell EJ, McCartney RA, Basquill D, et al. Antibody capture ELISA for the rapid diagnosis of enterovirus infections in patients with aseptic meningitis. J Med Virol 1986;19:213.

Bell EJ, Ross CAC, Grist NR. Echo 9 infection in pregnant women with suspected rubella. J Clin Pathol 1975;28:267.

Bendig JWA, O'Brien PS, Muir P, et al. Enterovirus sequences resembling coxsackievirus A2 detected in stool and spleen from a girl with fatal myocarditis. J Med Virol 2001;64:482.

Bergman I, Painter MJ, Wald ER, et al. Outcome in children with enteroviral meningitis during the first year of life. J Pediatr 1987;110:705.

Berkovich S, Rodriguez-Torres R, Lin J-S. Virologic studies in children with acute myocarditis. Am J Dis Child 1968;115:207.

Berlin LE, Rorabaugh ML, Heldrich F, et al. Aseptic menin-gitis in infants less than two years of age: diagnosis and etiology. J Infect Dis 1993;168:888.

Berry PJ, Nagington J. Fatal infection with echovirus 11. Arch Dis Child 1982;57:22.

Biggs DD, Toorkey BC, Carrigan DR, et al. Disseminated echovirus infection complicating bone marrow trans-plantation. Am J Med 1990;88:421.

Blotzer JW, Myers AR. Echovirus associated polyarthritis. Report of a case with synovial fluid and synovial histo-logic characterization. Arthritis Rheum 1978;21:978.

Bodian D. Histopathological basis of clinical findings in poliomyelitis. Am J Med 1949;6:563.

Bodian D. A reconsideration of the pathogenesis of poliomyelitis. Am J Hyg 1952;55:414.

Bodian D. Emerging concept of poliomyelitis infection. Science 1955;122:105.

Boring WD, Zu Rhein GM, Walker DL. Factors influencing host-virus interactions: II. Alteration of Coxsackie virus infection in adult mice by cold. Proc Soc Exp Biol Med 1956;93:273.

Boyd MT, Jordan SW, Davis LE. Fatal pneumonitis from congenital echovirus type 6 infection. Pediatr Infect Dis J 1987;6:1138.

Byington CL, Taggart EW, Carroll KC, et al. A polymerase chain reaction–based epidemiologic investigation of the incidence of nonpolio enteroviral infections in febrile and afebrile infants 90 days and younger. Pediatrics 1999;103.

Caldera R, Sarrut S, Mallet R, et al. Existetil des complica-tions cardiaques de la vaccine? Sem Hop Paris 1961;37:1281.

Camargo PR, Snitcowsky R, da Luz PL, et al. Favorable effects of immunosuppressive therapy in children with dilated cardiomyopathy and active myocarditis. Pediatr Cardiol 1995;16:61.

Caro V, Guillot S, Delpeyroux F, et al. Molecular strategy for "serotyping" of human enteroviruses. J Gen Virol 2001;82:79.

Centers for Disease Control and Prevention. Fatal mumps myocarditis in England. MMWR Morb Mortal Wkly Rep 1980;27:425.

Centers for Disease Control and Prevention. Enterovirus surveillance–United States, 1990. MMWR Morb Mortal Wkly Rep 1990; 39:788.

Centers for Disease Control and Prevention. Nonpolio enterovirus surveillance—United States, 1993-1996. MMWR Morb Mortal Wkly Rep 1997;46:748.

Centers for Disease Control and Prevention. Progress toward the global interruption of wild poliovirus type 2 transmission, 1999. Morb Mort Wk Rep 1999;48:736.

Centers for Disease Control and Prevention. Poliomyelitis prevention in the United States. MMWR Morb Mortal Wkly Rep 2000a;49:1.

Centers for Disease Control and Prevention. Enterovirus surveillance—United States, 1997-1999. MMWR Morb Mortal Wkly Rep 2000b;49:913.

Centers for Disease Control and Prevention. Circulation of a type 2 vaccine-derived poliovirus—Egypt, 1982-1993. MMWR Morb Mortal Wkly Rep 2001a;50:41.

Centers for Disease Control and Prevention. Public health dispatch: acute flaccid paralysis associated with circulating vaccine-derived poliovirus—Philippines, 2001. MMWR Morb Mortal Wkly Rep 2001b;50:874.

Centers for Disease Control and Prevention. Outbreak of poliomyelitis—Dominican Republic and Haiti, 2000. MMWR Morb Mortal Wkly Rep 2000c;49:1094.

Centers for Disease Control and Prevention. Poliomyelitis—Madagascar, 2002. MMWR Morb Mortal Wkly Rep 2002a;51:622.

Centers for Disease Control and Prevention. Enterovirus surveillance—United States, 2000-2001. MMWR Morb Mortal Wkly Rep 2002b;51:1047.

Centers for Disease Control and Prevention. Progress toward global eradication of poliomyelitis, 2001. MMWR Morb Mortal Wkly Rep 2002c; 51:253.

Chalhub E, Devivo D, Siegel BA, et al. Coxsackie A9 focal encephalitis associated with acute infantile hemiplegia and porencephaly. Neurology 1977;27:574.

Chambon M, Delage C, Bailly J-L, et al. Fatal hepatic necrosis in a neonate with echovirus 20 infection: use of the polymerase chain reaction to detect enterovirus in liver tissue. Clin Infect Dis 1997;24:523.

Chan KY, Iwahara M, Benson LN, et al. Immunosuppressive therapy in the management of acute myocarditis in children: a clinical trial. J Am Coll Cardiol 1991;17:458.

Cheeseman SH, Hirsch MS, Keller EW, et al. Fatal neonatal pneumonia caused by echovirus type 9 (letter). Am J Dis Child 1977;131:1169.

Cheever FS. Multiplication of Coxsackie virus in adult mice exposed to Roentgen radiation. J Immunol 1953;71:431.

Cherry JD, Jahn CL. Herpangina. The etiologic spectrum. Pediatrics 1965;36:632.

Cherry JD, Jahn CL. Virologic studies of exanthems. J Pediatr 1966;68:204.

Cherry JD, Lerner AM, Klein JO, et al. Coxsackie A9 infections with exanthems with particular reference to urticaria. Pediatrics 1963;31:819.

Chitsike I, van Furth R. Paralytic poliomyelitis associated with live oral poliomyelitis vaccine in child with HIV infection in Zimbabwe: case report. Br Med J 1999;318:841.

Chow LH, Beisel KW, McManus BM. Enterovirus infection of mice with severe combined immune deficiency: evidence for direct viral pathogenesis of myocardial injury. Lab Invest 1992;66:24.

Chow M, Baltimore D. Synthetic peptides from four separate regions of the poliovirus type 1 capsid protein VP1 induce neutralizing antibodies. Proc Natl Acad Sci USA 1985;82:910.

Christopher S, Theogaraj S, Godbole S, et al. An epidemic of acute hemorrhagic conjunctivitis due to coxsackievirus A24. J Infect Dis 1982;146:16.

Chumakov MP, Voroshilova MK, Shindarov L, et al. Enterovirus 71 isolated from cases of poliomyelitis-like disease in Bulgaria. Arch Virol 1979;60:329.

Clements GB, Galbraith DN, Taylor KW. Coxsackie B virus infection and onset of childhood diabetes. Lancet 1995;346:221.

Codd MB, Sugrue DD, Gersh BJ, et al. Epidemiology of idiopathic dilated and hypertrophic cardiomyopathy. A population-based study in Olmsted County, Minnesota, 1975-1984. Circulation 1989;80:564.

Committee on the ECHO Viruses, National Foundation for Infantile Paralysis, Enteric cytopathogenic human orphan viruses. Science 1955;122:1187.

Couch RB, Douglas RG, Lindgren KM, et al. Airborne transmission of respiratory infection with coxsackievirus A type 21. Am J Epidemiol 1970;91:78.

Craighead JE. The role of viruses in the pathogenesis of pancreatic disease and diabetes mellitus. Prog Med Virol 1975;19:162.

Craighead JE, Huber SA, Sriram S. Animal models of picornavirus-induced autoimmune disease: their possible relevance to human disease. Lab Invest 1990;63:432.

Craighead JE, Mahoney EM, Carver DH, et al. Orchitis due to coxsackie virus group B, type 5. N Engl J Med 1962; 267:498.

Curnen EC, Shaw EW, Melnick JL. Disease resembling nonparalytic poliomyelitis associated with virus pathogenic for infant mice. JAMA 1949;141:894.

Dagan R. Nonpolio enteroviruses and the febrile young infant: epidemiologic, clinical, and diagnostic aspects. Pediatr Infect Dis J 1996;15:67.

Dagan R, Hall CB, Powell KR, et al. Epidemiology and laboratory diagnosis of infection with viral and bacterial pathogens in infants hospitalized for suspected sepsis. J Pediatr 1989;115:351.

Dagan R, Jenista J, Menegus MA. Association of clinical presentation, laboratory findings, and virus serotypes with the presence of meningitis in hospitalized infants with enterovirus infection. J Pediatr 1988;113:975.

Dagan R, Menegus MA. A combination of four cell types for rapid detection of enteroviruses in clinical specimens. J Med Virol 1986;19:219.

Dahlquist GG, Ivarsson S, Lindberg B, et al. Maternal enteroviral infection during pregnancy as a risk factor for childhood IDDM. Diabetes 1995;44:408.

Dalakas M, Illa I. Post-polio syndrome: concepts in clinical diagnosis, pathogenesis, and etiology. Adv Neurol 1991;56:495.

Dalldorf G, Gifford R. Susceptibility of gravid mice to coxsackie virus infection. J Exp Med 1954;99:21.

Dalldorf G, Sickles G. An unidentified, filtrable agent isolated from the feces of children with paralysis. Science 1948;108:61.

Davis LE, Bodian D, Price D, et al. Chronic progressive poliomyelitis secondary to vaccination of an immunodeficient child. N Engl J Med 1977;297:241.

de Brito Bastos NC, de Carvalho ES, Schatzmayr H, et al. Antipoliomyelitis program in Brazil: a serologic study of immunity. Bull Pan Am Health Org 1974; 8:54.

Dechamps C, Peigue-Lafeuille HH, Laveran H, et al. Four cases of vesicular lesions in adults caused by enterovirus infections. J Clin Microbiol 1988;26:2182.

de Leeuw N, Melchers WJG, Balk AHMM, et al. No evidence for persistent enterovirus infection in patients with end-stage idiopathic dilated cardiomyopathy. J Infect Dis 1998;178:256.

De Renck J, De Coster W, Inderadjaja N. Acute viral polymyositis with predominant diaphragm involvement. J Neurol Sci 1977;33:453.

Dery P, Marks MI, Shapera R. Clinical manifestations of coxsackievirus infections in children. Am J Dis Child 1974;128:464.

Deseda-Tous J, Byatt PH, Cherry JD. Vesicular lesions in adults due to echovirus 11 infections. Arch Dermatol 1977;113:1705.

Disney ME, Howard EM, Wood BSB. Bornholm disease in children. Brit Med J 1953;1:1351.

Domok I, Balayan MS, Fayinka OA, et al. Factors affecting the efficacy of live poliovirus vaccine in warm climates. Bull World Health Org 1974;51:333.

Drew JH. Echo 11 virus outbreak in a nursery associated with myocarditis. Aust J Pediatr 1973;9:90.

Drucker NA, Colan SD, Lewis AB, et al. g-Globulin treatment of acute myocarditis in the pediatric population. Circulation 1994;89:252.

Enders JF, Weller TH, Robbins FC. Cultivation of the Lansing strain of poliomyelitis virus in cultures of various human embryonic tissue. Science 1949;109:85.

Farmer K, MacArthur BA, Clay MM. A follow-up study of 15 cases of neonatal meningoencephalitis due to coxsackie virus B5. J Pediatr 1975;87:568.

Feigin RD, Shackelford PG. Value of repeat lumbar puncture in the differential diagnosis of meningitis. N Engl J Med 1973;289:571.

Feldman AM, McNamara D. Myocarditis. N Engl J Med 2000;343:1388.

Fox JP. Epidemiological aspects of coxsackie and echo virus infections in tropical areas. 7th International Congress on Tropical Medicine and Malaria, vol 3, Rio de Janeiro, 1964. Francis T, Napier JA, Voight RB, et al. Evaluation of the 1954 Field Trial of Poliomyelitis Vaccine. Final Report: Vaccine Evaluation Center, Department of Epidemiology, University of Michigan, 1957.

Friedrich MG, Strohm O, Schulz-Menger J, et al. Contrast media-enhanced magnetic resonance imaging visualizes myocardial changes in the course of viral myocarditis. Circulation 1998;97:1802.

Frisk G, Nilsson E, Tuvemo T, et al. The possible role of coxsackie A and echo viruses in the pathogenesis of type I diabetes mellitus studied by IgM analysis. J Infect 1992;24:13.

Frothingham TE. ECHO virus type 9 associated with three cases simulating meningococcemia. N Engl J Med 1958;259:484.

Fujioka S, Koide H, Kitaura Y, et al. Molecular detection and differentiation of enteroviruses in endomyocardial biopsies and pericardial effusions from dilated cardiomyopathy and myocarditis. Am Heart J 1996;131:760.

Fukuyama Y, Ando T, Yokota J. Acute fulminant myoglobinuric polymyositis with picornavirus-like crystals. J Neurol Neurosurg Psychiatry 1977;40:775.

Galama JMD, de Leeuw N, Wittebol S, et al. Prolonged enteroviral infection in a patient who developed pericarditis and heart failure after bone marrow transplantation. Clin Infect Dis 1996;22:1004.

Gamble DR, Kinsley ML, Fitzgerald MG, et al. Viral antibodies in diabetes mellitus. Br Med J 1969;3:627.

Garg A, Shaiu J, Guyatt G. The ineffectiveness of immunosuppressive therapy in lymphocytic myocarditis: an overview. Ann Intern Med 1998;129:317.

Gatmaitan BG, Chason JL, Lerner AM. Augmentation of the virulence of murine coxsackievirus B-3 myocardiopathy by exercise. J Exp Med 1970;131:1121.

Gauntt CJ. Roles of the humoral immune response in coxsackievirus-B-induced disease. In Tracy S, Chapman NM, Mahy BWJ (eds). The Coxsackie B Viruses. Vol 223. Berlin: Springer, 1997.

Gear JHS, Measroch V. Coxsackievirus infection of the newborn. Prog Med Virol 1973;15:42.

Geer J. Coxsackie virus infections in Southern Africa. Yale J Biol Med 1961;34:289.

Gelfand HM. The occurrence in nature of the Coxsackie and ECHO viruses. Prog Med Virol 1961;3:193.

Gelfand HM, Holgium AH, Marchetti GE, et al. A continuing surveillance of enterovirus infections in healthy children in six United States cities. I. Viruses isolated during 1960 and 1961. Am J Hyg 1963;78:358.

Gelfand HM, LeBlanc DR, Fox JP, et al. Studies on the development of natural immunity to poliomyelitis in Louisiana. III. The serologic response to commercially produced "Salk vaccine" of children totally or partially susceptible to poliovirus infection. Am J Hyg 1959;70:303.

Georgieff MK, Johnson DE, Thompson TR, et al. Fulminant hepatic necrosis in an infant with perinatally acquired echovirus 21 infection. Pediatr Infect Dis J 1987;6:71.

Giacca M, Severini GM, Mestroni L, et al. Low frequency of detection by nested polymerase chain reaction of enterovirus ribonucleic acid in endomyocardial tissue of patients with idiopathic dilated cardiomyopathy. J Am Coll Cardiol 1994;24:1033.

Gilbert GL, Dickson KE, Waters M-J, et al. Outbreak of enterovirus 71 infection in Victoria, Australia, with a high incidence of neurologic involvement. Pediatr Infect Dis J 1988;7:484.

Gladish R, Hofmann W, Waldherr R. Myocarditis and insulitis in coxsackievirus infection. Z Kardiol 1976;65:835.

Glasgow LA, Balduzzi P. Isolation of coxsackie virus group A, type 4, from a patient with hemolytic uremic syndrome. N Engl J Med 1965;273:754.

Gleason RE, Kahn CB, Funk IB, et al. Seasonal incidence of insulin-dependent diabetes in Massachusetts, 1964-1973. Int J Epidemiol 1982;11:39.

Godeny EK, Gauntt CJ. Murine natural killer cells limit coxsackievirus B3 replication. J Immunol 1987;139:913.

Godtfredsen A, Hansen B. A case of mild paralytic disease due to ECHO virus type 11. Acta Pathol Microbiol Scand 1961;53:111.

Gondo K, Kusuhara K, Take H, et al. Echovirus type 9 epidemic in Kagoshima, southern Japan: seroepidemiology and clinical observation of aseptic meningitis. Pediatr Infect Dis J 1995;14:787.

Gordon RB, Lennette EH, Sandrock RS. The varied clinical manifestations of coxsackie viral infections. Arch Intern Med 1959;103:63.

Grasso M, Arbustini E, Silini E, et al. Search for coxsackievirus B3 RNA in idiopathic dilated cardiomyopathy using gene amplification by polymerase chain reaction. Am J Cardiol 1992;69:658.

Greenberg M, Abramson H, Cooper HM, et al. The relation between recent injections and paralytic poliomyelitis in children. Am J Public Health 1952;42:142.

Griffin LD, Kearney D, Ni J, et al. Analysis of formalin-fixed and frozen myocardial autopsy samples for viral genome in childhood myocarditis and dilated cardiomyopathy with endocardial fibroelastosis using polymerase chain reaction (PCR). Cardiovasc Pathol 1995;4:3.

Grist NR, Bell EJ. Coxsackieviruses and the heart. Am Heart J 1969;77:295.

Grist NR, Bell EJ. Enteroviral etiology of the paralytic poliomyelitis syndrome. Arch Environ Health 1970;21:382.

Grist NR, Bell EJ. A six-year study of coxsackievirus B infections in heart disease. J Hyg 1974;73:165.

Grist NR, Bell EJ. The epidemiology of enteroviruses. Scott Med J 1975;20:27.

Grist NR, Bell EJ, Assad F. Enteroviruses in human disease. Prog Med Virol 1978;24:114.

Grumbach IM, Heim A, Pring-Akerblom I, et al. Adenoviruses and enteroviruses as pathogens in myocarditis and dilated cardiomyopathy. Acta Cardiol 1999;54:83.

Gyorkey F, Cabral GA, Gorkey PK, et al. Coxsackievirus aggregates in muscle cells of polymyositis patient. Intervirology 1978;10:69.

Halfon N, Spector SA. Fatal echovirus type 11 infections. Am J Dis Child 1981;135:1017.

Hall CB, Cherry JD, Hatch MH, et al. The return of Boston exanthem: echovirus 16 infections in 1974. Am J Dis Child 1977;131:323.

Hall CE, Cooney MK, Fox JP. The Seattle Virus Watch Program. I. Infection and illness experience of Virus Watch families during a community-wide epidemic of echovirus type 30 aseptic meningitis. Am J Public Health 1970;60:1456.

Hanlon P, Hanlon L, Marsh V, et al. Serological comparisons of approaches to polio vaccination in the Gambia. Lancet 1987;1:800.

Harjulehto T, Aro T, Hovi T, et al. Congenital malformations and oral poliovirus vaccination during pregnancy. Lancet 1989;1:771.

Hartig PC, Madge GE, Webb SR. Diversity within a human isolate of coxsackie B4: relationship to viral-induced diabetes mellitus. J Med Virol 1983;11:23.

Haynes RE, Cramblett HG, Kronfol HJ. Echovirus 9 meningoencephalitis in infants and children. JAMA 1969;208:1657.

Helfand RF, Gary Jr HE, Freeman CY, et al. Serologic evidence of an association between enteroviruses and onset of type 1 diabetes mellitus. J Infect Dis 1995;172:1206.

Helfand RF, Khan AS, Pallansch MA, et al. Echovirus 30 infection and aseptic meningitis in parents of children attending a child care center. J Infect Dis 1994;169:1133.

Helin M, Savola J, Lapinleimu K. Cardiac manifestations during a coxsackie B5 epidemic. Br Med J 1968;ii:97.

Hertenstein JR, Sarnat HB, O'Connor DM. Acute unilateral oculomotor palsy associated with ECHO 9 viral infection. J Pediatr 1976;89:79.

Hildebrandt HM, Massab HF, Willis PW. Influenza virus pericarditis. Am J Dis Child 1962;104:579.

Hill AB, Knowelden J. Inoculation and poliomyelitis: a statistical investigation in England and Wales in 1949. Br Med J 1950;2:1.

Hiltunen M, Hyoty H, Knip M, et al. Islet cell antibody seroconversion in children is temporally associated with enterovirus infections. J Infect Dis 1997;175:554.

Ho M, Chen E-R, Hsu K-H, et al. An epidemic of enterovirus 71 infection in Taiwan. N Engl J Med 1999;341:929.

Honig EI, Melnick JL, Isacson P, et al. A endemiological study of enteric virus infections. Poliomyelitis, Coxsackie, and orphan (ECHO) viruses isolated from normal children in 2 socio-economic groups. J Exp Med 1956;103:247.

Horstmann DM. Acute poliomyelitis. Relation of physical activity at the time of onset to the course of the disease. JAMA 1950;142:236.

Horstmann DM, Paul JR. The incubation period in human poliomyelitis and its implications. JAMA 1947;135:11.

Howlett JG, Somlo F, Kalz F. A new syndrome of parotitis with herpangina caused by the Coxsackie virus. CMAJ 1957;77:5.

Huber SA, Job LP, Woodruff JF. In vitro culture of coxsackievirus group B, type 3 immune spleen cells on infected endothelial cells and biological activity of the cultured cells in vivo. Infect Immun 1984; 43:567.

Huff JC, Hierholzer JC, Farris WA. An "outbreak" of juvenile diabetes mellitus: consideration of a viral etiology. Am J Epidemiol 1974;100:277.

Hughes RO, Roberts C. Hand, foot, mouth disease associated with coxsackie A9 virus. Lancet 1972;2:751.

Imrle CW, Ferguson JC, Sommerville RG. Coxsackie and mumps virus infection in a prospective study of acute pancreatitis. Gut 1977;18:53.

Ion-Neldescu N, Dobrescu A, Strebel PM, et al. Vaccine-associated paralytic poliomyelitis and HIV infection (letter). Lancet 1994;343:51.

Ishiko H, Shimada Y, Yonaha M, et al. Molecular diagnosis of human enteroviruses by phylogeny-based classification by use of the VP4 sequence. J Infect Dis 2002;185:744.

Ishiko H, Takeda N, Miramura K, et al. Phylogenetically different strains of a variant of coxsackievirus A24 were repeatedly introduced but discontinued circulating in Japan. Arch Virol 1992;126:179.

James WD, Odom RB, Hatch MH. Gianotti-Crosti-like eruption associated with coxsackievirus A16 infection. J Am Acad Dermatol 1982;6:862.

Javett SN, Heymann S, Mundel B, et al. Myocarditis in the newborn infant: a study of an outbreak associated with coxsackie group B virus infection in a maternity home in Johannesburg. J Pediatr 1956;48:1.

Jehn UW, Fink MW. Myositis, myoglobinemia, and myoglobinuria associated with enterovirus echo 9 infection. Arch Neurol 1980;33:457.

Jenista JA, Dalzell LE, Davidson PW, et al. Outcome studies of neonatal enterovirus infection. Ped Res 1984a;18:230A.

Jenista JA, Powell KA, Menegus MA. Epidemiology of neonatal enterovirus infection. J Pediatr 1984b;104:685.

Jin O, Sole MJ, Butany JW, et al. Detection of enterovirus RNA in myocardial biopsies from patients with myocarditis and cardiomyopathy using gene amplification by polymerase chain reaction. Circulation 1990;82:8.

John TJ, Christopher S. Oral polio vaccination of children in the tropics. II. Antibody response in relation to vaccine virus infection. Am J Epidemiol 1975;102:414.

John TJ, Jayabal P. Oral polio vaccination of children in the tropics: I. The poor seroconversion rates and the absence of viral interference. Am J Epidemiol 1972;96:263.

Johnson RT, Portnoy B, Rogers NG, et al. Acute benign pericarditis: virologic study of 34 patients. Arch Intern Med 1961;108:823.

Johnston JM, Overall JC. Intravenous immunoglobulin in disseminated neonatal echovirus 11 infection. Pediatr Infect Dis J 1989;8:254.

Kaplan MH, Klein SW, McPhee J, et al. Group B coxsackievirus infections in infants younger than three months of age: a serious childhood illness. Rev Infect Dis 1983;5:1019.

Kaplan AS, Melnick JL. Oral administration of coxsackie viruses to newborn and adult mice. Proc Soc Exp Biol Med 1951;76:312.

Kaufman DL, Erlander MG, Clare-Salzler M, et al. Autoimmunity to two forms of glutamate decarboxylase in insulin-dependent diabetes mellitus. J Clin Invest 1992;89:283.

Kawai C. From myocarditis to cardiomyopathy: mechanisms of inflammation and cell death: learning from the past for the future. Circulation 1999;99:1091.

Kew O, Morris-Glasgow V, Landaverde M, et al. Outbreak of poliomyelitis in Hispaniola associated with circulating type 1 vaccine-derived poliovirus. Science 2002;296:356.

Kew OM, Pallansch MA, Nottay BK, et al. Genotypic relationships among wild polioviruses from different regions of the world. In Brinton MA, Heinz RX (eds). New Aspects of Positive-Strand RNA Viruses. Washington, D.C.: American Society for Microbiology, 1990:357.

Kew OM, Sutter RW, Nottay BK, et al. Prolonged replication of a type 1 vaccine-derived poliovirus in an immunodeficient patient. J Clin Microbiol 1998;36:2893.

Khatib R, Chason JL, Silberberg BK, et al. Age-dependent pathogenicity of group B coxsackieviruses in Swiss-Webster mice: infectivity for myocardium and pancreas. J Infect Dis 1980;141:394.

Kibrick S. Current status of coxsackie and ECHO viruses in human disease. Prog Med Virol 1964;6:27.

Kim-Farley RJ, Rutherford G, Lichfield P, et al. Outbreak of paralytic poliomyelitis, Taiwan. Lancet 1984;2:1322.

King AMQ, Brown F, Christian P, et al. Picornaviridae. In Van Regenmortel MHV, Fauquet CM, Bishop DHL (eds). Seventh Report of the International Committee on Taxonomy of Viruses. New York: Academic Press, 2000.

Kinney JS, McCray E, Kaplan JE, et al. Risk factors associated with echovirus 11 infection in a newborn nursery. Pediatr Infect Dis J 1986;5:192.

Klapper PE, Bailey AS, Longson M, et al. Meningoencephalitis caused by coxsackievirus group B type 2: diagnosis confirmed by measuring intrathecal antibody. J Infect 1984;8:227.

Knox AW. Influence of pregnancy in mice on the course of infection with murine poliomyelitis virus. Proc Soc Exp Biol Med 1950;73:520.

Kogon A, Spigland I, Frothingham TE, et al. The Virus Watch Program: a continuing surveillance of viral infections in metropolitan New York families. Am J Epidemiol 1969;89:51.

Kono R. Apollo 11 disease or acute hemorrhagic conjunctivitis: a pandemic of a new enterovirus infection of the eyes. Am J Epidemiol 1975;101:383.

Koontz CH, Ray CG. The role of coxsackie group B virus infections in sporadic myopericarditis. Am Heart J 1971;82:750.

Koprowski H. Immunization against poliomyelitis with living attenuated virus. Am J Trop Med Hyg 1956;5:440.

Krober MS, Bass JW, Powell JM, et al. Bacterial and viral pathogens causing fever in infants less than 3 months old. Am J Dis Child 1985;139:889.

Krugman RD, Hardy GE, Sellers C. Antibody persistence after primary immunization with trivalent oral poliovirus vaccine. Pediatrics 1977;60:80.

Kuban KC, Ephros MA, Freeman RL, et al. Syndrome of opsoclonus-myoclonus caused by coxsackie B3 infection. Ann Neurol 1983;13:69.

Kuhl U, Lauer B, Souvatzoglu M, et al. Antimyosin scintigraphy and immunohistologic analysis of endomyocardial biopsy in patients with clinically suspected myocarditis—evidence of myocardial cell damage and inflammation in the absence of histologic signs of myocarditis. J Am Coll Cardiol 1998;32:1371.

Kujala G, Newman JH. Isolation of echovirus type 11 from synovial fluid in acute monocytic arthritis. Arthritis Rheum 1985;28:98.

Lake AM, Lauer BA, Clark JC, et al. Enterovirus infections in neonates. J Pediatr 1976;89:787.

Landsteiner K, Popper E. Mikroscopische präparate von einem menschlichen und zwei affenrückemarken. Wein Klin Wschr 1908;21:1830.

Lansky LL, Krugman S, Huq G. Anicteric coxsackie B hepatitis. J Pediatr 1979;94:64.

Lasch EE, Abed Y, Abdulla K, et al. Successful results of a program combining live and inactivated poliovirus vaccines to control poliomyelitis in Gaza. Rev Infect Dis 1984;6:467.

Latham RD, Mulrow JP, Virmani R, et al. Recently diagnosed idiopathic dilated cardiomyopathy: incidence of myocarditis and efficacy of prednisone therapy. Am Heart J 1989;117:876.

Lauer B, Niederau C, Kuhl U, et al. Cardiac troponin T in patients with clinically suspected myocarditis. J Am Coll Cardiol 1997;30:1354.

Lee KJ, McCrindle BW, Bohn DJ, et al. Clinical outcomes of acute myocarditis in childhood. Heart 1999;82:226.

Leggiadro RJ, Chwatsky DN, Zucker SW. Echovirus 3 infection associated with anicteric hepatitis. Am J Dis Child 1982;136:744.

Lennette EH, Magoffin R, Knouf EG. Viral central nervous system disease: an etiologic study conducted at the Los Angeles County General Hospital. JAMA 1962;179:687.

Lepow ML, Carver DH, Wright HT, et al. A clinical, epidemiologic and laboratory investigation of aseptic meningitis during the four-year period, 1955-1958. I. Observations concerning etiology and epidemiology. N Engl J Med 1962a;266:1181.

Lepow ML, Coyne N, Thompson LB, et al. A clinical, epidemiologic and laboratory investigation of aseptic meningitis during the four-year period, 1955-1958. II. The clinical disease and its sequelae. N Engl J Med 1962b;266:1188.

Lerner AM, Klein JO, Levin HS, et al. Infections due to coxsackie virus group A, type 9, in Boston, 1959, with special reference to exanthems and pneumonia. N Engl J Med 1960;263:1265.

Liao O, Sindhwani R, Rojkind M, et al. Antibody-mediated autoimmune myocarditis depends on genetically determined target organ sensitivity. J Exp Med 1995;181:1123.

Lin K-H, Chern C-L, Chu P-Y, et al. Genetic analysis of recent Taiwanese isolates of a variant of coxsackievirus A24. J Med Virol 2001;64:269.

Lindenbaum JE, Van Dyck PC, Allen RG. Hand, foot and mouth disease associated with coxsackievirus group B. Scand J Infect Dis 1975;7:161.

Linnemann CC, Steichen J, Sherman WG, et al. Febrile illness in early infancy associated with ECHO virus infection. J Pediatr 1974;84:49.

Lipschultz SE, Easley KA, Orav EJ, et al. Left ventricular structure and function in children infected with human immunodeficiency virus: the prospective P2C2 HIV Multicenter Study. Circulation 1998;97:1246.

Lonnrot M, Salminen K, Knip M, et al. Enterovirus RNA in serum is a risk factor for beta-cell autoimmunity and clinical type 1 diabetes: a prospective study. J Med Virol 2000;61:214.

Lum LCS, Wong KT, Lam SK, et al. Fatal enterovirus 71 encephalomyelitis. J Pediatr 1998;133:795.

Marier R, Rodriguez W, Chloupek RJ, et al. Coxsackievirus B5 infection and aseptic meningitis in neonates and children. Am J Dis Child 1975;129:321.

Martin AB, Webber S, Fricker FJ, et al. Acute myocarditis. Rapid diagnosis by PCR in children. Circulation 1994;90:330.

Martino TA, Liu P, Petric M, et al. Enteroviral myocarditis and dilated cardiomyopathy: a review of clinical and experimental studies. In Rotbart HA (ed). Human Enterovirus Infections. Washington, D.C.: ASM Press, 1995.

Mason JW, O'Connell JB, Herskowitz A, et al. A clinical trial of immunosuppressive therapy for myocarditis. N Engl J Med 1995;333:269.

McBean AM, Thoms ML, Albrecht P, et al. The serologic response to oral polio vaccine and enhanced potency inactivated polio vaccines. Am J Epidemiol 1988;128:615.

McCarthy RE, III, Boehmer JP, Hruban RH, et al. Long-term outcome of fulminant myocarditis as compared with acute (nonfulminant) myocarditis. N Eng J Med 2000;342:690.

McKinney RE, Katz SL, Wilfert CM. Chronic enteroviral meningoencephalitis in agammaglobulinemic patients. Rev Infect Dis 1987;9:334.

Mease PJ, Ochs HD, Wedgewood RJ. Successful treatment of echovirus meningoencephalitis and myositis-fasciitis with intravenous immune globulin therapy in a patient with X-linked hypogammaglobulinemia. N Engl J Med 1981;304:1278.

Meehan WF, Bertrand CA. Ventricular tachycardia associated with echovirus infection. JAMA 1970;212:1701.

Melnick JL. Enterovirus 71 infections: a varied clinical pattern sometimes mimicking poliomyelitis. Rev Infect Dis 1984;6:S387.

Melnick JL. Discovery of the enteroviruses and the classification of poliovirus among them. Biologicals 1993;21:305.

Melnick JL. Enteroviruses: polioviruses, coxsackieviruses, echoviruses, and newer enteroviruses. In Fields BN, Knipe DM, Howley PM, et al (eds). Fields Virology. Philadelphia: Lippincott-Raven, 1996.

Melnick JL, Ledinko N. Social serology: antibody levels in a normal young population during an epidemic of poliomyelitis. Am J Hyg 1951;54:354.

Melnick JL, Shaw EW, Curnen EC. A virus from patients diagnosed as nonparalytic poliomyelitis or aseptic meningitis. Proc Soc Exp Biol Med 1949;71:344.

Melnick JL, Wimberly IL. Lyophilized combination pools of enterovirus equine antisera. New LBM pools prepared from reserves of antisera stored frozen for two decades. Bull World Health Org 1985;63:543.

Meyer HM, Johnson RT, Crawford IP, et al. Central nervous system syndromes of viral etiology. A study of 713 cases. Am J Med 1960;29:334.

Miller GD. Hand-foot-and-mouth disease. JAMA 1968;203:827.

Mills EL. Mononuclear phagocytes in the newborn: their relation to the state of relative immunodeficiency. Am J Pediatr Hematol Oncol 1983;5:189.

Minor TE, Allen CI, Tsiatis AA, et al. Human infective dose determinations for oral poliovirus type 1 vaccine in infants. J Clin Microbiol 1981;13:388.

Mirkovic RR, Schmidt NJ, Yin-Murphy M, et al. Enterovirus etiology of the 1970 Singapore epidemic of acute conjunctivitis. Intervirology 1974;4:119.

Miyamura K, Tanimura M, Takeda N, et al. Evolution of enterovirus 70 in nature: all isolates were recently derived from a common ancestor. Arch Virol 1986;89:1.

Modlin JF. Fatal echovirus 11 disease in premature neonates. Pediatrics 1980;66:775.

Modlin JF. Perinatal echovirus infection: insights from a literature of 61 cases of serious infection and 16 outbreaks in nurseries. Rev Infect Dis 1986;8:918.

Modlin JF. Neonatal enterovirus infections. In Baker C (ed). Neonatal Infections, vol 5. Philadelphia: Saunders, 1994.

Modlin JF, Bowman M. Perinatal transmission of coxsackie B3 virus in a murine model. J Infect Dis 1987;156:21.

Modlin JF, Crumpacker CS. Coxsackie B1 virus infection in the pregnant mouse and transmission to the fetus. Infect Immun 1982;37:222.

Modlin JF, Dagan R, Berlin LE, et al. Focal encephalitis with enterovirus infections. Pediatrics 1991;88:841.

Modlin JF, Polk BF, Horton P, et al. Perinatal echovirus 11 infection: risk of transmission during a community outbreak. N Engl J Med 1981;305:368.

Montgomery J, Gear J, Prinsloo FR, et al. Myocarditis of the newborn: an outbreak in a maternity home in southern Rhodesia associated with coxsackie group-B virus infection. S Afr Med J 1955;29:608.

Moore M. Enteroviral disease in the United States. J Infect Dis 1982;146:103.

Morens DM, Pallansch MA. Epidemiology. In Rotbart H (ed). Human Enterovirus Infections. Washington, D.C.: American Society for Microbiology, 1995.

Moritsugu Y, Sawada K, Hinohara M, et al. An outbreak of type 25 echovirus infection with exanthem in an infant home near Tokyo. Am J Epidemiol 1968;87:599.

Mostoufizadeh G, Lack EE, Gang DL, et al. Postmortem manifestations of echovirus 11 sepsis in five newborn infants. Hum Pathol 1983;14:819.

Muir P, Nicholson F, Illavia SJ, et al. Serological and molecular evidence of enterovirus infection in patients with end-stage dilated cardiomyopathy. Heart 1996;76:243.

Murphy AM, Simmul R. Coxsackie B4 virus infections in New South Wales during 1962. Med J Aust 1964;2:443.

Myaux JA, Unicomb L, Besser RE, et al. Effect of diarrhea on the humoral response to oral polio vaccination. Pediatr Infect Dis J 1996;15:204.

Nagington J, Wreghitt TG, Gandy G. Fatal echovirus 11 infections in outbreak in special-care baby unit. Lancet 1978;ii:725.

Nathanson N, Martin JR. The epidemiology of poliomyelitis: enigmas surrounding its appearance and disappearance. Am J Epidemiol 1979;110:672.

Neva FA. A second outbreak of Boston exanthem disease in Pittsburgh during 1954. N Engl J Med 1956;254:838.

Neva FA, Femster RF, Gorbach IJ. Clinical and epidemiological features of an unusual epidemic exanthem. JAMA 1954;155:544.

Norder H, Bjerregaard L, Magnius LO. Homotypic echoviruses share aminoterminal VP1 sequence homology applicable for typing. J Med Virol 2001;63:35.

Noren GR, Staley NA, Bandt CM, et al. Occurrence of myocarditis in sudden death in children. J Forensic Sci 1977;22:188.

Norwitz MS, Moore GT. Acute infectious lymphocytosis: an etiologic study of an outbreak. N Engl J Med 1968;279:399.

Oberste MS, Maher K, Flemister MR, et al. Comparison of classic and molecular approaches for the identification of untypable enteroviruses. J Clin Microbiol 2000;38:1170.

Oberste MS, Maher K, Kilpatrick DR, et al. Typing human enteroviruses by partial sequencing of VP1. J Clin Microbiol 1999;37:1288.

O'Neil KM, Pallansch MA, Winkelstein JA, et al. Chronic group A coxsackievirus infection in agammaglobulinemia: demonstration of genomic variation of serotypically identical isolates persistently excreted from the same patient. J Infect Dis 1988;157:183.

Onorato IM, Markowitz LE, Oxtoby MJ. Childhood immunization, vaccine-preventable diseases and infection with human immunodeficiency virus. Pediatr Infect Dis J 1988;7:588.

Onorato IM, Morens DM, Schonberger LB, et al. Acute hemorrhagic conjunctivitis caused by enterovirus type 70: an epidemic in American Samoa. Am J Trop Med Hyg 1985;34:984.

Oregan S, Robitaille P, Mongeau J, et al. The hemolytic-uremic syndrome associated with echo 22 infection. Clin Pediatr 1980;19:125.

Otatume S, Addy PA-K. Ecology of enteroviruses in tropics. I. Circulation of enteroviruses in healthy infants in tropical urban areas. Jpn J Microbiol 1975;19:201.

Paffenbarger RS, Wilson VO. Previous tonsillectomy and current pregnancy as they affect risk of poliomyelitis. Ann NY Acad Sci 1955;61:856.

Parks WP, Queiroga LT, Melnick JL. Studies of infantile diarrhea in Karachi, Pakistan. II. Multiple virus isolations from rectal swabs. Am J Epidemiol 1967;85:469.

Parrott RH, Ross S, Burke FG, et al. Herpangina: clinical studies of a specific infectious disease. N Engl J Med 1951;245:275.

Patriarca PA, Wright PF, John TJ. Factors affecting the immunogenicity of oral poliovirus vaccine in developing countries. Rev Infect Dis 1991;13:926.

Paul JR. History of Poliomyelitis. New Haven, Conn: Yale University Press, 1971.

Peters ACB, Vielvoye GJ, Versteeg J, et al. Echo 25 focal encephalitis and subacute hemichorea. Neurology 1979;29:676.

Pevear DC, Fancher MJ, Felock PJ, et al. Conformational change in floor of the human rhinovirus canyon blocks adsorption to HeLa cell receptors. J Virol 1989;63:2002.

Poyry T, Kinnunen L, Kapsenberg J, et al. Type 3 poliovirus/Finland/1984 is genetically related to common Mediterranean strains. J Gen Virol 1990;71:2535.

Pozzetto B, Gaudin OG, Aouni M, et al. Comparative evaluation of immunoglobulin M neutralizing antibody response in acute-phase sera and virus isolation for the routine diagnosis of enterovirus infection. J Clin Microbiol 1989;27:705.

Pozo F, Casas I, Tenorio A, et al. Evaluation of a commercially available reverse transcription-PCR assay for diagnosis of enteroviral infection in archival and prospectively collected cerebrospinal fluid specimens. J Clin Microbiol 1998;36:1741.

Price RA, Garcia JH, Rightsel WA. Choriomeningitis and myocarditis in an adolescent with isolation of coxsackie B5 virus. Am J Clin Pathol 1970;53:825.

Rabin ER, Hassan SA, Jenson AB, et al. Coxsackie virus B3 myocarditis in mice. Am J Pathol 1964;44:775.

Rager-Zisman B, Allison AC. The role of antibody and host cells in the resistance of mice against infection by coxsackie B-3 virus. J Gen Virol 1973;19:329.

Ramos-Alverez M, Olarte J. Diarrheal diseases of children. Am J Dis Child 1964;107:218.

Ramos-Alvarez M, Sabin AB. Characteristics of poliomyelitis and other enteric viruses recovered in tissue culture from healthy American children. Proc Soc Exp Biol Med 1954;87:655.

Rantakallio P, Leskinen M, Von Wendt L. Incidence and prognosis of central nervous system infections in a birth cohort of 12,000 children. Scand J Infect Dis 1986;18:287.

Rantala H, Uhari M. Occurrence of childhood encephalitis: a population-based study. Pediatr Infect Dis J 1989;8:426.

Ray CG, Tucker VL, Harris DJ, et al. Enteroviruses associated with the hemolytic-uremic syndrome. Pediatrics 1970;46:378.

Read SJ, Kurtz JB. Laboratory diagnosis of common viral infections of the central nervous system by using a single multiplex PCR screening assay. J Clin Microbiol 1999;37:1352.

Rewers M, Atkinson M. The possible role of enteroviruses in diabetes mellitus. In Rotbart HA, (ed). Human Enterovirus Infections. Washington, D.C.: American Society for Microbiology, 1995.

Rewers M, LaPorte R, Walczak M, et al. Apparent epidemic of insulin-dependent diabetes mellitus in midwestern Poland. Diabetes 1987;36:106.

Rice SK, Heinl RE, Thornton LL, et al. Clinical characteristics, management strategies, and cost implications of a statewide outbreak of enterovirus meningitis. Clin Infect Dis 1995;20:931.

Robertson HE, Acker MS, Dillenberg HO, et al. Community-wide use of a "balanced" trivalent oral poliovirus vaccine (Sabin). Can J Public Health 1962;53:179.

Robertson SE, Traverso HP, Drucker JA, et al. Clinical efficacy of a new, enhanced-potency, inactivated poliovirus vaccine. Lancet 1988;1:897.

Robinson CR, Doane FW, Rhodes AJ. Report of an outbreak of febrile illness with pharyngeal lesions and exanthem. CMAJ 1958;79:615.

Roden VJ, Cantor HE, O'Connor DM, et al. Acute hemiplegia of childhood associated with coxsackie A9 viral infection. J Pediatr 1975;86:56.

Rorabaugh ML, Berlin LE, Heldrich F, et al. Aseptic meningitis among infants less than two years of age: acute illness and neurologic complications. Pediatrics 1993;92:206.

Rorabaugh ML, Berlin LE, Rosenberg L, et al. Absence of neurodevelopmental sequelae from aseptic meningitis. Baltimore, Md: Society for Pediatric Research, 1992.

Rosen L, Melnick J, Schmidt NJ, et al. Subclassification of enteroviruses and ECHO virus type 34. Arch Ges Virusforsch 1970;30:89.

Rotbart HA. Pleconaril therapy of potentially life-threatening enterovirus infections. 36th Annual Meeting of the Infectious Disease Society of America, Denver, Colo, 1998. Rotbart HA. Pleconaril treatment of enterovirus and rhinovirus infections. Infect Med 2000;17:488.

Rotbart HA. Treatment of picornavirus infections. Antivir Res 2002;53:83.

Rotbart HA, Ahmed A, Hickey S, et al. Diagnosis of enterovirus infection by PCR of multiple specimen types. Pediatr Infect Dis J 1997;16:409.

Rotbart H, Brennan PJ, Fife KH, et al. Enterovirus meningitis in adults. Clin Infect Dis 1998;27:896.

Rotbart HA, Kinsella JP, Wasserman RL. Persistent enterovirus infection in culture-negative meningoencephalitis: demonstration by enzymatic amplification. J Infect Dis 1990;161:787.

Rotbart HA, Sawyer MH, Fast S, et al. Diagnosis of enteroviral meningitis by using PCR with a colorimetric microwell detection assay. J Clin Microbiol 1994;32:2590.

Rotbart HA, Webster ADB. Treatment of potentially life-threatening enterovirus infections with pleconaril. Clin Infect Dis 2001;32:228.

Rueckert RR. Picornaviridae and their replication. In Fields BN, Knipe DM (eds). Virology. New York: Raven Press, 1990.

Russell SJM, Bell EJ. Echoviruses and carditis. Lancet 1970;i:784.

Rytel MW, Kilbourne ED. Differing susceptibility of adolescent and adult mice to non-lethal infection with coxsackievirus B3. Proc Soc Exp Biol Med 1971;137:443.

Sabin AB. Pathogenesis of poliomyelitis: reappraisal in light of new data. Science 1956;123:1151.

Sabin AB. Properties and behavior of orally administered attenuated poliovirus vaccine. JAMA 1957;164:1216.

Sabin AB. Oral polio vaccine: history of its development and use and current challenge to eliminate poliomyelitis from the world. J Infect Dis 1985;151:420.

Sabin AB, Krumbiegel ER, Wigand R. ECHO type 9 virus disease. Am J Dis Child 1958;96:197.

Sainani GS, Krompotic E, Slodki SJ. Adult heart disease due to the coxsackie virus B infection. Medicine 1968;47:133.

Salk JE. Studies in human subjects on active immunization against poliomyelitis. I. A preliminary report of experiments in progress. JAMA 1953;151:1081.

Sanders DY, Cramblett HG. Viral infections in hospitalized infants. Am J Dis Child 1968;116:251.

Sawyer M, Holland D, Aintablian N, et al. Diagnosis of enteroviral central nervous system infection by polymerase chain reaction during a large community outbreak. Pediatr Infect Dis J 1994;13:177.

Sawyer MH, Saez-Llorenz X, Aviles CL, et al. Oral pleconaril reduces the duration and severity of enteroviral meningitis in children. Pediatric Academic Societies Annual Meeting, San Francisco, 1999.

Schiff GM, Sherwood JR. Clinical activity of pleconaril in an experimentally induced coxsackievirus A21 respiratory infection. J Infect Dis 2000;181:20.

Schiraldi O, Iandolo E. Polymyositis accompanying coxsackie virus B2 infection. Infection 1978;6:32.

Schmidtke M, Gluck B, Merkle I, et al. Cytokine profiles in heart, spleen, and thymus during the acute stage of experimental coxsackievirus B3-induced chronic myocarditis. J Med Virol 2000;61:518.

Schwimmbeck PL, Huber SA, Schultheiss H-P. Roles of T cells in coxsackievirus B-induced disease. In Tracy S, Chapman NM, Mahy BWJ (eds). The Coxsackie B Viruses, vol 223. Berlin: Springer, 1997.

Sells CJ, Carpenter RL, Ray CG. Sequelae of central-nervous-system enterovirus infections. N Engl J Med 1975;293:1.

Selzer G. Transplacental infection of the mouse fetus by coxsackie virus. Isr J Med Sci 1969;5:125.

Shafran SD, Halota W, Gilbert D, et al. Pleconaril is effective for enterovirus meningitis in adolescents and adults: a randomized placebo-controlled multicenter trial. 39th Interscience Conference on Antimicrobial Agents and Chemotherapy, San Francisco, 1999.

Shimizu C, Rambaud C, Cheron G, et al. Molecular identification of viruses in sudden infant death associated with myocarditis and pericarditis. Pediatr Infect Dis J 1995;14:584.

Shindarov LM, Chumakov MP, Voroshilova MK, et al. Epidemiological, clinical, and pathophysiological characteristics of epidemic poliomyelitis-like disease caused by enterovirus 71. J Hyg Epidemiol Microbiol Immunol 1979;23:284.

Simoes EA, John TJ. The antibody response of seronegative infants to inactivated poliovirus vaccine of enhanced potency. Develop Biol Stand 1986;14:127.

Singer JI, Mauer PR, Riley JP, et al. Management of central nervous system infections during an epidemic of enteroviral aseptic meningitis. J Pediatr 1980;96:559.

Smith SC, Ladenson JH, Mason JW, et al. Elevations of cardiac troponin I associated with myocarditis: experimental and clinical correlates. Circulation 1997;95:163.

Smith WG. Adult heart disease due to the coxsackie virus group B. Br Heart J 1966;28:204.

Smith WG. Coxsackie B myopericarditis in adults. Am Heart J 1970;80:34.

Solimena M, De Camilli P. Coxsackieviruses and diabetes. Nat Med 1995;1:25.

Spector SA, Straube RC. Protean manifestations of perinatal enterovirus infection. West J Med 1983;138:847.

Speer ME, Yawn DH. Fatal hepatoadrenal necrosis in the neonate associated with echovirus types 11 and 12 presenting as a surgical emergency. J Pediatr Surg 1984;19:591.

Steigman AJ, Lipton MM. Fatal bulbospinal paralytic poliomyelitis due to ECHO 11 virus. JAMA 1960;174:178.

Steinhoff MC. Viruses and diarrhea—a review. Am J Dis Child 1978;132:302.

Stevens KM. Estimate of molecular equivalent of antibody required for prophylaxis and therapy of poliomyelitis. J Hyg 1959;57:198.

Strebel PM, Sutter RW, Cochi SL, et al. Epidemiology of poliomyelitis in the United States one decade after the last reported case of indigenous wild virus-associated disease. Clin Infect Dis 1992;14:568.

Strikas RA, Anderson LJ, Parker RA. Temporal and geographic patterns of isolates of nonpolio enteroviruses in the United States. J Infect Dis 1986;153:346.

Sumaya CV, Corman LI. Enteroviral meningitis in early infancy: significance in community outbreaks. Pediatr Infect Dis J 1982;3:151.

Sutter RW, Patriarca PA, Suleiman AM, et al. Attributable risk of DTP (diphtheria and tetanus toxoids and pertussis vaccine) injection in provoking paralytic poliomyelitis during a large outbreak in Oman. J Infect Dis 1992;165:444.

Sutter RW, Prevots DR. Vaccine-associated paralytic poliomyelitis among immunodeficient persons. Infect Med 1994;11:426.

Sutton GC, Harding HB, Truehart RP, et al. Coxsackie B4 myocarditis in an adult: successful isolation of virus from ventricular myocardium. Aerospace Med 1967;38:66.

Sutton GC, Tobin JR, Fox RT, et al. Study of the pericardium and ventricular myocardium: exploratory mediastinoscopy and biopsy in unexplained heart disease. JAMA 1963;185:786.

Swartz TA, Roumiantzeff M, Peyron L, et al. Use of a combined DTP-polio vaccine in a reduced schedule. Dev Biol Stand 1986;65:159.

Sylvest E. Epidemic Myalgia: Bornholm Disease. London: Oxford University Press, 1934.

Talsma M, Vegting M, Hess J. Generalized Coxsackie A9 infection in a neonate presenting with pericarditis. Br Heart J 1984;52:683.

Technical Consultative Group to the World Health Organization on the Global Eradication of P. "Endgame" issues for the global polio eradication initiative. Clin Infect Dis 2002;34:72.

Toce SS, Keenan WJ. Congenital echovirus 11 pneumonia in association with pulmonary hypertension. Pediatr Infect Dis J 1988;7:360.

Trabelsi A, Grattard F, Nejmeddine M, et al. Evaluation of an enterovirus group-specific anti-VP1 monoclonal antibody, 5D8/1, in comparison with neutralization and PCR for rapid identification of enteroviruses in cell culture. J Clin Microbiol 1995;33:2454.

Ursing B. Acute pancreatitis in coxsackie B infection. Br Med J 1973;iii:524.

Van der Sar A. Acute infectious lymphocytosis with echovirus type 25. West Indian Med J 1979;28:185.

Vermont State Department of Public Health. Infantile Paralysis in Vermont. Brattleboro, Vt: Vermont Printing Co, 1924.

von Reyn CF, Clements CJ, Mann JM. Human immunodeficiency virus infection and routine childhood immunisation. Lancet 1987;ii:669.

Voroshilova MK, Chumakov MP. Poliomyelitis-like properties of AB-IV-coxsackie A7 group of viruses. Prog Med Virol 1959;2:106.

Warin JF, Davies JBM, Sanders FK, et al. Oxford epidemic of Bornholm disease, 1951. Br Med J 1953;i:1345.

Webster ADB, Rotbart HA, Warner T, et al. Diagnosis of enterovirus brain disease in hypogammaglobulinemic patients by polymerase chain reaction. Clin Infect Dis 1993;17:657.

Weiner LB, Rotbart HA, Gilbert DL, et al. Treatment of "enterovirus" meningitis with pleconaril (VP 63843), an antipicornavirus agent. 37th Interscience Conference on Antimicrobial Agents and Chemotherapy, Toronto, 1997.

Weinstein L, Aycock WL, Feemster RF. Relation of sex, pregnancy, and menstruation to susceptibility in poliomyelitis. N Engl J Med 1951; 245.

Weiss LM, Liu XF, Chang KL, et al. Detection of enteroviral RNA in idiopathic dilated cardiomyopathy and other human cardiac tissues. J Clin Invest 1991a;90:156.

Weiss LM, Movahed LA, Billingham ME, et al. Detection of coxsackievirus B3 RNA in myocardial tissues by polymerase chain reaction. Am J Pathol 1991b;138:497.

Weller TH, Enders JF, Buckingham M, et al. Etiology of epidemic pleurodynia: study of two viruses isolated from typical outbreak. J Immunol 1950;65:337.

Welliver RC, Cherry JD. Aseptic meningitis and orchitis associated with echovirus 6 infection. J Pediatr 1978;92:239.

Wenner HA, Abel D, Olson LC, et al. A mixed epidemic associated with echovirus types 6 and 11. Am J Epidemiol 1981;114:369.

Whitley RJ, Cobbs CG, Alford CA, et al. Diseases that mimic herpes simplex encephalitis. JAMA 1989;262:234.

World Health Organization Collaborative Study Group on Oral Poliovirus Vaccine. Effect of diarrhea on seroconversion to oral poliovirus vaccine. 32nd Interscience Conference on Antimicrobial Agents and Chemotherapy, Anaheim, Calif, 1992.

Wickman I. Beiträge zur Kenntnis der Heine-Medinschen Krankheit (Poliomyelitis Acuta und Verwandter Erkrankungen). Berlin: Karger, 1907.

Wiles HB, Gillette PC, Harley RA, et al. Cardiomyopathy and myocarditis in children with ventricular ectopic rhythm. J Am Coll Cardiol 1992;20:359.

Wilfert CM, Lauer BA, Cohen M, et al. An epidemic of echovirus 18 meningitis. J Infect Dis 1975;131:75.

Willems WR, Hornig C, Bauer H, et al. A case of coxsackie A9 virus infection with orchitis. J Med Virol 1978;3:137.

Woodruff J. Lack of correlation between neutralizing antibody production and suppression of coxsackie B-3 replication in target organs: evidence for involvement of mononuclear inflammatory cells in host defense. J Immunol 1979;123:31.

Woodruff JF. Viral myocarditis. Am J Pathol 1980; 101:427.

Woodruff JF, Kilbourne ED. The influence of quantitated post-weanling undernutrition on Coxsackievirus B-3 infection of adult mice: I. Viral persistence and increased severity of lesions. J Infect Dis 1970;121:137.

Woodruff JF, Woodruff JJ. Involvement of T lymphocytes in the pathogenesis of coxsackievirus B3 heart disease. J Immunol 1974;113:1726.

Wreghitt TG, Gandy GM, King A, et al. Fatal neonatal echo 7 virus infection (letter). Lancet 1984;ii:465.

Wright HT, Landing BH, Lennette EH, et al. Fatal infection in an infant associated with coxsackie virus group A, type 16. N Engl J Med 1963;268:1041.

Wyatt HV. Poliomyelitis in hypogammaglobulinemics. J Infect Dis 1973;128:802.

Yerly S, Gervaix A, Simonet V, et al. Rapid and sensitive detection of enteroviruses in specimens from patients with aseptic meningitis. J Clin Microbiol 1996;34:199.

Yoon JW. The role of viruses and environmental factors in the induction of diabetes. Curr Top Microbiol Immunol 1990;164:95.

Yoon JW, Austin M, Onodera T, et al. Virus-induced diabetes mellitus: isolation of a virus from the pancreas of a child with diabetic ketoacidosis. N Engl J Med 1979;300:1173.

Yow DM, Melnick JL, Blattner JR, et al. Enteroviruses in infantile diarrhea. Am J Hyg 1963;77:283.

Zhang A, Nanni RG, Oren DA, et al. Three-dimensional structure-activity relationships for antiviral agents that interact with picornavirus capsids. Sem Virol 1992;3:453.

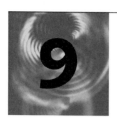

9 EPSTEIN-BARR VIRUS INFECTIONS

BEN Z. KATZ AND GEORGE MILLER

Epstein-Barr virus (EBV) was discovered in the 1960s in cell lines derived from African Burkitt's lymphomas (Epstein et al., 1964), malignant conditions that develop in patients who are not otherwise globally immunodeficient. Today this virus is well recognized as the etiologic agent of infectious mononucleosis. Extensive virologic and serologic evidence also implicates EBV as the cause of various lymphoproliferative disorders such as large cell lymphomas and lymphocytic interstitial pneumonia in immunosuppressed patients (Andiman et al., 1985).

INFECTIOUS MONONUCLEOSIS

Infectious mononucleosis is the typical, symptomatic, primary EBV infection seen in the otherwise healthy host. Infectious mononucleosis is an acute infectious disease occurring predominantly in older children and young adults. It is characterized clinically by fever, exudative or membranous pharyngitis, generalized lymphadenopathy, and splenomegaly. Characteristically, the peripheral blood shows an absolute increase in the number of atypical lymphocytes, and the serum has a high titer of heterophil antibody. Specific EBV antibodies are detected early in the illness and persist thereafter.

History

Infectious mononucleosis was first described as "glandular fever" by Pfeiffer in 1889. The term *infectious mononucleosis* was used by Sprunt and Evans (1920) in their description of hematologic changes in six young adults with a clinical syndrome characterized by a mononuclear leukocytosis. A diagnostic serologic test based on the association of heterophil antibody and mononucleosis was described by Paul and Bunnell (1932). This nonspecific test was made more specific by the development of differential absorption tests by Davidsohn (1937) (Table 9-1) and considerably simpler and more rapid (but occasionally less specific) by the more recent slide agglutination tests. The association of infectious mononucleosis with EBV was described by Henle et al. (1968) 4 years after the virus was discovered.

Etiology

Although discovery of the causative agent of infectious mononucleosis eluded the efforts of competent investigators for many years, the assumption was that it was a virus. A report by Henle et al. (1968) provided evidence of a relationship between the herpesvirus now known as EBV and infectious mononucleosis.

In 1968 Niederman et al. detected antibodies against EBV in patients with infectious mononucleosis by means of an indirect immunofluorescence test. In 24 patients with infectious mononucleosis, antibodies that were absent in preillness specimens appeared early in the disease, rose to peak levels within a few weeks, and remained at high levels during convalescence. These antibodies were distinct from heterophil antibodies.

Subsequent studies by Niederman et al. in 1970 and Sawyer et al. in 1971 provided additional evidence indicating that EBV is the cause of infectious mononucleosis. The evidence that supports this concept is as follows: (1) EBV antibody is absent before onset of illness, appears during illness, and persists for many years thereafter; (2) clinical infectious mononucleosis occurs only in persons lacking antibody, and it fails to occur when antibody is present; (3) EBV has been isolated from the pharynx and saliva of patients with infectious mononucleosis during their illness and for many months thereafter (Miller et al., 1973); and (4) cultured

TABLE 9-1	Heterophil Antibody Reactions in Normal and Infectious Mononucleosis (IM) Sera	
	AGGLUTINATION OF SHEEP RED BLOOD CELLS AFTER ABSORPTION WITH	
In the presence of	*Guinea pig kidney cells*	*Beef red blood cells*
Some normal human sera	−	+
Most IM sera	+ + +	−

lymphocytes from patients who have had infectious mononucleosis will form continuous cell lines in vitro that contain the EBV genome and express EBV antigens.

EBV is a member of the herpesvirus group. As is true for other herpesviruses, EBV can exist in a quiescent (latent) or actively replicating (lytic) state. Mature infectious particles are 150 to 200 nm in diameter, with a lipid-containing envelope surrounding an icosahedral nucleocapsid. The genome is composed of approximately 172,000 base pairs of double-stranded DNA. The entire nucleotide sequence of one strain is known (Baer et al., 1984). Within the viral particle and when the virus is lytically replicating, the genome is linear; within latently infected cells the genome is a circular extrachromosomal plasmid (Adams and Lindahl, 1975). In some cells EBV DNA also is integrated into the host cell chromosome (Matsuo et al., 1984).

In vitro the virus has a narrow host range, infecting B lymphocytes of human or other primate origin. However, in vivo the virus can be found in T lymphocytes, the epithelial elements of the buccal mucosa, the salivary glands, the tongue, and the ectocervix, as well. Within the mouth both parotid ductal epithelium and oropharyngeal squamous epithelial cells harbor EBV DNA and are sites of viral replication and release (Morgan et al., 1979; Sixbey et al., 1984; Wolf et al., 1984).

A number of viral antigen systems have been characterized, including viral capsid antigen (VCA), EB nuclear antigen (EBNA), membrane antigen (MA), and an early antigen (EA) complex, consisting of a diffuse component (D) and a restricted component (R). Each of these antigen systems is composed of a number of distinct viral gene products. For example, there are six different known EBNA genes. Antibodies to these different antigen systems can be demonstrated by a variety of techniques, including indirect immunofluorescence, immunoblotting, and enzyme-linked immunosorbent assay (ELISA).

Pathology

The generalized nature of infectious mononucleosis becomes apparent when the pathologic aspects of the disease are studied. Grossly, there may be diffuse enlargement of the lymphoid tissues, manifested by lymphadenopathy, splenomegaly, and pharyngeal lymphoid hyperplasia. Histologically, focal mononuclear infiltrations involve lymph nodes, spleen, tonsils, lungs, heart, liver, kidneys, adrenal glands, central nervous system (CNS), and skin. Bone marrow hyperplasia develops regularly, and in some instances small granulomas are present.

The lymphoid hyperplasia of infectious mononucleosis is not diagnostic; it can be seen in other conditions. Most of the hyperplasia involves T cells in the paracortical areas of the lymph node; however, in some instances there may be pronounced hyperplasia of B cells in the germinal follicle. The lymphoid hyperplasia is thought to consist of several distinct components. A few proliferating B cells are infected by EBV; they represent less than 0.1% of the circulating mononuclear cells in the acute phase of uncomplicated infectious mononucleosis. Other proliferating B cells may be "polyclonally activated" by the EBV infection but may not themselves contain EBV. The majority of the proliferating cells, represented by the atypical lymphocytes present in the blood, are reactive T cells (usually cytotoxic or suppressor, CD8+) and natural killer (NK) cells; they are not EBV-infected B lymphocytes (Pattengale et al., 1974). The proliferating T cells induce generalized lymph node hyperplasia and infiltrate many organs.

Thus it is the immune response against the virus that provides many of the pathologic conditions seen in acute infectious mononucleosis. Purtilo (1981) called these atypical lymphocytes "combatants in an immune struggle." Some of these cytotoxic T cells have the specific ability to eliminate EBV-infected B cells (Svedmyr and Jondal, 1975). Others suppress activation of EBV-infected B cells (Tosato et al.,

1979). Recent evidence indicates that CD4+ T-cells play a major role in inhibiting proliferation of B cells recently infected by EBV (Nikiforow et al., 2001). NK cells may also eliminate EBV-infected cells (De Waele et al., 1981). Antibodies, especially neutralizing antibodies, may play a role in limiting acute infectious mononucleosis as well, by limiting the spread of extracellular virus and participating in antibody-dependent cellular cytotoxicity (ADCC). It has been proposed that when this complex and finely tuned immunoregulatory mechanism fails, chronic or fatal EBV infection results. For example, if cytotoxic or suppressor T cells fail to eliminate infected B cells, excessive lymphoproliferation may occur. If, on the other hand, NK or cytotoxic T-cell activity is excessive, extensive B-cell death with resultant agammaglobulinemia may result (Andiman, 1984).

In the normal individual the extensive lymphoproliferation subsides, but the virus nevertheless persists in a latent state in the lymphoid compartment. Approximately one in a million peripheral blood mononuclear cells harbors EBV in the healthy EBV-seropositive individual (Rocchi et al., 1977).

Epidemiology

Although EBV infection is worldwide in distribution, clinical infectious mononucleosis is observed predominantly in developed countries, principally among adolescents and young adults. Seroepidemiologic surveys have revealed a gradual acquisition of antibody with age so that 50% to 90% of persons are antibody-positive by young adult life. The overall incidence of clinical infectious mononucleosis is approximately 50 per 100,000 persons per year in the general population of the United States; however, the incidence of mononucleosis in susceptible college students is approximately 5,000 per 100,000 persons, 100 times higher than in the general population (Niederman et al., 1970). The total EBV infection rate in college students is estimated to be at least twice as high (approximately 12,000 per 100,000 yearly), indicating that at least as many subclinical infections occur as overt infections. The so-called subclinical infections may be truly inapparent infections or atypical EBV-induced diseases such as thrombocytopenia, hemolytic anemia, pneumonitis, or rash (Andiman, 1979; Andiman et al., 1981).

Epidemiologic factors that have a significant effect on the host response to EBV infection include age, socioeconomic status, and geographic location. Infection during infancy and childhood is usually clinically inapparent, perhaps because of the immaturity of the immunologic responses of children (Sumaya, 1977). Clinical infectious mononucleosis is generally seen only in adolescents and young adults (Evans et al., 1968). In developing countries of the world, exposure to EBV occurs at a very early age. In these countries most older children and adolescents are immune to the virus. Therefore infectious mononucleosis is rare. In the United States, infection also occurs at an early age in individuals in low socioeconomic groups who live in crowded conditions with poor hygiene.

Many seroepidemiologic studies have confirmed that infectious mononucleosis is only moderately contagious, even in family settings. Henle and Henle (1970) found evidence of spread in 3 of 8 families (37.5%), and Fleischer et al. (1981) found spread in 7 of 36 susceptible contacts (19%). However, EBV infection appears to spread more efficiently under the conditions that exist in certain day-care nurseries (Pereira et al., 1969) and orphanages (Tischendorf et al., 1970).

The most likely modes of transmission are oral-salivary spread in children and close intimate contact (kissing) in young adults (Hoagland, 1955; Evans, 1960). Cell-free infectious virus is carried in saliva (Morgan et al., 1979). Prolonged pharyngeal excretion of EBV for periods up to several months after clinical infectious mononucleosis has been demonstrated (Miller et al., 1973; Niederman et al., 1976). Approximately 15% to 20% of immune individuals excrete small amounts of EBV in saliva at any one point in time. Patients undergoing immunosuppression have an increased frequency (>50%) of oropharyngeal excretion of larger amounts of virus (Strauch et al., 1974). If saliva is concentrated, virus can be found in up to 100% of normal individuals (Yao et al., 1985). Thus the virus may never be truly "latent" in oropharyngeal elements but, instead, may be present as a chronic, low-grade, productive infection. The infection can also be transmitted by transfusion of blood that is contaminated with EBV-infected lymphocytes (Gerber et al., 1969; Blacklow et al., 1971).

Clinical Manifestations

The incubation period has been estimated as 4 to 6 weeks on the basis of contact infections (Hoagland, 1984). After blood transfusion, heterophil-positive infectious mononucleosis has been shown to develop 5 weeks later (Blacklow et al., 1971; Turner et al., 1972).

The disease may begin abruptly or insidiously with headache, fever, chills, anorexia, and malaise, followed by lymphadenopathy and severe sore throat. The clinical picture is extremely variable in severity and duration. The disease in children is generally mild; in adults it is more severe and has a more protracted course.

Fever. The temperature usually rises to 39.4° C (103° F) and gradually falls over a variable period, averaging 6 days. In a severe case it is not unusual for temperatures to hover between 40° and 40.6° C (104° and 105° F) and to persist for 3 weeks or more, after which low-grade fevers may persist for several more weeks. Children are more likely to have low-grade fever throughout the course or to be afebrile.

Lymphadenopathy. Shortly after onset of illness, the lymph nodes rapidly enlarge to a variable size of approximately 1 to 4 cm. The nodes are typically tender, tense, discrete, and firm.

Any chain of lymph nodes may become enlarged, but the cervical group is most commonly involved. In addition, the following nodes are commonly affected: axillary, inguinal, epitrochlear, popliteal, mediastinal, and mesenteric. Massive mediastinal lymph node enlargement has been observed. Mesenteric lymphadenopathy frequently has been confused with acute appendicitis. Lymph node enlargement gradually subsides over a period of days or weeks, depending on the severity and extent of involvement.

Tonsillopharyngitis. Sore throat is one of the cardinal symptoms of the disease. The tonsils are usually enlarged and reddened, and more than 50% develop exudate. Thick grayish-white, shaggy, membranous tonsillitis is a common finding and may persist for 7 to 10 days. During the first week, small petechiae are present on the palate in approximately one third of patients. In the past many patients referred to physicians for treatment of "diphtheria" because of the appearance of the throat proved to have infectious mononucleosis.

Splenomegaly. Moderate enlargement of the spleen occurs in approximately 50% of cases.

In rare instances enlargement may be followed by rupture, causing hemorrhage, shock, and death if it is not recognized. Rutkow (1978) reviewed 107 reports of splenic rupture in patients with infectious mononucleosis and concluded that only 18 ruptures were truly spontaneous; most followed trauma.

The triad of lymphadenopathy, exudative pharyngitis, and splenomegaly in a febrile patient is typical but not pathognomonic of infectious mononucleosis. Other manifestations of the disease include hepatitis, skin eruptions, pneumonitis, myocarditis, pericarditis, and CNS involvement.

Hepatitis. Liver involvement occurs relatively frequently in patients with infectious mononucleosis. Hepatomegaly is present in 10% to 15% of cases, but moderately abnormal hepatic isoenzymes are found in more than 80% of patients tested. Frank jaundice develops in less than 5% of cases and is usually mild; however, hyperbilirubinemia is reported in 25% of patients. Hepatitis may provoke such symptoms as anorexia, nausea, and vomiting.

Rash. In cases of infectious mononucleosis that are well documented clinically and serologically, the incidence of dermatitis is 3% to 19% (Bernstein, 1940; Contratto, 1944; Milne, 1945; Press et al., 1945; McCarthy and Hoagland, 1964). The rash, when present, is usually located on the trunk and arms; rarely, it may present solely as palmar dermatitis (Petrozzi, 1971). It appears during the first few days of illness, lasts 1 to 6 days, and is usually erythematous, macular, and papular or morbilliform. Sometimes, urticarial or scarlatiniform eruptions are seen (Press et al., 1945; McCarthy and Hoagland, 1964; Cowdrey and Reynolds, 1969). Occasionally, erythema multiforme, cold-induced urticaria, and acrocyanosis may be associated with infectious mononucleosis (Barth, 1981; Hughes and Burrows, 1993). Rarely, the rash may be petechial, vesicular, or hemorrhagic, but other more common and more serious causes of such rashes should be considered before they are ascribed to infectious mononucleosis.

In 1967 Pullen et al. and Patel nearly simultaneously observed an increased incidence of skin rashes in patients with infectious mononucleosis who were given ampicillin. The copper-colored rash begins 5 to 10 days after the drug is begun, mainly over the trunk. It then develops into an extensive, generalized (including the palms and soles), macular, and papular pruritic eruption. It can last up to a week, with desquamation persisting for several more days. At its peak the rash is confluent over exposed areas and pressure points and more marked extensor surfaces. A faint macular rash sometimes is seen on the palatal and buccal mucosae. This rash may also be seen with the administration of ampicillin derivatives, such as amoxicillin (Mulroy, 1973), and other penicillins, such as methicillin (Fields, 1980). This rash does not represent a hypersensitivity to ampicillin; the drug may be used again once the infectious mononucleosis has subsided (Nazareth et al., 1972; Levene and Baker, 1968; McKenzie et al., 1976).

Pneumonitis. A small percentage of patients with infectious mononucleosis develop a paroxysmal cough, with a clinical picture and roentgenograms indistinguishable from those of atypical pneumonia. Pleural effusion also may develop. Hilar adenopathy is often observed in patients with extensive lymphoid hyperplasia.

Nervous system involvement. During the past three decades there have been increasing numbers of reports of CNS involvement in patients with infectious mononucleosis. These manifestations have been observed in the adult age group and also in children. The neurologic syndromes have included aseptic meningitis, encephalitis, the "Alice in Wonderland" syndrome, acute hemiplegia, infectious polyneuritis (Guillain-Barré syndrome), cranial nerve palsies, optic neuritis, peripheral neuropathy, transverse myelitis, acute cerebellar ataxia, dysautonomia, and CNS lymphoma. Demyelinating disease may follow cases of acute infectious mononucleosis (Connelly and Demitt, 1994; Matoba, 1990; Bray et al., 1992, Besnard et al., 2000).

■ **Case 1** A 10-year-old African-American boy with generalized lymphadenopathy, splenomegaly, typical blood picture, and positive heterophil antibody titer developed encephalitis during the course of his infection. He had headache, vomiting, and drowsiness that progressed to stupor. The cerebrospinal fluid showed pleocytosis with a predominance of lymphocytes and an elevated protein level. His sensorium gradually improved, and he made an uneventful recovery.

■ **Case 2** A 12-year-old Caucasian girl with a classic picture of infectious mononucleosis developed weakness of both lower and upper extremities, with absent reflexes. Spinal fluid findings showed albuminocytological dissociation characteristic of the Guillain-Barré syndrome, no cells, and a protein of 300 mg/dl. The paralysis cleared completely within 6 weeks. The diagnosis of infectious mononucleosis was confirmed by a typical blood smear and positive result of heterophil antibody test.

In general, the neurologic manifestations depend on the site of involvement, which may be anywhere in the CNS. The majority of patients recover completely, although fatalities have been associated with encephalitis.

Complications

Rupture of the spleen. Rupture of the spleen is a serious but, fortunately, rare complication of infectious mononucleosis. It has been attributed to an extensive lymphocytic and mononuclear cell infiltrate that presumably causes stretching and weakening of the capsule and trabeculae. Consequently, minor trauma to the splenic area or sudden increases in intraabdominal pressure may precipitate rupture. In rare instances it may develop spontaneously following progressive intrasplenic hyperplasia. The presence of this complication should be suspected in any patient who suddenly develops abdominal pain on the left side and signs of peritoneal irritation, hemorrhage, and shock (Rutkow, 1978).

Hematologic complications. The development of epistaxis, petechial and ecchymotic skin lesions, and hematuria, combined with thrombocytopenia, prolonged bleeding time, and poor clot retraction, is characteristic of thrombocytopenic purpura; recovery is the rule (Clarke and Davies, 1964). Other rare hematologic complications include hemolytic anemia, aplastic anemia, agranulocytosis, and agammaglobulinemia (Grierson and Purtilo, 1987).

An acute hemophagocytic syndrome resembling malignant histiocytosis in infants and children has been linked to EBV infection (Okano and Gross, 1996). Presenting symptoms include fever, hepatosplenomegaly, pancytopenia, and disseminated intravascular coagulation; hemophagocytosis is found on examination of bone marrow. The mortality rate ranges from 30% to 40%. The syndrome is associated with many infections, although EBV is the most common. EBV-associated hemophagocytic syndrome is more common in the Far East (e.g., Taiwan and Japan). Recent evidence suggests that the pathogenesis of this syndrome is related to macrophage hyperactivity initially directed against EBV-infected T and B lymphocytes (Lay et al., 1997). There is clinical overlap between this syndrome and the X-linked lymphoproliferative syndrome (Seemayer et al., 1995). Measuring the amount of EBV DNA in the peripheral blood via polymerase chain reaction (PCR) technology may prove useful for monitoring patients who develop complications following EBV-induced infectious mononucleosis (van Laar, et al., 2002).

Cardiac complications. Electrocardiographic changes during the course of infectious mononucleosis have been reported in adults. These are usually the only manifestations of cardiac involvement. However, there have been several reports of pericarditis and myocarditis characterized by severe chest pain and typical electrocardiographic findings (Hudgins, 1976; Butler et al., 1981).

Miscellaneous. Orchitis may occur rarely in association with infectious mononucleosis. In one case report (Ralston et al., 1960) the testicular involvement was bilateral; in another report (Wolnisty, 1962) it was unilateral. The orchitis subsided in 2 to 4 weeks. Renal failure, arthritis, rhabdomyolysis, pancreatitis, proctitis, ocular involvement, genital ulcers, biliary obstruction, and gall bladder hydrops have also been (rarely) reported (Koutras, 1983; Dinulos et al., 1994; Mayer et al., 1996; Osamah et al.,

1995; Hudson and Perlman, 1998; Barlow et al., 2000; Slobod et al., 2000).

Diagnosis

The diagnosis of infectious mononucleosis is usually made on the basis of (1) suggestive clinical features; (2) typical blood picture; (3) positive heterophil agglutination antibody test; and (4) ancillary laboratory findings, such as specific antibodies to EBV antigens. Younger children, especially, may have EBV infection with symptoms not characteristic of infectious mononucleosis and with negative heterophil antibody titers. In such instances measurement of specific EBV antibody against EBV antigens is required for diagnosis (Evans et al., 1975; Rapp and Hewetson, 1978). Examination and test results from a patient with mononucleosis seen early in the illness are illustrated in Fig. 9-1.

Clinical features. A history of fever associated with lymphadenopathy, exudative pharyngitis, and splenomegaly should suggest infectious mononucleosis as a diagnostic possibility. The following laboratory tests are not specific but are helpful in establishing the diagnosis.

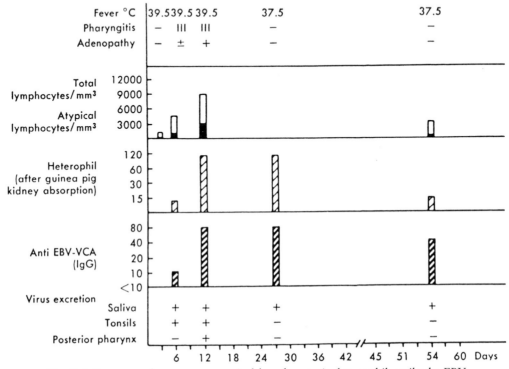

Fig. 9-1 Sequence of symptoms, atypical lymphocytosis, heterophil antibody, EBV antibody (anti-EBV–VCA), and EBV oral excretion in a patient with mononucleosis seen early in the illness. (From Niederman JC et al.: N Engl J Med 1976; 294:1355.)

Blood tests. An absolute increase in the number of atypical lymphocytes is a characteristic finding during some stages of the disease. In a blood smear these cells usually represent 10% or more of the field. These so-called Downey cells vary markedly in size and shape. With Wright's stain the cytoplasm is dark blue and vacuolated, presenting a foamy appearance; the nucleus is round, bean shaped, or lobulated and contains no nucleoli. The white blood cell count is variable. During the first week of the disease there may be leukopenia, but commonly there is leukocytosis with a predominance of lymphocytes. The white blood cell count may be so elevated that the presence of leukemia is suspected. In an occasional immunodeficient patient, infectious mononucleosis can progress to frank leukemia; in this instance all the primitive blasts in the circulation are EBV-transformed B cells (Robinson et al., 1980).

Atypical lymphocytes are not specific for infectious mononucleosis. They may be observed in a variety of clinical entities, including infectious hepatitis, rubella, primary atypical pneumonia, allergic rhinitis, asthma, and other diseases. Morphologically, the atypical cells in these other conditions are indistinguishable from those seen in infectious mononucleosis. Quantitatively, however, there is a difference; in infectious mononucleosis there are usually more than 10% atypical cells, whereas these other conditions usually have a lower percentage of atypical cells.

Heterophil antibodies. Heterophil antibodies were the first serologic markers discovered that could reasonably confirm the diagnosis of infectious mononucleosis. Heterophil antibody tests are still used more frequently than any of the virus-specific assays. Most sera of patients with infectious mononucleosis cause sheep red blood cells to agglutinate after they have been absorbed with guinea pig kidney antigens but not after absorption with bovine red blood cells. The reverse is often true of normal sera (see Table 9-1). The heterophil antibody responsible for this differential absorption in infectious mononucleosis is principally of the IgM class, appears during the first or second week of illness, and disappears gradually over 3 to 6 months. In a group of 166 patients studied by Niederman (1956) the heterophil antibody test was positive in 38% during the first week, in 60% during the second week, and in approx-imately 80% during the third week after onset of symptoms.

Sheep cell agglutinins are not specific for infectious mononucleosis. They occur in a number of other conditions, such as serum sickness, viral hepatitis, rubella, leukemia, and Hodgkin's disease. Low titers can also be demonstrated in the serum of some normal persons. Usually the absorption tests serve to distinguish these agglutinins from the heterophil antibodies of infectious mononucleosis. In general, the agglutinin titer is also higher in patients with infectious mononucleosis than in those with other conditions; an unabsorbed heterophil antibody titer above 1:128 and 1:40 or greater after absorption is considered significant.

A rapid slide test using equine red blood cells stabilized by formaldehyde has been evaluated as a diagnostic test for infectious mononucleosis. In 1965 Hoff and Bauer reported a high degree of correlation with the standard heterophil antibody test. They described the following advantages: (1) low incidence of false reactions; (2) high degree of specificity for infectious mononucleosis antibody; (3) great rapidity (2 minutes); and (4) ease of performance. This rapid test is a valuable diagnostic aid in clinical practice. Other rapid slide tests have become available, using the same principle of the absorbed heterophil agglutination but using equine or bovine erythrocytes that are citrated or formalinized. All have shown a specificity of 90% to 98% in most studies (Rapp and Hewetson, 1978).

Antibody titers to specific EBV antigens. Although infectious mononucleosis occurs only in previously seronegative individuals, IgG antibody to the VCA is usually already detectable early in the course of the illness. The acute illness may be diagnosed if VCA-specific IgM is present in serum, but this assay is difficult to perform and may yield false-positive reactions because of rheumatoid factors in blood. VCA-IgM responses disappear after several months, whereas VCA-IgG levels persist for life, albeit at more modest titers than are present during acute disease. Antibodies to the EA complex, associated with viral replication, are present in 70% to 80% of patients during acute disease and usually disappear after 6 months, although these antibodies may be detectable in healthy individuals for years after infectious mononucleosis (Horwitz et al.,

1985). EBNA appears more slowly, taking from 1 to 6 months to become detectable. The antibody response to EBNA (EBNA-1) is more delayed (Niederman and Miller, 1986). Testing acute and convalescent sera for titer rises to EBNA-1 can be a useful diagnostic procedure, although this test is not readily available clinically. A positive anti-VCA titer and a negative anti-EBNA titer are diagnostic of a primary EBV serologic response such as occurs in infectious mononucleosis. All late convalescent sera from healthy individuals contain EBNA antibodies. A diagram showing the sequence of development and persistence of these antibodies to EBV is shown in Fig. 9-2.

Detection of the virus. Biologically active virus can be isolated from saliva, peripheral blood, or lymphoid tissue by means of its ability to immortalize cultured human lymphocytes, usually from umbilical-cord blood. Occasionally, lymphoid cell lines can be grown directly from blood or lymph nodes. This assay is time consuming (6 to 8 weeks) and requires specialized tissue-culture facilities that are not generally available.

Viral antigens representative of the latent life cycle of the virus can be found in lymphoid tissues, in nasopharyngeal carcinoma tumors, and occasionally in the peripheral blood if the level of leukoviremia is high enough. During the acute phase of mononucleosis, approximately 1% or less of the circulating peripheral blood lymphocytes contain EBNA.

The most specific method of demonstrating EBV in pathologic material is nucleic acid hybridization. Three general techniques have been used: (1) Southern hybridization, which is capable of distinguishing the specific portions of EBV DNA that are present in the lesions; (2) in situ hybridization, which identifies the cells that contain EBV DNA or RNA; and (3) PCR, which amplifies EBV nucleic acid present in the tissue. Probes for nucleic acid detection methods are made from cloned EBV DNA fragments prepared by recombinant DNA techniques or from synthetic oligonucleotides. The probes are labeled by radioactive or nonisotopic methods.

The sensitivity of the Southern hybridization technique under the best conditions is approximately 10^5 EBV genomes, and more often approximately 10^6 genomes. This sensitivity is sufficient to detect EBV DNA in immunocompromised patients, where many copies of EBV DNA reside in each cell. However, it is not sensitive enough to detect EBV DNA regularly in peripheral blood of mononucleosis patients, in which only a few cells harbor EBV DNA. PCR is highly sensitive; it can detect approximately

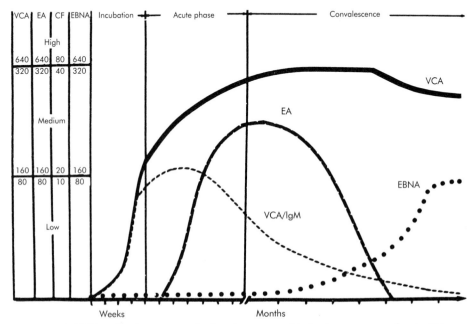

Fig. 9-2 EBV antibody response during the course of infectious mononucleosis. *EA,* Early antigen; *VCA,* viral capsid antigen; *EBNA,* EB nuclear antigen. (From de Thé G: In Klein G: Viral oncology, New York: Raven Press, 1980.)

10^4 genomes or less; therefore, in most cases of acute infectious mononucleosis, EBV DNA can be detected in the blood by PCR. Nucleic acid hybridization methods can be used as a rapid assay for salivary excretion of EBV.

Southern hybridization can determine whether patients are infected with the same or different viruses (Katz et al., 1988). Probes from regions of the genome near the termini provide additional information about whether the EBV is monoclonal or multiclonal (Raab-Traub and Flynn, 1986). Furthermore, the same probes can distinguish between latent and lytically replicating forms of EBV DNA. Using these techniques, it has been found that many EBV-associated lymphoproliferative diseases contain lytically replicating forms of EBV DNA (Katz et al., 1989).

In situ hybridization for the abundant EB virus–encoded small RNAs (EBERs) is a specific and sensitive technique for detection of EB viral gene expression in pathologic specimens (Howe and Steitz, 1986). EBER in situ hybridization permits the determination of the number and type of infected cells in paraffin-embedded tissues (Hamilton-Dutoit and Pallesen, 1994; Barletta et al., 1993).

Differential Diagnosis

Infectious mononucleosis is a notorious mimic of many other diseases. Lymphadenopathy, splenomegaly, and exudative tonsillitis are common manifestations of a number of entities. The following conditions are often confused with infectious mononucleosis.

Streptococcal tonsillitis or pharyngitis. This condition is suggested by fever, sore throat, exudative tonsillitis, and cervical adenitis. An increase in the number of polymorphonuclear leukocytes, positive culture from a throat swab specimen, and prompt therapeutic response to penicillin all point to a streptococcal cause.

Diphtheria. The membranous tonsillitis of infectious mononucleosis frequently resembles diphtheria. The diagnosis is confirmed by positive culture.

Blood dyscrasias. Blood dyscrasias, particularly leukemia, are suggested by the lymphadenopathy, splenomegaly, and increase in number of peripheral blood atypical lymphocytes. Laboratory tests, including bone marrow aspiration, establish the true diagnosis, although distinguishing these entities pathologically can occasionally be difficult.

Rubella. Rubella is commonly associated with a 2- to 4-day period of malaise and lymphadenopathy preceding the appearance of the rash. Rubella has a milder course, and frequently there is a history of exposure. A definite diagnosis of rubella can be established by evidence of a rise in the level of specific antibodies.

Measles. Measles, which is less frequently confused with infectious mononucleosis, is easily identified by the pathognomonic Koplik's spots. In doubtful cases a diagnosis of measles can be confirmed by demonstration of a rise in the level of measles antibodies.

Viral hepatitis. This disease may be clinically indistinguishable from infectious mononucleosis with jaundice. Specific serologic tests can confirm a diagnosis of hepatitis A, B, or C.

Cytomegalovirus infection. A mononucleosis-like syndrome characterized by fever, splenomegaly, and atypical lymphocytes occurs in some patients with acute cytomegalovirus infection. These patients have a negative heterophil agglutination determination and no evidence of recent EBV infection. Culture of urine or blood (buffy coat) or direct detection of antigen should be positive for cytomegalovirus.

Acquired toxoplasmosis with lymphadenopathy. Toxoplasmosis infection may be clinically indistinguishable from infectious mononucleosis. It is characterized by generalized lymphadenopathy, chiefly of the cervical group, and occasionally by pharyngeal involvement and exanthem. These patients have a negative heterophil and a positive toxoplasma antibody determination.

Infectious mononucleosis may also simulate Hodgkin's disease, scarlet fever, secondary syphilis, typhoid fever, rickettsial diseases, and many others.

Prognosis

In general, the prognosis for patients with infectious mononucleosis is excellent. Severe cases may be followed by long periods (6 to 12 months) of asthenia (White et al., 1998; Buchwald et al., 2000; White et al., 2001). Spontaneous rupture of the spleen, which is very rare, is fatal if it is not recognized and treated promptly (Farley et al., 1992). Deaths reported in infectious mononucleosis have also resulted from CNS complications, secondary bacterial infection following neutropenia, myocarditis, X-linked lymphoproliferative disease, and hemophagocytic syndrome.

Treatment

Infectious mononucleosis is a self-limited disease, and treatment is chiefly supportive. Antimicrobial drugs are not effective and do not alter the course of the infection. Bed rest is indicated in the acute stage of the disease. Aspirin or nonsteroidal antiinflammatory agents can usually control the pain or discomfort caused by the enlarged lymph nodes and pharyngeal involvement. In severe cases codeine or meperidine (Demerol) may be required.

Corticosteroid therapy has been reported to have a beneficial effect in certain situations. Severe symptoms referable to the throat and enlarged lymph nodes improve within 24 hours of corticosteroid therapy in many instances; if there is no response, tonsillectomy may be considered (Stevenson et al., 1992). In a well-controlled study of 132 patients with severe uncomplicated mononucleosis, Bender (1967) observed a significant decrease in the duration of fever; it persisted for an average of 1.4 days in the 66 corticosteroid-treated patients and an average of 5.6 days in the 66 matched control patients. Steroids may be considered for treatment of severe cases characterized by hematologic complications, marked toxemia, progressive tonsillar enlargement leading to airway encroachment, and evidence of neurologic or cardiac complications. Steroids are not recommended for treatment of mild cases of infectious mononucleosis because the long-term effects of intervention on the normal immune response to EBV are unknown. There are reports of neurologic or septicemic complications following steroid use (Waldo, 1981; Gold et al., 1995).

Sports should be avoided until the patient's spleen size has returned to normal (American Academy of Pediatrics, 2001). Rupture of the spleen often requires surgery. Transfusions, treatment for shock, and splenectomy can be lifesaving measures.

Acyclovir, ganciclovir, and foscarnet inhibit EBV DNA polymerase and thus block the lytic (but not the latent) phase of EBV replication; ganciclovir can also inhibit EBV-immortalization of B lymphocytes, and foscarnet can reduce the number of EBV copies in laboratory cell lines. All three agents inhibit viral DNA synthesis (represented by linear DNA) leading to virion production, but they have no effect on the number of latent (circular) genomes (Colby et al., 1980, Crumpacker, 1996; Oertel, 1999). Acyclovir and ganciclovir are nucleoside analogs that are preferentially incorporated into viral DNA through the action of the EBV thymidine kinase; foscarnet inhibits EBV DNA polymerase via a different mechanism.

When given to patients with infectious mononucleosis, acyclovir given with or without steroids reduces the level of oropharyngeal viral replication during the period of administration (Ernberg and Andersson, 1986; Tynell et al., 1996). However, after cessation of treatment, replication returns to previously high levels. During acyclovir treatment there is little or no reduction in the number of EBV-infected B cells found in the peripheral circulation. Acyclovir has minimal effects on the symptoms of mononucleosis as well, and therefore is not recommended for the treatment of patients with this disease.

OTHER EBV-ASSOCIATED DISEASES
X-Linked Lymphoproliferative Syndrome: Duncan's Disease

A spectrum of clinical manifestations of EBV infections in patients with recognized or presumed immunologic impairment has been reported. X-linked lymphoproliferative disease (XLP) was described in kindred males by Bar et al. in 1974 and Purtilo et al. in 1977; the disease causes severe and often fatal infectious mononucleosis, with death occurring after 1 or 2 weeks from hemorrhage, hepatic failure, or bacterial superinfection. This sex-linked recessive genetic disorder has variable phenotypic expression. Boys who survive EBV infection may subsequently develop a variety of hematologic complications, such as agammaglobulinemia, hypergammaglobulinemia, agranulocytosis, aplastic anemia, and malignancy. The mean age of 100 of these boys at death was approximately 6 years (Purtilo et al., 1982). The underlying genetic problem appears to be a mutation in a gene located on the X chromosome (Xq24) called *SAP*, an acronym for SLAM (signaling lymphocyte activation molecule)-associated protein. This genetic mutation leads to an ineffective cytotoxic T-cell and/or natural killer cell response to EBV as the result of defective T-lymphocyte signal pathways (Seemayer et al., 1995; Coffee et al., 1998; Sayos et al., 1998; Bottino et al., 2001). This disease may be difficult to diagnose because many patients have low or undetectable serologic responses to EBV despite infection; this is true of EBV infections in the setting of other immunodeficiencies as well (Andiman et al., 1985; Katz et al., 2001). Many such patients experience lymphocytosis, hepatic necrosis, and hemophagocytosis; EBV DNA and EBERs are found in liver or bone marrow by molecular hybridization techniques.

Rarely, cases of classic infectious mononucleosis in apparently normal girls have evolved into monoclonal or polyclonal lymphomas (Robinson et al., 1980; Abo et al., 1982). These patients presumably have undiagnosed immunoregulatory disorders with an abnormal immune response to EBV, which results in chronic or malignant disease following primary EBV infection.

EBV Infections in Transplant Patients

There is serologic and virologic evidence for reactivation of latent EBV in conjunction with immunosuppressive therapy (Strauch et al., 1974). Such reactivation, as well as primary EBV infection in this setting, may be associated with a spectrum of clinical manifestations, including benign or fatal lymphoproliferative disorders or non-Hodgkin's lymphomas (Ho et al., 1988). Thus it is not surprising that a variety of EBV-associated lymphoproliferative syndromes have been described in patients who have received kidney, heart, bone marrow, liver, or thymus transplants under cover of immunosuppressive therapy.

At least three factors are thought to contribute to the pathogenesis and timing of these lymphoproliferative syndromes: (1) the dosage, duration, and number of immunosuppressive drugs, particularly cyclosporin A or tacrolimus (FK506); (2) whether the patient is undergoing primary or reactivated EBV infection; and (3) the use of antibody to T cells (especially OKT3 antibody) as an immunosuppressive agent to maintain the graft or, in the case of bone marrow transplantation, to prevent graft-versus-host disease, in conjunction with the use of a T-cell-depleted allogeneic bone marrow (Martin et al., 1984). The latter scenario is often associated with lymphomas arising in donor cells, which can be detected through the presence of markers such as a sex chromosome or mitochondrial DNA polymorphism (Schubach et al., 1982). Chronic antigenic stimulation caused by the engrafted cells was thought to play a role in pathogenesis of EBV-associated lymphomas in recipients of allogeneic transplants; however, EBV-associated B-cell lymphomas have been described in recipients of autologous marrow transplant as well (Ho et al., 1985; Ho et al., 1988).

Posttransplant lymphoproliferative lesions display the same latent EBV gene products observed in B cells immortalized in vitro. Hanto et al. (1981) estimated an incidence of 1% (12 per 1,119) for lymphomas and other lymphoproliferative disorders among recipients of renal transplants. The incidence of lymphomas among heart-transplant patients in the Stanford series was 5% (9 per 182). The frequency of lymphomas in patients receiving transplantation of allogeneic T cell–depleted bone marrow may be as high as 15% to 20%. Nucleic acid hybridization is the principal technique used to demonstrate an association of EBV with these tumors. More recently, PCR has been used to demonstrate that patients who develop lymphoproliferative disease generally have viral loads that are several logs higher than those of patients who do not (Rowe et al., 2001). Discontinuation of cyclosporin A or tacrolimus therapy with or without concomitant antiviral therapy is accompanied by remission of the lymphoproliferative disease in 30% to 50% of cases; whether to reduce immunosuppression in asymptomatic transplant recipients with high viral loads is currently unknown. Chemotherapy and interferon-α have also been used (Swinnen, 1992; Benkerrou et al., 1993). There has been a report of a cure following bone marrow transplantation and treatment with etoposide (Pracher et al., 1994). A recent, highly encouraging strategy in recipients of allogeneic bone marrow transplants of adoptive immunotherapy involves the transfusion of donor EBV-specific cytotoxic T cells (Rooney, 1995). Anti–B cell antibodies (rituximab) have also been used for treatment (Oertel, 2000; Cook et al., 1999; Kuehnle et al, 2000); anti-B cell antibodies and ganciclovir have been used pre-emptively to treat asymptomatic patients with high viral loads as well (van Esser et al., 2002; Farmer et al., 2002).

EBV-Associated Diseases in AIDS Patients

Patients with acquired immunodeficiency syndrome (AIDS) develop four different EBV-associated lesions: (1) lymphomas; (2) lymphocytic interstitial pneumonitis (LIP); (3) oral "hairy" leukoplakia of the tongue; and (4) leiomyosarcoma.

Lymphomas. AIDS predisposes to EBV-associated lymphomas of several histologic types, including classic Burkitt's lymphoma with its associated chromosome abnormality and c-*myc* protooncogene translocation (Leder et al., 1976). However, many cases of Burkitt's lymphoma occurring in AIDS patients do not contain EBV (as is generally true of Burkitt's lymphoma outside the endemic regions) (Subar et al., 1988). Several other types of EBV-associated lymphomas, including CNS lymphoma and diffuse polyclonal or oligoclonal B-cell lymphoma found in extranodal sites such as the gut, are common complications of AIDS. CNS lymphoma is due to proliferation of EBV-infected B cells in an immunologically privileged site. It occurs infrequently in otherwise healthy individuals but is more common in immunosuppressed patients with AIDS (or those receiving organ transplants [Hochberg et al., 1983]). EBV is invariably present in CNS lymphoma (MacMahon et al., 1991).

Lymphocytic interstitial pneumonitis. LIP is a polyclonal lymphoproliferative process (Joshi et al., 1987) seen mainly in children with AIDS. The occurrence of LIP correlates with lymphoproliferative activity (i.e., lymphadenopathy and parotitis) elsewhere in the body. It initially is seen as a subacute or chronic pulmonary process (e.g., with dyspnea on exertion and clubbing) rather than as acute pneumonitis. It is characterized by a reticulonodular pattern on chest radiography (Rubinstein et al., 1986). Histologically, lung biopsies of these lesions reveal mature lymphoid follicle formation in the lung, including germinal centers, and infiltration with plasmacytoid cells. Up to 80% of the lesions are associated with EBV DNA (Andiman et al., 1985), and patients, when compared with matched controls, often have evidence of a primary or reactivated EBV serologic response (Katz et al., 1992). LIP may regress with acyclovir treatment or a low dose of corticosteroids given every other day (Pahwa, 1988). The lesions tend to worsen concomitant with other pulmonary infections.

Oral hairy leukoplakia. Oral hairy leukoplakia, which clinically resembles thrush, is seen principally on the lateral surface of the tongues of homosexual men with AIDS. Pathologically, the lesions resemble flat warts. Lytic EBV DNA replication and production of mature virions have been documented within the epithelial cells of these lesions, which regress with acyclovir treatment (Greenspan et al., 1985; Resnick et al., 1988).

Leiomyosarcoma. Leiomyosarcomas are malignant cancers of smooth muscle that are rare in childhood. Five cases in children with AIDS (and five cases in liver-transplant recipients) have been found to be EBV associated. The tumors were monoclonal or oligoclonal. There has been no report of an EBV-associated leiomyosarcoma in an immunocompetent host, thus strengthening the case for an association between immunosuppression and EBV-associated malignancy (McClain, 1995; Lee, 1995).

Congenital Infection

Occasionally, infants with birth defects believed to be secondary to congenital EBV infection have been described. One infant manifested bilateral congenital cataracts, cryptorchidism, hypotonia, and mild micrognathia. A "celery stalk" appearance of long bones was noted radiologically, similar to the condition seen with congenital rubella (Goldberg et al., 1981). A report by Icart et al. (1981) described more than 700 pregnant women with serologic evidence of EBV infection during pregnancy. Their pregnancies were three times more likely to result in early fetal death, premature labor, or delivery of an infant who would become ill. Until further data are available, however, it is difficult to know whether these associations are real or coincidental. One prospective study of 4,063 pregnant women during 4,108 gestations failed to show any intrauterine EBV infections (Fleisher and Bologonese, 1984).

Chronic Active EBV Infections

Rarely, patients have a true chronic active infection with EBV. In these patients there are numerous objective clinical and laboratory findings of major organ involvement, including pneumonitis, hepatitis, sicca syndrome, neuropathy, cardiomyopathy and uveitis, and a variety of hematologic abnormalities, such as neutropenia, eosinophilia, and thrombocytopenia (Schooley et al., 1986; Sato-Matsumura et al., 2000). These patients have prolonged, severe relapsing courses lasting more than 6 months, occasionally with a fatal outcome. In some instances, death has been associated with respiratory failure caused by interstitial pneumonitis; in other instances it has been linked to diffuse T-cell lymphomas associated with EBV DNA (Jones et al., 1988). The pathogenesis of this syndrome is not clear, but it possibly is due to increased EBV replication, because patients often have extremely high levels of EBV in affected tissues and antibody to the EBV replicative antigens VCA and EA. Characteristically, these patients also have low or absent antibody to the EBNAs. Some of these patients have selective absence of antibody to EBNA-1 (Miller et al., 1987).

Several families have been described in which this syndrome has occurred in several members (Joncas et al., 1984). The pathogenesis of this familial form of chronic active EBV infection is also unclear. One hypothesis is that mechanisms involved in the restriction of viral replication are deficient, either at the cellular level or at the immune level. A deficiency of killer cells that participate in ADCC has been suggested. That it is difficult to identify transforming virus in the saliva of some of the patients has prompted the alternative hypothesis that they are infected with nontransforming, lytic EBV variants.

Chronic Fatigue Syndrome

Chronic active EBV infection should not be confused with a "neuromyasthenic," "polymyalgic," or "chronic fatigue" syndrome (Fukuda et al., 1994). In most patients, EBV is not the causative agent of this syndrome, although some patients have elevations of antibody titers to EAs, a few patients lack antibody to EBNA-1 (Jones et al., 1985; Katz et al., 1989), and some patients do experience prolonged fatigue following mononucleosis (White et al., 1998; Buchwald et al., 2000; White et al., 2001). The symptoms of chronic fatigue syndrome include fatigue, chronic pharyngitis, tender lymph nodes, headaches, myalgia, and arthralgias. The symptoms are recurrent and prolonged, but no fatalities have been described. The natural history is variable, although children and adolescents have a better prognosis than adults.

BIBLIOGRAPHY

American Academy of Pediatrics Committee on Sports Medicine and Fitness. Medical conditions affecting sports participation. Pediatrics 2001;107:1205-1209.

Abo W, Takada K, Kamada M, et al. Evolution of infectious mononucleosis into EBV carrying monoclonal malignant lymphoma. Lancet 1982;1:1272-1275.

Adams A, Lindahl T. Epstein-Barr virus genomes with properties of circular DNA molecules in carrier cells. Proc Natl Acad Sci USA 1975;72:1477-1481.

Anderson Lund BM, Bergen T. Temporary skin reactions to penicillins during the acute stage of infectious mononucleosis. Scand J Infect Dis 1975;7:21-28.

Andiman WA. The Epstein-Barr virus and EB virus infections in childhood. J Pediatr 1979;95:171-182.

Andiman WA. Epstein-Barr virus–associated syndromes: a critical reexamination. Pediatr Infect Dis J 1984;3:198-203.

Andiman WA, Eastman R, Martin K, et al. Opportunistic lymphoproliferations associated with Epstein-Barr viral DNA in infants and children with AIDS. Lancet 1985; 1390-1393.

Andiman WA, Markowitz RI, Horstmann DM. Clinical, virologic, and serologic evidence of Epstein-Barr virus infection in association with childhood pneumonia. J Pediatr 1981;99:880-886.

Baer R, Bankier AT, Biggin MD, et al. DNA sequence and expression of the B95-8 Epstein-Barr virus genome. Nature 1984;310:207-211.

Bar RS, DeLor CJ, Clauben KP, et al. Fatal infectious mononucleosis in a family. N Engl J Med 1974;290:363-367.

Barletta JM, Kingma DW, Ling Y, et al. Rapid in situ hybridization for the diagnosis of latent Epstein-Barr virus infection. Mol Cell Probes 1993;7:105-109.

Barlow G, Kilding R, Green ST. Epstein-Barr virus infection mimicking extrahepatic biliary obstruction. J R Soc Med 2000;93:316-318.

Barth JH. Infectious mononucleosis (glandular fever) complicated by cold agglutinins, cold urticaria, and leg ulceration. Acta Derm Venereol (Stockh) 1981;61:451.

Bender CE. The value of corticosteroids in the treatment of infectious mononucleosis. JAMA 1967;199:97.

Benkerrou M, Durandy A, Fischer A. Therapy for transplant-related lymphoproliferative diseases. Hematol Oncol Clin North Am 1993;7:467-475.

Bernstein A. Infectious mononucleosis. Medicine 1940;19:85-159.

Besnard M, Faure C, Fromont-Hankard G, et al: Intestinal pseudo-obstruction and acute pandysautonomia associated with Epstein-Barr virus infection. Am J Gastroenterol 2000;95:280-284.

Blacklow NR, Watson BK, Miller G, Jacobson BM. Mononucleosis with heterophile antibodies and EB virus infection. Acquisition by an elderly patient in a hospital. Am J Med 1971;51:549-552.

Bottino C, Falco M. Parolini S, et al. NTB-A, a novel SG2D1A-associated surface molecule contributing to the inability of natural killer cells to kill Epstein-Barr virus-infected B cells in x-linked lymphoproliferative disease. J Exp Med 2001;194(3):235-246.

Bray PF, Culp KW, McFarlin DE, et al. Demyelinating disease after neurologically complicated primary Epstein-Barr virus infection. Neurology 1992;42:278-282.

Brichacek B, Hirsch I, Sibl O, et al. Association of some supraglottic laryngeal carcinomas with EB virus. Int J Cancer 1983;32:193-197.

Buchwald DS, Rae TD, Katon WJ, et al. Acute infectious mononucleosis: characteristics of patients who report failure to recover. Am J Med 2000;109:531-537.

Butler T, Pastore J, Simon G, et al. Infectious mononucleosis myocarditis. J Infect 1981;3:172-175.

Clarke BF, Davies SH. Severe thrombocytopenia in infectious mononucleosis. Am J Med Sci 1964;248:703-708.

Coffee AJ, Brooksbank RA, Brandau O, et al. Host response to EBV infection in X-linked lymphoproliferative disease results from mutations in an SH2-domain encoding gene. Nat Genet 1998;20:129-135.

Colby BM, Shaw JE, Elion GB, Pagano JS. Effect of acyclovir [9-(2-hydroxyethoxymethyl)guanine] on Epstein-Barr virus DNA replication. J Virol 1980;34:560-568.

Conant MA. Hairy leukoplakia. A new disease of the oral mucosa. Arch Dermatol 1987;123:585-587.

Connelly KP, DeWitt D. Neurologic complications of infectious mononucleosis. Pediatr Neurol 1994;10:181-184.

Contratto AN. Infectious mononucleosis: a study of one-hundred and ninety-six cases. Arch Intern Med 1944;73:449-459.

Cook RC, Connors JM, Gascoyne RD, et al. Treatment of post-transplant lymphoproliferative disease with rituximab monoclonal antibody after lung transplantation. Lancet 1999;354:1698-1699.

Cowdrey SC, Reynolds JS. Acute urticaria in infectious mononucleosis. Ann Allergy Asthma Immunol 1969;27:182.

Crumpacker CS. Ganciclovir. N Engl J Med 1996;335:721-729.

Davidsohn I. Serologic diagnosis of infectious mononucleosis. JAMA 1937;108:289.

De Waele M, Thielemans C, Van Camp BKG. Characterization of immunoregulatory T cells in EBV-induced infectious mononucleosis by monoclonal antibodies. N Engl J Med 1981;304:460-462.

Dinulos J, Mitchell DK, Egerton J, Pickering LK. Hydrops of the gall bladder associated with Epstein-Barr virus infection. Pediatr Infect Dis J 1994;13:924-929.

Epstein MA, Achong BG, Barr YM. Virus particles in cultural lymphoblasts from Burkitt's lymphoma. Lancet 1964;1:702-703.

Ernberg I, Andersson J. Acyclovir efficiently inhibits oropharyngeal excretion of Epstein-Barr virus in patients with acute infectious mononucleosis. J Gen Virol 1986;67:2267-2272.

Evans AS. Infectious mononucleosis in University of Wisconsin students. Report of five-year investigation. Am J Hyg 1960;71:342.

Evans AE, Niederman J, Cenabre LC, et al. A prospective evaluation of heterophile and Epstein-Barr virus-specific IgM antibody tests in clinical and subclinical infectious mononucleosis: specificity and sensitivity of the tests and persistence of antibody. J Infect Dis 1975;132:546.

Evans AS, Niederman JC, McCollum RW. Seroepidemiologic studies of infectious mononucleosis with EB virus. N Engl J Med 1968;279:1121-1127.

Farmer DG, McDiarmid SV, Winston D, et al. Effectiveness of aggressive prophylactic and preemptive therapies targeted against cytomegaloviral and Epstein-Barr viral disease after human intestinal transplantation. Transplantation Proceedings 2002;34:948-949.

Farley DR, Zietlow SP, Bannon MP, et al. Spontaneous rupture of the spleen due to infectious mononucleosis. Mayo Clin Proc 1992;67:846-853.

Fields DA. Methicillin rash in infectious mononucleosis (letter). West J Med 1980;133:521.

Fleisher G, Bolognese R. Epstein-Barr virus infections in pregnancy: a prospective study. J Pediatr 1984;104:374-379.

Fleisher GR, Pasquariello PS, Warren WS, et al. Intrafamilial transmission of Epstein-Barr virus infections. J Pediatr 1981;98:16-19.

Fukuda K, Straus SE, Hickie I, et al. The chronic fatigue syndrome. Ann Intern Med 1994;121:953-959.

Gerber P, Walsh JN, Rosenblum EN, Purcell RH. Association of EB-virus infection with the post-perfusion syndrome. Lancet 1969;1:593-596.

Gold WL, Kapral MK, Witmer MR, et al. Postanginal septicemia as a life-threatening complication of infectious mononucleosis. Clin Infect Dis 1995;20:1439-1440.

Goldberg GN, Fulginiti VA, Ray CG, et al. In utero EBV (infectious mononucleosis) infection. JAMA 1981;246:1579-1581.

Greenspan D, Greenspan JS, Conant M, et al. Oral "hairy" leucoplakia in male homosexuals: evidence of association with both papillomavirus and a herpes-group virus. Lancet 1984;2:831-834.

Greenspan JS, Greenspan D, Lennette ET, et al. Replication of Epstein-Barr virus within the epithelial lesions of oral "hairy" leukoplakia, and AIDS-associated lesion. N Engl J Med 1985;313:1564-1571.

Grierson H, Purtilo DT. Epstein-Barr virus infections in males with X-linked lymphoproliferative syndrome. Ann Intern Med 1987;106:538-545.

Hamilton-Dutoit SJ, Pallesen G. Detection of Epstein-Barr virus small RNAs in routine paraffin sections using non-isotopic RNA/RNA in situ hybridization. Histopathology 1994;25:101-111.

Hanto DW, Frizzera G, Purtilo DT, et al. Clinical spectrum of lymphoproliferative disorders in renal transplant recipients and evidence for the role of the Epstein-Barr virus. Cancer Res 1981;41:4253-4261.

Henle G, Henle W. Observations on childhood infections with the Epstein-Barr virus. J Infect Dis 1970;121:303.

Henle G, Henle W, Diehl V. Relation of Burkitt's tumor–associated herpes-type virus to infectious mononucleosis. Proc Natl Acad Sci USA 1968;59:94.

Ho M, Jaffe R, Miller G, et al. The frequency of Epstein-Barr virus infection and associated lymphoproliferative syndrome after transplantation and its manifestations in children. Transplantation 1988;45:719-727.

Ho M, Miller G, Atchison RW, et al. Epstein-Barr virus infections and DNA hybridization studies in posttransplantation lymphoma and lymphoproliferative lesions: the role of primary infection. J Infect Dis 1985;152:876-886.

Hoagland RJ. The transmission of infectious mononucleosis. Am J Med Sci 1955;229:262.

Hoagland RJ. The incubation period of infectious mononucleosis. Am J Public Health 1984;54:1699-1705.

Hochberg FH, Miller G, Schooley RJ, et al. Central-nervous system lymphoma related to Epstein-Barr virus. N Engl J Med 1983;309:745-748.

Hoff G, Bauer S. A new rapid slide test for infectious mononucleosis. JAMA 1965;194:351.

Horwitz CA, Henle W, Henle G, et al. Long term serological follow-up of patients for Epstein-Barr virus after recovery from infectious mononucleosis. J Infect Dis 1985;151:1150-1153.

Howe JG, Steitz JA. Localization of Epstein-Barr virus–encoded small RNAs by in situ hybridization. Proc Natl Acad Sci USA 1986;83:9006-9010.

Hudgins JM. Infectious mononucleosis complicated by myocarditis and pericarditis. JAMA 1976;235:2626.

Hudson LB, Perlman SE. Necrotizing genital ulcerations in a premenarcheal female with mononucleosis. Obstet Gynecol 1998;92:642-644.

Hughes J, Burrows NP. Infectious mononucleosis presenting as erythema multiforme. Clin Exp Dermatol 1993;18:373-374.

Icart J, Didier J, Dalens M, et al. Prospective study of Epstein-Barr virus (EBV) infection during pregnancy. Biomedicine 1981;34:160-163.

Joncas JH, Ghibu F, Blagdon M, et al. A familial syndrome of susceptibility to chronic active Epstein-Barr virus infection. CMAJ 1984;130:280-285.

Jones JF, Ray CG, Minnich LL, et al. Evidence for active Epstein-Barr virus infection in patients with persistent, unexplained illnesses: elevated anti-early antigen antibodies. Ann Intern Med 1985;102:1-7.

Jones JF, Shurin S, Abramowsky C, et al. T-cell lymphomas containing Epstein-Barr viral DNA in patients with chronic Epstein-Barr virus infections. N Engl J Med 1988;318:733-741.

Joshi VV, Kauffman S, Oleske JM, et al. Polyclonal polymorphic B-cell lymphoproliferative disorder with prominent pulmonary involvement in children with acquired immune deficiency syndrome. Cancer 1987;59:1455-1462.

Katz BZ, Andiman WA. Chronic fatigue syndrome. J Pediatr 1988;113:944-947.

Katz BZ, Berkman AB, Shapiro ED. Serologic evidence of active Epstein-Barr virus infection in Epstein-Barr virus–associated lymphoproliferative disorders in children with acquired immunodeficiency syndrome. J Pediatr 1992;120:228-232.

Katz BZ, Niederman JC, Olson BA, Miller G. Fragment length polymorphisms among independent isolates of Epstein-Barr virus from immunocompromised and normal hosts. J Infect Dis 1988;157:299-308.

Katz BZ, Raab-Traub N, Miller G. Latent and replicating forms of Epstein-Barr virus DNA in lymphomas and lymphoproliferative diseases. J Infect Dis 1989;160:589-598.

Katz BZ, Salimi B, Kim S, et al. Epstein-Barr virus burden in adolescents with systemic lupus erythematosus. Pediatr Infect Dis J 2001;20:148-153.

Koutras A. Epstein-Barr virus infection with pancreatitis, hepatitis, and proctitis. Pediatr Infect Dis J 1983;2:312-313.

Kuehnle I, Hulls MH, Liu Z, et al: CD20 monoclonal antibody (rituximab) for therapy of Epstein-Barr virus lymphoma after hematopoietic stem-cell transplantation. Blood 2000;95:1502-1505.

Lay J-D, Tsao C-J, Chen J-Y, et al. Upregulation of tumor necrosis factor-alpha gene by Epstein-Barr virus and activation of macrophages in Epstein-Barr virus–infected T cells in the pathogenesis of hemophagocytic syndrome. J Clin Invest 1997;100:1969-1979.

Leder P, Battery J, Lenoir G, et al. Translocations among antibody genes in human cancer. Science 1976;222:765-771.

Lee ES, Locker J, Nalesnik M, et al. The association of Epstein-Barr virus with smooth muscle tumors occurring after organ transplantation. N Engl J Med 1995;332:19-25.

Levene G, Baker H. Drug reactions: ampicillin and infectious mononucleosis. Br J Dermatol 1968;80:417-421.

MacMahon EME, Glass JD, Hayward SD, et al. Epstein-Barr virus in AIDS-related primary central nervous system lymphoma. Lancet 1991;338:969-973.

Martin PJ, Shulman HM, Schubach WH, et al. Fatal EBV-associated proliferation of donor B cells following treatment of acute graft-versus-host-disease with a murine monoclonal anti-T cell antibody. Ann Intern Med 1984;101:310.

Matoba AY. Ocular disease associated with Epstein-Barr virus infection. Arch Ophthalmol 1990;35:145.

Matsuo T, Heller M, Petti L, et al. Persistence of the entire Epstein-Barr virus genome integrated into human lymphocyte DNA. Science 1984;226:1322-1325.

Mayer HB, Wanke CA, Williams M, et al. Epstein-Barr virus-induced infectious mononucleosis is complicated by acute renal failure. Clin Infect Dis 1996;22:1009-1018.

McCarthy JT, Hoagland RJ. Cutaneous manifestations of infectious mononucleosis. JAMA 1964;187:153-154.

McClain KL, Leach CT, Jenson HB, et al. Association of Epstein-Barr virus with leiomyosarcomas in young people with AIDS. N Engl J Med 1995;332:12-18.

McKenzie H, Parratt D, White RO. IgM and IgG antibody levels to ampicillin in patients with infectious mononucleosis. Clin Exp Immunol 1976;26:214-221.

Miller G, Grogan E, Rowe D, et al. Selective lack of antibody to a component of EB nuclear antigen in patients with chronic active Epstein-Barr virus infection. J Infect Dis 1987;156:26-35.

Miller G, Niederman JC, Andrews LL. Prolonged oropharyngeal excretion of Epstein-Barr virus after infectious mononucleosis. N Engl J Med 1973;288:229.

Milne J. Infectious mononucleosis. N Engl J Med 1945;233:727.

Morgan DG, Miller G, Niederman JC, et al. Site of Epstein-Barr virus replication in the oropharynx. Lancet 1979;2:1154-1157.

Mulroy R: Amoxicillin rash in infectious mononucleosis (letter). Br Med J 1973;1:554.

Nazareth I, Mortimer P, McKendrick GD. Ampicillin sensitivity in infectious mononucleosis: temporary or permanent? Scand J Infect Dis 1972;4:229-230.

Niederman JC. Heterophil antibody determination in a series of 166 cases of infectious mononucleosis listed according to various stages of the disease. Yale J Biol Med 1956;28:629.

Niederman JC, Evans AS, Subrahmanyan MS, McCollum RW. Prevalence, incidence, and persistence of EB virus antibody in young adults. N Engl J Med 1970;282:361.

Niederman JC, McCollum RW, Henle G, Henle W. Infectious mononucleosis: clinical manifestations in relation to EB virus antibodies. JAMA 1968;203:205.

Niederman JC, Miller G. Kinetics of the antibody response to BamHI-K nuclear antigen in uncomplicated infectious mononucleosis. J Infect Dis 1986;154:346-349.

Niederman JC, Miller G, Pearson MA, et al. Infectious mononucleosis: Epstein-Barr virus shedding in saliva and oropharynx. N Engl J Med 1976;294:1355.

Nikiforow S, Bottomly K, Miller G. CD4+ T-cell effectors inhibit Epstein-Barr virus induced B-cell proliferation. J Virol 2001;75:3740-3752.

Oertel SH, Ruhnke MS, Anagnostopoulos I, et al. Treatment of Epstein-Barr virus-induced posttransplant lymphoproliferative disorder with foscarnet alone in an adult after simultaneous heart and renal transplantation. Transplantation 1999;67:765-767.

Oertel SHK, Anagnostopoulos I, Bechstein WO, et al. Treatment of posttransplant lymphoproliferative disorder with the anti-CD20 monoclonal antibody rituximab alone in an adult after liver transplantation. Transplantation 2000; 69:430-432.

Okano M, Gross TG. Epstein-Barr virus-associated hemophagocytic syndrome and fatal infectious mononucleosis. Am J Hematol 1996;53:111-115.

Osamah H, Finkelstein R, Brook JG. Rhabdomyolysis complicating acute Epstein-Barr virus infection. Infection 1995;23:119-120.

Pahwa S. Human immunodeficiency virus infection in children: nature of immunodeficiency, clinical spectrum, and management. Pediatr Infect Dis J 1988;7(suppl):61-71.

Pallesen G, Hamilton-Dutoit SJ, Zhou X. The association of Epstein-Barr virus (EBV) with T-cell lymphoproliferations and Hodgkin's disease. Adv Cancer Res 1993;62:179-239.

Patel BM. Skin rash with infectious mononucleosis and ampicillin. Pediatrics 1967;40:910-911.

Pattengale PK, Smith RW, Perlin E. Atypical lymphocytes in acute infectious mononucleosis. Identification by multiple T and B lymphocyte markers. N Engl J Med 1974;291:1145.

Paul JR, Bunnell WW. The presence of heterophile antibodies in infectious mononucleosis. Am J Med Sci 1932;183:90.

Pereira MS, Blake JM, Macrae AD. EB virus antibody at different ages. Br Med J 1969;4:526.

Petrozzi JW. Infectious mononucleosis manifesting as a palmar dermatitis. Arch Dermatol 1971;104:207.

Pfeiffer E. Drüsenfieber. Jahrb Kinderheilkd 1889;29:257.

Pracher E, Panzer-Grumayer ER, Zoubeck A, et al. Successful bone marrow transplantation in a boy with X-linked lymphoproliferative syndrome and acute severe infectious mononucleosis. Bone Marrow Transplant 1994;13:655-658.

Press JH, et al. Infectious mononucleosis: a study of 96 cases. Ann Intern Med 1945;22:546.

Pullen H, Wright N, Murdock, JM. Hypersensitivity reactions to antimicrobial drugs in infectious mononucleosis. Lancet 1967;2:1176.

Purtilo DT. Malignant lymphoproliferative diseases induced by Epstein-Barr virus in immunodeficient patients, including X-linked, cytogenetic, and familial syndromes. Cancer Genet Cytogenet 1981;4:251-268.

Purtilo DT, DeFlorio D, Hutt LM, et al. Variable phenotypic expression of an X-linked recessive lymphoproliferative syndrome. N Engl J Med 1977;297:1077-1081.

Purtilo DT, Sakamoto K, Barnabei V, et al. Epstein-Barr virus–induced diseases in boys with the X-linked lymphoproliferative syndrome (XLP). Am J Med 1982;73:49-56.

Raab-Traub N, Flynn K. The structure of the termini of the Epstein-Barr virus as a marker of clonal cellular proliferation. Cell 1986;47:883-889.

Ralston LS, Saiki AK, Powers WT. Orchitis as a complication of infectious mononucleosis. JAMA 1960;173:1348.

Rapp CE Jr, Hewetson JF. Infectious mononucleosis and the Epstein-Barr virus. Am J Dis Child 1978;132:78.

Ray CG, Gall EP, Minnich LL, et al. Acute polyarthritis associated with active Epstein-Barr virus infection. JAMA 1982; 248:2990-2993.

Resnick L, Herbst JS, Ablashi DV, et al. Regression of oral hairy leukoplakia after orally administered acyclovir therapy. JAMA 1988;259:384-388.

Robinson JE, Brown N, Andiman W, et al. Diffuse polyclonal B-cell lymphoma during primary infection with Epstein-Barr virus. N Engl J Med 1980;302:1293-1297.

Rocchi G, Felici A, Ragona G, Heinz A. Quantitative evaluation of Epstein-Barr virus-infected mononuclear peripheral blood leukocytes in infectious mononucleosis. N Engl J Med 1977;296:132.

Rooney CM, Smith CA, Ng CYC, et al. Use of gene-modified virus-specific T lymphocytes to control Epstein-Barr virus–related lymphoproliferation. Lancet 1995;345:9-13.

Rowe DT, Webber S, Schauer EM, et al. Epstein-Barr virus load monitoring: its role in the prevention and management of post-transplant lymphoproliferative disease. Transpl Infect Dis 2001;3:79-87.

Rubinstein A, Morecki R, Silverman B, et al. Pulmonary disease in children with acquired immune deficiency syndrome and AIDS-related complex. J Pediatr 1986;108: 498-503.

Rutkow IM. Rupture of the spleen in infectious mononucleosis. Arch Surg 1978;113:718.

Sato-Matsumura KC, Matsumura T, Kobayashi H, et al. Marked swollen erythema of the face together with sicca syndrome as a sign for chronic active Epstein-Barr virus infection. Br J Dermatol 2000;143:1351-1353.

Sawyer RN, Evans AS, Niederman JC, McCollum RW. Prospective studies of a group of Yale University freshmen: I. occurrence of infectious mononucleosis. J Infect Dis 1971;123:263.

Sayos J, Wu C, Morra M, et al. The X-linked lymphoproliferative-disease gene product SAP regulates signals induced through the co-receptor SLAM. Nature 1998;395:462-469.

Schooley RT, Carey RW, Miller G, et al. Chronic Epstein-Barr virus infection associated with fever and interstitial pneumonitis. Clinical and serologic features and response to antiviral chemotherapy. Ann Intern Med 1986;636-643.

Schubach WH, Hackman R, Neiman PE, et al. A monoclonal immunoblastic sarcoma in donor cells bearing Epstein-Barr virus genomes following allogeneic marrow grafting for acute lymphoblastic leukemia. Blood 1982;60:180-187.

Seemayer TA, Gross TG, Egeler RM, et al. X-linked lymphoproliferative disease. Pediatr Res 1995;38:471-478.

Sixbey JW, Nedrud JG, Raab-Traub N, et al. Epstein-Barr virus replication in oropharyngeal epithelial cells. N Engl J Med 1984;310:1225-1230.

Slobod KS, Sandlund JT, Spregel PH, et al. Molecular evidence of ocular Epstein-Barr virus infection. Clin Infect Dis 2000;31:184-188.

Sprunt TP, Evans FA. Mononuclear leukocytosis in reaction to acute infections ("infectious mononucleosis"). Bull Johns Hopkins Hosp 1920;31:410.

Stevenson SS, Webster G, Stewart IA. Acute tonsillitis in the management of infectious mononucleosis. J Laryngol Otol 1992;106:989-991.

Strauch B, Siegel N, Andrews LL, Miller G. Oropharyngeal excretion of Epstein-Barr virus by renal transplant recipients and other patients treated with immunosuppressive drugs. Lancet 1974;1:234.

Subar M, Neri A, Inghirami G, et al: Frequent c-*myc* oncogene activation and infrequent presence of Epstein-Barr virus genome in AIDS-associated lymphoma. Blood 1988;72:667-671.

Sumaya CV. Primary Epstein-Barr virus infections in children. Pediatrics 1977;59:16.

Svedmyr E, Jondal M. Cytotoxic effector cells specific for B cell lines transformed by EBV are present in patients with infectious mononucleosis. Proc Natl Acad Sci USA 1975;7:1622-1626.

Swinnen LD. Posttransplant lymphoproliferative disorder. Leuk Lymphoma 1992;6:289-297.

Tischendorf P, Shramek GJ, Balagtas RC, et al. Development and persistence of immunity to Epstein-Barr virus in man. J Infect Dis 1970;122:401.

Tosato G, Magrath I, Koski I, et al. Activation of suppressor T cells during Epstein-Barr virus-induced infectious mononucleosis. 1979;301:1133-1137.

Turner AR, MacDonald RN, Cooper BA. Transmission of infectious mononucleosis by transfusion of preillness plasma. Ann Intern Med 1972;77:751-753.

Tynell E, Aurelius E, Brandell A, et al. Acyclovir and prednisilone treatment of acute infectious mononucleosis. J Infect Dis 1996;174:324-331. (Erratum in J Infect Dis 1996;174:678).

van Esser JWJ, Niesters HGM, von der Holt B, et al. Prevention of Epstein-Barr virus-lymphoproliferative disease by molecular monitoring and preemptive rituximab in high-risk patients after allogenic stem cell transplantation. Blood 2002;99:4364-4369.

van Laar JAM, Buysse CMP, Vossen ACTM, et al. Epstein-Barr viral load assessment in immunocompetent patients with fulminant infectious mononucleosis. Arch Int Med 2002;162:937-939.

Waldo RT. Neurologic complications of infectious mononucleosis after steroid therapy. South Med J 1981;74:1159-1160.

White PD, Thomas JM, Amess J, et al. Incidence, risk and prognosis of acute and chronic fatigue syndromes and psychiatric disorders after glandular fever. Br J Psychiatry 1998;173:475-481.

White PD, Thomas JM, Kangro HO, et al. Predictions and associations of fatigue syndromes and mood disorders that occur after infectious mononucleosis. Lancet 2001;358:1946-1954.

Wolf H, Haus M, Wilmes E. Persistence of Epstein-Barr virus in the parotid gland. J Virol 1984;51: 795-798.

Wolnisty C. Orchitis as a complication of infectious mononucleosis: report of a case. N Engl J Med 1962;266:88.

Yao QY, Rickinson AB, Epstein MA. A reexamination of the Epstein-Barr virus carrier state in healthy seropositive individuals. Int J Cancer 1985;35:35-42.

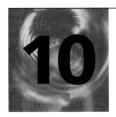

EYE INFECTIONS

GONZALO VICENTE AND BARRETT KATZ

The spectrum of clinical abnormalities of the child's eye is different than that of the adult eye. The child's eye is subject to the same infectious processes as the adult's, but it also is subject to unique events that can unfold into ocular disease. Whether contracted in utero because of maternal infection or via exposure to infectious agents transmitted through the placenta or present in the birth canal or elsewhere, pediatric infectious diseases are ubiquitous and problematic. This chapter presents an overview of the ways in which the child's eye and periorbital tissue react to more common infectious agents. Because almost any tissue type within, around, and behind the eye can be a site for infectious disease, the information presented here is organized by site of infection. Although infectious processes are not neatly compartmentalized, this organizational framework allows the clinician to begin to appreciate the range of infectious processes that can affect the visual system and its anatomic neighbors during the pediatric years. The descriptions begin with disorders affecting the most anterior anatomic structures and progress to structures located posteriorly (i.e., they start with the lids and end with the retina).

EXTERNAL EYE DISEASES
Preseptal Cellulitis

Cellulitis is an infection of the dermis and underlying tissue; when it occurs in tissue surrounding the orbit and eye, it becomes problematic for the eye itself. Cellulitis of the lids generally occurs with a localized infection of the lid, with associated trauma, or in association with an upper respiratory infection. The lid is commonly swollen and erythematous. Septal and preseptal cellulitis should be clinically differentiated, because their prognosis and treatments may differ. Also referred to as *periorbital cellulitis*, preseptal cellulitis affects the lid only anterior to the orbital septum, a fibrous structure that extends from the bony rim and inserts on the tarsal plate. This structure serves to limit the spread of microbes from progressing posteriorly and generally prevents a preseptal process from progressing to orbital involvement. Vision, pupils, and eye motility are expected to be normal. Localized unilateral edema of the eyelid and periorbital tissues is the hallmark of this process. When the process occurs anterior to the septum, there is no proptosis. Fever, pain, tenderness, discharge, and edema may be present. The extent of the erythema is a useful measure for following the clinical course of the disease. Warm compresses will help mobilize the subcutaneous fluid. Administration of an antibiotic ointment and oral antibiotics for 10 days is generally useful. Hospitalization for intravenous administration of antibiotics should be considered in the following situations:

- The patient is in a toxic state or is under the age of 5 years.
- Poor compliance with a regimen of oral antibiotics is expected.
- There has been no improvement after 2 days of oral antibiotic administration.
- Infection with *Haemophilus influenzae* is suspected (skin will have a purplish hue), and the patient is therefore at higher risk for secondary meningitis.

Preseptal Cellulitis Secondary to Penetrating Trauma

The history and examination of the patient will reveal the nature of the sustained trauma. Commonly, defined borders and a tender subcutaneous plaque mark the extent of localized infection. A likely causative agent is *Streptococcus erysipelatis*, a β-hemolytic streptococcus. Again, warm compresses, antibiotic ointment, and oral antibiotics with gram-positive coverage are the mainstays of therapy. A tetanus booster should be considered if penetrating trauma has occurred in an area endemic for tetanus.

Necrotizing Fasciitis

Necrotizing fasciitis is unique among the localized lid infections. It is characterized by a thrombosing infection that extends rapidly along the subcutaneous avascular tissue planes. It has been referred to as *flesh-eating disease* and may lead to toxic shock syndrome, with mortality rates reaching 30%. Even with prompt treatment, necrotizing fasciitis may lead to eschar formation during the fifth to seventh days of healing. These scars often will require correction through plastic surgery of the eyelids. Signs and symptoms include local numbness, disproportionate pain, a rose to blue-gray discoloration, and possibly bullae, necrosis, and eschar formation. *Streptococcus pyogenes* is the inciting organism in older children, whereas in newborns it is *Staphylococcus aureus*. Prompt recognition and administration of intravenous antibiotics are essential. If the infection continues to spread despite the use of intravenous antibiotics for 24 hours, then surgical débridement must be considered (Marshal et al., 1997). When an eschar is present or a focal necrotizing reaction is observed, the bite of an insect such as a brown recluse (*Loxosceles reclusa*) or black widow (*Latrodectus mactans)* spider should be considered (Seal et al., 1998).

Impetigo

Impetigo is a superficial bacterial infection of the epidermis commonly seen in children less than 6 years of age. Poor hygiene may be a risk factor. The infection is thought to have a contagious element. Commonly, red maculae develop and aggregate into vesicles that crust over as they age. Impetigo may spread centripetally; satellite lesions with a clear center can be observed. Etiologic agents include *S. aureus* and β-hemolytic *S. pyogenes*. Administration of bacitracin ointment or oral antibiotics such as dicloxacillin is instituted, along with efforts to keep adjacent tissues clean. Improved hygiene limits spread to other patients.

Herpetic Preseptal Cellulitis

Cellulitis can have a viral origin. The virus group most commonly responsible for cellulitis is the herpesvirus family. Viral cellulitis can occur as a primary or a recurrent infection. (See the discussion of herpetic keratitis later in this chapter.)

The hallmark of viral cellulitis is the presence of telltale vesicular changes typical of viral exanthems. Topical antiviral agents are often used, and topical antibiotic ointments are applied as prophylaxis against secondary infection.

Noninfectious Causes of Preseptal Cellulitis

Preseptal cellulitis also can be caused by blepharochalasis, a recurrent inflammation of the lids seen mostly in young females; by an insect bite; by angioedema; or by lid inflammation secondary to a corneal abrasion, ulcer, or conjunctivitis secondary to allergies or adenovirus. Lid swelling may be seen as a manifestation of adjacent viral conjunctivitis in young children. A membrane is commonly present in such an aggressive conjunctivitis, and, when present, can help differentiate this condition (Ruttum et al., 1996).

Hordeolum

An *internal* hordeolum (chalazion) is a lipogranuloma of the meibomian gland within the tarsal plate. It usually results from an obstruction of the gland duct and is recognized as a localized area of induration on the lid, removed from the lid margin (Plates 2-4). An external hordeolum (stye) is a pyogenic infection of the ciliary follicle at the lid margin, associated with inflammation of the glands of Zeis or Moll (Plate 5). An *external* hordeolum can drain or point anteriorly through the skin. Both of the above may be referred to as *sties*. The differentiation is not critical, because treatment is the same in both cases. Hordeolum can become a more chronic process and evolve into pyogenic granuloma. A more rapidly growing granulomatous process may be seen following surgery or trauma (Plate 6). When such a focal area of edema occurs within the plastic period of the central nervous system (CNS), the child is at risk for amblyopia if the lesion occludes the visual angle. Amblyopia becomes a possible complication if the swollen lid blocks visual input or compresses the eye, causing irregular astigmatism. Warm compresses three times a day for 2 weeks generally alleviate the signs and symptoms of hordeola. Antibiotic ointments may be used; their inclusion is controversial, but they may decrease the bacterial load of surrounding tissue. Incision and drainage may be needed if there is no resolution after the above treatment regimen has been followed. Focal injections of long-acting steroids have also been employed to shrink these lesions before resorting to surgical excision. Hordeolum are benign and usually self-limited. The associated infection rarely spreads beyond the lid.

Dacryoadenitis

Dacryoadenitis is an inflammation of the lacrimal gland. The inflamed lacrimal gland deforms the upper lid into a characteristic S shape. Local erythema is common, as are pain and induration. Dacryoadenitis can be caused by the following:

- Infection with Epstein-Barr virus (EBV)
- Mumps
- *S. aureus* infection
- *Streptococcus pneumoniae* infection
- Brucellosis
- Tuberculosis (TB) (Wright, 1995; Anonymous, 1999-2000; Rhem et al., 2000; Madhukar et al., 1991; Bekir et al., 2000)

Therapy for dacryoadenitis varies according to the cause. In cases of acute dacryoadenitis due to EBV, administration of systemic steroids improves recovery (Aburn et al., 1996).

Dacryocystitis

Dacryocystitis is an inflammation of the lacrimal duct or its sac. It is usually associated with a nonpatent or obstructed lacrimal sac or a ruptured dacryocystocele that occludes tear drainage. Obstructed lacrimal sacs are common in infants and usually resolve by 9 to 12 months of age. However, recurrent infections may warrant earlier intervention. Signs and symptoms may include epiphora (tearing), chronic conjunctivitis, swelling, tenderness, and erythema localized to the medial canthal area overlying the lacrimal sac. Discharge may be expressed through puncta at the medial lid margin. Noninvasive neuroimaging can be helpful in recognizing a mass that obstructs tear drainage and serves to differentiate a dacryocystocele from an inferior encephalocele.

Treatment for dacryocystitis. For chronic dacryocystitis, nasolacrimal duct (NLD) probing is performed on an outpatient basis. The timing of such probing and whether sedation should be used are subjects of continuing controversy. Topical antibiotics are often applied if the dacryocystitis is judged to be severe.

For acute dacryocystitis, treatment varies with setting and age of the patient. For neonates, treatment involves NLD probing and nasal endoscopy for excision of the intranasal cyst. If the dacryocystitis is associated with preseptal cellulitis, treatment includes NLD probing and administration of oral antibiotics. If the condition is associated with an orbital abscess, inferior orbitotomy is required to drain the abscess, along with NLD probing and stent placement. Finally, if the dacryocystitis follows facial trauma treatment includes dacrocystorhinostomy with stent placement (Campolattaro et al., 1997).

Canaliculitis

The canaliculus is the horizontal, proximal 10-mm portion of the lacrimal drainage system that connects the punctum to the lacrimal sac. It, too, may be affected by infectious processes, and it declares its involvement characteristically. Canaliculitis is associated with a gritty feel to the canaliculus on palpation, chronic conjunctivitis, epiphora, and localized swelling of the canaliculus; yellow, grainy discharge from a pouting lower punctum may be seen. New diagnostic techniques include use of 20-MHz ultrasound to image the highly reflective sulfur granules in the canal and to localize the site of obstruction and involvement (Tost et al., 2000). The most common pathogens are *Actinomyces israelii* and *Streptothrix* species. Other pathogens include *Arachnia propionica* and *Fusobacterium* species. Topical antibiotics, such as penicillin, erythromycin, and tetracycline, are commonly prescribed. If antibiotics fail to resolve the condition, surgical removal of canaliculiths and irrigation may become necessary (Weinberg et al., 1977; McKellar, 1997).

Blepharitis

Blepharitis is a chronic inflammation of the eyelid margin. It may have associated folliculitis and inflammation of the underlying hair structures. Blepharitis causes erythema, irritation, and crusting of eyelashes, typically without discharge. The infection may be confined to the lateral canthus, where the upper and lower lids join, and be localized and angular rather than a diffuse marginal process, as is the case with *Moraxella* angular blepharitis (Plate 7).

Blepharitis may be caused by any of the following:

- Viruses—herpes simplex virus (HSV; Plate 8), herpes zoster virus (HZV), human papillomavirus (HPV; blepharitis results from formation of papillomatous lesions
- Bacteria—*S. aureus*, *Propionibacterium acnes*, *Moraxella* species
- Mites—*Demodex folliculorum*
- Lice—*Phthirus pubis*; phthiriasis palpebrarum (crab lice and their products can cause a chronic follicular blepharoconjunctivitis)

P. pubis may be found in the eyelashes because pubic hair has a diameter similar to that of the lashes, and thus the louse can latch onto either.

Noninfectious conditions such as atopy may cause blepharitis in young adults (although atopy is more likely to involve corneal disease). It is important to note that such noninfectious conditions can exist in the presence of concurrent superimposed infections (e.g., *Candida* infection, especially in ulcerative blepharitis). Patients with atopy are also more susceptible to certain bacterial infections, given their defect in cell-mediated immunity and possible IgA antibody, and thus have a predisposition to this chronic lid change (Huber-Spitzy et al., 1992). Therapy consists of improved lid hygiene, warm compresses, and lid scrubs with diluted baby shampoo. Oral tetracyclines have been used in adults, but in children oral erythromycin may be a safer option (Meisler et al., 2000). An ointment of 0.25% physostigmine will inhibit the respiratory enzymes of lice and can be applied topically to treat lice infections.

Molluscum Contagiosum

Molluscum contagiosum is a local infection of the lid caused by a poxvirus. It is spread by direct or indirect contact with this DNA virus. Molluscum contagiosum can lead to chronic conjunctivitis caused by chronic shedding of viral particles. Histopathologic examination of the lesion shows typical eosinophilic intracytoplasmic inclusions (Henderson-Patterson bodies) (Wright, 1995). Molluscum contagiosum is typically present as a small, pale, waxy, umbilicated mass seemingly attached to the lid (Plate 9). There may be numerous lesions, especially in immunodeficient patients. When viral particles are shed onto the conjunctiva, a chronic follicular conjunctivitis results, with punctate epithelial erosions. This infection is self-limited, resolving after months to years. The lid lesion may be treated by excising, freezing, or curetting its central portion.

Kaposi's Sarcoma

Pediatric patients with AIDS can have this superficial tumor involving lid or conjunctival tissue. Children under the age of 5 years may be especially susceptible (Amir, 2001). This tumor is caused by human herpesvirus 8. The lesions begin as focal nontender erythema and progress to darker elevated typical lesions. Localized lid deformities occur and cause entropion (lid margin turned inward) or ectropion (lid margin turned outward). Generally these are managed with observation; consideration is given to resection or more aggressive treatment if the lesion occludes the visual axis and poses a risk for amblyopia. Kaposi's sarcoma is less common since the use of aggressive therapy for human immunodeficiency virus (HIV); the introduction of highly active antiretroviral therapy (HAART) has decreased the incidence as well as the size of lesions. Topical, intralesional, or systemic chemotherapy includes alitretinoin gel, liposomal daunorubicin, liposomal doxorubicin, paclitaxel, and interferon-α, and vinblastine. Cryotherapy and radiation have been used, as well (Dezube, 2000; Shimomura et al., 2000).

ORBITAL CELLULITIS

Orbital cellulitis is uncommon. The condition is more serious than preseptal infections because of the proximity and easy access to venous drainage and the cavernous sinus, and hence the potential for spread to orbital structures and the intracranial space. Orbital cellulitis involves the soft tissues posterior to the orbital septum, which extends from the periosteum of the orbital rim to the tarsal plate. Ethmoidal sinusitis is an overwhelming etiologic contributor, occurring in perhaps >90% of such cases. Also, because the sinuses develop over time, orbital sinusitis is a disease that affects children over the age of 5 years. When it occurs, orbital cellulitis can extend through the very thin lamina papyracea. In the preantibiotic era, such infections commonly caused death as a result of intracranial extension and complications. Although underlying sinusitis is the most common cause of orbital infections in the pediatric population, other causes include extension of infections or injuries in the dental or eyelid areas and hematogenous spread. Lid edema is common. Such edema may have a purplish discoloration in cases caused by *H. influenzae* infection. The erythema may extend only to the bony rim of the orbit, where the septum originates. The eye itself may be proptotic, causing corneal exposure because of poor lid closing; the conjunctiva may be injected and swollen; ocular motility may be restricted, and all fields of gaze may be associated with pain. Vision may be affected, and a relative pupillary afferent defect can be present when the optic nerve and its fibers are involved, compressed, or rendered ischemic. Orbital cellulitis is the most common cause of proptosis in children. Other, less common causes include capillary hemangioma, retrobulbar hemorrhage, emphysema following trauma, thyroid disease, gliomas, rhabdomyosarcoma, neuroblastoma, and metastasis (Sindhu et al., 1998). The most typical presentation of orbital cellulitis is lid swelling seen in isolation; diagnosis is made by exclusion (Uzcategui et al., 1998).

A worrisome complication of orbital cellulitis is cavernous sinus thrombosis. Venous blood may drain out of the orbit anteriorly through the external facial artery, or posteriorly, and thus carry pathogens to the cavernous sinuses and intracranial structures. Because several cranial nerves course through the cavernous sinus, this condition may then cause a cranial neuropathy localized to nerves III, IV, V1, V2, and VI. The motility problems may be out of proportion to the degree of proptosis seen. Conjunctival and ocular vessels may appear congested, because of obstruction of venous spaces and impeded venous return. Pain and tenderness may be present or absent. Since bilateral orbital cellulitis is extremely rare, bilateral cranial nerve involvement should raise the suspicion of a process within each cavernous sinus, as they are anatomically connected (Taylor, 1997).

Bacterial Orbital Cellulitis

H. influenzae used to be the most common pathogen prior to the use of *H. influenzae* vaccines. *H. influenzae* infection still occurs in children, especially in those who have not been vaccinated (Ambati et al., 2000; Donahue et al., 1998). However, the most common pathogens of orbital cellulitis now are members of the *Streptococcus* species, although inciting

pathogens vary with age and immune status of the patient, as shown below:

- Neonates: *S. aureus* and gram-negative bacilli
- Age 6 months to 5 years: *S. pneumoniae* and *H. influenzae*
- Older than 5 years: *S. aureus*, *S. pyogenes*, and *S. pneumoniae*
- Immunocompromised patients: gram-negative organisms (Taylor, 1997).

Overall, children under the age of 9 years will have only one aerobic pathogen. Older children may have multiple, complex infections. Posttraumatic orbital cellulitis patients have a higher incidence of anaerobic gas-forming pathogens such as *Clostridium perfringens*. Evaluation of the patient with orbital cellulitis includes blood cultures, complete blood count (CBC) with differential count, and orbital scanning (coronal and axial) with and without contrast to search for abscesses, sinus involvement, muscle inflammation, and foreign bodies. Conjunctival swab cultures have not been shown to be useful. If no meningitic signs are present a lumbar puncture for cerebrospinal fluid (CSF) cultures may not be useful (Ciarallo et al., 1993). If optic nerve function is compromised, surgical drainage is urgently required. The treatment for orbital cellulitis with or without an abscess consists of hospitalization for systemic antibiotics, with daily reevaluation of vision, motility, proptosis, and possible corneal exposure due to incomplete lid closure. The presence or absence of a relative afferent defect should be monitored to gauge optic nerve involvement, and intraocular pressure should be measured to gauge expansion. Nasal decongestants are helpful if there is an associated sinusitis. If any of the above signs or symptoms worsen or fail to improve after 48 hours, then surgical therapy should be considered. Reimaging to look for developing abscesses may be necessary (Rubin et al., 1989; Souliere et al., 1990).

Other processes to consider include orbital pseudotumor or fungal infection. If the patient continues to improve during a 7-day course of intravenous antibiotics, the patient may be discharged and switched to oral antibiotics for 10 additional days, with frequent follow-up visits. Consultations with specialists in otorhinolaryngology, ophthalmology, and neurology are often required and make for a combined evaluation that addresses the underlying infection, its cause, and its most important sequelae.

Fungal Orbital Cellulitis

When immunocompromised patients or those having poorly controlled diabetes with a history of diabetic ketoacidosis present with lid or orbit inflammation, the diagnosis of an underlying fungal infection (most commonly mucormycosis) is presumed until another diagnosis proves to be correct. Because fungal orbital processes can lead to rapid development of blindness and death by rapid intracranial extension and ischemic necrosis, a fungal process must be considered early in patients with diabetes with a seemingly orbital infection. Urgent surgical débridement of infected or necrotic tissue is often considered, as intravenous amphotericin is begun. Also, control of predisposing factors and correction of metabolic problems becomes imperative (Taylor, 1997).

Parasitic Orbital Cellulitis

Parasites also may occasionally cause orbital infections. Causes of parasitic orbital inflammation include hydatid cyst (dog tapeworm [*Echinococcus granulosus*]; Seal et al., 1998) and cysticercosis. Cysticercosis is infection with a cestode (*Taenia solium*) that may be acquired by drinking fresh water that contains the organism, or by ingesting undercooked, infected pork.

An isolated orbital myositis involving just one extraocular muscle may occur. Weakness of that muscle, deficits of ductions, pain with movement, and conjunctival hyperemia over the affected muscle's insertion can be seen. Extrusion of cysts may cause conjunctival inflammation (Raina, 1996). Treatment includes albendazole 15 mg/kg daily.

Postsurgical Orbital Cellulitis

Orbital cellulitis following strabismus surgery is quite rare, but may occur. Predisposing factors include unsuspected sinusitis, excessive eye rubbing, and poor hygiene. The most common pathogen is *S. aureus*. Clinical signs of postoperative cellulitis include marked swelling and pain, often appearing after a normal initial postoperative follow-up examination. Oral and intravenous antibiotics are employed, with the same caveats and considerations that apply to any orbital cellulitis and its therapy (Kivlin et al., 1995).

Noninfectious Causes of Orbital Cellulitis

Orbital pseudotumor affects the pediatric population. Fully 5% to 15% of all new cases have been reported to occur in children. Orbital pseudotumor is an idiopathic inflammatory condition of orbital tissue characterized by unilateral or bilateral proptosis, fullness, diplopia, lid swelling, and ductional deficits. It may cause pain, taking the form of a myositis that affects only one muscle. The conjunctiva will be inflamed only over the affected muscle, which will have palsy. This condition is extremely responsive to steroids (Mottow et al., 1978; Pollard et al., 1996).

Neoplastic causes of orbital cellulitis include lymphomas, rhabdomyosarcoma, neuroblastoma metastasis, and sphenoidal ridge meningiomas, which can all occur within the periorbita and resemble orbital infections.

CONJUNCTIVITIS

The conjunctiva is a mobile, thin, superficial epithelial layer. It is a mucous membrane. It contains superficial blood vessels. The palpebral portion of the conjunctiva extends from the lid margin to the sulcus or fornix, and its bulbar portion extends from the sulcus to the corneal limbus. Composed of epithelial cells, Langerhans cells, and occasional dendritic melanocytes, the conjunctiva serves as a protective covering for the external ocular surface and blends into the more specialized covering of the cornea. Inflammations of the cornea (called *keratitis*) are separated from those of the conjunctiva (called *conjunctivitis*), although the two conditions often occur simultaneously.

In children, conjunctival inflammation is a nonspecific generic response to a multitude of inciting insults that include infection, foreign bodies, uveitis, and even glaucoma. Most acute conjunctival infections in children are of bacterial origin, often occurring in the winter months; 20% may be of viral origin. Clinically, acute conjunctivitis is differentiated from a more chronic process, as etiologies of and therapies for the two conditions differ. Causes of acute conjunctivitis include the expected disease processes; chronic conjunctivitis can be caused by blepharitis, allergy, folliculosis, chlamydia, or ligneous changes. Although conjunctivitis resulting from all causes is usually self-limited, antibiotics are often employed in both viral and bacterial conjunctivitis, and steroids are considered. However, topical steroids and steroid-antibiotic combinations should not casually be dispensed, as steroids may exacerbate an undiagnosed herpetic infection. It must be remembered, too, that a red injected conjunctiva may be associated with deeper sources of inflammation or disease process, such as iritis, glaucoma, or uveitis (Taylor, 1997).

Bacterial Conjunctivitis

Bacterial conjunctivitis may affect one or both eyes. Presenting symptoms may include red, injected (hyperemic) conjunctiva; discharge may be watery or purulent (Plate 10). Matted eyelids are common. Pseudomembranes may be present; they do not cause bleeding when removed (Plate 11). True membranes occur, as well; these are fibrin coagulated exudates attached to inflamed conjunctiva, which cause bleeding if removed. This differentiation between pseudomembranes and true membranes is not as important as once thought, because both have similar etiologies (i.e., infection with β-hemolytic streptococcus, gonococcus, *Corynebacterium diphtheriae*). *Neisseria gonorrhoeae* is commonly considered first for neonatal conjunctivitities, that is, those occurring within the first month of life. When conjunctivitis occurs within the first 2 days of life, *Neisseria* must be considered. If infection with this organism is suspected, early treatment is imperative to prevent rapid corneal ulceration and penetration. Signs of *Neisseria* conjunctivitis include a hyperacute, purulent, yellow-green discharge (Plate 12).

Pseudomonas aeruginosa conjunctivitis secondary to *Pseudomonas* infection may be seen in premature and low–birth-weight infants. It may or may not be associated with invasive eye disease; however, more serious is the possibility (40%) of developing systemic complications including bacteremia, meningitis, brain abscess, and death (Shah, 1998).

Other bacterial pathogens include *Haemophilus influenzae*, *Borrelia burgdorferi* (the causative agent of Lyme disease), *S. pneumoniae*, *S. aureus*, *Listeria monocytogenes* (associated with farmyard dust, and the causative agent of the condition known as *farmer's eye*) (Seal et al., 1998), and *C. diphtheriae* (associated with pseudomembranes). The antibiotic treatment is entirely dependent on the suspected causative agent and its presumed sensitivities. Topical therapy often suffices, but systemic therapy must included for the more aggressive organisms (e.g., *Neisseria*, *Pseudomonas*). For hyperacute infections, eye lavages and intravenous antibiotics are employed (Taylor, 1997; Gross, 1997).

Chlamydia Infection

Chlamydia infections may be the leading cause of preventable infectious blindness in the world. Chlamydia is an obligate intracellular parasite, because of its lack of respiratory enzymes. Intracytoplasmic inclusion bodies are visible within infected tissue when viewed by light microscopy, and will fluoresce under ultraviolet light. When chlamydia infection affects the eye, its active inflammatory and scarring stage begins in the preschool age. Blindness occurs after age of 40, secondary to repeated childhood and adult bacterial infections and associated recurrent trauma. The cornea becomes opaque from lid-induced trauma, secondary to trichiasis and conjunctival scarring. Risk factors for the spread and persistence of chlamydia infection include poor facial hygiene, living environment that is endemic for the infection, presence of trachoma in siblings, and familial cattle ownership (West et al., 1996).

Serotypes A, B, Ba, and C are transmitted by black flies and are associated with trachoma. Serotypes D through K cause a keratoconjunctivitis also known as *trachoma inclusion conjunctivitis* or *adult chlamydial ophthalmia*. The former is seen in infants at birth; the latter is usually seen in young adults. Chlamydial ophthalmia may be sexually transmitted or passed along through fomites such as towels at swimming pools. Associated signs include urethritis. Types A through K can cause neonatal pneumonia, as well. Subtype L causes lymphogranuloma venereum, a supportive inguinal adenitis.

Presenting symptoms of acute chlamydial bacterial conjunctival infections may include irritation, ocular discharge, and redness. These infections can be bilateral or unilateral. Inferior palpebral follicles and large superior tarsal follicles can lead to Arlt's line, a diagnostic clue when seen as a longitudinal linear scarring of the conjunctiva (Plate 13). Limbal infiltrates of the cornea (Plate 14, *A*) then unfold into Herbert's pits (Plate 14, *B*), seen at the superior limbus, another characteristic sign that suggests chlamydia infection. These must be differentiated from those limbal infiltrates seen in staphylococcal hypersensitivity that are usually but not always located along the inferior corneal limbus. In the late chronic stages of chlamydia infection, the conjunctival scarring can cause inward rotation of the lid (entropion) and lash line (trichiasis) leading to recurrent corneal abrasions, infection, thinning, and scarring and result in blindness (Plate 15). A mild preauricular adenopathy (PAN) may also be present (Huber-Spitzy et al., 1992). Therapy includes prophylaxis (facial hygiene, available clean water); acute infections are treated with oral and topical antibiotics, over months. For chronic sequelae, corrective lid surgery to repair trichiasis may be necessary (Tadtara, 2001).

Viral Conjunctivitis

Epidemic keratoconjunctivitis. Epidemic keratoconjunctivitis is an adenoviral infection that is not uncommon and is extremely contagious. It usually occurs bilaterally, with one eye becoming affected first, followed by involvement of the second eye within 48 hours. It is associated with lid swelling; the bulbar conjunctivae are dramatically edematous. The patient complains of photophobia. The infection is most contagious within the first 7 days. The virulence of the organism upon ocular tissue can lead to permanent corneal, conjunctival, and punctal scarring. Peak symptoms occur days 5 to 7 after exposure. Viral conjunctivitis is often associated with a preceding upper respiratory tract infection. This virus may cause significant bilateral or unilateral lid swelling and mimic a cellulitis, especially in patients under 2 years of age. Though watery mucous discharge is common, purulent discharge may be seen. The following are associated with epidemic keratoconjunctivitis: foreign body sensation, PAN, photophobia, conjunctival membrane formation, conjunctival injection, subconjunctival hemorrhages, and conjunctival follicles (Plate 16). Infants, however, cannot form follicles, so when viral conjunctivitis occurs in an infant population it is nonfollicular. The cornea may initially show a diffuse epithelial keratitis that develops into subepithelial opacities in the 2 weeks following infection. Chronic infection is rare, but it may lead to the formation of symblepharon and tear drain obstruction, especially if membranes are present. The usual causative organisms are adenovirus types 8, 11, and 19.

Therapy is merely supportive—artificial tears, cool compresses, and transmission prevention. As with many virus infections, this is self-limited. If corneal opacities or blurred vision persist, steroids are sometimes employed. Topical steroids are safe only in the presence of the following:

- A membrane or pseudomembranes
- Marked foreign body sensation or chemosis
- Decreased visual acuity secondary to epithelial keratitis.

Differentiating adenoviral conjunctivitis from a herpetic infection has clinical import, as steroids will cause a significant worsening of a herpetic keratitis. Herpetic disease usually is unilateral, may involve skin vesicles and corneal dendrites, and does not occur as an epidemic. Topical interferon has not been shown to be effective in minimizing symptoms in the infected eye; however, it may decrease symptomatic infection of the other eye (Adams, 1984).

Pharyngeal conjunctival fever. This variant viral infection is known as *swimming pool conjunctivitis*. It is self-limiting with no permanent sequelae. Presenting symptoms include a nonpurulent follicular conjunctivitis, pharyngitis, fever, diarrhea, rash, and lymphadenopathy. The causative organism is adenovirus type 3 or 7. Therapy is merely supportive—artificial tears, cool compresses, and transmission prevention. As with most viral infections, it is self-limited, with resolution occurring in 2 to 3 weeks.

Hemorrhagic conjunctivitis. Hemorrhagic conjunctivitis is composed of a subset of presumedly viral infections that lead to subconjunctival hemorrhages (Plate 17). It derives its name from the often-dramatic hemorrhagic changes that occur within the conjunctivae. It is extremely contagious and may have associated punctate epithelial keratitis. The causative agents are picornaviruses (enterovirus 70 or coxsackievirus A24). Again, therapy is palliative; the condition is self-limited, with an average duration of about 10 days.

Human papilloma virus. HPV may affect periorbital tissue and generate a fleshy, vascular, often pedunculated growth arising from the conjunctiva. Pathogens include subtypes 6 and 11, which cause pedunculated papillomas, and subtypes 16 and 18, which cause sessile lesions. Many of these lesions have spontaneous remission, but others are chronic. Surgery is generally the mainstay of treatment. There is a high recurrence rate after excision; other methods include diathermy and cryotherapy. Orally administered

H$_2$ receptor blockers such as cimetidine work as a suppressor T-cell inhibitor and have shown potential in dermatology and in the conjunctiva to eliminate or reduce the papillomas.

Herpes simplex blepharoconjunctivitis. A primary herpes simplex infection can cause blepharoconjunctivitis (lid and conjunctiva); corneal disease will occur perhaps 67% of the time. It is thought that a dormant infection is established and can reactivate from within the trigeminal ganglion with clinical effects that are expressed along any branch of the fifth cranial nerve. The diagnosis of herpetic disease is based on clinical findings. Additional laboratory tests may include Giemsa staining of conjunctival scraping (showing multinucleated cells) or Papanicolaou staining (showing intranuclear eosinophilic inclusion bodies). Vesicular rash in the surrounding periorbital area may be present. It is the corneal involvement and its characteristic dendritic lesions with bulbar ends that become pathognomonic. Newborns with type 2 HSV infection can develop fatal encephalitis. HSV type 1 is seen above the umbilicus, and type 2 below; type 1 occurs in children, and type 2 in newborns, where it has a vertical transmission from the mother's birth canal.

Topical antiviral agents are employed, often for several weeks, until signs improve. Topical antibiotic ointment is also used on the skin lesions, presumably to prevent superinfection. Warm soaks to the affected skin become symptomatically effective.

Herpes zoster conjunctivitis. Zoster conjunctivitis is more rare in children than adults, although it can follow a more systemic infection or autoinoculation from skin lesions. Therapy includes steroids drops and systemic acyclovir.

Varicella (chicken pox) conjunctivitis. Vesicles, ulcerations, and internal ophthalmoplegia are the hallmark of varicella conjunctivitis. Acyclovir is commonly used; also, erythromycin ointment is applied to the skin vesicles to prevent secondary bacterial infection.

Newcastle disease virus. Newcastle disease virus is usually seen in those exposed to chickens or in those who handle them. It causes a nonspecific follicular conjunctivitis. This conjunctivitis is self-limited, lasting 7 to 10 days. Artificial tears and cool compresses may alleviate symptoms.

Molluscum contagiosum. Molluscum contagiosum is caused by a poxvirus and can result in a chronic conjunctivitis due to shedding of viral particles from an umbilicated wartlike lesion on the lid directly into the bulbar conjunctivae. Infected cells will have eosinophilic inclusion bodies, visible histologically. This infection itself is self-limited, resolving after months to years. The lid lesion, however, may be treated by excising, freezing, or curetting its central portion.

Less common causes of viral conjunctivitis. The following diseases also can cause viral conjunctivitis:
• Infectious mononucleosis (EBV)
• Influenza
• Measles
• Mumps
• Rubella

Parinaud's oculoglandular syndrome. Parinaud's oculoglandular syndrome is a unilateral, usually self-limited conjunctivitis associated with a focal nodule of the tarsal plate characterized by swelling and perhaps ptosis. This may be associated with regional lymphadenopathy and a characteristic neuroretinitis. Clinical signs and symptoms develop 7 to 14 days after exposure to a specific antigen. The syndrome is associated with severe preauricular adenopathy, unilateral conjunctival granulomas, large follicles, photophobia, foreign body sensation, conjunctival swelling, and external signs of inflammation. Systemic symptoms include fever, chills, general malaise, anorexia, and lymphadenitis (Plate 18). Possible causes of oculoglandular fever include the following:
• Cat-scratch disease (*Bartonella henselae* infection)
• *Francisella tularensis* infection
• Infectious mononucleosis (Mumps)
• TB
• *Yersinia pseudotuberculosis* infection
• *Mycobacterium leprae* infection
• Infection with *Treponema pallidum* (causative agent of syphilis)
• Lymphogranuloma venereum (chlamydia)
• Coccidioidomycosis
• Chancroid

Most infections are self-limited, without permanent sequelae. Antibiotics specific to each causative agent may be used, although the effects of treatment on eye changes are unproved. Some, but not all, studies recommend the removal of conjunctival granulomas to accelerate resolution (Conrad, 2001; Rhee, 1999; Carithers, 1985).

Fungal Conjunctivitis

Fungal infections of the conjunctival tissue in childhood are extremely rare; however, an adjunctive conjunctivitis may be present with a fungal keratitis.

Parasitic Conjunctivitis

Leeches must be considered in a child with a history of fresh water swimming or in the differential diagnosis of iris prolapse (Alcelik, 1997). Leishmaniasis, resulting from the bite of the sand fly vector, causes eyelid ulcer, blepharitis, granulomatous conjunctivitis, uveitis, and subcutaneous lymphangitis (Zijlstra et al., 2001). Loiasis (African eye worm), caused by *Loa loa* (a subcutaneous or subconjunctival migrating nematode that enters the host through the bite of a *Chrysops* or mango fly), has been reported to affect conjunctival tissue. Fly larvae that inhabit the nostrils of sheep can invade human tissues. Infections with *Thelazia* capillaris and *T. californiensis* (associated with birds) are seen in the Middle East and California (Seal et al., 1998). Fly larvae may be removed if visible after application of topical anesthetic. Therapy is directed at the removal of worm, and diethylcarbamazine may be used (Johnson et al., 1993). Steroids may alleviate inflammation.

Phlyctenular Conjunctivitis

Phlyctenular keratoconjunctivitis is characterized by a yellowish-white nodule seen within a focal area of inflamed conjunctival tissue. Its hallmark is a discrete, raised, irritating, unilateral phlyctenule lesion with surrounding hyperemia (Plate 19). Many cases are presumed to be bacterial in origin; causes include infection with *S. aureus*, adenovirus, or herpes virus, candidiasis, and lymphogranuloma venereum. TB can be a causative agent, especially in malnourished children aged 5 to 10 years. For nontuberculous phlyctenular conjunctivitis, topical antibiotics and artificial tears are employed. It is usually self-limited and resolves without sequelae, although corneal scarring is possible with aggressive limbal infections. If TB is suspected, then systemic therapy is warranted.

Noninfectious Causes of Conjunctivitis

Allergy. Conjunctivitis due to allergy is often associated with itching rather than irrita-tion. Affected children often blink constantly or rub their eyes. Lids may be thickened, as well as darkened. The conjunctiva may appear milky or pale; conjunctivitis due to allergy is associated with watery or mucoid discharge and pseudomembranes. Superior palpebral conjunctival papillae can be present (Plate 20). The condition may be vernal, or seasonal, with giant papillae and thick, ropy, dirty white discharge.

Chemicals. External irritants are a common source of conjunctivitis seen in childhood. Overchlorinated pool water, irritation from hair sprays, mace, rebound conjunctival injection due to chronic use of topical decongestant, vasoconstricting over-the-counter medication, and preservatives such as thimerosal or benzalkonium chloride (used in eye drops) can all cause dramatic conjunctival changes (Soparkar, 1997).

Contact lenses. Inflammation of the conjunctiva may occur in contact lens wearers, with formation of large papillae in upper palpebral conjunctiva. This is referred to as *giant papillary conjunctivitis.*

Reiter's syndrome. Reiter's syndrome is an immunologically based clinical triad of iritis, urethritis, and seronegative lower extremity arthritis; it can be seen with an associated conjunctivitis and punctate subepithelial keratitis.

Stevens-Johnson syndrome (erythema multiforme major). This is an acute systemic disorder that has both skin and mucous membrane signs and symptoms. Common causes are infections and medicines, which presumably trigger an acute hypersensitivity reaction. Patients may have a membranous or pseudomembranous conjunctivitis. This may lead to a secondary infection by *S. aureus,* scarring of the conjunctival fornices (symblepharon), destruction of the mucin-producing conjunctival cells leading to chronic dry eyes, and corneal scarring. Changes can be dramatic and may include a bilateral desquamative conjunctivitis with areas of focal necrosis.

Kawasaki disease. Kawasaki disease is a mucocutaneous lymph node process, presumably a systemic vasculitis of unknown (though possibly viral) etiology. It is associated with the characteristic conjunctival changes of bilateral hyperemia and hemorrhagic conjunctivitis seen without discharge, following a fever. Affected patients may have bilateral conjunctival injection before systemic signs and symptoms. Many patients also have an acute anterior uveitis. An infectious etiology is highly likely but has not been isolated.

Ligneous Conjunctivitis

Ligneous conjunctivitis is a disorder of the pediatric age group that begins with redness and watering of the eyes. An acute conjunctivitis follows. It is an idiopathic disorder associated with fibrinous "wood-like" plaques seen overlying conjunctival tissue.

Ophthalmia nodosa. This focal conjunctival granuloma is caused by the hairs of caterpillars or arachnids.

Mechanical irritation and exposure. Any insult to adjacent tissues can cause an inciting conjunctival inflammation, from ectropion to floppy eyelid syndrome.

Atopic keratoconjunctivitis. Atopy commonly has ocular involvement; up to 42% of patients with atopic dermatitis have ocular signs and symptoms. This includes blepharoconjunctivitis, keratoconjunctivitis, and cataracts. Altered immunity makes these patients more susceptible to herpes simplex keratitis and *Staphylococcus* blepharitis. Conjunctival and corneal scarring may occur (Garrity et al., 1984).

NEONATAL CONJUNCTIVITIS

Purulent conjunctival discharge within the first 28 days of life indicates neonatal infection. Ophthalmia neonatorum is seen less frequently since the advent of prophylactic use of silver nitrate 1%. Known as Credé's method, it does not protect against viral or chlamydial infections. Because this agent can cause chemical conjunctivitis, erythromycin ointment has also been tried as a prophylactic agent but may not work as well as silver nitrate. Some studies suggest no difference among silver nitrate, erythromycin, and tetracycline ointment in the prophylactic treatment for chlamydial or gonococcal conjunctivitis. Use of povidone-iodine solutions may increase, because they are microbicidal for bacteria, fungi, viruses, and protozoa. Good prenatal screening and treatment of the mother offers the best prophylaxis for the neonate (Zanoni et al., 1992; Hammerschlag et al., 1989; Benevento et al., 1990; Wutzler et al., 2000). Culture is imperative for proper etiologic identification.

Gonococcal Neonatal Conjunctivitis

Gonococcal conjunctivitis is a sight-threatening infection when it occurs in the neonatal period,

because this gram-negative intracellular diplococci can easily penetrate the cornea. Onset is generally between 2 and 5 days after birth. A very purulent discharge is the sine qua non of this entity (see Plate 12). Corneal ulceration may occur within hours. Diagnosis is made as the organism grows out on chocolate media cultures. Systemic therapy is imperative. Patients are hospitalization and given hourly eyewashes with normal saline until discharge is eliminated. This reduces the bacterial load and forces hourly monitoring of the cornea.

Inclusion Conjunctivitis

Chlamydia trachomatis serotypes D to K are the most common chlamydial pathogens in neonatal conjunctivitis. Onset occurs between fourth and fifteenth days of life. Patients will have a papillary reaction at this age, as infants cannot form follicles. Watery or mucous discharge along with a pseudomembrane may be present (pseudomembranes differ from membranes in that they do not cause bleeding when removed). Therapy includes systemic and topical antibiotics. Most neonatal chlamydial infections are self-limiting, without permanent sequelae, but treatment may lessen the risk of scarring and accelerate healing.

P. Aeruginosa Neonatal Conjunctivitis

Pseudomonas infections are a relatively common cause of conjunctivitis in preterm and low birth weight infants. They can rapidly progress systemically, with or without local invasive eye infection. Bilateral or unilateral purulent conjunctivitis with or without corneal involvement seen a few weeks after birth suggests infection with *Pseudomonas*. Average onset occurs 17 days following birth. Positive bacteremia occurs in approximately one third of cases. Gram-negative rods are seen on staining of corneal scrapings. Ultraviolet light may cause fluorescence of *Pseudomonas* pigment on the cornea (Shah, 1998). Systemic and topical antibiotics are recommended as soon as cultures are taken. Other bacterial causative agents include *S. aureus* (onset 5 days), *Streptococcus* species, and *Haemophilus aegyptius* (onset >5 days).

Herpetic Neonatal Conjunctivitis

When seen in neonates, herpetic conjunctivitis is likely to result from infection with HSV type 2. Its onset generally is 3 to 15 days after birth.

This infection is seen with vesicular blepharitis, conjunctivitis, and, more rarely, corneal involvement. The maternal history of previous genital herpes is expected. In a study of neonatal herpes by Whitley et al., 70% of maternal infections were asymptomatic. If infection with HSV type 2 is suspected, immediate ophthalmic and neurologic consultations are indicated, because HSV type 2 has been associated with chorioretinitis and encephalitis (Whitley et al., 1980). Topical agents for conjunctivitis and keratitis are used in association with systemic agents for intraocular or disseminated disease (Nelson, 1998).

Noninfectious Chemical Neonatal Conjunctivitis

A chemically induced conjunctival inflammation can occur with the use of silver nitrate drops, which are applied prophylactically at birth. Onset usually occurs in the first day of life. Mild conjunctivitis is the rule, with some watery discharge. It does not become purulent and is self-limited, resolving after a few days. Therapy consists of careful observation to distinguish this condition from an infectious one.

CORNEAL INFECTIONS

The cornea is a thin (0.5-mm), transparent, avascular structure that is optically clear; its clarity is essential for sight, and so any infection of this tissue becomes vision threatening. When changed by inflammation, scarring, or perforation, the cornea loses its transparency. Any level of the cornea may be involved in infection—epithelium, stroma, or endothelium. Any inflammation within corneal tissue is considered a keratitis. Typically, corneal infections are associated with an epithelial staining defect and an area of opacity representing an inflammatory infiltrate.

Scrapings from the cornea should be obtained prior to commencing antibiotic treatment for confirmatory diagnosis. For ulcers smaller than 2 mm, proper cultures may be difficult to obtain. Workup for bacterial infections includes chocolate agar cultures from corneal scrapings obtained with a sterile kimura spatula. If the infection is fungal in origin, workup involves Gomori's methenamine silver stain and Sabouraud dextrose agar. For *Acanthamoeba infections,* workup includes Periodic Acid Schiff (PAS) staining, Giemsa or calcofluor white staining, and *Escherichia coli* overlay culture. Workup of viral infection involves viral media, although diagnosis is mostly clinical.

A corneal biopsy may be necessary when patients fail to respond to treatment of presumed herpetic or bacterial disease. Microbiologic evaluation is often more sensitive than histopathologic evaluation (Alexadrakis, 2000).

Bacterial Keratitis

Common risk factors for bacterial keratitis are foreign body exposure, contact lens use, and corneal abrasion (Plate 21). Keratitis is associated with foreign body sensation, pain, photophobia, stromal infiltrates, and overlying epithelial defects that are visible with fluorescein staining. Patients with pneumococcal and *Pseudomonas* infection may have a mucopurulent discharge and hypopyon (a collection of white blood cells in the anterior chamber) (Plate 22, *A*). Well-defined stromal infiltrates are seen with *S. aureus* infections (Plate 22, *B*).

Common bacterial pathogens include *S. pneumoniae, S. aureus, Staphylococcus epidermidis, P. acnes, Serratia* species, *Corynebacterium* species, *P. aeruginosa,* and *Nocardia asteroides.*

Chronic and improper use of contact lenses is associated with increased prevalence of corneal ulcers. Patients who wear contact lenses for prolonged periods of time, especially those who sleep in contact lenses, cause chronic hypoxia to the corneal epithelium, rendering it susceptible to infection. Gram-negative organisms, such as *Pseudomonas* species, are more common causative organisms (Plate 23). Treatment must take into consideration the potential for this causative organism. A contact lens–related ulcer, infection, or abrasion should never be patched, as this might conceal a rapidly worsening *Pseudomonas* ulceration (Liesegang, 1997; Cutter et al., 1996; Schein et al., 1990).

Chlamydial keratitis. Chlamydial keratitis occurs concurrently with superior conjunctival disease. Multiple, small, perilimbic infiltrates are seen, usually in the superior half of the cornea. (See the discussion of chlamydial conjunctivitis.)

Postpenetrating keratoplasty infections. Postpenetrating keratoplasty infections usually begin at the donor-host interface. Predisposing risk factors include immunosuppression, exposed or loose corneal suture, graft failure, persistent epithelial defect, and Stevens-Johnson syndrome (Akova, 1999).

M. Leprae infection (leprosy, or Hansen's disease). Ocular declarations of leprosy may be seen in children, although half the incidences occur in adults (Plates 24 and 25). An association with vitamin A–deficiency keratopathy often complicates this infection (Plate 26). Ocular declarations of leprosy include prominent corneal nerves and a poor blink reflex. Other, less frequently occurring signs include cataracts, uveitis, and decreased corneal sensation. Lagophthalmos (poor lid closure) occurs early in children (Plates 27 and 28). Neurotrophic keratopathy is seen in patients with Hansen's disease. For this reflex to protect and maintain the corneal epithelium, the patient must have good corneal sensation and proper lid closure. Altered corneal sensation leads to a decrease in blinking frequency. Lubrication and tear production are decreased because of poor feedback to the lacrimal gland nerves. Because of a decrease in growth factors from corneal nerves, there may be poor corneal epithelial healing. Poor lid closure causes dryness and exposure, leading to corneal thinning, scarring, and recurrent suprainfection. Therapy is systemic and local and involves surgical correction of lagophthalmos, use of adhesive tape to assist with lid closure, and constant corneal lubrication.

Mycobacterium Tuberculosis keratoconjunctivitis. Mycobacterium infection may be associated with a herpeticlike vesicular rash that does not respond to antiviral agents but may resolve with antituberculosis treatment (Aclimados, 1992).

Keratitis associated with an infected lacrimal sac (dacryocystitis). Keratitis often is seen with infection of the lacrimal sac. It is often monobacterial, most commonly caused by infection with *S. pneumoniae* (Aasuri, 1999). (See discussion of lid infections.)

Syphilitic interstitial keratitis. Keratitis can occur in association with a congenital or acquired infection such as syphilis, and, when it is, it can be associated with an interstitial keratitis characterized by prominent corneal vessels growing within corneal stroma. This type of keratitis usually has neovascularization during its active phase; these blood vessels become ghost vessels when the lesion is inactive. These vessels can bleed and cause an intrastromal hemorrhage. Associated signs include photophobia, redness, pain, corneal edema, decreased corneal sensation, uveitis, and small nummular stromal infiltrates (Azimi, 1999). (See discussion of TORCH syndrome.)

Treatment for bacterial keratitis. Treatment for infection with gram-negative organisms includes fluoroquinolone and erythromycin versus fortified tobramycin-cefazolin drops. If causative organisms are gram positive, aminoglycosides and erythromycin are administered. If the infection is associated with syphilis, treatment includes aqueous penicillin, and possibly steroids, a dilating agent, and corneal transplant for chronic central scars.

Topical scrapings and cultures from the patient with cornea infections are useful before therapy is initiated (Garg, 1999).

Staphylococcus hypersensitivity keratitis. This condition is associated with concurrent bacterial blepharitis. The patient's immune system reacts, with bacterial antigens forming multiple perilimbal white infiltrates, usually along the inferior corneal limbus (where the inferior lid rests). These corneal infiltrates are often close to the sclera, but a clear zone exists between the infiltrates and the limbus (Plate 29). Patients may complain of severe light sensitivity, pain, and foreign body sensation. Therapy consists of good lid hygiene, warm compresses, and administration of erythromycin or bacitracin. Oral erythromycin has been shown to be effective in pediatric patients who are difficult to treat with the above methods. In adults, oral tetracycline is part of the regimen, but because of its dental side effects, it is not recommended in children (Meisler, 2000).

Viral Keratitis

HSV infection. An infection by this virus may result in permanent or recurrent corneal scarring, making it one of the leading indications for corneal transplants in the United States. Type 1 HSV is commonly seen in children, and type 2 in newborns, where it is vertically transmitted via the birth canal. This double-stranded DNA virus is ubiquitous. A dormant infection from within the trigeminal ganglion can recur along any branch of cranial nerve V, no matter which branch had the primary infection. Given the possibility of permanent sequelae, children suspected of having herpetic corneal infection should be referred immediately to an ophthalmologist. Recurrence in the eye is common—up to 18% for epithelial or stromal infections within the following 18 months. The risk of recurrence increases with each subsequent attack, leading to permanent scarring and corneal irregularity. The primary infection may be asymptomatic or may appear as a vesicular rash on the skin after exposure to someone with an active lesion. Other symptoms such as pain, photophobia, and blurred vision may be present. Any corneal layer may be involved at any time.

Some layers of the cornea and adjacent tissues may be preferentially affected.

Epithelial keratitis. Superficial corneal involvement is the most common presentation. Epithelial keratitis can appear as dendrites on the superficial cornea, with raised edges that stains with rose bengal, and terminal bulbs. These may coalesce into a geographic pattern, especially if this condition is confused with an adenovirus infection and treated with topical steroids. Dendrites usually measure 1 to 2 mm or less. They are difficult to see without a slit lamp and fluorescein staining (Plates 30-36).

Stromal keratitis. Deeper infections within the cornea offer a worse prognosis, with a tenfold higher rate of recurrence compared with epithelial infections. Disciform stromal keratitis is a deep annular infiltrate also known as a *Wesley ring*. It is a sign of a delayed hypersensitivity reaction and may lead to limbal vasculitis, which, if severe, may in turn lead to the formation of a dellen (a localized thinning of the cornea). Necrotic stromal keratitis has a cheesy stromal infiltrate. Interstitial keratitis occurs when the corneal infiltrates develop neovascularization and may be caused by an immune complex Ag-Ab hypersensitivity.

Endotheliitis. Endotheliitis is a unique change that occurs when keratitic precipitates are deposited on the endothelial surface, the deepest layer of the cornea in contact with the anterior chamber and its aqueous.

Trabeculitis. Inflammation of the trabecular meshwork, the main aqueous drainage of the eye at the junction of the iris and cornea, may lead to elevated intraocular pressure.

Iridocyclitis. As a stromal keratitis involves the uveal layers of the eye (iris and ciliary body), the aqueous, the anterior chamber, and the cornea share in the inflammatory response.

Multilayered trophic metaherpetic keratitis. A sterile ulcer secondary to poor healing seen as a result of decreased corneal sensation may develop, with persistent epithelial defects.

Given this infection's morbidity, treatment is complicated and lengthy. The Herpetic Eye Disease Study was a large, multicentered, double-masked placebo-controlled randomized clinical trial that evaluated best available treatments for this infection. It showed that oral acyclovir can decrease the incidence of recurrence of stromal and epithelial keratitis from 32% to 19% when compared with placebo. Oral acyclovir does not prevent epithelial disease from becoming the more serious stromal or iris type. The benefit of acyclovir is greatest for patients who have had prior recurrent stromal disease. It is effective for iridocyclitis only when used with steroids (Herpetic Eye Disease Study Group, 2000; Herpetic Eye Disease Study Group, 2001). There is also a role for acyclovir in neonates with widespread herpes simplex and in immunosuppressed children. In one trial, topical steroids decreased the progression and shortened the duration of keratouveitis when used concurrently with topical antiviral agents (Wilhelmus et al., 1994). Débridement of affected epithelial cells does not lead to faster healing when compared with topical antiviral agents (trifluridine, acyclovir, or vidarabine), although there may be a role for using both methods. Faster recovery has been reported when antiviral agents are used in combination with topical interferon (Wilhelmus, 2000). Topical antiviral agents should not be used chronically for more than 2 weeks because they delay epithelial healing. In patients with keratouveitis, topical steroids and dilating drops may be used to alleviate iritis symptoms.

Herpes zoster ophthalmicus. Zoster infections are usually seen after reactivation of the varicella virus and transmission along the ophthalmic branch of the trigeminal nerve. A unilateral vesicular rash following the dermatome of V1 is common. If vesicles are present at the side or tip of the nose (Hutchinson's sign) there is a 50% likelihood of corneal involvement (because it indicates involvement of the nasociliary branch the trigeminal nerve). Corneal pseudodendrites can appear upon the epithelium. Rose bengal stain will show the affected epithelial cells. These dendrites are similar in size to those of HSV but do not have terminal bulbs (Plates 37 and 38) The two most common eye findings in herpes zoster ophthalmicus are anterior uveitis and a nummular keratitis, with granular subepithelial deposits just below

Bowman's layer, seen with a halo of stromal haze. A severe complication may be a corneal neurotrophic ulcer due to poor corneal sensation and loss of corneal reflexes. Corneal disease may cause permanent vision loss. Further visual loss is seen with accompanying optic neuritis, glaucoma, posterior scleritis and orbital apex syndrome, or acute retinal necrosis (ARN). (See the discussions of retinitis and optic neuritis.) In cases with poor corneal sensation, frequent lubrication is essential to prevent ulcer and scar formation. Patching or tarsorrhaphy (suturing lids closed) may be necessary. As always, care should be taken when patching a the eye of a child under the age of 10 years to avoid occlusion amblyopia. Topical antibiotic ointment may be used on the affected skin to prevent secondary bacterial infection. Antiviral agents are commonly employed. Cycloplegic drops can be used to dilate the pupil and alleviate symptoms associated with iritis. Steroids are rarely useful (Harding, 1993).

Adenovirus keratitis. For information regarding adenovirus keratitis, see the discussion of viral conjunctivitis.

EBV keratitis. EBV can cause punctate epithelial lesions, and so on occasion will be associated with a mild nummular keratitis (Plate 39).

Fungal Keratitis

Keratitis caused by fungal antigens must be considered when the patient history includes organic material trauma, extended contact lens wear, or immunosuppression or when ulcers do not respond to antibiotic therapy.

Etiologies include *Aspergillus* species infection (more common in dry climates); *Candida albicans* infection (gray-white infiltrate with sharp borders, occurring typically in a cornea with previous disease); filamentous keratitis (dry raised infiltrate with feathery hyphate edges or a rough texture); and *Fusarium* species infection (more common in humid, tropical climates) (Plate 40).

Therapy includes topical natamycin 2.5%, amphotericin, or, if these are unavailable, chlorhexidine gluconate 0.2%. Oral ketoconazole is often employed as well (Garg, 2000; Rahman, 1998; Rosa, 1994)

Parasitic Keratitis

Acanthamoeba infection is associated with a wet, organic, rural trauma, and contact lens wear. Because chlorine is ineffective against *Acanthamoeba* cysts, the risk of *Acanthamoeba* infection in patients increases if they store or clean their contact lenses in tap water or if they are used in hot tubs or natural springs. These infections are often misdiagnosed, leading to delayed therapy. Diagnosis may, in fact, necessitate a corneal biopsy. Refractile cystic structures visible on microscopic analysis of corneal scrapings are noted with *Acanthamoeba* and seen between the epithelial cells. Rapid diagnosis is now possible with fluorescent antibody staining (Epstein, 1986). This keratitis is associated with severe pain, a foreign body sensation, radial perineuritis, snowstorm infiltrates, ring infiltrates, keratitis punctate, and pseudodendritic ulcers. In addition to antibiotics, corneal transplant may be needed in cases of central scarring; even with successful surgery, there is a risk of recurrence.

ENDOPHTHALMITIS

Endophthalmitis is, by definition, an inflammation that involves all the inner tissues of the eye, that is, the vitreous, retina, and uveal layers. Intraocular infections may emanate from bacteria, fungi, and parasites. Organisms may reach ocular tissue directly, follow surgery, or be seeded from a blood-borne source. Signs of infection within the eye may then manifest throughout multiple layers of the eye, presenting as a hypopyon (see Plate 22).

Endogenous Endophthalmitis

Eyelid swelling, purulent discharge, redness, corneal edema, hypopyon, vitritis, poor red reflex, poor vision, and pain are commonly associated with endophthalmitis.

Bacterial endophthalmitis. Bacterial endophthalmitis is most commonly seen in patients with preexisting medical conditions such as diabetes mellitus, gastrointestinal disorders, hypertension, cardiac disorders, or malignancy. Gram-positive organisms, most commonly streptococci and staphylococci, account for up to two thirds of infections. The most frequent sources of seeding of these infections are underlying endocarditis and the gastrointestinal tract. Vision is commonly damaged following even healed endophthalmitis. Treatment includes vitrectomy, intravitreal antibiotics, and systemic antibiotics. Visual and anatomic prognosis is usually poor, despite aggressive antibacterial therapies (Tsai et al., 2000; Okada et al., 1994).

Fungal endophthalmitis. A fungal source for endophthalmitis is suggested when multiple vitreous abscesses appear as "a string of pearls" or when there is an associated choroiditis. Most cases of fungal endophthalmitis occur in immunocompromised hosts; their signs of inflammation may be variable (Vose et al., 2001). *C. albicans* is the most common fungal pathogen. Risk factors for fungal endophthalmitis include the following:

- Deep tissue infection
- Low birth weight
- History of prematurity
- History of immunosuppression
- Parenteral feeding
- Prolonged intravenous access
- C. albicans fungemia
- History of intravenous drug use

Because of the widespread use of antifungal agents in patients with systemic fungal infections, endogenous fungal endophthalmitis has become rare. Recent studies report the presence of a more limited chorioretinal infection without spread into the vitreous in up to 9% of patients with known fungemia. An ophthalmic examination of dilated eyes is warranted in patients with the risk factors listed above, even though ocular findings usually do not change the course of therapy (Enzenauer et al., 1992; Stern et al., 2001, Donahue et al., 1994, Scherer et al., 1997).

Aspergillus infections of the inner eye can occur in the severely immunocompromised host. The presenting sign is a large unifocal area of chorioretinitis. Although histoplasmosis can cause endophthalmitis, it more typically is seen as focal chorioretinal scars, called *histo spots*. Vitritis is usually not present. The prognosis depends on location; peripheral lesions are asymptomatic, and macular lesions affect vision. Central lesions have devastating effects on vision if they are associated with chorioretinal neovascularization. For fungal infections, visual prognosis depends on the site of the initial choroiditis. Extended course of oral fluconazole following vitrectomy without intravitreal amphotericin B appears to be successful (Smiddy, 1998; Essman et al., 1997).

Exogenous Endophthalmitis

Traumatic endophthalmitis. Traumatic endophthalmitis can occur as sequelae of globe trauma. Risk factors for developing endophthalmitis following exogenous trauma include the following:

- Retained foreign body
- Rural setting
- Delay in primary wound closure (>24 hours)
- Disruption of the crystalline lens

Prompt wound closure, pars plana vitrectomy, and intravitreal and systemic antibiotics are the treatments of choice (Reynolds et al., 1997; Boldt et al., 1989; Foster et al., 1996; Thompson et al., 1993).

Postoperative endophthalmitis. Endophthalmitis can result from the entrance of an organism into the eye during intraocular surgery. Bacterial infections usually manifest within 4 days of surgery, often after a normal first postoperative visit. Lethargy, conjunctival inflammation, eyelid swelling, or fever can accompany signs of ocular infection. Vitritis with or without hypopyon is seen. The most common bacteria cultured from patients with postoperative endophthalmitis are *S. pneumoniae, H. influenzae,* and *S. aureus* (Simon et al., 1992). Predisposing factors are thought to be nasolacrimal gland obstruction and upper respiratory infection.

UVEITIS

The uveal tissue is composed of the vascular subretinal choroid, posteriorly, and the ciliary body and iris, anteriorly. Uveal inflammation (associated with inflammation of the surrounding aqueous or vitreous fluid) is seen in a variety of infections. The inflammation is referred to as *granulomatous* (involving epitheleoid cells deposited as dense plaques on the corneal endothelium; Plate 41) or *nongranulomatous* (lymphocytic and plasma cells with smaller punctate keratitic precipitates present on the endothelium.)

Etiology

Infectious granulomatous uveitis. Possible causes of infectious granulomatous uveitis include toxoplasmosis (see the discussion of retinitis); Lyme disease (B. burgdorferi is the causative agent); TB (see the discussion of retinitis); syphilis (uveitis is the most common ocular manifestation; Tamesis et al., 1990); and cytomegalovirus (CMV) infection.

Noninfectious causes. Noninfectious causes of granulomatous uveitis include Vogt-Koyanagi-Harada syndrome; sarcoidosis; multiple sclerosis; sympathetic ophthalmitis; phacoanaphylactic uveitis; and HLA-B27 associated anterior uveitis.

INFECTIONS OF THE OPTIC NERVE
Viral and Postviral Optic Neuritis

Optic neuritis is a generic term referring to a presumed inflammation of the optic nerve resulting in the signs of optic nerve dysfunction: loss of central vision, dyschromatopsia, a relative afferent relative pupillary defect, and visual field change. Sometimes, the specific inciting event for an optic neuritis can be uncovered; usually, it cannot. Viral etiology is suspected when a prodromal viral disease occurs within 2 weeks of onset of symptoms. Coronaviruses have been thought to be a causative factor in some cases of optic neuritis, but a recent study does not support their role (Dessau et al., 1999). The average age of onset of optic neuritis in children is 10 years. It is unilateral 40% of the time and bilateral in 60% of pediatric cases. If only one eye is affected, the visual prognosis may be better; also, the visual outcome in children with optic neuritis is usually better than in adults (Roussat et al., 2001; Lana-Peixoto et al., 2001; Brady et al., 1999), although some studies disagree (Morales et al., 2000). The overall risk of developing multiple sclerosis following optic neuritis is thought lower in children (20% to 26%).

As with adults, the optic disc in childhood optic neuritis may appear mildly swollen (66%) or normal on physical exam. Children may have concurrent neurologic signs of meningoencephalitis. Optic neuritis should remain a diagnosis of exclusion; its evaluation in the pediatric age group may necessitate a fat-suppressed gadolinium-enhanced MRI and CSF analysis. Therapies vary and may include intravenous steroids, followed by oral taper. Immunomodulatory agents (interferon-β-1b [Betaseron], interferon-β-1a [Avonex], and copolymer-1 [Copaxone]) are used in adults but their efficacy has not been proven in treating children.

Herpes zoster optic neuritis. Ocular herpes can spread and cause inflammation directly to the optic nerve. This infection carries a poor visual prognosis for return of normal vision and commonly unfolds with ensuing optic atrophy (Tunis et al., 1987). As with adults, the optic disc may appear swollen (66%) or normal. Optic neuritis may occur weeks after the onset of the vesicular rash and other initial signs and symptoms of herpetic eye disease.

Optic neuritis associated with sinusitis. Much of the older literature has suggested an association between optic neuritis and underlying sinusitis; many doubt the reality of this association. Radiologic studies have shown an increased incidence of paranasal sinus inflammatory changes in patients with optic neuritis. If a patient has an atypical headache and an optic neuritis, neuroimaging may be warranted not only to rule out an intracranial process but also to document any treatable paranasal sinus disease (Ergene et al., 2000; Moorman et al., 1999).

Vaccination-related optic neuritis. In childhood, optic neuritis may follow inoculations for measles or rubella or administration of BCG vaccine. Epidemiologic evidence for many of these associations has been disputed, so the cause and effect relationship between vaccination and optic neuritis remains controversial; an immunologically modulated pathophysiology rather than a direct effect of true infection has been postulated (Shaw et al., 1988; Stevenson et al., 1996; Ray et al., 1996; Yen et al., 1991).

Other causes of optic neuritis. Other reported infectious causes of optic neuritis include the following:

- Lyme disease
- TB
- *Cryptococcus* infection
- Toxoplasmosis
- Toxocariasis
- CMV infection
- HIV infection
- Coccidiomycosis

NEURORETINITIS

As an optic neuritis is an inflammation of the nerve, so a retinitis is an inflammation of the underlying retina. Optic nerve head swelling itself is a papillitis (anterior optic neuritis); when it occurs with retinal (macular) exudates, typically shaped in a stellate pattern, it is referred to as a *neuroretinitis*, implying changes in both nerve and retina (Plate 42). Epiretinal membrane formation is a rare late sequela. Focal retinal phlebitis may be a presenting sign. Patients complain of poor vision; the finding of a macular star is diagnostic. The diagnosis is a clinical one; a focused history that includes recent travel, consumption of uncooked foods, sexual contacts, and animal exposure often reveals the suspected pathogen. Laboratory evaluation depends on the history but may include complete blood count; determination of erythrocyte sedimentation rate;

bacterial, fungal, or viral cultures; antinuclear tests' measurement of angiotensin-converting enzyme levels; anti–double stranded DNA; C3; serology for syphilis or Lyme disease; screening for histoplasmosis, brucellosis, chlamydia, HIV, toxoplasmosis, EBV, or viral hepatitis B and C; and a tuberculin skin test.

Cat-scratch disease is thought to be a common cause of childhood neuroretinitis. Serology for IgM, and IgG for *B. henselae* may be positive in up to 64% of such neuroretinitis patients. If suspicion is high but serology is inconclusive, a polymerase chain reaction looking for *B. henselae* DNA obtained from an affected lymph node may be helpful. Nearly half of all cases of childhood neuroretinitis remain "idiopathic."

Cat-Scratch Neuroretinitis

Cat-scratch disease may be a common pediatric diagnosis; it is a rare case that affects the eye. Findings in this subacute lymphadenitis, which is caused by a rickettsial infection, typically include a swollen nerve and macular star, both presumed to be secondary to *B. henselae* or *Afipia felis* infection. The patient's history often involves a cat scratch weeks prior to onset or the known presence of a kitten within the proband's household. Systemic antibiotics are often employed, although with little documented effect on visual outcomes.

Other Infectious Causes of Neuroretinitis

Neuroretinitis may be caused by the following infectious conditions:

- Brucellosis
- HIV infection
- EBV infection
- Hepatitis B
- Hepatitis C
- Mumps
- HSV infection
- Chlamydia
- Leptospirosis
- *Rickettsia typhi* infection
- Toxoplasmosis
- Syphilis
- TB
- Histoplasma capsulatum

Treatment varies according to infectious agent suspected (Labalette et al., 2001; Suhler et al., 2000; Canzano et al., 2001; Ray et al., 2001; Mclean et al., 1992).

Diffuse Unilateral Subacute Neuroretinitis

Diffuse unilateral subacute neuroretinitis (DUSN) is a unique neuroretinitis caused by direct infiltration of the eye by a parasitic worm, usually within the subretinal space. Disc and retinal edema may be present, yet remarkably few inflammatory changes combine to cause decreased vision. A migrating nematode (whose activity is increased by the light of a direct ophthalmoscope) may be seen within and below the retina.

The condition is usually unilateral. An overlying vitritis can be seen. Retinal pigment disruption, vessel attenuation, optic nerve atrophy, and depressed electroretinogram readings are late complications of this condition. DUSN is presumed to be caused by a subretinal helminthic infection. The exact agent has not been determined. *Baylisascaris* (the raccoon ascarid) is a likely agent of origin for the large nematode variant. Other agents of origin may include *Toxocara canis*, or a *Paragonimus* (lung fluke), or *Alaria*. Therapy is often curative of the infection, although visual prognosis may remain poor. Focal argon green laser photocoagulation of the worm can be employed. Therapies with ivermectin and thiabendazole have not been generally successful. Newer systemic agents offer more promise (Casella et al., 1998; de Souza, 1999; Goldberg et al., 1993; Seal et al., 1998).

INFECTIONS OF THE RETINA
Acute Retinal Necrosis

ARN is a unilateral retinal wipeout that has been reported, rarely, in children. Herpesvirus is usually suspected (herpes simplex type 1 or 2 or herpes zoster); the condition may be seen in immunocompetent or immunosuppressed individuals. Patients come to attention because of visual loss, symptoms of retinal detachment (flashing lights, new floaters, curtain defect), and signs of retinal disease. Initially focal, peripheral areas of white, thickened retina and vitritis are seen, followed by growing areas of necrotic retina unfolding into retinal detachment. Optic neuritis and uveitis may be seen late in the course. A vesicular rash periorbitally may precede the eye finding by several days. ARN may be bilateral 60% of the time, especially if the patient has AIDS. Given the high risk of retinal detachment and poor prognosis without treatment, a prophylactic laser retinopexy barrage around the affected area with high dose antiviral agents is recommended to prevent progression and to protect the fellow eye from infection (Crapotta et al., 1993; Palay et al., 1991).

Progressive Outer Retinal Necrosis

Progressive outer retinal necrosis (PORN) is presumed to be a variant of herpetic retinal necrosis in patients with AIDS. It preferentially affects outer retinal layers (photoreceptors) and has a very poor outcome, even with treatment. PORN is associated with unilateral decreased vision and multifocal deep opacities, usually in the periphery, that progress to confluence and retinal detachment. There is minimal vitritis, perhaps because of the patients' immunodeficiency (CD4 is typically <130/mm^3). Herpes zoster virus is thought to be responsible. As with ARN, high-dose systemic antiviral therapy and retinopexy are used. Visual prognosis is guarded (Engstrom et al., 1994; Pavesio et al., 1995).

CMV Retinitis

CMV retinitis is seen in patients with severe immunocompromise (CD4 <50; e.g., 20% of patients with terminal AIDS). It is sometimes the first presenting sign of AIDS. Poor visual prognosis is a result of the high incidence of retinal detachments, rather than a direct effect of the infecting organism. Incidence has decreased in western countries since the advent of HAART therapies. It is interesting to note that this retinitis is remarkably responsive to proper antimicrobial agents. Poor vision, symptoms of retinal detachment (flashing lights, curtain defects, and floaters), and the characteristic focal retinitis marked by blood and cotton-wool spots are the hallmark of CMV changes. Impressive necrotizing retinopathy with multiple retinal hemorrhages occur, a condition called *pizza pie retinitis*. Treatment includes weekly intravitreal injections of ganciclovir or intravitreal implants; foscarnet, too, is a remarkably effective agent. If a retinal detachment is present, surgical repair may include vitrectomy, oil placement in the vitreous cavity, and intraoperative endolaser retinopexy (Marx et al., 1996; Hodge et al., 1996; Sison et al., 1991).

HIV Retinitis

It is thought that the HIV agent itself may cause a primary, mostly benign, retinal infection; vision may not be affected, unless the optic nerve itself is involved. Cotton-wool spots (nerve fiber layer infarcts) are present, along with small hemorrhagic areas within the superficial retina. When a primary optic neuropathy occurs, the disc itself is swollen, and optic nerve function compromised. Systemic antiretroviral drug regimens are employed.

Tuberculous Chorioretinitis

A combined infection of the choroid and retina is common in some conditions, tubercule infection being the prototypical example. Spread to the eye is typically hematogenous, from miliary lung disease. Tuberculous chorioretinitis should be suspected when an anterior uveitis fails to improve with treatment with topical steroids and retinal and choroidal changes are seen posteriorly. The most common eye finding in patients with TB is choroiditis, with overlying small focal lesions or one large tubercule; any part of the eye may be affected, however. Acute or chronic anterior granulomatous or nongranulomatous uveitis and a hypopyon may be present with a dense vitritis, papillitis, or vasculitis. Ocular findings may be present in as many of 18% of culture-positive TB patients; the incidence is even higher in patients with HIV. Treatment is systemic, often with careful use of steroids. Care must be taken with antituberculin medicines, as several are known to cause an optic neuropathy (Helm et al., 1993; Bouza, 1997; Psilas et al., 1991).

Syphilis Retinitis

Childhood syphilis may be associated with a focal inflammation of retina. A retinitis, chorioretinitis, optic neuritis, vasculitis, or vitritis may occur.

Pneumocystis Carinii Retinitis

Pneumocystis can be seen in immunocompromised hosts and usually signifies disseminated infection. Sight may not be affected. Lesions are usually yellow to pale in color, are at the level of the choroid, and are clustered within the posterior pole. Their size varies from 300 to 3,000 fm. No retinal necrosis is expected. Systemic antibiotics should be used, not necessarily for the eye infection, but rather to treat the disseminated *Pneumocystis* infection (Shami et al., 1991).

Lyme or *Borrelia* Retinitis

Borrelia infection may cause a retinal vasculitis, retinal hemorrhages, optic neuritis, choroidal lesions, and an exudative serous retinal detachment. The lesions may be multifocal, resembling acute posterior multifocal placoid pigment epitheliopathy, or APMPPE. Antibiotics administered in early stages afford best results (Bodine et al., 1992; Suttorp-Schulten et al., 1993).

Brucellosis Retinitis

Brucella abortus from cows or *B. melitensis* from goats may cause inflammatory changes within the retina. Nonspecific changes occur, with inflammation observed in deep and superficial retina; only the history suggests the cause of the disorder. Systemic antibiotics are employed (Seal et al., 1998).

Toxoplasmosis Retinitis

Toxoplasmosis is seen in patients with or without immunocompromise. When seen in the setting of AIDS, it may be confused clinically with CMV, and diagnosis may be possible only by evidence of response to antiparasitic therapy or when diagnosis is confirmed by retinal biopsy. *Toxoplasma gondii* is a common cause of posterior uveitis, the signature of its infection. Patients may experience poor vision, leukokoria (Plate 43), floaters, disc edema, and photophobia. Densely opaque lesions with smooth nongranular borders are seen (Plate 44); they usually have adjacent satellite lesions. A uveitis with aqueous and vitreous inflammatory reactions is present. The characteristic "light in the fog" description of this entity refers to the appearance of the lesions or the optic nerve as they are seen through the dense vitritis. Immunocompromised patients typically have bilateral, multifocal lesions without evidence of old scarring. A necrotizing retinopathy may be seen. It is similar to CMV but without the typical CMV retinal hemorrhages. In immunocompetent patients, the retinitis is usually seen as an old chorioretinal scar that may occur with a newer, fresher, more yellow, acute lesion.

In immunocompetent patients the disease is typically self-limited and does not require treatment unless lesions are near the macula or optic nerve, or if they are associated with severe vitritis. For more threatening infections, in the compromised patient, pyrimethamine, sulfadiazine, tetracycline, spiramycin, trimethoprim and sulfamethoxazole (Bactrim), and clindamycin have been used. Topical or oral steroids may be used after the antimicrobial treatments are initiated. Reactivation of the disease may occur in immunocompromised patients after the cessation of therapy (Holland et al., 1988; Holland et al., 1991; Opremcak et al., 1992).

Cysticercosis Retinitis

Posterior inflammation in the vitreous or subretinal space is said to occur in 13% to 46% of infected patients. Live larvae undulating within the eye have been reported. *T. solium* tapeworm larvae are the putative agent. Therapy may involve surgical removal of the worm, praziquantel 50mg/kg/day, or laser photocoagulation. Death of the larvae may cause severe worsening of inflammation.

Ocular Larva Migrans Syndrome

Infection with T. canis causes ocular larva migrans syndrome (OLM). Human transmission of this disease comes from eating contaminated food or handling puppies, dogs' feces, or infected dirt. It is most commonly seen in 5- to –10-year-olds. This canine ascarid is shed in the feces of all puppies. Poor vision from inflammation and fibrosis stemming from chorioretinal lesions can lead to epiretinal membrane formation and tractional retinal detachments, and endophthalmitis. Choroidal neovascular membranes may be a late complication. *T. canis* nematode larvae are the causative agent. This is the same agent that causes a more systemic disease, visceral larva migrans (VLM; Sabrosa et al., 2001). Unlike VLM, which produces more systemic and immunologic effects, OLM is localized to the eye, and thus serum immunologic studies such as anti-*Toxocara* IgG and Western blot analysis are not as helpful in diagnosis. Recent studies show that 400 mg of oral albendazole given twice per day, combined with steroids, may potentially suppress the inflammatory reaction to the dead larvae (Barisani-Asenbauer et al., 2001). Other studies propose the use of diethycarbamazine or single dose ivermectin (Seal et al., 1998).

Onchocerciasis Retinitis (River Blindness)

Onchocerca volvulus is endemic in parts of Central and South America and Africa. The filariae gain entry through the bite of a female black fly of the *Simulium* genus. The filariae then grow under the skin and release millions of microfilariae. These reach the eye either directly or hematogenously. They do not cause significant inflammation while the parasite is alive, but typically signs and symptoms worsen with treatment and death of the parasite. This is known as the *Mazzotti reaction*. Stromal keratitis, glaucoma, uveitis, optic neuritis, chorioretinitis, disturbance in the retinal pigment epithelium, vascular sheathing, and subretinal fibrosis and vision loss occurring in an endemic area are the signatures of river blindness. Up to a third of patients with systemic disease may have intraocular filariae, which may be visible within the anterior chamber. Annual ivermectin as a single dose is preferred in children above the age of 5 years, as it decreases parasitic load by killing only the microfilariae and thus produces less acute inflammation, especially when used concurrently with steroids (Newland et al., 1991; Dadzie et al., 1991).

SCLERITIS

The sclera—the outermost coat of the eye—can serve as a site of infection. Scleritis is associated with severe pain, local or diffuse inflammation, and engorged deeper immobile vessels. Scleritis usually occurs in conjunction with granulomatous systemic conditions such us sarcoidosis, TB, syphilis, Lyme disease, and infection with *P. aeruginosa*. Therapy depends on the cause of the scleritis (Helm et al., 1997). Topical and systemic corticosteroids and nonsteroidal antiinflammatory agents have been used.

CONGENITAL INFECTIONS (TORCH)

TORCH syndrome consists of infection with toxoplasmosis, other agents, rubella, cytomegalovirus, or herpes simplex. Intrauterine and perinatal infections of the eye can cause acute or delayed damage, both directly and by teratogenic effect. For most congenital infections, the earlier in pregnancy a fetus is affected, the higher the risk and the worse the prognosis. This is also true for congenital infections that affect the eye. As with any congenital disorder affecting sight, signs may have a delayed presentation (e.g., strabismus, amblyopia, or nystagmus). In addition, a congenital infection may prevent complete development of the macula and be a limiting factor in vision.

Toxoplasmosis

Toxoplasmosis may have many hosts. Maternal risk factors include ingestion of raw meat and exposure to cats' feces. Most primary maternal infections are asymptomatic. A mother born with congenital toxoplasmosis is not at risk for transmission to her fetus. This parasite has an affinity for the CNS, and therefor involves the retina. Most (80%) of congenitally infected infants have ocular involvement, with a bilateral local necrotizing retinitis and secondary choroiditis forming a flat-pigmented scar. New lesions will be elevated and white, with characteristic satellite foci. Optic neuritis may be an associated finding. Persistence of the anterior vascular capsule of the lens is said to occur.

For acute infections in women who seroconvert during pregnancy, pyrimethamine, sulfadiazine, folinic acid, and steroids are said to decrease the risk of severe sequelae in the infant, although with no impact on the maternal-fetal transmission rate. The infection may reactivate, even after appropriate therapy. There exist case reports of congenital transmission from mothers who became infected before conception (Vogel et al., 1996; Roberts et al., 2001; Foulon et al., 1999). Treatment for infants is similar to maternal treatment.

Rubella (German Measles)

The incidence of this disease has decreased markedly since the introduction of the rubella vaccine. However, many women of reproductive age worldwide remain at risk. There are differing opinions as to whether there is a significant association between gestational time of infection and individual ocular effects. Ocular disease is the most frequent manifestation in the congenital rubella syndrome (78% of cases). Anterior segment disease includes corneal opacities, microphthalmos, chronic nongranulomatous iridocyclitis, glaucoma, iris hypoplasia, persistence of the anterior vascular capsule of the lens, and cataract (which may begin microscopically and thus remain undetected until slit-lamp examination). Posterior segment disease includes bilateral retinal pigment degeneration with a characteristic salt-and-pepper appearance. Fortunately this retinal change rarely affects visual function (Givens et al., 1993; Freij et al., 1988). Evaluation should include IgM antibody determination and pharyngeal swab cultures. If a congenital cataract is present, it is urgent that surgery be performed to reduce the risk of amblyopia. Glaucoma also must be addressed immediately. No specific treatment for systemic congenital rubella has been established; treatment is primarily supportive (Epps et al., 1995).

Cytomegalic Inclusion Disease

Congenital CMV infection comes from viremia occurring within the mother, after primary exposure. Reinfection or reactivation is less common. Perhaps 1% of all newborns are infected, so this is a very common congenital infection. Approximately 15% of these infants have retinochoroiditis, but only 10% are symptomatic. A bilateral process with retinal necrosis and secondary granulomatous choroiditis is typically seen. In the acute setting, retinal hemorrhages and white opacities are observed. In later stages, atrophy of retina and retinal pigment epithelium occur. Persistence of the anterior vascular capsule of the lens occurs. Evaluation should include serology for IgM and viruses from body fluids and computed tomographic scan to search for periventricular calcifications. No specific treatment for systemic congenital CMV has been formally established, although both ganciclovir and foscarnet have been used. Treatment is primarily supportive (Epps et al., 1995).

Herpes Simplex Virus

As opposed to the other TORCH infections, neonatal transmission of HSV occurs perinatally, from the maternal cervix at birth, not through maternal viremia. There is a 50% risk of transmission from mothers with known vaginal infections. Typically HSV type 2 is the causative virus, but case reports exist of perinatal transmission of HSV type 1 (Glover et al., 1987). Congenital HSV can cause a necrotizing retinitis, with massive yellow-white exudates and overlying vitreous reaction, keratoconjunctivitis, cataracts, and persistence of the anterior vascular capsule of the lens. Diagnosis is clinical but may be confirmed by virus isolation from body fluids. Therapy includes acyclovir, vidarabine, topical agents, and débridement if an epithelial keratitis exists; delivery is by cesarian section as a prophylactic measure in a mother known to have the infection (Bale et al., 1992).

Syphilis

Neonatal transmission occurs through hematologous spread from maternal infection with the spirochete *Treponema pallidum*. Interestingly, the longer the mother has had syphilis, the lower the risk of fetal infection. Uveitis and keratitis may be acute in patients aged 5 to 25 years who were born with congenital syphilis. Pain, photophobia, neovascularization

of the cornea, glaucoma, and poor vision may be presenting signs. Chorioretinitis with a typical salt-and-pepper granularity, narrowed retinal vessels, optic atrophy, and pseudo–retinitis pigmentosa–like changes are seen. Diagnosis is a clinical one and may be confirmed with dark-field microscopy, Venereal Disease Research Laboratory (VDRL) slide test, and fluorescent treponemal antibody absorption (FTA-ABS) test. Therapy remains a challenge, with systemic aqueous penicillin G commonly employed.

ACKNOWLEDGMENTS

The authors wish to acknowledge Dr. Joseph Pasternak, Dr. Thomas Clinch, Dr. Sanjoy Chowdry, Dr. Howard Savage, and Dr. Mohamad Jaafar for assistance and contributions in the preparation of this chapter and its illustrations.

BIBLIOGRAPHY

Aasuri M. Co-occurrence of pneumococcal keratitis and dacryocystitis. Cornea 1999;18:273-276.

Aburn NS, et al. Infectious mononucleosis presenting with dacryoadenitis. Ophthalmology 1996;103:776-778.

Aclimados WA. Tuberculous keratoconjunctivitis. Br J Ophthalmol 1992;76:175-176.

Adams CP. Interferon treatment of adenoviral conjunctivitis. Am J Ophthalmol 1984;98:429-432.

Akova Y. Microbial keratitis following penetrating keratoplasty. Ophthalmic Surg Lasers 1999;30:449-455.

Alcelik T. Ocular leech infestation in a child. Am J Ophthalmol 1997;124:110-112.

Alexadrakis G. Corneal biopsy in the management of progressive microbial keratitis. Am J Ophthalmol 2000;129:571-576.

Ambati BK et al. Periorbital cellulitis before and after the advent of *Haemophilus influenzae* type B vaccine. Ophthalmology 2000;107:1450-1453.

Amir. H. Kaposi's sarcoma before and during a human immunodeficiency virus epidemic in Tanzanian children. Pediatr Infect Dis J 2001;20:518-521.

Azimi P. Interstitial keratitis in a 5 year old. Pediatr Infect Dis J 1999;18:299.

Bale JF Jr, et al. Congenital infections and the nervous system. Pediatr Clin North Am 1992;39:669-690.

Barisani-Asenbauer T, et al. Treatment of toxocariasis with albendazole. J Ocul Pharmacol Ther 2001;17:287-294.

Bekir NA, et al. *Brucella melitensis* dacryoadenitis: a case report. Eur J Ophthalmol 2000;10:259-261.

Benevento WJ, et al. The sensitivity of *Neisseria gonorrhoeae*, *Chlamydia trachomatis*, and herpes simplex type II to disinfection with povidone-iodine. Am J Ophthalmol 1990;109:329-333.

Bodine SR, et al. Multifocal choroiditis with evidence of Lyme disease. Ann Ophthalmol 1992;24:169-173.

Boldt HC, et al. Rural endophthalmitis. Ophthalmology 1989;96:1722-1726.

Bouza E. Ocular tuberculosis. A prospective study in a general hospital. Medicine 1997;76:53-61.

Brady K, et al. Optic neuritis in children: clinical features and visual outcome. J AAPOS 1999;3:98-103.

Campolattaro BN, et al. Spectrum of pediatric dacryocystitis: medical and surgical management of 54 cases. J Pediatr Ophthalmol Strabismus 1997;34:143-153.

Canzano JC, et al. Pars plana vitrectomy for epiretinal membrane secondary to cat scratch neuroretinitis. Retina 2001;21:272-273.

Carithers HA. Cat-scratch disease. An overview based on a study of 1,200 patients. Am J Dis Child 1985;139:1124-1133.

Casella A, et al. Antihelminthic drugs in diffuse unilateral subacute neuroretinitis. Am J Ophthalmol 1998;125:109-111.

Ciarallo LR, et al. Lumbar puncture in children with periorbital and orbital cellulitis. J Pediatr 1993;122:355-359.

Conrad DA. Treatment of cat-scratch disease. Curr Opin Pediatr 2001;13:56-59.

Crapotta JA, et al. Visual outcome in acute retinal necrosis. Retina 1993;13:208-213.

Cutter GR, et al. The clinical presentation, prevalence, and risk factors of focal corneal infiltrates in soft contact lens wearers. CLAO J 1996;22:30-37.

Dadzie KY, et al. Changes in ocular onchocerciasis after two rounds of community-based ivermectin treatment in a holo-endemic onchocerciasis focus. Trans R Soc Trop Med Hyg 1991;85:267-271.

de Souza E. Diffuse bilateral subacute neuroretinitis: first patient with documented nematodes in both eyes. Arch Ophthalmol 1999;117:1349-1351.

Dessau R, et al. Coronaviruses in spinal fluid of patients with acute monosymptomatic optic neuritis. Acta Neurol Scand 1999;100:88-91.

Dezube BJ. New therapies for the treatment of AIDS-related Kaposi sarcoma. Curr Opin Oncol 2000;12:445-449.

Donahue SP, et al. Intraocular candidiasis in patients with candidemia. Clinical complications derived from a prospective multicenter study. Ophthalmology 1994;101:1302-1309.

Donahue SP, et al. Preseptal and orbital cellulitis in childhood. A changing microbiologic spectrum. Ophthalmology 1998;105:1902-1905.

Dua H. Non-*Acanthamoeba* amebic keratitis. Cornea 1998;17:675-677.

Engstrom RE, et al. The progressive outer retinal necrosis syndrome. A variant of necrotizing herpetic retinopathy in patients with AIDS. Ophthalmology 1994;101:1488-1502.

Enzenauer RW, et al. Screening for fungal endophthalmitis in children at risk. Pediatrics 1992;90:451-457.

Epps RE, et al. TORCH syndrome. Semin Dermatol 1995;14:179-186.

Epstein R. Rapid diagnosis of *Acanthamoeba* keratitis from corneal scrapings using indirect fluorescent antibody staining. Arch Ophthalmol 1986;104:1318-1321.

Ergene E, et al. Acute optic neuritis: association with paranasal sinus inflammatory changes on MRI. J Neuroimaging 2000;10:209-215.

Essman TF, et al. Treatment outcomes in a 10-year study of endogenous fungal endophthalmitis. Ophthalmic Surg Lasers 1997;28:185-194.

Foster RE, et al. Useful visual outcome after treatment of *Bacillus cereus* endophthalmitis. Ophthalmology 1996;103:390-397.

Foulon W, et al. Treatment of toxoplasmosis during pregnancy: a multicenter study of impact on fetal transmission and children's sequelae at age 1 year. Am J Obstet Gynecol 1999;180:410-415.

Freij BJ, et al. Maternal rubella and the congenital rubella syndrome. Clin Perinatol 1988;15:247-257.

Garg P. Ciprofloxacin-resistant *Pseudomonas* keratitis. Ophthalmology 1999;106:1319-1323.

Garg P. Keratomycosis: clinical and microbiologic experience with dematiaceous fungi. Ophthalmology 2000;107:574-580.

Garrity JA, et al. Ocular complications of atopic dermatitis. Can J Ophthalmol 1984;19:21-24.

Givens KT, et al. Congenital rubella syndrome: ophthalmic manifestations and associated systemic disorders. Br J Ophthalmol 1993;77:358-363.

Glover MT, et al. Congenital infection with herpes simplex type I. Pediatr Dermatol 1987;4:336-340.

Goldberg MA, et al. Diffuse unilateral subacute neuroretinitis. Morphometric, serologic, and epidemiologic support for *Baylisascaris* as a causative agent. Ophthalmology 1993;100:1695-1701.

Gross R. A comparison of ciprofloxacin and tobramycin in bacterial conjunctivitis in children. Clin Pediatr (Phila) 1997;36:435-444.

Hammerschlag MR, et al. Efficacy of neonatal ocular prophylaxis for the prevention of chlamydial and gonoccal conjunctivitis. N Engl J Med 1989;320:769-772.

Harding SP. Management of ophthalmic zoster. J Med Virol 1993;suppl 1:97-101.

Helm C, et al. Ocular tuberculosis. Surv Ophthalmol 1993;38:229-256.

Helm C, et al. Combination intravenous ceftazidime and aminoglycosides in the treatment of pseudomonal scleritis. Ophthalmology 1997;104:838-843.

Herpetic Eye Disease Study Group. Oral acyclovir for herpes simplex virus eye disease: effect on prevention of epithelial keratitis and stromal keratitis. Arch Ophthalmol 2000;118:1030-1036.

Herpetic Eye Disease Study Group. Predictors of recurrent herpes simplex virus keratitis. Cornea 2001;20:123-128.

Hodge WG, et al. Once-weekly intraocular injections of ganciclovir for maintenance therapy of CMV retinitis: clinical and ocular outcome. J Infect Dis 1996;174:393-396.

Holland GN, et al. Ocular toxoplasmosis in patients with the acquired immunodeficiency syndrome. Am J Ophthalmol 1988;106:653-667.

Holland GN, et al. Current practices in the management of ocular toxoplasmosis. Am J Ophthalmol 1991;111:601-610.

Huber-Spitzy V, et al. Treatment of ocular chlamydial infection: comparison of tetracyclines and norfloxacin. Ophthalmologica 1992;205:62-68.

Huber-Spitzy V, et al. Ulcerative blepharitis in atopic patients—Is *Candida* species the causative agent? Br J Ophthalmol 1992;76:272-274.

Johnson A, et al. Microbiology and immunology, ed 2. Harwal Publishing: Malvern, Penn, 1993.

Kivlin J, et al. Periocular infection after strabismus surgery. The periocular infection study group. J Pediatr Ophthalmol Strabismus 1995;32:42-49.

Labalette P, et al. Cat scratch disease neuroretinitis diagnosed by PCR approach. Am J Ophthalmol 2001;132:575-576.

Lana-Peixoto M, et al. The clinical profile of childhood optic neuritis. Arq Neuropsiquiatr 2001;59:311-317.

Liesegang TJ. Contact lens-related microbial keratitis. Part I. Epidemiology. Cornea 1997;16:125-131.

Madhukar K, et al. Tuberculosis of the lacrimal gland. J Trop Med Hyg 1991;94:150-151.

Marshall DH, et al. Periocular necrotizing fasciitis: a review of five cases. Ophthalmology 1997;104:1857-1862.

Marx JL, et al. Use of ganciclovir implant in the treatment of recurrent cytomegalovirus retinitis. Arch Ophthalmol 1996;114:815-820.

McKellar M. Cast-forming *Actinomyces israelii* canaliculitis. Aust NZ J Ophthalmol 1997;25:301-303.

Mclean DR, et al. Neurobrucellosis: clinical and therapeutic features. Clinical Infect Dis 1992;15:582-590.

Meisler D, et al. Oral erythromycin treatment for childhood blepharokeratitis. J AAPOS 2000;4:379-380.

Moorman C, et al. Is sphenoid sinus opacity significant with optic neuritis? Eye 1999;13:76-82.

Morales D, et al. Optic neuritis in children. J Pediatr Ophthalmol Strabismus 2000;37:254-259.

Mottow L, et al. Idiopathic inflammatory orbital pseudotumor in childhood. I. Clinical characteristics. Arch Ophthalmol 1978;96:1410-1417.

Nelson L (ed). Harley's Pediatric Ophthalmology, ed 4. Philadelphia: Saunders, 1998.

Newland HS, et al. Ocular manifestations of onchocerciasis in a rain forest area in West Africa. Br J Ophthalmol 1991;75(3):163-169.

Okada AA, et al. Endogenous bacterial endophthalmitis. Report of a ten-year retrospective study. Ophthalmology 1994;101:832-838.

Opremcak EM, et al. Trimethoprim-sulfamethoxazole therapy for ocular toxoplasmosis. Ophthalmology 1992;99:920-925.

Palay DA, et al. Decrease in the risk of bilateral acute retinal necrosis by acyclovir therapy. Am J Ophthalmol 1991;112:250-255.

Pavesio SE, et al. Progressive outer retinal necrosis (PORN) in AIDS patients: a different appearance of varicella-zoster retinitis. Eye 1995;9:271-276.

Pollard Z, et al. Acute rectus muscle palsy in children as a result of orbital myositis. J. Pediatr 1996;128:230-233.

Psilas K, et al. Antituberculosis therapy in the treatment of peripheral uveitis. Ann Ophthalmol 1991;23:254-258.

Rahman, M. Randomised trial of 0.2% chlorhexidine gluconate and 2.5% natamycin for fungal keratitis in Bangladesh. Br J Ophthalmol 1998;82:919-925.

Raina, U. Spontaneous extrusion of extraocular cysticercus cysts. Am J Ophthalmol 1996;121:438-441.

Ray CL, et al. Bilateral optic neuropathy associated with influenza vaccination. J Neuroophthalmol 1996;16:182-184.

Ray S, et al. Neuroretinitis. Int Ophthalmic Clin 2001;41:83-102.

Reynolds DS, et al. Endophthalmitis after penetrating ocular trauma. Curr Opin Ophthalmol 1997;8:32-38.

Rhee D (ed). The Wills Eye Manual, ed 3. Philadelphia: Lippincott Williams & Wilkins, 1999.

Rhem MN, et al. Epstein-Barr virus dacryoadenitis. Am J Ophthalmol 2000;129:372-375.

Roberts F, et al. Histopathologic features of ocular toxoplasmosis in the fetus and infant. Arch Ophthalmol 2001;119:51-58.

Rosa RH. The changing spectrum of fungal keratitis in south Florida. Ophthalmology 1994;101:1005-1013.

Roussat B, et al. Acute optic neuritis in children: clinical features and treatment. A study of 28 eyes in 20 children. J Fr Ophtalmol 2001;24:36-44.

Rubin SE, et al. Medical management of orbital subperiosteal abscess in children. J Pediatr Ophthalmol Strabismus 1989;26:21-27.

Ruttum M, et al. Adenovirus conjunctivitis mimics preseptal and orbital cellulitis in young children. J Pediatr 1996;128:230-233.

Sabrosa NA, et al. Nematode infections of the eye: toxocariasis and diffuse unilateral subacute retinitis. Curr Opin Ophthalmol 2001;12:450-454.

Schein OD, et al. Ulcerative keratitis in contact lens wearers. Incidence and risk factors. Cornea 1990;9(suppl 1):S55-S58.

Scherer WJ, et al. Implications of early systemic therapy on the incidence of endogenous fungal endophthalmitis. Ophthalmology 1997;104:1593-1598.

Seal D, et al. Ocular Infection Investigation and Treatment in Practice. St. Louis: Mosby, 1998.

Shah S. Complications of conjunctivitis caused by *Pseudomonas aeruginosa* in a newborn intensive care unit. Pediatr Infect Dis J 1998;17:97-102.

Shami MJ, et al. A multicenter study of *Pneumocystis* choroidopathy. Am J Ophthalmol 1991;112:15-22.

Shaw FE, et al. Postmarketing surveillance for neurologic adverse events reported after hepatitis B vaccination. Experience of the first three years. Am J Epidemiol 1988;127:337-352.

Shimomura S, et al. Local treatment of AIDS-associated bulky Kaposi's sarcoma in the head and neck region. Auris Nasus Larynx 2000;27:335-338.

Sison RF, et al. CMV retinopathy as the initial manifestation of AIDS. Am J Ophthalmol 1991;112:243-249.

Simon J, et al. Recognized scleral perforation during eye muscle surgery: incidence and sequelae. J Pediatr Ophthalmol Strabismus 1992;29:273-275.

Sindhu K, et al. Etiology of childhood proptosis. J Paediatr Child Health 1998;34:374-376.

Smiddy WE. Treatment outcomes of endogenous fungal endophthalmitis. Curr Opin Ophthalmol 1998;9:66-77.

Soparkar C. Acute and chronic conjunctivitis due to over-the-counter ophthalmic decongestants. Arch Ophthalmol 1997;115:34-38.

Souliere CR Jr, et al. Selective non-surgical management of subperiosteal abscess of the orbit: computerized tomography and clinical course as indication for surgical drainage. Int J Pediatr Otorhinolaryngol 1990;19:109-119.

Stern JH, et al. Recurrent endogenous candidal endophthalmitis in a premature infant. J AAPOS 2001;5:50-51.

Stevenson VL, et al. Optic neuritis following measles/rubella vaccination in two 13 year old children. Br J Ophthalmol 1996;80:1110-1111.

Suhler E, et al. Prevalence of serologic evidence of cat scratch disease in patients with neuroretinitis. Ophthalmology 2000;107:871-876.

Suttorp-Schulten MS, et al. Long term effects of ceftriaxone treatment on intraocular Lyme borreliosis. Am J Ophthalmol 1993;116:571-575.

Tadtara KF. Trachoma: a review. J Chemother 2001;13(suppl 1):18-22.

Tamesis RR, et al. Ocular syphilis. Ophthalmology 1990;97:1281-1287.

Taylor D. Pediatric Ophthalmology, ed 2. London: Blackwell Science, 1997.

Thompson JT, et al. Infectious endophthalmitis after penetrating injuries with retained intraocular foreign bodies. National eye trauma system. Ophthalmology 1993;100:1468-1474.

Tost F, et al. Clinical diagnosis of chronic canaliculitis by 20-MHz ultrasound. Ophthalmologica 2000;214:433-436.

Tsai Y, et. al. Pediatric endogenous endophthalmitis. J Formos Med Assoc 2000;99:435-437.

Tunis SW, et al. Acute retrobulbar neuritis complicating herpes zoster ophthalmicus. Ann Ophthalmology 1987;19:453-456.

Uzcategui N, et al. Clinical practice guidelines for the management of orbital cellulitis. J Pediatr Ophthalmol Strabismus 1998;35:73-79.

Vogel N, et al. Congenital toxoplasmosis transmitted from an immunologically competent mother infected before conception. Clin Infect Dis 1996;23:1055-1060.

Vose M, et al. Candida endophthalmitis: an unusual complication of intravenous access. Postgrad Med J 2001;77:119-120.

Weinberg RJ, et al. Fusobacterium in presumed *Actinomyces* canaliculitis. Am J Ophthalmol 1977;84:371-374.

West SK, et al. Risk factors for constant, severe trachoma among preschool children in Kongwa, Tanzania. Am J Epidemiol 1996;143:73-78.

Whitley RJ, et al. The natural history of herpes simplex virus infection of the mother and newborn. Pediatrics 1980;66:489-494.

Wilhelmus KR, et al. Herpetic Eye Disease Study. A controlled trial of topical corticosteroids for herpes simplex stromal keratitis. Ophthalmology 1994;101:1883-1895.

Wilhelmus, KR. The treatment of herpes simplex virus epithelial keratitis. Trans Am Ophthalmol Soc 2000;98:505-532.

Wright K. Pediatric Ophthalmology and Strabismus. St. Louis: Mosby, 1995.

Wutzler P, et al. Virucidal and chlamydicidal activities of eye drops with povidone-iodine liposome complex. Ophthalmic Res 2000;32:118-125.

Yen MY, et al. Bilateral optic neuritis following BCG vaccination. J Clin Neuroophthalmol 1991;11:246-249.

Zanoni D, et al. A comparison of silver nitrate with erythromycin for prophylaxis against ophthalmia neonatorum. Clin Pediatr (Phila) 1992;31:295-298.

Zijlstra EE, et al. Leishmaniasis in Sudan. Tran R Soc Trop Med Hyg 2001;95(suppl 1):S27-S58.

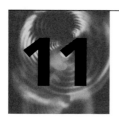

FUNGAL INFECTIONS IN CHILDHOOD

MARGARET K. HOSTETTER

In the normal child, fungal infection is a relatively uncommon event; however, if the child's defenses are compromised by prematurity, destruction or penetration of the epithelial barrier, or neutrophil deficiency or dysfunction, fungal infections carry increasing morbidity and risk of mortality. This chapter distinguishes between fungal infections seen in normal children and those more prevalent in compromised hosts. Because the chapter is not meant to be an all-inclusive review, the reader is referred to more detailed compendia when necessary. Management of fungal infections in normal children is summarized in Table 11-1.

FUNGAL INFECTIONS IN NORMAL CHILDREN
Superficial Fungal Infections

Dermatophytes. Infections with the dermatophytes *Trichophyton, Microsporum,* and *Epidermophyton* are the major causes of superficial dermatophyte infections including tinea corporis, tinea pedis, and tinea cruris. These conditions are typically acquired by direct contact with infected humans or animals or, in the case of the geophilic dermatophytes, from exposure to soil.

Tinea corporis (ringworm) may present as papulosquamous, vesicular, or granulomatous disease. In papulosquamous disease, an erythematous papule enlarges to become a marginated lesion with a scaly border and a central clearing. Minute vesicles may be seen at the advancing edge. The vesicular form is differentiated from the papulosquamous form by the presence of firm vesicles on the base of the lesion. Granulomatous disease is seen uncommonly, usually in immunocompromised children or after treatment with topical steroids. This type of tinea corporis manifests as firm, nontender nodules with overlying crust or plaque. Infrequently, this presentation can be seen in postpubertal girls as a consequence of shaving the legs.

Tinea pedis (athlete's foot) is facilitated by maceration of the skin and a moist pedal environment occurring with sweating or repeated exposure to standing water, as in locker rooms. Peeling of the skin and fissures between the toes are occasionally accompanied by vesicles or small bullae. The diagnosis is confirmed by the appearance of hyphae in scrapings from affected skin that are mounted in 20% potassium hydroxide and examined microscopically.

Tinea cruris (jock itch) occurs most frequently in adolescent and young adult males but has also been reported in females who wear tight-fitting costumes or exercise clothes. The infection appears as a red to reddish brown macular rash spread over the perineum and inner thighs. Lesions have well-demarcated borders, often with vesicular lesions. Although the appearance is dramatic, the lesions are not painful.

These three forms of dermatophyte infection can all be treated with topical antifungal therapy administered once to twice daily for 14 to 21 days. For tinea pedis and tinea cruris, the addition of drying agents such as Burow's solution (aluminum acetate) can accelerate healing of weeping or maturated skin. Topical antifungal agents useful for these conditions include the imidazoles (miconazole) and the allylamines (terbinafine). Steroids are generally contraindicated, and systemic therapy is unnecessary for all but the granulomatous form of tinea corporis.

Superficial Infections Requiring Systemic Therapy

Dermatophytes. Dermatophytic infection of the scalp, tinea capitis, presents most frequently as painless hair loss in a primary school-aged child. *Trichophyton tonsurans* has become the

TABLE 11-1	Fungal Infections in Normal Children	
Disease	*Causative organisms*	*Treatment*
Superficial Fungal Infections Requiring Topical Therapy		
Tinea corporis (ringworm)	*Epidermophyton*	Topical antifungal creams
Tinea cruris (jock itch)	*Microsporum*	(corporis or cruris) or
Tinea pedis (athlete's foot)	*Trichophyton*	powders (cruris or pedis):
		nystatin, terbinafine,
		clotrimazole or miconazole
Diaper dermatitis	*Candida albicans*; other species rarely	Topical antifungal creams: nystatin, clotrimazole, or miconazole
Superficial Fungal Infections Requiring Systemic Therapy		
Tinea capitis	*Trichophyton tonsurans* most	Griseofulvin 10 mg/kg/day
Tinea unguium	common; *Microsporum* spp. less so	microsized or 15 mg/kg/day ultramicrosized PO × 6 weeks
		Fluconazole (6 mg/kg/d), itraconazole (5 mg/kg/d), or terbinafine (62.5-250 mg/d) PO × 4 weeks
Locally Invasive Infections		
Vulvovaginitis	*C. albicans*; other species	Nystatin or clotrimazole troches
Laryngitis	less common	for vaginitis
		Oral fluconazole for vaginitis, laryngitis
Asymptomatic histoplasmosis	*Histoplasma capsulatum*	No treatment necessary
Allergic sinusitis or bronchopulmonary aspergillosis (ABPA)	*Aspergillus fumigatus* or *flavus*	No treatment necessary; some favor corticosteroids for ABPA
Systemic Disease		
Blastomycosis Cutaneous Pulmonary	*Blastomyces dermatitidis*	Parenteral amphotericin B, 1.0 mg/kg/d
Coccidioidomycosis	*Coccidioides immitis*	Parenteral amphotericin B, 1.0 mg/kg/d
Histoplasmosis Symptomatic pulmonary disease Disseminated disease	*H. capsulatum*	Parenteral amphotericin B, 1.0 mg/kg/d

dominant cause over the past 10 years and may present some diagnostic confusion because its presentation is typically more indolent (Rasmussen and Ahmed, 1978). Broken hair shafts, patchy alopecia, and the absence of tenderness or other systemic signs should suggest the diagnosis, once trichotillomania has been ruled out.

Organisms causing tinea capitis are sometimes differentiated as involving either the ectothrix of the hair shaft (*Microsporum canis* and *Microsporum audouinii*) or the endothrix (*T. tonsurans*). Species infecting the outside of the hair shaft (ectothrix) fluoresce yellow-green under the Wood's lamp, but species invading the inner hair shaft (endothrix) do not generate fluorescence. Although most cases are treated as a result of clinical diagnosis, hair shafts can be sent for culture and also examined microscopically after immersion in 20% potassium hydroxide.

This disorder requires systemic therapy and is unlikely to resolve with topical antifungal agents. Griseofulvin administered once a day in a dose of 15 mg/kg/day (maximum 1 gram) in micronized form or 10 mg/kg/day (maximum 750 mg) in ultramicronized form has a lengthy record of success, but resolution typically requires a course of 6 weeks or more (Gan et al., 1987; Martinez-Roig et al, 1988). Absorption is enhanced when the drug is taken with whole milk. Patients should be monitored periodically for neutropenia. Recent controlled trials indicate that allylamines, imidazoles, or triazoles may also be effective. A study comparing 6 weeks of therapy with griseofulvin at 20 mg/kg micronized preparation with 4 weeks of terbinafine, itraconazole, or fluconazole found no difference in efficacy between griseofulvin and terbinafine (92% to 94%) but slightly decreased efficacy for itraconazole and fluconazole (84% to 86%). These differences were statistically significant (Gupta et al., 2001).

A substantial percentage of children may go on to develop a kerion, a form of tinea capitis marked by severe inflammation, including boggy, erythematous, and edematous skin accompanied by seemingly purulent drainage and crusted lesions of the scalp. Fever, lymphadenopathy, and leukocytosis are often present; rarely there may be an underlying staphylococcal infection as well. Despite its alarming appearance, kerion is not tender to palpation. Some experts believe that infection with *T. verrucosum*, a zoophilic dermatophyte acquired from infected farm animals, is especially likely to induce kerion (Schwartz, 1983; Stocker et al., 1977). Treatment again includes griseofulvin, as described above. There is no indication that intralesional steroids accelerate the healing process (Ginsburg et al., 1987).

Candida species. Superficial mucosal infections may also occur with *Candida* species, *C. albicans* being the most common. In most series, approximately 80% of full-term infants are colonized with *Candida* species after the first 3 to 4 weeks of age as a consequence of vertical transmission (Baley, 1991). Adherent patches of pearly white, curdlike material on the buccal or gingival mucosa overlie areas of mild erosion that appear when the lesions are scraped away. In normal infants, thrush readily resolves with 7 to 10 days of therapy with nystatin solution administered as 1 cc to the inside of each cheek twice a day; if the lesions fail to resolve or recur, consideration should be given to the possibility of a T-cell immunodeficiency such as human immunodeficiency virus (HIV) infection.

The second most common cutaneous infection with *Candida* species is diaper dermatitis, which typically appears during the second to fourth month of life. Weeping, brightly erythematous lesions with a scalloped border and distant satellites are quite distinctive. Topical antifungal creams containing clotrimazole, miconazole, or nystatin are prescribed.

Other forms of superficial candidal infection including glossitis or angular cheilosis may appear after routine courses of oral antibiotics. Prolonged exposure to water (e.g., as seen in bartenders or dishwashers) may develop candidal onychomycosis, a form of nail infection that is notoriously difficult to eradicate without prolonged courses of oral antifungal agents. Persistent intertrigo should suggest diabetes.

Locally Invasive Infections

Candida species. Three forms of locally invasive candidal infection occurring in otherwise normal children are vulvovaginitis, laryngeal candidiasis, and chronic draining otitis externa. Vulvovaginitis appears virtually exclusively in postpubertal females and may be a consequence of diabetes mellitus or the use of corticosteroids, immunosuppressive agents, or birth control pills. The use of oral tetracycline for treatment of acne is also a risk factor. *C. albicans* is the most common cause. Presenting signs and symptoms of the disease include a curdlike, cheesy, or mucoid discharge from the vagina accompanied by dysuria, vulvar burning, and intense pruritus. Biopsies in women and in animals infected with *C. albicans* show invasion of the superficial layers of the vaginal mucosa with both blastospores and filamentous forms. Relapsing or recurrent infections are common even in normal women. Treatment requires the use of vaginal troches containing azoles or oral therapy with these same agents (clotrimazole, miconazole, or fluconazole). Vaginal creams are not thought to be as effective as troches.

Laryngeal candidiasis is an uncommon complication of inhalational steroid use that typically has a hoarse voice as the presenting sign (Wang et al., 1997; Williams et al., 1983). The diagnosis is made by direct observation of cheesy, curdlike material on the vocal chords. Treatment typically requires oral antifungal therapy.

The child with a chronic draining ear after prolonged courses of broad-spectrum antibiotics or the use of otic drops and steroids for treatment of chronic otitis media should be cultured for *Candida* species. Therapy for 1 to 2 months with oral fluconazole or another agent to which the isolate is susceptible typically leads to resolution unless the process has extended to the mastoid, in which case surgical débridement and parenteral therapy with amphotericin B will be required.

Aspergillus species. Only two types of non-invasive aspergillosis appear in normal children: allergic bronchopulmonary aspergillosis and allergic sinusitis. As ubiquitous fungi, *Aspergillus* species readily colonize the airways of normal hosts and can cause a syndrome of wheezing, sputum production, pulmonary infiltrates, and hypersensitivity. Sputum contains both eosinophils and fungal elements, typically hyphae. Many patients have antecedent asthma; approximately 10% of patients with cystic fibrosis may also be affected (Brueton et al., 1980). Virulence factors precipitating this cascade are not understood, but treatment typically involves several weeks of prednisolone, 0.5 to 1.0 mg/kg/day. Amphotericin B is not recommended, but some studies have shown a benefit to the use of itraconazole (Wilson and Gibson, 2001). No prospective studies have proven that chronic steroids are beneficial over the long term, unless the course is complicated by recurrent disease or deteriorating pulmonary function.

Allergic sinusitis parallels this process in the upper respiratory tract, although infections with *Alternaria* and *Curvularia* have also been implicated. Patients typically have a long history of recurrent sinusitis, sinus surgery, and nasal polyps. A clinical hallmark of the disease is the finding of dark plugs in nasal discharge. Laboratory findings include peripheral eosinophilia, elevated serum immunoglobulin E (IgE), IgE antibodies specific for the colonizing fungus, and positive results of a skin test for fungal antigens.

Although erosion of bone may occasionally be demonstrable on computed tomographic (CT) scan, this process is not invasive. The mainstay of treatment is surgical débridement of obstructed sinuses; some experts use oral corticosteroids postoperatively, but the duration of therapy and a potential role for oral antifungal agents have not been defined. Successful therapy is correlated with a decrease in IgE levels.

Histoplasmosis. Pulmonary histoplasmosis is a common condition in the endemic regions of the Ohio and Mississippi River Valleys. In more than 90% of children, acquisition of the organism is not associated with symptoms. Symptomatic infections with histoplasmosis develop in only 5% of infected individuals, and 90% of these have a self-limited, flulike illness with fever, malaise, mild cough, and nonpleuritic chest pain that resolves within 2 weeks. Fewer than 5% of symptomatic individuals go on to develop more dramatic symptoms, including reticulonodular infiltrates, hilar adenopathy, severe respiratory distress, or pericardial effusions. These patients will require parenteral amphotericin B. Children with mild to moderate pulmonary infection, arthritis, erythema nodosum, or pericarditis do not require antifungal therapy. Children with an overwhelming exposure, symptoms lasting longer than a month, compression granulomata in the chest or mediastinum, or progressive disseminated histoplasmosis require treatment with amphotericin B.

Locally Invasive Disease Requiring Systemic Therapy

Blastomycosis. Infections with *Blastomyces dermatididis* occur predominantly in normal children in the Mississippi and Ohio River basins, the Missouri River basin, areas of Western New York, areas of Eastern Ontario, and regions along the St. Lawrence River. There is some geographic overlap with regions where histoplasmosis is endemic. Both pulmonary and extrapulmonary manifestations of this fungus occur in normal children. The full spectrum of pulmonary disease from mild illness to overwhelming respiratory failure has been documented; in some children, a chronic process leads to night sweats, weight loss, and chest pain that mimic tuberculosis or neoplasms. Radiographic images are typically dramatic, with one or more lobes of the lung completely obliterated. This disease requires at least 4 to 6 weeks of parental therapy with amphotericin B.

Extrapulmonary manifestations of blastomycosis include wartlike, verrucous lesions of the skin, oropharynx, or larynx as well as acute or subacute osteomyelitis. Genitourinary tract disease typically does not occur in children. Diagnosis requires isolation and culture of the fungus from the lesions; the most specific serologic test demonstrates a rise in antibodies directed against a 120-kDa surface protein, but this test is still a research tool (Klein and Jones, 1990). Parental therapy with amphotericin B is recommended if severe pulmonary signs and symptoms are severe, at least for initial therapy over 3 to 4 weeks. Studies in adults have shown that itraconazole at 200 to 400 mg/kg/day is effective therapy if continued for 6 months. Monotherapy with itraconazole may be acceptable for moderately ill patents, but only if close follow-up can be assured (Dismukes et al., 1992).

Coccidioidomycosis. Infections ascribable to *Coccidioides immitis* occur most frequently in the southwest, Mexico, and Central and South America. Approximately two thirds of infected patients have subclinical disease; the remainder have self-limited, primary pulmonary infections. As with blastomycosis, fewer than 5% of patients have severe pulmonary disease, and fewer than 1% experience disseminated disease. Neonates and young infants are at increased risk for the latter form of the disease, as are otherwise normal African Americans, Native Americans, and Hispanics. This disease is occurring with greater frequency among immunocompromised patients as well (p. 198). Both pulmonary and extrapulmonary manifestations, such as osteomyelitis, arthritis, meningitis, and cutaneous disease, require amphotericin B at least for initial therapy for 4 to 6 weeks; meningitis requires both systemic and intrathecal amphotericin B. Sufficiently large, prospective studies to determine optimal dose, optimal duration of treatment, and outcome for use of the azoles have not been performed. Diagnosis requires culture of the organism from tissue, but observation of spherules with 2 to 5-μm endospores can be diagnostic if infected tissue and body fluids are examined with 20% potassium hydroxide preparations. Complement fixation antibody titers increasing beyond 1:256 are thought by many to predict disseminated disease (Oldfield et al., 1997).

Histoplasmosis. Fewer than 0.2% of children infected with histoplasmosis will manifest a severe form of pulmonary disease. Infants under 1 year of age can develop massive infection of the reticuloendothelial system with hep-atosplenomegaly, failure to thrive, and pancy-topenia (Little et al., 1959; Tesh et al., 1964). Otherwise normal children with these manifestations require systemic therapy with amphotericin B.

FUNGAL INFECTIONS IN THE COMPROMISED HOST
Forms of Compromise

Breaching or erosion of the epithelial barrier by burns, the placement of central venous catheters, or the implantation of peritoneal dialysis catheters can compromise the normal protective functions of the skin. Deficiencies in neutrophil number (neutropenia after chemotherapy) or function (children with chronic granulomatous disease or myeloperoxidase deficiency) can also predispose to fungal disease. Broad compromise of host defenses in premature infants, especially those of very low birth weight (less than 1,000 g) predisposes these infants to infections with bacteria, viruses, or yeasts; typically, the first fungal infection occurs at a mean of 30 days, usually in the aftermath of a bacterial illness (Leibovitz et al., 1992: Baley et al., 1984). In contrast, the more circumscribed T-cell dysfunction in the DiGeorge syndrome or HIV infection often leads to recurrent fungal disease. Because *Candida* species are the most common cause of fungal infections in the compromised host, their many-faceted presentations are discussed first. Management strategies for opportunistic fungal infections in the immunocompromised host are discussed in Table 11-2.

Candida infections specific to the nursery

Congenital candidiasis, a rare entity, manifests as diffuse erythema and neutrophilia in the full-term infant within 24 hours of birth (Fig. 11-1) and is often mistaken for staphylococcal scalded skin syndrome, particularly when desquamation ensues after 36 to 48 hours (Johnson et al., 1981; Whyte et al., 1982; Wolach et al., 1991). In the premature infant the disease may be accompanied by a pustular rather than a macular erythema (Fig. 11-2) as well as by life-threatening pulmonary infection. In both premature and full-term newborns, the disease is thought to arise from silent ascension of *Candida* species from the vagina to the amniotic fluid. Diagnosis in the infant with skin manifestations can be made by gram strain of skin swab or fluid from a pustule; rarely the

TABLE 11-2	Fungal Infections in the Compromised Child	
Disease	Causative organisms	Treatment
Candida Infections		
Congenital candidiasis	*Candida albicans*; other species rarely	Topical antifungal creams (nystatin or clotrimazole) in full-term infants Parenteral amphotericin B, 1.0 mg/kg/d in the premature infant

Candiduria
  Cystitis
  Pyelonephritis
  Mycetoma
	C. albicans; other species less common	Fluconazole, 6 mg/kg/d for cystitis
		Parenteral amphotericin B, 1.0 mg/kg/d for pyelonephritis or mycetoma
		Mycetoma may also respond to fluconazole, 6 mg/kg/d, or surgical treatment if recalcitrant

Candidemia	*C. albicans*; *Candida parapsilosis* in nurseries; other species emerging	Parenteral amphotericin B, 1.0 mg/kg/d× 14 days after eradicated from blood culture Remove central venous catheter
Hepatosplenic candidiasis	*C. albicans*; other species less common	Parenteral amphotericin B, 1.0 mg/kg/d × months
Disseminated candidiasis	*C. albicans*; other species emerging	Parenteral amphotericin B, 1.0 mg/kg/d × 4-6 weeks at least Liposomal preparations may be required in patients with renal compromise
Vulvovaginitis Laryngitis	*C. albicans*; other species less common	Nystatin or clotrimazole troches for vaginitis; Oral fluconazole for vaginitis, laryngitis
Asymptomatic histoplasmosis	*Histoplasma capsulatum*	No treatment necessary
Allergic sinusitis or bronchopulmonary aspergillosis (ABPA)	*Aspergillus fumigatus* or *Aspergillus flavus*	No treatment necessary; some favor corticosteroids for ABPA
Other Fungal Infections		

Aspergillosis
  Cutaneous
  Sinusitis
	A. fumigatus and *A. flavus*; *Aspergillus niger* and *Aspergillus terreus* rarely	Parenteral amphotericin B, 1.0-1.5 mg/kg/d
		Consider addition of itraconazole, 5-12 mg/kg/d

Invasive pulmonary		Parenteral amphotericin B
Cerebral		Parenteral amphotericin B
Emerging mycoses	*Rhizopus, Mucor, Cunninghamella*	Parenteral amphotericin B, 1.0-1.5 mg/kg/d
Zygomycosis		Surgical resection may benefit patients with mucormycosis and phaeohyphomycosis
Fusariosis	*Fusarium solani, Fusarium moniliforme, Fusarium oxysporum*	*Fusarium* spp. and *P. boydii* are frequently resistant to amphotericin B
Pseudallescheriosis	*Pseudallescheria boydii*	
Penicilliosis	*Penicillium marneffei*	
Phaeohyphomycosis	*Alternaria, Curvularia*	
Trichsporonosis	*Trichosporon beigelii*	

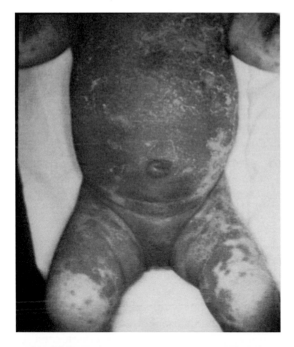

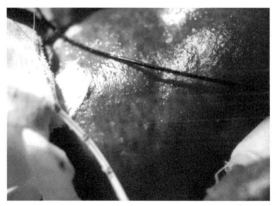

Fig. 11-2 Premature infant with congenital candidiasis. Note papular involvement. (Courtesy Dr. Jeffrey McKinney, Division of Infectious Diseases, Yale University School of Medicine, New Haven, Conn.)

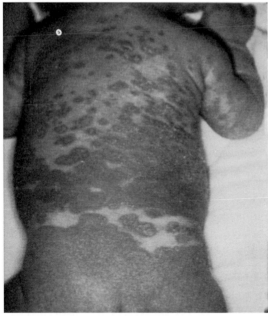

Fig. 11-1 Full-term infant with congenital candidiasis. Note extensive desquamation. (Courtesy Dr. Catherine M. Bendel, Division of Neonatology, University of Minnesota, Minneapolis, Minn.)

organism must be cultured from the placenta. Results of blood cultures are usually negative.

In the full-term infant, the process will typically resolve with a week of therapy with topical antifungal agents such as nystatin or clotrimazole cream. In the premature infant, parenteral amphotericin B is required, although

the prognosis is uniformly poor because of pulmonary involvement (Bendel and Hostetter, 1994).

Candiduria

Typically encountered in patients with diabetes or in hospitalized patients with indwelling urinary catheters, candiduria may represent colonization, lower tract infection, or upper tract disease, the latter encompassing both pyelonephritis and renal candidiasis as a consequence of disseminated candidal infection.

Funguria, a rare event, is found in only 0.1% of urine cultures (Guze and Harley, 1957). However, in patients with indwelling urinary catheters, approximately 26% of proven infections are caused by Candida species (Platt et al., 1986). Coexisting risk factors include diabetes mellitus, the use of antibiotics, female sex, immunosuppression, extremes of age, and urinary stasis (Lundstrom and Sobel, 2001). In a multicenter study, *C. albicans* was isolated in 51.8% of patients with funguria; *Candida glabrata* was second (15.6%) (Kauffman et al., 2000).

Asymptomatic colonization of urinary catheters, stents, or nephrostomy tubes is difficult to distinguish from true infection without additional testing, often including blood cultures in the febrile patient. Pyuria may indicate urethral irritation from the catheter, cystitis, or pyelonephritis. Similarly, the number of organisms in the cultured specimen is often not helpful, given the propensity of *Candida* species to multiply rapidly in urine. In the absence of fever, pyuria, or colony counts greater than 10^3, true infection is unlikely, and treatment other than removal of the catheter is not required. Some experts recommend treatment in renal transplant recipients, in premature newborns, and in neutropenic patients; under these circumstances 4 to 6 mg/kg/day of fluconazole (200 mg/day in adults) has been employed (Lundstrom and Sobel, 2001). Because considerably fewer than 10% of candiduric patients develop candidemia, treatment should be undertaken only if a second urinary specimen is positive. The optimal treatment regimen is unknown.

Although candiduria is common in patients with indwelling urinary catheters, cystitis is an uncommon event. Symptoms are indistinguishable from cystitis ascribable to bacteria. Oral fluconazole at 4 to 6 mg/kg/day (200 mg/day for children weighing more than 40 kg) is generally preferable to amphotericin B bladder washes (50 mg amphotericin B per liter of fluid). Studies in adults have shown that *Candida* species resistant to fluconazole may be susceptible to 5-fluorocytosine (5-FC) as monotherapy (25 mg/kg/day) or to intravenous amphotericin B in a dose of 0.3 mg/kg/day, (Fischer et al., 1987), but the latter regimen has not been tried in children. The upper urinary tract should be imaged in febrile patients because of the likelihood of unsuspected obstruction.

Positive blood cultures accompanying candiduria may indicate ascending pyelonephritis or renal candidiasis. Ascending pyelonephritis appears in the setting of obstructive nephropathy ascribable to fungus balls in the collecting system or to operative stents. Systemic antifungal therapy for 2 to 6 weeks with fluconazole (6 mg/kg/day) or amphotericin B, 0.7-1.0 mg/kg/day, must be coupled with relief of obstruction in order to ensure resolution. Amphotericin B doses should not be reduced in the presence of renal compromise, but further deterioration of renal function can be expected (Bennett, 1974a; Bennett, 1974b). Although liposomal preparations of amphotericin B may be viewed as a panacea under these circumstances, recent clinical evidence indicates that some formulations may fail to penetrate the kidney, thereby leading to recalcitrant infection (Lundstrom and Sobel, 2001; Hell et al., 1999).

Hematogenous seeding of the kidneys as a consequence of disseminated candidiasis must be treated with high-dose parenteral amphotericin B, 1.0 to 1.5 mg/kg/day. Fluconazole has also proven effective in adults, but prospective studies are lacking in children.

Candidemia

Candidemia occurs when *Candida* species enter the bloodstream. Recent literature (Nucci and Anaissie, 2001) points to the intestinal tract, rather than the skin, as the most likely source, at least in adults, although one might argue that the premature newborn delivered by cesarian section may not readily acquire flora from vertical transmission.

Risk Factors in Susceptible Populations

The neonate. Approximately 6% of infants weighing less than 1,500 grams will become infected with Candida species during their hospitalization (Stoll et al., 1996). This incidence reflects both the prevalence of colonization and the relative influence of other risk factors in this population. The incidence of candidemia in infants weighing more than 2,500 grams is tenfold less; candidemia in these infants is typically related to congenital anomalies, especially of the gastrointestinal tract (Rabalais et al., 1996).

In a large multicenter study of 2,157 patients, approximately 23% of premature infants in six neonatal intensive care units (NICUs) were colonized with *Candida* species during their course of stay in the nursery. In colonized infants, *C. albicans* occurred most frequently (62%), with *Candida parapsilosis* present in 32% (Saiman et al., 2001). The presence of central venous catheters and the use of intravenous lipids were risk factors for colonization with *C. albicans*, whereas colonization with *C. parapsilosis* was independently associated with the use of H_2 blockers. Only 5% of health-care workers' hands were positive for *C. albicans*, while 19% carried *C. parapsilosis*. Nonetheless, carriage rates did not correlate with NICU site-specific rates of infant colonization (Saiman et al., 2001).

Risk factors for candidemia in the colonized premature infant include gestational age less than 32 weeks, 5-minute Apgar score less than 5, shock, disseminated intravascular coagulation, prior use of intralipid or parenteral nutrition, the presence of central venous catheters, use of H_2 blockers, intubation, or length of stay >7 days (Saiman et al., 2000). It is interesting to note that colonization of the gastrointestinal tract antedated candidemia in 43% of cases, suggesting that for the neonate, other sources of colonization may contribute to the risk of candidemia.

Patients with disorders of neutrophil number or function. In the neutropenic patient, duration of antibiotic therapy and number of previous bacterial infections are additional risk factors. In bone marrow–transplant recipients, the increased duration of granulocytopenia and total body irradiation as part of the preparative regimen are independent associations in the colonized patient (Verfaillie et al., 1991). More than 85% of cancer or transplant patients have central venous catheters, and peripheral blood cultures are sometimes used to distinguish line sepsis from true candidemia.

Children with chronic granulomatous disease stand at increased risk of candidal infections because the molecular defect precludes intracellular killing of catalase-positive organisms (Boxer and Morganroth, 1987; Gaither et al., 1987; Cohen et al., 1981; Kim et al., 1969). Defective nonoxidative killing accounts for the increased susceptibility of patients with neutrophil myeloperoxidase deficiency (Ludviksson et al., 1993).

In each of these susceptible populations candidemia is the most common presenting condition, with *C. albicans* again the leading species. Treatment requires removal of an intravascular catheter, if present; prospective studies have repeatedly demonstrated increased morbidity and mortality in candidemic patients whose catheters are retained (Eppes et al., 1989; Karlowicz et al., 2000; Leibovitz et al., 1992; Mermel, 2000). In premature infants, candidemia ascribable to *C. albicans* is associated with poorer outcomes than those caused by any other species (Faix, 1992). At least 50% of premature newborns with candidemia ascribable to *C. albicans* had concomitant meningitis (Faix, 1992). The duration of fungemia may be prolonged for more than 7 days in over 30% of patients (Chapman and Faix, 2000).

Systemic antifungal therapy with parenteral amphotericin B is the treatment of choice. Clinical experience has validated the use of relatively short courses of therapy for 10 to 14 days after blood cultures become negative in those patients whose catheters are promptly removed (Donowitz and Hendley, 1995).

Disseminated Candidiasis

The most dreaded complication of candidemia is disseminated candidiasis, in which the organism spreads from the bloodstream to tissues throughout the body, including meninges, eyes, heart valves, lungs, kidneys, or bones. In these patients, most of whom exhibit severe neutropenia or posttransplant immunosuppression, mortality approaches 30% despite the rapid institution of antifungal therapy. Prophylaxis of bone marrow–transplant patients with fluconazole has remarkably decreased the incidence of this complication (Goodman et al., 1992); however, at least two reports have found an increase in azole-resistant species such as *C. krusei* or *C. glabrata* (Wingard et al., 1991; Cesaro et al., 1993).

Among premature newborns, disseminated infection occurs in at least 6% to 10% (Stoll et al., 1996). A recent study in a single nursery of 100 premature newborns weighing less than 1,000 grams showed that a 6-week regimen of prophylactic intravenous fluconazole in a dose of 3 mg/kg divided every third day for 2 weeks, then every other day for 2 weeks, then every day for 2 weeks reduced both colonization and infection in the treatment group. In particular, 10 infants in the placebo group had *Candida* species isolated from blood (6), blood and urine (2), or urine only (2); in the treatment group there were no systemic infections (Kaufman et al., 2001).

Diagnosis requires the isolation of *Candida* species from blood or otherwise sterile tissue in a colonized patient. Patients with candidemia should be evaluated for lesions in the retina (endophthalmitis) and kidney at the very least; these complications occur in approximately 10% of premature newborns (Noyola et al., 2001), but no study has systematically examined their occurrence in older patients. Many experts recommend routine echocardiograms for those patients with intravascular catheters in place. Concurrent candidal meningitis is a rare occurrence outside the newborn period, where some studies have found a prevalence approaching 50% (Faix, 1992).

Treatment necessitates the removal of intravascular catheters and the rapid institution of parenteral amphotericin B in doses of 1 to 1.5 mg/kg/day (Mermel et al., 2001; Rex et al., 2000). No more than 24 hours should elapse before the fungemic patient is receiving a dose of 0.7 to 1 mg/kg/day. Older protocols favoring smaller increments in daily dosing are inefficacious because of the overwhelming immunosuppression induced by modern regimens.

A rise in creatinine occurs in more than 80% of patients receiving amphotericin B (Lundstrom and Sobel, 2001; Bennett, 1974a). Patients experiencing a twofold increase in creatinine, evidence of tubular compromise, or renal tubular acidosis may benefit from one of the liposomal amphotericin B preparations. In particular, Ambisome has been well tolerated at doses ranging from 7.5 to 22.5 mg/kg/day (Walsh et al., 2001) in trials in adults. Ambisome has also been used in neonates (Juster-Reicher et al., 2000; Weitkamp et al., 1998). However, some liposomal preparations may be too large to penetrate the kidney; at least three cases of persistent renal candidiasis have failed to resolve until treatment was changed from a liposomal preparation (Abelcet) to amphotericin B desoxycholate (Hell et al., 1999).

Patients with concomitant candidal meningitis may benefit from the addition of 5-fluorocytosine (FC) in doses up to 100 mg/kg/day; levels of 5-FC should be kept under 25 µg in order to avoid bone marrow suppression or hepatotoxicity. Although 5-FC should never be used alone because of the rapid development of resistance, its ability to penetrate the CSF makes it an ideal adjunct in cases of meningitis. No data from in vitro or in vivo studies suggest that the combination of amphotericin B and an azole is superior to amphotericin B alone.

Hepatosplenic Candidiasis

Hepatosplenic candidiasis, a chronic form of disseminated candidiasis that arises as neutropenia resolves, has been associated with fever and infected abscesses in the liver or spleen detected by CT or magnetic resonance imaging (Thaler et al., 1988; Pastakia et al., 1988). This process is thought to involve silent seeding of the liver and spleen during the period of neutropenia. Because of intermittent courses of antifungal agents during phases of neutropenia, cultures from abscesses are negative approximately 75% of the time, although fungal elements may be visualized on wet mount. Prolonged courses of systemic amphotericin B (0.5 mg/kg/day) often extending for 6 months or more are required for resolution or calcification of the lesions (Semelka et al., 1992; Sallah et al., 1998; Walsh et al., 1995). If the patient has received amphotericin B during the period of neutropenia immediately preceding recognition of the infection, the dose of amphotericin B should be increased to 0.75 to 1.0 mg/kg/day,

and 5-FC should be added. Progressive or refractory infection may require the use of liposomal preparations of amphotericin B, fluconazole, or itraconazole.

Opportunistic Fungi

Other opportunists also infect the compromised host. Presentations are varied, and management strategies are complex. For an excellent discussion, the reader is referred to a review (Gaur and Flynn, 2001). *Aspergillus fumigatus* and *Aspergillus flavus* are the most common species in invasive pulmonary aspergillosis and in the disseminated form of this disease, which may extend to bones or brain as well. Both of these manifestations are seen only in immunocompromised patients, as is rhinocerebral aspergillosis or isolated cerebral abscess. Invasive pulmonary infection occurs as a consequence of inhalation of conidia from the environment during prolonged neutropenia. Procedures such as CT may be required in order to visualize the pleural-based nodules that are the hallmark of this disease. Because the fungus is virtually never cultured from the bloodstream, diagnosis is typically delayed without biopsy of lung tissue; isolation of the organism from bronchoalveolar lavage is helpful when it has tested positive, but the sensitivity is low (approximately 60%). Therapy with systemic amphotericin B at 1.5 mg/kg/day or with high doses of liposomal preparation (e.g., Ambisome at greater than 15 mg/kg/day) is often unavailing, especially if neutrophils do not return.

Cutaneous aspergillosis occurs far more frequently in the immunocompromised host, but rare reports have involved normal children whose skin was damaged by severe abrasions, as in auto accidents, or by contaminated dressings.

Locally invasive and systemic infections due to *Mucormycosis* and other emerging pathogens such as *Fusarium, Petriellidium boydii, Alternaria*, or *Curvularia* may also occur in the immunocompromised host (Gaur and Flynn, 2001). Resistance of amphotericin B occurs frequently with fungi such as *Fusarium solani* and *Penicillium marneffei*, and other fungicidal agents are unfortunately lacking. Surgical excision of disease localized to lung or kidneys may prove helpful in decreasing fungal burden in immunocompromised hosts and may be essential if drug resistance is encountered. A detailed discussion of presentation, treatment, and outcomes in these relatively rare fungal infections is presented elsewhere.

FUNGAL INFECTIONS IN HIV DISEASE

Fungal infections in HIV-infected children are both a diagnostic hallmark and a complication of the disease (Pirofski, 2001). Children exhibiting these infections typically have markedly reduced cellular immune function and may have, as accompanying risk factors, nutritional compromise, presence of intravascular catheters, damage or disruption of epithelial barriers in the skin or the intestine, and antibiotic-induced changes of the bacterial microflora. Although invasive fungal infections in HIV-infected children are much less common than in adults, disease attributable to commensal organisms like *Candida*, ubiquitous fungi such as *Aspergillus* or *Cryptococcus neoformans*, and endemic fungi such as *Histoplasma capsulatum*, *C. immitis*, and *P. marneffei* have all been described. Lengthening life span ascrib-

able to the use of highly active antiretroviral therapy means that more children will likely be exposed to these consequences. Current treatment regimens are summarized in Table 11-3.

Infections with *Candida* Species

As commensals of the gastrointestinal tract, *Candida* species are typically acquired by vertical transmission from the mother at or around the time of birth. Numerous prospective studies have emphasized that at least 80% of full-term infants are colonized with *Candida* by 3 to 4 weeks of age (Baley, 1991) and as many as 30% of adults may be colonized (Lundstrom and Sobel, 2001). The organism typically resides quiescently in the gastrointestinal tract unless the function of T lymphocytes or neutrophils is compromised.

In contrast to the predilection for candidemia or disseminated disease in the neutropenic host, HIV-infected children with a deficiency in T-lymphocyte function typically

---

TABLE 11-3   Fungal Infections in the HIV-infected Child

Disease	Causative organisms	Treatment
Candida Infections		
Mucocutaneous candidiasis	*Candida albicans*; other species emerging	Fluconazole, 6 mg/kg/d PO
Esophagitis	*C. albicans*; other species emerging	Parenteral amphotericin B, 1.0 mg/kg/d
Disseminated candidiasis	*C. albicans*; other species emerging	Parenteral amphotericin B, 1.0 mg/kg/d Remove central venous catheter
Other Fungal Infections		

Cryptococcosis
  Pulmonary
  Meningoencephalitis
	Cryptococcus neoformans	Parenteral amphotericin B, 1.0 mg/kg/d PLUS flucytosine 100 mg/kg/d for induction, then fluconazole 12 mg/kg/d PO for maintenance

Aspergillosis	*Aspergillus fumigatus, Aspergillus flavus*	Parenteral amphotericin B, 1.5 mg/kg/d PLUS itraconazole 5-12 mg/kg/d PO
Coccidioidomycosis	*Coccidioides immitis*	Fluconazole 8-12 mg/kg/d for localized disease; parenteral amphotericin B, 1.0 mg/kg/d for disseminated disease
Histoplasmosis Penicilliosis	*Histoplasma capsulatum* *Penicillium marneffei*	Parenteral amphotericin B, 1.0 mg/kg/d for localized disease; add itraconazole, 5-12 mg/kg/d PO for disseminated disease

have mucocutaneous candidiasis of the oropharynx or the esophagus as a presenting sign.

Oropharyngeal candidiasis manifests as expanding plaquelike lesions that extend throughout the oral cavity and must be differentiated from Epstein-Barr virus–associated hairy leukoplakia. Esophageal candidiasis may occur contiguously with oral disease or as an isolated phenomenon, either asymptomatic or symptomatic. Painful swallowing or retrosternal chest pains are typical manifestations. Therapies for oropharyngeal candidiasis in HIV-infected children include nystatin, amphotericin B suspension, or fluconazole, the latter agent now the drug of choice. Children whose esophageal symptoms fail to respond to parenteral amphotericin B should be evaluated for the presence of concomitant herpes simplex or cytomegalovirus.

The incidence of candidemia in HIV infected children is approximately 6% to 7%, and the presence of a central venous catheter and concomitant bacteremia are the predominant risk factors (Pirofski, 2001). Prolonged prophylaxis with oral ketoconazole or fluconazole was associated with 50% of the cases of disseminated candidiasis in another study. Although occurring only rarely, in HIV-infected children, the presence of candidemia or disseminated candidiasis should be treated with parenteral amphotericin B and prompt removal of the central venous catheter.

Cryptococcosis

Infection with *C. neoformans*, a ubiquitous intracellular yeast, is associated with use of corticosteroids, lymphoproliferative disease, and late stage HIV infection (Pirofski, 2001). Acquisition of the organism in early childhood has been documented by seroprevalence studies, and both cellular and humoral arms of immune defense of the immune system are involved in host defense. The prevalence of *Cryptococcus* in HIV-infected children is approximately 1%. Infection with the organism manifests as meningoencephalitis, cryptococcemia, or disseminated cryptococcosis. The median age of onset in two studies is between and 8 and 11.8 years (Pirofski, 2001), suggesting that prolonged survival associated with improved antiretroviral viral therapy may make cryptococcosis a more common complication of pediatric HIV disease.

Diagnosis requires positive cultures from blood or cerebrospinal fluid. Positive cryptococcal antigen titers can be a helpful adjunct, but the diagnosis should not be discarded if the antigen titers are negative. Recommendations for treatment are derived from adult regimens and include induction therapy with parenteral amphotericin B and 5-FC, followed by fluconazole (12 mg/kg/day) for consolidation and maintenance therapy.

Aspergillosis

Aspergillus species are acquired by inhalation of the mold from soil or water. The major risk factor for disseminated aspergillosis is defects in neutrophil number or function, but cellular immunity and steroid therapy are additional risk factors. Although the prevalence of aspergillosis in HIV-infected children is extremely low at less than 1%, manifestations of infection include invasive pulmonary aspergillosis and central nervous system disease. Diagnosis requires the presence of branching hyphae on Gomori's methenamine silver stain of involved tissue. Blood cultures are virtually always negative, but isolation from bronchoscopy in children with infiltrates, consolidation, or pleural nodules on chest radiograph or CT scan is extremely helpful. Treatment includes amphotericin B at doses up to 1.5 mg/kg/day, with itraconazole at 5 to 12 mg/kg/day used concomitantly or secondarily for maintenance. On the basis of regimens employed for chronic granulomatous disease, the use of interferon-α white blood cell transfusions, or granulocyte colony-stimulating factor has been proposed, but the efficacy has not been demonstrated in HIV-infected children.

Histoplasmosis, coccidiomycosis, and penicilliosis are uncommonly encountered outside of areas of edemicity. Histoplasmosis is found most frequently in the Ohio and Mississippi River Valley, coccidiomycosis in the southwestern United States, and *P. marneffei* in Southeast Asia and China. In the HIV-infected patient, histoplasmosis may manifest as acute pulmonary disease, cavitary lung disease, or disseminated disease, the latter an AIDS-defining infection. Diagnosis requires culture of the organism from bone marrow, blood, respiratory secretions, or deep tissue. Antigen detection in urine or serum may be helpful in diagnosis and for monitoring the response to therapy. Parenteral amphotericin B at doses up to 1 mg/kg/day with the addition of itraconazole (5 to 12 mg/kg/day) is required. Daily itraconazole prophylaxis is effective in preventing relapse. Fluconazole has no activity.

The focus of coccidioidal disease in HIV-infected children is the lung, with fever and dyspnea the presenting complaints. Chest x-rays most frequently show diffuse, bilateral, reticulonodular infiltrates. Diagnosis requires culture of the organism from sputum, bronchoalveolar lavage fluid, or tissue. Blood cultures are virtually never positive. The incidence of disseminated coccidioidomycosis is increasing in adults with HIV infection, but only one study has evaluated the infection in immunocompromised children, and this was prior to the onset of the HIV epidemic. Disease localized to one lung can be treated with fluconazole in doses of 8 to 12 mg/kg/day, but disseminated disease requires amphotericin B in doses up to 1.0 mg/kg/day.

Penicilliosis is now frequently recognized in HIV-infected individuals from Southeast Asia whose presenting symptoms are fever, cough, and papular skin lesions with central umbilications similar to molluscum contagiosum. The organism can be isolated from blood or skin lesions, bone marrow, or lymph node biopsies. Characteristic skin lesions should prompt the initiation of therapy with amphotericin B in doses up to 1.0 mg/kg/day. For disseminated disease, itraconazole (5 to 12 mg/kg/day) is the treatment of choice. Unfortunately, disease due to *P. marneffei* is unresponsive to therapy in approximately 20% of HIV-infected patients, and responders relapse with disappointing frequency (Shenep JL Flynn PM, 1997).

BIBLIOGRAPHY

Baley JE. Neonatal candidiasis: the current challenge. Clin Perinatol 1991;18:263-280.

Baley JE, Kliegman RM, Fanaroff AA. Disseminated fungal infections in very low–birth-weight infants: clinical manifestations and epidemiology. Pediatrics 1984;73:144-152.

Bendel CM, Hostetter M. Systemic candidiasis and other fungal infections in the newborn. Semin Pediatr Infect Dis 1994;5:35-41.

Bennett JE. Chemotherapy of systemic mycoses (first of two parts). N Engl J Med 1974a;290:30-32.

Bennett JE. Chemotherapy of systemic mycoses (second of two parts). N Engl J Med 1974b;290:320-332.

Boxer LA, Morganroth ML. Neutrophil function disorders. Dis Mon 1987;33:681-780.

Brueton MJ, Ormerod LP, Shah KJ, Anderson CM. Allergic bronchopulmonary aspergillosis complicating cystic fibrosis in childhood. Arch Dis Child 1980;55:348-353.

Cesaro S, Rossetti F, Perilongo G, et al. Fluconazole prophylaxis and *Candida* fungemia in neutropenic children with malignancies. Haematologica 1993;78:249-251.

Chapman RL, Faix RG. Persistently positive cultures and outcome in invasive neonatal candidiasis. Pediatr Infect Dis J 2000;19:822-7.

Cohen MS, Isturiz RE, Malech HL, et al. Fungal infection in chronic granulomatous disease. The importance of the phagocyte in defense against fungi. Am J Med 1981;71:59-66.

Dismukes WE, Bradsher RW Jr, Cloud GC, et al. Itraconazole therapy for blastomycosis and histoplasmosis. The National Institute for Allergy and Infectious Diseases (NIAID) Mycoses Study Group. Am J Med 1992;93:489-497.

Donowitz LG, Hendley JO. Short-course amphotericin B therapy for candidemia in pediatric patients. Pediatrics 1995;95:888-891.

Eppes SC, Troutman JL, Gutman LT. Outcome of treatment of candidemia in children whose central catheters were removed or retained. Pediatr Infect Dis J 1989;8:99-104.

Faix RG. Invasive neonatal candidiasis: comparison of albicans and parapsilosis infection. Pediatr Infect Dis J 1992;11:88-93.

Fischer JF, Hicks BC, Dipiro JT. Efficacy of a single intravenous dose of amphotericin B in urinary tract infections caused by *Candida*. J Infect Dis 1987;156:685-687.

Gaither TA, Medley SR, Gallin JI, Frank MM. Studies of phagocytosis in chronic granulomatous disease. Inflammation 1987;11:211-227.

Gan VN, Petruska M, Ginsburg CM. Epidemiology and treatment of tinea capitis: ketoconazole vs griseofulvin. Pediatr Infect Dis J 1987;6:46-49.

Gaur A, Flynn P. Emerging fungal infections in the immunocompromised host. Semin Pediatr Infect Dis 2001;12:279-287.

Ginsburg CM, Gan VN, Petruska M. Randomized controlled trial of intralesional corticosteroid and griseofulvin vs griseofulvin alone for treatment of kerion. Pediatr Infect Dis J 1987;6:1084-1087.

Goodman JL, Winston DJ, Greenfield RA, et al. A controlled trial of fluconazole to prevent fungal infections in patients undergoing bone marrow transplantation. N Engl J Med 1992;326:845-851.

Gupta AK, Adam P, Dlova N, et al. Therapeutic options for the treatment of tinea capitis caused by *Trichophyton* species: griseofulvin versus the new oral antifungal agents, terbinafine, itraconazole, and fluconazole. Pediatr Dermatol 2001;18:433-438.

Guze LB, Harley LD. Fungus infections of the urinary tract. Yale J Biol Med 1957;30:292-305.

Hell W, Kern T, Klouche M. Failure of a lipid amphotericin B preparation to eradicate candiduria: preliminary findings based on three cases. Clin Infect Dis 1999;29:686-687.

Johnson DE, Thompson TR, Ferrieri P. Congenital candidiasis. Am J Dis Child 1981;135:273-275.

Juster-Reicher A, Leibovitz E, Linder N, et al. Liposomal amphotericin B (AmBisome) in the treatment of neonatal candidiasis in very low birth weight infants. Infection 2000;28:223-226.

Karlowicz MG, Hashimoto LN, Kelly RE Jr, Buescher ES. Should central venous catheters be removed as soon as candidemia is detected in neonates? Pediatrics 2000;106:E63.

Kauffman CA, Vazquez JA, Sobel JD, et al. Prospective multicenter surveillance study of funguria in hospitalized patients. The National Institute for Allergy and Infectious Diseases (NIAID) Mycoses Study Group. Clin Infect Dis 2000;30:14-18.

Kaufman D, Boyle R, Hazen KC, et al. Fluconazole prophylaxis against fungal colonization and infection in preterm infants. N Engl J Med 2001;345:1660-1666.

Kim MH, Rodey GE, Good RA, et al. Defective candidacidal capacity of polymorphonuclear leukocytes in chronic granulomatous disease of childhood. J Pediatr 1969;75:300-303.

Klein BS, Jones JM. Isolation, purification, and radiolabeling of a novel 120-kD surface protein on *Blastomyces dermatitidis* yeasts to detect antibody in infected patients. J Clin Invest 1990;85:152-161.

Leibovitz E, Iuster-Reicher A, Amitai M, Mogilner B. Systemic candidal infections associated with use of peripheral venous catheters in neonates: a 9-year experience. Clin Infect Dis 1992;14:485-491.

Little J, Bruce J, Andrews H, et al. Treatment of disseminated infantile histoplasmosis with amphotericin B. Pediatrics 1959;24:1-3.

Ludviksson BR, Thorarensen O, Gudnason, et al. *Candida albicans* meningitis in a child with myeloperoxidase deficiency. Pediatr Infect Dis J 1993;12:162-164.

Lundstrom T, Sobel J. Nosocomial candiduria: a review. Clin Infect Dis 2001;32:1602-1607.

Martinez-Roig A, Torres-Rodriguez JM, Bartlett-Coma A. Double blind study of ketoconazole and griseofulvin in dermatophytoses. Pediatr Infect Dis J 1988;7:37-40.

Mermel LA. Prevention of intravascular catheter-related infections. Ann Intern Med 2000;132:391-402.

Mermel LA, Farr BM, Sherertz RJ, et al. Guidelines for the management of intravascular catheter-related infections. Clin Infect Dis 2001;32:1249-1272.

Noyola DE, Fernandez M, Moylett EH, Baker CJ. Ophthalmologic, visceral, and cardiac involvement in neonates with candidemia. Clin Infect Dis 2001;32:1018-1023.

Nucci M, Anaissie E. Revisiting the source of candidemia: skin or gut? Clin Infect Dis 2001;33:1959-1967.

Oldfield EC III, Bone WD, Martin CR, et al. Prediction of relapse after treatment of coccidioidomycosis. Clin Infect Dis 1997;25:1205-1210.

Pastakia B, Shawker TH, Thaler M, et al. Hepatosplenic candidiasis: wheels within wheels. Radiology 1988;166:417-421.

Pirofski L. Fungal infections in children with human immunodeficiency virus infection. Semin Pediatr Infect Dis 2001;12:288-295.

Platt R, Polk BF, Murdock B, Rosner B. Risk factors for nosocomial urinary tract infection. Am J Epidemiol 1986;124:977-985.

Rabalais GP, Samiec TD, Bryant KK, Lewis JJ. Invasive candidiasis in infants weighing more than 2,500 grams at birth admitted to a neonatal intensive care unit. Pediatr Infect Dis J 1996;15:348-352.

Rasmussen JE, Ahmed AR. *Trichophyton* reactions in children with tinea capitis. Arch Dermatol 1978;114:371-372.

Rex JH, Walsh TJ, Sobel JD, et al. Practice guidelines for the treatment of candidiasis. Infects Diseases Society of America. Clin Infect Dis 2000;30:662-678.

Saiman L, Ludington E, Dawson JD, et al. Risk factors for *Candida* species colonization of neonatal intensive care unit patients. Pediatr Infect Dis J 2001;20:1119-1124.

Saiman L, Ludington E, Pfaller M, et al. Risk factors for candidemia in Neonatal Intensive Care Unit patients. The National Epidemiology of Mycosis Survey study group. Pediatr Infect Dis J 2000;19(4):319-24.

Sallah S, Semelka R, Kelekis N, et al. Diagnosis and monitoring response to treatment of hepatosplenic candidiasis in patients with acute leukemia using magnetic resonance imaging. Acta Haematol 1998;100:77-81.

Schwartz ME. Barn itch. Am Fam Physician 1983;27:149-153.

Semelka RC, Shoenut JP, Greenberg HM, Bow EJ. Detection of acute and treated lesions of hepatosplenic candidiasis: comparison of dynamic contrast-enhanced CT and MR imaging. J Magn Reson Imaging 1992;2:341-345.

Shenup JL, Flynn PM. Pulmonary fungal infections in immunocompromised children. Curr Opin Pediatr 1997;9:213-218.

Stocker WW, Richtsmeier AJ, Rozycki AA, Baughman RD. Kerion caused by *Trichophyton verrucosum*. Pediatrics 1977;59:912-915.

Stoll BJ, Gordon T, Korones SB, et al. Late-onset sepsis in very low birth weight neonates: a report from the National Institute of Child Health and Human Development Neonatal Research Network. J Pediatr 1996;129:63-71.

Tesh R, Shacklette M, Diercks F, Hirschl D. Histoplasmosis in children. Pediatrics 1964;56:894-903.

Thaler M, Pastakia B, Shawker TH, et al. Hepatic candidiasis in cancer patients: the evolving picture of the syndrome. Ann Intern Med 1988;108:88-100.

Verfaillie C, Weisdorf D, Haake R, et al. *Candida* infections in bone marrow transplant recipients. Bone Marrow Transplant 1991;8:177-184.

Walsh TJ, Goodman JL, Pappas P, et al. Safety, tolerance, and pharmacokinetics of high-dose liposomal amphotericin B (AmBisome) in patients infected with *Aspergillus* species and other filamentous fungi: maximum tolerated dose study. Antimicrob Agents Chemother 2001;45:3487-3496.

Walsh TJ, Whitcomb PO, Revankar SG, Pizzo PA. Successful treatment of hepatosplenic candidiasis through repeated cycles of chemotherapy and neutropenia. Cancer 1995;76:2357-2362.

Wang JN, Liu CC, Huang TZ, et al. Laryngeal candidiasis in children. Scand J Infect Dis 1997;29:427-429.

Weitkamp JH, Poets CF, Sievers R, et al. *Candida* infection in very low–birth-weight infants: outcome and nephrotoxicity of treatment with liposomal amphotericin B (AmBisome). Infection 1998;26:11-15.

Whyte RK, Hussain Z, deSa D. Antenatal infections with *Candida* species. Arch Dis Child 1982;57:528-535.

Williams AJ, Baghat MS, Stableforth DE, et al. Dysphonia caused by inhaled steroids: recognition of a characteristic laryngeal abnormality. Thorax 1983;38:813-821.

Wilson W, Gibson A: Azoles for allergic bronchopulmonary aspergillosis associated with asthma (Cochrane Review). Cochrane Database Syst Rev 2001;4.

Wingard JR, Merz WG, Rinaldi MG, et al. Increase in infection among patients with bone marrow transplantation and neutropenia treated prophylactically with fluconazole. N Engl J Med 1991;325:1274-1277.

Wolach B, Bogger-Goren S, Whyte R. Perinatal hematological profile of newborn infants with *Candida* antenatal infections. Biol Neonate 1991;59:5-12.

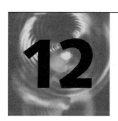

INFECTIONS OF THE GASTROINTESTINAL TRACT

LARRY K. PICKERING AND THOMAS G. CLEARY

Acute infectious gastroenteritis is one of the most common infectious diseases of humans, ranking second to acute respiratory tract infections as a worldwide cause of morbidity. In developing areas of the world, diarrhea is a significant cause of death in infants. Young children in developing countries experience approximately 1.5 billion episodes of diarrhea and 3.5 million associated deaths each year (Bern et al., 1992; Claeson and Merson, 1990). In the United States 20 to 35 million episodes of diarrhea occur every year, resulting in 2.1 to 3.7 million physician visits. In addition, an average of 220,000 children younger than 5 years of age with diarrhea are hospitalized in the United States, and approximately 125 deaths occur each year as a result of gastroenteritis (Cicirello and Glass, 1994). Approximately 76 million cases of foodborne illness in all ages occur per year in the United States, of which 300,000 manifest as acute diarrhea (Mead et al., 1999). Hospitalization and outpatient care for pediatric diarrhea result in direct costs of more than $2 billion per year, with additional indirect costs to families (Avendano et al., 1993). The usual clinical syndrome is characterized by various combinations of nausea, vomiting, abdominal cramps, and diarrhea; fever and dehydration also may be present. Occasionally, systemic manifestations occur, including bacteremia, neurologic manifestations, and immune-mediated extraintestinal manifestations of enteric infections.

Practice guidelines for management of infectious diarrhea have been published by the Infectious Diseases Society of America (IDSA) (Guerrant et al., 2001). Other evidence-based recommendations include guidelines for management of acute gastroenteritis in young children developed by the American Academy of

Pediatrics (American Academy of Pediatrics, 1996); guidelines on acute diarrhea in adults (DuPont et al., 1997); a primer for physicians dealing with diagnosis and management of foodborne illness developed jointly by the American Medical Association (AMA), the Centers for Disease Control and Prevention (CDC), the U.S. Food and Drug Administration (FDA) and the U.S. Department of Agriculture (Centers for Disease Control and Prevention, 2001); and guidelines for prevention of opportunistic infections among human immunodeficiency virus (HIV)–infected persons developed by the U.S. Public Health Service (USPHS) and the IDSA (Centers for Disease Control and Prevention, 2002b); (Table 12-1). The causative agents include bacteria, viruses, and parasites (Box 12-1). Bacterial and viral causes of diarrhea are reviewed in this chapter; parasitic causes of diarrhea are discussed in Chapter 13.

BACTERIAL GASTROENTERITIS

Bacterial agents associated with diarrhea that are discussed include *Aeromonas* species, *Campylobacter* species, *Clostridium difficile*, *Escherichia coli*, *Salmonella* species, *Shigella* species, *Vibrio cholerae*, and *Yersinia enterocolitica*. Some of these bacterial pathogens are identified routinely in microbiology laboratories, whereas others require specialized media or growth conditions. Fluid replacement is critical in all persons with diarrhea, and appropriate antimicrobial therapy may favorably alter the course of illness associated with some enteropathogens.

Etiology

Many bacteria are associated with diarrhea in humans (Box 12-1) and vary in importance according to host factors, including immune status, geography, epidemiologic considerations,

TABLE 12-1   Evidence-based Medical Data Sources for Diarrheal Disease

Guideline	Organization
Diarrhea in adults[*]	American College of Gastroenterology
Acute gastroenteritis in children[†]	American Academy of Pediatrics
Diarrhea practice guidelines[‡]	Infectious Diseases Society of America
Primer on foodborne disease[§]	American Medical Association
	Centers for Disease Control and Prevention
	Food and Drug Administration
	U.S. Department of Agriculture
Prevention opportunistic infections[‖]	Infectious Diseases Society of America
	U.S. Public Health Service

[*]DuPont HL, Practice Parameters Committee of the American College of Gastroenterology. Guidelines on acute diarrhea in adults. Am J Gastroenterol 1997;92:1962-1975.
[†]American Academy of Pediatrics, Subcommittee on Acute Gastroenteritis. Practice parameter: the management of acute gastroenteritis in young children. Pediatrics 1996;97:424-436.
[‡]Guerrant RL, VanGilder T, Steiner TS, et al. Practice guidelines for the management of infectious diarrhea. Infectious Diseases Society of America. Clin Infect Dis 2001;32:331-350.
[§]Centers for Disease Control and Prevention. Diagnosis and management of foodborne illnesses: a primer for physicians. MMWR 2001;50:1-69.
[‖]Centers for Disease Control and Prevention. Guidelines for preventing opportunistic infections among HIV-infected persons 2002. MMWR 2002b;51:1-52.

and virulence mechanisms. Organisms are discussed here in alphabetic order.

Aeromonas *species.* Aeromonas species are composed of gram-negative bacilli that are found in soil and fresh and brackish water worldwide. These organisms are associated with several disease states in humans, including soft-tissue infections, bacteremia, and gastroenteritis. The association of *Aeromonas* species with gastroenteritis is controversial, but evidence shows that *A. hydrophila, A. caviae,* and *A. veronii* are associated with gastroenteritis (Janda and Abbott, 1998). *Aeromonas* species possess several colonization factors and elaborate a large number of extracellular enzymes, including enterotoxins that are thought to play a prominent role in *Aeromonas*-associated gastroenteritis (Sears and Kaper, 1996).

Campylobacter *species.* Campylobacter species are composed of gram-negative bacilli that are recognized as one of the most frequent causes of acute bacterial diarrhea throughout the world (Allos, 2001; Jimenez et al., 1999) and are one of the most frequently identified organism in the FoodNet program (Centers for Disease Control and Prevention, 2002a). *C. jejuni* is a major cause of bacterial diarrhea in the United States, but other species—including *C. coli, C. fetus, C. lari, C. hyointestinalis,* and *C. upsaliensis*—also have been associated with diarrhea and occasionally with invasive disease

in humans. Animals, specifically poultry and cattle, are the reservoirs of *C. jejuni,* which generally is associated with foodborne disease. In most laboratories *C. coli* is identified as *C. jejuni. C. fetus* is an uncommon cause of disease in humans, but when infection occurs this organism produces fever, bacteremia, and meningitis, usually in immunocompromised hosts and neonates.

Clostridium difficile. *C. difficile* is a spore-forming gram-positive anaerobic bacillus that produces two exotoxins: toxin A, an enterotoxin, and toxin B, a cytotoxin. The organism causes gastrointestinal tract infections in humans that range in severity from asymptomatic colonization to severe diarrhea, pseudomembranous colitis, toxic megacolon, colonic perforation, and death (Bartlett, 1994; Gerding et al., 1995; Kelly et al., 1994). Toxin-producing *C. difficile* frequently is recovered from stools of asymptomatic infants during their first year of life, among whom 25% to 65% may be colonized; colonization rates decrease to 0% to 5% in older children and adults. Toxigenic *C. difficile* is a cause of antibiotic-associated diarrhea in adults, but the role of *C. difficile* in childhood illness, especially in infants, remains controversial (Cerquetti et al., 1995; Mitchell et al., 1995b). *C. difficile* can be isolated from soil and frequently is present in the hospital environment.

BOX 12-1

ETIOLOGY OF ACUTE GASTROENTERITIS

Bacteria

Aeromonas spp.
Bacillus cereus
Campylobacter jejuni
Campylobacter coli
Clostridium difficile
Clostridium perfringens
Escherichia coli
Plesiomonas shigelloides
Salmonella spp.
Shigella spp.
Vibrio cholerae
Vibrio parahaemolyticus
Yersinia enterocolitica

Viruses

Enteric adenovirus (types 40 and 41)
Astrovirus
Caliciviruses
Rotavirus

Parasites

Protozoa
Cryptosporidium parvum
Cyclospora cayetanensis
Entamoeba histolytica
Giardia lamblia
Isospora belli
Microsporida *(Enterocytozoon bieneusi,
    Encephalitozoon intestinalis)*
Helminths
Capillaria philippinensis
Schistosoma spp.
Strongyloides stercoralis
Trichinella spiralis
Trichuris trichiura

Escherichia coli. *E. coli* is a gram-negative bacillus that commonly inhabits the intestine and ordinarily causes no clinical symptoms. Although isolation of *E. coli* is not difficult, recognition of pathogenic strains is complex because of the multiple factors that enable this organism to cause disease and the methods needed to establish a diagnosis. Specific recognition of pathogenic strains is accomplished readily in research or reference laboratories; therefore laboratory confirmation of gastrointestinal tract disease caused by *E. coli*, other than *E. coli* O157:H7, generally is not available.

In 1951 *E. coli* organisms were shown as serologically heterogeneous by Kauffman, who divided the species into various somatic groups. *E. coli* possesses O (somatic) antigens, H (flagellar) antigens, and K (capsular) antigens. The serotype, which is a chromosomally determined characteristic, depends on these antigens.

E. coli strains that cause diarrhea currently are grouped according to their pathogenic phenotype(s) (Nataro and Kaper 1998). The provisional classification includes Shiga toxin–producing *E. coli* (STEC), which elaborates toxins that inhibit protein synthesis; enterotoxigenic *E. coli* (ETEC), which elaborates enterotoxins; enteroinvasive *E. coli* (EIEC), which invades the intestinal epithelium; enteropathogenic *E. coli* (EPEC), which demonstrates epithelial adherence and produces attaching and effacing lesions; and enteroaggregative *E. coli* (EAEC), which demonstrates a stacked-brick adherence to epithelial cells (Table 12-2). These categories of *E. coli* are associated with different epidemiologic patterns and clinical syndromes.

Shiga Toxin–Producing *E. coli*. Infection with STEC produces bloody diarrhea and may

---

TABLE 12-2	*E. coli* Associated with Diarrhea

Classification	Pathogenic mechanism
Shiga toxin–producing *E. coli* (STEC)	Attaching and effacing lesion
	Shiga toxins
Enterotoxigenic *E. coli* (ETEC)	Heat-stable (ST) and heat-labile (LT) (cholera-like)
	enterotoxins that cause fluid loss
	Adhesins
Enteroinvasive *E. coli* (EIEC)	Invasion of intestinal cells
	Invasion plasmid is closely related to invasion plasmid of
	Shigellae
Enteropathogenic *E. coli* (EPEC)	Adhesins with production of attaching and effacing lesions
Enteroaggregative *E. coli* (EAEC)	Adhesins

progress to hemolytic-uremic syndrome (HUS). STEC also are referred to as *verotoxin E. coli* and *enterohemorrhagic E. coli* (EHEC). The most common STEC serotype in the United States is *E. coli* O157:H7, although many other STEC serotypes have been recognized worldwide. STEC produces Shiga toxin 1 (Stx 1), which is identical to the cytotoxin produced by *Shigella dysenteriae* type 1; a related toxin that is immunologically distinct and is called Shiga toxin 2 (Stx 2); and variants of these toxins that are related closely to Stx 2. Shortly after this class of *E. coli* was recognized, the distinctive hemorrhagic colitis associated with these organisms was shown to be complicated by development of HUS (Karmali et al., 1983). Although other causes for HUS exist, the majority of HUS cases are associated with STEC infection. Cattle are the most important animal reservoir of STEC, although many other animals can carry these organisms; humans also may serve as a reservoir for person-to-person transmission.

Enterotoxigenic *E. coli*. ETEC produces plasmid-encoded enterotoxins (Sears and Kaper, 1996). Although belonging to specific serogroups, ETEC organisms are not identified routinely by serotyping. The heat-labile enterotoxin (LT) and heat-stable enterotoxin (ST) produced by ETEC are characterized in Table 12-3. LT, like cholera toxin, activates adenylate cyclase. ST activates guanylate cyclase, with a resulting increase in cyclic guanosine monophosphate (cGMP). Both LT and ST cause production of watery diarrhea without blood or mucus. Many of the ETEC strains possess specific adhesion factors enabling them to colonize the small intestine. Such colonization factor antigens contribute to disease production by these toxigenic bacteria. Colonization factors appear in electron microscopy as filamentous structures that often resemble fimbriae. ETEC cause disease in all ages, especially in infants and children living in developing countries, travelers from developed to developing countries, and victims of outbreaks of foodborne disease in the United States.

Enteroinvasive *E. coli*. EIEC organisms produce intestinal tract disease by their ability to penetrate and multiply within the intestinal epithelial cells. These enteroinvasive *E. coli* organisms resemble shigella in this respect and cause either a dysentery-like illness or watery diarrhea. Although these *E. coli* organisms tend to include certain serologic groups, serotyping to identify these organisms generally is not performed. Infections generally occur in adults; foodborne outbreaks have been reported (Olsen et al., 2000).

Enteropathogenic *E. coli*. Infection with EPEC is associated with both sporadic and epidemic diarrhea in infants, especially in developing countries. EPEC refers to those organisms that cause disease but do not produce LT or ST, do not have the genes coding for these toxins, and are not enteroinvasive. EPEC infection causes a distinct histopathologic lesion (referred to as the *attaching or effacing lesion*) in human intestine that involves destruction of microvilli and close adherence of bacteria to the membrane of the enterocyte with caplike pedestals upon which the bacteria rests. The genes responsible for this phenotype have been defined (Nataro and Kaper, 1998).

Enteroaggregative *E. coli*. EAEC has been associated with acute and chronic diarrhea in developing countries and in adults with traveler's diarrhea. Chronic persistent diarrhea is especially likely to be due to EAEC (Nataro and Kaper, 1998). EAEC organisms are defined by their aggregative or "stacked-brick" pattern of appearance in HEp-2 cell assays. Virulence mechanisms of EAEC remain poorly understood.

Salmonellae. The various terminologies used to classify salmonellae are confusing (Brenner, 2000). The two species of salmonella are *S. choleraesuis*, which includes six subspecies that contain almost all the serotypes pathogenic for humans, and *S. bongor*. Because *S. choleraesuis* refers to both a species and a serotype, the species designation *S. enterica* is recommended. Currently, *Salmonella* nomenclature is frequently shortened (e.g., *S. enterica* subspecies *enterica* serotype *typhimurium* can be shortened to *S. typhimurium*). During 2001, 40,495 *Salmonella* isolates and 368 cases of typhoid fever were reported to the CDC (Centers for Disease Control and Prevention, 2003). Of the known serotypes, the three most commonly reported were *S. typhimurium*, *S. enteritidis*, and *S. newport*, accounting for 50% of the isolates. Salmonellal gastroenteritis occurs throughout life but is most common in the first year. Reptiles—including turtles, snakes, lizards, and iguanas—have certain serotypes, such as *S. marina*, *S. poano*, *S. chameleon*, and *S. arizonae*, adapted to them. *S. typhi* and *S. paratyphi* are

TABLE 12-3 Diarrhea-associated Toxins

Characteristics of organism toxin	VIBRO CHOLERAE	ESCHERICHIA COLI		SHIGA TOXIN
	Cholera toxin	Labile toxin (LT)	Stable toxin (ST)	(Stx 1, Stx 2)
Molecular weight (MW)	85,600	73,000	2,000	71,000
Immunogenic	Yes	Yes	No	Yes
Genetic control of toxin	Chromosome Bacteriophage	Plasmid	Plasmid	Phage in STEC Chromosome in *S. dysenteriae*
Multimeric protein (A and B subunits)	Yes	Yes	No	Yes
A and B synthesized separately and then associated	Yes	Yes	—	Yes
B subunit binds to cell	Yes	Yes	—	Yes
Cell receptor	GM_1, ganglioside	GM_1, ganglioside	100,000 MW protein (not GM_1)	Galactose-α 1-4; galactose-β 1-4; glucose ceramide (Gb3)
Internalization	By noncoated surface microinvaginations	By noncoated surface microinvaginations	Unknown	By receptor-mediated endocytosis through coated pits
Subunit with enzymatic activity	Yes	Yes	—	Yes
Intracellular target site	Inner-surface plasma membrane	Inner-surface plasma membrane	Inner-surface plasma membrane	Cytosol
Action	Modification of plasma membrane enzymes	Modification of plasma membrane enzymes	Modification of plasma membrane enzymes	Cleaves adenine residue from membrane 28S ribosomal RNA
Enzyme affected	Activation of adenylate cyclase	Activation of adenylate cyclase	Activation of guanylate cyclase	Blocks attachment site for EF 1-dependent aminoacyl tRNA binding
Mode of action	NAD-dependent ADP ribosylation of GTP-binding compartment of adenylate cyclase	NAD-dependent ADP ribosylation of GTP-binding compartment of adenylate cyclase	Unknown	A1-catalyzed inactivation of the 28S ribosomal subunit
Site of action	Small intestine epithelium	Small intestine epithelium	Small intestine epithelium	Small and large intestine
Physiologic action	Absorption Secretion	Absorption Secretion	Absorption Secretion	Probably causes fluid loss through injury to enterocytes with decreased absorption

ADP, Adenosine diphosphate; *GTP*, guanosine triphosphate; *EF*, elongation factor; *NAD*, nicotinamide-adenine dinucleotide; *STEC*, Shiga toxin-producing *E. coli*; *Stx 1*, Shiga toxin 1; *Stx 2*, Shiga toxin 2.

highly adapted to humans and have no other natural hosts. For all other *Salmonella* strains a wide range of domestic and wild animals serve as reservoirs. Numerous outbreaks of disease due to salmonellae have been associated with contaminated food products (Olsen et al., 2000).

Shigellae. Four main serogroups compose the genus *Shigella*. Each group includes a number of types that are distinguished by biochemical and serologic criteria: group A, *S. dysenteriae*; group B, *S. flexneri*; group C, *S. boydii*; and group D, *S. sonnei*. Group D accounts for approximately 80% of the episodes of shigellosis in the United States. *S. boydii* and *S. dysenteriae* are uncommon causes of diarrhea in the United States.

The human intestinal tract is the natural habitat of shigellae. A specific virulence plasmid is necessary for the epithelial-cell invasiveness manifested by shigellae. *S. dysenteriae* type 1 (Shiga bacillus) produces a protein synthesis–inhibiting toxin (Shiga toxin) (Bartlett et al., 1986). Other shigellae make little or no Shiga toxin. STEC produce a toxin either essentially identical to Shiga toxin (Stx 1) or less closely related (Stx 2). Shiga toxin recognizes a receptor, globotriaosylceramide (Gb3), in sensitive cells and is translocated by endocytosis to the cytoplasm, where it blocks protein synthesis. The only significant reservoir of shigellae is humans, although primates may become infected. Infection may occur from person-to-person contact and through contaminated food and water. Infection is most common from 6 months to 10 years of age.

Vibrio cholerae. *V. cholerae* O1 and O139 consist of gram-negative bacilli that may cause sudden, profuse, watery diarrhea that can progress to rapid dehydration, acidosis, and death. The biotypes of *V. cholerae* O1 (classic and El Tor) each include organisms of Inaba, Ogawa, and (rarely) Hikojima serotypes. All clinical isolates of *V. cholerae* O1 from the United States have been biotype El Tor, serotype Inaba. Most strains were acquired outside the United States, with the remainder isolated from people who had eaten contaminated raw and undercooked shellfish from the Gulf of Mexico. In South America an epidemic of cholera caused by El Tor biotype *V. cholerae* O1 began in 1991.

In 1992 large-scale epidemics of cholera were reported in India and Bangladesh. The causative agent was *V. cholerae* O139. This organism elaborates the same cholera toxin but differs from the O1 strains in the lipopolysaccharide structure. Cholera strains that are not classified as O1 or O139 are referred to as *non-O1 strains* (nonagglutinating or noncholera *Vibrio*). These strains generally do not elaborate enterotoxin, are not associated with large outbreaks, and occasionally cause sporadic disease. The reservoirs of *V. cholerae* are humans and copepods and other zooplankton in brackish water or estuaries. *V. cholerae* O1 and O139 produce a heat-labile enterotoxin that activates adenylate cyclase and catalyzes the formation of cyclic adenosine monophosphate (AMP), which results in the secretion of fluid and electrolytes into the lumen of the intestine.

Other *Vibrio* species associated with acute diarrheal illness include *V. hollisae*, *V. parahaemolyticus*, *V. furnissii*, *V. fluvialis*, and *V. mimicus*. Clinical manifestations of infection with *V. parahaemolyticus* are gastroenteritis (59%), wound infection (34%), and septicemia (5%) (Daniels et al., 2000). *V. vulnificus* has been associated with gastroenteritis following ingestion of raw oysters, although this organism generally is associated with wound infection and may produce a severe and fatal illness in patients who are immunocompromised (Centers for Disease Control and Prevention, 1996c).

Yersinia *species.* The genus *Yersinia* includes *Y. pestis*, *Y. pseudotuberculosis*, *Y. enterocolitica*, and other environmental species that are rarely human pathogens. *Y. enterocolitica* is a gram-negative bacillus that is an uncommon cause of diarrhea, mesenteric adenitis, and extraintestinal infection in the United States. *Y. pseudotuberculosis* has been associated with abdominal pain. Fifty serotypes and several biotypes and phage types of *Y. enterocolitica* have been reported and inhabit the intestinal tract of many animals and birds and survive in fresh water. Strains pathogenic for humans vary by geographic location and include strains in serotypes 0:3, 0:4, 0:8, 0:9, 0:13, 0:18, 0:20, and 0:21, and biotypes 1, 2, 3, and 4. Serotypes causing diseases may vary in different geographic areas; types 0:3 and 0:8 are responsible for most outbreaks in the United States. Outbreaks have been reported following ingestion of contaminated milk or food such as chitterlings. Laboratory personnel must be alerted to the possibility that this organism is being considered as a potential pathogen so that appropriate selective media can be used for isolation. Animals, especially pigs, are the principal reservoir of *Y. enterocolitica*.

Some reports suggest that other bacteria, such as *Listeria monocytogenes*, cause diarrhea (Hof, 2001, Aureli et al., 2000).

Epidemiology

Bacterial enteropathogens are transmitted by the fecal-oral route, either through contaminated food or water or by person-to-person spread. The mode of transmission depends on the organism and the immune status of the host. In immunocompetent hosts a large inoculum is necessary for infection with virtually all bacteria, generally requiring ingestion of over 10^6 organisms. Shigellae are an exception, with 10 to 100 organisms transmitting infection. In addition, a low inoculum of STEC can produce disease. *S. typhi*, *S. paratyphi*, and shigellae are inhabitants of only the human intestinal tract, whereas the other bacterial enteric pathogens have animal hosts and can be transmitted to humans by contact with contaminated materials.

Major categories of diarrhea caused by enteric pathogens include illness acquired as a result of the following: (1) exposure to child-care settings or hospitals, (2) foodborne or waterborne disease, (3) exposure to antimicrobial agents, (4) travel, or (5) exposure to animals (e.g., pets). In addition, immunosuppressed hosts are susceptible and may have more severe manifestations of disease. Children who attend child-care centers have a significantly greater risk of diarrheal illness than age-matched children not in child-care centers (Holmes et al., 1996; Reves et al., 1993). Diarrheal illnesses are common in less developed countries as a consequence of increased urbanization (crowding), decreasing incidence of breast-feeding, large numbers of refugees from civil disruption, lack of clean water and food, and presence of malnutrition.

Children less than 6 years of age are particularly at risk for diarrhea associated with *Aeromonas* species (Janda and Abbott, 1998). Outbreaks of diarrhea caused by *Aeromonas* species in child-care centers also have been reported (de la Morena et al., 1993; Sempertegui et al., 1995), but volunteers who have been fed the organism have not become ill.

C. jejuni is an important cause of diarrhea worldwide. Disease occurs in all age groups, with the highest incidence in children under 5 years of age and young adults. Most farm animals; meat sources; poultry carcasses; and many pet dogs and cats, especially the young, harbor this organism. Transmission occurs from ingestion of undercooked chicken and pork, contaminated food and water, and unpasteurized milk. Transmission also can occur from contact with infected pets (puppies and kittens) and farm animals. Person-to-person spread appears to be uncommon; outbreaks have been reported, including outbreaks of *C. upsaliensis* in child-care centers (Goossens et al., 1995). The incubation period is 2 to 5 days, with a range of up to 10 days.

Spores of *C. difficile* are acquired from the environment or by fecal-oral transmission from colonized individuals. Colonization rates can reach 50% in asymptomatic neonates and infants but decline to less than 5% in children over 2 years of age and in adults. Risk factors for disease are administration of antimicrobial therapy, repeated enemas, prolonged nasogastric tube insertion, and intestinal tract surgery, all of which alter the normal intestinal flora and allow *C. difficile* to proliferate. Hospitals are reservoirs for *C. difficile*, and child-care centers also may be a source. The incubation period is unknown.

STEC is recognized as a cause of sporadic diarrhea and has been associated with many outbreaks. STEC outbreaks associated with undercooked beef, especially ground beef, are a major health problem. Outbreaks caused by contaminated water, unpasteurized milk, apple cider, sprouts, lettuce, salad dressings, and salami have been reported (Centers for Disease Control and Prevention, 1996a; Keene et al., 1994; Centers for Disease Control and Prevention, 2001; Olsen et al., 2000). Person-to-person transmission of *E. coli* O157:H7 has been described in child-care centers, custodial institutions, families, and hospitals (Belongia et al., 1993). The incubation period is 3 to 4 days, with a range up to 10 days. ETEC causes disease primarily in infants less than 18 months of age in developing nations and in adult travelers (Gorbach et al., 1975). Contaminated food, and less often water, are thought to be the major modes of transmission. Person-to-person transmission is uncommon. The incubation period is 1 to 3 days. EPEC causes outbreaks of disease, especially in infants in nurseries, through contaminated instruments or other contaminated aspects of the environment or through health-care personnel. EPEC is uncommon in the United States but remains a major cause of acute and persistent diarrhea in many developing countries. EIEC organisms are a rare cause of infantile diarrhea in the United States. EIEC are transmitted through contaminated food, and outbreaks have been described. EAEC has been recognized as a cause of diarrhea in infants in developing countries and in travelers to these locales. Some strains may cause chronic diarrhea in infants.

Disease resulting from *Salmonella* is reported worldwide. Humans usually ingest salmonellae from contaminated food, including meat; dairy products, including ice cream; poultry products, especially eggs (Centers for Disease Control and Prevention, 1996b); vegetables, including sprouts; and fruit. Organisms are present on the surface of meat; thus any conditions favoring multiplication enhance the possibility of disease production. Animals are infected and perpetuate the infection among themselves, easily contaminating other animals during transport. Selected *Salmonella* serotypes frequently are associated with transmission from reptiles such as iguanas, snakes, lizards, and turtles (Ackman et al., 1995). A large U.S.-wide foodborne outbreak of *S. enteritidis* occurred in 1994 following national distribution of ice cream that had been contaminated by transport of ice cream mix in the same tanker trailers used for transport of unpasteurized eggs (Hennessy et al., 1996). Consumption of raw fruits and vegetables contaminated during slicing has been reported. An estimated 2 million cases of *Salmonella* gastroenteritis occur per year in the United States, with the rates of infection being highest in infants and young children. Nosocomial transmission within hospitals, nursing homes, and institutions results from cross-contamination involving personnel, equipment, and aerosol (Novak and Feldman, 1979). In regions where sewage disposal and water purification are inadequate, enteric infections are frequent, and the likelihood of spread is enhanced. *S. typhi* and *S. paratyphi* are exclusively human pathogens, with most cases in the United States occurring following foreign travel, especially to the Indian subcontinent. The incubation period is 3 to 21 days, depending on the inoculum ingested and the health and immune status of the patient.

Communicability of disease resulting from shigellae depends on human fecal material transmitting infection either through person-to-person contact or through food and water. The highest incidence of shigellae is in children 1 to 4 years of age, particularly during the warm season, with illness uncommon in infants under 6 months of age. In one study, 50% of children infected with shigellae were asymptomatic (Guerrero et al., 1994). Large outbreaks of infection are related to contaminated food or water or can occur in conditions of crowding where personal hygiene is poor, such as in jails, child-care centers, custodial institutions, and refugee camps. Infection can occur following ingestion of 10 to 100 organisms. The incubation period is 1 to 4 days, with a range of up to 7 days.

Cholera has caused devastating worldwide pandemics, with perpetual endemic disease occurring in India and Bangladesh. An epidemic of cholera began in Peru in January 1991 and subsequently has spread to several other countries in Latin America. Cases have been identified in the United States over the past decade and are related to eating shellfish from the Gulf of Mexico or to travel to South America. Most reported cases of cholera in the United States are imported or follow ingestion of raw or inadequately cooked seafood from polluted waters. El Tor organisms can persist in water for long periods of time. Carriage and excretion of the organism usually last several weeks but may last longer. In endemic areas, cholera is a disease of childhood, although infants less than 1 year old usually are spared. When epidemics reach previously unaffected countries, persons of all ages are infected. The *V. cholerae* O139 epidemics in Asia have occurred predominantly in adults. Presumably, *V. cholerae* O1 exposure during childhood does not protect against O139 exposure later in life. Because the cholera toxins of *V. cholerae* O1 and O139 are immunologically and genetically identical, this indicates that preexisting antitoxin antibody does not provide protection against *V. cholerae* O139 infections (Cholera Working Group, 1993; Nair et al., 1994). The incubation period is 2 to 3 days, with a range of up to 5 days.

Y. enterocolitica infection affects all age groups, but most episodes occur in infants and children in whom a spectrum of illness occurs, including gastroenteritis. Some geographic variation in recognized disease in the United States occurs for reasons that are not clear. The highest isolation rates have been reported during the cold season in areas with temperate climates, including the United States, Canada, and Northern Europe. Outbreaks of disease have been traced to contaminated food, including milk, tofu, and pork chitterlings (Lee et al., 1990). Pathogenic strains most commonly are isolated from raw pork or pork products. Persons with excessive iron storage syndromes have increased susceptibility to *Yersinia* bacteremia.

Pathogenesis and Pathology

The intestinal tract has a number of nonimmunologic defense mechanisms that help form a barrier against infection (Grady and Keusch, 1971). The indigenous flora are present in numbers up to 10^{11} organisms per gram of stool in the large bowel. Competition for substrate plus other environmental alterations including decreased pH or production of antibacterial substances probably contribute to which organisms succeed in causing disease. Antibiotics alter growth of indigenous flora and may contribute to colonization by enteric pathogens.

Secretions containing glycoconjugates such as mucin may diminish bacterial adherence to epithelial cells both mechanically and by competition at receptor sites. Normal peristalsis expels nonadherent organisms. Gastric acid inhibits growth of many bacteria, and lysozyme and bile salts in the intestinal tract hinder growth of many bacteria. Immunologic defense mechanisms include secretory IgA, production of which is dependent on antigen exposure to the local intestinal surface. The secretory piece of IgA increases resistance of these antibodies to protease; thus this class of antibody best withstands the environment of the lumen of the bowel. Antibody binds toxins and bacteria, thus preventing adsorption, and may be bactericidal in combination with complement and lysozyme.

Malabsorption or profuse watery isotonic diarrhea is caused by dysfunction of the small intestine. *V. cholerae* is the prototype of organisms that cause profuse malabsorption because of the effects of their enterotoxins on intestinal cells. In other instances, such as dysentery, the colon or the terminal ileum are invaded by bacteria. *Shigella* species constitute the prototype of invasive organisms causing dysentery. The mucosal invasion and disruption are visible as ulcerations and result in the presence of blood and mucus in stool.

Diarrhea can be categorized as inflammatory or noninflammatory, resulting from virulence mechanisms of enteropathogens. Inflammatory diarrhea occurs following adherence, invasion, or cytotoxin production by bacteria. Noninflammatory diarrhea occurs as a result of adherence, enterotoxin production by bacteria, or loss of villous cells caused by enteric viruses. Bacterial pathogens must be able to adhere in the intestinal mucosa to cause disease, establishing the adhesins of the bacteria as a critical part of virulence.

Bacteria produce one or more of four types of toxins: enterotoxins, cytoskeleton-altering toxins, cytotoxins, and toxins with neural activity (Sears and Kaper, 1996). Enterotoxins stimulate net intestinal secretion without histologic evidence of intestinal damage. Cytoskeleton-altering toxins produce an alteration in cell shape without inducing significant cell injury. Cytotoxins produce cellular damage, as documented by gross findings such as intestinal hemorrhage, light-microscopic evidence of intestinal damage, or cellular injury. Toxins with neural activity include those that involve release of one or more neurotransmitters from the enteric nervous system or alter smooth-muscle activity in the intestine.

Aeromonas species produce several colonization factors and enterotoxins, which are the primary virulence factors identified in aeromads. Two broad groups of *Aeromonas* enterotoxins (cytolytic and cytotonic) are recognized. The cytolytic enterotoxin is the more common enterotoxin and is a beta hemolysin referred to as *aerolysin*.

C. jejuni has the potential to invade epithelial cells and produce dysentery. In addition, several major toxins have been reported to be produced by some *C. jejuni* strains associated with diarrheal disease. These toxins include a heat-labile enterotoxin, a cytolethal distending toxin, other cytotoxins, and a HEp-2 elongating toxin. Consistent association between the toxins and clinical disease is lacking.

E. coli causes disease by several mechanisms, as described previously. The toxins of STEC are Stx 1 or verocytotoxin 1 (VT1), and Stx-2 or verocytotoxin 2 (VT2). Stx-2 is immunologically distinct from Stx-1 but is genetically and mechanistically closely related. Other closely related variant toxins, some of which have been studied extensively, also exist. These toxins work like Shiga toxin produced by *S. dysenteriae* type 1. The primary site of histopathologic conditions is the colon.

Approximately 40% to 50% of ETECs produce only ST, 30% to 40% produce ST and LT, and 20% to 30% produce only LT. Disease may be associated with production of either or both enterotoxins produced by ETEC. Stools are watery and often of large volume, as occurs in a mild case of cholera.

The ability of EIEC to invade cells is due to virulence genes present on a 140-megadalton plasmid. This invasion contributes to the dysentery associated with infection by EIEC. Some EIECs produce an enterotoxin referred to as *Shigella* enterotoxin 2 or *EIEC* enterotoxin, which may play a role in the watery diarrhea associated with EIEC infections.

The adherent but noninvasive EPEC organisms colonize the small intestine and produce a distinctive histopathologic lesion, which involves destruction of microvilli and close adherence of the bacteria to the membrane of the enterocyte, which results in a cuplike pedestal formation on which each bacterium rests. This classic lesion is referred to as the attaching-effacing (AE) lesion and requires the presence of several virulence genes. EAEC strains have been reported to produce three toxins that potentially are able to stimulate intestinal secretion, the best characterized of which is EAEC heat-stable enterotoxin 1 (EAST1).

Salmonellae produce disease by adhering to and then penetrating intestinal mucosal cells by endocytosis (mucosal translocation) before reaching the lamina propria. Bacterial proliferation occurs in the lamina propria and mesenteric nodes. Penetration is rapid, and macrophage engulfment without killing has been demonstrated. The terminal ileum and cecum are maximally involved, and neutrophilic inflammation is apparent in these locations. Peyer's patches and the mesenteric nodes may be enlarged. Salmonellae survive in an intracellular location and gain access to the reticuloendothelial system, and are thus protected from antibody and some antimicrobial agents. This intracellular location may contribute to prolonged carriage and excretion of the organism. *S. typhi* elicits a mononuclear cell response in the lamina propria. *S. typhi* and *S. paratyphi* traverse the mucosa and are more likely to cause bacteremia than other *Salmonella* species.

Nontyphoidal salmonella serotypes, including *S. typhimurium*, usually cause watery diarrhea. The pathogenesis of the secretory response to salmonella infection is uncertain. Although several enterotoxins are produced by various salmonella strains, their role in disease is not well defined. Water and electrolyte transport abnormalities accompany experimental salmonella infections.

Shigella species are recognized primarily for causing dysentery, although watery diarrhea more characteristic of small bowel involvement is a frequent occurrence. *Shigella* organisms invade colonic epithelium through M cells then spread laterally from cell to cell. In addition to invasion, *S. dysenteriae* type 1 produces Shiga toxin, which inhibits protein synthesis in eukaryotic cells.

The severe diarrhea caused by *V. cholerae* is produced by the O1 and O139 serogroups. The rapidly dehydrating noninflammatory diarrhea results from the organisms' ability to produce a heat-labile enterotoxin referred to as *cholera toxin*. The toxin production of this organism is coded by chromosomal DNA (Table 12-3) (Holmgren, 1981). Nontoxigenic *V. cholerae* can acquire the cholera toxin gene by infection by a filamentous bacteriophage that carries the cholera toxin gene. The bacteriophage gains entry to the *V. cholerae* cell by way of pili, which also function as adhesion molecules in the intestine. Once the bacteriophage gains entry to the *V. cholerae* cell, the cholera toxin gene is incorporated into the bacterial chromosome, and the cell can produce cholera toxin (Waldor and Mekalanos, 1996). This toxin has provided a wealth of information about the structure and function of enterotoxins and about the pathogenesis of diarrheal diseases. This protein exotoxin activates adenylate cyclase and catalyzes the formation of cyclic AMP (cAMP), resulting in the secretion of fluid into the lumen of the intestinal tract. The toxin has two component parts. The B subunit binds to a receptor, GM_1 ganglioside, present on the surface of intestinal cells. The A subunit of the toxin penetrates the cell and must gain access to the interior to catalyze the adenosine diphosphate (ADP) ribosylation of guanosine triphosphate (GTP)–binding protein. This results in activation of adenylate cyclase and conversion of adenosine triphosphate (ATP) to cAMP. The increased concentration of intracellular cAMP activates electrolyte transport with water from the extracellular fluid to the lumen of the intestinal tract. Secretion then exceeds fluid absorption.

Increased cAMP also inhibits the transport of sodium and chloride from the lumen of the gut across the brush border and into the cell, with decreased absorption as membrane permeability in the villus cell is diminished. Glucose-coupled sodium and water transport into cells occurs by an independent mechanism that is unaltered. Thus oral electrolyte solution can still be absorbed from the intestine.

Y. enterocolitica produces several disease syndromes, including watery diarrhea, ulcerative enterocolitis, and mesenteric adenitis not associated with diarrhea. *Y. enterocolitica* infection mimics the mucosal translocation and bacterial proliferation in nodes and lamina propria described for *Salmonella* species. Strains of *Y. enterocolitica* possess adherence mechanisms and produce heat-stable enterotoxins thought to be important in the pathogenesis of the watery diarrhea syndrome.

Clinical Manifestations

Clinical manifestations that occur following infection with an enteropathogen include signs and symptoms related to the gastrointestinal tract, systemic manifestations, and complications that may be intestinal or extraintestinal in origin.

Aeromonas species. *Aeromonas* species have been associated with a variety of intestinal and extraintestinal infections (Janda, 1998). A wide spectrum of gastrointestinal tract symptoms may occur, but the most common manifestation is an acute, self-limited, watery diarrhea. A dysenteric illness is less common.

C. jejuni. *C. jejuni* may produce enteric disease ranging from watery diarrhea to dysentery. *C. jejuni* is often excreted without producing symptoms. Infected individuals may manifest diarrhea, abdominal pain, chills, and fever. Abdominal pain can mimic that associated with appendicitis. Blood, mucus, and fecal leukocytes may be present in stool, resembling the illness produced by shigellae. Organisms may be excreted for 2 to 3 weeks in untreated persons. Most patients recover in less than 1 week, but 20% have a relapse or prolonged or severe ill-

ness, which may mimic inflammatory bowel disease. *C. jejuni* has caused bacteremia in children with immunodeficiency, in malnourished children, and in neonates (Reed et al., 1996). Immunoreactive complications include reactive arthritis, Guillain-Barré syndrome, Fisher syndrome, Reiter's syndrome, and erythema nodosum.

E. coli. STEC produces a variety of clinical syndromes that begin with nausea, vomiting, severe abdominal pain, and watery diarrhea that may progress to bloody diarrhea and hemorrhagic colitis over several days. Only 30% of patients have fever as part of this syndrome. Although bloody diarrhea is the most distinctive manifestation of STEC infection, nonspecific watery diarrhea and asymptomatic infections also occur. HUS follows EHEC enteritis in approximately 10% of patients, and thrombotic thrombocytopenia purpura is a postdiarrheal complication in adults (Pickering et al., 1994; Wong et al., 2000).

ETEC strains are an important cause of traveler's diarrhea and diarrheal illness in children in developing countries (DuPont, 1997). ETEC strains produce watery diarrhea without blood or mucus. The severity of illness following ETEC infection varies from mild to severe, with up to 10 to 20 stools per day. Disease is self-limited, lasting 3 to 5 days in an immunocompetent host, but severe dehydration may occur in infants. The disease is a malabsorptive diarrhea with watery stools without blood or white blood cells, and low-grade fever may be present.

EIEC can produce either dysentery with blood and mucus in stools or watery diarrhea. Onset of fever, nausea, cramps, and tenesmus may be rapid. The clinical manifestations of dysentery are similar to those produced by shigellae. EIEC disease is uncommon in infants.

EPEC characteristically infects infants and children younger than 2 years of age, particularly in developing countries, and has caused numerous outbreaks of acute and chronic infantile diarrhea worldwide. These organisms are of particular importance in tropical countries and developing nations where crowding and poor hygiene occur. EPEC-associated diarrheal illness is uncommon in older children and adults. Frequent, green, slimy stools are produced, usually without blood or fecal leukocytes. Diarrhea may be severe and can result in dehydration.

EAEC has been recognized, primarily in infants and young children in the developing world, as a cause of both acute and chronic diarrhea. Data suggest that these organisms may be common enteropathogens of early childhood.

Salmonella *species.* Infection with salmonellae have been associated with several clinical syndromes: (1) acute gastroenteritis, which is most common; (2) enteric fever; (3) septicemia with or without localized infections; and (4) inapparent infection and carrier state (Saphra and Winter, 1957). The clinical manifestations of these syndromes often overlap.

Gastroenteritis. Salmonella gastroenteritis occurs throughout life but is most common in the first year, decreases during childhood, and remains constant throughout the adult years (Centers for Disease Control and Prevention, 2003). Illness varies in severity from mild to severe in all groups. Nausea, vomiting, and diarrhea are associated with severe abdominal cramps and tenderness. Fever and prostration may be pronounced. Chills and weakness are common. Stools are numerous and may contain mucus and blood. Bloody diarrhea is observed often in young children but is uncommon in adults. In approximately 50% of the patients, the temperature falls to normal within 1 or 2 days, and recovery is uneventful. In others the disease may last 1 week or more. Protracted or recurrent diarrhea occurs and may represent a secondary consequence of mucosal invasion and destruction of the epithelium. In severe infections, shock with cyanosis, hypothermia, and circulatory collapse, which precedes death, may occur. In some patients, gastroenteritis is followed by septicemia or by signs of localization. Metastatic foci are more likely to occur in patients with sickle cell disease, infants less than 6 months of age, and in immunocompromised persons such as those with acquired immunodeficiency syndrome (AIDS) (Centers for Disease Control, 1992).

Enteric Fever. Although infections caused by *Salmonella* species constitute a serious public health problem, those caused by *S. typhi* have become relatively infrequent in the United States. The number of cases of typhoid fever reported in the United States during the last two decades rarely has exceeded 500 per year (Centers for Disease Control and Prevention, 2003).

The onset of symptoms of typhoid fever in most cases is gradual, with fever, headache, malaise, and loss of appetite. The typical course in an adult is illustrated in Figure 12-1. The temperature rises in a steplike manner for 2 to 7 days to an average of approximately 40° C (104° F) and characteristically remains at this level for 3 to 4 weeks in the absence of specific antimicrobial therapy. The pulse rate is slow relative to the fever. Diarrhea is present in some patients, although constipation may persist throughout infection. Either manifestation may be accompanied by abdominal tenderness, distention, and pain. In the early stages of illness, discrete rose-colored spots may be scattered over the trunk, especially the abdomen. The spleen is enlarged in most patients. Severely ill

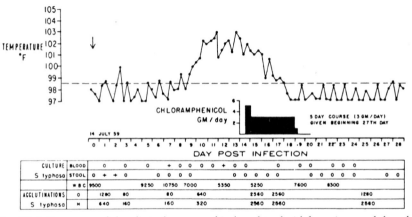

Fig. 12-1 Summary of the clinical course of induced typhoid fever in an adult volunteer. Therapy consisted of two 5-day courses of chloramphenicol separated by a 1-week interval. (From Hornick RB, et al. N Engl J Med 1970;283:686.)

patients may become delirious or stuporous. The white blood cell count, as a rule, shows leukopenia.

Typhoid fever in children in the first 2 years of life exhibits certain differences from the clinical course in adults (Hornick et al., 1970). The diagnosis in infancy is often made by chance isolation of *S. typhi* from stools or blood in infants in whom the onset is often abrupt, with high fever, vomiting, convulsions, and meningeal signs. The slow pulse rate is not a frequent finding. Rose spots occur less commonly than in adults. Leukocytosis is the rule, and the white blood cell count may be as high as 20,000 to 25,000 cells/μL, but neutrophils rarely exceed 60% to 70%. The spleen usually is palpable. The course of the disease is short, rarely persisting more than 2 weeks. The mortality rate in infancy is low when appropriate therapy is administered. *Salmonella* species other than *S. typhi* may produce a disease with all the manifestations of typhoid fever, including persistent fever; intestinal tract symptoms; rose spots; leukopenia; and positive cultures of blood, stool, and urine (Hohmann, 2001).

Septicemia With or Without Localized Infection. *Salmonella* species also are responsible for a disease characterized by intermittent fever, chills (in adults), anorexia, and loss of weight. The characteristic features of typhoid fever are absent. Stool cultures usually are negative, although blood cultures yield the causative organism. A focus of infection is identified in approximately one fourth of patients with bacteremia. The acute focal process may be directly or indirectly connected with the intestinal tract and may cause appendicitis, cholecystitis, peritonitis, or salpingitis. Hematogenous spread of organisms may result in foci of infection in the brain, skin, lungs, spleen, middle ear, bone, or joints. Meningitis is caused by a variety of salmonella types and occurs principally in young infants, with a high morbidity rate. The urinary tract also can be involved. Osteomyelitis and pyarthrosis, caused by many serotypes, can occur in any bone, but the long bones, spine, and ribs are affected most commonly. Pneumonia usually is accompanied by a high temperature and often terminates fatally. This manifestation occurs almost exclusively in elderly patients, many of whom suffer from unrelated medical problems.

Inapparent Infection and the Carrier State. Asymptomatic infection with salmonellae occurs in an estimated 0.2% of people, as documented by positive stool cultures in the absence of clinical illness. Some of these persons have had known contact with symptomatic persons or are being investigated because of a recognized source of contaminated food. Persons who have been infected usually excrete organisms for weeks to months. Carriers of *S. typhi*, especially those with abnormal gall bladders, may excrete organisms for years.

Shigella *species.* Mild illness with transient diarrhea is a common manifestation of shigella infection. Persons with mild infection have watery diarrhea or loose stools for a few days, with mild or absent constitutional symptoms. The classic clinical picture of bacillary dysentery is characterized by severe abdominal pain, tenesmus, and constitutional symptoms with frequently passed stools containing mucus and blood. Patients with moderately severe disease may have an abrupt onset with fever, abdominal pain, vomiting, and then diarrhea. Stools occur 7 to 12 times daily, are watery, green, or yellow, and contain mucus and undigested food. Disease may progress with development of all of the features of dysentery. Acute symptoms may persist for 7 to 10 days, and meningismus, delirium, and convulsions may accompany dysentery caused by shigella infection. Bacteremia is uncommon but may occur in persons who are immunocompromised or malnourished. The most severe illness occurs most frequently in young infants, in the elderly, and in debilitated persons. Sequelae of shigella infection include toxic megacolon; hemolytic uremic syndrome associated only with *S. dysenteriae* type 1; reactive arthropathy (Reiter's syndrome), which generally occurs 2 to 5 weeks following the dysenteric illness in persons genetically predisposed; and fulminant toxic encephalopathy.

V. cholerae. Infection with *V. cholerae* results in a spectrum ranging from asymptomatic excretion to mild to moderate diarrhea to severe, dehydrating illness. Asymptomatic infection is much more common than clinical illness. Severe illness in adults may be characterized by rapid fluid loss in excess of 20 L per 24 hours. Profound shock and death can occur within a day if fluid replacement is not instituted. The acutely ill patient usually appears in a shocklike state, with soiling of clothes by excessive fecal discharge. The feces usually are clear and without odor, contain flecks of mucus that impart a "rice-water" appearance, and have high concentrations of sodium and bicarbonate. Vomiting without nausea, described as effortless, usually follows the onset of diarrhea. The skin of the hands may have a characteristic appearance resembling wrinkled "washer woman's hands" in persons with severe dehydration. Fever, if present, is low grade, or the patient may develop hypothermia.

Y. enterocolitica. Clinical manifestations of infection with *Y. enterocolitica* depend on the age and immune status of the host. Watery diarrhea is a common manifestation of *Y. enterocolitica.* Infection with this organism also can produce a dysentery syndrome, most often occurring in young children. Older children and adolescents may develop acute mesenteric adenitis or ileitis that mimics acute appendicitis and includes diarrhea, fever, right lower quadrant tenderness, abdominal pain, and leukocytosis. Acute bacteremia with metastatic foci, including involvement of the liver and spleen, occurs in elderly adults or immunocompromised hosts. Postinfectious sequelae include erythema nodosum and reactive arthritis, most often in adults. Patients with β-thalassemia and iron overload are at an increased risk for severe yersiniosis.

Diagnosis and Differential Diagnosis

Demographic and epidemiologic data, clinical manifestations, immune status of the host, and knowledge of virulence mechanisms of enteropathogens provide the framework for establishing the cause of enteric infection using microscopy, culture, rapid diagnostic tests, and specialized laboratory tests (Box 12-2). Examination of stool for the presence of leukocytes and blood provides insight into whether the organism is invasive or produces a cytotoxin. Stool cultures cannot be justified for all patients with acute diarrhea. When culture is indicated, the specimen should be inoculated onto culture plates that can detect *Campylobacter* species, STEC, *Salmonella* species, and Shigella species. Selective media or testing may be necessary for *V. cholerae, Y. enterocolitica, C. difficile* and many food-borne pathogens. Laboratory confirmation of *E. coli*–associated disease generally is not available in most diagnostic laboratories because detection of toxins or invasive properties requires cell cultures, animal models, gene probes, polymerase chain reaction (PCR) testing or other specific assays. Serotyping of *E. coli* in diarrheal outbreaks in infants is potentially helpful for recognition of EPEC but is more helpful in outbreak evaluation than in the diagnostic evaluation of a single infant. *E. coli* O157:H7 should be suspected if non–sorbitol fermenting *E. coli* are present; confirmation in a reference laboratory is necessary. All laboratories should include a sorbitol-MacConkey agar plate as part of routine stool culture to screen for non–sorbitol fermenting *E. coli* O157:H7. If present, these organisms should be confirmed by serologic testing.

S. typhi frequently is detected in blood cultures during the first 2 weeks of illness. When enteric fever is suspected, blood and bone marrow must be obtained for culture. In patients not from endemic areas serologic tests may be helpful if they are positive but generally are not useful. The leukocyte count is usually 10,000 to 15,000 cells/μL, with a slight increase in number of polymorphonuclear cells. Leukopenia found in the enteric fever type of infection is seldom seen in the gastroenteric form. Positive blood cultures are more frequent in infants less than 6 months of age and occasionally occur in older persons, especially in the presence of severe infections. Stool cultures usually yield salmonellae during the acute phase of the disease and often for weeks to months thereafter. Symptoms subside despite continued colonization of the gastrointestinal tract with the organism.

Most clinical microbiology laboratories include specific media for culture of stool at 42°C in a reduced-oxygen, high–carbon dioxide environment to enable isolation of *C. jejuni* and *C. coli.* Identification of other *Campylobacter* species from stool requires specialized media and filtration techniques that are not generally used in most diagnostic laboratories.

V. cholerae presents diagnostic problems in the United States, where it is an uncommon pathogen. The unprepared laboratory may miss the diagnosis. If *V. cholerae* is suspected, laboratory personnel should be alerted, which will increase the likelihood of a correct diagnosis. *V. cholerae* grows rapidly on certain alkaline-enrichment media, such as thiosulfate citrate bile salts sucrose (TCBS) agar, which has a pH greater than 6.0. The organisms can be distinguished from other enteric bacteria on TCBS agar by the fact that they form characteristic opaque yellow colonies. Suspect colonies are

---

BOX 12-2

DIAGNOSTIC METHODS FOR BACTERIAL ENTERIC PATHOGENS

Nonspecific Tests

Microscopy
Fecal lactoferrin assay
Fecal leukocytes
Stool occult blood
Complete blood count

Routine Screening Culture

Enteric agar media
   Differential media (e.g., MacConkey [MAC], eosin methylene blue [EMB])
   Moderately selective media (e.g., Hektoen enteric [HE], xylose-lysine-desoxycholate [XLD], Salmonella-
     Shigella [SS])
Enrichment broth
Sorbitol-MAC agar

Organism-Specific Identification

Organism	Media or method
Salmonella	Brilliant green or bismuth sulfite agar
Campylobacter	Skirrow's formula, Campy-BAP, Butzler's formula, Preston's formula
Aeromonas	BAP, MAC, EMB
Vibrio	Thiosulfate-citrate-bile-salt-sucrose (TCBS) agar, *V. cholerae* O1 antisera
Yersinia	Cefsulodin-irgasan-novobiocin (CIN) agar
Clostridium difficile	Cycloserine–cefoxitin–fructose–egg yolk (CCFA) anaerobically, *C. difficile* toxin EIA
Enterohemorrhagic *E. coli*	Sorbitol MAC, O157 antisera, H7 antisera

---

confirmed serologically by agglutination with specific antisera. Isolated specimens of *V. cholerae* O1 and O139 should be confirmed and tested for production of cholera toxin. For *Y. enterocolitica*, laboratory personnel must be alerted to use specific media to facilitate growth and recognition of this organism. *C. difficile* toxins are identified by use of enzyme immunoassay (EIA).

Complications

Complications associated with acute infectious bacterial diarrhea are those that occur during the acute episode, which include dehydration, bacteremia, and metastatic foci, and those that occur after the acute episode, which may be immune mediated. The severity of acute bacterial gastroenteritis is correlated best with fluid and electrolyte loss and the extent of dehydration. Most infections are self-limited and localized to the gastrointestinal tract; however, significant dehydration and even death can occur, especially in young, elderly, and immunocompromised patients. Replacement fluids have diminished the morbidity rate for all diarrheal illnesses, and specific antibiotics have contributed to effective therapy of several of these entities. In developing nations in which nutrition is poor, diarrheal illnesses often contribute to protein-calorie malnutrition, growth failure, and susceptibility to additional pathogens.

Salmonella suppurative foci such as meningitis, pyarthrosis, and osteomyelitis occur infrequently. The patient may have an altered mental status, with a spectrum of effects including delirium, stupor, and aphasia. It is important to ascertain if direct invasion of the central nervous system has occurred in the presence of such signs and symptoms. Fortunately, intestinal tract perforation and hemorrhage are rare in the United States even with *S. typhi*, primarily because infections are diagnosed rapidly and treated appropriately. These complications characteristically occur after 2 weeks of untreated disease. Relapse may occur in 15% to 20% of persons treated for *S. typhi* and does so usually within 10 to 18 days of withdrawal from antibiotics. Chronic carriage of *S. typhi* has been attributed to chronic infection of the gallbladder.

Complications of *C. jejuni* enteritis include Reiter's syndrome, reactive arthritis, Guillain-Barré syndrome, and erythema nodosum (Rees et al., 1995). Reactive arthritis also has been associated with *Salmonella, Shigella, C. difficile*, and *Yersinia* infections. *Y. enterocolitica* rarely can cause chronic and recurrent enteric symptoms, which respond to antibiotic therapy, as well as erythema nodosum. Septicemic illness is potentially severe and has occurred in immunocompromised hosts. The nonsuppurative arthritis usually is self-limited and usually lasts a few months.

Prognosis

Prognosis generally is dependent on the age and nutritional status of the patient and the presence of an underlying disease or condition. The vast majority of intestinal tract infections are self-limited, with no complications occurring and complete recovery expected. The very young, the elderly, and those with protein-calorie malnutrition or underlying disease such as HIV are at risk for complications or prolonged illness (Centers for Disease Control, 1992). Overall, fatality from any of these agents seldom exceeds 1% when health-care delivery is adequate.

Treatment

Therapy of children with gastroenteritis includes fluid and electrolyte replacement and maintenance; maintenance of dietary intake; specific therapy with antimicrobial agents; and infrequent use of nonspecific therapy, including antidiarrheal compounds.

Infants, children, and adults with gastroenteritis require fluid replacement. Oral hydration with fluid containing carbohydrates and electrolytes has significantly reduced the morbidity and mortality from diarrheal disease. The AAP and the CDC have made similar recommendations for management of acute diarrhea in children (Duggan et al., 1992; Provisional Committee on Quality Improvement, 1996). Oral rehydration therapy is the preferred treatment of fluid and electrolyte losses caused by diarrhea in children with mild to moderate dehydration. Children who have diarrhea and who are not dehydrated should continue to be fed age-appropriate diets (Brown et al., 1994; Snyder, 1994). Children who require rehydration should be fed age-appropriate diets as soon as they have been rehydrated. Typically, reintroduction of diet can occur 8 to 12 hours after initiation of oral rehydration. Breast-feeding should be resumed as soon as possible, preferably immediately after rehydration. Antimotility agents, opiates, bismuth subsalicylate, and adsorbents are not recommended for treatment of diarrhea in children 1 month to 5 years of age (American Academy of Pediatrics, 1996). Probiotic compounds have been shown to be effective in the treatment and prevention of diarrhea due to several enteric pathogens, but their role has not been fully delineated (Van Niel et al., 2002).

Hospitalization usually is not necessary unless a fluid deficit of ≥5% has occurred and rehydration cannot be provided through oral solutions. *V. cholerae* causes the most rapid losses, and replacement may be an emergency. Since glucose-coupled electrolyte and water transport across the epithelium are unaltered by the various toxins, it is possible to replace fluids orally. Replacement fluids should not be prepared by parents without medical supervision, since hypernatremia is a risk of inappropriately prepared fluid and electrolyte solutions. Fluid replacement using the World Health Organization (WHO) formulation, mixed and used as recommended (Hayani et al., 1992), or one of the premixed fluid and electrolyte replacement solutions is preferred. The WHO has recommended a change in the WHO oral rehydration solution to contain less salt and carbohydrate (World Health Organization, 2002).

Specific antimicrobial therapy (Table 12-4) is administered to select patients with gastroenteritis to abbreviate the clinical course and decrease excretion of the causative organism (Pickering and Cleary, 2002). A stool culture should be obtained when antimicrobial therapy is anticipated, and susceptibility testing of any suspected pathogen should be performed to ensure that appropriate therapy is being given. Changing susceptibility patterns and an increase in antimicrobial resistance often make the initial selection of an antimicrobial agent difficult (Pickering, 1996).

TABLE 12-4	Antimicrobial Therapy for Bacterial Organisms Causing Gastroenteritis
Organism	Antimicrobial agent
Campylobacter jejuni[*]	Erythromycin or azithromycin or ciprofloxacin[*]
Clostridium difficile	Metronidazole or vancomycin
Escherichia coli	
EPEC, ETEC, EIEC	Trimethoprim-sulfamethoxazole (TMP/SMX) or ciprofloxacin[*]
EAEC	Uncertain
STEC	Not indicated
Salmonella gastroenteritis[*]	None (cefotaxime, ceftriaxone ampicillin, TMP/SMX, or chloramphenicol, for bacteremia and other sites of infection)
Salmonella typhi[*] (typhoid fever)	Chloramphenicol, TMP/SMX, ampicillin, ceftraxione, or cefotaxime
Shigella species[*]	Azithromycin, ciprofloxacin,[*] ceftriaxone, cefotaxime nalidixic acid; TMP/SMX for susceptible strains
Vibrio cholerae O1	Doxycycline or tetracycline or TMP/SMX
Vibrio cholerae O139	Doxycycline or tetracycline
Yersinia enterocolitica	
Gastroenteritis	None
Bacteremia[*]	TMP/SMX, tetracycline, aminoglycoside, cefotaxime, or ciprofloxacin[*]

[*]Ciprofloxacin or ofloxacin can be used for nonpregnant women over 17 years old.

The course of nontyphoid *Salmonella* infection is not altered by antibiotics, and excretion of the organisms may be prolonged by their use. Routine antibiotic therapy is not of benefit for most children with salmonella gastroenteritis, with possible exceptions being infants, immunocompromised patients, and persons with severe episodes. Patients with salmonella infections in sites other than the intestinal tract also should be treated with antimicrobial agents (Pickering and Cleary, 2002).

Shigella, *V. cholerae*, ETEC, *C. jejuni*, and *C. difficile* infections generally are treated with antibiotics when the patient is symptomatic and the organism has been identified. Excretion of the organism is shortened, and therapy may alter disease. At present it is unclear whether antibiotics decrease the severity of illness or complications with *Y. enterocolitica* or EAEC. Therapy for patients with STEC is not recommended (Wong, et al., 2000); however, appropriately conducted studies are needed to clarify the risks and benefits of antibiotic therapy of patients with *E. coli* O157:H7 enteritis (Safdar et al. 2002).

Preventive Measures

Preventive measures include hand washing, education, breast-feeding, proper food preparation and hygiene, knowledge of risks of animal exposure and travel, immunization, and interaction with public health officials when illness occurs. Interruption of fecal-oral spread is essential for diminishing transmission of enteric pathogens. If hospitalized, individual patients should be isolated during an illness. Strict hand washing should be initiated, as should appropriate processing or disposal of contaminated materials. Guidelines for prevention of enteric infections in persons infected with HIV are applicable to all children and include information about potential exposures due to food and water, pets, and travel (Centers for Disease Control and Prevention, 2002b). Guidelines for avoidance of illness from foodborne and waterborne exposure are available (Centers for Disease Control and Prevention, 2001).

To prevent infection with *S. typhi* and *Shigella* species, which are exclusively human pathogens, as well as other enteropathogens, and to reduce the incidence of disease, the following measures should be taken: (1) sanitary disposal of human feces; (2) purification and protection of water supplies; (3) pasteurization of milk and milk products; (4) strict sanitary supervision of preparation and serving of all foods; (5) proper refrigeration of food and milk; (6) exclusion of persons with diarrhea from handling food; (7) avoidance of eating raw or undercooked food, including eggs, meat, and poultry; (8) avoidance of contact with reptiles and ill animals; (9) use of appropriate precautions when traveling to developing countries; (10) hand washing (the importance of which should be stressed); and (11) irradiation of food (Tauxe, 2001).

Reducing the spread of enteric pathogens where animal reservoirs play an important role is more complex. Animal reservoirs are probably responsible for the majority of human salmonella infections in the United States. Poultry and milk products often are implicated, either directly or indirectly, with contamination of meat-processing areas, markets, or kitchens. By-products of the meat-packing industry (e.g., fertilizer or bone meal) perpetuate infection in animals. Prevention of salmonella infections in humans depends on interrupting transmission. The task of controlling salmonellosis among animals and preventing the spread of infection to people is enormous. The consumption of raw or undercooked eggs should be avoided, and all egg products must be stored and prepared as recommended. Households with young children or immunosuppressed individuals should not keep reptiles as pets because of the risk of zoonotic salmonellosis. Continued surveillance is needed to identify and eliminate the multiple sources of infection.

Immunization

S. typhi vaccine is the only vaccine available in the United States to prevent infection with diarrhea-producing organisms. The previously available vaccines against *V. cholerae* and rotavirus were removed from the market in 2000.

Typhoid immunization is not recommended routinely in the United States but is recommended for persons with occupational exposure, those traveling to endemic areas, persons living in areas of high endemicity, and household members of known carriers. Two vaccines are available to U.S. civilians: (1) an orally administered, live, attenuated vaccine using *S. typhi* strain Ty21a given in three to four doses, 2 days apart, which is not recommended for children younger than 6 years of age; and (2) a parenteral vaccine containing the capsular polysaccharide Vi antigen given in a single dose and not recommended for children younger than 2 years of age (Levine and Noriega, 1994).

Several vaccine candidates are in various stages of clinical testing.

VIRAL GASTROENTERITIS
Etiology

Acute viral gastroenteritis affects all age groups, may occur in either sporadic or epidemic form, and is responsible for a large proportion of diarrhea for which an etiologic agent cannot be defined. Most illnesses are self-limited, and in immunocompetent hosts recovery is complete. If severe dehydration occurs, morbidity and mortality may be substantial. The four viral agents that have been established as causes of childhood gastroenteritis are discussed below (Table 12-5). Several of the viruses that have been identified in stool are shown in Fig. 12-2. Each of these viruses has a distinct appearance on immunoelectron microscopy, of which size is one characteristic.

Enteric adenoviruses. Adenoviruses are DNA viruses that include 47 distinct serotypes that cause disease in humans. Types 40 and 41, and rarely 31, have been associated with gastroenteritis (Brandt et al., 1985). The enteric adenoviruses are 70 to 80 nm in diameter, nonenveloped, and contain double-stranded DNA.

Astroviruses. Astroviruses, which were first described in 1975, are nonenveloped, single-stranded RNA viruses 28 to 30 nm in diameter, with a characteristic five- or six-pointed star appearance when seen by electron microscopy. The single-stranded RNA genome encodes

---

TABLE 12-5 Diagnostic Methods for Enteric Viral Pathogens

Organism	Routine identification	Research or reference methods	Approximate size (nm)
Enteric adenovirus	EM, EIA*	PCR, culture, restriction enzyme analysis	70-80
Astrovirus	EM, EIA*	RT-PCR, culture	28-30
Caliciviruses	EM	EIA, RT-PCR	35-39
Rotavirus	EM, EIA*	RT-PCR, electropherotyping	70

EIA, Enzyme immunoassay; *EM*, electron microscopy; *RT-PCR*, reverse transcriptase–polymerase chain reaction.
*Assays are available commercially.

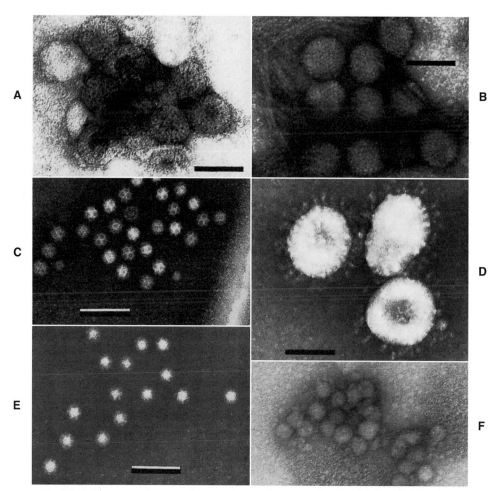

Fig. 12-2 Electron microscopic appearance of viruses visualized in stool. All micrographs are printed with a bar representing 100 nm to illustrate differences in size. **A,** Rotavirus; **B,** adenovirus; **C,** calicivirus; **D,** coronavirus; **E,** astrovirus; **F,** small round virus. (**A, B,** and **F** courtesy Miller SE, Duke University, Durham, North Carolina; **C** and **E,** courtesy Szymanski MT, Hospital for Sick Children, Toronto; **D,** courtesy Bradley DW, Centers for Disease Control and Prevention, Atlanta.)

three structural proteins and is approximately 7.2 Kb long. Eight antigenic types have been described.

Caliciviruses. Caliciviruses are singlestranded RNA viruses that are closely related to picornaviruses. Four calicivirus genera have been described, including noroviruses or "Norwalk-like" viruses (NLVs), "Sapporo-like viruses" (SLVs), vesivirus, and lagovirus (Green et al, 2000). NLVs and SLVs cause gastroenteritis in humans and also are called human caliciviruses (HuCV). Vesivirus and lagovirus mainly infect animals. Two morphologies of calicivirus, typical and atypical, have been described. SLVs have the typical calicivirus morphology that reveals the "star of David"

(Fig. 12-2, *C*) appearance similar to many animal caliciviruses. The surface structure of NLVs is smooth and usually does not reveal the "star of David" appearance. To distinguish them from SLVs, the NLVs also were referred to as "small round structured viruses" (SRSVs). Before the Norwalk virus was cloned in 1990 (Jiang et al., 1990), individual members were named after their location of discovery.

The Norwalk virus was first described from an outbreak of gastroenteritis that occurred in Norwalk, Ohio, in 1969. A bacteria-free filtrate from a stool specimen produced gastroenteritis in several volunteers, and stools from the infected individuals could be serially passed in additional volunteers. In 1972 immune electron microscopic examination using serum from a symptomatic patient demonstrated 27-nm particles in an infectious stool filtrate (Fig. 12-2) (Dolin et al., 1972; Kapikian et al., 1972). These viruses cannot be cultivated in cell culture, thus hindering acquisition of information about their epidemiology and properties.

Rotaviruses. In 1973 rotavirus particles were visualized in a duodenal biopsy by electron microscopy (Bishop et al., 1973; Kapikian et al., 1974). Rotaviruses currently are recognized as the single most common agent causing diarrhea in infants from 6 to 24 months of age in the United States. Rotaviruses also cause diarrhea in many other animal species.

Rotaviruses consist of an 11-segment genome of double-stranded RNA. The genome of this 70- to 75-nm virus is located within the inner core, and each gene segment codes for a separate viral protein (Estes and Cohen, 1989; Prasad et al., 1990). Rotavirus groups A through F have been described, but only groups A, B, and C have been identified in humans. Group A rotaviruses are common causes of gastroenteritis in children, but the significance of groups B and C has not been fully defined. The group designation of rotavirus is determined by VP6. Group A rotaviruses can be classified further into serotypes, which are determined by VP7 glycoprotein (G type) and VP4 protease-cleaved hemagglutinin (P type). There are 14 serotypes of group A rotaviruses, 7 of which (G types 1, 2, 3, 4, 8, 9, and 12) have been identified in humans. Serotypes 1 through 4 are the major causes of human disease.

Other viruses. Additional viruses including coronaviruses, pestiviruses, Breda viruses, parvoviruses, toroviruses, picornaviruses and picobirnavirus have been implicated as a cause of human gastroenteritis with varying degrees of supporting evidence.

Epidemiology

Enteric adenovirus types 40 and 41 are widespread and cause endemic diarrhea and outbreaks of diarrhea in hospitals, orphanages, and child-care centers (Van et al., 1992). These viruses infect all age groups (Kotloff et al., 1989), with antibody prevalence studies showing that more than 50% of children are seropositive by the third or fourth year of life. Infection appears to occur all year. The mode of transmission is fecal-oral and the incubation period lasts from 3 to 10 days. Enteric aden-

oviruses cause 2% to 22% of pediatric diarrhea in inpatients or outpatients. Enteric adenoviruses are a more important cause of viral gastroenteritis in infants less than 6 months of age than in older children (Bates et al., 1993). Children admitted to a hospital with enteric adenovirus infection are more likely to have diarrhea for more than 5 days but less likely to be febrile or dehydrated than children with rotavirus infection (Grimwood et al., 1995). Asymptomatic infection is common, and asymptomatic excretion after illness may last for several weeks (Van et al., 1992).

Astrovirus has been associated with diarrhea worldwide and has been linked to outbreaks of diarrhea in schools, pediatric wards, geriatric care facilities, and child-care centers, implicating person-to-person transmission (Mitchell et al., 1995a). Illness occurs mainly in children less than 4 years of age and in the elderly. More than 80% of adults have antibodies against the virus. Astrovirus has been associated with food-borne outbreaks. Asymptomatic infection is common, and asymptomatic excretion after an illness may last for several weeks. The incubation period is 1 to 4 days.

HuCVs are distributed worldwide. Serosurveillance indicates that children acquire antibody against NLVs at an early age and the antibody prevalence continues to increase throughout the school years to adulthood. Seroprevalance is higher in developing countries (Jiang, et al., 1995). NLVs may contribute 60%, and SLVs 40%, of HuCV-associated sporadic diarrhea episodes in children.

Studies in child-care centers show that calicivirus-associated diarrhea and asymptomatic infection are both widespread (Matson et al., 1990). The major public health concern about NLVs is their ability to cause large foodborne and waterborne outbreaks of gastroenteritis (Olsen, 2000). The outbreaks have occurred in schools, recreation camps, cruise ships, nursing homes, and restaurants. Outbreaks result from contaminated water or ice and ingestion of inadequately cooked contaminated shellfish, salads, and cake frosting (Barwick et al., 2000; Olsen et al., 2000). The incubation period usually ranges from 24 to 48 hours.

Rotavirus infection occurs most frequently during the cooler months of the year in temperate climates, but in tropical areas, infection occurs throughout the year. Rotavirus appears first in the Southwestern United States in

November and moves to the Northeast by March or April of each year. Infection with group A rotaviruses most frequently occurs in children 6 to 24 months of age. Infections in neonates are often asymptomatic, and both asymptomatic and symptomatic reinfections are common (Velazquez et al., 1996). Incidence rates in community-based and child-care center studies in this age group range from 0.2 to 0.8 episodes per child per year (Brandt et al., 1979; Kapikian et al., 1976). Rotaviruses cause up to 50% of the episodes of diarrhea requiring hospitalization in infants and children and are common causes of outbreaks in children in child-care centers (Bartlett et al., 1988; O'Ryan et al., 1990) and hospitals. Rotavirus results in 55,000 hospitalizations per year, 20 to 40 deaths per year, and over $1 billion per year in health-care costs in the United States (Glass et al., 1996). Serotypes 1 and 3 are the most frequently isolated serotypes from children with rotavirus diarrhea in the United States (Matson et al., 1990a). Rotaviruses can be excreted for several days before and for up to 10 days after diarrhea occurs, with the quantity of virus highest early in the course of illness (Pickering et al., 1988). Transmission occurs through the fecal-oral route. The incubation period ranges from 1 to 3 days.

Pathogenesis and Pathology

Caliciviruses are transmitted by the fecal-oral route. Infected volunteers have had detectable virus in their stools during the first 72 hours after the onset of illness. Infection with these agents results in delayed gastric emptying, although the gastric mucosa is morphologically normal. Microscopic broadening and blunting of the villi in the jejunum are apparent. The mucosa remains histologically intact, but there is a mononuclear cell infiltration. Small-intestinal enzyme studies showed decreased amounts of the enzymes measured.

Rotavirus is excreted in extraordinarily high concentrations early in the course of the illness, with as many as 10^{11} particles per gram of feces. Rotavirus particles have been visualized by electron microscopy in intestinal epithelial cells, aspirated duodenal secretions, and feces of infected persons. In addition, rotavirus has been detected in the liver and kidneys of children with immunodeficiencies (Gilger et al., 1992). Morphologically, shortening and blunting of the villi of the duode-

num and upper small intestine accompany acute illness (Schreiber et al., 1973). The microvilli of the absorptive cells are distorted, and other cells have swollen mitochondria. Rotavirus particles infect the mature enterocytes located in the middle and upper villous epithelium. This destruction of the mature enterocyte is associated with a decrease in the surface area of the intestine and decreased production of one or more mucosal disaccharidases. The destroyed infected cells are replaced by immature cells, resulting in a deficit in glucose-facilitated sodium transport. Diarrhea then results from decreased absorption secondary to the altered ion transport. Complete recovery has been confirmed by biopsy as early as 4 weeks after the episode of diarrhea. Although rotaviruses encode an enterotoxin, NSP4, the significance of this toxin is uncertain (Ball et al., 1996).

Astroviruses have been detected in symptomatic infections in the low villous epithelium and in macrophages of the lamina propria. Short-term monosaccharide intolerance and prolonged cow's milk intolerance have been reported.

Clinical Manifestations

Enteric adenoviruses cause diarrhea that lasts 6 to 9 days and may be associated with emesis and fever. Diarrhea is watery without blood or fecal leukocytes. Persistent lactose intolerance has been reported. Diarrhea caused by enteric adenovirus can last longer than other types of viral gastroenteritis. Asymptomatic infection is common.

Diarrhea caused by astroviruses usually occurs in children and in the elderly. Symptoms include low-grade fever, malaise, nausea, vomiting, and watery diarrhea that usually lasts 4 days. Vomiting is less common than with other viruses. Cow's milk intolerance has been reported following infection. Asymptomatic infection is common.

Most patients who sustain calicivirus infections have nausea, vomiting, headache, malaise, abdominal cramps, and diarrhea. Fever and chills are less common. The symptoms last from 12 to 24 hours. The disease lasts for 3 to 4 days, is self-limited, and does not cause chronic infection. Stools usually are not bloody and do not contain mucus or cells. Transient lymphopenia has been observed in volunteers challenged with these agents.

Acute infections caused by rotavirus are characterized by an abrupt onset of watery diarrhea that characteristically is not associated with blood or mucus in the stool. The mean duration of illness in immunocompetent hosts is 5 to 7 days, but chronic infection can occur in immunodeficient children, and disease can be more severe in malnourished hosts. Vomiting is often present before or after onset of diarrhea. Dehydration and metabolic acidosis are common and may necessitate hospitalization. Rotaviruses are responsible for at least one half of the cases of infantile diarrhea requiring hospitalization. Rotaviruses have been associated with liver damage in immunodeficient hosts. In children in child-care centers, asymptomatic infections represent up to 50% of all rotavirus infections (O'Ryan et al., 1990). Recurrent infections are common in children in child-care centers and in other settings in which exposure is frequent (Velazquez et al., 1996).

Diagnosis and Differential Diagnosis

The clinical differentiation of viral gastroenteritis from gastroenteritis due to bacteria or protozoa may be difficult. Various epidemiologic factors such as season and age, as well as clinical manifestations, may be helpful. Viral gastroenteritis rarely is associated with bloody diarrhea. Laboratory support is needed to substantiate a clinical diagnosis. The most widely used assays for detection of a viral enteropathogen are electron microscopy, immune electron microscopy, EIA, latex agglutination, gel electrophoresis, culture of the virus, PCR, and reverse transcriptase–PCR (RT-PCR). Different assays currently are used for each virus (Table 12-5). Commercial EIAs are available for detection of rotavirus, enteric adenoviruses, and astrovirus.

Electron microscopy initially was used to detect enteric adenoviruses, but commercially available assays that use monoclonal antibodies in EIA techniques are available (Van et al., 1992). Enteric adenoviruses can be cultivated in special cell lines. Restriction enzyme analysis is the definitive method used for classifying individual isolates.

Astroviruses grow in human colonic carcinoma cells in the presence of trypsin. Electron microscopy, immune electron microscopy, immunofluorescence of cell culture, EIA (Herrmann et al., 1990), and RT-PCR (Mitchell

et al., 1995a) can be used as detection methods. These methods currently are available in research laboratories. RT-PCR and genome sequencing have been used for epidemiologic studies.

Neither NLVs nor SLVs can be cultivated in cell culture or passed in animal models, which hampers study of these viruses. Following cloning and sequencing of NV in 1990, two major types of assays for diagnosis of HuCVs have been developed. One type is used to detect viral antigens or antibodies against the antigens through recombinant EIAs, and the other is used to detect the viral RNA through RT-PCR (Jiang, 1992). Neither type of assay depends on a clinical source for reagents.

For detection of rotavirus in stool specimens the original diagnostic technique of electron microscopy is still used as the single method available to identify all of the viral pathogens, including group A and non–group A rotavirus. EIA and latex agglutination assays are more readily available and detect group A rotaviruses (Yolken et al., 1978). As a general rule, latex agglutination tests have shown as high a specificity but a lower sensitivity than EIA (Dennehy et al., 1988). Electropherotyping is a valuable means of studying the epidemiology of rotavirus infection, but it is not used as a diagnostic test. Oligonucleotide probes and RT-PCR tests have been used in research settings (Gouvea et al., 1990). Serologic assays for total antibody to rotavirus or serotype-specific response are useful to substantiate an infection but currently are not useful diagnostic tests during the acute course of an infection.

Complications

Severe dehydration as a consequence of vomiting and diarrhea is the major complication of viral gastroenteritis, especially in young infants and elderly debilitated adults. Immunocompromised patients may have prolonged viral shedding and symptoms of diarrhea caused by viral enteropathogens.

Prognosis

In general, the prognosis with any of these viral infections of the intestinal tract is excellent. The illness is self-limited and usually lasts for 1 to 4 days. Immunocompromised patients can experience unremitting symptoms or fatal disease.

Treatment

The general principles of rehydration therapy are the same as those described for bacterial gastroenteritis (American Academy of Pediatrics, 1996). There is no specific antiviral therapy for any of the viral enteropathogens. Oral rehydration should be used for most children, except those who are severely dehydrated and cannot tolerate oral feedings due to shock, coma, or ileus.

Preventive Measures

Appropriate hygiene and frequent hand washing are necessary for interruption of the fecal-oral spread of these agents. Careful food preparation measures must be enforced to reduce spread by contaminated food and water (Centers for Disease Control and Prevention, 2001; Barwick et al., 2000; Olsen et al., 2000).

Hospital isolation measures must be followed to prevent nosocomial diarrhea. Hospitalized patients with diarrhea should be isolated using contact precautions (Garner, 1996). The prevention of rotavirus infection would be a major contribution to reducing the morbidity and mortality of acute infectious gastroenteritis. Therefore it is expected that immunization will make a major contribution toward this goal.

Immunizations

Ultimate prevention of most cases of viral gastroenteritis depends on safe and effective vaccines. The greatest progress in this area has been with development of rotavirus vaccines. Unfortunately the first rotavirus vaccine licensed by the FDA in the United States was associated with an increased rate of intussusception, resulting in withdrawal from the market in 2000, 14 months after licensure (Murphy et al., 2001). Other candidate vaccines are undergoing testing.

BIBLIOGRAPHY

Ackman DM, Drabkin P, Birkhead G, Cieslak P. Reptile-associated salmonellosis in New York state. Pediatr Infect Dis J 1995;14:955-959.

Allos BM. *Campylobacter jejuni* infections: update of emerging issues and trends. Clin Infect Dis 2001;32:1201-1206.

American Academy of Pediatrics, Subcommittee on Acute Gastroenteritis. Practice parameter: the management of acute gastroenteritis in young children. Pediatrics 1996;97:424-436.

Aureli P, Fiorucci GC, Caroli D, et al. An outbreak of febrile gastroenteritis associated with corn contaminated with *Listeria monocytogenes*. N Engl J Med 2000;342:1236-1241.

Avendano P, Matson DO, Long J, et al. Costs associated with office visits for diarrhea in infants and toddlers. Pediatr Infect Dis J 1993;12:897-902.

Ball JM, Tian P, Seng CO, et al. Age-dependent diarrhea induced by a rotaviral non-structural glycoprotein. Science 1996;272:101-104.

Bartlett AV, Prado D, Cleary TG, Pickering LK. Production of shigatoxin and other enterotoxins by serogroups of *Shigella*. J Infect Dis 1986;154:996-1002.

Bartlett AV, Reves RR, Pickering LK. Rotavirus in infant-toddler day-care centers: epidemiology relevant to disease control strategies. J Pediatr 1988;113:435-441.

Bartlett JG. *Clostridium difficile*: history of its role as an enteric pathogen and the current state of knowledge about the organism. Clin Infect Dis 1994;18:S265-S272.

Barwick RS, Levy DA, Craun GF, et al. Surveillance for waterborne disease outbreaks—United States, 1997-1998. MMWR 2000;49:1-35.

Bates PR, Bailey AS, Wood DJ, et al. Comparative epidemiology of rotavirus, subgenus F (types 40 and 41) adenovirus, and astrovirus gastroenteritis in children. J Med Virol 1993;39:224-228.

Belongia EA, Osterholm MT, Soler JT, et al. Transmission of *Escherichia coli* O157:H7 infection in Minnesota child day-care facilities. JAMA 1993;269:883-888.

Bern C, Martines J, de Zoysa I, Glass RI. The magnitude of the global problem of diarrhoeal disease: a 10-year update. Bull World Health Org 1992;70:705-714.

Bishop RF, Davidson GP, Holmes IH, Ruck BJ. Evidence for viral gastroenteritis. N Engl J Med 1973;289:1096-1097.

Brandt CD, Kim HW, Rodriguez WJ, et al. Adenovirus and pediatric gastroenteritis. J Infect Dis 1985;151:437-443.

Brandt CD, Kim HW, Yolken RH, et al. Comparative epidemiology of two rotavirus serotypes and other viral agents associated with pediatric gastroenteritis. Am J Epidemiol 1979;110:243-254.

Brenner FW, Villar RG, Angulo FJ, et al. Salmonella nomenclature. J Clin Microbiol 2000;38:2465-2467.

Brown KH, Peerson JM, Fontaine O. Use of nonhuman milks in the dietary management of young children with acute diarrhea: a meta-analysis of clinical trials. Pediatrics 1994;93:17-27.

Centers for Disease Control. 1993 Revised classification system for HIV infection and expanded AIDS surveillance case definition for AIDS among adolescents and adults. MMWR 1992;41:1-19.

Centers for Disease Control and Prevention. The management of acute diarrhea in children: oral rehydration, maintenance and nutritional therapy. MMWR 1992;41:1-20.

Centers for Disease Control and Prevention. Lake-associated outbreak of *Escherichia coli* O157:H7-Illinois, 1995. MMWR 1996a;45: 437-439.

Centers for Disease Control and Prevention. Outbreaks of *Salmonella* serotype *Enteritidis* infection associated with consumption of raw shell eggs: United States, 1994-1995. MMWR 1996b;45:737-742.

Centers for Disease Control and Prevention. *Vibrio vulnificus* infections associated with eating raw oysters: Los Angeles, 1996. MMWR 1996c;45:621-624.

Centers for Disease Control and Prevention. Diagnosis and management of foodborne illnesses: a primer for physicians. MMWR 2001;50:1-69.

Centers for Disease Control and Prevention. Preliminary Foodnet data on the incidence of foodborne illnesses—selected sites, United States, 2001. MMWR 2002a;51:325-329.

Centers for Disease Control and Prevention. Guidelines for the preventing opportunistic among HIV-infected persons 2002. MMWR 2002b; 51:1-52.

Centers for Disease Control and Prevention. Summary of notifiable diseases—United States, 2001. MMWR 2003;50:1-108.

Cerquetti M, Luzzi I, Caprioli A, et al. Role of *Clostridium difficile* in childhood diarrhea. Pediatr Infect Dis J 1995;14:598-603.

Cholera Working Group, International Centre for Diarrhoeal Diseases Research, Bangladesh. Large epidemic of cholera-like disease in Bangladesh caused by *Vibrio cholerae* O139 synonym Bengal. Lancet 1993;342:387-390.

Cicirello HG, Glass RI. Current concepts of the epidemiology of diarrheal diseases. Semin Pediatr Infect Dis 1994;5:163-167.

Claeson M, Merson MH. Global progress in the control of diarrheal diseases. Pediatr Infect Dis J 1990;9:345-355.

Daniels NA, MacKinnon L, Bishop R, et al. *Vibrio parahaemolyticus* infections in the United States, 1973-1998. J Infect Dis 2000;181:161-162.

de la Morena ML, Van R, Singh K, et al. Diarrhea associated with *Aeromonas* species in children in day-care centers. J Infect Dis 1993;168:215-218.

Dennehy PH, Gauntlett DR, Tente WE. Comparison of nine commercial immunoassays for the detection of rotavirus in fecal specimens. J Clin Microbiol 1988;26:1630-1634.

Dolin R, Blacklow NR, DuPont H, et al. Biological properties of Norwalk agent of acute infectious nonbacterial gastroenteritis. Proc Soc Exp Biol Med 1972;140:578-583.

Duggan C, Santosham M, Glass RI. The management of acute diarrhea in children: oral rehydration, maintenance, and nutritional therapy: Centers for Disease Control and Prevention. MMWR 1992;41:1-20.

DuPont HL, Capsuto EG. Persistent diarrhea in travelers. Clin Infect Dis 1996;22:124-128.

DuPont HL, Practice Parameters Committee of the American College of Gastroenterology. Guidelines on acute diarrhea in adults. Am J Gastroenterol 1997;92:1962-1975.

Estes MK, Cohen J. Rotavirus gene structure and function. Microbiol Rev 1989;53:410-449.

Garner JS. Guideline for isolation precautions in hospitals. Infect Control Hosp Epidemiol 1996;17:53-80.

Gerding DN, Johnson S, Peterson LR, et al. *Clostridium difficile*–associated diarrhea and colitis. Infect Control Hosp Epidemiol 1995;16:459-477.

Gilger MA, Matson DO, Conner ME, et al. Extraintestinal rotavirus infections in children with immunodeficiency. J Pediatr 1992;120:912-917.

Glass RI, Kilgore PE, Holman RC, et al. The epidemiology of rotavirus diarrhea in the United States: surveillance and estimates of disease burden. J Infect Dis 1996;174 (suppl 1):S5-S11.

Goossens H, Giesendorf AJ, Vandamme P, et al. Investigation of an outbreak of *Campylobacter upsaliensis* in day-care centers in Brussels: analysis of relationships among isolates by phenotypic and genotypic typing methods. J Infect Dis 1995;172:1298-1303.

Gorbach SL, Kean BH, Evans DG, et al. Travelers' diarrhea and toxigenic *Escherichia coli*. N Engl J Med 1975;292:933-936.

Gouvea V, Glass RI, Woods P, et al. Polymerase chain reaction amplification and typing of rotavirus nucleic acid from stool specimens. J Clin Microbiol 1990;28:276-282.

Grady GF, Keusch GT. Pathogenesis of bacterial diarrheas. N Engl J Med 1971;285:831-900.

Green KY, Ando T, Balayan MS, et al. Taxonomy of the caliciviruses. J Infect Dis 2000:181(suppl 2):S322-S330.

Grimwood K, Carzino R, Barnes GL, Bishop RF. Patients with enteric adenovirus gastroenteritis admitted to an Australian pediatric teaching hospital from 1981 to 1992. J Clin Microbiol 1995;33:131-136.

Guerrero L, Calva JJ, Morrow AL, et al. Asymptomatic *Shigella* infections in a cohort of Mexican children younger than two years of age. Pediatr Infect Dis J 1994;13:597-602.

Guerrant RL, VanGilder T, Steiner TS, et al. Practice guidelines for the management of infectious diarrhea. Infectious Diseases Society of America. Clin Infect Dis 2001;32:331-350.

Hayani KC, Ericsson CD, Pickering LK. Prevention and treatment of diarrhea in the traveling child. Semin Pediatr Infect Dis 1992;3:22-32.

Hennessy TW, Hedberg CW, Slutsker L, et al. A national outbreak of *Salmonella enteritidis* infections from ice cream. N Engl J Med 1996;334:1281-1286.

Herrmann JE, Nowak NA, Perron-Henry DM, et al. Diagnosis of astrovirus gastroenteritis by antigen detection with monoclonal antibodies. J Infect Dis 1990;161:226-229.

Hof H. *Listeria monocytogenes*: a causative agent of gastroenteritis? Eur J Clin Microbial Infect Dis 2001;20:369-373.

Hohmann EL. Nontyphoidol salmonettosis. Clin Infect Dis 2001;32: 263-269.

Holmes SJ, Morrow AL, Pickering LK. Child care practices: effects of social changes on epidemiology of infectious diseases and antibiotic resistance. Epidemiol Rev 1996;18:10-28.

Holmgren J. Actions of cholera toxin and the prevention and treatment of cholera. Nature 1981;292:413-417.

Hornick RB, Greisman SE, Woodward TE, et al. Typhoid fever: pathogenesis and immunologic control. N Engl J Med 1970;283:739-746.

Janda JM, Abbott SL. Evolving concepts regarding the genus *Aeromonas*: an expanding panorama of species, disease presentations, and unanswered questions. Clin Infect Dis 1998;27:332-344.

Jiang X, Cubitt D, Hu J, et al. Development of an ELISA to detect MX virus, a human calicivirus in the snow mountain agent genogroup. J Gen Virol 1995;76:2739-2747.

Jiang X, Graham D, Wang K, et al. Norwalk virus genome cloning and characterization. Science 1990;250:1580-1583.

Jiang X, Matson DO, Velazquez FR, et al. Study of Norwalk-related viruses in Mexican children. J Med Virol 1995;47:309-316.

Jiang X, Wang J, Graham DY, et al. Detection of Norwalk virus in stool by polymerase chain reaction. J Clin Microbiol 1992;30:2529-2534.

Jimenez SG, Heine RG, Ward RB, et al. *Campylobacter upsaliensis* gastroenteritis in childhood. Pediatr Infect Dis J 1999;18:998-992.

Kapikian AZ, Kim HW, Wyatt RG, et al. Reovirus-like agent in stools: association with infantile diarrhea and development of serologic tests. Science 1974;185:1049-1053.

Kapikian AZ, Kim HW, Wyatt RG, et al. Human reovirus-like agent as the major pathogen associated with "winter" gastroenteritis in hospitalized infants, young children, and their contacts. N Engl J Med 1976;294:965-972.

Kapikian AZ, Wyatt RG, Dolin R, et al. Visualization by immune electron microscopy of a 27-nm particle associated with acute infectious nonbacterial gastroenteritis. J Virol 1972;10:1075-1081.

Karmali MA, Petric M, Steele BT, Lin C. Sporadic cases of hemolytic uremic syndrome associated with faecal cytotoxin and cytotoxin producing *E. coli* in stools. Lancet 1983;1:619-620.

Keene WE, McAnulty JM, Hoesly FC, et al. A swimming-associated outbreak of hemorrhagic colitis caused by *Escherichia coli* O157:H7 and *Shigella sonnei*. N Engl J Med 1994;331:579-584.

Kelly CP, Pothoulakis C, LaMont JT. *Clostridium difficile* colitis. N Engl J Med 1994;380:256-261.

Kotloff KL, Losonsky GA, Morris JG, et al. Enteric adenovirus infection and childhood diarrhea: an epidemiologic study in three clinical settings. Pediatrics 1989; 84:219-225.

Lee LA, Gerber AR, Lonsway DR, Smith JD. *Yersinia enterocolitica* O:3 infections in infants and children, associated with the household preparation of chitterlings. N Engl J Med 1990;322:984-987.

Levine MM, Noriega F. Current status of vaccine development for enteric diseases. Semin Pediatr Infect Dis 1994;5:245-250.

Matson DO, Estes MK, Burns JW, et al. Serotype variation of human group A rotaviruses in two regions of the United States. J Infect Dis 1990a;162:605-614.

Matson DO, Estes MK, Tanaka T, et al. Asymptomatic human calicivirus infection in a day-care center outbreak. Pediatr Infect Dis J 1990b;9:190-196.

Mead PS, Slutskerl, Dietz V, et al. Food related illness and death in the United States. Emerg Infect Dis 1999;5:607-625.

Mitchell DK, Monroe SS, Jiang X, et al. Virologic features of an astrovirus diarrhea outbreak in a day-care center revealed by reverse transcriptase-polymerase chain reaction. J Infect Dis 1995a;172:1437-1444.

Mitchell DK, Van R, Mason EH, et al. Prospective study of infection with *Clostridium difficile* in children given amoxicillin/clavulanate for otitis media. Pediatr Infect Dis J 1995b;15:514-519.

Murphy TV, Gargiullo PM, Massoudi MS, et al. Intussusception among infants given and oral rotavirus vaccine. N Engl J Med 2001;344:564-572.

Nair GB, Ramamurthy T, Bhattacharya SK, et al. Spread of *Vibrio cholerae* O139 Bengal in India. J Infect Dis 1994;169:1029-1034.

Nataro JP, Kaper JB. Diarrheagenic *Escherichia coli*. Clin Microbiol Rev 1998;11:142-201.

Novak R, Feldman S. Salmonellosis in children with cancer: review of 42 cases. Am J Dis Child 1979;133:298-300.

Olsen SJ, MacKinon LC, Goulding JS, et al. Surveillance for foodborne disease outbreaks—United States, 1993-1997. MMWR 2000;49:1-51.

O'Ryan ML, Matson DO, Estes MK, et al. Molecular epidemiology of rotavirus in children attending day-care centers in Houston. J Infect Dis 1990;162:810-816.

Pickering LK. Emerging antibiotic resistance in enteric bacterial pathogens. Semin Pediatr Infect Dis 1996;7:272-280.

Pickering LK, Bartlett AV, Reves RR, Morrow AL. Asymptomatic excretion of rotavirus before and after rotavirus diarrhea in children in day-care centers. J Pediatr 1988;112:361-365.

Pickering LK, Cleary TG. Therapy for diarrheal illness in children. In Blaser MJ, Smith PD, Raudin JI, et al. (eds). Infections of the Gastrointestinal Tract. New York, NY: Raven Press, 2002, 1223-1240.

Pickering LK, Obrig TG, Stapleton FB. Hemolytic uremic syndrome and enterohemorrhagic *Escherichia coli*. Pediatr Infect Dis J 1994;13:459-475.

Prasad BVV, Burns JW, Mariette E, et al. Localization of VP4 neutralization sites in rotavirus by three-dimensional cryoelectron microscopy. Nature 1990;343:476-479.

Reed RP, Friedland IR, Wegerhoff FO, et al. *Campylobacter* bacteremia in children. Pediatr Infect Dis J 1996;15:345-348.

Rees JH, Soudain SE, Gregson NA, Hughes RAC. *Campylobacter jejuni* infection and Guillain-Barré syndrome. N Engl J Med 1995;333:1374-1379.

Reves RR, Morrow AL, Bartlett AV, et al. Child day-care increases the risk of clinic visits for acute diarrhea and diarrhea due to rotavirus. Am J Epidemiol 1993;137:97-107.

Safdar N, Said A, Gangnon RE, et al. Risk of hemolytic uremic syndrome after antibiotic treatment of *Escherichia coli* O157:H7 enteritis. A meta-analysis. JAMA 2002; 288:996-1001.

Saphra I, Winter JW. Clinical manifestations of salmonellosis in man. An evaluation of 7,779 human infections identified at the New York Salmonella Center. N Engl J Med 1957;256:1128.

Schreiber DS, Blacklow NR, Trier JS. The mucosal lesion of the proximal small intestine in acute infections nonbacterial gastroenteritis. N Engl J Med 1973;288:1318-1323.

Sears CL, Kaper JB. Enteric bacterial toxins: mechanisms of action and linkage to intestinal secretion. Microbiol Rev 1996;60:167-215.

Sempertegui F, Estrella B, Egas J, et al. Risk of diarrheal disease in Ecuadorian day-care centers. Pediatr Infect Dis J 1995;14:606-612.

Snyder J. The continuing evolution of oral therapy for diarrhea. Semin Pediatr Infect Dis 1994;5:231-235.

Tauxe RV. Food safety and irradiation: protecting the public from foodborne infections. Emerg Infect Dis 2001;7:516-521.

Van Niel CW, Feudtner C, Garrison MM, et al. *Lactobacillus* therapy for acute infectious diarrhea in children: a meta-analysis. Pediatrics 2002;109:678-684.

Van R, Wun C, O'Ryan MC, et al. Outbreaks of human enteric adenovirus types 40 and 41 in Houston day-care centers. J Pediatr 1992;120:516-521.

Velazquez FR, Matson DO, Calva JJ, et al. Rotavirus infection in infants as protection against subsequent infections. N Engl J Med 1996;335:1022-1028.

Waldor MK, Mekalanos JJ. Lysogenic conversion by a filamentous phage encoding cholera toxin. Science 1996;272:1910-1914.

World Health Organization. New formulation for oral rehydration salts will save millions of lives: number of deaths and severity of illness will be reduced. Available at: http//www.who.int/inf/en/pr-2002-35.html. Accessed August 2002.

Wong CS, Jelacic S, Habeeb RL, et al. The risk of the hemolytic uremic syndrome after antibody treatment of *Escherichia coli* O157:H7 infections. N Engl J Med 2000;342:1930-1936.

Yang S, Leff MG, McTague D, et al. Multistate surveillance for food handling, preparation and consumption behaviors associated with foodborne diseases: 1995 and 1996 BRFSS food-safety questions. MMWR 1998;47:33-57.

Yolken RH, Wyatt RG, Zissis G, et al. Epidemiology of human rotavirus types 1 and 2 as studied by enzyme-linked immunosorbent assay. N Engl J Med 1978;229:1156-1161.

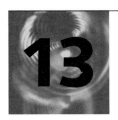

HELMINTH INFECTIONS

PETER J. HOTEZ

GLOBAL MORBIDITY OF HELMINTH INFECTIONS

Helminth infections are often considered to be the most common infectious diseases of humankind. The World Health Organization (WHO) estimates that 2 billion people are infected worldwide with one or more different species of soil-transmitted helminths (*Ascaris, Trichuris*, and hookworms) or schistosomes. Approximately 400 million of these helminth infections occur in school-age children. Together, the soil-transmitted helminths (STHs) and schistosomes account for an estimated 40% of the global morbidity from all infectious agents exclusive of the malaria parasite *Plasmodium falciparum*. The STHs and schistosomes are primarily important causes of parasitic diseases in the developing nations of the tropics and subtropics. With the exception of *Enterobius* (pinworm) and *Toxocara* (zoonotic dog ascarid), the STHs are not considered important indigenous causes of parasitic disease among children living in North America and Europe. Toxocariasis is the most prevalent and potentially serious helminth infection in temperate climates. Tapeworm infections are also common in temperate climates, the most serious of which is the pork tapeworm, *Taenia solium*, the etiologic agent of neurocysticercosis (NCC). NCC has emerged as an important cause of pediatric epilepsy in North America. This chapter focuses on the major helminths of children both in temperate climates and in the developing world, the STH infections, schistosomiasis, and NCC.

SOIL-TRANSMITTED HELMINTH (INTESTINAL NEMATODE) INFECTIONS

The intestinal nematodes are often referred to as *geohelminths* or STHs in reference to their requirement to develop in the external environment, frequently the soil, during a portion of their life cycle. The WHO currently favors the term *STH* to describe the "unholy trinity" of *Ascaris lumbricoides, Trichuris trichiura*, and the hookworms (*Necator americanus* and *Ancylostoma duodenale*), which are devastating pathogens for children living in developing countries. *Toxocara canis* is an important STH in temperate climates. Although the pinworm *Enterobius vermicularis* is not, strictly speaking, an STH, it often occurs during coinfection with STHs and therefore will be discussed here.

STH infections occur among every age group, but school-age children (between the ages of 5 and 14 years) are particularly susceptible to acquiring heavy STH worm burdens with *Ascaris, Trichuris*, and *Enterobius* (Hotez, 2000). With the exception of hookworm infection, which can cause high worm burdens in adults and even the elderly (Gandhi et al., 2001; Bethony et al., 2002), children typically suffer greater morbidity from STHs compared with less heavily infected adults. It is not known whether the predisposition to high STH burdens during childhood has a genetic, immunologic, or behavioral basis. Nevertheless, an increasing body of evidence suggests that children chronically infected with these worms suffer from deficits in their physical growth, intelligence, and cognition (Drake et al., 2000). Therefore the STHs have attracted the attention of a new generation of experts interested in the vigor and well being of children from less-developed countries. Increasingly, the WHO and other international agencies have looked to anthelminthic deworming programs as much for their value in improving educational school performance as for their value in improving health.

Ascariasis and Trichuriasis

In North America, transmission of *A. lumbricoides* (large roundworm) and *T. trichiura* (whipworm) no longer occurs commonly in the United States and Canada, although both infections are highly endemic to Mexico and Central America. Transmission of both infections still occurs to some extent in Eastern Europe. Ascariasis and trichuriasis are the most common infections in the tropics and subtropics, each occurring in at least 1 billion people. In China alone, it is estimated that 530 million people harbor *A. lumbricoides* and 212 million harbor *T. trichiura* (Hotez et al., 1997). Although *Ascaris* and *Trichuris* each produce different diseases in children, it is sometimes possible to treat them together because they share the following common features:

- Both STHs are not directly infectious to humans, but instead require a period of time in which the eggs incubate in the environment before they become infectious. *Ascaris* and *Trichuris* eggs are notoriously hardy to environmental extremes, a feature that permits them to survive in urban as well as rural areas. For this reason it is common to see urban children living in the slums of large cities such as Mexico City and Guatemala City infected with these parasites. It has been reported that ascaris eggs can be recovered from the paper currency in some less-developed countries. This is in contrast to hookworm, which more typically relies on rural agricultural practices for its survival.
- *Ascaris* and *Trichuris* organisms in the adult stages live in the intestine, although they occupy distinct niches. *A. lumbricoides* inhabits small intestine, and *T. trichiura* inhabits the colon.
- Resistance and immunity to *Ascaris* and *Trichuris* organisms are inadequate in childhood, so children harbor greater numbers of worms than adults (i.e., children appear to be more predisposed to heavy infections).
- Even among infected children the STHs exhibit aggregated distributions in endemic areas, so many children harbor small numbers of adult worms (light and moderate infections), whereas a significant minority of children harbor large number of worms (heavy infections). Moderately and heavily infected children develop the greatest amount of disease in terms of severity.
- Moderate and heavy infections produce similar chronic sequelae, namely physical growth retardation and stunting (Hall, 1993), as well as intellectual, cognitive, and behavioral deficits (Drake et al., 2000).
- Adult female *Ascaris* and *Trichuris* worms produce large numbers of eggs that pass out with the fecal stream. A specific diagnosis of both STH infections is established by identifying the characteristic eggs on fecal exam.
- The benzimidazoles (BZs) albendazole (400 mg once, or more for heavy infections) and mebendazole (100 mg twice a day for 3 days) are equally effective against *Ascaris* and *Trichuris* infections (Table 13-1). The BZs do not have proven safety in children under 2 years of age, although they have been used extensively in young children in less-developed countries (Biddulph, 1990; Cowden and Hotez, 2000). The WHO recommends use of either BZ (especially albendazole because of its efficacy in a single dose) for deworming children in school-based programs. Because the BZs are embryotoxic and teratogenic in laboratory animals, it is advised to weigh the risks versus benefits for these agents. BZs should be avoided in children with blood dyscrasias or preexisting liver disease. Pyrantel pamoate is a second-line drug available in liquid suspension (11 mg/kg [maximum 1 g]), which is suitable for the treatment of *A. lumbricoides* infection (administered in a single dose), but not for *T. trichiura* infection. Oxantel (not available in the United States) is suitable for the treatment of trichuriasis; in some countries it is formulated in a liquid preparation with pyrantel pamoate.

There are also important distinctions between *Ascaris* and *Trichuris*. The whipworm *T. trichiura* has the simplest life cycle among the STHs. Humans become infected with *T. trichiura* by ingesting the embryonated eggs. The larvae hatch in the intestine and penetrate the columnar epithelium. The adult worms reside in the large intestine, where their finely attenuated anterior end creates epithelial tunnels in the mucosa, while their larger posterior end protrudes into the lumen of the large intestine. By this process the adult whipworm disrupts the normal architecture of the colonic epithelium and elicits inflammation. Heavily infected children develop either a *Trichuris* dysentery syndrome (TDS) or *Trichuris* colitis

TABLE 13-1   **First-line Treatment Recommendations for Common Parasitic Diseases of Childhood[*][†]**

Disease	Drug	Dosage
Enterobiasis	Mebendazole	100 mg PO given once; repeat in 2 weeks
	Albendazole[‡]	400 mg PO given once; repeat in 2 weeks
Ascariasis	Mebendazole	100 mg PO bid. × 3 days
	Albendazole[‡]	400 mg PO given once
Trichuriasis	Mebendazole	100 mg PO bid × 3 days
	Albendazole[‡]	400 mg PO given once
Hookworm	Mebendazole	100 mg PO bid. × 3 days
	Albendazole[‡]	400 mg PO given once
Toxocariasis	Albendazole[‡]	400 mg PO bid. × 5 days[‡]
Dipylidiasis	Praziquantel	5-10 mg/kg PO given once
Diphyllobothriasis	Praziquantel	5-10 mg/kg PO given once
Taeniasis	Praziquantel	5-10 mg/kg PO given once
Hymenolepiasis (*Hymenolepis diminuta*)	Praziquantel	5-10 mg/kg PO given once
Hymenolepiasis (*Hymenolepis nana*)	Praziquantel	25 mg/kg PO given once
Cysticercosis	Albendazole	15 mg/kg/day (max 800 mg) in 2 doses × 8-30 days; can be repeated as necessary[§]
Schistosomiasis		
Schistosoma haematobium	Praziquantel	40 mg/kg/day in 2 doses × 1 day
Schistosoma japonicum	Praziquantel	60 mg/kg/day in 3 doses × 1 day
Schistosoma mansoni	Praziquantel	40 mg/kg/day in 2 doses × 1 day

[*]Based on agents available in the United States (Medical Letter, 2002).
[†]Discussions about these agents are available in the text.
[‡]Albendazole is an approved drug but is considered investigational for this condition by the U.S. Food and Drug Administration
[§]Some studies indicate that praziquantel is equivalent to albendazole; corticosteroids and anticonvulsants may be indicated. Cimetidine may need to be coadministered to increase absorption.

(Bundy and Cooper, 1989). Children with TDS have severe diarrhea with blood and mucus that can result in emaciation and anemia. Mucosal swelling of the rectum can cause an urge to bear down as if stool were present; protracted tenesmus may cause rectal prolapse (Bundy and Cooper, 1989; Despommier et al., 1995). Children with *Trichuris* colitis develop chronic malnutrition, short stature, anemia of chronic disease, and even finger clubbing. Similarities between *Trichuris* colitis and other forms of inflammatory bowel disease such as Crohn's disease and ulcerative colitis have been reported (Bundy and Cooper, 1989). Children with either TDS or *Trichuris* colitis often respond well to specific anthelminthic treatment; afterward they frequently experience impressive catch-up growth.

As with whipworm, humans become infected with *A. lumbricoides* when they ingest embryonated eggs. However, the similarity to the whipworm life cycle ends there, as the emerging larva penetrates the small intestine and enters through the circulatory system before it reaches the lungs. Eosinophilia occurs as the larvae migrate through the tissues. The pulmonary migrations of *A. lumbricoides* larvae elicit a Löffler's-like pneumonia consisting of eosinophilic pulmonary infiltrates and wheezing. After molting in the lung, the larvae are coughed and swallowed, thereby allowing the larvae to enter into the gastrointestinal tract. In the small intestine the larvae become adult worms that grow to lengths of more than 30 cm. *Ascaris* adversely affects the nutritional status of children, resulting in growth retardation (Crompton, 1992). In large numbers, the worms become entangled in a bolus to cause acute intestinal obstruction. Frequently this requires surgical intervention. The adult worms may also migrate into the biliary tree to cause hepatobiliary and pancreatic ascariasis

(Basavaraju and Hotez, 2003). These processes can be precipitated by the administration of certain irritants, possibly including generalized anesthesia.

Hookworm (*Necator* and *Ancylostoma*)

Like *Ascaris* and *Trichuris*, the two major human hookworms, *N. americanus* and *A. duodenale*, are important STHs of children, in whom they cause iron deficiency and protein malnutrition (Hotez, 1989). An estimated 1 billion infections occur worldwide, with 194 million cases in China alone (Hotez et al., 1997). Unlike the other two members of the "unholy trinity," however, the hookworms are also significant health problems of adults and the elderly. In some regions, there are distinct epidemiologic differences between the hookworms and other STHs. For instance, in China and Southeast Asia it is common to see almost a direct linear relationship between hookworm infection intensity and increasing age, so that the highest hookworm burdens occur among individuals over the age of 50, whereas the highest *Ascaris* and *Trichuris* worm burdens occur in children (Gandhi et al., 2001; Bethony et al., 2002). Another major difference between *Ascaris* and *Trichuris* versus hookworm is that the eggs of hookworms hatch when they are deposited in the soil. This requires relatively precise conditions of moisture and shade that are usually met only in agriculturally intensive rural areas. There is a strong relationship between endemic hookworm and the farming of certain crops such as tea (India), sweet potatoes and corn (China), coffee (Central and South America), and rubber (Africa). After hatching, the emerging hookworm larvae molt twice to become third-stage infective larvae, which either penetrate through the skin (*A. duodenale* and *N. americanus*) or are ingested (*A. duodenale*). Eosinophilia arises as the larvae migrate through the lungs and other tissues. Ultimately, the larvae gain entry into the intestine, where they molt and grow into adult hookworms. The adult hookworms attach to the mucosal and submucosal layers of the small intestine and lacerate villus capillaries to cause local intestinal hemorrhage–some of the blood is directly ingested by the parasite. Therefore, iron deficiency and anemia are the major features of moderate and heavy hookworm infections. Chronic hookworm anemia of childhood results in physical and mental growth retardation (Hotez, 1989; Hotez and Pritchard, 1995). The BZ anthelminthic agents albendazole and mebendazole (in the doses described for treatment of *Ascaris* and *Trichuris* infections) are the treatments of choice for hookworm. However, children and adults often mount a poor immune response to hookworms, so that they remain susceptible to the infection even after receiving anthelminthic chemotherapy (Albonico et al., 1995; Hotez et al., 1996). For that reason BZs have frequently failed to control hookworm in highly endemic areas. As an alternative or complementary approach to control, the possibility of developing an anti-hookworm vaccine is under investigation (Hotez et al., 1999). An infantile form of infection with *A. duodenale* has been described that causes failure to thrive, melena, and profound anemia. It has been conjectured that infants may sometimes acquire *A. duodenale* larvae by ingesting them in the breast milk from mothers who harbor developmentally arrested larvae.

Toxocariasis

T. canis infection resulting in either visceral larva migrans (VLM) or ocular larva migrans (OLM) is a major zoonosis in the United States, Europe, and Japan. Accidental infection with the eggs of this canine ascarid results in significant extraintestinal symptomatology when the larval stages of the parasite migrate through viscera after they fail to complete their development in an aberrant human host. Most commonly humans acquire VLM or OLM by ingesting *T. canis* eggs shed in the feces of dogs harboring the adult worms (Hotez, 1995). In many parts of the United States the prevalence of toxocariasis is almost 100% in puppies less than 6 months of age (Hermann et al., 1973). Children between the ages of 1 and 4 years often come into contact with *T. canis* eggs while playing in sandboxes and on playgrounds that were contaminated by a family pet or stray dog. For that reason, VLM is typically a disease of toddlers and young children (Hotez, 1993). In contrast, OLM more commonly occurs in older children.

Because most of the clinical cases of toxocariasis go undiagnosed, there are no precise estimates for the number of cases in the United States (Schantz, 1989). As Schantz (1989) has pointed out, the prevalence of larva migrans is probably high based on the large number of serum samples that are sent annually to state and local health departments (and forwarded to the Centers for Disease Control and Prevention [CDC]) from patients with a presumptive diagnosis of toxocariasis. The CDC receives an estimated 2,600 to 3,500 specimens every year, of which about 25% to 33% test positive (Schantz, 1989). At least 10,000 individuals in the United States are believed to suffer from toxocariasis (Stehr-Green and Schantz, 1987). The widespread environmental contamination with *T. canis* eggs from some 55 million dogs maintained as pets and another 60 to 80 million unknown dogs in the United States (Elliot et al., 1985; Stehr-Green and Schantz, 1987), together with the intimate play of children with pets, have combined to facilitate relatively high rates of pediatric toxocariasis in the United States, Europe, and Japan (Schantz, 1989; Schantz, 1991; Petithory et al., 1994; Uga and Kataoka, 1995). In the United States and its associated commonwealths, the seroprevalence of toxocariasis is highest in Puerto Rico and in the Southeast (Schantz, 1989). Among some populations of socioeconomically disadvantaged African-American children the seroprevalence approaches 30% (Herrmann et al., 1985), and among Hispanic children attending a hospital-based primary care clinic in Massachusetts the seroprevalence was reported to be 16% (Bass et al., 1987). Although a proportion of these children live in rural areas, the seroprevalence in inner cities is also high. For instance, the prevalence of toxocariasis among Hispanic children living in Bridgeport, Connecticut may exceed 50% (Sharghi et al., 2001). Of interest is the association between plumbism and *T. canis* infection. Banked sera from inner-city children with elevated serum lead levels have been found to be associated with a high seroprevalence of toxocariasis (Marmor et al., 1987). It has been suggested that the habit of pica (geophagia) is a risk factor for both clinical entities.

The ingestion of *T. canis* eggs can result in any one of three distinct diseases syndromes— VLM, OLM, and covert toxocariasis—all of which occur predominantly in children (Hotez, 1993; Hotez, 1995; Sharghi et al., 2000).

As noted earlier, VLM is primarily a disease of young children. Each ingested *T. canis* egg releases a larva, which invades the intestinal mucosa and migrates through viscera where it both causes mechanical destruction and elicits host inflammation. Eosinophils are a predomi-

nant leukocyte involved in the inflammatory responses to the parasite. Classic VLM occurs after the eggs hatch in the gastrointestinal tract and as the larvae migrate through the lungs to cause a pneumonitis, the liver to cause a hepatitis, and the brain to cause a cerebritis. *Toxocara* cerebritis can cause neuropsychiatric disturbances, and there is even some evidence to suggest that *T. canis* is an important etiologic agent of occult epilepsy (Arpino et al., 1990; Nelson et al., 1990). Infected children usually have a leukocytosis, persistent eosinophilia, hyperglobulinemia, and increased serum isohemagglutinins. In addition to identifying the characteristic clinical manifestations, a diagnosis of VLM can be confirmed by enzyme-linked immunosorbent assay (ELISA) that measures specific antibody against *T. canis* larval or egg antigens. ELISA testing on sera from children with a presumptive diagnosis of toxocariasis (with a sensitivity of 85% and a specificity of 92% at a dilution of greater than 1:16) is available from Parasitic Disease Consultants (Tucker, Georgia) or from the CDC. Some newer information suggests that albendazole offers promise in the therapy of VLM (Hotez, 1995). For instance, Sturchler et al. (1989) showed that patients receiving a 5-day treatment course of albendazole (10 mg/kg/day in two divided doses) improved, relative to patients who received treatment with an older anthelminthic drug, thiabendazole. Albendazole in doses of 400 mg twice a day for 3 to 5 days have also been suggested (Medical Letter, 2000). Because mebendazole is poorly absorbed outside of the gastrointestinal tract, high doses may be required to achieve a therapeutic effect in the viscera. In an adult patient, Bekhti (1984) reported success using 1 g of mebendazole 3 times a day for 21 days. Possible concerns about the use of high-dose BZs in young children have been discussed previously in this chapter.

The majority of patients infected with *Toxocara* remain asymptomatic. However, it has been suggested that some of these individuals, in fact, have a covert form of toxocariasis (Sharghi et al., 2000; Sharghi et al., 2001). The presenting signs of these patients include only partial manifestations of VLM, including eosinophilia and wheezing. Covert toxocariasis should be suspected in any child with asymptomatic eosinophilia. It has been further suggested that covert toxocariasis may be linked to asthma in some children. The association between *T. canis* infection and asthma has been better established in Europe than in North America (Sharghi et al., 2001), although the full association with asthma has yet to be explored.

Patients with OLM often have no systemic involvement. Instead, older children (between the ages of 5 and 10 years) are infected with larvae that appear to exclusively invade the retina to cause posterior pole and peripheral pole larval tracks and granulomas. The basis for this phenomenon is not known. However, because there is little systemic (extraocular) involvement the child with OLM does not typically have an eosinophilia. For similar reasons, immunodiagnostic testing on children with OLM is often not helpful. Indeed, only 45% of clinically diagnosed OLM patients have anti-*Toxocara* antibody titers greater than 1:32 (Schantz et al., 1979). Therefore, the diagnosis of OLM requires the skill of an ophthalmologist familiar with the characteristic peripheral and posterior pole retinal lesions in a child with a unilateral loss in visual acuity and/or a strabismus (frequently an exotropia). For patients with macular detachment, improvements have been observed after vitrectomy in association with adjunct anthelminthic chemotherapy.

Enterobiasis

Infection with the human pinworm, *E. vermicularis*, is a common pediatric problem in the United States. There are no precise recent estimates for the prevalence of enterobiasis; it was reported in 1941 that 19% of the children visiting an outpatient clinic at Children's Hospital Boston were infected with pinworms (Weller and Sorenson, 1941). Some investigators believe that pinworm is not nearly as common as it once was (Vermund and MacLeod, 1988; Vermund, 2000), although it still occurs in North American elementary schools and daycare centers (Crawford and Vermund, 1987). Embryonated eggs of *E. vermicularis* are infectious to humans shortly after being deposited in the perianal area by adult female pinworms. Human enterobiasis results when the eggs are ingested through oral contact with contaminated fingers or fomites (night clothing and bed linen). The eggs may also be swallowed if they become airborne and associate with household or schoolroom dust particles. Finally, autoinfection resulting from eggs attached to the fingernails (acquired by the child during scratching in an effort to relieve perianal pruritus) represents a significant number of cases.

The larvae that are liberated from eggs in the gastrointestinal tract migrate to the jejunum and ileum, where they develop into adult male and female pinworms. The adult worms live in the cecum and proximal colon. After mating, the adult female pinworms migrate out and onto the perianal area where they deposit their eggs.

Generally speaking, the larval and adult pinworms do not elicit significant pathology in the large intestine. Liu et al. (1995), however, reported a case of severe eosinophilic colitis in an 18-year-old homosexual male who acquired a massive inoculum of *E. vermicularis* presumably by direct anal-oral contact. In other rare instances, the adult pinworm may migrate into the appendix or other ectopic sites to cause acute abdominal symptoms that may require surgical intervention (Dalimi and Khoshzaban, 1993). By far the major clinical feature of pediatric enterobiasis is intense perianal itching (pruritus ani) caused by host inflammation to migrating adult pinworms and their eggs. Bacterial superinfection may exacerbate this process. In girls, migrating pinworms may enter the vagina to cause a vaginitis or even introduce bacteria into the genitourinary tract to cause urinary tract infections (Simon, 1974).

Because pinworm eggs, unlike other intestinal nematode eggs, are not found in the feces, a specific diagnosis of enterobiasis is made on the basis of their recovery from the perianal area. This is usually accomplished by applying adhesive tape first to the perianal skin and then onto a microscope slide. Some investigators believe that the time of highest yield for pinworm egg recovery is early in the morning before a bath or bowel movement.

The goal for treating pediatric enterobiasis is the eradication of adult pinworms. Usually a single dose of mebendazole (100 mg), albendazole (400 mg), or pyrantel pamoate (11 mg/kg [maximum 1 g]) is adequate for this purpose (Medical Letter, 2000). However, because newly ingested eggs may be refractory to the anthelminthic agent, a second dose is required after 2 weeks to eliminate newly developed adult pinworms. A frequent problem reported by physicians and nurses is the recurrence of enterobiasis in a child despite two treatment doses of a specific anthelminthic agent. Almost always, this phenomenon occurs as a consequence of reinfection. Therefore it is important that the pediatrician repeat a diagnostic examination in order to confirm this. It is also recommended that all members of a household be treated for pinworm infection and that, at the time of treatment, underwear, bedclothes, and towels be laundered in hot water.

TREMATODE (FLUKE) INFECTIONS: SCHISTOSOMIASIS

Large numbers of snail-borne trematodes infect humans throughout the world (especially in East Asia), but schistosomiasis is by far the most important pediatric fluke infection. More than 200 million individuals worldwide are infected with one of the three major species of schistosomes: *Schistosoma mansoni*, *Schistosoma haematobium*, and flukes of the *Schistosoma japonicum* complex. School-age children have a predisposition to high schistosome worm burdens similar to their propensity to acquire heavy *Ascaris* and *Trichuris* infections. The prevalence and intensity of schistosomiasis typically peak during adolescence (McGarvey, 2000). Increasing evidence suggests that schistosomes, like the STHs, impair growth and cognition. All three major schistosome infections are water-borne because of their absolute requirement for a snail intermediate host. The relationship between schistosomes in the juvenile stages and their snail hosts has evolved in an intricate manner, so that each schistosome species has rather precise requirements for a particular snail host species. In fact, the geography of human schistosomiasis depends on the availability of the appropriate snail. Upon exiting the snail intermediate host, larval schistosomes known as cercariae have the ability to swim and penetrate human skin. Human schistosomiasis occurs in association with water contact. Following larval development, the adult schistosomes establish in the vasculature of either the mesenteric veins that drain the intestines (*S. mansoni* and *S. japonicum*) or the bladder plexus (*S. haematobium*). Much of the morbidity in schistosomiasis results from the eggs that escape the vasculature to cause microhemorrhages. The eggs then enter the surrounding tissues, where they elicit granuloma formation and fibrosis.

S. mansoni is the only species of schistosome endemic in the Western Hemisphere, especially in Brazil and some parts of the Caribbean.

S. mansoni infections also occur commonly in Africa. The eggs are equipped with a lateral spine that facilitates rupture out of the vasculature and into the intestine, where they cause bloody diarrhea and intestinal fibrosis. Many of the eggs also become swept into the portal veins and liver, causing hepatic fibrosis. Chronic heavy infections during childhood result in hepatosplenomegaly, physical growth stunting, and reduced muscle mass. Some of these effects are reversible following anthelminthic therapy with praziquantel. *S. mansoni* infections are diagnosed by identifying the characteristic eggs through fecal examination or rectal biopsy.

The major human schistosomes of the. *japonicum* complex include *S. japonicum* and *S. mekongi*. The majority of cases of *S. japonicum* occur along the Yangtze River and its tributaries in China, where an estimated 750,000 cases occur (Hotez et al., 1997). Major endemic foci also occur in the Philippines. *S. mekongi* is a closely related species that uses a different snail intermediate host; infections occur near the Mekong River and its tributaries in Southeast Asia. *S. japonicum* has had an important influence on the history of modern China and is believed to be partly responsible for preventing a Communist takeover of Taiwan after 1949 by aborting amphibious assaults that were launched from the mainland. At one time *S. japonicum* was known as "the fluke that saved Formosa." During the Great Leap Forward between 1958 and 1960, Mao Tsetung is believed to have mobilized hundreds of thousands of peasants in order to combat schistosomiasis by having them bury snails or remove them individually by sticks. On average, *S. japonicum* produces greater numbers of eggs than *S. mansoni*; this results in more significant intestinal and hepatosplenic disease. Occasionally *S. japonicum* eggs enter the lungs to produce pulmonary schistosomiasis and ultimately cor pulmonale. In addition, eggs of this species have been reported to enter the brain and spinal cord and cause cerebral schistosomiasis and transverse myelitis, respectively. Heavy acute infections with *S. japonicum* can produce a serious systemic febrile illness known as *Katayama fever* (named after the Katayama Valley in Japan). It is believed that this syndrome was responsible for incapacitating Mao's troops in preparation for their invasion of Taiwan. Less commonly, a syndrome similar to Katayama fever occurs during heavy acute *S. mansoni* infections. In both the Philippines and in China, a dose-relationship between the intensity of *S. japonica* infection and body size and nutritional status has been uncovered (McGarvey, 2000). Some of these findings are reversible following anthelminthic chemotherapy with praziquantel. A similar relationship may exist between infection and cognition. Infection is diagnosed either through fecal examination or rectal biopsy. *S. japonica* is the only major human schistosome with significant animal reservoirs such as water buffalo, cattle, and pigs. This zoonotic feature of *S. japonicum* infection has led to the suggestion that it might be possible to vaccinate significant animal reservoirs in order to interrupt transmission to humans (Liu et al., 1998).

S. haematobium infection is endemic in Africa and the Middle East and is a significant cause of bladder disease and hematuria in these regions. Long-standing infections lead to bladder fibrosis and sometimes even squamous metaplastic changes. There is a strong epidemiologic link between chronic *S. haematobium* infection and squamous carcinoma of the bladder. In Egypt, squamous carcinoma is more common than adenocarcinoma as the leading form of bladder cancer. As in other types of schistosomiasis, chronic *S. haematobium* infections during childhood result in physical growth retardation, as well as reduced school performance. Praziquantel is the treatment of choice. Diagnosis is established by identifying the characteristic terminal-spined eggs on urinalysis or by recovering the eggs on a filter.

In regions where children are coinfected with STHs and schistosomes, there is increasing recognition that deworming with both albendazole and praziquantel will provide short-term benefit with respect to catch-up physical growth, improved physical fitness, and improved school performance. The recently established Partnership for Parasite Control (PPC) of the WHO is conducting longitudinal studies to evaluate whether frequent and regular administrations of albendazole and praziquantel significantly improve the health and education of children living in endemic developing countries, particularly in Africa. Of concern is the sustainability of such programs, given that there is no apparent immunity to posttreatment reinfection among these children and that in highly endemic areas, twice or even thrice yearly treatments may be required throughout childhood.

CESTODE (TAPEWORM) INFECTIONS
Adult Tapeworm Infections

Despite their large size, adult tapeworms in the intestine of a child do not usually cause severe symptoms or pathology. All the major species of human tapeworms are composed of an intestinal attachment organ known as a scolex (with suckers, hooks, or grooves) and a chain of egg-containing proglottid segments known as the strobila. Tapeworm species identification is made either by recovering the scolex or, in some cases, by examining the proglottid segments and eggs in a fecal sample. Praziquantel is the drug of choice for the treatment of tapeworm infections, having largely replaced niclosamide. For all of the major tapeworm infections except *Hymenolepis nana*, praziquantel is administered in a single dose (5 to 10 mg/kg). The major tapeworm infections of children are discussed in the following sections.

Dipylidiasis. The dog tapeworm *Dipylidium caninum* is acquired by ingesting the cysticercoid larval stage contained within a flea of the genus *Ctenocephalides*. Young children, although often asymptomatic, may experience diarrhea, anorexia, and abdominal pain (Chappell et al., 1990).

Diphyllobothriasis. The fish tapeworm *Diphyllobothrium latum* was at one time endemic among the Scandinavian immigrant populations of Minnesota and Michigan. A related parasite, *D. alascense* occurs among the Inuit. Both tapeworms are acquired by ingesting raw fish; fish become infected when they ingest another crustacean intermediate host containing the larval stage of the parasite. The most dramatic clinical feature of diphyllobothriasis is vitamin B_{12} deficiency, at times leading even to megaloblastic anemia.

Hymenolepiasis. Two major species of the genus *Hymenolepis*, *Hymenolepis diminuta* and *H. nana*, are pathogens of humans. Heavy infections with these small tapeworms may cause diarrhea, nausea, anorexia, and abdominal pain (Hamrick et al., 1990). *H. nana*, the dwarf tapeworm, has the interesting feature of being able to complete all of its life cycle stages from egg to adult tapeworm in humans without requiring an intermediate host. To eradicate the intermediate life cycle stages of *H. nana* that occur in humans, it may be necessary to administer praziquantel in a larger dose (25 mg/kg, once) than necessary for other adult human tapeworm infections.

Taeniasis. Infections with either the cattle tapeworm, *Taenia saginata*, or the pork tapeworm, *T. solium*, are usually asymptomatic despite their enormous size. However, severe pathology may result when humans serve as the intermediate host of *T. solium*, resulting in NCC (see the following section). To prevent household transmission of neurocysticercosis, individuals identified by fecal exam as harboring adult *T. solium* in their intestine should be treated with praziquantel.

Neurocysticercosis

In contrast to the benign cestode infections that result when humans serve as the definitive hosts for large tapeworms, far more serious disease occurs in humans who serve as intermediate hosts for the larval stages of tapeworms. Human cysticercosis occurs through the ingestion of eggs of *T. solium* as a consequence of contact with feces from an individual who harbors the pork tapeworm in the intestine. Once *T. solium* eggs are ingested they liberate oncospheres in the duodenum, where they can invade the intestinal mucosa and enter the circulation. From there they disseminate to the muscles and grow into cysticerci. NCC occurs when cysticerci enter the brain and eyes. NCC is an important emerging infection in the United States, occurring predominantly among families of immigrants from endemic regions of Latin America and Asia. In these countries, family members become infected with the adult tapeworm through ingestion of raw or uncooked pork and then shed *T. solium* eggs in their feces. Children acquire cysticercosis usually through exposure to *T. solium* eggs from immigrant family members or immigrant domestic workers in the household (Schantz et al., 1992). In the United States, NCC is currently one of the most common parasitic disease of the central nervous system (St. Geme et al., 1993) and a leading cause of epilepsy among Hispanic children living in Los Angeles and other cities along the Mexican border (Richards et al., 1985).

Cysticerci can live for months or years undisturbed in the brain. The pathogenic sequence of events leading to NCC is initiated when the cysticercus (a trilaminated "bladder worm" with an invaginated scolex) elicits a vigorous host inflammatory response that includes lymphocytes, plasma cells, and eosinophils. The obser-

vation that inflammation is often greatest around dying cysticerci has significant implications for appropriate specific anthelminthic treatment strategies (see the following section). Host inflammatory responses surrounding dying cysticerci in the brain can trigger seizure foci. Children with "simple" NCC often present with a solitary inflamed parenchymal mass lesion in association with partial seizures followed by secondary generalization (Mitchell and Crawford, 1988). On contrast-enhanced computed tomography (CT) this type of lesion demonstrates pronounced ring enhancement. Children can also have multiple or extra-parenchymal lesions leading to "complicated" NCC. Some investigators believe that complicated disease results from prolonged reexposure in endemic areas. In addition to having multiple cysts these children may also have increased intracranial pressure, meningoencephalitis, arachnoiditis, and hydrocephalus.

Diagnostic imaging with either CT or magnetic resonance imaging (MRI) is usually necessary to diagnose NCC. Although either CT or MRI is considered nearly equivalent for this purpose (both modalities require the use of contrast media for complete assessment) there are also some circumstances that might lead the physician to choose one or the other modality (St. Geme et al., 1993). For instance, CT is superior to the MRI for detecting characteristic calcification patterns found in certain types of granulomas, whereas MRI is superior for detecting subarachnoid cysts in the posterior fossa, cysts in the cisterns around the brain stem, intraventricular cysts, and cerebral edema (St. Geme et al., 1993). MRI is more sensitive for detecting intraparenchymal cysts. For confirmation of clinical and radiographic presumptive diagnostic tests, antibodies to cysticercus antigen can be measured in the serum using an enzyme-linked immunotransfer blot (EITB) assay, available from the CDC or through a private laboratory (Specialty Laboratories, Inc., Los Angeles, Calif.) (St. Geme et al., 1993). The EITB assay is 100% specific, although it has poor sensitivity for children with a solitary lesion, possibly as low as 30% (Di Pentima and White, 2000). A scoring system with major criteria (neuroradiologic lesions, positive EITB, cigar-shaped calcifications on soft tissue x-rays) and minor criteria (presence of subcutaneous nodules, punctate calcifications on radiographic studies, and clinical manifestations of intracranial lesions during treatment with anticysticercal drugs) has been proposed (Di Pentima and White, 2000); the combination of two major and one minor criteria, or one major and two minor criteria, plus a history of exposure are considered diagnostic (Di Pentima and White, 2000). Finally, a fecal examination may reveal the presence of *T. solium* eggs, which could predispose the patient to autoinfection, as well as identify potential family or domestic household carriers.

There is some controversy regarding the optimal treatment for a child with a solitary parenchymal ring-enhancing lesion; such a child may not benefit from specific anthelminthic chemotherapy that targets an already dying larval worm, because these cysts may spontaneously resolve. Anticonvulsants alone may be sufficient for these children, because many remain seizure free after their discontinuation (Mitchell and Crawford, 1988). In the majority of patients, lesions will disappear without sequelae, the seizures will cease, and the imaging studies will normalize (Di Pentima and White, 2000). For these patients, anticonvulsants may be tapered approximately 2 years following therapy (Di Pentima and White, 2000). Others investigators, however, have argued that specific anthelminthic therapy is necessary to eliminate potentially undetected cysts (St. Geme et al., 1993). Certainly, for multiple cysts and other forms of "complicated" NCC, anthelminthic chemotherapy should be considered. These conditions include active extraparenchymal NCC and ventricular NCC (Di Pentima and White, 2000). Both albendazole and praziquantel have been well studied for the treatment of NCC and are effective for this purpose. Albendazole (15 mg/kg/day in 2 doses for 8 to 30 days, repeated as necessary, particularly for ventricular and subarachnoid disease) has been shown to be marginally better than praziquantel in terms of cyst resolution and clinical improvement (St. Geme et al., 1993). Patients with a single or fewer than three parenchymal cysts have been also shown to benefit from a short, 3- to 7-day course of albendazole (Alarcon et al., 1989). Albendazole metabolite levels are not significantly affected by corticosteroids or anticonvulsants (Di Pentima and White, 2000). Therapy with praziquantel (50 mg/kg/day in 3 doses for 15 days [Medical Letter, 2000]) is also acceptable, but it should be administered together with cimetidine, particularly when praziquantel is administered with

corticosteroids and anticonvulsants that promote first-pass metabolism (Di Pentima and White, 2000). Among the contraindications for specific anthelminthic therapy is their use for patients with cysticercal encephalitis, in whom the drugs can exacerbate inflammation and cerebral edema, potentially inducing herniation and death (Di Pentima and White, 2000). Uncontrolled elevated intracranial pressure from extraparenchymal disease also contraindicates use of anthelminthic therapy. Prior to anthelminthic therapy, patients should undergo ophthalmologic examination in order to rule out ocular cysticercosis. It has been reported that sight-threatening inflammation can develop during therapy, although some patients with ocular cysticercosis have been successfully treated with albendazole (Di Pentima and White, 2000).

In addition to anticonvulsant therapy, anti-inflammatory adjunct therapy with corticosteroids can be critical for patients undergoing cysticidal therapy who experience headache, vomiting, or seizures (St. Geme et al., 1993) or who are at risk for increasing their intracranial pressure during therapy. These children usually require hospitalization. For complicated NCC it is advisable to manage patients in consultation with a neurosurgeon in anticipation of possible elevations in intracranial pressure, for the management of hydrocephalus, and for the possible need for cerebrospinal fluid diversion, surgical decompression, or ventriculoperitoneal shunting. Family members or domestic household contacts found to harbor *T. solium* tapeworms should be treated with a single dose of praziquantel as described previously.

BIBLIOGRAPHY

Alarcon F, Escalante L, Duenas G, et al. Neurocysticercosis: short course of treatment with albendazole. Arch Neurol 1989;46:1231-1236.

Albonico M, Smith PG, Ercole E, et al. Rate of reinfection with intestinal nematodes after treatment of children with mebendazole or albendazole in a highly endemic area. Trans R Soc Trop Med Hyg 1995;89:538-541.

Arpino C, Castelli Gattinara G, Piergili D, Curatolo P. *Toxocara* infection and epilepsy in children: a case-control study. Epilepsia 1990;31:33-36.

Basavaraju S, Hotez PJ. Gastrointestinal and surgical complications of ascariasis. Infections in Medicine. In press.

Bass JL, Mehta KA, Glickman LT, et al. Asymptomatic toxocariasis in children. Clin Pediatr (Phila) 1987;26:441-446.

Bekhti A. Mebendazole in toxocariasis. Ann Intern Med 1984;28:24-28.

Bethony J, Chen JZ, Lin SX et al. Emerging epidemiological patterns of Necator hookworm infections in Asia. Trop Med Int Health 2002; submitted

Biddulph J: Mebendazole and albendazole for infants. Pediatr Infect Dis J 1990;9:373.

Bundy DAP, Cooper ES. Trichuris and trichuriasis in humans. Adv Parasitol 1989;28:107-173.

Chappell CL, Enos JP, Penn HM. Dipylidium caninum, an underrecognized infection in infants and children. Pediatr Infect Dis J 1990;9:745.

Cowden J, Hotez P. Mebendazole and albendazole treatment of geohelminth infections in children and pregnant women. Pediatr Infect Dis J 2000; 19:659-660.

Crawford FG, Vermund SH. Parasitic infections in day care centers. Pediatr Infect Dis J 1987;6:744.

Crompton DWT. Ascariasis and childhood malnutrition. Trans R Soc Trop Med Hyg 1992;86:577-579.

Dalimi A, Khoshzaban F. Comparative study of two methods for the diagnosis of Enterobius vermicularis in the appendix. J Helminthol 1993;67:85-86.

Despommier DD, Gwadz RW, Holez PJ. Parasitic diseases, ed 3, Springer-Verlag.

Di Pentima MC, White AC. Neurocysticercosis: controversies in management. Semin Pediatr Infect Dis 2000;11:261-268.

Drake LJ, Jukes MCH, Sternberg RJ, Bundy DAP. Geohelminth infections (ascariasis, trichuriasis, and hookworm): cognitive and developmental impacts. Semin Pediatr Infect Dis 2000;11:245-251.

Elliot DL, Tolle SW, Goldberg L, Miller JB. Pet-associated illness. N Engl J Med 1985;313:985-995.

Gandhi NS, Chen JZ, Khoshnood K, et al. Epidemiology of *Necator americanus* hookworm infections in Xiulongkan Village, Hainan Province, China: high prevalence and intensity among middle-aged and elderly residents. J Parasitol 2001;87:739-743.

Hall A. Intestinal parasitic worms and the growth of children. Trans R Soc Trop Med Hyg 1993;87:241-242.

Hamrick HJ, Bowdre JH, Church MT. Rat tapeworm *(Hymenolepis diminuta)* infection in a child. Pediatr Infect Dis J 1990;9:216.

Hermann N, Glickman LT, Schantz PM, et al. Seroprevalence of zoonotic toxocariasis in the United States: 1971-1973. Am J Epidemiol 1985;122:890-896.

Hotez PJ. Hookworm disease in children. Pediatr Infect Dis J 1989;8:516-520.

Hotez PJ. Visceral and ocular larva migrans. Semin Neurol 1993;13:175-179.

Hotez PJ. *Toxocara canis.* In Burg FD, Wald ER, Ingelfinger JR, Polin RA (eds). Gellis and Kagan's Current Pediatric Therapy, ed 15. Philadelphia: Saunders, 1995.

Hotez PJ. Pediatric geohelminth infections: trichuriasis, ascariasis, and hookworm infections. Semin Pediatr Infect Dis 2000;11:236-241.

Hotez PJ, Feng Z, Xu LQ, et al. Emerging and reemerging helminthiases and the public health of China. Emerg Infect Dis 1997;3:303-310.

Hotez PJ, Ghosh K, Hawdon JM, et al. Experimental approaches to the development of a recombinant hookworm vaccine. Immunol Rev 1999;171:163-171.

Hotez PJ, Hawdon JM, Cappello M, et al. Molecular approaches to vaccinating against hookworm disease. Pediatr Res 1996;40:515-521.

Hotez PJ, Pritchard DI. Hookworm infection. Sci Am 1995;272:68-75.

Liu LX, Chi J, Upton MP, Ash LP. Eosinophilic colitis associated with larvae of the pinworm Enterobius vermicularis. Lancet 1995;346:410-412.

Liu SX, Song GC, Xu YX, et al. Progress in the development of an effective vaccine against schistosomiasis in China. Int J Infect Dis 1998;2:176-180.

Marmor M, Glickman L, Shofer F, et al. *Toxocara canis* infection of children: epidemiologic and neuropsychologic findings. Am J Public Health 1987;77:554-559.

McGarvey ST. Schistosomiasis: impact on childhood and adolescent growth, malnutrition, and morbidity. Semin Pediatr Infect Dis 2000;11:269-274.

Medical Letter on Drugs and Therapeutics. Drug for parasitic infections. Medical Letter 2002 (April).

Mitchell WG, Crawford TO. Intraparenchymal cerebral cysticercosis in children: diagnosis and treatment. Pediatrics 1988;82:76-82.

Nelson J, Frost JL, Schochet SS. Unsuspected cerebral *Toxocara* infection in a fire victim. Clin Neuropathol 1990;9:106-108.

Petithory J-C, Beddok A, Quedoc M. Zoonoses d'origine ascaridienne: les syndromes de larva migrans viscéral. Bull Acad Natl Med 1994;178:635-647.

Richards FR, Schantz PM, Ruiz-Tiben E, Sorvillo FJ. Cysticercosis in Los Angeles County. JAMA 1985;254:3444-3448.

Schantz PM. *Toxocara* larva migrans now. Am J Trop Med Hyg 1989;41:21-34.

Schantz PM. Parasitic zoonoses in perspective. Int J Parasitol 1991;21:161-170.

Schantz PM, Meyer D, Glickman LT. Clinical serologic and epidemiologic characteristics of ocular toxocariasis. Am J Trop Med Hyg 1979;28:24-28.

Schantz PM, Moore AC, Munoz JL, et al. Neurocysticercosis in an Orthodox Jewish community in New York City. N Engl J Med 1992;327:692-695.

Sharghi N, Schantz PM, Caramico L, et al. Environmental exposure to *Toxocara* as a possible risk factor for asthma: a clinic-based case-control study. Clin Infect Dis 2001;32:E111-E116.

Sharghi N, Schantz P, Hotez PJ. Toxocariasis: an occult cause of childhood neuropsychological deficits and asthma. Semin Pediatr Infect Dis 2000;11:257-260.

Simon RD. Pinworm infestation and urinary tract infection in young girls. Am J Dis Child 1974;128:21-22.

St. Geme JW III, Maldonado YA, Enzmann D, et al. Consensus: diagnosis and management of neurocysticercosis in children. Pediatr Infect Dis J 1993;12:455-461.

Steele M, Kuhls T, Nida K, et al. Infect Immun 1995;63:3840-3845.

Stehr-Green JK, Schantz PM. The impact of zoonotic diseases transmitted by pets on human health and the economy. Vet Clin North Am Small Anim Pract 1987;17: 1-15.

Sturchler D, Schubarth P, Gualzata M, et al. Thiabendazole v. albendazole in treatment of toxocariasis: a clinical trial. Ann Trop Med Parasitol 1989;83:473-478.

Uga S, Kataoka N. Measures to control *Toxocara* egg contamination in sandpits of public parks. Am J Trop Med Hyg 1995;52:21-24.

Vermund SH. Pinworm (*Enterobius vermicularis*). Semin Pediatr Infect Dis 2000;11:252-256.

Vermund SH, MacLeod S. Is pinworm a vanishing infection? Laboratory surveillance in a New York City medical center from 1971 to 1986. Am J Dis Child 1988;142:566-568.

Weller TH, Sorenson CW. Enterobiasis: its incidence and symptomatology in a group of 505 children. N Engl J Med 1941;224:143-146.

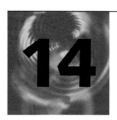

14

HAEMOPHILUS INFLUENZAE TYPE B

DENNIS A. CLEMENTS

*H*aemophilus influenzae type b (HIB) is a small, pleomorphic, nonmotile gram-negative bacterium that is naturally a parasite only of humans. Its name derives from the mistaken identification by Pfeiffer in 1892 that it was responsible for the influenza pandemic and from the fact that it requires two factors from blood for growth. *H. influenzae* is easily divided into encapsulated forms, which cause invasive disease (discussed in this chapter), and unencapsulated forms, which Pfeiffer had identified in the airways of those dying from influenza. The unencapsulated forms typically cause mucosal disease (otitis media, bronchitis, and conjunctivitis), except in aged, immunosuppressed, malnourished, or premature individuals, in whom they may cause invasive disease.

HIB was once the most common bacterial pathogen to cause meningitis in children in countries where nationwide reporting of diseases is established (Box 14-1). In 1978 HIB was estimated to have caused 46% of all bacterial meningitis (10,000 cases) in the United States, regardless of age. In addition, it caused an equal number of other invasive diseases, such as buccal and periorbital cellulitis, pneumonia, arthritis, epiglottitis, and pericarditis. This disease burden is equivalent to that caused by paralytic polio in the United States in the 1950s (Cochi et al., 1988).

Since the introduction of HIB vaccine in 1987 the incidence of HIB disease in the United States has decreased 97% among children <5 years of age. The disease incidence in persons >5 years of age has not changed and remains about 0.4 per 100,000. Non-type b *H. influenzae* disease in children <5 years of age has decreased slightly but is now more common than known type b disease (Centers for Disease Control and Prevention, 1998).

ETIOLOGY

HIB organisms are gram-negative coccobacilli or filamentous rods, hence the descriptive term *pleomorphic*. They grow on chocolate agar, where they have a glistening, semitransparent appearance. They are further identified by the requirement for X (hemin or other porphyrins) and V (coenzyme nicotinamide adenine dinucleotide) factors for growth on blood agar. (A more sensitive test for the X factor requirement is to test the ability of *H. influenzae* to convert delta aminolevulinic acid to porphyrin.) Other tests such as the production of indole from tryptophan and detection of β-galactosidase (ONPG test) activity are also useful in discriminating *H. influenzae* from other *Haemophilus* species.

A more rapid method of identifying type b organisms is to use type b antiserum on a slide with the unidentified organism. If agglutination does not occur, one can be sure that the organism is not a type b. However, if agglutination does occur, it is possible that the organism is a type b. False positive results are frequent because of cross-reactivity of antigens and because of autoagglutination by nontypable strains.

Another method for selective identification of type b organisms is to use antiserum agar as described by Michaels and Stonebraker (1975). A suitable clear nutrient agar is prepared containing hyperimmune HIB antiserum (produced in burros). When this selective medium is inoculated with appropriate specimens, a halo of agglutination is observed around each HIB colony after 24 to 48 hours. This is a very sensitive method for detecting colonization and also allows for a quantitative assay.

Typable and nontypable *H. influenzae* can be divided into biotypes by the presence or absence of three enzyme activities: urease,

---

BOX 14-1

A BRIEF HISTORY

1892	Pfeiffer erroneously identified *Haemophilus influenzae* as the causative agent in the lungs of patients dying during the influenza pandemic.
1930	Margaret Pittman described 6 serotypes (a through f) of encapsulated *H. influenzae* based on antigenic differences in their capsular polysaccharides.
1935	Fothergill and Wright described an inverse relationship between the age of HIB disease and the serum level of bactericidal antibody against *H. influenzae* type b (HIB).
1944	Alexander demonstrated that hyperimmune sera protected rabbits against developing meningitis when inoculated with HIB.
1950	The use of chloramphenicol markedly decreased the mortality from infection resulting from HIB.
1970	Schneerson purified the HIB polysaccharide capsule component polyribosyl-ribotyl phosphate (PRP), to be used as a vaccine immunogen.
1974	Peltola demonstrated that PRP was immunogenic in children over 18 months of age in a vaccine trial of 100,000 children in Finland.
1984	Kayhty reported a 90% protective vaccine efficacy in children older than 18 months in the 1974 Finnish HIB trial.
1985	PRP vaccine was licensed in the United States to be given to children >2 years of age.
1980s	PRP was conjugated with various proteins to increase its immunogenicity in children less than 18 months of age.
1985-1987:	A controlled trial of PRP-D given in the first 6 to 12 months of life in Finland was shown to be protective.
1987	PRP-D was licensed for use in the United States in children who had reached 18 months of age.
1990	HbOC and PRP-OMP were licensed for use in children as young as 2 months in the United States.
1993	PRP-T and DTP-HbOC combination vaccines were licensed in the United States.
1995	Multiple reports showed decreased HIB disease to 5% to 10% of previous levels in the United States.
1996	Increased incidence of HIB was shown in Alaskan Eskimos.
1998-1999	*H. influenzae* type a disease with virulence factor similar to that of HIB was found in Utah.

---

ornithine decarboxylase, and production of indole from tryptophan (Kilian, 1976). This system divides *H. influenzae* organisms into eight (I to VIII) groups, but 90% of type b organisms are biotype I. Hence, this has proved to be of little epidemiologic use for type b organisms. Unencapsulated *H. influenzae*, however, show a much wider distribution of biotypes, and this technique is more useful in epidemiologic studies of nontypable disease.

The polysaccharide capsule of *H. influenzae* is an important virulence factor. The type b capsule consists of a repeating polymer of five carbon sugar units, ribose, and ribitol phosphate. The cell envelope includes lipo-oligosaccharide (LOS) and outer-membrane proteins (OMP). Pili or fimbriae extend from the outer membrane, but their presence appears to be variable. They apparently mediate the

attachment of HIB to epithelial cells, which is essential to establish colonization but perhaps disadvantageous in the blood.

H. influenzae was invariably sensitive to ampicillin until the early 1970s, when resistance resulting from the production of a plasmid-mediated β-lactamase was first described. At present 15% to 50% of HIB isolates are β-lactamase producers, depending on geographical location (Wenger et al., 1990). Resistance to chloramphenicol because of plasmid-mediated chloramphenicol acetyltransferase production has also been described.

There has been keen interest in determining which subtypes of HIB cause invasive disease. This was explored in the United States by Barenkamp et al. (1983). They reported that a high proportion of cases (84%) of invasive HIB disease is caused by only a few OMP subtypes

(1H, 44%; 3L, 28%; and 1L, 12%), but there was no specificity of disease by subtype. They also reported that subtype prevalence varies over time. Subtype 2L accounted for 22% of cerebrospinal fluid (CSF) and blood isolates during the years 1977 through 1980 but only 4% in 1981 and 1982. In Holland, van Alphen et al. (1987) documented that 80% to 90% of HIB organisms causing invasive disease in Europe are OMP subtype 3L (van Alphen subtype 1) and that 83% of the isolates from Iceland are subtype 2L (van Alphen subtype 2). Takala et al. (1989) reported that one subtype (van Alphen 1c), which has been rarely isolated elsewhere, causes very little epiglottitis, compared with meningitis, in Finland. Thus there is suggestive evidence that virulence may vary with OMP subtype.

Attempts have also been made to categorize HIB isolates by LOS typing because LOS subtypes are more varied, which could increase their value as an epidemiologic tool. Unfortunately, LOS patterns of individual isolates appear to be unstable during storage, and, in the animal model, LOS expression by an individual clone may vary according to environmental conditions.

Newer techniques such as multilocus enzyme electrophoresis (ET) and clonotyping attempt to identify HIB isolates by differences in single enzyme loci or DNA sequence changes, respectively. Most isolates with the same ET pattern belong to the same OMP and LOS subtypes, suggesting homogeneity of isolates. Musser et al. (1988) showed that HIB strains could be separated into three genetic groups or "clonotypes," each of which is associated with a restricted group of OMP subtypes, suggesting limited clonal ancestry of HIB. One clonotype was predominant in Europe, but all three were found in the United States.

PATHOGENESIS

HIB, a natural infection only in humans, is spread by respiratory secretions. However, most colonized children do not become ill, and carriage alone does not necessarily induce an antibody response. Type b strains may persist in the airway for prolonged periods, thus increasing the opportunity for transmission. Animal models indicate that, in the minority in whom disease occurs, invasion through the mucosa into the blood is facilitated by mucosal damage (viral infection, trauma, and so on) or increased

numbers of mucosal organisms. After penetration into the bloodstream, they are protected from phagocytosis by their capsules and multiply while disseminating to the meninges, epiglottis, or synovial surfaces. The patient may become symptomatic at any time after bacteremia occurs. The predilection of HIB for the epiglottis is not understood, but it is known that blood colony counts in patients with epiglottitis are considerably lower than those in patients with meningitis.

CLINICAL MANIFESTATIONS
Meningitis

The pathology of meningitis is discussed in Chapter 21. HIB appears to have associated subdural effusions more than other causes of bacterial meningitis. The slow resolution of these effusions, some of which may be empyemas, has led to debate about the length of time these patients should be treated and whether surgical intervention is necessary. The persistence of bacterial cell products (particularly LOS) in the subdural space is thought to be responsible for prolonged fever in some of these patients.

Cellulitis

Buccal cellulitis occurs principally in children less than 18 months of age and may be related to bottle feeding. It can appear overnight in an otherwise healthy child. It often has a violaceous hue or it can appear erysipeloid. HIB can often be cultured from the blood or a saline aspirate of the cheek. Due consideration should be given to whether the child might have another focus of infection, particularly if blood cultures are positive. Other bacterial causes need to be considered, particularly in the older child or if there is an associated facial abrasion.

Orbital cellulitis (Figure 14-1) can be a medical emergency. It is usually an extension of an ethmoid sinusitis, and, if there is proptosis of the eye or paralysis of eye movement, decompression of the orbit is mandatory. This disease needs to be distinguished from "preseptal," or periorbital, cellulitis (Figure 14-2), which is a cellulitis of the eyelid and contiguous structures but which does not compromise the blood supply or the movement of the eye (Goldberg et al., 1978).

Epiglottitis

In epiglottitis manifestation the epiglottis is acutely edematous and erythematous. HIB can

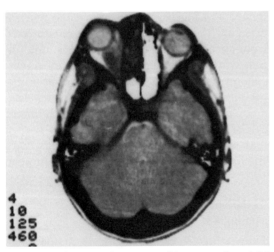

Fig. 14-1 Computed tomographic scan of a child with orbital cellulitis. Proptosis of the eye and involvement of deeper structures is evident.

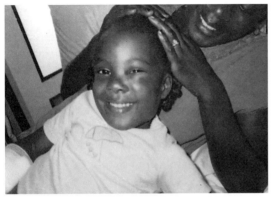

Fig. 14-2 Child recovering from a case of HIB preseptal (periorbital) cellulitis.

often be cultured from the surface of the pharynx, as well as from the blood. Some investigators feel that there may be an allergic component to this disease, which accounts for the extremely rapid course (as few as 4 to 6 hours) with which this disease often manifests. Children appear to be in a toxic state, but more strikingly they hold their heads forward trying to keep their airway patent. A short period of intubation with appropriate antibiotic treatment reverses this process quickly.

Septic Arthritis

HIB may cause septic arthritis in the young child. It is clinically indistinguishable from the disease caused by *Staphylococcus aureus*. Large joints—the hip in particular—are involved. It is important to have adequate drainage when large joints are affected, both for organism

identification and for healing. Latex agglutination tests on fluid from the joint space may be positive for HIB. If the child is very young, it is important to consider whether there is a contiguous osteomyelitis.

Pneumonia

The incidence of this infection is truly unknown. Many children are probably inadvertently treated when they are given antibiotics for other upper-respiratory illnesses, such as otitis media or sinusitis. Children with documented meningitis, pericarditis, or epiglottitis may have pneumonia as well. A definitive diagnosis is hampered in many cases because of the inability to obtain a positive diagnosis. One British study suggested that positive results of an HIB latex agglutination test in children with pneumonia may not be accurate (Isaacs, 1989). Thus many children in the past may have been falsely assumed to have HIB pneumonia. HIB cultured from the blood in a patient with clinical or roentgenographic pneumonia can be considered confirmatory. It has been reported that as many as 90% of patients with HIB pneumonias will have a pleural reaction and effusion.

Pericarditis

Although infrequent, this disease manifestation is frightening because of its rapidity of onset and lack of clinical symptoms. Respiratory distress in a child who is in a toxic state and has a normal chest roentgenogram are often the only symptoms. The child may have an underlying pneumonia or meningitis, and this disease process has been reported to occur in children who are on antibiotic treatment. Echocardiography followed by pericardiocentesis and appropriate antibiotic therapy are indicated. Copious pericardial exudate often persists for several days after therapy is initiated.

Bacteremia

Children who appear to be in a toxic state but have no focus of infection may have HIB bacteremia, which is diagnosed with a positive blood culture.

DIAGNOSIS

The isolation of HIB from a normally sterile body site is the method of diagnosis of choice in all diseases. HIB bacteremia, for instance, is always diagnosed with the isolation of HIB from the blood. However, there are limitations to this otherwise optimal standard. Occasionally a child may be given an antibiotic for treatment of a less severe disease before manifesting clinical meningitis. If the clinical history is compatible with meningitis and there are CSF changes (low sugar, high protein, and increased number of neutrophils) and a CSF latex agglutination test that is positive for HIB, most would agree that the child should be assumed to have HIB meningitis. If the results of the CSF latex agglutination test are negative, however, even if the urine antigen test results are positive, it is unlikely that this patient should be considered to have HIB meningitis if HIB does not grow from the CSF culture. If HIB grows from the CSF culture and the CSF is otherwise benign, it should be assumed that the child has HIB meningitis and that the disease was detected at an early stage.

A positive diagnosis for HIB is often difficult in a patient with cellulitis because clinicians are often reluctant to aspirate from the inflamed tissue. If blood cultures are positive for HIB or if the clinical picture is compatible with this diagnosis and the urine latex test is positive for HIB, the diagnosis can be assumed to be correct. Where there are no positive results, it is prudent to treat with an antibiotic that would also be effective for *S. aureus* infections.

If an aspirate is performed in septic arthritis, it will often confirm the bacterial cause of the infection, but if it is not performed then the physician must rely on the results of blood cultures and/or urine latex tests. If the child is already receiving an oral antibiotic, the same previously discussed difficulties that occur if cultures are negative also must be taken into consideration here. It is extremely important, however, that if there is doubt about the cause of the arthritis the patient be treated with antibiotics (and surgical drainage, if indicated) that would be effective against *S. aureus* infections, as well as against HIB infections.

Pericarditis always requires drainage, and, if the drainage is performed early in the course of disease, a positive culture for HIB from the fluid or blood is likely. If, however, the child has been on antibiotics and cultures are negative, a latex agglutination test that is positive for HIB from the pericardial fluid or urine would be useful.

Pneumonia remains the most difficult of all the infections to document, because there is question about the meaning of positive latex agglutination tests in these patients (see the

previous discussion). A positive blood culture or positive results of a latex agglutination test from pleural fluid may be confirmatory, but these tests may not have positive results even if performed.

Laboratory Tests

Gram stain and culture are the tests of choice to document infection. However, prior antibiotic treatment often makes blood cultures sterile. CSF cultures are less critically affected, particularly by the prior use of oral antibiotics, and thus may still be positive. Additionally, diseases with localized infection (arthritis and epiglottitis) have a lower level of bacteremia, and positive cultures may be missed if an inadequate volume of blood is taken for culture.

Several methods of antigen detection are useful even when the organisms have been made nonviable by antibiotics. The most popular and sensitive is the latex particle agglutination test, which uses anti-PRP antibody on latex particles that agglutinate in the presence of PRP antigen. This results of this test may be negative, however, if there is an overabundance or, alternately, a shortage of PRP antigen. It is also occasionally falsely positive for HIB as a result of cross-reactivity with some *Escherichia coli*, *Streptococcus pneumoniae*, *S. aureus*, and *Neisseria meningitidis* strains. Nevertheless, a positive latex test, in the presence of a strongly suggestive clinical course, is useful.

DIFFERENTIAL DIAGNOSIS
Meningitis

In the developed world the most common cause of meningitis in children between the ages of 3 months and 3 years was once HIB. The disease is indistinguishable from other causes of meningitis by clinical signs and symptoms alone. Chapter 21 deals with clinical symptoms so they are not discussed here. With the advent of HIB immunization in children as young as 2 months old in the United States, HIB as a cause of meningitis decreased 95%. *N. meningitidis* and *S. pneumoniae* are now the leading causes of meningitis in this age group. (CDC, Division of Bacterial and Mycotic diseases, 2002). HIB meningitis can be differentiated from the previously mentioned causes of bacterial meningitis preferably by the results of CSF culture or by a blood culture positive for HIB in conjunction with a compatible CSF picture. A urine latex test that is positive for HIB with a compatible clinical course and CSF analysis would also be acceptable. Other possible diagnoses include *Streptococcus agalactiae* (group B streptococcus) or *Listeria monocytogenes* in infants, and tuberculosis (TB) meningitis or aseptic meningitis in a child of any age. TB meningitis typically has a CSF lymphocytosis, increased protein, and decreased glucose. Aseptic meningitis may have a CSF pleocytosis and slightly elevated protein level, but the glucose level is usually within normal limits.

Epiglottitis

The presenting symptoms for epiglottitis include upper-airway obstruction and a toxic-looking appearance. Symptoms often appear rapidly, frequently in just a few hours. In areas where epiglottitis is common, it is customary to visualize the epiglottis with an anesthesiologist or intensivist present so that the child can be immediately intubated if necessary. At the time of intubation the epiglottis is cherry red and swollen, and it is useful to swab the epiglottis for bacterial culture. If the epiglottis is not typical in appearance (for epiglottitis) but the child requires intubation, it is useful to send the swab for viral culture. Most viral causes of a similar clinical-appearing syndrome have other symptoms of a respiratory infection (e.g., cough, coryza, conjunctivitis) and have a longer period of recovery. Children whose presenting symptoms include drooling and positioning the head forward to facilitate air entry occasionally have other red and swollen pharyngeal structures (uvula or posterior pharynx); cultures from the blood or mucosal surfaces of these children often grow HIB.

There is evidence that virtually all cases of epiglottitis in young children, as determined by inspection of the epiglottis during intubation, are caused by HIB. HIB was isolated from 114 of 123 (93%) blood cultures collected from epiglottitis patients in a study in Melbourne, Australia, and no other pathogens were isolated (Gilbert et al., 1990). When the diagnosis is not bacteriologically confirmed, it is usually because appropriate specimens have not been taken.

Pneumonia

The diagnosis of HIB pneumonia is difficult because blood cultures may not be positive for HIB, as a result of prior antibiotic therapy or an associated low level of bacteremia. If there is a pleural effusion, aspiration of fluid for culture

or latex agglutination may provide a positive result. However, the value of only a urine latex test that is positive for HIB is debatable, as previously mentioned. The presence of a significant effusion suggests that the pneumonia may be caused by HIB: up to 90% of HIB pneumonias have effusions (compared with only 10% for *S. pneumoniae*) in some reports. Drainage of a large effusion may not be required for recovery, unless there is an empyema, but usually speeds the healing process.

Septic Arthritis

This disease manifestation is assumed to be secondary to seeding synovial surfaces subsequent to bacteremia. Large joints, particularly the hip, are most commonly affected and should be surgically drained to avoid permanent damage. If the child was febrile and/or irritable before diagnosis, he or she may already be taking an antibiotic, and thus blood cultures may be negative for HIB. If there is a small antigen load in the blood or if the urine is dilute, then results of the urine latex test may be negative as well. In this case only an aspirate of the joint for culture and latex agglutination may permit a diagnosis. In the absence of a positive culture it is prudent to treat for a possible *S. aureus* septic arthritis, as well, because it is common in the same age group and the symptoms are identical. If the child is very young it is important to determine whether there is a contiguous osteomyelitis.

Cellulitis

Cellulitis of the face or around the orbit (periorbital) often develops rapidly. There is some suggestion that facial cellulitis may be associated with maxillary sinusitis or bottle feeding. These superficial skin infections are markedly different from the deep orbital tissue infection, "orbital" cellulitis, that commonly has an associated ipsilateral ethmoid sinusitis. Computed tomographic (CT) imaging may be required to distinguish the difference, since the eyelid is often too swollen to allow inspection of eye movement. The inability to move the eye suggests "orbital" infection, and decompression of the orbit is often required to avoid permanent sequelae. A positive microbiologic diagnosis can be made in these infections only if theblood culture or aspirate from the infected tissue is positive for HIB. A positive result from a urine latex test alone is suggestive and, some would believe, sufficient. However, if the diagnosis is uncertain, treatment to cover *S. aureus, S. pneumoniae,* and *Streptococcus pyogenes* would be prudent.

COMPLICATIONS

Most of the complications of HIB disease are found in the youngest patients who have meningitis. This is not unexpected. The youngest children often have the most fulminant disease and the fewest focal symptoms to alert parents and physicians of their diagnosis before the disease progresses to meningitis, the consequences of which necessarily affect the brain.

Subdural Fluid

Subdural effusions are frequently associated with HIB meningitis. Some of these effusions probably represent subdural empyemas, and there is debate about which of these require surgical drainage. It would seem appropriate to treat with antibiotics and perform serial CT scans, or other appropriate imaging procedures, to document whether the effusion or empyemas will resolve on their own. Children with these fluid collections often have persistent fever, which is compatible with the presence of persistent HIB antigen (particularly LOS) in the subdural space, causing the febrile reaction. Subdural fluid HIB antigen tests in some patients are positive for as long as a month after initial treatment, although cultures of the fluid are sterile.

Hearing Loss

The most common sequela of HIB disease is hearing loss, which has been reported in 5% to 15% of cases. It appears that prior treatment of the child with oral antibiotics may actually increase the incidence of hearing loss—probably by decreasing bacteremia and hence symptoms but masking a smoldering central nervous system (CNS) infection. There is also evidence that the early treatment of meningitis with steroids decreases the incidence of hearing loss in some patients. If this finding is verified, it will be useful in preventing significant morbidity in these children.

Intellectual Functioning

A sizable minority of children (5% to 20%) will have significant intellectual impairment after HIB meningitis. In the United States, as compared with other developed nations, there are more sequelae after HIB disease, but the median and mean age of patients with meningitis is younger in the United States, which may predispose patients to more complications. In addition, there have been studies that look at more subtle measurements of intellectual functioning in the United States. It has been reported that a disturbingly high percentage (up to 40%) of patients have "soft" intellectual problems, such as the inability to concentrate or specific learning disabilities when compared with their siblings or peers (Sell, 1987). With the advent of preventive immunization the incidence of all of these sequelae should decrease.

PROGNOSIS

In the United States the death rate from HIB disease is approximately 3% of those known to be infected (Wenger et al., 1990). Meningitis carries the highest death rate, since it occurs in the youngest children and affects the brain. Mental retardation, hearing loss, and mild neurologic abnormalities have also been described; the rates of each are dependent on the population examined and the intensity of investigation.

IMMUNITY

The protective role of PRP antibodies was first demonstrated by Fothergill and Wright in 1933. They noted an increased incidence of HIB disease when maternal antibody began to wane at 4 to 6 months of age. Like other polysaccharide antigens, PRP is T-cell independent and thus does not induce immunologic memory; the ability to respond to PRP with production of antibody (particularly IgG2) is not acquired until about 18 to 24 months old. Thus the greatest period of susceptibility to disease is between 4 and 24 months old, which is the peak incidence of disease in the United States. This lack of response to polysaccharide antigen is also responsible for the susceptibility of these children to *N. meningitidis* and *S. pneumoniae* infections. Immunization for the prevention of these diseases has necessitated the conjugation of the polysaccharide to a protein moiety to induce the infant immune system to make antibody to the polysaccharide and thus protect itself. This is discussed at the end of the chapter.

It is therefore apparent that children who acquire HIB infection at an early age may not mount an immunologic response. Therefore, even children who have had HIB disease should be vaccinated with the conjugate vaccine.

EPIDEMIOLOGIC FACTORS

The HIB nasopharyngeal carriage rate is generally less than 5%, but most children have acquired antibody to PRP by the age of 5 years without becoming ill, suggesting exposure to HIB or cross-reacting polysaccharides of other organisms. Disease is more common in children living under crowded conditions such as in day-care centers or inner-city areas. Although there is seasonal variation in disease, clear-cut epidemics have not been described.

Before the advent of conjugate HIB vaccine, the incidence and type of disease varied by country, but approximately 90% to 95% of disease occurred before the age of 5, regardless of location. The case attack rate per 100,000 children less than 5 years of age was 50 to 60 in Australia and Scandinavia and 60 to 130 in the United States. In certain ethnic groups such as Alaskan Eskimos, American Indians, and Australian aboriginals, the case attack rate was as high as 400 per 100,000 children less than 5 years old (1% to 2% of all children). When the incidence was high (e.g., in Alaskan Eskimos), the median age of disease was low (6 months), and epiglottitis was rare. In Australia and Finland, where the incidence of disease was lower, the median age was higher (27 months) and 30% to 40% of the disease was epiglottitis.

The differences in incidence of disease in different locations may be a result of genetic, as well as environmental, factors. Alaskan Eskimos in the same environment as non-Eskimos had a higher incidence of HIB disease, despite apparently adequate antibody levels. In addition, black Americans without the Km1 allotype had a higher incidence of disease than did black Americans with this allotype.

Population-based epidemiologic studies in Australia, Finland, and the United States before widespread use of conjugate vaccine demonstrated differences in the case attack rates for all invasive HIB disease and, in particular, in the relative frequency of the major clinical manifestations, namely, meningitis and epiglottitis (Table 14-1). A comprehensive study from Australia showed that the annual case attack rate of invasive HIB infections was 58.5 per 100,000 in children less

than 5 years old and almost two thirds (64%) of cases occurred in children over 18 months old (Gilbert et al., 1990). Meningitis (mean age, 20 months) and epiglottitis (mean age, 36 months) each accounted for approximately 40% of infections (attack rates of 23 per 100,000 each). Interestingly, attack rates for Haemophilus influenzae disease in Australian aboriginal children were reported to be 450 per 100,000, which is similar to that found in Alaskan natives. Population-based studies from Finland showed that the HIB case attack rate (52 per 100,000) and proportion of cases of meningitis (46%) and epiglottitis (29%) were similar to those in Australia (Takala, 1989). The attack rate for HIB disease was higher in the United States, even in populations that are primarily white. Studies from the United States estimated that the overall HIB attack rate was 60 to 100 per 100,000, of which approximately 60% were meningitis and 5% to 15% were epiglottitis.

In general, meningitis occurs at an earlier age than epiglottitis, so populations with a higher proportion of cases of meningitis have a lower mean age overall of HIB disease. In addition, populations with higher HIB attack rates also have a lower mean age of meningitis relative to those populations with lower attack rates. Thus a lower mean age of disease is relative to HIB disease incidence and disease manifestations (Figure 14-3). One could hypothesize that there is a pool of susceptible young children that gradually diminishes over time, coincident with the maturation of the immune system. If the environment provides for early exposure to the HIB organism, then there is an increased frequency of meningitis. If exposed later, they are less likely to become diseased even if infected, and their diseases are more likely to be localized. However, this hypothesis is still unproved.

Sex Distribution

Generally, the sex distribution for HIB disease manifestations—except pneumonia and epiglottitis—is equal. There is perhaps a small predominance of males when all studies are considered, but it is small. The distribution for epiglottitis is, however, unequivocally dominated by males. Most studies show a 1.5 to 2.0:1 male/female ratio. In studies of HIB pneumonia there is a predominance of males (2:1), but, as previously mentioned, complete case

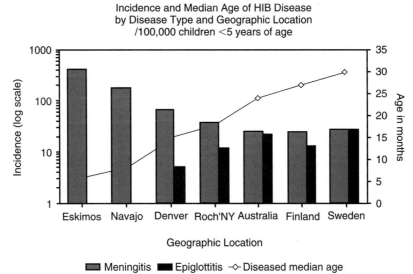

Fig. 14-3 Median age by country by disease type. (Modified from Clements DA, Gilbert GL: Aust NZ J Med 1990;20:828-834.)

TABLE 14-1	Estimated Incidence of Invasive *Haemophilus influenzae* Type b Disease

| | ANNUAL RATE/100,000 CHILDREN <5 YR OF AGE | | |
Population/place	*Meningitis*	*Epiglottitis*	*Mean age (mo)*
Alaskan natives	601	5	10
Australia (aboriginal)	450	0	7
Navajo Indians	152	0	8
United States (average)	19-69	5-15	8-15
Sweden	27	28*	30
Finland	26	13	28
Australia	25	23*	27
England	18	9	24

Modified from Clements DA, Gilbert GL: Aust NZ J Med 1990;20:828-834 and Broome CV: Pediatr Infect Dis J 1987;6:779-782.
*Includes patients with clinically, but not bacteriologically, confirmed epiglottitis (of which >95% of cases probably result from HIB).

ascertainment for pneumonia is questionable, which may (or may not) bias this finding.

Age Distribution

HIB disease is primarily a disease of children between 3 months and 5 years old. Most disease manifestations, except epiglottitis, are concentrated in the younger ages. Epiglottitis, although varying in incidence in different populations, seems to have a median age of disease of between 2 and 3 years (compared with 12 to 18 months for most other disease manifestations). The reason for this difference in age distribution is not known. Except for epiglottitis, the incidence of HIB disease is inversely proportional to the level of anti-PRP antibody measured in children's serum.

The age distribution of HIB disease is best demonstrated by data from Australia, where the incidence of epiglottitis is common. Data from the United States give similar age distributions, except the meningitis cases tend to occur even earlier in life. It is instructive to see that the overall distribution of disease is dependent on the predominant disease manifestations. Most other causes of HIB disease have an age distribution similar to that of meningitis (Figures 14-4 and 14-5).

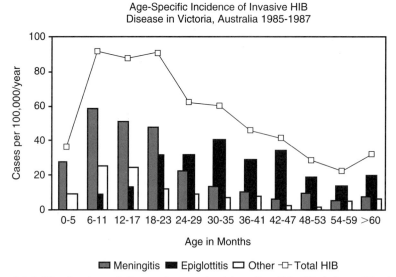

Fig. 14-4 Distribution of disease by age in Australia. (Modified from Ward JI, Cochi S: In Plotkin SA, Mortimer EA [eds]. Vaccines, ed 1. Philadelphia: Saunders, 1988.)

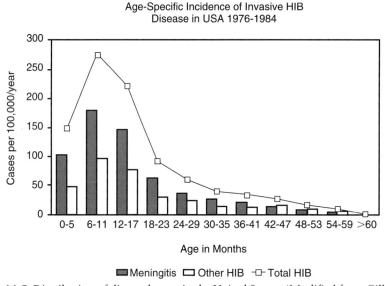

Fig. 14-5 Distribution of disease by age in the United States. (Modified from Gilbert GL, et al.: Pediatr Infect Dis J 1990;9:252-257.)

Seasonal Incidence and Year-to-Year Variation

There appears to be very little year-to-year variation in HIB disease incidence in countries where HIB disease has been systematically followed (Finland and Australia). There is, however, a seasonal variation. HIB is least common in the summer months; the disease clusters around the winter months. Some investigators have shown a bimodal fall-spring distribution, but others have shown that winter is the most common time.

RISK FACTORS

Infection rates depend on host susceptibility and exposure to the infectious agent. Protection from HIB disease in the first few months of life is provided by maternal antibody; thereafter the risk is relatively high until the child can mount an antibody response to HIB polysaccharide antigen, which develops gradually over the first few years of life.

Two studies from the United States have reported that crowded conditions increase the risk of HIB disease (Cochi et al., 1986; Istre et al., 1985). Crowding can result from smaller or fewer rooms per family unit or an increased number of persons per family. Attendance at day-care centers also appears to increase the risk of HIB disease, and children with HIB infection are more likely to have siblings who attend day care or school. Breast-feeding appears to be protective, but children who breast-feed may be less likely to be exposed to environments where there is a large number of other children. After controlling for number of siblings and residence size, family income does not seem to be a risk factor for disease.

Family members of children with HIB disease are often HIB carriers, particularly siblings aged 3 to 6 years. In an Australian study in which day-care exposure and siblings were risk factors for HIB disease, the risk of disease by attending day care was modified by whether the child had siblings, suggesting that day care has an effect similar to an increased number of siblings. Both of these measures are probably related to crowding or the potential for organism transmission.

Some unknown genetic factors may increase the risk of HIB disease. Aboriginals, Eskimos, and American Indians have a particularly high incidence of HIB disease. The environmental exposure may be the predominant determinant in the setting of a homogeneous genetic background. Black Americans who lack the Km1 immunoglobulin allotype have an increased incidence of HIB disease. Reasons for this increase in disease rate are unknown.

TREATMENT

Until 1974 HIB was universally susceptible to ampicillin. Beginning in that year, sporadic reports of resistance to ampicillin began to appear. Chloramphenicol, which had not been routinely used except in children known to be allergic to ampicillin, became commonly used. The advent of second-generation cephalosporins, such as cefuroxime, provided another possible treatment for HIB disease in the subsequent years, but variable CNS penetration and treatment failures precluded their use. At present, with 15% to 50% of HIB producing β-lactamase, the antibiotics of choice are the third-generation cephalosporins cefotaxime (100 to 150 mg/kg/day divided q6h)

and ceftriaxone (50 to 75 mg/kg/day divided q12h). These two antibiotics have very low minimum inhibitory concentrations against all HIB, regardless of whether they produce β-lactamase. Some clinicians have concluded that ampicillin can be used if the HIB organism isolated does not produce β-lactamase, but HIB isolates both sensitive and resistant to ampicillin have been recovered from the same patient on occasion.

Although chloramphenicol is infrequently used at present, it is important to note that there are recent reports of resistance to this antibiotic as a result of the ability of some HIB organisms to produce chloramphenicol acetyltransferase.

PREVENTIVE MEASURES
Immunization

PRP alone. In 1974 100,000 Finnish children were immunized with either unconjugated PRP or with meningococcal group A vaccine in a trial to prevent an outbreak of meningococcal A disease. In the 4 years after vaccination there were 20 cases of HIB disease in children over 18 months of age in the group that received meningococcal vaccine and only two cases in the PRP vaccine group—90% vaccine efficacy (Peltola et al., 1984). Protective efficacy for the polysaccharide antigen was not demonstrated in children less than 18 months of age. In an attempt to overcome the inability of the polysaccharide antigen alone to protect the youngest children, PRP was subsequently conjugated to several proteins to better stimulate antibody production and convert the immunogen to a T-cell–dependent antigen.

In spite of the limitations of the use of PRP alone as an immunogen to children over 2 years of age, it was judged to be cost effective and was licensed for use in the United States in 1985. Because PRP is at least partially effective in children between 18 and 24 months, it was also recommended at that time that high-risk children (those attending day-care centers and close contacts of cases) in the 18- to 24-month age group be vaccinated, with the proviso that they be vaccinated again at 24 months of age.

Replacement immunoglobulin therapy and the 1974 vaccine trials suggested that an anti-PRP antibody level above 0.15 µg/ml would be protective. However, because antibody levels fall over time, a higher level (>1.0 µg/ml) after immunization was postulated to be required for sustained protection. In addition, in children less than 6 months of age, levels of anti-PRP antibody acquired prenatally from the mother are falling, which complicates the assessment of vaccine immunogenicity.

Complicating these findings is the fact that in Finnish children over 18 months of age, PRP immunization was shown to be 90% protective against HIB disease in 1974. However, when licensed in the United States for children over 2 years of age, vaccine efficacy averaged only 60%, estimated by several retrospective case-control studies (Ward et al., 1988). This may have been a result of differences in populations or possibly the differences in use of vaccine under controlled versus uncontrolled conditions. Nevertheless, it gives reason to be cautious when extrapolating results of vaccine trials from one population to another.

PRP conjugate vaccines. After unsuccessful attempts to enhance PRP immunogenicity by changing the PRP polymer length and mixing PRP with DTP or pertussis vaccine, PRP was conjugated (covalently linked) to one of several protein carriers, including a mutant diphtheria toxin (PRP-CRM—Lederle-Praxis); diphtheria toxoid (PRP-D—Connaught Laboratories); an outer membrane protein of *Neisseria meningitidis* (PRP-OMP–Merck, Sharp, and Dohme); and tetanus toxoid (PRP-T—Mérieux). The amount of specific antibody produced (IgG1, IgG2, and IgM) after immunization depends on the method of conjugation and the age of the child. It is not clear whether a level of 1.0 μg/ml of anti-PRP antibody is required in response to T-cell–dependent vaccines in order to maintain protection. A lower antibody level may be protective if there is a prompt anamnestic response to a second PRP exposure as a result of vaccine or natural infection.

PRP-D. PRP-D contains PRP conjugated to diphtheria toxoid with a 6-carbon spacer (Connaught Laboratories). In children over 14 months of age, one 20-μg (PRP) dose gives antibody levels >1 μg/ml in 67% of children. For children between 9 and 15 months, two doses were required to achieve the same levels. In younger children, antibody produced is primarily IgM and thus relatively short-lived, whereas proportionately higher levels of IgG are produced in older children. Nevertheless, the antibody levels achieved are considerably higher than those with PRP alone, even in the youngest age groups. In children less than

6 months of age, even three injections may fail to achieve levels greater than 1 μg/ml, and levels decline rapidly in the subsequent year. A booster dose of the conjugate or PRP vaccine alone at 18 months produces a good response. These data encouraged the use of this vaccine in two efficacy trials; one in Alaska and the other in Finland.

In 1985 the PRP-D vaccine was given to Finnish children in a three-dose schedule at 3, 5, and 7 months of age. The protective efficacy was 83% for one injection, 90% for two injections, and 100% for three injections. However, the antibody response was relatively poor in children less than 7 months of life; invasive disease occurs less often in this age group in Finnish children. The same vaccine was also used in a trial in Alaskan children but was not protective. A genetic or environmental factor may contribute to the early mean age of disease in Alaskan children and, because of the poor antibody response in the youngest children, may have been responsible for the difference in vaccine efficacy reported. Until recently, PRP-D was still the most commonly commercially available conjugate HIB vaccine in Europe. It has never been widely used in the United States.

HbOC. Low–molecular-weight oligosaccharides of PRP are coupled to a mutant variant of diphtheria toxin in this Lederle-Praxis vaccine. This was the first conjugate vaccine to be licensed for use in children at 2 months of age in the United States. There is little antibody response to the initial dose of vaccine at 2 months of age, but there is a brisk and sustained antibody response to subsequent doses of vaccine. As in all conjugate vaccines, there are almost no side effects to vaccination. The present recommendation for vaccination includes three doses of vaccine (preferably 2 months apart) by 6 months of age and a booster at 15 months of age.

PRP-OMP. Merck and Company have conjugated PRP to a protein from group B *N. meningitidis.* This vaccine is immunogenic with the first dose given. Its demonstrated efficacy in the Navajo population (even after 1 dose), where there is a very early median age of HIB disease, was particularly impressive. The only case of disease (arthritis) in the immunized group was in a child who was over a year of age and who had failed to receive her booster immunization. It was subsequently licensed for use in children as young as 2 months of age.

It requires two immunizations (preferably 2 months apart) in the first 6 months of life and a booster at 12 months.

Response to subsequent doses of vaccine is less than to HbOC and, although it appears to be T-cell dependent, it does not boost to the same level as the other licensed product. However, there is an extremely good antibody response to the first dose of vaccine. There are no significant side effects associated with this vaccine.

PRP-T. PRP-T is composed of high–molecular-weight PRP covalently linked to a formalin-detoxified tetanus toxin. Active surveillance for adverse events after immunization shows some mild local and systemic reactions, similar to those of the other conjugate HIB vaccines. Of 107,000 infants who received vaccine in Finland, only 43 adverse events were noted; 33 were reported after the first dose, 8 after the second, and 2 after the booster dose. Most reactions occurred in children who received the DTP vaccine at the same time. Immunogenicity from the vaccine is high, with 90% to 95% of recipients having anti-PRP antibody levels above 1 μg/ml after the third dose. This vaccine (compared with other conjugate PRP vaccines) reportedly yields the highest percentage of children with anti-PRP antibodies above 1 μg/ml after the primary series (Fritzell and Plotkin, 1992).

Mixed-conjugate vaccine administration. Although each conjugate HIB vaccine is tested before approval in many children, children in clinical trials all receive the same manufacturer's vaccine for the series. In "the real world," families move and health providers change vaccine brands because of supply problems or price differences. Several studies have looked at whether there is a difference in anti-PRP antibody production if different conjugate vaccines are used during the third and fourth series of immunizations. To date, none have shown any decreased immunogenicity because of changing vaccine sources during the series; in fact, there is a subtle suggestion that some mixed-brand strategies actually enhance anti-PRP antibody production. It is obviously not feasible to design a mixed strategy to be routinely given to children, so researchers must accept at least that there are no untoward effects if patients receive mixed-brand conjugate HIB vaccines during the series.

Neonatal immunization. Studies assessing the preterm and newborn's response to conjugate HIB vaccines are few but support that infants with a gestational age of at least 28 weeks respond adequately (although not optimally) to vaccination at 2, 4, and 6 months of chronologic age. Children less than 28 weeks have less response and may need a different strategy (such as delay to 3, 5, and 7 months of age). The number of studies is small, however, and each study has used only one vaccine brand, so further analysis is needed. To date, though, it is preferable to immunize infants of 28 weeks or greater gestation with conjugate HIB vaccination on the regularly suggested schedule.

Prenatal maternal immunization. One study of approximately 100 mothers, half of whom received HIB vaccine in the last trimester (one third PRP, two thirds conjugate PRP) demonstrated significant increase in the infant's anti-PRP level in cord blood (17 to 29 μg/ml versus 0.29 μg/ml). This may be a reasonable strategy in populations that have very early HIB disease (Alaskan Eskimos) or where vaccination of infants is problematic. The effect of this increased antibody level on subsequent infant HIB immunization is unclear at this time.

CHEMOPROPHYLAXIS

There has been considerable controversy about the use of rifampin to prevent secondary cases of HIB. There is sufficient evidence that rifampin, taken orally, will markedly decrease the carrier rate of HIB in the pharynx (estimates are as high as 95%) and thereby reduce secondary or coprimary cases if it is administered soon after the discovery of the primary case. What is not clear is the advantage this has in stopping the spread of disease. Several studies show that family members or close contacts often carry the organism in the throat, which is presumably where the diseased child obtains the infection. However, unless there is another susceptible child in the environment, rifampin treatment may be of little use. At present the recommendations are to treat all members of a family, including the patient, with rifampin (20 mg/kg per day, max 600 mg) once daily for 4 days if there is another child less than 48 months of age in the home. Treatment of contacts at day-care centers should be individualized, but, in general, prophylaxis at day care is no longer routinely recommended. In fact,

HIB immunization is an admission requirement for entry to day care, so the need for prophylaxis should not be a concern.

Two approaches other than immunization have been taken to decrease disease incidence in populations where the median age of patients with HIB disease is very low. Maternal immunization with HIB before delivery has been performed in Navajo Indians, a measure that boosts the mother's anti-PRP IgG levels. In addition, newborns of Navajo mothers have received repeated doses of intramuscular immunoglobulin to boost IgG levels. Both of these strategies have had some effect on increasing anti-PRP antibody in the newborn, but the advent of conjugated HIB vaccines that can be given at 2 months of age may have obviated the use of these therapies.

HIB Disease Epidemiology Since the Inception of HIB Vaccine

HIB disease has decreased markedly since the licensure of the HIB vaccine. Interestingly, there was a decrease in the disease incidence in children less than 18 months of age (in addition to the expected decrease in children over 18 months of age) when the vaccine was first given to 18-month-old children. This was in spite of the fact that there did not seem to be a decreased oral-pharyngeal HIB colonization rate after vaccination. Subsequently, when the conjugate HIB vaccines were licensed and given, there was a further decrease in the HIB disease rate and concomitant decrease in the oral HIB colonization rate (suggesting less ability to spread infection). At present the HIB disease rate in the United States has been reduced 95% to 97% depending on the population measured (Figure 14-6) (Adams et al., 1993; Michaels and Ali, 1993; Murphy et al., 1993, Centers for Disease Control and Prevention, 1998). In Alaskan Eskimos the disease incidence initially decreased 90% (but this has included passive immunoglobulin therapy also) (Singleton et al., 1994) but then increased again when the vaccine used was changed from one brand to another. The exact cause of the resurgence of the disease is unknown. It is hypothesized that it is either due to a decreased immunogenicity of the first dose of vaccine by one of the manufacturers or by an increased HIB carrier state in the population (Galil, 1999). However, a study by Perdue et al. (2000) showed a decrease in HIB disease in children older than 10 years of age,

suggesting that HIB carrier states actually decreased. Singleton et al. (2000), though, concluded that the HIB-OMP vaccine should be used minimally as the first dose of HIB vaccine in Alaskan Eskimos to increase immunogenicity and decrease carriage in this highly susceptible population with the first dose.

There has also been some concern that there may be emergence of other typeable *H. influenzae* bacteria secondary to the decrease in HIB disease. There have been some reports of increasing frequency of infections with *H. influenzae* type f, but the most striking increase has been in a report from Utah, where in a 10-month period five cases of *H. influenzae* type a were reported (Adderson, 2001). None had been reported in the previous 7 years. Four of the cases had meningitis and one had purpura fulminans—diseases similar to those caused by HIB in the past. The median age of infection was 12 months. Three of the cases were caused by a strain with a deletion mutation similar to that found in HIB.

A new concern is that the welcome decrease in HIB disease has made it unusual for those training in pediatrics to have experience with what was once a common disease. This is similar to the decrease in experience and awareness that has occurred with measles, mumps, rubella, and now varicella. However, this is not such a high price to pay for what has been a great cause of morbidity and mortality in young children.

• • •

The recommendations of the Advisory Committee on Immunization Practices (ACIP) for the use of HIB vaccines have not been updated since published in MMWR 1993;42 (RR-13): 8-12) (see below). Recommendations for use of combination vaccines are made in Table 14-2.

RECOMMENDATIONS FOR HIB VACCINATION
General
All infants should receive a conjugate HIB vaccine (separate or in combination with DTP [TETRA-MUNE™]), beginning at age 2 months (but not earlier than 6 weeks). If the first vaccination is delayed beyond age 6 months, the schedule of vaccination for previously unimmunized (Table 14-3) and immunized (Table 14-4) children should be followed. When possible, the HIB conjugate vaccine used at the first vaccination should be used for all subsequent vaccinations in the

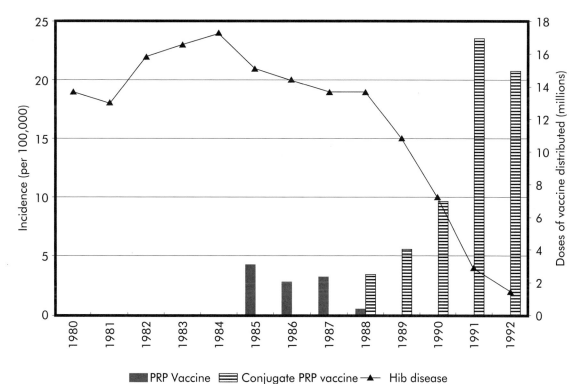

Fig. 14-6 *Haemophilus influenza* type b meningitis incidence in children <5 years of age and (PRP) vaccine doses distributed by year in the United States. Modified from data supplied by CDC, Atlanta, Ga.

TABLE 14-2	Combination Vaccines Containing HIB Conjugate Vaccines (USA)	
Licensed vaccine	*Trade name*	*Manufacturer*
HbOC+DTP	TETRAMUNE™	Lederle Laboratories
PRP-T+DTP	ActHIB/DTP™	Pasteur Mérieux/Connaught Laboratories
PRP-T+DtaP	TriHIBit™ (4th dose booster only)	Connaught Laboratories
PRP-OMP+HepB	COMVAX™ (not less than 6 weeks of age)	Merck and Company

primary series. When either HIB vaccines or TETRAMUNE™ is used, the vaccine should be administered intramuscularly using a separate syringe and administered at a separate site from any other concurrent vaccinations.

HbOC or PRP-T

Previously unvaccinated infants aged 2 to 6 months should receive three doses of vaccine administered 2 months apart, followed by a booster dose at age 12 to 15 months, at least 2 months after the last vaccination. Unvaccinated children ages 7 to 11 months should receive two doses of vaccine,

2 months apart, followed by a booster dose at age 12 to 18 months, at least 2 months after the last vaccination. Unvaccinated children ages 12 to 14 months should receive two doses of vaccine, at least 2 months apart. Any previously unvaccinated child aged 15 to 59 months should receive a single dose of vaccine.

PRP-OMP

Previously unvaccinated infants ages 2 to 6 months should receive two doses of vaccine administered at least 2 months apart. Although PRP-OMP induces a substantial antibody response after one

TABLE 14-3	Schedule for HIB Conjugate Vaccine Administration Among Previously Unvaccinated Children

Vaccine	Age at first vaccination (mo)	Primary series	Booster
HbOC/PRP-T*	2-6	3 doses, 2 mo apart	12-15 mo
	7-11	2 doses, 2 mo apart	12-18 mo
	12-14	1 dose	2 mo later
	15-59	1 dose	—
PRP-OMP	2-6	2 doses, 2 mo apart	12-15 mo
	7-11	2 doses, 2 mo apart	12-18 mo
	12-14	1 dose	2 mo later
	15-59	1 dose	—
PRP-D	15-59	1 dose	—

*TETRAMUNE™ may be administered by the same schedule for primary immunization as HbOC/PRP-T (when the series begins at 2 to 6 months of age). A booster dose of DTP or DTaP should be administered at 4 to 6 years of age, before kindergarten or elementary school. This booster is not necessary if the fourth vaccinating dose was administered after the fourth birthday. See ACIP statement for information on use of DTP and contraindications for use of pertussis vaccine (44).
—Not applicable.

dose, all children should receive all recommended doses of PRP-OMP. Because of the substantial antibody response after one dose, it may be advantageous to use PRP-OMP vaccine in populations that are known to be at increased risk for disease during early infancy (e.g., Alaskan Natives). A booster dose should be administered to all children at 12 to 15 months of age at least 2 months after the last vaccination. Unvaccinated children ages 7 to 11 months should receive two doses of vaccine, 2 months apart, followed by a booster dose at 12 to 18 months of age, at least 2 months after the last dose. Unvaccinated children ages 12 to 14 months should receive two doses of vaccine, 2 months apart. Any previously unvaccinated child 15 to 59 months of age should receive a single dose of vaccine.

PRP-D

One dose of PRP-D may be administered to unvaccinated children aged 15 to 59 months. This vaccine may be used as a booster dose at 12 to 18 months of age following a two- or three-dose primary series, regardless of the vaccine used in the primary series. This vaccine is not licensed for use among infants because of its limited immunogenicity and variable protective efficacy in this age group.

Tetramune™

This combination vaccine TETRAMUNE™ may be used for routine vaccination of infants, beginning at age 2 months, to prevent diphtheria, tetanus, pertussis, and invasive HIB disease. Previously unvaccinated infants aged 2 to 6 months should receive three doses administered at least 2 months apart. An additional dose should be administered at 12 to 15 months of age, after at least a 6-month interval following the third dose. Alternatively, acellular DTP and HIB vaccine can be administered as separate injections at 12 to 15 months of age. Acellular DTP is preferred for doses four and five of the five-dose DTP series. For infants who begin both HIB and DTP vaccinations late (after 2 months of age), TETRAMUNE™ may be used for the first and second doses of the vaccine series. However, because delay in initiation of the DTP series does not reduce the number of required doses of DTP, additional doses of DTP without HIB are necessary to ensure that all four doses are administered. Infants ages 7 to 11 months who have not previously been vaccinated with DTP or HIB vaccines should receive two doses of TETRAMUNE™, administered at least 2 months apart, followed by a dose of DTP vaccine 4 to 8 weeks after the second dose of TETRAMUNE™. An additional dose of DTP and HIB vaccines should then be administered: DTP vaccine at least 6 months after the third immunizing dose against diphtheria, tetanus, and pertussis; and HIB vaccine at 12 to 18 months of age, at least 2 months after the last HIB dose.

TETRAMUNE™ may be used to complete an infant immunization series started with any HIB vaccine (licensed for use in this age group) and with any DTP vaccine if both vaccines are to be administered simultaneously. Completion of the primary series using the same HIB vaccine, however, is preferable. Conversely, any DTP vaccine may be used to complete a series initiated with TETRAMUNE™ (see the general ACIP statement on Diphtheria, Tetanus and Pertussis: Recommendations for Vaccine Use and Other Preventive Measures [44] for further information).

Other considerations for HIB vaccination

Other considerations for HIB vaccination are discussed in the following section:

1) Although an interval of 2 months between doses of HIB vaccine in the primary series is recommended, an interval of 1 month is acceptable, if necessary.

2) Unvaccinated children aged 15 to 59 months may be administered a single dose of any one of the four HIB conjugate vaccines or TETRAMUNE™ (if both HIB and DTP vaccines are indicated).

3) After the primary infant vaccination series is completed, any of the four licensed HIB conjugate vaccines (or TETRAMUNE™ if both HIB vaccine and DTP vaccine are indicated) may be used as a booster dose at age 12 to 15 months.

4) The primary vaccine series should preferably be completed with the same HIB conjugate vaccine. If, however, different vaccines are administered, a total of three doses of HIB conjugate vaccine is adequate. Any combination of HIB conjugate vaccines that is licensed for use among infants may be used to complete the primary series.

5) Infants born prematurely should be vaccinated according to the schedule recommended for other infants, beginning at age 2 months.

6) HIB conjugate vaccines may be administered simultaneously with DTP (or DTaP) vaccine, OPV, IPV, MMR, influenza, and hepatitis B vaccines. TETRAMUNE™ may be administered simultaneously with OPV, IPV, MMR, influenza, and hepatitis B vaccines.

7) Because natural infection does not always result in the development of protective anti-PRP antibody levels (*45*), children <24 months of age who develop invasive HIB disease should receive HIB vaccine as recommended in the schedule. These children should be considered unimmunized, and vaccination should start as soon as possible during the convalescent phase of the illness.

8) HIB vaccine is immunogenic in patients with increased risk for invasive disease, such as those with sickle-cell disease (*46*), leukemia (*47*), human immunodeficiency virus (HIV) infection (*48,49*), and in those who have had splenectomies (*50*). However, in persons with HIV infection, immunogenicity varies with stage of infection and degree of immunocompromise. Efficacy studies have not been performed in populations with increased risk of invasive disease (see the general ACIP statement on Use of Vaccines and Immune Globulins in Persons with Altered Immunocompetence [*51*]).

9) Children who attend day care are at increased risk for HIB disease. Therefore, efforts should be made to ensure that all day care attendance <5 years of age are fully vaccinated.

10) Rifampin chemoprophylaxis for household contacts of a person with invasive HIB disease is no longer indicated if all contacts ages <4 years are fully vaccinated against HIB disease. A child is considered fully immunized against HIB disease following a) at least one dose of conjugate vaccine at ≥15 months of age, b) two doses of conjugate vaccine at 12 to 14 months of age, or c) two or more doses of conjugate vaccine at <12 months of age, followed by a booster dose at ≥12 months of age. In households with one or more infants <12 months of age (regardless of vaccination status) or with a child aged 1 to 3 years who is inadequately vaccinated, all household contacts should receive rifampin prophylaxis following a case of invasive HIB disease that occurs in any family member. The recommended dose is 20 mg/kg as a single daily dose (maximal daily dose 600 mg) for 4 days. Neonates (<1 month of age) should receive 10 mg/kg once daily for 4 days.

Adverse reactions

Adverse reactions to each of the four HIB conjugate vaccines are generally uncommon. Swelling, redness, and/or pain have been reported in 5% to 30% of recipients and usually resolve within 12 to 24 hours. Systemic reactions such as fever and irritability are infrequent. Available information on side effects and adverse reactions suggests that the risks for local and systemic events following TETRAMUNE™ administration are similar to those following concurrent administration of its individual component vaccines (i.e., DTP and HIB vaccines), and may be due largely to the pertussis component of the DTP vaccine (*52*).

Surveillance regarding the safety of TETRAMUNE™, PRP-T, and other HIB vaccines in large-scale use aids in the assessment of vaccine safety by identifying potential events that may warrant further study. The Vaccine Adverse Events Reporting System (VAERS) of the U.S. Department of Health and Human Services encourages reports of all serious adverse events that occur after receipt of any vaccine.* Invasive HIB disease is a reportable condition in 43 states. All health-care workers should report any case of invasive HIB disease to local and state health departments.

Contraindications and precautions

Vaccination with a specific HIB conjugate vaccine is contraindicated in persons known to have experienced anaphylaxis following a prior dose of that vaccine. Vaccination should be delayed in children with moderate or severe illnesses. Minor illnesses

---

*Questions about reporting requirements, completion of report forms, or requests for reporting forms should be directed to VAERS at 1-800-822-7967.

TABLE 14-4	HIB Vaccination Schedules for Children With a Lapse in Administration	
Current age	*Prior vaccination history*	*Recommendations*
7-11 mo	1 dose	1 dose 7-11 mo, booster >12-15 mo
7-11 mo	2 doses HbOC or PRP-T	1 dose 7-11 mo, booster >12-15 mo
12-14 mo	1 dose before 12 mo	2 doses of any licensed conjugate HIB vaccine
12-14 mo	2 doses before 12 mo	1 dose of any licensed conjugate HIB vaccine
15-59 mo	Any incomplete schedule	1 dose of any licensed HIB conjugate vaccine

Modified from 2000 AAP Redbook
All doses should be separated by 2 months.

(e.g., mild upper-respiratory infection) are not contraindications to vaccination.

Contraindications and precautions of the use of TETRAMUNE™ are the same as those for its individual component vaccines (i.e., DTP or HIB) (see the general ACIP statement on Diphtheria, Tetanus, and Pertussis: Recommendations for Vaccine Use and Other Preventive Measures [44] for more details on the use of vaccines containing DTP).

BIBLIOGRAPHY

Adams WG, Deaver KA, Cochi SL, et al. Decline of childhood *Haemophilus influenzae* type b (HIB) disease in the HIB vaccine era. JAMA 1993;269:221-226.

Adderson EE, Byington CL, Spencer L, et al. Invasive Serotype a *Haemophilus influenzae* infections with a virulence genotype resembling *Haemophilus influenzae* type b: emerging pathogen in the vaccine era? Pediatrics 2001;108:18.

Barenkamp SJ, Granoff DM, Pittman M. Outer membrane protein subtypes and biotypes of *Haemophilus influenzae* type b: relation between strains isolated in 1934-1954 and 1977-1980. J Infect Dis 1983;148:1127.

Broome CV. Epidemiology of *Haemophilus influenzae* type b infections in the United States. Pediatr Infect Dis J 1987;6:779-782.

Centers for Disease Control and Prevention. Recommendations of the Advisory Committee on Immunization Practices (ACIP) for the use of HIB vaccines. MMWR 1993;42:1-15.

Centers for Disease Control and Prevention. Progress toward elimination of *Haemophilus influenzae* type b disease among infants and children: United States 1987-1997. MMWR 1998;47:993-998.

Clements DA, Gilbert GL. Immunization for the prevention of *Haemophilus influenzae* type b infections: a review. Aust NZ J Med 1990;20:828-834.

Cochi SL, Fleming DW, Hightower AW, et al. Primary invasive *Haemophilus influenzae* type b disease: a population-based assessment of risk factors. J Pediatr 1986;108:887-896.

Cochi SL, O'Mara D, Preblud SR. Progress in *Haemophilus* type b polysaccharide vaccine use in the United States. Pediatrics 1988;81:166-168.

Fritzell B, Plotkin S. Efficacy and safety of a *Haemophilus influenzae* type b capsular polysaccharide-tetanus protein conjugate vaccine. J Pediatr 1992;121:355-362.

Galil K, Singleton R, Levine OS, et al. Reemergence of invasive *Haemophilus influenzae* type b disease in a well-vaccinated population in remote Alaska. J Infect Dis 1999;179:101-106.

Gilbert GL, Clements DA, Broughton S. *Haemophilus influenzae* type b infections in Victoria, Australia 1985-87: a population based study to determine the need for immunization. Pediatr Infect Dis J 1990;9:252-257.

Goldberg F, Berne AS, Oski FA. Differentiation of orbital cellulitis from preseptal cellulitis by computed tomography. Pediatrics 1978;62:1000-1005.

Isaacs D. Problems in determining the etiology of community-acquired childhood pneumonia. Pediatr Infect Dis J 1989;8:143-148.

Istre CR, Conner JS, Broome CV, et al. Risk factors for primary invasive *Haemophilus influenzae* disease: increased risk from day-care attendance and school-age household members. J Pediatr. 1985;106:190-195.

Kilian M. A taxonomic study of the genus *Haemophilus* with the proposal of a new species. J Clin Micro 1976; 93:9-62.

Michaels RH, Ali O. A decline in *Haemophilus influenzae* type b meningitis. J Pediatr 1993;122:407-409.

Michaels RH, Stonebraker FE, Robbins JB. Use of antiserum agar for detection of *Haemophilus influenzae* type b in the pharynx. Pediatr Res 1975;9:513-516.

Moxon ER. Virulence genes and prevention of *Haemophilus influenzae* infections. Arch Dis Child 1985;60:1193-1196.

Murphy TV, White KE, Pastor P, et al. Declining incidence of *Haemophilus influenzae* type b disease since introduction of vaccination. JAMA 1993;269:246-248.

Musser JM, Granoff DM, Pattison PE, Selander RK. A population genetic framework for the study of invasive diseases caused by serotype b strains of *Haemophilus influenzae*. Proc Natl Acad Sci USA 1985;82:5078-5082.

Musser JM, Kroll JS, Moxon ER, Selander RK. Clonal populations structure of encapsulated *Haemophilus influenzae*. Infect Immun 1988;56:1837-1845.

Perdue DG, Bulkow LR, Gellin BG, et al. Invasive *Haemophilus influenzae* disease in Alaskan residents aged 10 years and older before and after infant vaccination programs. JAMA 2000;283:3089-3094.

Peltola H, Kayhty H, Virtanen M, Makela PH. Prevention of *Haemophilus influenzae* type b bacteremic infections with the capsular polysaccharide vaccine. N Engl J Med 1984;310:1566-1569.

Sell SH. *Haemophilus influenzae* type b meningitis: manifestations and long-term sequelae. Pediatr Infect Dis J 1987;6:775-778.

Singleton R, Bulkow LR, Levin OS, et al. Experience with the prevention of invasive *Haemophilus influenzae* type b disease by vaccination in Alaska: the impact of persistent oropharyngeal carriage. J Pediatr 2000;137:313-320.

Singleton RJ, Davidson NM, Desmet IJ, et al. Decline of Haemophilus influenzae type b disease in a region of high risk: impact of passive and active immunization. Pediatr Infect Dis J 1994;13:362-367.

Takala AK, Eskola J, Peltola H, Mäkelä PH. Epidemiology of invasive *Haemophilus influenzae* type b disease among children in Finland before vaccination with *Haemophilus influenzae* type b conjugate vaccine. Pediatr Infect Dis J 1989;8:297-302.

Takala AK, van Alphen L, Eskola J, et al. *Haemophilus influenzae* type b strains of outer membrane subtypes 1 and 1c cause different types of invasive disease. Lancet 1987;2:647-650.

van Alphen L, Geelen L, Jonsdottir K, et al. Distinct geographical distribution of HIB subtypes in Western Europe. J Infect Dis 1987;156:216-218.

Ward JI, Broome CV, Harrison LH, et al. *Haemophilus influenzae* type b vaccines: lessons for the future. Pediatrics 1988;81:886-892.

Ward JI, Cochi S. *Haemophilus influenzae* vaccines. In Plotkin SA, Mortimer EA (eds). Vaccines, ed 1. Philadelphia: Saunders, 1988.

Wenger JD, Hightower AW, Facklam RR, et al. Bacterial meningitis in the United States, 1986: report of a multistate surveillance study. J Infect Dis 1990;162:1316-1323.

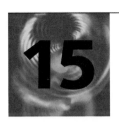

15

HERPES SIMPLEX VIRUS INFECTIONS

PAULA W. ANNUNZIATO

Herpes simplex viruses (HSV) are among the most widely disseminated infectious agents of humans. The ubiquity of these viruses is not generally appreciated because they often do not produce overt disease. However, the various clinical syndromes caused by HSV in infants and children—particularly, neonatal infections, gingivostomatitis, encephalitis, and infections in the immunocompromised—are clinically significant problems.

ETIOLOGY

A member of the herpesvirus group, HSV is composed of an inner core containing linear double-stranded DNA, surrounded concentrically by an icosahedral capsid of approximately 100 nm, an amorphous layer termed the *tegument*, and an outer envelope composed of lipids and glycoproteins. Enveloped HSV particles range in size from 150 to 200 nm. HSV usually is considered the prototype of the human herpesviruses, and cytomegalovirus (CMV), varicella-zoster virus (VZV), and Epstein-Barr virus (EBV) resemble it in morphologic appearance. The two antigenic types of HSV, types 1 (HSV-1, designated human herpesvirus 1) and 2 (HSV-2, designated human herpesvirus 2), contain DNA with 50% homology (Nahmias and Dowdle, 1968). The two types can be distinguished by the following means: (1) restriction enzyme analysis of the DNA (Buchman et al., 1978; Buchman et al., 1979); (2) antigenic structure determined by Western blotting (Growdon et al., 1987); and (3) certain antibody determinations (see the following paragraphs). Subtypes of HSV-1 and HSV-2 can be further distinguished by analysis of viral DNA with restriction enzymes (Buchman et al., 1978; Buchman et al., 1979; Corey, 1982). Subtypes differ in less than 10% of their DNA, and they do not show significant antigenic variation, so they can be distinguished from one another only by DNA analysis.

HSV DNA encodes for a number of structural and nonstructural viral proteins and glycoproteins (g). As with all of the herpesviruses, replication occurs in a regulated cascading sequence, with immediate early alpha genes controlling subsequent transcription and translation of early beta and late gamma gene products (Roizman and Knipe, 2001). Alpha genes encode proteins that initiate viral transcription, beta genes control synthesis of proteins and enzymes such as thymidine kinase necessary for viral replication, and gamma genes encode structural proteins of HSV, including the glycoproteins. There are at least 10 envelope glycoproteins of HSV: gB, gC, gD, gE, gG, gH, gI, gK, gL, and gM. These glycoproteins are antigenic and therefore play an important role in generating immune responses by the infected host. They also play important roles in viral infectivity. Some glycoproteins (gB, gC, gD, gH, and gL) mediate viral attachment to and penetration of host cells; gC binds to the C3b component of complement, and gE binds to the Fc portion of IgG.

The relative importance of immune responses to each of the glycoproteins and to nonstructural proteins for protection of the host is the subject of much investigation. Infection with one HSV does not result in immunity to the other type, but there is some indication that partial protection is induced against HSV-2 infection when there is preexisting immunity to HSV-1 (Boucher et al., 1990; Breinig et al, 1990).

Antibody responses to each type of HSV cannot be distinguished by commercially available antibody assays, but they may be detected by Western blot, using known strains of HSV-1 and HSV-2 as antigens. Antibodies to types 1 and 2 can also be distinguished by using gG as the antigen in an immunologic antibody assay such as enzyme-linked immunosorbent assay (ELISA), since gG is distinct for each type of HSV (Whitley, 2001). Soon, gG-based ELISAs are expected to be available for clinical use.

HSV is readily transmitted to a variety of animals. Animal models are useful for studying viral latency and the effects of antiviral drugs. Tissue cultures infected with HSV show cytopathic effects characterized by degeneration and clumping of the cells and the presence of typical intranuclear inclusion bodies and multinucleated giant cells. Infection in tissue cultures is at first focal, reflecting cell-to-cell viral spread, and then generalized throughout a culture, reflecting release of infectious virus into supernatant media.

HSV-1 has been associated chiefly with nongenital infections of the mucous membranes of the mouth, lips, and eyes and of the central nervous system (CNS). HSV-2 most commonly has been associated with genital and neonatal infections. There are no strict anatomic barriers; HSV-1 can cause genital and neonatal infection, and HSV-2 can infect the oral mucosa.

All of the herpesviruses share the characteristic of becoming latent after primary infection; the virus may subsequently reactivate periodically and produce clinical symptoms in certain individuals. The phenomenon of latent infection permits long-term persistence of the virus within the host and potential future transmissibility to others. For both HSV-1 and HSV-2 the site of latency is the sensory ganglia. Presumably, HSV reaches the ganglia during primary infection when the sensory nerve endings, as well as the skin or mucous membranes, are invaded by the virus. Based on studies in animals, HSV is thought to reach the ganglia by retrograde axonal transport. Various factors such as fever, sunlight, stress, and trauma may trigger a recurrent infection, but at times no stimulus is apparent. Surgical transection of the trigeminal nerve frequently results in the appearance of herpetic vesicles in the facial skin. In studies of ganglia obtained at autopsy from patients with no clinical evidence of HSV infection at death, HSV-1 or HSV-2 was isolated in tissue culture by cocultivation techniques from approximately 50% of trigeminal ganglia and 15% of sacral ganglia (Baringer, 1974; Baringer and Swoveland, 1973).

There is no morphologic or antigenic evidence of the presence of HSV in latently infected ganglia; however, limited amounts of viral RNA are detectable. During latent infection there is consistent expression of RNA that is transcribed in the opposite orientation to and overlapping part of the alpha gene encoding a viral protein termed the *infected cell protein 0* (ICP0). This RNA is referred to as the *latency-associated transcript* (LAT); its role in latency remains puzzling despite extensive investigation (Bloom et al., 1996; Croen et al., 1987; Farrell et al., 1991; Garber et al., 1997; Krause et al., 1995; Leib et al., 1989; Perng et al., 1994; Thompson and Sawtell, 2001; Steiner et al., 1989; Stevens et al., 1988; Thompson and Sawtell 2000; Thompson and Sawtell, 1997).

Immunologic factors have long been hypothesized to control reactivation of HSV, since immunocompromised patients are at high risk to develop reactivation syndromes, but no specific abnormal or absent immunologic reactions have been consistently implicated. In general, HSV can reactivate despite specific humoral and cell-mediated immunity. The following cells or cell-mediated immune reactions may play roles in host defense against HSV: macrophages, cytotoxic T cells, natural killer (NK) cells, antibody-dependent cellular cytotoxicity (ADCC), and cytokines released as a result of antigenic stimulation of lymphocytes and macrophages (Corey and Spear, 1986). Antibody may play a role by neutralization of virus and participation in ADCC. It seems most likely that host immune responses determine the extent to which reactivated HSV is able to multiply and cause disease, whereas the phenomena of virus latency and reactivation are probably regulated by multiple factors including expression of cell proteins in the neuron and suppression of HSV protein expression.

PATHOLOGY

The characteristic lesion caused by HSV on the skin is a vesicle and on the mucous membranes is an ulcer. The epidermis but not the dermis is usually involved so that scarring after healing is uncommon. Invaded epithelial cells are destroyed by the virus and the associated inflammatory response of the host, sparing an intact superficial cornified layer that covers the vesicle; in the ulcer this upper layer is not present. Cells invaded by HSV demonstrate the following characteristics: coalescence to form multinucleated giant cells, nuclear degeneration, ballooning, and intranuclear inclusions. Cells in deeper tissues characteristically exhibit hemorrhagic necrosis. A biopsy specimen of a herpetic vesicle showing eosinophilic intranuclear inclusions and giant cells is shown in Plate 45, *E*.

CLINICAL MANIFESTATIONS OF PRIMARY INFECTIONS

Primary infections are defined as those that occur in individuals with no preexisting antibody to HSV. The clinical manifestations of primary herpetic infections are determined by a variety of factors including (1) the portal of entry of the virus and (2) host factors such as age, immune competence, and integrity of the cutaneous barrier. The various clinical entities that may be encountered are listed in Figure 15-1. The most common recognized HSV infection in children is acute gingivostomatitis. The other diseases are relatively uncommon or rare. The incubation period for primary infection is approximately 6 days, with a range of 2 to 20 days. The host-parasite relationship for HSV is shown in Figure 15-1. Primary infection of a susceptible host is frequently inapparent for both HSV-1 and HSV-2 (Boucher et al., 1990; Breinig et al., 1990; Brock et al., 1990; Langenberg et al., 1989; Strand et al., 1986). Patients with asymptomatic HSV-2 infections of the genital tract are as likely to subsequently shed virus as are those with histories of symptomatic disease (Wald et al., 2000). Clinically apparent primary infections may be characterized by a vesicular eruption, fever, and other constitutional symptoms. Recurrent clinical infections usually are characterized by a localized vesicular eruption and absence of constitutional symptoms. The primary infection can be asymptomatic, and recurrent infections can be symptomatic. Alternatively, the primary infection may be symptomatic with asymptomatic recurrences, or there may be any other combination of symptomatic and asymptomatic infections (Corey and Spear, 1986; Langenberg et al., 1989; Strand et al., 1986). Because of this phenomenon, it is impossible to

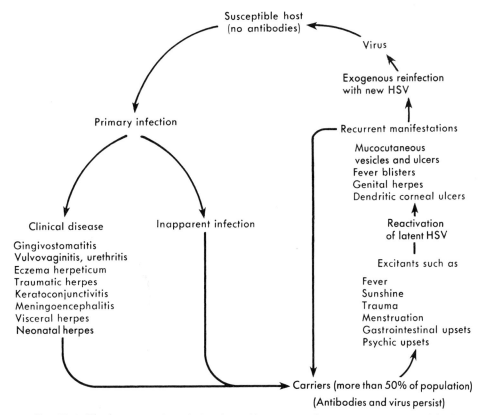

Fig. 15-1 The host-parasite relationship of herpes simplex virus in man. (Modified from Blank H, Rake G: Viral and rickettsial diseases of the skin, eye, and mucous membranes of man, Boston: Little, Brown, 1955.)

differentiate between primary and recurrent HSV infections on clinical grounds alone.

Acute Herpetic Gingivostomatitis

Acute herpetic gingivostomatitis almost always is caused by HSV-1. Most children have no symptoms during their primary infection with the virus; an estimated 5% develop clinically apparent gingivostomatitis. Primary infection of the mucous membranes of the mouth occurs most often in the 1- to 4-year age group and occasionally in adolescents and adults. The illness begins with the abrupt onset of fever (39.4° to 40.6° C; 103° to 105° F), irritability, anorexia, and sore mouth. Along with these constitutional symptoms, striking lesions appear on the oral mucous membranes and the oropharynx. The gums are swollen, reddened, and friable and bleed very easily (Plate 45, A and B). White 2- to 3-mm plaques or shallow ulcers with red areolae develop on the buccal mucosa, tongue, palate, and fauces. The lesions usually appear in the mouth first; occasionally, however, they may develop first on the tonsils and subsequently progress forward. The regional anterior cervical lymph nodes become enlarged and tender. Satellite vesicular lesions around the mouth are not uncommon. Infants with gingivostomatitis who are thumb suckers can also infect the thumb (or other fingers) by self-inoculation.

The disease varies considerably in severity and duration. It may be extremely mild, with a paucity of lesions, low-grade fever, and minimal constitutional symptoms. Under these circumstances, the patient improves within 5 to 7 days. On the other hand, an occasional infant is desperately ill with high fever, extensive hemorrhagic mouth lesions, evidence of dehydration and acidosis, and a course that does not abate until the tenth to fourteenth day.

Acute Herpetic Vulvovaginitis

Acute herpetic vulvovaginitis is usually a sexually transmitted infection. An exception is vulvovaginitis that is an unusual manifestation of HSV-1 infection in children secondary to auto-inoculation from gingivostomatitis (Krugman, 1952). In infants and children who develop isolated vulvovaginitis caused by HSV, the virus should be typed, since the possibility of child abuse must be considered if HSV-2 is isolated. Vulvovaginitis caused by HSV-2 is not uncommon in sexually active adolescents and adults.

The counterpart of this disease in sexually active males is penile ulcers and vesicles caused by HSV. The spectrum of disease is similar to that of herpetic gingivostomatitis, with a high percentage of asymptomatic infections (Corey and Spear, 1986; Brock et al., 1990; Johnson et al., 1989; Strand et al., 1986). According to data from the Centers for Disease Control and Prevention, 22% of those sampled between 1988 and 1994 were seropositive for HSV-2, but only 3% reported having genital herpes (Fleming et al., 1997). Symptomatic patients often complain of dysuria, and children may refuse to void. The perineal area is usually reddened, edematous, and studded with painful, shallow, white ulcers 2 to 4 mm in diameter. Many of these lesions coalesce to form larger ulcers (Plate 45, C). The regional inguinal lymph nodes are enlarged and tender. Fever and constitutional symptoms subside within 5 to 7 days, and nonmucosal lesions become crusted by the tenth to fourteenth day. Healing is complete without scarring by the end of the third week.

Eczema Herpeticum (Kaposi's Varicelliform Eruption)

Eczema herpeticum, a manifestation of herpetic infection of the skin, was first described by Kaposi in 1887. It is characterized by vesicular and crusting eruptions superimposed on atopic eczema or chronic dermatitis (Lynch et al., 1945). Primary infection usually is more severe than secondary infection. This disease starts abruptly with high fever (40° to 40.6° C; 104° to 105° F), irritability, and restlessness, followed by the appearance of crops of vesicles concentrated chiefly on the eczematous skin. In areas of broken skin there may be ulcers and weeping, with a hemorrhagic component. A smaller number of lesions may involve the normal skin. The lesions may appear in crops over a period of 7 to 9 days, then rupture and become crusted within a few days. Thus, as the disease progresses in some children, it may resemble varicella.

Like other herpetic infections, this disease varies considerably in severity from extremely mild to potentially rapidly fatal, especially if it is primary. Severe cases have been related to deficient cell-mediated immunity to HSV (Vestey et al., 1989). Extensive areas of weeping, oozing skin may be associated with severe fluid loss and with bacterial superinfection.

Traumatic Herpetic Infections

Traumatic herpetic infections of the skin are similar to eczema herpeticum except that they are localized rather than generalized. The site of an abrasion, burn, or break in the skin may be infected with HSV. The source of the virus may be a sympathetic parent or caretaker who tried to reassure the child by "kissing [the injury site] better." HSV also may be transmitted during athletic activities, such as wrestling, in which there are both skin trauma and close physical contact with others. Vesicular lesions that develop at the site of inoculation may be associated with fever, constitutional symptoms, and regional lymphadenopathy. Another form is due to trauma to a nerve that is latently infected with HSV, with resultant reactivation of the virus. These syndromes may be difficult to differentiate clinically.

Acute Herpetic Keratoconjunctivitis

Primary herpetic infections of the eye are relatively rare. Fever and constitutional symptoms are associated with keratoconjunctivitis and preauricular adenopathy. Usually the infection is unilateral. The cornea has a hazy appearance, and the patient may be unable to close the eyelid (Plate 45, *D*). A purulent and membranelike exudate is present. The skin around the eye may exhibit discrete vesicles. The eye usually clears completely in 2 weeks if the infection is confined chiefly to the conjunctiva. Superficial corneal involvement is characterized by the formation of typical dendritic ulcers. These infections may cause a serious impairment of sight. Deep infections such as keratitis disciformis, hypopyon keratitis, and iridocyclitis are almost always accompanied by significant scarring.

Acute Herpetic Encephalitis and Meningoencephalitis

Primary infection of the CNS is an unusual manifestation of HSV infection in children. Infection of the CNS with HSV-2 beyond the neonatal period (often in conjunction with genital HSV) in an otherwise healthy individual is almost always associated with a self-limited form of meningitis rather than encephalitis, although it may occasionally cause a serious illness (Boucquey et al., 1990). An estimated 15% of patients with primary genital HSV infection will have mild concomitant meningitis (Kohl, 1988).

In contrast, HSV-1 typically causes a rapidly progressive, fatal type of encephalitis, with death after 1 to 2 weeks in approximately 70% of patients who are untreated. There are few reports of cases of benign HSV-1 meningitis (Rathore et al., 1996). The clinical manifestations of 113 biopsy-proved cases of HSV encephalitis are listed in Table 15-1. The

TABLE 15-1   Historical Findings and Signs at Presentation of 113 Patients With Biopsy-proved Herpes Simplex Encephalitis

Characteristics	Number/total	Percent
Historical Findings		
Altered consciousness	109/112	97
Fever	101/112	90
Personality change	62/87	71
Headache	89/110	81
Vomiting	51/111	46
Recurrent herpes labialis	24/108	22
Memory loss	14/59	24
Signs and Presentation		
Dysphasia	58/76	76
Autonomic nervous system dysfunction	53/88	60
Ataxia	22/55	40
Seizures	43/112	38
Hemiparesis	41/107	38

Modified from Whitley RJ, et al: JAMA 1982b;247:318.

encephalitis frequently may be localized in the frontotemporal area, simulating a mass lesion, or it may be widespread, involving both cerebral hemispheres. The cerebrospinal fluid (CSF) usually shows pleocytosis with a predominance of lymphocytes. Computed tomography (CT) and magnetic resonance imaging (MRI) often can be used to localize the affected area of the brain (Kohl et al., 1988; Schroth et al., 1987).

Approximately one third of patients with herpes encephalitis experience a primary infection, but there is no known clinical difference between primary and secondary HSV infection in this instance (Whitley, 1994). The virus is believed to reach the brain either by the hematogenous route, from olfactory neurons of the respiratory mucosa, or from infected ganglia. Immunocompromised patients are not at increased risk to develop this form of HSV infection (Kohl et al., 1988).

Neonatal HSV Infections

HSV infections in premature and newborn infants are usually caused by HSV-2, most often the consequence of primary maternal genital HSV-2 infection during the last trimester of pregnancy. Characteristically, the mother's genital infection is asymptomatic, she delivers vaginally, and the infant is unwittingly exposed to the virus during delivery. Less commonly, the infant is infected by HSV-1 secondary to primary maternal gingivostomatitis at term (Amortegui et al., 1984) or exposure to someone else with HSV infection, such as a father or grandparent. The reported incidence of neonatal herpes is 1 in 2,500 to 5,000 live births (Whitley and Lakeman, 1995).

The presence of specific antibodies in an infant is likely to play at least some role in protection after exposure (Sullender et al., 1988). To a large extent, this may account for the observation in prospective studies that the rate of infection during primary maternal HSV-2 infection is approximately 50%, whereas during recurrent infection it is less than 8%. In this report none of the 34 infants born vaginally to women with recurrent HSV at delivery were later found infected; all had detectable neutralizing antibodies to HSV-2 (Prober et al., 1987). Similarly, high titers of ADCC antibodies at presentation in HSV-infected neonates have not been associated with disseminated infections. High titers of ADCC antibodies are seen in babies who have been exposed to HSV but have

not been infected or have had only localized infections (Kohl et al., 1989; Kohl, 1991).

Rarely, infants may be infected in utero with either HSV-1 or HSV-2 during an episode of maternal viremia that may or may not have been clinically apparent (Florman et al., 1973; Hutto et al., 1987). The spectrum of congenital disease varies from chronic to fulminant; some infants have died within days of birth, and others have survived with severe neurologic sequelae. Most have evidence of acute, chronic, or recurrent skin infections with HSV. Infants with zosteriform rashes present at birth may have had HSV infection (Music et al., 1971; Rabalais et al., 1990).

The clinical picture of full-blown neonatal herpes is well recognized. At the end of the first week of life the infant develops fever or hypothermia, progressively increasing icterus, hepatosplenomegaly, and vesicular skin lesions. Anorexia, vomiting, lethargy, respiratory distress, cyanosis, and circulatory collapse may follow. Untreated, the outcome is frequently fatal. The presence of skin vesicles is helpful in distinguishing neonatal herpes from other infections; however, skin lesions are absent in approximately 20% of affected babies. In infants without rash, neonatal HSV infection should be considered when there are signs and symptoms of bacterial meningitis but no bacterial cause can be identified (Arvin et al., 1982) and when there is an interstitial pneumonic process beginning at approximately 4 days of age. Infected infants are usually also febrile and thrombocytopenic and have evidence of liver involvement (Anderson, 1987; Hubbell et al., 1988). Fulminant hepatitis has also been described as the initial symptom of neonatal HSV (Benador et al., 1990). One study has reported HSV infection of the CNS in an infant who did not develop symptoms until he was 2 months old, when he developed a skin lesion caused by HSV-2 (Thomas et al., 1989).

Whitley et al. (1980) classified neonatal HSV into three presenting groups on the basis of their experience with 95 proved cases. These groups include (1) disseminated disease (hepatitis, pneumonia, or disseminated intravascular coagulation, with or without CNS involvement) in 51%; (2) isolated CNS involvement in 32%; and (3) disease localized to the eye, skin, or mouth in 17%. Untreated, the mortality rates were 85%, 50%, and 0%, respectively (Whitley et al., 1980)

HSV in Immunocompromised Hosts

In the immunocompromised host, HSV infections may show two unusual courses: (1) disseminated disease may occur with widespread dermal, mucosal, and visceral involvement; or (2) disease may remain localized but with a greatly prolonged course, persisting for periods as long as 9 months with indolent, often painful ulcerative lesions (Schneidman et al., 1979). These two forms of the infection appear more likely in patients whose T-lymphocyte function is depressed. In immunocompromised patients both primary and recurrent HSV infections may be severe.

Other Illnesses Associated With HSV

Other illnesses associated with HSV include infection of the fingers (herpetic whitlow) (Gill et al., 1988); pharyngitis (Corey et al., 1983); respiratory infection, including epiglottitis (Bogger-Goren, 1987; Schwenzfeier and Fechner, 1976); lymphadenitis with lymphangitis (Sands and Brown, 1988; Tamaru et al., 1990); parotitis (Arditi et al., 1988); and erythema multiforme (Arditi et al., 1988; Brown et al., 1987a), which may result from hypersensitivity of the host to HSV. All are either unusual or rare in children.

RECURRENT INFECTIONS

Recurrent herpetic infections are more common than clinically apparent primary infections. The most common type is herpes labialis, the well-known fever sore that is manifested by vesicular lesions at the corner of the mouth. Other recurrent lesions may appear on any part of the skin or mucous membranes. As indicated before, these are generally less severe than primary infections and not associated with constitutional symptoms. Two exceptions to this general rule are HSV encephalitis, which may be a primary or secondary infection, and severe HSV in the immunocompromised patient, which may be recurrent and yet severe (Corey and Spear, 1986).

DIAGNOSIS

Infection with HSV should be suspected in a patient who develops fever, constitutional symptoms, and a vesicular exanthem or enanthem. The diagnosis can be confirmed by (1) isolation of virus from local lesions, (2) demonstration of viral antigens or DNA in skin lesions or CSF, (3) serologic tests showing a significant rise in the level of antibodies during convalescence from a primary infection, and (4) histologic evidence of type A intranuclear inclusion bodies and multinucleated giant cells in infected tissue.

Isolation of Virus and Viral Antigen Tests

HSV can be cultivated in a variety of cell cultures; inoculation of these cultures produces cytopathic changes that are usually evident within 24 to 48 hours. Cultures with suspected infection can be stained with fluorescein-labeled monoclonal antibodies so that identification and simultaneous typing of HSV can be performed rapidly and the results made available to the clinician. Cultures are now available in many hospital laboratories, because HSV is rather easy to propagate and grows rapidly. Culture is superior to Papanicolaou and Tzanck smears, since the latter tests are nonspecific and may yield false-positive and false-negative reactions.

Smears from skin or mucous membrane lesions for direct staining with fluorescein-tagged monoclonal antibodies are very useful for rapid diagnosis. For preparing smears, vigorous swabbing of an open ulcer or ruptured vesicle should be performed to include epithelial cells that harbor the virus in the specimen. An ELISA that identifies HSV antigens in samples from lesions with sensitivity equal to that of culture may be used for rapid identification of HSV, although it will not distinguish between types 1 and 2 (Baker et al., 1989; Dascal et al., 1989).

Diagnosis is often difficult when HSV encephalitis or pneumonia is suspected. In the latter case, smears of tracheal or bronchial secretions may be submitted to the diagnostic laboratory, but positive results may reflect asymptomatic shedding of virus from the oral cavity and upper respiratory tract rather than true infection. When CNS infection is suspected, skin lesions may or may not be present; in any case they offer no specific diagnostic clues. To make a certain diagnosis of herpes encephalitis, a brain biopsy may be required. At present, performing a brain biopsy for diagnosis of HSV encephalitis is controversial. Proponents cite its diagnostic sensitivity and specificity, low rate of complications, and ability to limit the use of the antiviral acyclovir (ACV) to patients with proven disease (Hanley et al., 1987; Whitley et al, 1982b). Opponents cite the risk of complications of the procedure, delay in ACV therapy, potential for false-negative results, and lack of serious toxicity of ACV (Fishman, 1987; Wasiewski and Fishman, 1988). When a brain biopsy can be performed readily and safely, it may be worth the small risk of complications (approximately 2%), although polymerase chain reaction (PCR) detection of HSV DNA in CSF is supplanting brain biopsy for this indication (Guffond et al., 1994; Lakeman and Whitley, 1995; Rozenberg and Lebon, 1991; Troendle-Atkins et al., 1993). The reported incidence of false-negative results for biopsied brain specimens is approximately 4% (Kohl et al., 1988). CT scan and MRI can be used to localize the affected area of the brain, and an electroencephalogram (EEG) may provide nonspecific clues, such as periodic slow and sharp waves that suggest HSV encephalitis. The abnormalities of the CT scan in neonates with HSV probably will not be localized to the temporal or frontal lobes of the brain, as in herpes encephalitis in an older child, but more likely will be generalized. In patients with neonatal HSV of the CNS the CT scan is at times normal (Noorbehesht et al., 1987). Brain biopsy material can be cultured for virus or examined by immunohistochemistry for viral antigens or by electron microscopy. Demonstration of HSV by in situ hybridization in brain biopsy specimens has been reported (Bamborschke et al., 1990).

It is rare to isolate HSV from CSF of patients with either neonatal or postnatal HSV encephalitis, although it is more common to isolate the virus from the CSF of neonates. The presence of antibodies to HSV in CSF, if significantly greater in titer than the serum titer, is considered diagnostic of HSV encephalitis (Kahlon et al., 1987). These antibodies are not always detected early enough in the illness, however, to make this test useful in providing guidance about whether or not to institute antiviral therapy (Van Loon et al., 1989). An especially promising technique for diagnosis of HSV encephalitis is PCR (Lakeman and Whitley, 1995; Rowley et al., 1990). PCR assays amplify DNA that is detected with a molecular probe; this technique has been successful diagnostically in a number of patients early in the illness. It is specific, accurate, and rapidly performed, and has become widely used in the clinical setting.

The interest in diagnosing maternal HSV in pregnant women at term, especially in those with asymptomatic infections, has been great. It is now recognized, based on studies of over 6,000 pregnant women for whom cultures were performed before and at delivery, that performing maternal genital cultures for women who have a history of genital HSV is not only expensive but yields little useful information. Women who have had positive cultures during pregnancy are not likely to have positive cultures at delivery, and only a minority of infants at risk are identified if only women with a past history of genital herpes are evaluated (Arvin et al., 1986; Prober et al., 1988). PCR is a sensitive and specific procedure for identifying women with genital HSV at delivery (Hardy et al., 1990). However, PCR detects virus DNA rather than infectious virus particles, and studies have not yet addressed whether this is a useful procedure for predicting which infants will be infected with HSV. Careful physical exam at the onset of labor to detect genital lesions remains the best method in the clinical setting to identify women at risk of transmitting HSV to their infants.

Serologic Tests

Although neither as rapid nor as specific as demonstration of virus in lesions, testing paired samples of sera from the acute and convalescent phases of an illness for HSV antibodies may have diagnostic utility in limited settings. The levels of these antibodies begin to rise by the end of the first week of illness after a primary infection. Often, however, there is no rise in antibody titer with recurrent HSV infection, and these tests may yield false-positive results, since rising levels of antibodies to HSV may also be seen with VZV infections.

An ELISA method in which gG of HSV-1 and HSV-2 is used for the antigen is an important antibody test. With this assay, antibodies specific to either type of HSV can be measured; therefore it is possible to determine if an individual has been infected with either or both types of HSV (Corey and Spear, 1986; Johnson et al., 1989). This test is not yet available commercially.

Histologic Studies

The demonstration of acidophilic intranuclear inclusion bodies, multinucleated giant cells, and ballooning degeneration of the epithelial cells of a lesion from biopsy material reinforces the diagnosis of HSV. Immunofluorescence with specific antiserum or monoclonal antibodies is important to confirm a tissue diagnosis.

DIFFERENTIAL DIAGNOSIS
Acute Herpetic Gingivostomatitis

Acute herpetic gingivostomatitis can usually be recognized clinically without laboratory confirmation. The following diseases may be confused with it:

- *Herpangina.* The lesions of herpangina, caused by group A coxsackievirus, are clinically indistinguishable in appearance from those of HSV (Plate 45, *F*). However, the distribution of the lesions makes it possible to separate these two conditions. With herpangina, they usually are confined to the anterior fauces and soft palate, and gingivitis does not occur, whereas with herpetic infection, gingivitis is a typical manifestation.
- *Acute membranous tonsillitis.* Acute membranous tonsillitis secondary to streptococcal infection, EBV infection, diphtheria, and other infectious agents may simulate herpetic involvement of the tonsillar area. Invariably, herpetic lesions appear on the tongue, buccal mucosa, palate, and gingival tissues. Cultures and blood smears are the most helpful diagnostic laboratory procedures.
- *Thrush.* Thrush is generally not associated with fever and constitutional symptoms. Lesions are polymorphous elevated white plaques without ulceration.

Acute Herpetic Vulvovaginitis

Acute involvement of the skin of the perineal area may simulate herpetic vulvovaginitis. The following conditions are most commonly confused:

- *Ammoniacal dermatitis with secondary infection.* Fever and systemic symptoms are absent as a rule with this condition. The lesions extend onto the thighs and diaper area.
- *Gonorrheal and monilial vulvovaginitis.* Vesicular and ulcerative lesions are usually not present and the lesions can be identified by appropriate cultures.
- *Impetigo.* Lesions are usually present elsewhere, particularly on the nares and other sites readily scratched. Viral diagnostic procedures (see section on diagnosis) and bacterial cultures may provide helpful diagnostic information.

Eczema Herpeticum

Herpetic infection of eczematous skin lesions must be differentiated from the following conditions:

- *Eczema with secondary bacterial infection.* These lesions may resemble eczema herpeticum, but fever and constitutional symptoms are usually not present.
- *Varicella.* Varicella is not an unusually severe infection in children with eczema, and the rash does not become disseminated or confluent.
- *Eczema vaccinatum.* This disease may be almost impossible to distinguish clinically from eczema herpeticum, and the diagnosis requires the performance of laboratory procedures. Fortunately, however, eczema vaccinatum has become a disease of the past, since routine vaccination of children for smallpox is no longer performed.

Traumatic Herpes Infections

Traumatic herpetic infections may be confused with herpes zoster or with secondary bacterial infection of the site that has been traumatized. Performing methods of viral diagnosis of HSV may be necessary to make a certain diagnosis.

Acute Herpetic Keratoconjunctivitis

A variety of bacteria—including *Haemophilus* species, pneumococci, and staphylococci—and viruses such as picornaviruses, influenza viruses, rubeola, and adenoviruses may cause conjunctivitis. Adenovirus infection with enlargement of the preauricular lymph nodes may be an isolated phenomenon or may be accompanied by respiratory symptoms. Differentiation requires assessment of the history and accompanying symptoms and physical findings of the patient. Cultures and scrapings are often required to make the correct diagnosis.

Neonatal HSV

In infants with vesicular skin lesions HSV may be confused with varicella. Historical information concerning exposure to varicella or VZV is helpful. It may be necessary either to identify the viral antigen in the vesicular lesion or to perform a culture. In infants without skin lesions, neonatal HSV infection may be confused with bacterial sepsis, enteroviral infections, pneumonia, or meningitis. The average length of time until onset of pneumonia caused by group B beta-hemolytic streptococcus is 20 hours, whereas HSV pneumonia begins on average at 5 days (Hubbell et al., 1988). Appropriate empiric treatment and rapid diagnosis are important because early treatment improves the outcome. If skin lesions are not present, the diagnosis may be made by isolation of HSV from the mouth or conjunctiva or, more rarely, from the urine or CSF (Hammerberg et al., 1983). Occasionally it may be possible to isolate HSV from buffy coat cells if the infant has viremia (Golden, 1988). On rare occasions it is necessary to obtain a biopsy of the brain to diagnose infants with obvious CNS involvement and no skin lesions (Arvin et al., 1982; Koskiniemi et al., 1989). Infants with positive throat cultures only in the first 24 hours of life born vaginally to women with genital herpes have been reported (Prober et al., 1988). These infants appear to "carry" HSV briefly but are not actually infected.

HSV Encephalitis

Many other conditions mimic HSV encephalitis. These include vascular disease, brain abscess, other forms of viral encephalitis (enterovirus, mumps, EBV, measles, influenza, arbovirus), cryptococcal infection, tumor, toxic encephalopathy, Reye's syndrome, toxoplasmosis, tuberculosis, and lymphocytic choriomeningitis.

COMPLICATIONS

Bacterial complications rarely occur in a patient with acute gingivostomatitis. Dehydration and acidosis may result from the patient's refusal of fluids because of extensive and painful lesions in the mouth. Eczema herpeticum occasionally may become secondarily infected with bacteria, which may be a potential focus for the development of septicemia.

PROGNOSIS

The prognosis of patients with acute herpetic gingivostomatitis is excellent. Early therapy of eczema herpeticum is associated with a good prognosis. Extensive eczema herpeticum, neonatal HSV, and herpes simplex encephalitis are highly fatal if not treated with an antiviral drug. The prognosis of neonatal HSV and herpes encephalitis has improved since the development of antiviral drugs, particularly ACV.

As is true for many HSV infections, the prognosis for patients with neonatal herpes depends on the extent of the infection at the time antiviral therapy is begun. Early therapy improves the outcome, but progression of the disease (e.g., development of chorioretinitis) has been reported despite antiviral treatment. Poor prognosis has been associated with acute primary maternal disease at delivery, prematurity, visceral involvement, and EEG abnormalities (Koskiniemi et al., 1989). Collaborative studies (Whitley et al., 1991a; Whitley et al., 1991b) on 202 infants infected with HSV-1 or HSV-2 have revealed the following information. The death rate for patients who have been treated for disseminated HSV infection is approximately 60%, and for those treated for encephalitis it is approximately 15%. Approximately 60% of survivors of disseminated disease and 30% to 40% of those surviving encephalitis are developing normally at 1 year of age (Whitley and Hutto, 1985; Whitley et al., 1991a; Whitley et al., 1991b). The mortality after neonatal HSV infection limited to the skin, eye, or mouth is essentially nil, with approximately 10% having sequelae. Among infants with skin, eye, or mouth disease, those who experienced three or more recurrences of skin lesions during the first 6 months of life were at greater risk of neurologic impairment (Whitley et al., 1991a). The prognosis has been reported as better after HSV-1 than after HSV-2 neonatal encephalitis (Corey et al., 1988; Whitley et al., 1991a). For example, of 15 infants with HSV-2 encephalitis, only 23% were normal at 18 months of age, whereas of 9 who had encephalitis caused by HSV-1, all were normal at the same age. These infants had all been treated appropriately with vidarabine or ACV (Corey et al., 1988).

Treatment with ACV has also decreased the mortality and morbidity of herpes encephalitis beyond the neonatal period, and ACV therapy has proved to offer a better prognosis than vidarabine (Whitley et al., 1986). The mortality rate for 32 patients treated with ACV was approximately 30%, as compared with 54% in 37 who received vidarabine. Roughly 40% of ACV-treated patients were free of sequelae 6 months later, compared with only 14% of vidarabine-treated patients. The better the patient's condition is before initiation of therapy, particularly with regard to neurologic status, the better the outcome (Whitley and Hutto, 1985).

IMMUNITY

Many infants are born with HSV antibodies passively acquired from the mother. This passive immunity is somewhat protective, but it disappears by approximately 6 months of age. Active immunity in the form of long-lasting humoral and cellular immune responses develops after an apparent or inapparent primary infection with HSV. This immunity to HSV, however, is incomplete and does not necessarily protect against future exogenous herpetic infections or against recurrent endogenous herpetic infections, although the infection may be modified (Buchman et al., 1978). The virus may reactivate after latent infection, and reinfection may also occur. In addition, patients may have latent infection with more than one type of HSV (Whitley et al., 1982a). A prior infection with HSV-1 appears to attenuate the severity of subsequent infection with HSV-2 (Corey and Spear, 1986; Johnson et al., 1989).

Host factors important in defense have been analyzed best in infants. Although the presence of neutralizing antibodies in infants does not necessarily prevent disseminated infection, they may attenuate the illness considerably (Arvin et al., 1986; Sullender et al., 1987; Yeager et al., 1980). The functions of NK cells and T lymphocytes—including production of cytokines such as interleukin-2 and interferon—are all immature in infants, which appears to predispose infants to serious infection with HSV (Kohl, 1988; Kohl, 1989; Kohl et al., 1989; Sullender et al., 1987). In all probability, in the healthy child and adult, antibodies and cellular immunity act in concert in host defense against HSV.

EPIDEMIOLOGIC FACTORS

Herpetic infections are worldwide in distribution. In former times, HSV-1 was an infection of young children and most were infected before 6 years of age. In recent decades much of the population of industrialized societies escapes primary HSV-1 infection in the first decade of life; in these groups young adults are more likely to experience primary HSV-1 gingivostomatitis. For HSV-2 infections, as with other sexually transmitted diseases, the highest rate of infection is during the second and third decades.

Transmission of HSV is by intimate contact and can occur during periods of asymptomatic shedding as well as when recognized lesions are present. Infectious virus may be recovered from saliva, skin and mucosal lesions, and urine, all of which are potential sources. Although patients with recurrent lesions are infectious to others for a shorter period of time than those with primary infections, recurrent lesions and asymptomatic shedding are responsible for most episodes of transmission.

In an extensive study of the natural history of herpetic infection in 4,191 Yugoslavian children, the incidence of clinically apparent infection, primary herpetic gingivostomatitis, was 12%. The peak incidence according to age was in the second year of life, and there was no seasonal variation. Adults with herpetic lesions were the chief source of infection. Nine minor epidemics were observed. The incubation period was 2 to 12 days, with a mean of 6 days (Juretic, 1966). New genital HSV infections are more frequently symptomatic; in a prospective study of over 2,000 HSV-2 seronegative adults, the rate of HSV-2 infection was 5.1 cases per 100 person-years. Over 30% of newly acquired infections were symptomatic. Roughly half of new infections in women were symptomatic, whereas only about a quarter of new infections in men were symptomatic (Langenberg et al., 1989).

There has been a disturbing increase in HSV-2 infections in the United States during the last decades. A seroepidemiologic study of HSV-2 infection in 4,201 participants, in which a type-specific (gG) antibody assay was used between 1976 and 1980, revealed that 16.4% of the sampled U.S. population between 15 and 74 years of age had detectable antibodies to HSV-2. The prevalence of antibodies increased from less than 1% positive in children less than 15 years old to 20.2% in young adults. The highest prevalence of positive titers in elderly individuals was 19.7% in whites and 64.7% in blacks (Johnson et al., 1989). There was a 30% relative increase in HSV-2 seropositivity in the period between 1988 and 1994. During the latter study period, 22% of the sampled population over the age of 12 years had antibody to HSV-2 (Fleming et al., 1997). Increases in prevalence occurred in all age groups. As in the earlier study, the highest prevalence rates were in elderly individuals; 23% of whites over 70 years and 74% of blacks over 70 years were seropositive.

Neonatal HSV is usually acquired from a maternal genital source. Maternally transmitted

HSV infections in the perinatal period apparently are increasing in incidence (Sullivan-Bolyai et al., 1983b). Intrauterine infection has been reported but seems rare (Florman et al., 1973; Hutto et al., 1987; Stone et al., 1989). Delivery of an infant by cesarean section usually prevents neonatal infection if the fetal membranes remain intact or have been ruptured for less than 4 hours before delivery. Therefore, cesarean section is indicated for women with genital lesions present at the onset of labor. If genital lesions are present in a woman in preterm labor or with premature rupture of membranes, standard obstetric management should be followed. Cesarean section to prevent HSV transmission is not indicated for women without active genital lesions during labor. Most infants who develop neonatal HSV are born vaginally to mothers with no history or knowledge of genital HSV infection. Although an infant may be infected with HSV after exposure to a woman with recurrent HSV (Growdon et al., 1987), the high-risk situation for transmission is not in women with a history of recurrent genital HSV but in those with no history of this disease. Transmission to an infant is far greater after maternal primary infection than after maternal recurrent genital HSV.

The effects on the fetus of a first episode of genital herpes during pregnancy have been analyzed prospectively in a report of 29 women infected in various trimesters and their offspring (Brown et al., 1987b). This study confirmed the serious nature of primary, in contrast to secondary, infection during pregnancy. Of the 15 offspring in the first group, 3 were infected, and none of the 14 offspring of women with nonprimary disease were infected. The timing of maternal HSV infection relative to delivery of the infant also affects the risk of neonatal infection. Seroconversion occurred during gestation in 1.3% of 7,046 pregnant women at risk for developing HSV infection who were followed prospectively (Brown et al., 1997). In this group, none of the infants of mothers who seroconverted before delivery developed neonatal infection. Nine women in this study developed genital HSV infection near the time of delivery but did not have antibody to the genital HSV strain at delivery; four infants born to these mothers developed neonatal HSV infection.

Infants may on occasion be inadvertently infected through scalp monitors during delivery (Parvey and Ch'ien, 1980), during breastfeeding (Sullivan-Bolyai et al., 1983a), in intensive-care nurseries (Hammerberg et al., 1983), and from family members besides the mother (Yeager et al., 1983). The availability of molecular biologic techniques for viral "fingerprinting," using restriction endonucleases to evaluate the DNA of HSV isolates, has been invaluable in proving many of these transmissions.

TREATMENT

The treatment of mucocutaneous HSV beyond the neonatal period is chiefly supportive. Infants and small children with gingivostomatitis require careful observation for possible dehydration. Fluids should be given intravenously if necessary. Citrus fruit juices and other irritating liquids should be avoided. Cold drinks such as apple, pear, and peach juices often seem well tolerated. Treatment with intravenous ACV (10 mg/kg every 8 hours; Table 15-2) may be considered for children with extensive oral lesions who require IV fluids. ACV is relatively nontoxic; the main associated adverse effects include rash, gastrointestinal discomfort, and mild azotemia, which can be avoided by maintenance of good hydration. ACV is both an inhibitor of and a faulty substrate for viral DNA polymerase; because ACV requires phosphorylation by a viral enzyme to exert its antiviral effects, it is relatively nontoxic to uninfected cells that lack the enzyme. Approximately 20% of the oral formulation is absorbed by the gastrointestinal tract. ACV is marketed in topical, oral, and intravenous formulations. Topical ACV has very little use; it shortens the course of primary genital HSV from an average of 14 to 11 days.

Oral ACV for uncomplicated gingivostomatitis in children has not been extensively studied. Pharmacokinetic data support an oral dose of 24 mg/kg four times a day for children between the ages of 1 month and 2 years for the treatment of HSV (Tod et al., 2001). In a randomized double-blind placebo-controlled trial of 72 children between 1 and 6 years of age, children who were treated with ACV 15 mg/kg five times a day had lesions and difficulty eating and drinking for fewer days than those who received placebo (Amir et al., 1997). Treatment was initiated within 72 hours of onset of symptoms in this study. In a study of 174 nonimmunocompromised adults with oral herpes,

TABLE 15-2	Antiviral Dosing for Treatment of HSV Infections		
Drug	Pediatric dose	Adult dose	Comments
Acyclovir (ACV)	Oral dose: 20 mg/kg/dose q6-8 h	Oral dose: 400 mg q8h	Severe or potentially severe infections* are treated with IV dose which must be adjusted dose
200 mg/5 ml suspension	IV dose: 10-20 mg/kg/dose q8h	IV dose: 5-10 mg/kg/dose q8h	
200-mg capsule 800-mg tablet			
Famciclovir 500-mg tablet	None	250 mg PO q8h	
Valacyclovir	None	1000 mg PO q12hrs	
500-mg tablet 1-g tablet			
Foscarnet	40 mg/kg/dose IV q8h	40 mg/kg/dose IV q8h	For acyclovir-resistant HSV

*Potentially severe infections include but are not limited to neonatal HSV infections, HSV encephalitis, and first episode HSV infections in immunocompromised patients.

many of whom probably had secondary HSV, a dosage of 400 mg 5 times a day by mouth for 5 days hastened healing if therapy was begun in the very early stages of the illness (Spruance et al., 1990).

Genital HSV infections are treated with ACV, famciclovir, or valacyclovir. Oral ACV (200 mg 5 times a day for an adult; Table 15-2) is effective treatment, but the less frequent dosing schedules of famciclovir and valacyclovir make them desirable options in many situations. Valacyclovir and famciclovir are both prodrugs with good oral bioavailability. Valacyclovir is an ester of ACV; the recommended dosage for treatment of genital HSV infection is 1,000 mg orally twice a day for 5 days (Table 15-2). Famciclovir is metabolized to its active form, penciclovir. The dosage of famciclovir for the treatment of first episodes of genital HSV infection is 250 mg orally every 8 hours for 5 days and for recurrent episodes is 125 mg twice a day for 5 days (Table 15-2). Neither of these drugs is approved for use in children, and there are no pediatric suspensions available. They may be useful for the treatment of HSV infections in adolescents. Frequently recurring genital HSV can be suppressed by long-term oral administration of ACV (400 to 800 mg per day [two to four 200-mg capsules in divided doses]) (Gold and Corey, 1987; Guinan, 1986; Merz et al., 1988; Straus et al., 1989).

Children with herpetic keratoconjunctivitis should be treated with topical trifluridine; topical ophthalmic ACV ointment is not a licensed product in the United States. Children with conjunctivitis and mucosal or cutaneous lesions should also be treated with oral ACV. The care of children with this disease should be supervised by an ophthalmologist. However, some infants with neonatal HSV present with conjunctivitis; special consideration should be taken with infants less than 1 month old. They should receive intravenous ACV and topical ophthalmic ointment (Liesengang, 1988) and should be evaluated for systemic HSV infection. Recurrent ocular HSV infections should be prevented with long-term administration of oral ACV. In a randomized placebo-controlled trial, ACV 400 mg twice daily for 12 months suppressed recurrent infections (Table 15-3) (Herpetic Eye Disease Study Group, 1998).

Serious HSV infections such as encephalitis and neonatal HSV should be treated with intravenous ACV (10 to 20 mg/kg every 8 hours; Table 15-2) for 2 to 3 weeks. Immunocompromised children with severe mucocutaneous involvement should be given ACV 10 mg/kg every 8 hours, usually for 5 to 7 days. Children with profound immunosuppression may require a longer duration of therapy. Lower dosages should be used for children with renal compromise (Balfour and Englund, 1989).

TABLE 15-3	Doses of Antiviral Agents for Suppression of Recurrent HSV Infections[*]	
Drug	Pediatric dose	Adult dose
Acyclovir	Oral: 10-20 mg/kg/dose q8h	Oral: 200 mg q8h or 400 mg q12h
	IV: 5-10 mg/kg/dose q8h	IV: 5 mg/kg/dose q8h
Famciclovir	None	125-250 mg PO q12h
Valacyclovir	None	500 mg—1 g every day

[*]Doses may need to be adjusted upward if breakthrough lesions occur. Suppression therapy for patients with frequent recurrences should be discontinued annually to reassess the need for suppressive therapy. Suppression therapy in immunocompromised patients at high risk for recurrences should be continued until the high-risk period is over.

For both neonatal HSV and HSV encephalitis it is often necessary to begin therapy before a proved diagnosis, because the earlier treatment is begun, the better the outcome (Sullivan-Bolyai et al., 1986; Whitley and Hutto, 1985; Whitley et al., 1986). Treatment with ACV for 1 to 2 days before a diagnostic culture is obtained usually does not interfere with a positive result (Balfour and Englund, 1989). All babies under 1 month of age who have HSV infection must be treated intravenously, even if their symptoms are mild, because the incidence of progression to CNS or disseminated disease is more than 50% in babies in whom infection is localized to the skin, mouth, or eye.

Close follow-up of patients after treatment of neonatal HSV and HSV encephalitis is also critical, because relapses in both diseases have been reported (Brown et al., 1987a; Gutman et al., 1986; Kohl, 1988). In most instances of relapse, retreatment with ACV for several weeks is believed helpful, but it is not known whether additional therapy with orally administered ACV on a long-term basis adds any additional benefit. Relapse of HSV encephalitis caused by hypersensitivity to HSV, a form of postinfectious encephalitis, has been reported (Koenig et al., 1979). Relapse has also been reported after treatment for only 10 days (VanLandingham et al., 1988).

Resistance of HSV to ACV is a problem in some settings (Hirsch and Schooley, 1989). HSV may become resistant in three ways. Most commonly, it may cease producing thymidine kinase, the enzyme that phosphorylates ACV into an active antiviral compound. It may also produce either an altered form of thymidine kinase or an altered form of DNA polymerase (Balfour, 1989). Strains of HSV resistant to ACV have been found in immunocompromised patients (Englund et al., 1990) and, less com-

monly, in immunocompetent patients (Kost et al., 1993). These strains have limited ability to spread to others because they are also less invasive than ACV-sensitive strains of HSV. Resistance to ACV may arise rapidly in immunocompromised patients, and, although the ability to detect these strains remains a research tool, clinically useful methods to detect them are being developed (Englund et al., 1990). Currently the therapy of choice for serious HSV infections that do not respond to ACV is foscarnet (Safrin et al., 1991). Foscarnet inhibits HSV replication by acting directly on the virus DNA polymerase and does not require phosphorylation by the virus thymidine kinase. The dose of foscarnet for the treatment of HSV infections is 40 mg/kg/dose administered intravenously every 8 hours (Table 15-2). Adverse effects associated with the administration of foscarnet include renal toxicity, electrolyte disturbances, and CNS toxicity. HSV strains with altered DNA polymerase may be resistant to foscarnet, ACV, or both drugs. In some cases, therapy with both foscarnet and ACV may be successful (Straus et al., 1994).

PREVENTIVE MEASURES

Most herpetic infections are difficult to prevent. Children with eczema should avoid contact with others with HSV infections if possible. Infants whose mothers have active genital HSV during labor should be delivered by cesarean section, particularly if the membranes are intact or have been ruptured for less than 4 hours. Newborn infants should not have contact with persons with active herpes lesions.

Suppressive antiviral therapy should be considered for patients who experience frequent HSV recurrences or recurrences in sites that can be associated with significant morbidity such as ophthalmologic HSV infections. Suppressive therapy is also administered to immunocompromised patients at risk for severe HSV recurrences (Table 15-3).

The advantages of a successful herpes simplex vaccine are apparent; attempts to develop one are in progress, including efforts with subunit vaccines and with a live attenuated vaccine (Straus et al., 1994; Whitley, 2001). Recombinant gD and combination gD and gB vaccines are well tolerated and immunogenic in people without prior HSV-2 infection (Adria et al., 1995; Straus et al., 1993). Trials assessing the efficacy of both gB and gD vaccines have been disappointing, however, including recent trials of a combined subunit vaccine (Corey et al., 1999).

The effectiveness of administration of ACV to pregnant women who develop primary HSV to prevent infection of the infant is unknown. Data collected by the Acyclovir in Pregnancy Registry indicates that administration of ACV during pregnancy is safe (Centers for Disease Control and Prevention, 1993). ACV has been shown to decrease virus shedding (Wald et al., 1997) and have a desirable impact on the need for cesarean section (Braig et al., 2001; Scott et al., 1996). Studies have not shown whether maternal ACV prevents neonatal infection. It is also not known if administration of ACV to an infant delivered vaginally to a woman with active genital HSV is effective in preventing neonatal HSV. Therefore neither of these possible preventive strategies is recommended at this time. Clinicians caring for pregnant women who develop first episode genital HSV during the third trimester may wish to consider ACV therapy to suppress virus shedding at the time of delivery.

BIBLIOGRAPHY

Adria G, Langenberg M, Burke R, et al. A recombinant glycoprotein vaccine for herpes simplex type 2: safety and efficacy. Ann Intern Med 1995;122:889-898.

Amir J, Harel L, Smetana Z, Varsano I. Treatment of herpes simplex gingivostomatitis with acyclovir in children: a randomized double blind placebo controlled study. BMJ 1997;314:1800.

Amortegui A, Macpherson T, Harger J. A cluster of neonatal herpes simplex infections without mucocutaneous manifestations. Pediatrics 1984;73:194-198.

Anderson RD. Herpes simplex virus infection of the neonatal respiratory tract. Am J Dis Child 1987;141:274-276.

Arditi M, Shulman S, Langman C, et al. Probable herpes simplex type 1-related acute parotitis, nephritis, and erythema multiforme. Pediatr Infect Dis J 1988;7:427-428.

Arvin A, Hensleigh P, Prober C, et al. Failure of antepartum maternal cultures to predict the infant's risk of exposure to herpes simplex virus at delivery. N Engl J Med 1986;315:796-800.

Arvin A, Yeager A, Bruhn F, Grossman M. Neonatal herpes simplex infection in the absence of mucocutaneous lesions. J Pediatr 1982;100:715-721.

Baker D, Gonik B, Milch P, et al. Clinical evaluation of a new virus ELISA: a rapid diagnostic test for herpes simplex virus. Obstet Gynecol 1989;73:322-325.

Balfour H, Englund J. Antiviral drugs in pediatrics. Am J Dis Child 1989;143:1307-1316.

Bamborschke S, Porr A, Huber M, Heiss W. Demonstration of herpes simplex virus DNA in CSF cells by in situ hybridization for early diagnosis of herpes encephalitis. J Neurol 1990;237:73-76.

Baringer JR. Recovery of herpes simplex virus from human sacral ganglions. N Engl J Med 1974;291:828.

Baringer JR, Swoveland R. Recovery of herpes simplex virus from human trigeminal ganglions. N Engl J Med 1973;288:648-650.

Benador N, Mannhardt W, Schranz D, et al. Three cases of neonatal herpes simplex virus infection presenting as fulminant hepatitis. Eur J Pediatr 1990;149:555-559.

Bloom DC, Hill JM, Devi-Rao G, et al. A 348-pair region in the latency-associated transcript facilitates herpes simplex virus type 1 reactivation. J Virol 1996;70:2449-2459.

Bogger-Goren S. Acute epiglottitis caused by herpes simplex virus. Pediatr Infect Dis J 1987;6:1133-1134.

Boucher FD, Yasukawa LL, Bronzan RN, et al. A prospective evaluation of primary genital herpes simplex virus type 2 infections acquired during pregnancy. Pediatr Infect Dis J 1990;9:499-504.

Boucquey D, Chalon M-P, Sindic C, et al. Herpes simplex virus type 2 meningitis without genital lesions: an immunoblot study. J Neurol 1990;237:285-289.

Braig S, Luton D, Sibony O, et al. Acyclovir prophylaxis in late pregnancy prevents recurrent genital herpes and viral shedding. Eur J Obstet Gynecol 2001;96:55-58.

Breinig MK, Kingsley LA, Armstrong JA, et al. Epidemiology of genital herpes in Pittsburgh: serologic, sexual, and racial correlates of apparent and inapparent herpes simplex infections. J Infect Dis 1990;162:299-305.

Brock BV, Selke MA, Benedetti J, et al. Frequency of asymptomatic shedding of herpes simplex virus in women with genital herpes. JAMA 1990;263:418-420.

Brown Z, Ashley R, Douglas J, et al. Neonatal herpes simplex virus infection: relapse after initial therapy and transmission from a mother with an asymptomatic genital herpes infection and erythema multiforme. Pediatr Infect Dis J 1987a;6:1057-1061.

Brown Z, Vontver L, Benedetti J, et al. Effects on infants of a first episode of genital herpes during pregnancy. N Engl J Med 1987b;317:1246-1251.

Brown ZA, Selke S, Zeh J, et al. The acquisition of herpes simplex virus during pregnancy. N Engl J Med 1997;337:509-515.

Buchman TG, Roizman B, Adams G, Stover BH. Restriction endonuclease fingerprinting of herpes simplex virus DNA: a novel epidemiologic tool applied to a nosocomial outbreak. J Infect Dis 1978;138:488-498.

Buchman TG, Roizman B, Nahmias AJ. Demonstration of exogenous genital reinfection with herpes simplex virus type 2 by restriction endonuclease fingerprinting of viral DNA. J Infect Dis 1979;140:295-304.

Centers for Disease Control and Prevention. Pregnancy outcomes following systemic prenatal acyclovir exposure. MMWR Morb Mortal Wkly Rep 1993;42:806-809.

Corey L. The diagnosis and treatment of genital herpes. JAMA 1982;248:1041-1049.

Corey L, Adams HG, Brown ZA, Holmes KK. Genital herpes simplex infections: clinical manifestations, course, and complications. Ann Intern Med 1983;54:262-265.

Corey L, Langenberg AG, Ashley R, et al. Recombinant glycoprotein vaccine for the prevention of genital HSV-2 infection: two randomized controlled studies. JAMA 1999;282:331-340.

Corey L, Spear P. Infections with herpes simplex viruses. N Engl J Med 1986;314:686-691,749-757.

Corey L, Stone E, Whitley R, K M. Difference between herpes simplex virus type 1 and type 2 neonatal encephalitis in neurological outcome. Lancet 1988;1:1-4.

Croen KD, Ostrove JM, Dragovic LJ, et al. Latent herpes simplex virus in human trigeminal ganglia. N Engl J Med 1987;317:1427-1432.

Dascal A, Chan-Thim J, Morahan M, et al. Diagnosis of herpes simplex virus infection in a clinical setting by a direct antigen detection enzyme immunoassay. J Clin Microbiol 1989;27:700-704.

Englund J, Zimmerman M, Swierkosz E, et al. Herpes simplex virus resistant to acyclovir: a study in a tertiary care center. Ann Intern Med 1990;12:416-422.

Farrell MJ, Dobson AT, Feldman L. Herpes simplex virus latency-associated transcript is a stable intron. Proc Natl Acad Sci USA 1991;88:790-794.

Fishman R. No, brain biopsy need not be done in every patient suspected of having herpes simplex encephalitis. Arch Neurol 1987;44:1291-1292.

Fleming DT, McQuillan GM, Johnson RE, et al. Herpes simplex virus type 2 in the United States, 1976 to 1994. N Engl J Med 1997;37:1105-1111.

Florman AL, Gershon AA, Blackett PR, Nahmias AJ. Intrauterine infection with herpes simplex virus: resultant congenital malformations. JAMA 1973;225:129-132.

Garber DA, Schaffer PA, Knipe DM. A LAT-associated function reduces productive-cycle gene expression during acute infection of murine sensory neurons with herpes simplex virus type 1. J Virol 1997;71:5885-5893.

Gill M, Arlett J, Buchan K. Herpes simplex virus infection of the hand. Am J Med 1988;84:89-93.

Gold D, Corey L. Acyclovir prophylaxis for herpes simplex infection. Antimicrob Agents Chemother 1987;31:361-367.

Golden S. Neonatal herpes simplex viremia. Pediatr Infect Dis J 1988;7:425-426.

Growdon WA, Apodaca L, Cragun J, et al. Neonatal herpes simplex virus infection occurring in second twin of an asymptomatic mother. JAMA 1987;257:508-511.

Guffond T, Dewilde A, Lobert P, et al. Significance and clinical relevance of the detection of herpes simplex virus DNA by the polymerase chain reaction in cerebrospinal fluid from patients with presumed encephalitis. Clin Infect Dis 1994;18:744-749.

Guinan M. Oral acyclovir for treatment and suppression of genital herpes simplex virus infection. JAMA 1986;255:1747-1749.

Gutman L, Wilfert C, Eppes S. Herpes simplex virus encephalitis in children: analysis of cerebrospinal fluid and progressive neurodevelopmental deterioration. J Infect Dis 1986;154:415-421.

Hammerberg O, Watts J, Chernesky M, et al. An outbreak of herpes simplex virus type 1 in an intensive care nursery. Pediatr Infect Dis J 1983;2:290-294.

Hanley D, Johnson R, Whitley R. Yes, brain biopsy should be a prerequisite for herpes simplex encephalitis treatment. Arch Neurol 1987;44:1289-1290.

Hardy D, Arvin A, Yasukawa L, et al. Use of polymerase chain reaction for successful identification of asymptomatic genital infection with herpes simplex virus in pregnant women at delivery. J Infect Dis 1990;162:1031-1035.

Herpetic Eye Disease Study Group. Acyclovir for the prevention of recurrent herpes simplex virus eye disease. N Engl J Med 1998;339:300-306.

Hirsch MS, Schooley RT. Resistance to antiviral drugs: the end of innocence. N Engl J Med 1989;320:313-314.

Hubbell C, Dominguez R, Kohl S. Neonatal herpes simplex pneumonitis. Rev Infect Dis 1988;10:431-438.

Hutto C, Arvin AM, Jacobs R, et al. Intrauterine herpes simplex infections. Ann Intern Med 1987;110:97-101.

Johnson RE, Nahmias AJ, Magder LS, et al. A seroepidemiologic survey of the prevalence of herpes simplex virus type 2 infection in the United States. N Engl J Med 1989;321:7-12.

Juretic M. Natural history of herpetic infection. Helv Pediatr Acta 1966;21:356.

Kahlon J, Chatterjee S, Lakeman F, et al. Detection of antibody to herpes simplex virus in the cerebrospinal fluid of patients with herpes simplex encephalitis. J Infect Dis 1987;155:38-44.

Koenig H, Rabinowitz SG, Day E, Miller V. Post-infectious encephalomyelitis after successful treatment of herpes simplex encephalitis with adenine arabinoside. N Engl J Med 1979;300:1089-1093.

Kohl S. Herpes simplex virus encephalitis in children. Pediatr Clin North Am 1988;35:465-483.

Kohl S. The neonatal human's immune response to herpes simplex virus infection: a critical review. Pediatr Infect Dis J 1989;8:67-74.

Kohl S. Role of antibody-dependent cellular cytotoxicity in defense against herpes simplex virus infections. J Infect Dis 1991;13:108-114.

Kohl S, West MS, Loo LS. Defects in interleukin-2 stimulation of neonatal natural killer cytotoxicity to herpes simplex virus–infected cells. J Pediatr 1988;112:976-981.

Kohl S, West MS, Prober CG, et al. Neonatal antibody–dependent cellular cytotoxicity antibody levels are associated with the clinical presentation of neonatal herpes simplex virus infection. J Infect Dis 1989;160:770-776.

Koskiniemi M, Happonen MM, Jarvenpaa AL, et al. Neonatal herpes simplex virus infection: a report of 43 patients. Pediatr Infect Dis J 1989;8:30-35.

Kost RG, Hill EL, Tigges M, et al. Recurrent acyclovir-resistant genital herpes in an immunocompetent patient. N Engl J Med 1993;329:1777-1782.

Krause PR, Stanberry N, Bourne B, et al. Expression of the herpes simplex virus type 2 latency-associated transcript enhances spontaneous reactivation of genital herpes in latently infected guinea pigs. J Exp Med 1995;181:297-306.

Krugman S. Primary herpetic vulvovaginitis: report of a case; isolation and identification of herpes simplex virus. Pediatrics 1952;9:585.

Lakeman FD, Whitley RJ. Diagnosis of herpes simplex encephalitis: application of polymerase chain reaction to cerebrospinal fluid from brain-biopsied patients and correlation with disease. J Infect Dis 1995;171:857-863.

Langenberg A, Benedetti J, Jenkins J, et al. Development of clinically recognizable genital lesions among women previously identified as having "asymptomatic" herpes simplex virus type 2 infection. Ann Intern Med 1989;110: 882-887.

Leib DA, Bogard CL, Kosz-Vnenchak M, et al. A deletion mutant of the latency-associated transcript of herpes simplex virus type 1 reactivates from the latent state with reduced frequency. J Virol 1989;63:2893-2900.

Liesegang TJ. Ocular herpes simplex infection: pathogenesis and current therapy. Mayo Clin Proc 1988;63:1092-1105.

Lynch FW, Evans CA, Bolin VS, Steves RJ. Kaposi's varicelliform eruption: extensive herpes simplex as a complication of eczema. Arch Dermatol Syph 1945;51:129.

Merz GJ, Jones CC, Mills J, et al. Long-term acyclovir suppression of frequently recurring genital herpes simplex virus infection. JAMA 1988;260:201-206.

Music SI, Fine EM, Togo Y. Zoster-like disease in the newborn caused by herpes simplex virus. N Engl J Med 1971;284:24-26.

Nahmias A, Dowdle W. Antigenic and biologic differences in herpesvirus hominis. Prog Med Virol 1968;10:110.

Noorbehesht B, Enzmann DR, Sullender W, et al. Neonatal herpes simplex encephalitis: correlation of clinical and CT findings. Radiology 1987;162:813-819.

Parvey LS, Ch'ien LT. Neonatal herpes simplex virus infection introduced by fetal-monitor scalp electrodes. Pediatrics 1980;65:1150-1153.

Perng GC, Dunkel EC, Geary PA, et al. The latency-associated transcript gene of herpes simplex virus type 1 (HSV-1) is required for efficient in vivo spontaneous reactivation of HSV-1 from latency. J Virol 1994;68: 8045-8055.

Prober CG, Sullender WM, Yasukawa LL, et al. Low risk of herpes simplex virus infections in neonates exposed to the virus at the time of vaginal delivery to mothers with recurrent genital herpes simplex virus infections. N Engl J Med 1987;316:240-244.

Prober G, Hensleigh PA, Boucher FD, et al. Use of routine viral cultures at delivery to identify neonates exposed to herpes simplex virus. N Engl J Med 1988;318:887-891.

Rabalais GP, Yusk JW, Wilkerson SA. Zosteriform denuded skin caused by intrauterine herpes simplex virus infection. Pediatr Infect Dis J 1990;10:79-81.

Rathore MH, Mercurio K, Halstead D. Herpes simplex type 1 meningitis. Pediatr Infect Dis J 1996;15:824-828.

Roizman B, Knipe DM. Herpes simplex viruses and their replication. In: Knipe DM, Howley PM (eds). Fields Virology, vol 2. Philadelphia: Lippincott Williams and Wilkins, 2001.

Rowley AH, Whitley RJ, Lakeman FD, Wolinsky SM. Rapid detection of herpes-simplex-virus DNA in cerebrospinal fluid of patients with herpes simplex encephalitis. Lancet 1990;1:440-441.

Rozenberg F, Lebon P. Amplification and characterization of herpesvirus DNA in cerebrospinal fluid from patients with acute encephalitis. J Clin Micro 1991;29:2412-2417.

Safrin S, Crumpacker C, Chatic P, et al. A controlled trial comparing foscarnet with vidarabine for acyclovir-resistant mucocutaneous herpes simplex in the acquired immunodeficiency syndrome. N Engl J Med 1991;325:551-555.

Safrin S, Kemmerly S, Plotkin B, et al. Foscarnet-resistant herpes simplex virus infections in patients with AIDS. J Infect Dis 1994;169:193-196.

Sands M, Brown R. Herpes simplex lymphangitis. Arch Intern Med 1988;148:2066-2067.

Schneidman DW, Barr RJ, Graham JH. Chronic cutaneous herpes simplex. JAMA 1979;241:592.

Schroth G, Gawehn J, Thron A, et al. Early diagnosis of herpes simplex encephalitis by MRI. Neurology 1987;37: 179-183.

Schwenzfeier CW, Fechner RE. Herpes simplex of the epiglottis. Arch Otolaryngol 1976;102:374-375.

Scott LL, Sanchez PJ, Jackson GL, et al. Acyclovir suppression to prevent cesarean delivery after first-episode genital herpes. Obstet Gynecol 1996;87:69-73.

Spruance SL, Stewart JCB, Rowe N, et al. Treatment of recurrent herpes simplex labialis with oral acyclovir. J Infect Dis 1990;161:185-190.

Steiner I, Spivack JG, Lirette R, et al. Herpes simplex virus type 1 latency-associated transcripts are evidently not essential for latent infection. EMBO J 1989;8:505-511.

Stevens JG, Haarr L, Porter DD, et al. Prominence of the herpes simplex virus latency-associated transcript in trigeminal ganglia from seropositive humans. J Infect Dis 1988;158:117-123.

Stone KM, Brooks CA, Guinan ME, Alexander ER. National surveillance for neonatal herpes simplex virus infections. Sex Transm Dis 1989;16:152-156.

Strand A, Vahlne A, Svennerholm B, et al. Asymptomatic virus shedding in men with genital herpes infection. Scand J Infect Dis 1986;18:195-197.

Straus S, Corey L, Burke RL, et al. Placebo-controlled trial of vaccination with recombinant glycoprotein D of herpes simplex virus type 2 for immunotherapy of genital herpes. Lancet 1994;343:1460-1463.

Straus S, Seidlin M, Takiff H, et al. Effect of oral acyclovir treatment on symptomatic and asymptomatic virus shedding in recurrent genital herpes. Sex Transm Dis 1989;16:107-113.

Straus SE, Savarese B, Tigges M, et al. Induction and enhancement of immune responses to herpes simplex virus type 2 in humans by use of a recombinant glycoprotein D vaccine. J Infect Dis 1993;167:1042-1052.

Sullender WM, Miller JL, Yasukawa LL, et al. Humoral and cell-mediated immunity in neonates with herpes simplex virus infection. J Infect Dis 1987;155:28-37.

Sullender WM, Yasukawa LL, Schwartz M, et al. Type-specific antibodies to herpes simplex virus type 2 (HSV-2) glycoprotein G in pregnant women, infants exposed to maternal HSV-2 infection at delivery, and infants with neonatal herpes. J Infect Dis 1988;157:165-171.

Sullivan-Bolyai J, Fife KH, Jacobs RF, et al. Disseminated neonatal herpes simplex type 1 from a maternal breast lesion. Pediatrics 1983a;71:455-457.

Sullivan-Bolyai J, Hull HF, Wilson C, et al. Herpes simplex virus infection in King County, Washington. JAMA 1983b;250:3059-3062.

Sullivan-Bolyai JZ, Hull HF, Wilson C, et al. Presentation of neonatal herpes simplex virus infections: implications for a change in therapeutic strategy. Pediatr Infect Dis J 1986;5:309-331.

Tamaru J, Mikata A, Horie H, et al. Herpes simplex lymphadenitis. Am J Surg Pathol 1990;14:571-577.

Thomas EE, Scheifele DW, MacLean BS, Ashley R. Herpes simplex type 2 aseptic meningitis in a two-month-old infant. Pediatr Infect Dis J 1989;8:184-186.

Thompson RL, Sawtell NM. The herpes simplex virus type 1 latency-associated transcript gene regulates the establishment of latency. J Virol 1997;71:5432-5440.

Thompson RL, Sawtell NM. HSV latency-associated transcript and neuronal apoptosis. Science 2000;289:1651.

Thompson RL, Sawtell NM. Herpes simplex virus type 1 latency-associated transcript gene promotes neuronal survival. J Virol 2001;75:6660-6675.

Tod M, Lokiec F, Bidault R, et al. Pharmacokinetics of oral acyclovir in neonates and in infants: a population analysis. Antimicrob Agents Chemother 2001;45:150-157.

Troendle-Atkins J, Demmler GJ, Buffone GJ. Rapid diagnosis of herpes simplex virus encephalitis by using the polymerase chain reaction. J Pediatr 1993;123:376-380.

VanLandingham KE, Marsteller HB, Ross GW, Hayden FG. Relapse of herpes simplex encephalitis after conventional acyclovir therapy. JAMA 1988;259:1051-1053.

Van Loon AM, Van der Logt JTM, Heessen FWA, et al. Diagnosis of herpes simplex virus encephalitis by detection of virus-specific immunoglobulins A and G in serum and cerebrospinal fluid by using an antibody-capture enzyme-linked immunosorbent assay. J Clin Microbiol 1989;27:1983-1987.

Vestey JP, Howie SEM, Norval M, et al. Severe eczema herpeticum is associated with prolonged depression of cell-mediated immunity to herpes simplex virus. Curr Probl Dermatol 1989;18:158-161.

Wald A, Corey L, Cone R, et al. Frequent genital herpes simplex virus 2 shedding in immunocompetent women. J Clin Invest 1997;99:1092-1097.

Wald A, Zeh J, Selke S, et al. Reactivation of genital herpes simplex virus type 2 infection in asymptomatic seropositive persons. N Engl J Med 2000;342:844-850.

Wasiewski WW, Fishman MA. Herpes simplex encephalitis: the brain biopsy controversy. J Pediatr 1988;113:575-578.

Whitley R, Arvin A, Prober C, et al. A controlled trial comparing vidarabine with acyclovir in neonatal herpes simplex virus infection. N Engl J Med 1991a;324:444-454.

Whitley R, Arvin A, Prober C, et al. Predictors of morbidity and mortality in neonates with herpes simplex virus infections. N Engl J Med 1991b;324:450-454.

Whitley RJ. Herpes simplex virus infections of women and their offspring: implications for a developed society. Proc Nat Acad Sci USA 1994;91:2441-2447.

Whitley RJ. Herpes simplex viruses. In: Knipe DM, Howley PM (eds). Fields Virology, vol. 2. Philadelphia: Lippincott Williams and Wilkins, 2001.

Whitley RJ, Alford CA, Hirsch MS, et al. Vidarabine versus acyclovir therapy in herpes simplex encephalitis. N Engl J Med 1986;314:144-146.

Whitley RJ, Hutto C. Neonatal herpes simplex virus infections. Pediatr Rev 1985;7:119-126.

Whitley RJ, Lakeman FD. Herpes simplex virus infection of the central nervous system: therapeutic and diagnostic considerations. Clin Infect Dis 1995;20:414-420.

Whitley RJ, Lakeman FD, Nahmias AJ, Roizman B. DNA restriction-enzyme analysis of herpes simplex virus isolates obtained from patients with encephalitis. N Engl J Med 1982a;307:1060-1062.

Whitley RJ, Nahmias AJ, Visintine AM, et al. The natural history of herpes simplex virus infection of mother and child. Pediatrics 1980;66:489-494.

Whitley RJ, Soong S, Linneman CJ, et al. Herpes simplex encephalitis. JAMA 1982b;247:317-320.

Yeager A, Arvin AM, Urbani LJ, Kemp JA. Relationship of antibody to outcome in neonatal herpes simplex virus infections. Infect Immun 1980;29:532-538.

Yeager A, Ashley R, Corey L. Transmission of herpes simplex virus from father to neonate. J Pediatr 1983;103:905-907.

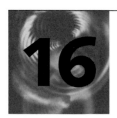

16 HUMAN HERPESVIRUS 6, 7, AND 8

CAROLINE BREESE HALL

*Unmasked within its cellular cache
    a microbe minuscule unknown;
Creator of the rose-like rash
    described by sages ages past.*

*Molecular techniques unfold
    its programmed, dark genomic soul,
Revealing its recondite hold
    on newly born to those now old.*

                                    CBH

HUMAN HERPESVIRUS 6

The sixth exanthematous disease of childhood, long of unknown ancestry, has now been recognized to be one of the manifestations of the sixth member of the human herpesvirus family, human herpesvirus 6 (HHV-6). With this has come the recognition that this virus, which causes roseola, like other members of its family has multiple personalities and potential import for individuals of all ages.

History

The first description of roseola may have been in Meigs and Pepper's *A Practical Treatise of the Diseases of Children* (Meigs and Pepper, 1870), wherein it is referred to as *roseola aestiva* or *roseola autumnalis*. In this textbook the exanthematous disease was described as "chilliness alternating with heat, with loss of strength and spirits, headache, restlessness, sometimes mild delirium and slight convulsive phenomena," and the rash of roses as "irregularly circular with rather large patches, at first of red, but soon changing to a deep rose color."

In 1910 Zahorsky described the first clear cases of roseola, and in 1941 Breese conducted the first prospective study of roseola cases. The epidemiologic and clinical description of these roseola cases from Breese's practice closely mimics those subsequently described for HHV-6. A decade later Kempe et al. (1950) described the

transmission of the agent of roseola via blood from one infant to another and to monkeys via both blood and nasal secretions. Although a viral etiology was suspected, the attempts at identification and isolation by Breese and subsequently by Kempe were unsuccessful.

HHV-6 was initially discovered by Salahuddin et al. in 1986 in adult patients with lymphoreticular diseases and human immunodeficiency virus (HIV) infection. Two years later Yamanishi et al. (1988) isolated the same virus from the blood of four infants with roseola infantum. Although this novel virus was found initially in the B-lymphocytes of adult immunocompromised patients, it was subsequently noted to have primary affinity for T lymphocytes, and its original appellation, human B lymphotrophic virus (HBLV), was changed to HHV-6.

Characterization

HHV-6 is a member of the Roseolovirus genus of the betaherpesvirus subfamily. Like other herpesviruses, HHV-6 possesses the characteristic electron-dense core and an icosahedral capsid, surrounded by a tegument and outer envelope, the location of the important glycoproteins and membrane proteins. The capsid of HHV-6, with a diameter of 90 to 110 nm, is assembled initially in the nucleus, where the tegument is acquired. Fully tegumented capsids of a diameter of 165 nm are subsequently released into the cytoplasm; the capsids then become enveloped by budding into cytoplasmic vesicles. The extruded virions have a diameter of about 200 nm. The replication of HHV-6 in peripheral blood mononuclear cells is slow and lytic and characterized by the formation of syncytia.

The double-stranded DNA genome of HHV-6 is approximately 160 base pairs (bp) in length, with a unique long (UL) segment of about

144,000 bp bracketed on each end by direct repeat elements of variable length (Pellett and Dominguez, 2001). The genome codes approximately 100 proteins; for most the function has been judged mainly on the homology with other closely related herpesviruses. Of note is that some of the coded proteins are homologous to potentially important immune mediators. Open reading frames U12 and U51 encode seven transmembrane receptor proteins homologous to chemokine receptors in humans, and U83 encodes a functional chemokine homolog. The tegument protein p100, a product of U11, is a major focus of the immune response to HHV-6. These proteins are likely to be important in the pathogenesis of HHV-6 by their mimicking the immune responses of the host, which may allow HHV-6 to escape elimination, resulting in the characteristic persistence of the virus.

A major component of the cellular receptor for HHV-6 is CD46, which is present on the surface of all nucleated cells, allowing HHV-6 to infect a wide range of cells. The mature CD4+ T cell is the prime target of HHV-6, but the virus may infect natural killer (NK) cells, gamma-delta T lymphocytes, monocytes, dendritic cells, astrocytes, and a variety of cell lines of T and B cells, megakaryocytes, and epithelial tissue, among others.

HHV-6 is composed of two closely related variants, HHV-6A and HHV-6B (Pellett and Dominguez, 2001). The genomic identity between strains from the two variants is generally high, about 95% in protein or nucleotides sequences in conserved genes. The ends of the genome, near the repetitive elements, tend to have greater divergence. The two variants, however, are distinct in terms of their cellular tropism, molecular and biologic characteristics, epidemiology, and clinical associations. Roseola and other primary infections with HHV-6 appear to be almost exclusively from variant B. The occurrence and circumstances of primary infection from variant A alone have yet to be determined. HHV-6A and HHV-6B are most closely related to human herpesvirus 7 (HHV-7) but share some amino acid similarities with human cytomegalovirus (CMV). HHV-6 has some serologic cross-reactivity with HHV-7, but not with other herpesviruses (Black and Pellett, 1999).

Epidemiology

Recent serologic studies of HHV-6 have highlighted the ubiquitous occurrence of HHV-6 infection in every country in which it has been studied. Acquisition of infection is usually in the first year or two of life, and in adults ≥95% possess antibody. In the United States, Japan, and other countries, HHV-6 infection is acquired during infancy, primarily at 6 to 18 months of age, with the mean age about 9 months (Figure 16-1). Infection occurs with amazing alacrity within a few months and correlates with the decline of maternal antibody (Figure 16-1). Prospective studies of over 5,000 children in Rochester, New York, have indicated that at birth essentially all infants possess passive maternal antibody, which declines over the next several months, reaching a nadir by 4 months, with a subsequent rapid increase in the proportion of seropositive infants to 18 months of age (Hall et al., 1994). Almost all children acquire infection by 3 years of age and remain seropositive throughout life. Although seroepidemiologic studies have shown some variation in HHV-6 seropositivity in different geographic areas, most show that HHV-6 infection is a ubiquitous infection acquired early in life, resulting in high seroprevalence rates in adults. In the United States and a number of other industrialized nations, almost all (depending on the assay employed) adults are seropositive (Braun et al., 1997).

The major modes of transmission of HHV-6 are incompletely defined. HHV-6 persists after primary infection in the blood, respiratory secretions, urine, and other anatomic sites. Presumably, the source of the rapid and complete acquisition of infection by the infant, therefore, is the asymptomatic shedding of HHV-6 in secretions of the care-givers and close contacts of the infant. Other modes of transmission also may be possible, including perinatal transmission. This possibility has been suggested by the detection of the HHV-6 genome in the cord blood and peripheral blood mononuclear cells of asymptomatic neonates (Hall et al., 1994). HHV-6 DNA has been detected in the cervical secretions of pregnant women, but its presence has not been confirmed in breast milk (Leach et al., 1994; Okuno et al., 1995).

The impact of HHV-6 infection, not suspected by the long-held clinical conceptions of roseola, is indicated by the proportion of acute emergency room visits for young children that HHV-6 engenders because of high fevers, toxicity, and seizures (Hall et al., 1994).

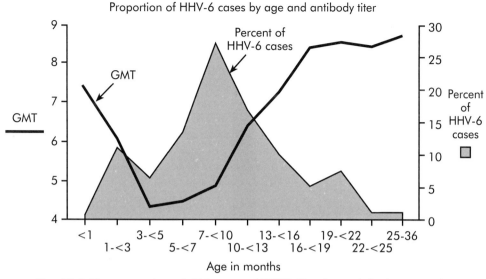

Fig. 16-1 The proportion of 335 cases of HHV-6B primary infection occurring according to age in months and in relation to their mean titer *(GMT)* ($\log_2$) of IgG antibody to HHV-6. The 335 cases of primary HHV-6 infection were identified by isolation of HHV-6 from the blood and by seroconversion from a prospective study of children less than 3 years of age with febrile illnesses who were brought to outpatient facilities at the University of Rochester Medical Center, Rochester, N.Y. (Some cases reported in Hall CB, et al: N Engl J Med 1994;331:432-438.)

Approximately 20% of the infants 6 to 12 months of age and 10% of the children in the first 2 years of life who were evaluated in Rochester, New York for acute infection were identified as having primary HHV-6 infection. The cost of evaluating these children places an appreciable burden on the healthcare system.

Immunity

The relative protection of infants against primary infection until maternal antibody declines indicates that serum antibody does provide protection, although it is not complete. Primary infection is characterized by viremia, which results in the production of neutralizing antibody and cessation of the viremia. Specific IgM antibodies are the first to appear, about 5 days from the onset of clinical symptoms. Within the subsequent 1 to 2 months, IgM antibodies decline and usually are no longer detectable. Specific IgG antibodies rise during the second and third weeks, with a subsequent increase in their avidity. HHV-6 IgG antibody generally persists for life, but at lower levels than during early childhood. Specific IgA antibodies have been identified in a few adult patients. Antibody levels may fluctuate subsequent to primary infection, possibly as a result of reacti-

vation of latent virus, and significant increases in antibody levels have been noted with the occurrence of other infections, especially closely related DNA viruses, such as HHV-7 and CMV (Pellett et al., 1992; Tanaka-Taya et al., 2000). Specific IgM antibodies may also be present in reactivated disease and are present in a small proportion of normal individuals (Suga et al., 1992). Normal children during the years after their primary infection may again exhibit fourfold rises in IgG antibody to HHV-6 (Hall et al., 1994). Although some of these significant antibody rises occurred during an acute infection with another agent, many remain unexplained, and most do not appear to be the result of reactivated latent HHV-6. Reinfection with HHV-6 of a different variant or strain is possible. Two different HHV-6B infections have been documented by genomic analysis in one infant (Dewhurst et al., 1992).

Cellular immunity appears important in the control of primary HHV-6 infection and subsequently in the maintenance of latency. The appearance of reactivated HHV-6 infection in patients who are immunosuppressed, which may be associated with clinical findings and sometimes with dissemination, is clinical evidence of the importance of cellular immunity.

In vitro studies have shown a proliferative response of peripheral blood mononuclear cells of healthy adults to HHV-6 (Wang et al., 1999). The acute stage of primary infection is associated with increased NK cellular activity, possibly via interleukin-15 (IL-15, and the induction of interferon (IFN)-α. In vitro replication is diminished with exogenous IFN-α. HHV-6 also induces IL-1β and tumor necrosis factor–α, suggesting that HHV-6 may modulate the immune response during primary infection and reactivation by the stimulation of host cell production of cytokines (Pellett et al., 2001).

Subsequent to primary infection, HHV-6 infection generally persists in a state of latency or chronic infection with the production of infectious virus. The components of the immune response important in controlling persistent infections are unclear. Reactivation of latent virus occurs in immunosuppressed patients but may occur even in normal individuals throughout life under conditions mostly unknown. HHV-6 DNA is frequently detected after primary infection in peripheral blood mononuclear cells and secretions of normal individuals, but the prime site of latent HHV-6 infection has not been well delineated. Experimental evidence suggests that HHV-6 may latently infect monocytes and macrophages of a variety of tissues, as well as early bone marrow progenitors from which reactivation may subsequently occur (Luppi et al., 1999).

Clinical Manifestations

Primary HHV-6 infections. Contact cases or the source for primary HHV-6 infection that occurs in an infant is almost always unknown, but the incubation period may be estimated from Kempe's studies (Kempe et al., 1950) to be approximately 10 days. Roseola is the most distinctive manifestation of primary HHV-6 infection and appears to be the major presentation of initial infection in Japan. In large studies of U.S. children evaluated in outpatient clinics and emergency facilities the classical manifestations of roseola are present only in about 15% to 20% of primary cases. Clinical manifestations are varied (Hall et al., 1994; Kusuhara et al., 1992). Most striking and characteristic is the abrupt onset of high fever, which tends to persist for 3 to 6 days. The peak fever over the first several days usually reaches 39° to 40° C, and approximately half of the patients have fevers above 40° C. The viremia

correlates with the febrile period and generally with the magnitude of the viral titer (Asano et al., 1991). The fever may be accompanied only by nonspecific signs and symptoms, including lethargy, anorexia, and toxicity, although many children appear relatively well considering the height of the fever. Such children are often diagnosed as having "nonspecific" or "viral" febrile illnesses, frequently with otitis. The latter diagnosis appears to be based mostly on the erythematous condition of the tympanic membranes, which commonly occurs in these young children. On follow-up, however, most of these children do not have the typical signs of otitis media and sequelae, such as middle-ear effusions. Although the initial presentation of children with primary HHV-6 infection engenders the diagnosis of a febrile illness of unknown etiology, approximately 20% to 25% have the primary diagnosis of gastroenteritis or respiratory illness (Table 16-1).

The physical findings accompanying primary HHV-6 infection may also be varied. Lymphadenopathy commonly is present in the

TABLE 16-1 Clinical Manifestations of Primary HHV-6 Infection in 335 Children <25 Months of Age[*]

Sign or symptom	Proportion of HHV-6 patients with sign or symptom (percentage)
Fever	100
Fever >39° C	88
Irritability	76
Lethargy	77
Lymphadenopathy (cervical, occipital)	74
Toxic appearance	68
Palpebral erythema	62
Inflamed tympanic membranes	55
Upper respiratory tract signs	41
Gastrointestinal signs (vomiting, diarrhea)	38
Rash	
During fever	11
At defervescence	21
Seizures	13

[*]From prospective study of children presenting to outpatient facilities at the University of Rochester, New York, with primary HHV-6 infection identified by isolation of HHV-6 from blood and seroconversion.

cervical region, particularly in the posterior occipital area, and becomes most prominent on the third or fourth day of the illness. The pharynx may be mildly injected, and sometimes an enanthema of small red maculopapular spots on the soft plate and uvula (Nagayama's spots) may be present. The palpebral conjunctivae also may be mildly inflamed and slightly edematous. As mentioned earlier, the tympanic membranes are frequently inflamed, in part because of the fever and mild catarrhal otitis.

Roseola (Exanthem Subitum). All of the aforementioned findings may be present in children with roseola. The typical course of roseola is similar to that just outlined, with the abrupt onset of high fever; nonspecific signs, especially irritability; cervical and posterior occipital lymphadenopathy; and the appearance of a rash with defervescence. Occasionally the rash appears before the fever has subsided completely and sometimes not until after the child has been afebrile for a day. The rash may be varied in appearance and is not distinctive for roseola. It may be evanescent, lasting only a few hours or remaining for 1 to 3 days. Characteristically the lesions are rose colored, as noted by Meigs and Pepper (1870); macular or maculopapular; and approximately 2 to 3 mm in diameter. The lesions fade on pressure, rarely coalesce, may be rubelliform or morbilliform, and are not pruritic. The rash usually is first noted on the trunk, with subsequent spread to the neck, upper extremities, face, and lower extremities. However, it may be more limited in distribution, occurring primarily on the trunk, neck, and face. The exanthem clears completely, leaving no pigmentation or desquamation.

Neonatal infection. Despite the general conception and observations for roseola, HHV-6 infection may occur in very young infants, including neonates. In Rochester approximately 15% of the primary HHV-6 infections studied were in infants in the first 8 weeks of life. The clinical manifestations of symptomatic primary HHV-6 infection in these young infants generally are similar to those of older infants, but may be milder. A febrile illness with no localizing signs is the most frequent presentation, but the fever tends to be lower than that of older infants.

Asymptomatic infection occurs, as indicated by the detection of HHV-6 DNA in the peripheral blood mononuclear cells at birth or in the subsequent neonatal period and may be more frequent in neonates than clinically manifest infection (Hall et al., 1994). The import of this remains unclear. In some, but not all of these infants, the HHV-6 DNA persists in the peripheral blood cells for variable periods, and subsequent development of clinical primary HHV-6 infection is possible. This may suggest that perinatal transmission of HHV-6 in some cases may be associated with less durable immunity.

Laboratory findings. The most distinctive laboratory finding to accompany primary HHV-6 infection is the course of the peripheral white blood cell (WBC) count. On initial presentation the total WBC count is diminished for age, usually about 8,000 cells/mm^3 (Fig. 16-2) (Hall et al., 1994). Subsequently, the total WBC count falls, reaching its nadir on days 3 and 4, and then rises toward normal, thus correlating with the febrile course. The peripheral lymphocyte count is most diminished, but the proportion of neutrophils also falls below the norm for age. Most other laboratory findings remain within normal limits. Sometimes the erythrocyte sedimentation rate or C reactive protein level may be elevated, but in most children these values remain within the normal range.

Diagnosis

Differential diagnosis. The clinical diagnosis of primary HHV-6 infection is difficult because of its varied manifestations, which may mimic many other infections. The abrupt onset of high fever and toxicity often suggests the diagnosis of sepsis or meningitis in the initial evaluation. Other viral infections, such as enteroviral and influenza infections, may have similar manifestations. The distinctive features of HHV-6 infection are the abrupt and initially persistent high fever, commonly 40° C or more, in an infant with the characteristic demographics, primarily age (between 6 and 18 months), without known contact. HHV-6 is also not seasonal, as are such viruses as enteroviruses and influenza. The subsequent characteristic pattern of development of lymphadenopathy, particularly posterior occipital nodes, and the pattern of the WBC count are not likely to be helpful initially. Roseola often may be diagnosed retrospectively once the typical course has been observed, and the rash has appeared at defervescence. Other viral diseases, such as echovirus 16 infection, may produce similar rubelliform or morbilliform rashes,

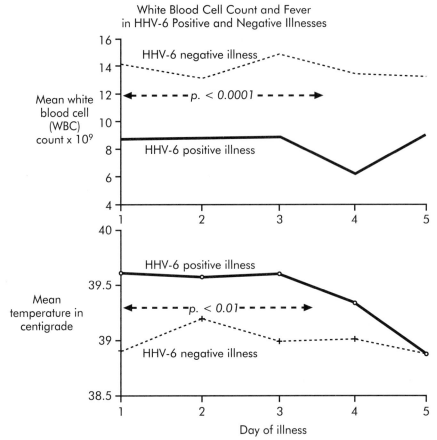

Fig. 16-2 Mean peripheral white blood cell count (WBC) (×10⁹) and temperature in 2,005 children under 3 years of age presenting with acute febrile illness to outpatient facilities at University of Rochester Medical Center. Compared are 285 children with primary HHV-6 illness and 1,720 children with illness resulting from other causes according to day of illness. (Unpublished data, plus data modified from Hall CB: Contemporary pediatrics 1996;13:45-47, and Hall CB: In Long SS, Prober CG, Pickering LK [eds]. Principles and practice of pediatric infectious diseases, 1997;1176-1181.)

occasionally on defervescence. Recently HHV-7 has been identified as causing some cases of roseola and other febrile illnesses, which may be indistinguishable clinically. HHV-7, however, tends to occur slightly later in life (Caserta et al., 1998; Tanaka et al., 1994).

Laboratory diagnosis. The laboratory diagnosis of primary HHV-6 infection currently remains problematic, requiring difficult or laboratory research techniques. The difficulty of diagnosis is further compounded by the persistent or latent nature of HHV-6. HHV-6 DNA may be detected in peripheral blood lymphocytes or in other sites by hybridization and polymerase chain reaction (PCR) assay or by Southern blot hybridization, which is generally

less sensitive than PCR. However, the detection of HHV-6 DNA in these sites does not necessarily indicate primary infection; most frequently it is persistent virus from previous infection and is not accompanied by concurrent viremia. Detection of HHV-6 DNA in plasma and determination of a high virus load offer higher sensitivity for detecting primary infection (≥90%), but these characteristics may also be present in patients with reactivation of HHV-6 (Chiu et al., 1998). A reverse-transcriptase PCR assay has recently been developed that reliably differentiates between latent and actively replicating HHV-6 (Norton et al., 1999; van den Bosch, 2001). These assays, however, are generally available only in research laboratories.

A number of serologic assays have been developed, including the immunofluorescence assay (IFA), anticomplement IFA, enzyme immunoassay (EIA), neutralization assays, immunoblot, and immunoprecipitation (Braun et al., 1997). The IFA and EIA are most frequently used and generally correlate with neutralization titers. Serologic diagnosis, however, has a number of drawbacks. First, it is rarely helpful in the time frame of clinical management when a convalescent serum is required. Specific IgM assays have been used as an indication of acute or reactivated infection, but not all children undergoing primary infection produce IgM antibodies, and approximately 5% of normal adults have detectable IgM antibodies to HHV-6 (Suga et al., 1992). Additionally, because essentially all adults possess antibody to HHV-6, the presence of specific antibody in a single sample is not meaningful. Furthermore, rises in titer may not indicate either new infection or reactivation. Cross-reacting antibodies with other DNA viruses, especially HHV-7, further confound the diagnosis (Black et al., 1996). Currently available serologic assays also are not able to differentiate between variant A and B infections. In normal children the diagnosis of primary HHV-6 infection therefore requires the detection of viremia (i.e., isolation of HHV-6 from the peripheral blood mononuclear cells) and a significant serologic rise. HHV-6 viremia occurs rarely in normal children other than with primary infection. Isolation of HHV-6, however, requires cocultivation with stimulated cord blood cells and subsequent identification techniques that are feasible only in research laboratories.

Complications

The major complications of primary HHV-6 infection involve the central nervous system (CNS). Roseola has long been observed to have occasional CNS manifestations such as seizures, bulging of the anterior fontanelle, meningoencephalitis or encephalitis, and hemiplegia, as noted in past case reports (Kimberlin, 1999). In most instances such CNS findings resolve, but long-term sequelae occasionally have been reported (Kimberlin, 1999). The most frequent complication of acute infection, however, is febrile seizures (Barone et al., 1995; Hall et al., 1994; Kimberlin, 1999; Suga et al., 2000). In a prospective study of over 200 children with primary HHV-6 infection, seizures occurred in 13%, with the highest rate in children 12 to 15 months of age, in whom 36% developed seizures, compared with only 13% of matched children with acute febrile illnesses not caused by HHV-6 (Hall et al., 1994). The seizures associated with primary HHV-6 infection are characteristic of febrile seizures in terms of age, occurring primarily after 6 months of age, but also have differentiating characteristics. Approximately half of the febrile seizures occurred after the first day of fever and tended to be prolonged or recurrent. Nevertheless, a subsequent study suggested that febrile seizures associated with HHV-6 infection have no worse, and possibly even better, prognosis than those not caused by HHV-6 infections (Jee et al., 1998).

HHV-6 DNA has been detected in the cerebrospinal fluid (CSF) of children with acute primary HHV-6 infection with or without CNS complications and subsequently in normal children with past HHV-6 infection. The significance of this is unclear, but some studies suggest that the presence of HHV-6 DNA in the CSF is associated with acute and long-term CNS sequelae (Caserta et al., 1994; Kimberlin, 1999; Kondo et al., 1993; Suga et al., 1993; Suga et al., 2000). One recent study has suggested that the febrile seizures associated with HHV-6 infection may be engendered by direct invasion of the CNS by HHV-6 rather than only by fever (Suga et al., 2000). Other studies have indicated that if HHV-6 DNA in the CSF is associated with neurologic symptoms, those neurologic findings tend to be variable and not diagnostic for HHV-6 infection, suggesting they could be related to other concurrent conditions (Studahl et al., 2000). HHV-6 DNA also may be frequently detected in brains of individuals dying of multiple causes (Luppi et al., 1994; Luppi et al., 1995). Whether HHV-6 invades the brain during primary infection with subsequent persistence and development of sequelae is unknown. In some cases of encephalitis in both children and adults, HHV-6 DNA in the CSF has been detected, but whether the encephalitic manifestations are a direct result of HHV-6 infection is unproved (Jones et al., 1994; McCullers et al., 1995; Yoshikawa et al., 1992).

HHV-6's frequent persistence in multiple sites, including peripheral white blood cells, brain, lymph nodes, secretions, and skin, portend the possibility of reactivation and complications subsequently. In normal children, little information currently exists about this possibility. In immunocompromised patients, however, reactivation with the detection and isolation of HHV-6 from multiple sites is frequent, and the role that HHV-6 plays in the course of illness in such patients is a subject of much recent interest and potential importance (Dockrell and Paya, 2001; Emery, 2001; Griffiths et al., 2000; Mendez et al., 2001). Bone marrow and solid organ transplant recipients have been examined in multiple studies for the occurrence of HHV-6 infection. These studies have shown that reactivation after transplant occurs frequently and tends to be early, in the first few weeks after transplantation. Most reactivations are asymptomatic or are associated with mild rash and fever. However, bone marrow suppression, delayed engraftment, and graft-versus-host disease have been also associated with the reactivation of HHV-6. Pneumonitis has also been reported to occur, but it is often difficult to associate clearly with HHV-6 infection, as other opportunistic infections concurrently present may produce similar findings. HHV-6 reactivation and disease in these immunocompromised patients have been correlated with the degree of immunosuppression, OKT3 use, and solid organ transplantation. The risk of HHV-6 reactivation appears to increase when infection with other related herpesviruses, especially CMV, is concurrently present. Indeed, the detection of reactivation from HHV-6, as well as HHV-7, has been shown to correlate with the viral load and severity of CMV infection. The association or interaction between HHV-6 and HIV infection may also be important. In vitro evidence suggests HHV-6 may be a cofactor in HIV infection, as it results in increased replication. Clinical studies have documented in HIV patients that HHV-6 may become viremic and correlates with a greater HIV load. However, progression of HIV disease has not been clearly shown.

HHV-6 has been linked with a number of other diverse diseases, mostly through case reports. HHV-6 has been suggested as a cause of chronic fatigue syndrome, but the evidence is controversial and the association tenuous. Other associated diseases include some forms of multiple sclerosis, multiple organ failure syndrome, pityriasis rosea, hepatitis, viral hemophagocytosis, idiopathic thrombocytic purpura, and drug hypersensitivity syndromes, among others. None of these has yet been proved to have a direct causal relationship to HHV-6 infection.

Therapy

A number of antiviral agents, especially ganciclovir and acyclovir, have been evaluated for treatment of HHV-6 infection, mostly in immunocompromised patients, but none has been consistently efficacious nor approved for therapeutic use (De Clerq et al., 2001). In vitro acyclic or carbocyclic analogs of guanosine, as well as non–guanosine-derived drugs, such as foscarnet, cidofovir, and brivudin, have been tested for their effect on the replication of HHV-6 in various assays (De Clerq et al., 2001). Among these agents the most effective with the greatest antiviral selectivity index was foscarnet, followed by two guanosine analog, S2242 and A-5021, and the cidofovir. These drugs, however, generally have associated toxicity and have been evaluated in only a few patients in uncontrolled studies. Prophylaxis with acyclovir has been attempted in allogenic bone marrow transplant recipients without benefit. Interferon-α and interferon-β have been shown to diminish HHV-6 replication experimentally, but have not been evaluated clinically.

Summary

With discovery of its etiology, the sixth exanthematous disease of old has assumed a new position as the sixth member of the herpesvirus family. HHV-6 primary infection manifests in varied, and not always benign, ways and places an appreciable burden on the health care of children in the first 2 years of life. The additional burden caused by reactivation of HHV-6 after primary infection in older children and adults remains unknown, but evidence suggests that in certain patients, such as the immunosuppressed, HHV-6 may play a direct or indirect role in the course of their disease.

HUMAN HERPESVIRUS 7

The seventh member of the herpesvirus family, HHV-7, was first identified in the cells from a healthy adult in 1990 by Frenkel and colleagues, who noted during their work with activated T cells an unusual cytopathic effect. Subsequent investigation by these and many other researchers have characterized HHV-7 as the member of the herpesvirus family that most closely resembles HHV-6 (Black, 1999; Gompels, 2000).

Characterization

HHV-7 is classified within the genus Roseolovirus within the subfamily Betaherpesvirinae, as is HHV-6. HHV-7 closely resembles HHV-6 morphologically, antigenically, and genomically. It contains a nucleocapsid containing DNA surrounded by a dense tegument and a lipid envelope. The genomes of HHV-6 and HHV-7 are colinear, and have a strong homology. HHV-7, however, is distinct antigenically; by a number of its biologic properties, such as cellular tropism, gene expression, and splicing pattern; and pathologically.

HHV-7 also primarily infects CD4+ T cells, but with a narrower cell tropism of CD4+ T cells than that seen with HHV-6, such as cord and peripheral blood mononuclear cells. In vitro it may be propagated in a continuous immature T-lymphoblastoid cell line, SupT-1, in which it induces a ballooning cytopathic effect. In humans, HHV-7 has been identified as being latent in CD4+ T lymphocytes.

In the epithelial cells of salivary glands it appears productive with viral shedding (Black and Pellett, 1999). Other tissues have recently been shown to contain HHV-7 antigen, such as skin, mammary glands, and lungs.

At least 20 proteins of HHV-7 have been identified, including 7 glycoproteins (Gompels, 2000). A phosphoprotein (pp85) is believed to be the main target of the human immune response. Since HHV-6 and HHV-7 have a close homology, human antibodies as well as monoclonal antibodies to HHV-7 have some cross-reactivity to those of HHV-6. In vitro, some T-cell clones raised against HHV-6 also have been shown to react to HHV-7 antigens.

Immunity

The immune response during HHV-7 primary infection is incompletely deciphered, but cellular immunity appears to be important, as with HHV-6. HHV-7 also enhances NK cell activity and IL-15. In the few patients with primary HHV-7 infection who have been studied, specific IgG antibody has been identified to rise significantly after the second week from the onset of infection (Caserta et al., 1998; Tanaka et al., 1994). Primary infection with HHV-7 may be associated with reactivation of HHV-6 infection in vitro in cells from normal individu-als with previous HHV-6 infection, suggesting that HHV-7 has a transacting function in the reactivation of HHV-6. Thus, primary HHV-7 may also be associated with significant serologic increases in response to HHV-6 infection.

Epidemiology

HHV-7 is also a ubiquitous infection of childhood but generally occurs somewhat later than HHV-6 and over a wider age range (Black and Pellett, 1999; Gompels, 2000; Lanphear et al., 1998). Seroprevalence studies indicate that most individuals in the United States have acquired HHV-7 infection by 6 to 10 years of age. HHV-7 is shed from the saliva in 95% or more of adults, indicating a high rate of previous infection and the consistent ability of HHV-7 to persist thereafter (Black and Pellett, 1999).

HHV-7 is most likely transmitted via the saliva of contacts in which the virus is actively replicating. However, why HHV-7 infection is not acquired earlier and more universally at younger ages is not clear. The virus is ubiquitous, and since it is found in the secretions of almost all adults, infant contact with it is likely early and constant. HHV-7 DNA has also been detected in the cellular fraction of about 10% of breast-milk samples collected shortly after delivery, and breast-fed infants have been shown to have a slightly greater rate of seropositivity to HHV-7 than those who were bottle-fed (Fujisaki et al., 1998). Nevertheless, HHV-7 infection is relatively rare in the first months of life. Furthermore, in children under 20 months of age, breast-feeding has been associated with a lower risk of early acquisition of HHV-7 antibody (Lanphear et al., 1998).

Clinical Manifestations

Little is known about the clinical manifestations of HHV-7. Primary infection with clinical disease has been rarely identified, despite prospective evaluation of a large group of children with varying febrile illnesses (Caserta et al., 1998). In the few cases described, HHV-7 primary infection may appear similar to HHV-6 infection and can be the cause of an occasional case of roseola or recurrent roseola (Black and Pellett, 1999; Caserta et al., 1998; Tanaka et al., 1994; Torigoe et al., 1995). HHV-7 may also be associated with a variety of nonspecific symptoms. Seizures may occur during the febrile period, and HHV-7 DNA has been detected in CSF (Portolani, 1998). HHV-7 has also been associated serologically with exanthematous illnesses appearing similar to those of rubella and measles (Black and Pellett, 1999).

The biologic and possible clinical manifestations associated with HHV-7 reactivation are perhaps the most interesting (Emery et al., 1999). The interaction of HHV-7 with other herpesviruses confounds deciphering the role HHV-7 may play in a variety of entities, especially those in immunocompromised hosts. Of particular recent interest is the effect of HHV-7 in transplant recipients (Dockrell and Paya, 2001; Emery, 2001). As with HHV-6, reactivation of HHV-7 is correlated with the degree of immunosuppression. The reactivation of HHV-7 is usually concurrent with that of HHV-6 and CMV. Whether it contributes to bone marrow suppression, graft-versus-host disease, or delayed engraftment, and associated clinical manifestations, is unclear. However, HHV-7 reactivation has been correlated in transplant patients with increased CMV detection, viral load, disease, and severity (Black and Pellett, 1999; Dockrell and Paya, 2001; Emery, 2001; Gompels, 2000).

In HIV-infected patients, reactivation of HHV-7 also has been documented to occur. However, modulation of the disease's progression or manifestations of HHV-7 infection has been suggested but not well confirmed. The frequency of HHV-7 detection in blood mononuclear cells and saliva from patients with HIV infection has been reported as increased, diminished, and similar to controls (DiLuca et al., 1995; Fabio et al., 1997; Lucht et al., 1998). In vitro HHV-7 and HHV-6 appear to have opposite effects on the replication of HIV (Black and Pellett, 1999; Gompels, 2000). Both HHV-7 and HIV infect T cells using the CD4 receptor. Addition of HHV-7 to HIV infected cells in vitro results in diminished replication of HIV, which in part may result from reciprocal interference between HHV-7 and HIV in infecting lymphocytes as well as phagocytes. These observations have suggested a potential prophylactic and therapeutic approach for controlling HIV infection.

A variety of other diseases have been associated with HHV-7 infection, but little information suggests the relationship is causal. HHV-7 may possibly act as a cofactor, but often it is probably no more than an innocent witness; its presence the result of the high frequency of persistence and shedding characteristic of HHV-7. One entity of recent interest is pityriasis rosea, which has been proposed to be a manifestation of HHV-7 reactivation. HHV-7 has been recovered in tissue culture from peripheral blood mononuclear cells of patients with pityriasis rosea, and HHV-7 DNA has been identified in their skin. However, other reports have questioned this association (Drago, 1997).

HHV-7 has also been reported, mostly through case reports, to be associated with syndromes similar to those seen with Epstein-Barr virus (EBV), such as mononucleosis and chronic infection, as well as hepatitis, encephalitis, and chronic fatigue syndrome.

Diagnosis

HHV-7 may be isolated from most normal individuals' saliva, in activated cord blood, or peripheral blood mononuclear cells. Although HHV-7 may be propagated in SupT-1 cells, this cell line cannot be used for primary isolation. Activated cord blood cells are preferred with subsequent adaptation in SupT-1 cells. Specific identification may be accomplished by detection of monoclonal antibodies to HHV-7.

Serologic diagnosis of HHV-7 is possible with a variety of tests, most frequently an EIA or IFA. Immunoblot and neutralizing assays have also been developed (Black and Pellett, 1999). The immunologic cross-reactivity between HHV-6 and HHV-7 necessitates that the cross-reacting HHV-6 antibodies be removed by adsorption with HHV-6 infected cell lysates. HHV-7 DNA may be detected by both nested and unnested PCR in saliva, peripheral blood mononuclear cells, and other body fluids. These assays have been developed further into multiplex and quantitative PCR assays.

In general, any of these tests alone does not differentiate primary infection from reactivation because of the high persistence of HHV-7 in various body sites after primary infection and its interaction with other herpesviruses, as mentioned previously. In normal children, isolation of HHV-7 from peripheral blood mononuclear cells during the acute illness plus demonstration of seroconversion generally indicates primary infection. Although IgM antibodies to HHV-7 have been identified, they cannot be used to indicate primary infection, as they also occur in healthy individuals with previous infection.

Therapy and Prevention

Currently no confirmed therapeutic or prophylactic modes exist for HHV-7, and with current understanding of this virus, their use would be rarely indicated. HHV-7 generally does not show the same sensitivity to the guanine analogs as HHV-6, indicating that HHV-7 lacks a thymidine kinase gene homologue. HHV-7, however, has been shown in vitro to be sensitive to an experimental guanosine analog, S2242 (De Clerq et al., 2001). Cidofovir, as well as several other experimental nucleoside phosphonates, have been shown in vitro to diminish HHV-7 replication (De Clerq et al., 2001; Gompels, 2000).

Summary

HHV-7, although closely related to its sibling, HHV-6, morphologically and genomically, is distinctively different in its biologic importance as a cause of illness in children. Currently much more knowledge exists about the virologic structure of this virus and its in vitro character than its personality, penchants, and potential in humans. Perhaps its most interesting characteristic is its varied but frequent interactions with other herpesviruses and its potential role as a cofactor or immune modulator of associated diseases, such as those affecting patients with HIV and those who are immunocompromised for other reasons.

HUMAN HERPESVIRUS 8

In 1872, Moritz Kaposi in Hungary first described an aggressive, pigmented sarcoma of the skin as idiopathic. This tumor is now well known, but Kaposi's sarcoma in the United States and other Western nations was rare, occurring in < 0.06 per 100,000 people, until the evolution of the AIDS epidemic. In the early 1980s, reports that homosexual men were being affected frequently by Kaposi's sarcoma began to appear; the reported incidence of these lesions subsequently increased to 15% to 20% of homosexual HIV-infected men.

Characterization

Although the etiology of Kaposi's sarcoma had been suspected as being viral for some time, the association with human herpesvirus 8 (HHV-8) and Kaposi's sarcoma was not made until Chang and colleagues (1994) discovered Kaposi's sarcoma–associated herpesvirus (KSHV). They identified two novel DNA fragments isolated from Kaposi's lesions that demonstrated homology to gammaherpesviruses. KHSV has now been classified as HHV-8 within the gamma-2 subgroup of herpesviruses, the Rhadinovirus group, which contains several other animal herpesviruses. The only other known human gammaherpesvirus, EBV, is classified as a gamma-1-herpesvirus. Subsequent characterization shows HHV-8 to have a large (165-kb) genome with 66 of the genes encoding conserved structural and replication proteins along with other genes (Schulz, 2000). Some possess close homology to human genes cyclin-D, bcl-2, and IL-6, which have a potential role in oncogenesis and the inhibition of apoptosis. Gene expression in Kaposi's sarcoma appears highly restricted, suggesting that most Kaposi's sarcoma cells are latently rather than lytically infected by HHV-8. Only recently have researchers been able to propagate HHV-8 in vitro. Most frequently used are continuous cell lines from HIV-associated body cavity lymphomas such as KSHV-EBV infected cells in which infection is mostly latent. In several other cell lines the latent HHV-8 infection may switch to a lytic infection.

Epidemiology

Marked variations occur in the distribution of HHV-8 infection in different geographic and socioeconomic settings. These mostly mirror the diverse incidence rates of classic Kaposi's sarcoma. Seroepidemiologic studies also generally reflect this, with the highest positivity occurring in Africa, especially Central Africa; with low rates in the United States, Japan, and in certain Northern-European countries; and with rates in between in most Mediterranean countries (Antman and Chang, 2000). The reported rates vary according to the assay used, but in blood donors the rate has been as high as 50% or more in various parts in of Africa and as low as 0.2% in Japan (Antman and Chang, 2000; Fujii, 1999; Schulz, 2000). In the United States seropositivity in blood donors is generally 10% but has been reported to be less than 5% when assays that detect the ORF-65 protein are used and as high as 25% when EIA is performed on purified virions. The highest risk group in the United States is homosexual men, who have rates of about 40% whether symptomatic or asymptomatic.

Transmission of HHV-8 may occur by several routes, although sexual transmission, as well as possibly transmission via saliva, appears to predominate in Western countries. This is based on the identification of HHV-8 in semen and on the epidemiologic data indicating the greater risk of Kaposi's sarcoma in HIV-infected homosexual men than in HIV-infected intravenous drug users or HIV-infected hemophiliacs (Moore and Chang, 1995). Additional routes of infection are indicated by the presence of HHV-8 DNA in saliva and peripheral blood lymphocytes and by the differences in geographic distribution and age. In Africa, where the endemic form of Kaposi's sarcoma exists, HHV-8 occurs commonly in childhood with a relatively high prevalence before the age of sexual activity. Perinatal transmission has also been shown to occur in Africa and has been suggested to occur in Western countries, such as Sardinia (Serraino et al., 2001). In those parts of Africa with high rates of infection in children, both horizontal and perinatal transmission appear to be important. In the United States, seropositivity in healthy children is generally not found but has been reported to occur in a few patients who are immunosuppressed, such as transplant recipients (Antman and Chang, 2000; Malekzadeh et al., 1987). However, in Egypt, HHV-8 infection has been recently reported in immunocompetent children (Andreoni and Sarmati, 2002). Transmission was suggested to occur via saliva of close contacts that contained HHV-8 DNA.

Clinical Manifestations

Primary infection in immunocompetent children has been rarely documented in areas with a low prevalence of HHV-8 infection, such as the United States. In many African countries with high rates of infection in the population, children are commonly infected. However, recently primary infection in healthy children in Egypt was reported, which was associated with an acute illness characterized by fever, a maculopapular rash, and pharyngeal involvement (Andreoni and Sarmati, 2002). Nevertheless, HHV-8 has been detected primarily in patients with Kaposi's sarcoma (plate 54), body cavity-based lymphomas, and multicentric Castleman's disease and in skin lesions of transplant patients. The causal role of HHV-8 in these lesions is supported by studies that show that the presence of HHV-8 in peripheral blood lymphocytes precedes and predicts the risk of developing Kaposi's sarcoma (Antman and Chang, 2000; Moore and Chang, 1995).

Primary infection with HHV-8 is usually asymptomatic. The clinical manifestations associated with HHV-8 infection are primarily those of Kaposi's sarcoma and result from reactivation under conditions of immunosuppression. The lesions of Kaposi's sarcoma are distinctive vascular, purplish nodules that may appear as isolated cutaneous and intraoral lesions; disease may also be more widespread, involving the lungs, biliary tract, and other viscera.

Four variants of Kaposi's sarcoma exist: the classic variant, the endemic form, the epidemic (HIV-associated) form, and the immunosuppression-associated form. The classic form generally affects only older men from Mediterranean and Eastern European countries. The disease is chronic and not aggressive, and long survival is usual. The endemic form, which occurs mostly in parts of Africa, especially Central Africa, affects both adults and children and is now one of the most frequent tumors occurring in children in these regions. This form of Kaposi's sarcoma is not associated with HIV infection and has manifestations in children in Africa that are different from those of the endemic form occurring in adults. The endemic form is typically a fatal lymphadenopathic disease, which usually is not accompanied by skin lesions. The epidemic form of Kaposi's sarcoma is the one that is closely associated with HIV infection and in the United States, primarily with homosexuality. The appearance of this form of Kaposi's sarcoma is generally a marker of an aggressive course and a poor prognosis.

HHV-8 infection has also been associated with other diseases, most of which have not been confirmed as being caused by HHV-8. One such entity is multiple myeloma, for which HHV-8 has been suggested as the cause, but not confirmed, although HHV-8 has been shown to induce proliferation of infected plasma cells. Other associations include sarcoidosis, cutaneous T-cell lymphomas, and basal and squamous cell carcinomas. Several case reports have suggested that HHV-8 may produce afebrile illnesses associated with lymphadenopathy, anemia, thrombocytopenia, and hepatitis in immunosuppressed patients (Oksenhendler et al., 1998).

Diagnosis

HHV-8 cannot be readily isolated in tissue culture. Thus, serologic and PCR assays have been used primarily to determine the presence of past and reactivated HHV-8 infection. Serologic assays are generally preferable as they are more sensitive than PCR. HHV-8 DNA may be detected in most Kaposi's sarcoma lesions, but in the mononuclear cells in peripheral blood, the viral loads are variable and often below the level detectable by PCR (Antman and Chang, 2000, Corchero et al., 2001). Serologic assays, predominately IFA, EIA, and immunoblot assays, have been developed to detect antibodies against HHV-8 antigens that are both latent, such as ORF 73, and lytic, such as ORF K8.1 and glycoprotein B (Corchero et al., 2001; Schulz, 1998). The antigens have been produced for these assays by recombinant expression, from primary effusion lymphoma (PEL) cell lines that contain the HHV-8 genome, and from purified virions. In general, assays based on lytic antigens are more sensitive than those based on latent antigens, and IFAs are more sensitive than EIAs. The lytic PEL-based IFAs have been considered most sensitive and are frequently used. However, some sera from normal subjects, including children, contain antibodies that are cross-reactive with HHV-8 antigens, which may result in false-positive reactions in lytic PEL-based IFAs. Recent improvements in these assays have avoided the problem and have been highly sensitive, using recombinant expressed K8.1 to which no cross-reactive antibodies exist (Corchero et al., 2001).

Prophylaxis and Therapy

No effective prophylactic agent for HHV-8 infection currently exists. The most effective means of prophylaxis in the United States is that associated with prevention of HIV infection. A number of therapeutic agents have been examined in vitro for their efficacy in diminishing replication of HHV-8 (De Clerq et al., 2001). Among these, cidofovir appears to have promise, along with an experimental guanosine analog, S2242. Ganciclovir is less effective but still moderately so, whereas acyclovir is ineffective. Therapy for Kaposi's sarcoma has included surgical excision for small singular lesions to more involved and combination therapies with surgery, radiation, and chemotherapy for more advanced disease. Interferon has been tried anecdotally via intralesional, subcutaneous, and intravenous administration. Since the course of Kaposi's sarcoma is highly associated with the degree of immunosuppression, the newer and more effective highly active antiretroviral therapy has offered benefit for patients with HIV infection and Kaposi's sarcoma.

Summary

HHV-8 has catapulted to importance with its increasing prevalence in immunocompromised patients in the United States. In parts of Africa, HHV-8 infection remains a major health-care burden, affecting both children and adults. Over the few years since the discovery of HHV-8, progress has been rapid in deciphering its virologic structure and function. Improved diagnostic assays have been pivotal in a greater understanding of its pathogenesis. Methods for control that are being concurrently explored include epidemiologic and therapeutic approaches and the potential for immunization.

BIBLIOGRAPHY

Agbalika F. Transient angiolymphoid hyperplasia and Kaposi's sarcoma after primary infection with human herpesvirus 8 in a patient with human immunodeficiency virus infection. N Engl J Med 1998;338:1585-1590.

Andreoni, M Sarmati L, et al. Primary human herpesvirus 8 infection in immunocompetent children. JAMA 2000;287:1295-1300.

Antman K, Chang Y. Kaposi's sarcoma. N Engl J Med 2000;342:1027-1038.

Asano Y, Nakashima T, Yoshikawa T, et al. Severity of human herpesvirus-6 viremia and clinical findings in infants with exanthem subitum. J Pediatr 1991;118:891-895.

Barone SR, Kaplan MH, Krilov LR. Human herpesvirus-6 infection in children with first febrile seizures. J Pediatr 1995;127:95-97.

Black J, Pellett P. Human herpesvirus 7. Rev Med Virol 1999;9:245-262.

Black JB, Schwarz TF, Patton JL, et al. Evaluation of immunoassays for detection of antibodies to human herpesvirus 7. Clin Diagn Lab Immunol 1996;3:79-83.

Braun D, Dominguez G, Pellett P. Human herpesvirus 6. Clin Microbiol Rev 1997;10:521-567.

Breese BB Jr. Roseola infantum (exanthem subitum). NY State J Med 1941;41:1854-1859.

Caserta MT, Hall CB, Schnabel K, et al. Neuroinvasion and persistence of human herpesvirus 6 in children. J Infect Dis 1994;170:1586-1589.

Caserta M, Hall C, Schnabel K, et al. Primary human herpesvirus 7 infection: a comparison of human herpesvirus 7 and human herpesvirus 6 infections in children. J Pediatr 1998;133:386-389.

Chang Y, Cesarman F, Pessin MS, et al. Identification of herpesvirus-like DNA sequences in AIDS-associated Kaposi's sarcoma. Science 1994;266:1865-1869.

Chiu SS, Cheung CY, Tse CY, et al. Early diagnosis of primary human herpesvirus 6 infection in childhood: serology, polymerase chain reaction, and virus load. J Infect Dis 1998;178:1250-1256.

Corchero J, Mar E-C, Spira T, et al. Comparison of serologic assays for detection of antibodies against human herpesvirus 8. Clin Diagn Lab Immunol 2001;8:913-921.

De Clerq E, Naesens L, De Bolle L, et al. Antiviral agents active against human herpesviruses HHV-6, HHV-7, and HHV-8. Rev Med Virol 2001;11:381-395.

Dewhurst S, Chandran B, McIntyre K, et al. Phenotypic and genetic polymorphisms among human herpesvirus-6 isolates from North American infants. Virology 1992;190:490-493.

DiLuca D, Mirandola P, Ravaioli T, et al. Human herpesviruses 6 and 7 in salivary glands and shedding in saliva of healthy and human immunodeficiency virus positive individuals. J Med Virol 1995;45:462-468.

Dockrell D, Paya C. Human herpesvirus-6 and -7 in transplantation. Rev Med Virol 2001;11:23-36.

Drago F, Ranieri E, Malaguti F, et al. Human herpesvirus 7 in pityriasis rosea. Lancet 1997;349:1367-1368.

Emery V. Human herpesvirus 6 and 7 in solid organ transplant recipients. Clin Infect Dis 2001;32:1357-1360.

Emery V, Atkins M, Bowen E, et al. Interactions between β-herpesviruses and human immunodeficiency virus in vivo: evidence for increased human immunodeficiency viral load in the presence of human herpesvirus 6. J Med Virol 1999;57:278-282.

Fabio G, Knight S, Kidd I, et al. Prospective study of human herpesvirus 6, human herpesvirus 7, and cytomegalovirus infections in human immunodeficiency virus–positive patients. J Clin Microbiol 1997;35:2657-2659.

Frenkel N, Schirmer EC, Wyatt LS, et al. Isolation of a new herpesvirus from human CD4+ T cells. Proc Natl Acad Sci USA 1990;87:748-752.

Fujii T, Taguchi H, et al. Seroprevalence of human herpesvirus 8 in human immunodeficiency virus 1-positive and human-immunodeficiency virus 1-negative population in Japan. J Med Virol 1999;57:159-162.

Fujisaki H, Tanaka-Taya K, Tanabe H, et al. Detection of human herpesvirus 7 (HHV-7) DNA in breast milk by polymerase chain reaction and prevalence of HHV-7 antibody in breast-fed and bottle-fed children. J Med Virol 1998;56:275-279.

Gompels U. Human herpesviruses 6 and 7. In Zuckerman A, Banatvala J, Pattison J (eds). Principles and Practice of Clinical Virology. Chichester, West Sussex, England: John Wiley & Sons, 2000.

Griffiths P, Clark D, Emery V. Betaherpesviruses in transplant recipients. J Antimicrob Chemother 2000;45:29-34.

Hall CB, Long CE, Schnabel KC, et al. Human herpesvirus-6 infection in children: prospective evaluation for complications and reactivation. N Engl J Med 1994;331:432-438.

Jee S, Long C, Hall C, et al. Risk of recurrent seizures after a primary human herpesvirus 6-induced febrile seizure. Pediatr Infect Dis J 1998;17:43-48.

Jones CMV, Dunn HG, Thomas EE, et al. Acute encephalopathy and status epilepticus associated with human herpesvirus-6 infection. Dev Med Child Neurol 1994;36:646-650.

Kempe HC, Shaw EB, Jackson JR, et al. Studies on the etiology of exanthema subitum (roseola infantum). J Pediatr 1950;37:561-568.

Kimberlin D. Neuroinvasion of human herpesviruses 6 and 7. Herpes 1999;3:60-63.

Kondo K, Nagafuji H, Hata A, et al. Association of human herpesvirus-6 infection of the central nervous system with recurrence of febrile convulsions. J Infect Dis 1993;167:1197-1200.

Kusuhara K, Ueda K, Miyazaki C, et al. Attack rate of exanthem subitum in Japan. Lancet 1992;340:482.

Lanphear B, Hall C, Black J, et al. Risk factors for the early acquisition of human herpesvirus 6 and human herpesvirus 7 infections in children. Pediatr Infect Dis J 1998;19:9.

Leach CT, Newton ER, McParlin S, et al.. Human herpesvirus-6 infection on the female genital tract. J Infect Dis 1994;169:1281-1283.

Lucht E, Brytting M, Bjerregaard L, et al. Shedding of cytomegalovirus and herpesvirus 6, 7, and 8 in saliva of human immunodeficiency virus type 1 infected patients and healthy controls. Clin Infect Dis 1998;27:134-141.

Luppi M, Barozzi P, Maiorana A, et al. HHV-6 in normal brain tissue. J Infect Dis 1994;169:943-944.

Luppi M, Barozzi P, Maiorana A, et al. Human herpesvirus-6: a survey of presence and distribution of genomic sequences in normal brain and neuroglial tumors. J Med Virol 1995;47:105-111.

Luppi M, Barozzi P, Morris C, et al. Human herpesvirus 6 latently infects early bone marrow progenitors in vitro. J Virol 1999;73:754-759.

Malekzadeh M, Church J, Siegel S, et al. Human immunodeficiency virus–associated Kaposi's sarcoma in a pediatric renal transplant recipient. Nephron 1987;42:62-65.

McCullers JA, Lakeman FD, Whitley RJ. Human herpesvirus 6 is associated with focal encephalitis. Clin Infect Dis 1995;21:571-576.

Meigs JF, Pepper W. A Practical Treatise of the Diseases of Children. Philadelphia: Lindsay and Blakiston, 1870.

Mendez J, Dockrell D, Espy M, et al. Human ß-herpesvirus interactions in solid organ transplant recipients. J Infect Dis 2001;183:179-184.

Moore PS, Chang Y. Detection of herpesvirus-like DNA sequences in Kaposi's sarcoma in patients with and those without HIV infection. N Engl J Med 1995;332:1181-1185.

Norton R, Caserta M, Hall C, et al. Detection of human herpesvirus 6 by reverse transcription-PCR. J Clin Microbiol 1999;37:3672-3675.

Oksenhendler E, Cazals-Hatem D, Schulz T, et al. Kaposi's sarcoma–associated herpesvirus (human herpesvirus-8). J Gen Virol 1998;79:1573-1591.

Okuno T, Oishi H, Hayashi K, et al. Human herpesvirus 6 and 7 in cervixes of pregnant women. J Clin Microbiol 1995;33:1968-1970.

Pellett P, Dominguez G. Human herpesviruses 6A, 6B, and 7 and their replication. In Knipe D, Howley P (eds). Fields Virology. Philadelphia: Lippincott Williams & Wilkins, 2001.

Pellett PE, Black JB, Yamamoto M. Human herpesvirus 6: the virus and the search for its role as a human pathogen. Adv Virus Res 1992;41:1-52.

Portolani M, Leoni S, Guerra A, et al. Human herpesvirus-7 DNA in cerebrospinal fluid. Minerva Pediatr 1998;50:39-44.

Salahuddin SZ, Ablashi DV, Marleham PD, et al. Isolation of a new virus, HBLV, in patients with lymphoproliferative disorders. Science 1986;234:596-601.

Schulz T. Kaposi's sarcoma-associated herpesvirus (human herpesvirus-8). Gen Virol 1998;79:1573-1591.

Schulz T. Kaposi's sarcoma-associated herpesvirus (human herpesvirus 8). In Zuckerman A, Banatvala J, Pattison J. Principles and practice of clinical virology. Chichester, West Sussex, England, 2000, John Wiley & Sons Ltd.: 167-186.

Serraino D, Locatelli M, Songini M, et al. Human herpesvirus-8 infection among pregnant women and their children: results from the Sardinia-IDDM Study 2 (letter). Int J Cancer 2001;91:740-741.

Studahl M, Hagberg L, Rekabdar E, et al. Herpesvirus DNA detection in cerebral spinal fluid: differences in clinical presentation between alpha-, beta-, and gamma-herpesviruses. Scand J Infect Dis 2000;32:237-248

Suga S, Suzuki K, Ihira M, et al. Clinical characteristics of febrile convulsions during primary HHV-6 infection. Arch Dis Child 2000;82:62-66.

Suga S, Yoshikawa T, Asano Y, et al. IgM neutralizing antibody responses to human herpesvirus 6 in patients with exanthem subitum or organ transplantation. Microbiol Immunol 1992;36:495-506.

Suga A, Yoshikawa T, Asano Y, et al. Clinical and virological analyses of 21 infants with exanthem subitum (roseola infantum) and central nervous system complications. Ann Neurol 1993;33:597-603.

Tanaka K, Kondo T, Torigoe S, et al. Human herpesvirus 7: Another causal agent for roseola (exanthem subitum). J Pediatr 1994;125:1-5.

Tanaka-Taya K, Kondo T, Nakagawa N, et al. Reactivation of human herpesvirus 6 by infection of human herpesvirus 7. J Med Virol 2000;60:284-289.

Torigoe S, Kumamoto T, Koide W, et al. Clinical manifestations associated with human herpesvirus 7 infection. Arch Dis Child 1995;72:518-519.

van den Bosch G, Locatelli G, Geerts L, et al. Development of reverse transcriptase PCR assays for detection of active human herpesvirus 6 infection. J Clin Microbiol 2001;39:2308-2310.

Wang FZ, Dahl H, Ljungman P, et al. Lymphoproliferative responses to human herpesvirus-6 variant A and variant B in healthy adults. J Med Virol 1999;57:134-139.

Yamanishi K, Okuno T, Shiraki K, et al. Identification of human herpesvirus 6 as a causal agent for exanthem subitum. Lancet 1988;1:1065-1067.

Yanagihara K, Tanaka-Taya K, Itagaki Y, et al. Human herpesvirus-6 meningoencephalitis with sequelae. Pediatr Infect Dis J 1995;14:240-241.

Yoshikawa T, Nakashima T, Suga S, et al. Human herpesvirus-6 DNA in cerebrospinal fluid of a child with exanthem subitum and meningoencephalitis. Pediatrics 1992;89:888-890.

Zahorsky J. Roseola infantilis. Pediatrics 1910;22:60-64.

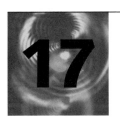

17

INFECTION IN THE IMMUNOINCOMPETENT CHILD

STEPHEN J. CHANOCK

Over the past three decades, major strides have been made in the prevention and treatment of infectious complications in children with defects in immune function. Two trends have contributed substantially to a decrease in morbidity and mortality in immunoincompetent children: an understanding of the types of infections associated with specific immune deficits, and the judicious use of an expanding therapeutic armamentarium. New antimicrobial agents and diagnostics techniques have improved the outlook for all children with breaches in immune function. The paradigms for treatment of immunoincompetent children have been investigated primarily in children undergoing cytotoxic therapy for cancer, which, in turn, have been applied to the care of children with severe primary immunodeficiencies or infection with the human immunodeficiency virus type 1 (HIV-1).

By definition, an immunoincompetent child has at least one significant alteration in host defense systems, which directly leads to an increased risk for infection with an opportunistic pathogen. Defects in host immunity can be (1) inherited, as in a primary immunodeficiency (e.g., chronic granulomatous disease or Wiskott-Aldrich syndrome); (2) secondary to an acquired infection (e.g., HIV-1); or (3) a consequence of therapeutic intervention (e.g., myelotoxic chemotherapy). The investigation of immunoincompetent children has traditionally linked patterns of infection with specific defects in host defenses. Most often, the presence of an opportunistic infection has been ascribed to the absence of or defect in an arm of host defenses (Figure 17-1). These associations have been instrumental in elucidating fundamental principles of immunology.

By definition, opportunistic infections occur in children with immune deficits with greater frequency and severity than in healthy children. The spectrum of potential pathogens includes viral, bacterial, fungal, and protozoan organisms (Table 17-1). Many opportunistic infections are ubiquitous and often colonize the skin and the respiratory and gastrointestinal (GI) tracts. As mentioned above, specific defects in host defense have been associated with susceptibility to particular pathogens; for instance, splenectomy increases the risk for infection with encapsulated bacteria. In many circumstances, particularly following chemotherapy or HIV-1 infection, more than one defect in immune function can be present and lead to either a succession of infections or, in rare circumstances, coinfection. Notably, infection can involve more than one site. Because the immunoincompetent child is at high risk for multiple infections, the astute clinician will be vigilant and pursue all signs and symptoms of possible infection (Tables 17-2 and 17-3).

The impact of infectious complications on quality of life and the cost of care are often overlooked. Children with defects in immune function frequently undergo costly tests and examinations and spend large blocks of time in medical facilities. Consequently, extensive evaluation and therapy can lead to acquisition of nosocomial infections. Furthermore, infection can delay therapy, and thus adversely impact outcome.

This chapter reviews advances in understanding the determinants for risk of infection in the immunoincompetent child, including alterations in host defenses and genetic and environmental risk factors, and discusses current diagnostic approaches and principles of therapy. The emphasis is on issues that surround the diagnosis, treatment, and prevention of infections in neutropenic children with cancer.

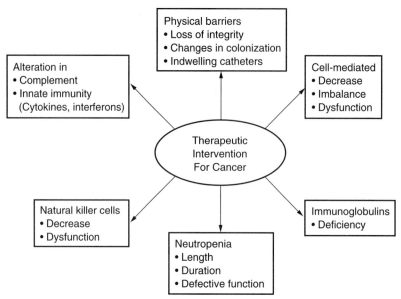

Fig. 17-1 Alterations in host defense systems in children undergoing therapy for cancer.

TABLE 17-1	Pathogens Associated With Specific Immune Deficits in Children With Cancer			
Alteration	*Bacteria*	*Fungi*	*Viruses*	*Parasites*
Neutropenia	Enteric gram-negative bacilli			
	Escherichia coli			
	Klebsiella pneumoniae			
	Enterobacter spp.			
	Citrobacter spp.			
	Pseudomonas aeruginosa			
	Gram-positive cocci			
	Staphylococcus aureus			
	S. non-*aureus*			
	Streptococci (alpha-hemolytic)			
	Enterococci (*Enterococcus faecium, Enterococcus faecalis*)			
	Anaerobes			
	Clostridium spp.			
	Bacteroides spp.			
Depressed cell-mediated immunity	*Legionella* spp.	*Candida* spp.	Varicella-zoster virus	*Toxoplasma gondii*
	Listeria monocytogenes	*Cryptococcus neoformans*	Herpes simplex virus	*Cryptosporidium* spp.
	Mycobacterium spp.	*Histoplasma capsulatum*	Cytomegalovirus	*Strongyloides* spp.
	Nocardia asteroides	*Pneumocystis carinii*	Epstein-Barr virus	

TABLE 17-1   Pathogens Associated With Specific Immune Deficits in Children With Cancer—Cont'd

Alteration	Bacteria	Fungi	Viruses	Parasites
Immunoglobulin deficiency	*Haemophilus influenzae* *Streptococcus pneumoniae* *S. aureus*		Enterovirus	*Giardia lamblia*
Splenectomy (including functional asplenia)	*S. pneumoniae* *H. influenzae* *Neisseria meningitidis* *Capnocytophaga* spp.			*Babesia* spp.
Mucositis (oral)	Streptococci α-Hemolytic Anaerobic	*Candida albicans*	Herpes simplex virus	
Skin	Gram-positive Staphylococci Streptococci *Corynebacterium* spp. *P. aeruginosa*	*C. albicans* *Aspergillus* spp. *Malassezia furfur* Zygomycetes		

TABLE 17-2   Modification of Empiric Therapy for Fever and Neutropenia

Cardiac instability	Broaden coverage (e.g., vancomycin, aminoglycoside, and new β-lactam)
Breakthrough bacteremia	Change antibiotics pending sensitivity testing of isolate
	Gram-positive: vancomycin
	Gram-negative: new β-lactam + aminoglycoside
Catheter-associated site	Add vancomycin
Severe gingivitis/mucositis	Add anaerobic coverage (clindamycin or metronidazole)
	Evaluate and cover for herpes simplex
Esophagitis	Anticandidal therapy
	Evaluate and cover for herpes simplex
Intraabdominal infection	Broaden coverage to include anaerobic organisms and enterococci
Anorectal infection	Add anaerobic coverage and consult surgeon for follow-up
Pulmonary infiltrate	
Focal	If neutrophil count is recovering: continue therapy and observe
	If persistently neutropenic: consider induced sputum, followed by bronchoscopy
Interstitial	Induced sputum followed by bronchoscopy, if indicated
	Consider broadening coverage to include trimethoprim-sulfamethoxazole and erythromycin
Persistent fever	Empiric antifungal therapy between days 4 and 7 with amphotericin B or voriconazole
	Daily blood cultures and close examination, including regular chest radiographs

This approach has evolved over the past 30 years and has served as an important template for supportive therapy for transplant recipients (both marrow and solid organ), primary immunodeficiencies, and HIV-1 infection. When appropriate, issues specific to an additional immunoincompetent group are addressed, to illustrate the spectrum of issues and the complexity of applying the current paradigms for care.

TABLE 17-3	Emerging Pathogens in the Immunoincompetent Child
Bacteria	Vancomycin-resistant enterococci
	Highly resistant gram-negative bacilli
	Aminoglycoside-resistant gram-negative bacilli
Fungi	*Fusarium* spp.
	Trichosporon spp.
	Paecilomyces spp.
	Scedosporium spp.
	Zygomycetes
	Rhizopus spp.
	Mucor spp.
	Absidia spp.
	Pigmented molds
Parasites	*Cryptosporidium* spp.

DEFECTS IN HOST DEFENSES ARE ASSOCIATED WITH INCREASED RISK FOR INFECTION

The most frequent reason for acquired immuno-incompetence in children is cancer therapy (see Figure 17-1). Infection is the major cause of morbidity and mortality in children with cancer and is most commonly associated with the loss of circulating neutrophils, known as *neutropenia*. There is a direct relationship between a depressed neutrophil count and risk for serious infection (Bodey et al., 1966; Pizzo, 1993). Risk is related directly to the depth and duration of neutropenia and not to the underlying disease (Kocak et al., 2002). There is an increased incidence of serious infection when the absolute neutrophil count falls below 500 cells/mm³. The risk is substantially higher when the absolute neutrophil count is below 100 cells/mm³. The longer the duration of neutropenia, the greater the risk for infection; the highest morbidity and mortality are observed when the duration of neutropenia approaches 3 weeks. In addition, the timing of neutropenia is also important. Severe infection is more likely to occur before or at the time of the nadir of neutropenia, whereas when children show signs of marrow recovery, the risk for serious infection is lower (Baorto et al., 2001; Griffin and Buchanan, 1992). It is also notable that comorbidity with, for example, cardiac, pulmonary, or renal insufficiency, increases the risk for infection, as does relapse of cancer, especially leukemia (Talcott et al., 1988).

Studies performed during the last three decades confirm that patients with an absolute neutrophil count less than 500 cells/mm³ constitute a population that requires urgent empiric therapy when they become febrile (Pizzo, 1993). Children with congenital agranulocytosis, cyclic neutropenia or autoimmune neutropenia are vulnerable to cutaneous infections but rarely to systemic or life-threatening infections (Chanock and Pizzo, 1996; Zeidler and Welte, 2002). This difference can be partly attributed to coexistent mucositis and, perhaps, additional cellular defects in children receiving myelotoxic chemotherapy (Lehrnbecher et al., 1997). Even children with HIV-1 infection who become neutropenic appear to carry a lesser risk for invasive bacterial and fungal infections (Chanock and Pizzo, 1996).

Qualitative defects in phagocytic cells can lead to infection with opportunistic infections. Inherited defects in chemotaxis, phagocytosis, or microbicidal activity have been described. Initially, clusters of similar opportunistic infections in family members called attention to potential immunodeficiency. Subsequent investigation has lead to the revelation of the molecular defects and the biochemical consequences. For instance, the study of chronic granulomatous disease (CGD) has lead to basic insights into the NADPH-oxidase enzyme system and its role in generating microbicidal oxygen radicals (Babior, 1999). CGD is an inherited disorder in which phagocytic cells are unable to generate a sufficient oxidative burst, resulting in defective killing of catalase-positive bacteria, particularly *Staphylococcus aureus*, but also opportunistic fungi such as *Aspergillus* species (Winkelstein et al., 2000). There are two forms of CGD based on patterns of inheritance: the X-linked form, which is most common (~70%), and autosomal recessive CGD, which is rarer (~30%) (Winkelstein et al., 2000). For some patients, recombinant interferon-γ decreases the number and severity of infections (International Chronic Granulomatous Disease Cooperative Study Group, 1991). Additional phagocytic disorders have been described (e.g., myeloperoxidase deficiency, leukocyte adhesion deficiency, Chédiak-Higashi syndrome, and Rac2 deficiency) in which specific defects predispose affected individuals to specific types of infection (Segal and Holland, 2000). For example, mutation in the interleukin-12 (IL-12) gene leads to severe mycobacterial infection

(Doffinger et al., 2002). Overall, most defects in phagocyte function predispose children to recurrent bacterial infections, particularly involving soft-tissue abscesses, dermatitis, adenitis, and sinopulmonary infections; however, it is notable that soft tissue infections can be difficult to diagnose and treat in neutropenic children (Johnston et al., 2001).

It is also notable that qualitative neutrophil defects have also been described in hematologic diseases, particularly, acute myelogenous leukemia and myelodysplastic syndromes. There is a wide spectrum of documented defects following cytotoxic agents and radiation therapy reviewed elsewhere (Lehrnbecher et al., 1997). Chemotherapeutic agents have been shown to inhibit phagocytosis, generation of superoxide, and in vitro microbicidal activity (Roilides et al., 1991; Roilides et al., 2003). Corticosteroids suppress phagocytic function, yet increase circulating neutrophils, through demargination and the apparent inhibition of apoptosis or programmed cell death. Still, the contribution of functional defects is not nearly as significant as the loss (or decrease) in circulating neutrophils, which is the most important risk factor for serious bacterial or fungal infection.

There are many causes for defective cell-mediated immunity in children. Classically, aberrant cellular immunity predisposes the patient to infections with intracellular organisms such as bacteria (e.g., *Salmonella* species, *Listeria* species, and *Mycobacterium* species); viruses (e.g., cytomegalovirus [CMV], herpes simplex virus [HSV], varicella-zoster virus [VZV], and Epstein-Barr virus); and fungi (e.g., *Histoplasma capsulatum, Cryptococcus neoformans*, and *Pneumocystis carinii*). Defects in cell-mediated immunity can be due to inherited deficiencies (e.g., severe combined immunodeficiency or Wiskott-Aldrich syndrome) or select immunosuppressive drugs (e.g., cyclosporin A or corticosteroids). However, HIV-1 infection has emerged as the most common cause of defective cell-mediated immunity (discussed in Chapter 1). Specific medications are notable for suppressing cell-mediated immunity. For instance, long-term use of corticosteroids increases the risk for infection with many of the pathogens listed above by depressing T-cell lymphocyte function, cytokine production, and redistribution of lymphocyte subpopulations (Cupps and Fauci, 1982; Sarlis et al., 2000). In addition, corticosteroids inhibit wound healing and neutrophil chemotaxis to sites of infection, thus masking the signs and symptoms of inflammation (Cupps and Fauci, 1982). Cyclosporin A is a potent immunosuppressive agent used to prevent rejection in solid organ–transplant patients or to control graft-versus-host disease in marrow-transplant patients, but it associated with significant immunosuppression, especially in concert with corticosteroids (Berenguer et al., 1995). It has a profound effect on CD4 lymphocytes and inhibits production of interleukin-2 (IL-2) and interferon-γ.

Intensive chemotherapy has significant effects on the number and distribution of T-cell subsets, leading to depletion of CD4 and CD8 lymphocytes (Mackall et al., 1994; Mackall et al., 1995). The effect may persist for months after completion of chemotherapy and is partly related to age and thymic activity. Older children possess less potential for thymic regeneration, resulting in delayed regeneration of T-cell subpopulations (Mackall et al., 1996). Though not as significant as HIV-1 infection, the loss of cell-mediated immunity can lead to an increased risk for opportunistic infections (Mackall et al., 1994). For instance, intensive chemotherapeutic regimens for solid tumors have been complicated by severe infections (namely, infection with viral pathogens and *P. carinii* pneumonia [PCP]) previously seen only in children with leukemia. This parallels the fundamental observation by Hughes and colleagues: in children with leukemia, the intensity of therapy is directly proportional to the risk for developing PCP (Hughes et al., 1975).

A frequently overlooked component of the host defense system is the anatomic integrity of the skin and mucosal surfaces. The presence of protective flora, together with a web of protective immune pathways (e.g., innate and cell-mediated systems), prevents initiation of infection. However, breakdown of the skin or loss of mucosal integrity can provide a point of entry for an opportunistic infection to access deep tissue or the bloodstream. Oral and GI mucosal surfaces can be disrupted by chemotherapeutic agents, which allow normal or hospital-acquired flora access to the bloodstream. Specifically, coinfection of disrupted surfaces (with HSV) can facilitate entry for bacterial or fungal pathogens, especially streptococcal and candidal species. The use of long-term, indwelling vascular catheters, while advantageous for repeated blood sampling and administration of intravenous infusions, poses a persistent risk for infection (Rackoff et al., 1999; Shaul et al., 1998). Local infiltration of the line site can lead to bacteremia and seeding of distant, sterile sites. Late vascular occlusion of central venous catheters (CVCs) is not always symptomatic, and can be the nidus for a blood-borne infection (Wilimas et al., 1998). On rare occasion, mechanical obstruction can require emergent surgical intervention; such obstruction can result from enlarged lymph nodes, an enlarging tumor mass, or scar tissue following surgical procedures or radiation therapy.

The loss of splenic function places children at high risk for serious infection with encapsulated bacteria, such as *Streptococcus pneumoniae, Haemophilus influenzae, Klebsiella* species, and *Neisseria meningitidis*. There is some debate about the relationship between the reason for asplenia and the risk for infection. It is has been observed that children who have undergone a posttrauma splenectomy are less likely to develop life-threatening infection because of splenic remnants that provide a modicum of functional activity. Still, most experts agree that the loss of the spleen as a result of surgery, radiation, or autoinfarct (e.g., sickle cell anemia) or a congenital absence of the spleen predisposes patients to serious infection with encapsulated bacteria. This also applies to children who have undergone marrow transplant, who probably have significant splenic dysfunction and appear to remain at risk for *S. pneumoniae* infection (Schutze et al., 2001).

In immunoincompetent children, the endogenous flora of the skin and GI tract can be altered by repeated hospitalization and frequent antibiotic therapy. Antibiotic-induced shifts in flora have substantial consequences for development of opportunistic infections. Uncommon pathogens can flourish and possibly infect the compromised host. Excessive use of broad-spectrum antibiotics can select for highly resistant bacterial pathogens, which can cause infections that are difficult to treat. Outcome with highly resistant bacteria is especially deleterious in the immunoincompetent child; for instance, morbidity and mortality are especially high in pediatric oncology patients infected with vancomycin-resistant enterococci (VRE). Alpha-streptococcal bacteremia can occur in children with severe mucositis, often superinfected with HSV (Bochud et al., 1994). Similarly, bacteremia with fastidious organisms, such as *Capnocytophaga* species, which are regular inhabitants of the oral cavity, can gain access to the bloodstream if there is significant mucositis. Bacteremia with gram-negative aerobes, anaerobes, enterococci, or other enteric pathogens (e.g., *Streptococcus bovis*) should prompt investigation of the GI tract as the source of infection.

INFECTIONS IN THE IMMUNOINCOMPETENT CHILD
Bacterial Infections

The most significant bacterial pathogens that infect immunoincompetent children arise from endogenous flora of the skin, respiratory tree, and GI tract. Over the past several decades, there have been gradual shifts in the distribution of isolated blood-borne pathogens in neutropenic children. Initially, gram-positive pathogens (e.g. staphylococci) predominated, but this was in the prechemotherapy era. With the advent of myelotoxic chemotherapeutic agents, the emergence of neutropenia as a central risk factor was accompanied by the emergence of gram-negative bacilli (e.g., *Escherichia coli, Klebsiella* species, and *Pseudomonas aeruginosa*) as the most common and dangerous blood isolates (Bodey et al., 1966). The use of broad-spectrum antibiotics and frequent hospitalizations contributed to the change in colonization patterns, which incidentally paralleled an increase in gram-negative isolates from the blood of febrile, neutropenic children. It is notable that not all children colonized with these pathogens developed serious infection. Because of the high mortality rate associated with infection with gram-negative organisms, particularly with *P. aeruginosa*, empiric antibiotics became the standard of care (Bodey et al., 1985). Recently, a disturbing trend has been noted: the emergence of gram-negative bacteria resistant to commonly used antibiotics (Aquino et al., 1995; Levy et al., 1996; Wehl et al., 1999).

In the 1980s, the incidence of infections with gram-negative organisms began to subside, and gram-positive bacteria emerged as the most common blood-born isolates (Pizzo et al., 1980; Wade et al., 1982). This trend has coincided with the use of antibiotics with a wider spectrum of activity (e.g., the third-generation cephalosporins and fluoroquinolones, the former for treatment and the latter for prevention), and the widespread use of indwelling CVCs. The majority of Silastic catheters have a permanent insertion site in the skin, which is frequently colonized by the same organisms that are associated with catheter-associated bacteremia (Salzman and Rubin, 1995). Most of the gram-positive bacterial isolates are also drawn from skin and GI flora. The spectrum of gram-positive pathogens includes the staphylococci (both coagulase-positive and coagulase-negative), α-hemolytic streptococci, and enterococci.

A disturbing trend has been the emergence of gram-positive bacteria that are highly resistant to commonly prescribed antibiotics (Bruckner et al., 2002) (see Table 17-3). This is a formidable challenge for treatment because of the paucity of active agents available. Over the past decade, both *Enterococcus faecalis* and *Enterococcus faecium* have acquired antibiotic resistance through plasmid-mediated and chromosomal-mediated mechanisms. Unfortunately, some enterococci are highly resistant to penicillins, aminoglycosides, and vancomycin. This has important implications for choosing antibiotics in general and, specifically, when enterococci are isolated. A worrisome increase in VRE was observed in intensive care units in the early 1990s (Centers for Disease Control and Prevention, 1993). Colonization with VRE was associated with previous antibiotic therapy, particularly with vancomycin, and the length of hospitalization. This trend was also noted on adult and pediatric oncology wards, where morbidity and mortality associated with VRE are high (Montecalvo et al., 1994; Rubin et al., 1992). Fecal colonization can persist for up to a year. In the child already colonized with VRE, persistent neutropenia is a risk factor for developing VRE infection (Henning et al., 1996). In response to this disturbing development, the Centers for Disease Control and Prevention have formally recommended that use of vancomycin be restricted, particularly on oncology and transplant wards (Centers for Disease Control and Prevention, 1993).

New, more intensive therapeutic strategies have further compromised host defenses beyond neutropenia and set the stage for life-threatening gram-positive infections. The syndrome of alpha-streptococcal sepsis is associated with rapid onset and high mortality (Bochud et al., 1994; Elting et al., 1992; Sotiropoulos et al., 1989). Risk factors for developing this dangerous infection include the use of high-dose cytosine arabinoside, severe mucositis, prophylactic use of fluoroquinolones, and persistent neutropenia (Bochud et al., 1994). The onset is heralded by fever, which can quickly lead to hypotension, shock, respiratory embarrass-ment, renal failure, and encephalopathy (Bochud et al., 1994; Elting et al., 1992; Sotiropoulos et al., 1989). Because isolates can be penicillin- and cephalosporin-resistant, vancomycin is appropriately recommended.

Infection with one or more anaerobes is distinctly unusual in the immunoincompetent child. Isolation of an anaerobe (usually *Bacteroides* species or *Clostridium* species) should prompt an evaluation of the GI tract, because anaerobic bacteremia is usually associated with a breach in the integrity of intestinal tract (Fainstein et al., 1989). Anaerobes are part of the normal flora and do not cause disease unless they gain access to the blood stream through an interruption in the integrity of the GI tract. On occasion, anaerobic bacteria can be isolated in polymicrobial bacteremia. Anaerobes can be associated with specific sites of infection, such as intraabdominal abscesses, peritonitis, and anorectal infections. Isolation of anaerobes from specific anatomic sites other than the blood is cumbersome and attempted only when there is sufficient suspicion.

Viral Infections

Over the last 30 years, there has been a growing appreciation of the importance of viral infections in immunoincompetent children. All children, whether immunoincompetent or not, are constantly exposed to common respiratory and GI viruses. Attempts to quantify the number of infections and the effect on immunoincompetent children have been hindered by insufficient methods for isolation and detection. Reliance upon serology is especially difficult in immunoincompetent children, many of whom cannot mount a sufficient antibody response. Still, surveys of infectious events in children undergoing cancer therapy have suggested that viral infections are common (Nakamura et al., 2000). The incidence of viral infections is higher during induction or relapse compared with remission (Wood and Corbitt, 1985). In fact, it is tempting to postulate that the majority of unexplained febrile, neutropenic episodes are due to viral infections. However, significant viral infections have not been closely associated with neutropenia per se. Severe viral infections are generally restricted to children with defects in cell-mediated immunity.

Infection with herpes group viruses can be severe and even life threatening. Herpes virus group infections are either primary or secondary processes. Most children have a primary infection with HSV, VZV, and CMV early in life, followed by latency. Infection recurs because of reactivation of the latent virus, which can be caused by cancer, chemotherapy (including treatment with corticosteroids), transplantation, or HIV infection. For example, in patients with leukemia who are seropositive for HSV (indicating prior infection), clinically significant reactivation occurs frequently. Most develop HSV mucositis, but on occasion dissemination leads to hepatitis, encephalitis, and pneumonitis. In marrow-transplant recipients, HSV reactivation is a major problem, because it can complicate care of the mouth and inhibit adequate oral intake.

The danger of primary VZV was first recognized in children with leukemia, many of whom subsequently developed pneumonitis, encephalitis, hepatitis, Reye's syndrome, and purpura fulminans. The pretreatment mortality rate was 7% to 14% (Feldman et al., 1975). The reactivated form of VZV is zoster, also known as *shingles*. Recurrent VZV can cause painful skin lesions, usually restricted to adjacent dermatomes, but cutaneous dissemination occurs in about a quarter of patients, and, on occasion, visceral spread can occur and, if untreated, constitute a life-threatening event.

CMV has emerged as one of the major pathogens in immunoincompetent children, particularly those undergoing transplantation (either marrow or solid organ). Primary CMV frequently occurs in the healthy child and is generally not a significant infection. On the other hand, primary infection in the immunoincompetent child can quickly deteriorate into a life-threatening event. Even reactivation of CMV is associated with significant morbidity. Transplant centers take great care to prevent primary exposure; measures include strict hand washing, use of irradiated blood products, and determination of the serologic status of donor and recipient. Prophylactic antiviral strategies initially used acyclovir, but ganciclovir has assumed the central role in preemptive therapy

in bone marrow–transplant patients at risk for CMV disease (Balfour et al., 1989; Schmidt et al., 1991). Overall, morbidity and mortality has decreased, but infection still occurs, at a later time—usually after conclusion of the preemptive ganciclovir.

Common respiratory viral infections (e.g., respiratory syncytial virus [RSV] infections, parainfluenza, influenza, and adenovirus infections) can result in significant morbidity and mortality in immunoincompetent children. Outbreaks on pediatric oncology wards are common, calling attention to the importance of scrupulous adherence to infection control protocols during peak season for highly contagious respiratory viruses (Englund et al., 1991; Harrington et al., 1992; Whimbey et al., 1995). What begins as an upper respiratory tract infection with RSV or parainfluenza can quickly spread to the lower tract, followed by severe pneumonia. A number of centers have observed RSV pneumonia in marrow-transplant recipients, especially in the acute posttransplant period (Lujan-Zilbermann et al., 2001). Adenovirus can cause a serious primary infection, primarily of the respiratory tract, but in the marrow recipient, debilitating hemorrhagic cystitis can be difficult to manage (Foster and Chanock, 2000). These trends underscore the importance of improved diagnostic techniques, which include rapid test kits and culture technologies. However, the diagnostic advances have not been matched by effective, new antiviral agents.

Fungal Infections

An increase in significant fungal infections has been observed in immunoincompetent children observed over the past 2 decades. Prolonged episodes of febrile neutropenia are associated with a high risk for fungal infection. In particular, the duration of neutropenia after initiation of antibiotics is a major risk factor for an invasive mycosis in the cancer patient (Wiley et al., 1990). This trend is not surprising, because dose intensification strategies have induced deeper and longer bouts of neutropenia. Documented invasive mycosis generally occurs as a secondary infection event during periods of prolonged neutropenia. Repeated use of antibacterial therapy, often coupled with antineoplastic therapy, significantly alters the balance of GI and skin flora, probably providing an advantage for the growth of opportunistic fungi (e.g., *Candida* species). In marrow-transplant recipients, the pattern for fungal infections is bimodal—early candidal infection and later, postengraftment pulmonary infections primarily with *Aspergillus* species (Hovi et al., 2000; Wald et al., 1997).

Most fungal infections in children with cancer are caused by *Candida* species. *C. albicans* is a normal inhabitant of the GI or skin flora, but with disruption of mucosal surfaces, dissemination can develop and lead to eventual infection of distant sterile sites (e.g., eyes, liver, spleen, and kidneys) (Guiot et al., 1994). Children with leukemia or lymphoma are prone to develop chronic disseminated candidiasis, which can cause persistent fever in the neutropenic child and is difficult to diagnose. Recent trends indicate that species other than *C. albicans*, such as *Candida parapsilosis*, are on the rise (Levy et al., 1998). Some attribute this to the widespread use of prophylactic fluconazole therapy in transplant and intensively treated patients (Wingard, 1994). Adding to this pressure is the chronic use of fluconazole for oropharyngeal candidiasis, a major problem in children with HIV-1 infection and severe combined immunodeficiency.

The second most frequent fungal pathogen is *Aspergillus* (Patterson et al., 2000) Although *Aspergillus fumigatus* is the most worrisome, other *Aspergillus* species can cause disease in immunoincompetent children; for instance, children with CGD develop infection with *Aspergillus niger*, *Aspergillus flavus*, and *Aspergillusterreus*. Many of the dangerous fungal pathogens are not normal microbial flora. Because *Aspergillus* invades the respiratory tract, nasal cultures have been studied and shown to have modest value (Aisner et al., 1979; Horvath and Dummer, 1996); some centers still make use of surveillance cultures, but the cost and efficacy are debatable. *Aspergillus* infection can be associated with nosocomial acquisition or environmental exposure. For example, *Aspergillus* outbreaks have been associated with aerosolization of spores during nearby construction. Extensive playing or gardening in mulch beds is not recommended, because of the risk for inhalation of spores.

Disturbing new trends suggest that additional fungi are on the increase in immunoincompetent children (see Table 17-3) (Groll and Walsh, 2001). For instance, outbreaks of *Fusarium* and *Trichosporon* species have been reported in the hospital setting. Infection with Zygomycetes and the dematiaceous molds have serious sequelae; because they are difficult to diagnose, treatment is often initiated late and the prognosis guarded. Recent evidence has suggested that *Fusarium*, a pathogen whose appearance is on the rise, might be water borne, with sources both in and out of the hospital. Therefore, the identification of one or more cases should prompt investigation (Anaissie et al., 2001).

It is also notable that endemic mycoses can be a major problem, particularly in children with an acquired immunodeficiency. Reactivation of any one of the following can complicate therapy: *C. neoformans*, *H. capsulatum*, *Coccidioides immitis*, and *Blastomyces dermatitidis*. However, it is important to be aware of the geographic distribution of endemic mycosis.

P. carinii was initially recognized as an opportunistic pulmonary pathogen in young immunoincompetent children suffering from severe malnutrition. Ribosomal RNA sequencing suggests that it should be classified with fungi, and not parasites, though some still dispute this conclusion (Edman et al., 1988). Nearly all children are exposed to *P. carinii* in the first years of life. Primary infection occurs in young children with HIV-1 infection or primary immunodeficiencies and in infants undergoing therapy for cancer. It is characterized by a high burden of cysts and carries a poorer prognosis in the very young, but with early diagnosis, preventive measures, and treatment, survival has improved (Centers for Disease Control and Prevention, 1995). In older children with cancer or HIV-1 infection, nearly all cases of PCP represent reactivation of infection (Grubman and Simonds, 1996). *P. carinii* infection can arise in children with cell-mediated immune deficits; in the preprophylaxis era, it was most commonly diagnosed during maintenance therapy in children with acute lymphoblastic leukemia (Hughes et al., 1977).

Parasitic Infections

Parasitic infections are rare in children with cancer who do not reside in an endemic area. Recent trends indicate an increase in the incidence of *Cryptosporidium* species in children attending day care, but outbreaks on the pediatric oncology ward are unusual. Infection with *Toxoplasma gondii* is distinctly rare in children, even among children with HIV-1 infection.

Severe infection with *Strongyloides stercoralis* occurs in conjunction with adult T-cell leukemia and human T-lymphotropic virus 1 infection, both of which are occasionally observed in adolescents living in the United States.

DIAGNOSTIC CONSIDERATIONS

Advances in the diagnostic modalities for evaluating the febrile neutropenic child have lead to earlier identification of infection, but they have not substantially altered the likelihood of finding a pathogen (Box 17-1). A site of infection is determined in roughly one third of pediatric oncology patients with fever and neutropenia. Because of the severe consequences of infection in a subset of the neutropenic child, fever should be investigated thoroughly in all children with neutropenia. Exceeding a threshold temperature of 38.5° C places the child at sufficiently high risk that prompt evaluation and hospitalization should occur. Even if a neutropenic child has three measured temperatures between 38.0° C and 38.4° C within a 24-hour period, admission and evaluation should take place. This algorithm, now codified for consistency in study designs, is driven by the experience of 30 years and the fact that there are no current highly sensitive markers (e.g., signs, symptoms, or measurements, namely, imaging or measured factors) for identifying the bacteremic child (Feld et al., 2002; Hughes et al., 1990; Hughes et al., 1997). For instance, in 1,001 febrile episodes that occurred in 324 pediatric and young adults, there were no reliable predictors for bacteremia (Pizzo et al., 1982b). The neutropenic child presents an added challenge to the clinician because inflammatory changes, often heralding infection, are notably depressed or absent, which is a particularly difficult problem if the neutropenia is profound (i.e., absolute neutrophil count less than 100).

The decision to admit a febrile, neutropenic child for treatment with antibiotics is based upon a presumed risk, one that can evolve over a short period of time. It is not a routine event, and treatment is initiated on the basis of information at the time of hospitalization (Box 17-1). However, the clinical status can rapidly change over hours to days, especially if the child remains neutropenic. Therefore, it is imperative that the child be evaluated twice a day and that particular attention be directed at serial examination of mucosal membranes and catheter sites. In many instances, modification of therapy is required because of isolation of a resistant organism or development of a site of infection.

At the time of admission for febrile neutropenia, two sets of blood cultures should be obtained before initiation of antibiotics and, if a CVC is present, all lumens should be sampled. Blood analysis should include serum electrolyte level and hepatic and renal function tests, which can be useful for monitoring organ dysfunction or toxicity related to medications. The administration of some antibiotics, such as the aminoglycosides or amphotericin B preparations, frequently alters renal function and therefore merits close monitoring. A chest radiograph is critical for monitoring care, because infiltrates can develop as neutropenia resolves.

For the majority of febrile episodes in nonneutropenic cancer patients, infection is the presumed cause of fever, but again in only a third is a source identified. Other reasons for fever include side effects of cytotoxic chemotherapy or supportive care drugs (e.g., antibiotics, such as vancomycin and phenytoin) and the underlying malignancy. Fever due to tumor burden occurs classically in children with leukemia. Nearly 50% of children experience significant fever at the time of presentation for diagnosis, but by the time maintenance therapy begins, tumor fever probably occurs less frequently (Nakamura et al., 2000). Evaluation should include consideration of common pediatric problems (e.g., otitis media, streptococcal pharyngitis). In the nonneutropenic child, empiric therapy should be reserved for high-risk situations, namely, the presence of a CVC or an internal prosthesis. After drawing blood cultures through each lumen, treatment with intravenous antibiotics can be administered on an inpatient or occasionally on an outpatient basis, with clear directives for follow-up. Infection of the implanted prostheses can be very difficult to eradicate and often requires surgical débridement and replacement.

New imaging techniques (e.g., computed tomography [CT] and magnetic resonance imaging [MRI]) have improved the ability to diagnose pneumonia or deep fungal infections, such as hepatosplenic candidiasis, at an earlier stage, particularly in the neutropenic child

---

BOX 17-1

DIAGNOSTIC EVALUATION OF FEBRILE, NEUTROPENIC CHILD

Initial Approach

History of recent exposures and activities
Complete examination, including oral, perirectal, and catheter-insertion sites
Blood tests
    Complete blood count
    Serum electrolyte levels
    Hepatic and renal function tests
Microbiologic analysis
    Blood cultures
        If central venous catheter is present, obtain culture specimen from each lumen
        If no catheter is present, perform peripheral blood cultures
    Urine culture
    Nasopharyngeal specimen
        Perform rapid-detection and culture techniques for common respiratory viruses
Chest radiograph
Additional imaging as indicated
    Abdomen: CT, MRI, or ultrasound
    Sinus: Radiography or CT
    Chest: CT

Follow-up

Assessment of temperature every 4 hours
Daily examination, including oral and perirectal regions
Complete blood count
Repeat blood cultures (if temperature > 38°-38.5° C) at least once every 24 hours
    Sample all lumens if catheter in place
Repeat radiograph if pulmonary symptoms are present

CT, Computed tomography; *MRI*, magnetic resonance imaging.

(Archibald et al., 2001). Flexible bronchoscopy and CT or ultrasound-guided percutaneous biopsy can provide critical sampling for microbiologic confirmation. The diagnostic armamentarium of the laboratory has increased the spectrum of rapid-detection tests, and improvements in culture techniques have accelerated the efficiency and speed of the laboratory (Kaditis et al., 1996; Walsh and Chanock, 1998). One must proceed with great caution in performing invasive studies in neutropenic children; the risk for iatrogenic complications is high.

New techniques for sampling circulating sentinel markers for severe infection are under active investigation (Oude Nijhuis et al., 2002). Theoretically, surrogate markers, primarily, immune response proteins, can detect impending infection earlier. For many years, the C-reactive protein has been used as a surrogate for significant inflammation associated with bacterial infection. Unfortunately, its sensitivity and specificity are inadequate to determine whether or not to administer antibiotics. Novel markers are under active investigation, and the preliminary results are promising. Further studies are needed to validate their usefulness in the clinical setting. These include measurements of circulating levels of interleukin-6, interleukin-8, interleukin-1, mannose-binding lectin, or the soluble Fc gamma receptor type III (Lehrnbecher et al., 1999; Soker et al., 2001).

The technique of using frequent surveillance cultures to identify possible infection in neutropenic patients has been extensively investigated. The approach has been applied to children at high risk (e.g., those undergoing a marrow transplant) before the onset of fever and during supportive care for children with fever and neutropenia. The results have not demonstrated clinical utility for clinical care. Moreover, these cultures are expensive and cumbersome.

Stratification of Risk in Febrile Neutropenic Children

The last 30 years have taught us that there are differences in the risk for infection in neutropenic children based on the depth and duration of neutropenia and, to a lesser extent, other factors. For nearly a decade, the field has concentrated on schema for stratification of risk. The purpose is to define a set of a priori criteria that could be used to determine whether treatment with antibiotics should be initiated and, if so, where and what class of antibiotics should be given. Moreover, the strategy is intended to identify those with bacteremia at presentation, which can be done with high accuracy given current models and techniques (Pappo and Buchanan, 1991; Rackoff et al., 1996). It is safe to say that the astute clinician can generally recognize the high- and low-risk circumstances, but the predictive value of applying the proposed approach is still far from established (Pappo and Buchanan, 1991). Talcott and colleagues first proposed two groups based on risk (Talcott et al., 1988). High-risk adult cancer patients experienced more serious morbidity and mortality if they had one or more of the following: (1) hospitalization at the time of new fever and neutropenia; (2) comorbidity (e.g., cardiovascular instability, uncontrollable pain, respiratory distress); (3) relapse (Talcott et al., 1988). Patients without any of the three appeared to have a better outcome, but a minority of them still experienced serious complications. Follow-up analytical approaches have concentrated on economic factors, days in hospital, and duration of antibiotic therapy. Subsequent attempts to apply these criteria in adults and children have met with mixed success, mainly because of small numbers (Alexander et al., 2002; Bash et al., 1994; Griffin and Buchanan, 1992; Lucas et al., 1996; Mullen and Buchanan, 1990; Mullen et al., 1999;Talcott et al., 1994). Similar criteria have been applied to children at low risk, who were subsequently discharged early according to the following: (1) evidence of marrow recovery (e.g., increasing monocytes); (2) blood cultures with no growth; (3) no fever; (4) improvement in a localized site of infection; (5) capability for return if fever recurred (Buchanan, 1993).

A number of single-institution studies have demonstrated the applicability of identifying high- and low-risk pediatric patients, but, to date, no center has shown the utility of this in a prospective study (Klaassen et al., 2000a and b; Petrilli et al., 2000). It is notable that the issue of assessing low-risk candidates leads directly to two distinct study questions: the efficacy of oral therapy, and the administration of therapy on an outpatient basis. For the former, hospital studies have shown equivalency between oral and intravenous antibiotics, but the results of studies in the outpatient setting are less compelling (Talcott and Finberg, 1999; (Freifeld et al, 1999).

Empiric Antibiotic Therapy

The judicious use of empiric antibiotics in febrile, neutropenic children has substantially decreased morbidity and mortality. The initial approach embraced a strategy that targeted the most dangerous pathogens—gram-negative bacilli, particularly *P. aeruginosa*. The choice of antibiotics should be based on the need (1) to achieve high serum bactericidal levels, (2) to provide broad coverage for the most likely pathogens, (3) to accomplish this with minimal toxicity, and (4) to decrease the likelihood of selecting for resistant bacteria. Early intervention improves outcome in patients who are already bacteremic at the time of presentation and still may prevent dissemination of an occult infection (Rackoff et al., 1996). The success of this approach has been tempered by several developments: a shift toward gram-positive pathogens, the emergence of highly resistant gram-positive (e.g., VRE) and gram-negative bacilli, and a steady increase in the incidence of invasive fungal infections. Despite 30 years of refining the algorithm for approaching the febrile, neutropenic patient, mortality for all such patients still hovers around 2%.

Antibacterial Therapy

A number of antibiotic regimens have been proposed for initial empiric antibacterial therapy in the febrile, neutropenic child. The choice should take into account the activity against pathogens likely to be encountered in neutropenic children, such as gram-negative (including *P. aeruginosa*) and gram-positive (e.g., staphylococci and streptococci) bacilli. An additional factor for consideration is the recent institutional history of blood isolates and, specifically, their antibiotic susceptibility patterns. Because recent trends have suggested that incidences of resistant bacteria are increasing, it is important to be aware of local trends so that appropriate changes can be made in the choice of antibacterial therapy.

Currently, the standard of care is to initiate broad-spectrum antibacterial agents at the first sign of fever and neutropenia. Many studies have been published evaluating the safety, toxicity profile, and local experience with one or more antibiotics. Randomized controlled studies have been published that validate the importance of choosing either monotherapy (e.g., ceftazidime or imipenem) or a combination of two agents (e.g., a β-lactam and an aminoglycoside). The differences between monotherapy and combination therapy are not significant overall. In fact, the data demonstrate that the approaches are equal with respect to survival. Differences are restricted to toxicity profiles or the need to modify therapy. The Working Committee of the Infectious Diseases Society of America updated guidelines in 1997 for the study and use of antibiotics in neutropenic patients (Hughes et al., 1990; Hughes et al., 1997).

The use of combination therapy was the standard practice at most institutions until the late 1980s. In many institutions, combination therapy is the first-line choice for febrile, neutropenic children (Cordonnier et al., 1997; Fleischhack et al., 2001). Initially, an aminoglycoside was combined with a carboxypenicillin (e.g., carbenicillin and ticarcillin) or a ureidopenicillin penicillin (e.g., azlocillin and piperacillin) to provide double coverage for gram-negative bacilli and provide synergy against these pathogens (EORTC, 1993). Attempts to use either the carboxypenicillins or ureidopenicillins alone were met with failure because of the rapid emergence of resistant organisms. Similarly, in the neutropenic patient, aminoglycoside monotherapy is also inadequate, because clinical and microbiologic failures frequently occur. Administration of aminoglycosides requires careful monitoring of serum levels to reduce renal toxicity, but even this has been simplified by the shift toward single-dose daily aminoglycoside therapy (Postovsky et al., 1997). If an aminoglycoside is to be used, the selection should be based on local antibiotic susceptibility patterns.

Monotherapy with either a third-generation cephalosporin (e.g., ceftazidime, cefepime and cefoperazone) or the carbapenem (e.g., imipenem-cilastatin and meropenem) has become a standard of care in many institutions (Chuang et al., 2002; Freifeld et al., 1995; Mustafa et al., 2001; Pizzo et al., 1986). In fact, a metaanalysis of ceftazidime studies concluded that it is equivalent to combination therapy (Sanders et al., 1992). In large, randomized studies, patients receiving monotherapy required more frequent modifications in therapy, especially if neutropenia lasted longer than 1 week. Monotherapy should be given judiciously, with full recognition of possible problems and complications. Caution should be used in choosing ceftazidime if there is a high incidence of infection with *Enterobacter* species and *Serratia* species (Chow et al., 1991); resistance to ceftazidime has been noted during therapy. Similarly, monotherapy with imipenem should not be used to treat *P. aeruginosa* because of the high likelihood of the development of resistance during therapy. In the National Cancer Institute randomized study comparing imipenem-cilastatin and ceftazidime, there was no clear difference in outcome, but a higher number of patients than expected in the imipenem group required modification of antibiotics secondary to nausea or diarrhea (Freifeld et al., 1995). Imipenem also lowers the seizure threshold in patients with central nervous system (CNS) disease (Karadeniz et al., 2000). The newer carbapenem, meropenem, has comparable efficacy to imipenem but a lower incidence of adverse effects (Boogaerts et al., 1995).

Combination oral therapy has been studied in hospitalized low-risk patients. Combinations of ciprofloxacin and ampicillin/sulbactam was found to be equivalent to intravenous ceftazidime (Freifeld et al., 1999). In the pediatric setting, single institution studies have confirmed the approach (Klaassen et al., 2000a and b). Other studies have reported similar success as continuation therapy (Park et al., 2003). Oral monotherapy, particularly with fluoroquinolones, has been investigated with mixed results (Bayston et al., 1989). Despite the initial enthusiasm for this class of antibiotics, it has not become the standard of care because of frequent breakthrough bacteremia and an association with the alpha-streptococci syndrome.

In response to the observed increase in gram-positive blood isolates, clinical studies turned toward evaluating vancomycin as part of the initial therapy for fever and neutropenia. The rationale was first proposed for children with an indwelling catheter or prosthesis only, but the studies have not conclusively supported this position. A retrospective analysis of 550 episodes of gram-positive bacteremias at the National Cancer Institute concluded that vancomycin can be reserved until a gram-positive bacteria is isolated and the antibiotic susceptibility pattern requires its use (e.g., for treatment of most coagulase-negative staphylococci) (Rubin et al., 1988). Overall, outcome was not adversely affected by waiting. Currently, there are insufficient data to recommend widespread use of vancomycin as part of first-line empiric therapy (Chanock and Pizzo 1996; Koya et al., 1998). The emergence of resistant gram-positive organisms (e.g., methicillin-resistant staphylococci and penicillin- and cephalosporin-resistant alpha-streptococci) in some institutions has challenged this view (Bruckner et al., 2002). The danger of providing empiric vancomycin to all febrile, neutropenic patients is that many are treated unnecessarily and the approach adds further selective pressure for the emergence of VRE (Adcock et al., 1999; Lin et al., 2000). Empiric vancomycin is appropriate in certain circumstances, such as in centers with a high incidence of alpha-streptococci or methicillin-resistant staphylococci or in patients with an internal prosthesis. In some centers, teicoplanin, which has a favorable toxicity profile and similar activity against gam-positive organisms, has been used and carries a similar risk for emergence of resistance (Sidi et al., 2000). In the febrile, neutropenic patient with cardiovascular instability, vancomycin should be considered in combination with an aminoglycoside and either a carbapenem or extended spectrum β-lactam.

New antibacterial agents have been developed to combat the increase in highly resistant gram-positive bacteria. Two new agents (e.g., quinupristin-dalfopristin and linezolid) have shown some promise, but this has been tempered by recent reports of resistance developing with therapy. Quinupristin-dalfopristin is a streptogramin, and has activity against vancomycin-resistant *E. faecium* but not E. *faecalis*; it also has activity against methicillin-resistant staphylococci and penicillin-resistant streptococci, but little effectiveness against gram-negative bacilli (Eliopoulos, 2003). Linezolid has an excellent bioavailability pro-

file, permitting oral therapy in some cases. Its activity is against both types of enterococci, but the emergence of resistant organisms with therapy has been reported. Extended-spectrum quinolones (e.g., clinafloxacin and trovofloxacin) have also been used anecdotally to treat resistant enterococci (Zaman et al., 1996).

Empiric Antifungal Therapy

The neutropenic child with persistent or recurrent fever despite broad-spectrum antibiotic therapy is at high risk for invasive fungal infection. Empiric therapy with a broad-spectrum antifungal antibiotic provides early therapy for clinically occult infection. Because the risk for serious infection persists with prolonged febrile neutropenia, empiric antifungal therapy can also provide prophylaxis against further infection in the high-risk setting (Pizzo et al., 1982a). At the first sign of new fever, or persistent fever, after 4 to 7 days, systemic antifungal therapy is begun, even if the patient had been receiving oral antifungal prophylaxis (EORTC, 1989). This approach has been embraced because of the high risk, estimated to be between 9% and 31% (EORTC, 1989; Pizzo et al., 1982a; Wiley et al., 1990).

Until recently, the best choice was desoxycholate amphotericin B administered at 0.5 mg/kg/day, which is sufficient for most *Candida* species, but not *Aspergillus* species or *Candida tropicalis*. Documented infection with these organisms should be treated with higher doses. The azoles, itraconazole and fluconazole, have been investigated in cancer and transplant patients; studies have not provided a strong rationale for using either of these agents, except in special circumstances (Boogaerts et al., 2001; Winston et al., 2000). The toxicity profile of amphotericin B is significant and includes problems with renal function and infusion-related complications (e.g., fever and chills), which can make the assessment of the already febrile, neutropenic patient more complex. New lipid formulations of amphotericin B have been approved for empiric antifungal therapy (Prentice et al., 1997; Walsh et al., 1999c); they are notable for decreased renal and infusional toxicity (Walsh et al., 1999b and c; Wong-Beringer et al., 1998). The data indicate comparable efficacy, but considerably less toxicity and a decrease in breakthrough fungal infections (Walsh et al., 1999c; Walsh et al., 2001). Indeed, the lipid formulations can be given in higher doses, which can be beneficial with infections that are difficult to treat (e.g., *Aspergillus* infection of the respiratory tract) (Walsh et al., 2001).

New antifungal agents, with more favorable toxicity profiles and extended spectrum of activity that includes *Aspergillus* have recently been approved. In a randomized study, a novel broad-spectrum triazole, voriconazole has comparable efficacy, but fewer proved and probable breakthrough infections and less toxicity, both infusional and renal (Walsh et al., 2002b). Already, it is widely used in many centers with comparable success. Voriconazole can be given orally or by intravenous route (Walsh et al., 2002a and b). It causes a unique toxicity, transient visual disturbances, and hallucinations. Voriconazole is related to the other triazoles (e.g., fluconazole and itraconazole), which have been used successfully in preventive strategies and treatment for many *Candida* species and *C. neoformans* infections. The echinocandins are a new class of antifungal agents with an excellent spectrum of activity and a favorable toxicity profile (Groll and Walsh, 2001). In a large, randomized study, caspofungin is at least as effective as amphotericin B for the treatment of invasive candidiasis (Mora-Duarte et al., 2002). New antifungal agents with excellent activity against *Aspergillus* and most *Candida* species represent a major development in the treatment of children with invasive fungal infections (Groll and Walsh, 2001). Because of the favorable toxicity profiles, it will be possible to treat patients earlier and perhaps change the approach toward empiric therapy and prophylaxis.

LENGTH AND MODIFICATION OF THERAPY

The decision to use empiric antibiotics raises a series of questions as to when to start, modify, and terminate antibiotic therapy. The first step in administering empiric antibiotics is to initiate broad coverage, taking into consideration specific findings and exposures. This phase lasts until the pretreatment cultures are available, at which time the clinical status of the patient is assessed over several days. It must be emphasized that once a neutropenic child is febrile, there is a substantial risk for further infectious events, such as progression or a secondary event. Empiric antibiotics do not protect the patient with persistent neutropenia

from secondary infections, which can be selected for by broad-spectrum antibiotic therapy. Institutions have advocated using vancomycin after 2 or 3 days of persistent fever, but this approach lacks supporting evidence and is strongly discouraged. Modification of therapy is required in many patients and constitutes a critical factor in the overall success of treatment (see Table 17-2). Usually antibiotic changes are made in response to the isolation of a pathogen or the recognition of a new site of infection (e.g., pneumonia or cellulitis). Close observation, both in hospital and after discharge, is necessary. It is worth noting that recurrent fever in the neutropenic child requires immediate evaluation and resumption of therapy (Jones et al., 1994).

If a pathogen or clinical site is defined, treatment should extend for as long as would be required to treat the infection in a nonneutropenic host *or* until resolution of neutropenia has been achieved. If there is any question, the longer duration is recommended. Termination of antibiotics for a defined focus of infection while the patient is still neutropenic creates high risk and is associated with relapse or progression of the primary infection. If a pathogen is isolated in a febrile neutropenic child, broad-spectrum antibiotic coverage should be continued until recovery of neutrophils is achieved, because the risk for subsequent infections does not subside until this point.

In low-risk patients with fever of unexplained origin who become afebrile within 72 to 96 hours and have no growth on pretreatment cultures, many physicians have advocated discontinuation of empiric antibiotics. A number of alternative approaches have been advocated for patients before full recovery of bone marrow has been achieved, including conversion to simplified intravenous antibiotics (e.g., daily ceftriaxone and amikacin in Europe), switch to oral antibiotics, or discontinuation of all therapy (EORTC, 1993). A number of publications have examined low-risk populations from single institutions. The safety of early discharge applies to most but not all patients. For example, in one study, nearly 10% of children required rehospitalization. Although many have embraced this approach, a large randomized study has yet to establish its equivalency or advantage over oral antibiotics administered in the hospital (Freifeld et al., 1999; Talcott and Finberg, 1999). Critical issues in monitoring, follow-up, and compliance make this difficult to study across institutions.

Duration of treatment should be longer in high-risk patients, especially those with comorbidity or expected prolonged feuer neutropenia (e.g., aplastic anemia). In patients who do not recover neutrophil counts within 7 to 10 days, a similar approach can be applied to the uncomplicated child with negative cultures and no evidence for prolonged fever; discontinue and observe closely. It is notable that the average time to defervescence in three large, randomized fever and neutropenia studies at the National Cancer Institute was about 3 days after initiation of empiric therapy. It has been demonstrated that discontinuing antibiotics after 7 days of empiric therapy in patients who remain febrile and neutropenic is associated with serious sequelae (Pizzo et al., 1979). The child with aplastic anemia represents a vexing problem. Duration of treatment for established bacterial infection should extend at least 7 days after the patient becomes afebrile. For fungal infections, the duration of therapy is long and should be determined by the clinical response to extended therapy.

PREVENTIVE STRATEGIES FOR THE NEUTROPENIC CHILD

Ever since the relationship between therapy-induced neutropenia and severe infection was recognized, deliberate strategies have been investigated to prevent infection by isolation measures, immunization strategies, and antibiotic prophylaxis. The rationale has been to suppress colonizing flora, which are responsible for the majority of serious infections. In the transplant setting, partial protection from infection has been achieved through cumbersome and expensive intervention, including complete isolation with laminar air flow, dietary restrictions, sterilization of all entering items, and use of oral nonabsorbable antibiotics. Otherwise, there are insufficient data to support the use of reverse isolation precautions or dietary manipulation on the pediatric oncology ward.

The use of prophylactic antibiotics to prevent bacterial infections in neutropenic patients has been extensively investigated. Two strategies have been employed to "globally" decontaminate the GI tract: the use of nonabsorbable antibiotics, and, more recently, the use of systemic fluoroquinolones. No discernible advantage has been demonstrated with nonabsorbable antibiotics. Furthermore, combinations of nonabsorbable antibiotics (e.g., vancomycin, polymyxin, gentamicin, and nystatin) are poorly tolerated and increase the risk for selecting resistant bacteria. Compliance is also a major problem in children, particularly because the preparations are unpalatable and have to be taken several times a day. Both nonabsorbable and systemic antibiotics are associated with significant GI side effects, such as diarrhea, cramps, and abdominal pain. Still, some centers use nonabsorbable antibiotics as part of an overall strategy to decontaminate both the environment and the patient during marrow transplantation. Previously, a series of studies evaluated the broad-spectrum antibacterial agent trimethoprim-sulfamethoxazole (TMP-SMX) but failed to demonstrate efficacy in the prevention of infection in the neutropenic host. Fluoroquinolones have been investigated because of their favorable bioavailability profile and activity against aerobic gram-negative organisms. The results have been mixed in neutropenic cancer patients. The number of infections caused by gram-negative bacteria can be reduced slightly, but the incidence of fever with neutropenia and intravenous antibiotic use was not affected significantly (Dekker et al., 1987; Karp et al., 1987). Long-term use of fluoroquinolones has been associated with the emergence of resistant gram-positive and gram-negative bacteria. In addition, prophylactic use of fluoroquinolones increases the risk for infection with α-hemolytic streptococci, especially in children receiving intensive cytosine arabinoside with severe mucositis. Because of this concern, the addition of penicillin or rifampin to a fluoroquinolone has been advocated to counter this trend. Many transplant centers choose to give fluoroquinolones, sometimes with penicillin or rifampin, if α-hemolytic streptococci have been a problem in the institution. This strategy is not recommended for children undergoing chemotherapy because of a paucity of data to support its general use.

There are several notable examples of the successful use of prophylactic antibiotics for select pathogens. TMP-SMX is effective in preventing PCP in children at risk (e.g., children with HIV-1 infection, those undergoing intensive therapy for leukemia, and solid tumor- and postengraftment marrow-transplant recipients) (Grubman and Simonds, 1996; Hughes et al.,

1977). Since the first report of successful chemoprophylaxis against PCP, further studies have shown that intermittent administration is protective and rarely interferes with antileukemic therapy (Hughes et al., 1977; Hughes et al., 1987). Similarly, the use of acyclovir reduces the incidence of recurrent HSV disease in patients receiving intensive chemotherapy or a marrow transplant (Saral et al., 1981). Acyclovir has little in vitro activity against CMV, yet it has been shown to reduce CMV infection in both marrow and renal transplant recipients (Balfour et al., 1989; Meyers et al., 1988). Ganciclovir has better activity against CMV and predictably has replaced acyclovir as the antiviral agent of choice for CMV prophylaxis in solid organ and marrow transplantation (Goodrich et al., 1994; Meyers et al., 1988; Schmidt et al., 1991). The use of preventive ganciclovir in marrow recipients has delayed the bulk of serious CMV infection to after 100 days, coincidentally the time for discontinuation of therapy.

Because of the emergence of invasive fungal infections as a major challenge in immunoincompetent children, the use of prophylactic antifungal agents has been extensively investigated. The use of systemic antifungal prophylaxis with the oral azole fluconazole has been shown to decrease fungal colonization and infection in adult marrow-transplant recipients in two randomized studies (Goodman et al., 1992; Marr et al., 2000; Slavin et al., 1993). This paradigm has been successfully applied to children undergoing marrow transplantation with comparable results. The data are less compelling for fluconazole or itraconazole prophylaxis in children receiving chemotherapy for leukemia or solid tumors (Menichetti et al., 1999; Rotstein et al., 1999; Winston et al., 1993). Even in the transplant setting, this intervention comes at the expense of the emergence of fungal pathogens that are less common and more difficult to treat (e.g., *Candida glabrata, Candida krusei*, and *Aspergillus* species) (Marr et al., 2000; Wingard et al., 1991). Fluconazole and itraconazole have also been used to successfully manage recurrent oral thrush, a major problem in children with HIV infection. Lastly, new agents, such as the new triazole (e.g., voriconazole) or an echinocandin (e.g., caspofungin) have shown promise for prophylaxis in the high-risk setting, (e.g., marrow trans-

plantation), but further studies are required (Walsh, 2002a).

IMMUNIZATION

Worldwide, the strategy of active immunization has dramatically reduced the burden of serious diseases, such as pertussis, measles, and *H. influenzae* type b infection. In the immuno-incompetent child, any one of these infections can be severe and life threatening. Because most children receive routine immunizations prior to the onset of immunosuppression, the dilemma of whether to administer booster injections is not difficult. Vaccines that are not attenuated can be given—for instance, booster diphtheria, tetanus, and pertussis can be given, but with the caveat that a partial response is expected. Generally, live attenuated vaccines (e.g., measles, mumps, and rubella) are contraindicated for the immunoincompetent child. Because the oral, live attenuated polio vaccine is no longer regularly recommended, there are no restrictions on vaccines given to healthy family members. The two exceptions to the restriction on live attenuated vaccines are the use of varicella-zoster vaccine in children receiving cancer therapy and measles in children with HIV-1 infection (American Academy of Pediatrics, 2000; Gershon et al., 1989). Measles, mumps, and rubella vaccine can be given to children with leukemia who are in remission more than 3 months after conclusion of chemotherapy. However, the overall immune status should be considered in the coordination with chemotherapy schedule. Children who undergo an allogeneic marrow transplant require reimmunization with all vaccines. They should be considered unimmunized and receive vaccines on schedule beginning at least 1 or 2 years after completion of therapy and in the absence of graft-versus-host disease. In the interim, many experts recommend use of passive immunization in high-risk settings (see below).

Lastly, routine immunizations, particularly with live-attenuated viral vaccines can be dangerous to young children with primary immunodeficiencies, particularly those characterized by significant cell-mediated defects. In fact, severe, adverse reactions can lead to establishment of the diagnosis. For instance, severe infection following administration of BCG, an attenuated vaccine, has been associated with an inherited defect in the interferon-γ or interleukin-12 pathways (Doffinger et al., 2002).

Passive immunization is a strategy for preventing serious infection in the immunoincompetent child. The history of administration of pooled serum immunoglobulins is closely linked to the successful management of hypogammaglobulinemic and agammaglobulinemic conditions. Regular use of immunoglobulin preparations has had a substantial impact on the care of children and adults with inherited immunodeficiencies. The lessons learned from this experience have readily been applied to other immunoincompetent children, such as those infected with HIV-1, those who have received marrow transplants, and those undergoing intensive chemotherapy. For these conditions, minimal published data are available to support intervention, particularly in children undergoing cancer chemotherapy.

Hyperimmune globulin, specific for a pathogen, has become an important component of the management of select infections, namely, VZV, CMV, and possibly RSV infection (especially in the marrow-transplant recipient). It is notable that pooled serum immunoglobulins contain high titers of antibodies to common viruses, such as adenovirus, CMV, measles, and RSV. Consequently, some experts recommend the use of hyperimmune globulin for prevention and treatment in the severely compromised host (e.g., allogeneic marrow-transplant recipient) (Reed et al., 1989). CMV immune globulin has been successfully used to manage discordant donor-recipient pairs in solid organ transplants (e.g., renal transplantation). Its application in marrow-transplant recipients has been widely embraced, and small studies have shown a benefit for either CMV globulin or pooled immunoglobulin therapy, given throughout the period of highest risk (e.g., immediate posttransplantation period) (Goodrich et al., 1994). It is notable that there are no controlled studies to support this intervention for the other viruses mentioned above. For instance, immunoincompetent children may benefit from administration of pooled human immune globulin during a community outbreak of measles.

Varicella-zoster immune globulin (VZIG) is used to contain outbreaks of VZV in immunoincompetent children and can be used to decrease morbidity and mortality in seronegative children. The timing of administration is critical; protection can be achieved if VZIG is administered within 72 to 96 hours of exposure, and protection lasts for 3 weeks. Further exposure after 3 weeks requires repetition of VZIG. Unlike the pooled immunoglobulin preparations, VZIG is administered intramuscularly. On occasion, commercial preparations of pooled immunoglobulins can be substituted for VZIG, when it is unavailable, or intramuscular therapy is contraindicated.

The generation of recombinant antibodies to specific pathogens or mediators of inflammation and sepsis represent exciting new additions to the therapeutic armamentarium. So far, a humanized form of a monoclonal antibody to RSV has shown great promise for prevention and in some cases, ameliorating treatment of pneumonia in the young at risk child. Current data support its use for RSV in high-risk premature infants. Experience with palivizumab has been extrapolated to high-risk older children (e.g., recipients of transplants, both solid and marrow; cardiac surgery patients; and, possibly, recipients of intensive chemotherapy) (Boeckh et al., 2001). Further studies are needed to determine the indications for using this therapy in high-risk children. Similarly, monoclonal antibodies directed against different components of bacteria or the host response (i.e., tumor necrosis factor or interleukin-1) have shown great promise, but definitive studies are needed before this therapy can be accepted as first-line therapy for sepsis.

RECOMBINANT GROWTH FACTORS AND CYTOKINES

A major advance in the supportive care of children with neutropenia is the development of recombinant hematopoietic growth factors. Two recombinant growth factors, granulocyte-macrophage colony-stimulating factor (GM-CSF) and granulocyte colony-stimulating factor (G-CSF), have been evaluated in clinical trials involving cancer and bone marrow–transplant patients. Both G-CSF and GM-CSF can accelerate granulopoiesis (resulting in a shortening of neutropenia) and augment microbicidal activity. G-CSF and GM-CSF delay neutrophil apoptosis (e.g., programmed cell death), resulting in a prolongation of the circulating half-life of neutrophils, which is critical in patients recovering from myeloablative therapy (Colotta et al., 1992). They also rapidly mobilize neutrophils for collection in anticipation of granulocyte transfusion, a modality that is once again used for profoundly neutropenic children with life-threatening infection (Bensinger et al., 1993; Cesaro et al., 2003; Chanock and Gorlin, 1996). G-CSF mobilized granulocyte transfusion therapy has also been used in children with aplastic anemia, because of an inability to recover neutrophils, and in CGD, to supplement qualitatively defective neutrophils. However, in both circumstances, it is reserved for particularly difficult cases (Stroncek et al., 1996). In addition, G-CSF mobilizes peripheral CD34 hematopoietic stem cells in sufficient quantity for marrow transplantation. The toxicity profiles for G-CSF and GM-CSF differ little; both can cause fever, myalgia, bone pain, and headache. In rare circumstances, children can develop a polyserositis with capillary leak syndrome.

Both G-CSF and GM-CSF have been widely used in oncology and marrow-transplant patients. In fact, some would argue that these expensive agents have been overused, even in the pediatric setting (Parsons et al., 2000). The American Society for Clinical Oncology has regularly convened a blue-ribbon panel to review the literature and recommend guidelines for use of G-CSF and GM-CSF (Box 17-2) (American Society of Clinical Oncology, 1994; American Society of Clinical Oncology, 1996). Use of these factors should be reserved for one of the following indications: (1) prevention of serious infection during chemotherapy-induced neutropenia of long duration in patients who are at high risk (estimated incidence ≥40% or a previous history of severe infection during neutropenia); (2) acceleration of neutrophil recovery in the treatment of an invasive fungal or bacterial infection in a profoundly neutropenic child; (3) stimulation of a donor for either marrow transplantation or granulocyte transfusion. G-CSF has been shown to decrease the incidence of febrile neutropenic episodes by about half in high-risk patients (i.e., in which the incidence of fever and neutropenia was at least 40% in the control group). In most studies, although not all, the use of preventive G-CSF or GM-CSF resulted in decreased hospitalizations and use of antibiotics, but there is little evidence to demonstrate a survival advantage or improved tumor response rate with use of these agents. There is no evidence to support the initiation of G-CSF or GM-CSF in the neutropenic oncology patient who is admitted for fever and neutropenia. In vitro, these agents enhance the microbicidal activity of neutrophils and monocytes, but the clinical importance of these observations is still unclear (Roilides et al., 2003). Nonetheless, many experts recommend their use in profoundly neutropenic children with life-threatening infection. Lastly, G-CSF and GM-CSF have proved to be beneficial in children with agranulocytosis (Kostmann's syndrome) and acquired severe neutropenia (either aplastic anemia or autoimmune neutropenia); long-term use sustains neutrophil counts at higher circulating levels and thereby decreases serious infectious complications.

BOX 17-2

RECOMMENDED USE OF RECOMBINANT HEMATOPOIETIC GROWTH FACTORS IN CHILDREN WITH CANCER

Prevention of infectious episodes in high-risk setting
    Begin administration shortly after completion of chemotherapy
    Continue until recovery of peripheral neutrophils is achieved
Adjunct therapy for documented, life-threatening infection (limited data)
    Rationale:
        Augment host defense
        Accelerate recovery of neutrophils
Mobilization of blood products
    Granulocytes from allogeneic donor
    Mobilization of CD34+ stem cells—allogeneic or autologous transplantation

CLINICAL SYNDROMES IN THE FEBRILE, NEUTROPENIC CHILD WITH CANCER
Pulmonary Infiltrates in the Immunoincompetent Child

The most common site of infection in the neutropenic child is the lung (Neville et al., 2002). Between the spectrum of pathogens and variability in radiographic findings, the clinician faces a formidable set of diagnostic and therapeutic challenges. In many instances, neutropenia can mask inflammation, resulting in a delay in the radiographic appearance of pneumonia. Recent advances in CT technology and flexible bronchoscopy, coupled with improved laboratory diagnostics are critical additions for evaluation of a child with respiratory symptoms (Walsh et al., 1999a). Upper respiratory tract symptoms can mask more serious lower tract disease. Consequently, induced sputum and bronchoscopy are sometimes indicated, even if the radiograph appears "normal." Early intervention translates into improved outcome, further supporting the need to aggressively investigate respiratory complaints, however, insignificant they appear at first.

Pneumonia in the immunoincompetent child can be divided into two major categories, focal and interstitial, both of which can evolve during and after neutropenia (Walsh et al, 1999a). The algorithms developed for the investigation and treatment of pneumonia are complex and require regular examination and repeat radiographs, primarily because lower tract disease can progress quickly in this setting.

The approach for treatment of the neutropenic child with a focal pulmonary infiltrate at the onset of fever is not significantly different from that for treatment of the nonneutropenic child. Empiric treatment should be initiated with broad-spectrum antibiotics that are effective against the common pediatric bacterial pathogens (e.g., *S. pneumoniae*, *H. influenzae*, *Chlamydia* species, and *Mycoplasma* species) and also against hospital-acquired gram-negative bacilli (e.g., *Klebsiella* species, *P. aeruginosa*, and *E. coli*). Antibiotics used for empiric therapy for fever and neutropenia are suitable for focal infiltrates, but an additional macrolide (e.g., erythromycin or azithromycin) should be considered to provide adequate coverage for "atypicals," which, on occasion, can include *Legionella* species. If the infiltrates progress despite antibacterial therapy, further diagnostic evaluation is necessary to investigate the possibility of infection with *Mycobacterium* species, *Nocardia* species, or invasive mycoses.

The presence of diffuse interstitial infiltrates in an immunoincompetent child calls for immediate evaluation. The differential diagnosis includes common respiratory pathogens, *Legionella* species, *Mycoplasma* species, and *P. carinii* in children not on a prophylactic regimen. PCP has nearly been eliminated in pediatric oncology patients with intermittent TMP-SMX therapy. Still, suspicion should be high, especially if there are issues related to compliance. In many instances, symptoms are not commensurate with radiographic changes. Common respiratory pathogens are often associated with upper respiratory tract symptoms (e.g., cough, congestion, coryza). A nasopharyngeal wash for respiratory viruses (e.g., RSV, parainfluenza, and influenza) should be performed. On the other hand, PCP often presents with a fever, dry cough, and significant hypoxemia but minimal radiographic changes. There should be a low threshold for performing an induced sputum examination to look for cysts. If both studies are not diagnostic, bronchoscopy should be considered. In nonneutropenic hosts with interstitial infiltrates who are unable to undergo bronchoscopy, an empiric trial of TMP-SMX and erythromycin should be considered.

Of the possible common respiratory viruses identified by nasopharyngeal wash, treatment is available for RSV. Marrow recipients are at high risk for fatal progression of RSV, the initial manifestation of which can involve upper respiratory symptoms, but which quickly can move into the lower tracts. The use of aerosolized ribavirin combined with immunoglobulin therapy (see prior discussion) has been used successfully in high-risk children (Boeckh et al., 2001). CMV pneumonitis occurs only in transplant recipients, and usually as either a reactivation post transplant or a primary infection. CMV can be isolated from a bronchoscopy by culture or pathologic evaluation of collected material. In some circumstances, the presence of a new interstitial infiltrate in a child with CMV antigenemia is sufficient evidence to begin treatment with either ganciclovir or foscarnet and immunoglobulin therapy (Emmanuel et al., 1988; Reed et al., 1988).

New infiltrates occurring in patients on antibiotic therapy can be separated into two groups: those that occur as marrow recovery is evident, and those that occur in patients who remain neutropenic. Patients with new infiltrates occurring at the time of marrow recovery have an excellent prognosis and rarely have a new pathogen identified. New infiltrates occurring in the persistently neutropenic child are more likely to represent a fungal infection, which carries a poorer prognosis. Fever, dry cough, hemoptysis, or pleuritic chest pains are associated with invasive *Aspergillus* infection. On occasion, the radiographic appearance shows a halo of air within a focal lesion. CT studies are the best method for confirming the presence of multiple infiltrates and often pick up cavitary lesions missed on radiographs (Walsh, 1999a). Detection of *Aspergillus* species in the lower respiratory tract through analysis of sputa, tracheal aspirations, or bronchoalveolar lavage fluid should be considered diagnostic, and therapy should be instituted immediately (Horvath and Dummer, 1996). Percutaneous biopsy guided by CT or ultrasound provides confirmation of diagnosis but is often contraindicated because of bleeding problems (e.g., low platelets). *Aspergillus* species in the respiratory tract in the nonneutropenic patient can represent colonization (Yu et al., 1986).

INDWELLING VENOUS CATHETER–ASSOCIATED INFECTION

A major advance in the care of immunoincompetent children has been the use of indwelling CVCs, which can be inserted through the skin or subcutaneously implanted. The reliance on CVCs has greatly facilitated the administration of medications and blood products while simplifying the repeated sampling of blood for tests in children who otherwise have poor venous access. However, the use of a CVC carries a risk for two major categories of complications: infection and thrombosis. The rates of infectious complications vary among institutions, but the national average is approximately 7 per 1000 catheter-days (O'Grady et al., 2002). Factors that influence differences in these rates include insertion techniques, frequency of access and flushing, maintenance care of the line site, patient populations, and institutional colonization patterns. Still, the risk for bacteremia is as high as 30% for the lifetime of the inserted catheter. About 60% of bacteremias occur in neutropenic children, indicating that local factors are important. The estimated risk for developing a catheter-associated bacteremia in a nonneutropenic child is about one tenth of that observed in neutropenic children (Hiemenz

et al., 1986). Polymicrobial infection is rare but suggests substantial problems in the care of the catheter (e.g., poor hygiene or unprotected swimming or bathing).

There are three types of infection associated with indwelling CVCs. The most significant is a blood-borne catheter-associated infection (e.g. bacteremia or fungemia). In many circumstances, systemic treatment can be administered with the line left in place, but in some circumstances, the line has to be removed. The pathogenesis of catheter-associated bacteremia suggests that one of several predisposing events has occurred: migration of skin flora at the exit site of the catheter resulting in catheter tip infection; contamination of the access point; infection of the subcutaneously tunneled portion of the tubing; attachment to the catheter during transient bacteremia; or a contaminated infusate. The second most common site of infection is the insertion site, which can often be treated with systemic antibiotic therapy directed at common skin pathogens (e.g., streptococci and staphylococci). Infection at the site of insertion tracking along the subcutaneous course is less common and is frequently difficult to eradicate without removal of the line.

There are several factors that influence the decision to treat with intravenous antibiotics in an effort to preserve the indwelling CVC. These include the type(s) of pathogens isolated and the presence of simultaneous infections of the tunnel site and distant sites at the time of diagnosis. In addition, the overall need for a CVC should be considered and can influence the decision to remove the CVC. Overall, the majority of catheter-associated bacteremias are caused by gram-positive cocci (e.g., staphylococci and streptococci), which often colonize the skin; coagulase-negative *Staphylococcus* is the most frequent isolate (Das et al., 1997). However, the frequently hospitalized child is at greater risk for colonization with gram-negative bacilli, which are often resistant to commonly used broad-spectrum antibiotics. Catheter-related bacteremia without evidence of a tunnel infection can be successfully treated without removing the catheter. Shortly after initiation of appropriate antibiotic therapy, blood cultures should be repeated to document clearing of the bacteremia. Intravenous antibiotics should be infused through each lumen or port on a regular schedule. Regular antibiotic flushes can be given to ensure adequate levels throughout the lumen of the line but at this time are not routinely recommended (Henrickson et al., 2000; O'Grady et al., 2002). Removal of the catheter should be considered if any one of the following is observed: cardiac instability (e.g., hypotension; positive blood cultures drawn after 48 hours of therapy with appropriate antibiotics; or evidence of a large thrombosis). Isolation of any one of the following pathogens should warrant removal of the line because eradication is unlikely: fungal pathogens (e.g., *Candida, Trichosporon,* or *Fusarium* species); *Bacillus cereus*; or *Mycobacterium* species, especially if there is tunnel site involvement (Cotton et al, 1987; Eppes et al., 1989; Walsh et al., 1999a).

Local infection, particularly along the tunneling of the catheter, can be a significant problem. Often, the first indication is minor erythema, tenderness, or induration. Intravenous antibiotics should be administered and the clinical course closely monitored, because in many cases the line has to be removed. Infection restricted to the insertion site with no clear evidence of extension along the subcutaneous tract can be treated on an outpatient basis if the child is nonneutropenic, if there is minimal tenderness, and if there is no evidence of abscess formation (e.g., purulent discharge). However, in the neutropenic child, parenteral antibiotics are required to achieve sufficiently high levels at the site of infection. Although a minor exit site infection in a nonneutropenic child may respond to oral antibiotics, intravenous antibiotics are required when there is evidence of significant erythema, tenderness, or purulent discharge. Similarly, any evidence of infection at the catheter site in a neutropenic patient warrants hospitalization and initiation of intravenous therapy with broad-spectrum antibiotics.

MUCOSITIS

The most common cause of disruption of mucosal membrane surfaces in children is cytotoxic chemotherapy. The same agents that depress circulating neutrophils often induce mucositis. On occasion, radiation therapy delivered to the oral-pharyngeal region can be associated with mucositis. *Mucositis* is a generic term applied to ulcerous lesions of the oral mucosa, and the condition can vary substantially in severity. In some cases it manifests as small oral ulcers, whereas in severe cases, its hallmark is sloughing of the oral and GI mucosa. On occasion, necrotizing gingivitis can develop and requires treatment with broad-spectrum antibacterial agents that are effective against anaerobic organisms. Infection with these organisms manifests as marginal or necrotizing gingivitis, characterized by a periapical line of erythema and exquisite tenderness. Significant mucositis can preclude adequate oral intake, leading to poor nutrition and dehydration. To date, preventive strategies have not been successful, but recent studies have provided sufficient reason to investigate the use of recombinant GM-CSF for prevention or perhaps treatment in high-risk patients (Fung and Ferrill, 2002).

Mucositis serves as a portal of entry for infection of the bloodstream. Pathogens that gain entry include oral flora, alpha-streptococci, lactobacilli, and other usually nonpathogenic bacteria, but also gram-negative bacilli and fungi, particularly in those who have been hospitalized or have been on antibiotics for extended periods of time.

It is difficult to distinguish oral thrush (candidiasis) from chemotherapy-induced mucositis; often the two conditions occur together. Chemotherapy-induced mucositis resolves temporally when the patient's neutrophil counts recover. Frequently, candidal lesions are treated with oral therapy, clotrimazole troches, or nystatin, but in severe cases, especially those complicated by esophagitis, an azole is required (e.g., fluconazole or voriconazole). Oral acyclovir is used successfully to treat HSV, but not infrequently, intravenous therapy is needed because of severe mouth discomfort. Many institutions have adopted preventive measures such as mouth rinses with chlorhexidine and oral hygiene protocols. Varying degrees of success have been reported for the reduction of the incidence and severity of mucositis.

INTRAABDOMINAL INFECTIONS

One of the most vexing challenges for the care of the immunoincompetent child is the evaluation of abdominal pain. Because there are many causes of abdominal pain, one has to weigh the severity of signs and symptoms in the context of the immune deficit(s). In the pediatric oncology patient who has received intensive chemotherapy, one has to consider antibiotic-related colitis, chemotherapy-induced mucositis, and anatomic disruption due to infiltrating tumor or severe infection. Moreover, children with neutropenia might not generate a brisk inflammatory response, resulting in a delay in the recognition of the signs and symptoms of deep infection. Disruption of mucosal integrity can extend throughout the GI tract, providing an entry point for sepsis or intraabdominal abscesses. It is difficult to distinguish these problems from appendicitis, which still occurs with regular frequency in immunoincompetent children. In the profoundly neutropenic child, a necrotic enteropathy develops in the terminal ileum, cecum or appendix. This is known as *typhlitis*, a condition that mimics an acute appendicitis (Skibber et al., 1987). The infection progresses rapidly and often requires surgical intervention, a high-risk procedure in the neutropenic child. Despite the fact that gram-negative bacilli are the most common pathogens seen in the necrotic tissue, bacteremia is observed in only a third of cases (Sloas et al., 1993). Imaging techniques such as CT and MRI are useful and classically demonstrate thickened bowel walls and, occasionally, free air in the bowel wall, a condition known as pneumotosis intestinalis. Indications for surgical intervention include perforation, uncontrolled bleeding, abscess formation, and septic shock (Shamberger et al., 1986; Skibber et al., 1987). If the signs and symptoms are recognized very early, broad-spectrum antibiotic therapy and conservative medical management can obviate the need for surgery (Schlatter et al., 2002).

A major complication of antibiotic therapy in the immunoincompetent child is antibiotic-associated pseudomembranous colitis. The pathogen responsible for this debilitating problem is the obligate anaerobe, *Clostridium difficile*, which is part of the normal fecal flora in 5% of healthy children. The carriage rate is probably higher in hospitalized children, particularly those receiving repeat courses of broad-spectrum antibiotics. Asymptomatic colonization rates are high in young infants but decrease with age. *C difficile* secretes two toxins: toxin A, an enterotoxin, and toxin B, which is detected in the laboratory by its cytopathic effect on tissue culture cell lines. Whereas the former, toxin A, most likely contributes to the acute symptoms, toxin B appears to affect the severity of disease (Burgner et al., 1997). There is a wide spectrum of clinical manifestations, which can range from asymptomatic bloody stools, to watery diarrhea (with or with-out blood), to abdominal pain and, in rare cases, toxic megacolon. Although nearly every available antibiotic and select chemotherapeutic agents have been reported to cause pseudomembranous colitis, ampicillin, cephalosporins, and clindamycin are the major culprits. Most cases of hospital acquired *C. difficile*–associated diarrhea are nosocomial (McFarland et al., 1989). The first line of treatment is oral metronidazole. Oral vancomycin should be reserved for cases that are not responsive to treatment with metronidazole. Relapses can be retreated with metronidazole with a high rate of success. Intravenous antibiotics are not recommended for treatment of symptomatic *C. difficile* infection.

ANORECTAL INFECTION

In general, healthy children rarely develop infection in the anorectal region. Children receiving chemotherapy are prone to develop serious infection in this region. Lesions in the rectal mucosa provide access to the bloodstream and also become the focal point for cellulitis and perirectal abscesses. As a consequence of neutropenia, the host inflammatory response is blunted and minimal symptoms and signs are apparent, making even superficial infection difficult to recognize. Therefore, the slightest discoloration or pain should be evaluated and antibiotic therapy initiated quickly. Since anorectal infections are often polymicrobial, including enterococci, gram-negative bacilli, and anaerobes, broad-spectrum antibiotic regimens that include anaerobic coverage should be considered. Surgical drainage should be restricted to advanced infection and avoided in the neutropenic host, since there is a high incidence of postoperative complications (Lehrnbecher et al., 2002a).

CNS INFECTION

Infection of the CNS is rare in the neutropenic child (Sommers and Hawkins, 1999). Typically, CNS infections develop in children who have undergone a neurosurgical procedure, especially the placement of an indwelling intraventricular device (ventriculoperitoneal shunt or Ommaya reservoir). Infectious complications of an Ommaya reservoir can usually be treated with the apparatus left in place. The primary pathogens are skin pathogens, staphylococci, and *Propionibacterium acnes*. Meningitis is rare in the immunoincompetent child, but on occasion infection with *C. neoformans* occurs, especially in children with impaired cellular immunity (e.g., after marrow transplantation or with HIV-1 infection) or in those in overt leukemic relapse. *Candida* meningitis is also possible, but again, rarely seen in pediatric oncology patients. Children with cell-mediated defects rarely develop toxoplasmosis, which is more common in adults.

URINARY TRACT INFECTION

Urinary tract infection (UTI) in the neutropenic child is rare. In surveys of common infectious complications of children undergoing therapy for acute leukemia, UTIs are distinctly unusual (Nakamura et al., 2000). Though considered a component of the evaluation of the newly febrile, neutropenic child, the likelihood of a positive urine culture is very small (Korzeniowski, 1991). The need to repeat urine cultures in persistently febrile, neutropenic children has not been established and is not recommended, unless there are specific signs and symptoms directing the evaluation toward this site. Renal abscess and hydronephrosis occasionally complicate a recent surgical intervention or progressive disease in the abdomen or pelvis.

CONCLUSION

It is anticipated that in the future genomics will provide further insight into risks for infection and possibly provide new strategies to prevent or treat infection, especially at earlier stages (Collins, 2003). Already, the field of genomics has provided the tools to dissect the complex genetics of common and uncommon diseases (Taylor et al., 2001). For instance, common genetic variants in the mannose-binding protein appear to be risk factors for developing infection in children with immunodeficiencies. Further studies have suggested that common variants (~35%) in the mannose-binding gene could predispose individuals to a greater likelihood of major infections—in both cancer and marrow-transplant patients (Mullighan et al., 2002; Neth et al., 2001). Similarly, variation in the interleukin-4 gene, a critical cytokine in Th1/Th2 balance, is associated with candidemia in patients with acute leukemia (Choi et al., 2003). This approach also is currently being applied in the field of pharmacogenomics, which seeks to use genetic variants to guide therapeutic intervention.

The last decades have seen an increase in the number of immunoincompetent children with acquired deficiencies (e.g., more children receiving intensive chemotherapy or having perinatally acquired HIV infection). Success in the past has been based on developing useful algorithms for diagnosis and treatment of infectious complications. The strategies have focused on early detection and intervention. The principles enumerated here are founded on the care of the febrile, neutropenic child, but there are still important challenges that lie ahead. These include (1) validation of a risk stratification schema that will have a sufficiently high predictive value to implement across centers; (2) sensitive and specific diagnostics for all pathogens; (3) new antimicrobial agents to combat recalcitrant pathogens and newly resistant pathogens; (4) preventive strategies designed to be effective before serious sequelae ensue. These goals will be achieved through a coordinated approach toward basic science and clinical research in this field, which will hopefully translate into strategies that diminish the duration and intensity of immune dysfunction and accelerate the immune recovery.

BIBLIOGRAPHY

Adcock KG, Akins RL, Farrington EA. Evaluation of empiric vancomycin therapy in children with fever and neutropenia. Pharmacotherapy 1999;19:1315.

Aisner J, Murillo J, Schimpff SC, et al. Invasive *Aspergillus* in acute leukemia: correlation with nose cultures and antibiotic use. Ann Intern Med 1979;90:4.

Alexander SW, Wade KC, Hibberd PL, et al. Evaluation of risk prediction criteria for episodes of febrile neutropenia in children with cancer. J Pediatr Hematol Oncol 2002; 24:38.

American Academy of Pediatrics. Immunization in special clinical circumstances. In Peter G (ed). 2000 Red Book: Report of the Committee on Infectious Diseases, ed 25. Elk Grove Village, Ill: American Academy of Pediatrics, 2000.

American Society of Clinical Oncology. American Society of Clinical Oncology recommendations for the use of hematopoietic colony–stimulating factors: evidence-based, clinical practice guidelines. J Clin Oncol 1994; 12:2471.

American Society of Clinical Oncology. Update of recommendations for the use of hematopoietic colony–stimulating factors: evidence-based clinical practice guidelines. J Clin Oncol 1996;14:1957.

Anaissie E, Kuchar RT, Rex J, et al. Isolation of pathogenic *Fusarium* species in a hospital potable water supply: Implications for risks to patient care and environmental health. Clin Infect Dis 2001;33:1871.

Archibald S, Park J, Geyer JR, et al. Computed tomography in the evaluation of febrile neutropenic pediatric oncology patients. Pediatr Infect Dis J 2001;20:5.

Aquino VM, Pappo A, Buchanan GR, et al. The changing epidemiology of bacteremia in neutropenic children with cancer. Pediatr Infect Dis 1995;14:140.

Balfour HH, Chase BA, Stapleton JJ, et al. A randomized, placebo-controlled trial of acyclovir for the prevention of cytomegalovirus disease in recipients of renal allografts. N Engl J Med 1989;320:1381.

Baorto EP, Aquino VM, Mullen CA, et al. Clinical parameters associated with low bacteremia risk in 1100 pediatric oncology patients with fever and neutropenia. Cancer 2001;92:909.

Babior BM. NADPH oxidase: an update. Blood 1999;93:1464.

Bash RO, Katz JA, Cash JV, Buchanan GR. Safety and cost effectiveness of early hospital discharge of lower risk children with cancer admitted for fever and neutropenia. Cancer 1994;74:189.

Bayston KF, Want S, Cohen J. A prospective, randomized comparison of ceftazidime and ciprofloxacin as initial empirical therapy in neutropenic patients with fever. Am J Med 1989;87:269.

Bensinger WI, Price TH, Dale DC, et al. The effects of daily recombinant human granulocyte colony-stimulating factor administration on normal granulocyte donors undergoing leukapheresis. Blood 1993;81:1883.

Berenguer J, Allende M, Lee J, et al. Pathogenesis of pulmonary aspergillosis: granulocytopenia versus cyclosporine and methylprednisolone-induced immunosuppression. Am J Respir Crit Care Med 1995;152:1079.

Bochud P, Eggiman P, Calandra T, et al. Bacteremia due to viridans *Streptococcus* in neutropenic patients with cancer: clinical spectrum and risk factors. Clin Infect Dis 1994;18:25.

Bodey GP, Buckley M, Sathe YS, Freireich EJ. Quantitative relationships between circulating leukocytes and infection in patients with acute leukemia. Ann Intern Med 1966;64:328.

Bodey GP, Jadeja L, Elting L. *Pseudomonas* bacteremia: a retrospective analysis of 410 episodes. Arch Intern Med 1985;145:1621.

Boeckh M, Berrey MM, Bowden RA, et al. Phase 1 evaluation of the respiratory syncytial virus–specific monoclonal antibody palivizumab in recipients of hematopoietic stem cell transplants. J Infect Dis 2001;184:350.

Boogaerts M, Winston DJ, Bow EJ, et al. Intravenous and oral itraconazole versus intravenous amphotericin B deoxycholate as empirical therapy for persistent fever in neutropenic patients with cancer who are receiving broad-spectrum antibacterial therapy: a randomized, controlled trial. Ann Intern Med 2001;135:412.

Boogaerts MA, Demuynck H, Mestdagh N, et al. Equivalent efficacies of meropenem and ceftazidime as empirical monotherapy of febrile neutropenic patients. J Antimicrob Chemother 1995;36:185.

Bowden RA, Sayers M, Flournoy N, et al. Cytomegalovirus immune globulin and seronegative blood products to prevent primary cytomegalovirus infection after marrow transplantation. N Engl J Med 1986;314:1006.

Browne MJ, Perek D, Dinndorf PA, et al. Infectious complications of intraventricular reservoirs in cancer patients. Pediatr Infect Dis J 1987;6:182.

Bruckner LB, Korones DN, Karnauchow T, et al. High incidence of penicillin resistance among alpha-hemolytic streptococci isolated from the blood of children with cancer. J Pediatr 2002;140:20.

Buchanan GR. Approach to treatment of the febrile cancer patient with low-risk neutropenia. *Hematol Oncol Clin North Am* 1993;7:919.

Burgner D, Siarakas S, Eagles G, et al. A prospective study of *Clostridium difficile* infection and colonization in pediatric oncology patients. Pediatr Infect Dis J 1997;16:1131.

Centers for Disease Control and Prevention. Recommendations for preventing the spread of vancomycin resistance. MMWR Recomm Rep 1993;4:1.

Centers for Disease Control and Prevention. Nosocomial enterococci resistant to vancomycin: United States, 1989-1993. MMWR Morb Mortal Wkly Rep 1993;42:597.

Centers for Disease Control and Prevention. 1995 revised guidelines for prophylaxis against *Pneumocystis carinii* pneumonia for children infected with or perinatally exposed to human immunodeficiency virus. MMWR Recomm Rep 1995;44:1.

Centers for Disease Control and Prevention. 1999 USPHS/IDSA guidelines for the prevention of opportunistic infections in persons infected with human immunodeficiency virus. Clin Infect Dis 2000a;30:S29.

Centers for Disease Control and Prevention. Guidelines for preventing opportunistic infections among hematopoietic stem cell transplant recipients. MMWR Recomm Rep 2000b;49:1

Cesaro S, Chinello P, Silvestro GD, et al. Granulocyte transfusions from G-CSF–stimulated donors for the treatment of severe infections in neutropenic pediatric patients with oncohematological diseases. Support Care Cancer 2003;11:101.

Chanock SJ, Gorlin JB. Granulocyte transfusions. Infect Dis Clin North Am 1996;10:327.

Chanock SJ, Pizzo PA. Infection prevention strategies for children with cancer and AIDS: contrasting dilemmas. J Hosp Infect 1995;30:197.

Chanock SJ, Pizzo PA. Fever in the neutropenic host. Infect Dis Clin North Am 1996;10:777.

Choi EH, Foster C, Taylor J, et al. Chronic disseminated candidiasis in adult acute leukemia is associated with a common IL4 promote haplotype in a pilot study. J Infect Dis 2003;187:1153.

Chow J, Fine M, Shales D, et al. Enterobacter bacteremia: clinical features and emergence of antibiotic resistance during therapy. Ann Intern Med 1991;115:585.

Chuang YY, Hung IJ, Yang CP, et al. Cefepime versus ceftazidime as empiric monotherapy for fever and neutropenia in children with cancer. Pediatr Infect Dis J 2002;21:203.

Collins FS, Green ED, Guttmacher AE, Guyer MS. A vision for the future of genomics research. *Nature* 2003;422:835.

Colotta F, Re F, Polentarutti N, et al. Modulation of granulocyte survival and programmed cell death by cytokines and bacterial products. Blood 1992;80:2012.

Cordonnier C, Herbrecht R, Pico JL, et al. Cefepime/amikacin versus ceftazidime/amikacin as empirical therapy for febrile episodes in neutropenic patients: a comparative study. The French Cefepime Study Group. Clin Infect Dis 1997;24:41.

Cotton DJ, Gill V, Hiemenz J. Bacillus bacteremia in an immunocompromised patient population: clinical features, therapeutic interventions, and relationship to chronic intravascular catheters. J Clin Microbiol 1987; 25:672.

Craft A, Reid M, Gardner P, et al. Virus infections in children with acute lymphoblastic leukemia. Arch Dis Child 1979;54:755.

Cupps TR, Fauci AS. Corticosteroid-mediated immunoregulation in man. Immunol Rev 1982;65:133.

Das I, Philpott C, George RH. Central venous catheter–related septicaemia in paediatric cancer patients. J Hosp Infect 1997;36:67.

Dekker AO, Rozenberg-Arska M, Verhoef J. Infection prophylaxis in acute leukemia: a comparison of ciprofloxacin with trimethoprim-sulfamethoxazole and colistin. Ann Intern Med 1987;106:7.

Doffinger R, Dupuis S, Picard C, et al. Inherited disorders of IL-12 and IFN gamma-mediated immunity: a molecular genetics update. Mol Immunol 2002;38:903.

Edman JC, Kovacs JA, Masur H, et al. Ribosomal RNA sequence shows *Pneumocystis carinii* to be a member of the fungi. Nature 1988;334:519.

Eliopoulos GM. Quinupristin-dalfopristin and linezolid: evidence and opinion. Clin Infect Dis 2003;36:473.

Elting LS, Bodey GP, Keefe BH. Septicemia and shock syndrome due to viridans streptococci: a case-control study of predisposing factors. Clin Infect Dis 1992;14:1201.

Emmanuel D, Cunningham I, Jules-Elysee K, et al. Cytomegalovirus pneumonia after bone marrow transplantation successfully treated with the combination of ganciclovir and high-dose intravenous immune globulin. Ann Intern Med 1988;109:777.

Englund JA, Anderson LJ, Rhame FS. Nosocomial transmission of respiratory syncytial virus in immunocompromised adults. J Clin Microbiol 1991;29:115.

EORTC, International Antimicrobial Therapy Cooperative Group. Empiric antifungal therapy in febrile granulocytopenic patients. Am J Med 1989;86:668.

EORTC, International Antimicrobial Therapy Cooperative Group. Efficacy and toxicity of single daily doses of amikacin and ceftriaxone versus multiple daily doses of amikacin and ceftazidime for infection in patients with cancer and granulocytopenia. Ann Intern Med 1993;119: 584.

Eppes SC, Troutman JL, Gutman LT. Outcome of treatment of candidemia in children whose central catheters were removed or retained. Pediatr Infect Dis J 1989; 8:99.

Fainstein V, Elting LS, Bodey GP. Bacteremia caused by nonsporulating anaerobes in cancer patients: a 12-year experience. Medicine 1989;68:151.

Feld R, Paesmans M, Freifeld A, et al. Methodology for clinical trials involving patients with cancer who have febrile neutropenia: updated guidelines of the Immunocompromised Host Society/Multinational Association for Supportive Care in Cancer, with Emphasis on Outpatient Studies. Clin Infect Dis 2002;35:1463.

Feldman S, Hughes WT, Daniel CB. Varicella in children with cancer: seventy-seven cases. Pediatrics 1975;56:388.

Fleischhack G, Schmidt-Niemann M, Wulff B, et al. Piperacillin, beta-lactam inhibitor plus gentamicin as empirical therapy of a sequential regimen in febrile neutropenia of pediatric cancer patients. Support Care Cancer 2001;9:372.

Foster CB, Choi EW, Chanock SJ. Adenovirus and marrow transplantation. Pediatr Pathol Mol Med 2000; 19:97-114.

Freidfeld A, Marchigiani D, Walsh T, et al. A double-blind comparison of empirical oral and intravenous antibiotic therapy for low-risk febrile patients with neutropenia during cancer chemotherapy. N Engl J Med 1999;341:305.

Freifeld AG, Walsh T, Marshall D, et al. Monotherapy for fever and neutropenia in cancer patients: a randomized comparison of ceftazidime versus imipenem. J Clin Oncol 1995;13:165.

Fung SM, Ferrill MJ. Granulocyte macrophage-colony stimulating factor and oral mucositis. Ann Pharmacother 2002;36:517.

Gershon AA, Steinberg SP, the Varicella Vaccine Collaborative Study Group of the National Institute of Allergy and Infectious Diseases. Persistence of immunity to varicella in children with leukemia immunized with live attenuated varicella vaccine. N Engl J Med 1989; 320:892.

Goodman JL, Winston DJ, Greenfield RA, et al. A controlled trial of fluconazole to prevent fungal infections in patients undergoing bone marrow transplantation. N Engl J Med 1992;326:845.

Goodrich JM, Boeckh M, Bowden R. Strategies for the prevention of cytomegalovirus disease after marrow transplantation. Clin Infect Dis 1994;19:287.

Griffin TC, Buchanan GR. Hematologic predictors of bone marrow recovery in neutropenic patients hospitalized for fever: implications for discontinuation of antibiotics and early hospital discharge. J Pediatr 1992;121:28.

Groll AH, Walsh TJ. Uncommon opportunistic fungi: new nosocomial threats. Clin Microbiol Infect 2001;7:8.

Groll AH, Walsh TJ. Caspofungin: pharmacology, safety and therapeutic potential in superficial and invasive fungal infections. Expert Opin Investig Drugs 2001;10:1545.

Grubman S, Simonds RJ. Preventing *Pneumocystis carinii* pneumonia in human immunodeficiency virus–infected children: new guidelines for prophylaxis. CDC, US Public Health Service, and the Infectious Disease Society of America. Pediatr Infect Dis J 1996;15:165.

Guiot HFL, Fibbe WE, van't Wout JW. Risk factors for fungal infections in patients with malignant hematologic disorders: implications for empirical therapy and prophylaxis. Clin Infect Dis 1994;18:525.

Harrington RD, Hooton RD, Hackman RC, et al. An outbreak of respiratory syncytial virus in a bone marrow transplant center. J Infect Dis 1992;165:987.

Henning KJ, Delencastre H, Eagan J, et al. Vancomycin-resistant *Enterococcus faecium* on a pediatric oncology ward: duration of stool shedding and incidence of clinical infection. Pediatr Infect Dis J 1996;15:848.

Henrickson KJ, Axtell RA, Hoover SM, et al. Prevention of central venous catheter–related infections and thrombotic events in immunocompromised children by the use of vancomycin/ciprofloxacin/heparin flush solution: A randomized, multicenter, double-blind trial. J Clin Oncol 2000;18:1269.

Hiemenz J, Skelton J, Pizzo PA. Perspective on the management of catheter-related infections in cancer patients. Pediatr Infect Dis 1986;5:6.

Horvath JA, Dummer S. The use of respiratory-tract cultures in the diagnosis of invasive pulmonary aspergillosis. Am J Med 1996;100:171.

Hovi L, Saarinen-Pihkala UM, Vettenranta K, et al. Invasive fungal infections in pediatric bone marrow transplant recipients: single center experience of 10 years. Bone Marrow Transplant 2000;26:999.

Hughes WT, Armstrong D, Bodey GP, et al. Guidelines for the use of antimicrobial agents in neutropenic patients with unexplained fever. J Infect Dis 1990;161:381.

Hughes WT, Armstrong D, Bodney GP, et al. 1997 Guidelines for the use of antimicrobial agents in neutropenic patients with unexplained fever. Clin Infect Dis 1997;25:551.

Hughes WT, Feldman S, Aur RJ, et al. Intensity of immunosuppressive therapy and the incidence of *Pneumocystis carinii* pneumonitis. *Cancer* 1975;36:2004.

Hughes WT, Kuhn S, Chaudhary S, et al. Successful chemoprophylaxis for *Pneumocystis carinii* pneumonitis. N Engl J Med 1977;297:1419.

Hughes WT, Rivera GK, Schell MJ, et al. Successful intermittent chemoprophylaxis for *Pneumocystis carinii* pneumonitis. N Engl J Med 1987;316:1627.

International Chronic Granulomatous Disease Cooperative Study Group. A controlled trial of interferon-γ to prevent infection in chronic granulomatous disease. N Engl J Med 1991;324:509.

Johnston DL, Waldhausen JH, Park JR. Deep soft tissue infections in the neutropenic pediatric oncology patient. J Pediatr Hematol Oncol 2001;23:443.

Jones GR, Konsler GK, Dunaway RP, et al. Risk factors for recurrent fever after the discontinuation of empiric antibiotic therapy for fever and neutropenia in pediatric patients with a malignancy or hematologic condition. J Pediatr 1994;124:703.

Kaditis AG, O'Marcaigh AS, Rhodes KH, et al. Yield of positive blood cultures in pediatric oncology patients by a new method of blood culture collection. Pediatr Infect Dis J 1996;15:615.

Karadeniz C, Oguz A, Canter B, et al. Incidence of seizures in pediatric cancer patients treated with imipenem/cilastatin. Pediatr Hematol Oncol 2000;17:585.

Karp JE, Merz WG, Hendricksen C, et al. Oral norfloxacin for prevention of gram-negative bacterial infections in patients with acute leukemia and granulocytopenia: a randomized, double-blind, placebo-controlled trial. Ann Intern Med 1987;106:1.

Klaassen RJ, Allen U, Doyle JJ. Randomized placebo-controlled trial of oral antibiotics in pediatric oncology patients at low-risk with fever and neutropenia. J Pediatr Hematol Oncol 2000a;22:405.

Klaassen RJ, Goodman TR, Pham B, et al. "Low-risk" prediction rule for pediatric oncology patients presenting with fever and neutropenia. J Clin Oncol 2000b;18:1012.

Klastersky J, Paesmans M, Rubenstein E, et al. The Multinational Association for Supportive Care in Cancer risk-index: a multinational scoring system for identifying low-risk febrile neutropenic cancer patients. J Clin Oncol 2000;18:3038.

Kocak U, Rolston KV, Mullen CA. Fever and neutropenia in children with solid tumors is similar in severity and outcome to that in children with leukemia. Support Care Cancer 2002;10:58.

Korzeniowski OM. Urinary tract infection in the impaired host. Med Clin North Am 1991;75:391.

Koya R, Andersen J, Fernandez H, et al. Analysis of the value of empiric vancomycin administration in febrile neutropenia occurring after autologous peripheral blood stem cell transplants. Bone Marrow Transplant 1998;21:923.

Lehrnbecher T, Foster C, Vázquez N, et al. Therapy-induced alterations in host defense in children receiving therapy for cancer. J Pediatr Hematol Oncol 1997;19:399.

Lehrnbecher T, Marshall D, Gao C, et al. A second look at anorectal infections in cancer patients in a large cancer institute: the success of early intervention with antibiotics and surgery. Infection 2002a;5:272.

Lehrnbecher T, Stanescu A, Kuhl J. Short courses of intravenous empirical antibiotic treatment in selected febrile neutropenic children with cancer. Infection 2002b;30:17.

Lehrnbecher T, Venzon D, de Haas M, et al. Assessment of measuring circulating levels of interleukin-6, interleukin-8, C-reactive protein, soluble Fc gamma receptor type III, and mannose-binding protein in febrile children with cancer and neutropenia. Clin Infect Dis 1999;29:414.

Levy I, Leibovici L, Drucker M, et al. A prospective study of gram-negative bacteremia in children. Pediatr Infect Dis J 1996;15:117.

Levy I, Rubin LG, Vasishta S, et al. Emergence of *Candida parapsilosis* as the predominant species causing candidemia in children. Clin Infect Dis 1998;26:1086.

Lin PL, Oram RJ, Lauderdale DS, et al. Knowledge of Centers for Disease Control and Prevention guidelines for the use of vancomycin at a large tertiary care children's hospital. J Pediatr 2000;137:694.

Lucas KG, Brown AW, Armstrong D, et al. The identification of febrile, neutropenic children with neoplastic disease at low risk for bacteremia and complications of sepsis. Cancer 1996;15:791.

Lujan-Zilbermann J, Benaim E, Tong X, et al. Respiratory virus infections in pediatric hematopoietic stem cell transplantation. Clin Infect Dis 2001;33:962.

Mackall CL, Bare CV, Titus JA, et al. Thymic-independent T cell regeneration occurs via antigen driven expansion of peripheral T cells resulting in a repertoire that is limited in diversity and prone to skewing. J Immunol 1996;156:4609.

Mackall CL, Fleisher TA, Brown M, et al. Lymphocyte depletion during treatment with intensive chemotherapy for cancer. Blood 1994;84:2221.

Mackall C, Fleisher T, Brown M, et al. Age, thymopoiesis, and CD4+ T-lymphocyte regeneration after intensive chemotherapy. N Engl J Med 1995;332:143.

Marr KA, Seidel K, Slavin MA, et al. Prolonged fluconazole prophylaxis is associated with persistent protection against candidiasis-related death in allogeneic marrow transplant recipients: long-term follow-up of a randomized, placebo-controlled trial. Blood 2000;96:2055.

McFarland LV, Mulligan ME, Kwok RYY, Stamm WE. Nosocomial acquisition of *Clostridium difficile* infection. N Engl J Med 1989;320:204.

Menichetti F, Del Favero A, Martino P, et al. Itraconazole oral solution as prophylaxis for fungal infections in neutropenic patients with hematologic malignancies: a randomized, placebo-controlled, double-blind, multicenter trial. Clin Infect Dis 1999;28:250.

Meyers JD, Reed EC, Shepp DH, et al. Acyclovir for prevention of cytomegalovirus infection and disease after allogeneic marrow transplantation. N Engl J Med 1988;318:70.

Montecalvo MA, Horowitz H, Gedris C, et al. Outbreak of vancomycin-, ampicillin-, and aminoglycoside-resistant *Enterococcus faecium* bacteremia in an adult oncology unit. Antimicrob Agents Chemother 1994;38:1363.

Mora-Duarte J, Betts R, Rotstein C, et al. Comparison of caspofungin and amphotericin B for invasive candidiasis. N Engl J Med 2002;347:2020.

Mullen CA, Buchanan GR. Early hospital discharge of children with cancer treated for fever and neutropenia. Identification and management of the low-risk patient. J Clin Oncol 1990;8:1998.

Mullen CA, Petropoulos D, Roberts WM, et al. Outpatient treatment of fever and neutropenia for low risk pediatric cancer patients. Cancer 1999;86:126.

Mullighan CG, Heatley S, Doherty K, et al. Mannose-binding lectin gene polymorphisms are associated with major infection following allogeneic hemopoietic stem cell transplantation. Blood 2002;99:3524.

Mustafa MM, Aquino VM, Pappo A, et al. A pilot study of outpatient management of febrile neutropenic children with cancer at low risk of bacteremia. J Pediatr 1996;128:847.

Mustafa MM, Carlson L, Tkaczewski I, et al. Comparative study of cefepime versus ceftazidime in the empiric treatment of pediatric cancer patients with fever and neutropenia. Pediatr Infect Dis J 2001;20:362.

Nakamura S, Gelber RD, Blattner S, et al. Long-term follow-up and infectious complications of therapy for acute lymphoblastic leukemia in children. Int J Pediatr Hematol Oncol 2000;6:321.

Neth O, Hann I, Turner MW, et al. Deficiency of mannose-binding lectin and burden of infection in children with malignancy: a prospective study. Lancet 2001;358:598.

Neville K, Renbarger J, Dreyer Z. Pneumonia in the immunocompromised pediatric cancer patient. Semin Respir Infect 2002;17:21.

O'Grady NP, Alexander M, Dellinger EP, et al. Guidelines for the prevention of intravascular catheter-related infections. The Hospital Infection Control Practices Advisory Committee, Center for Disease Control and Prevention. Pediatrics 2002;110:51.

Oude Nijhuis CSM, Daenen SMGJ, Vellenga E, et al. Fever and neutropenia in cancer patients: the diagnostic role of cytokines in risk assessment strategies. Crit Rev Oncol Hematol 2002;44:163.

Pappo AS, Buchanan GR. Predictors of bacteremia in febrile neutropenic children with cancer. Proc Am Soc Clin Oncol 1991;10:331.

Park JR, Coughlin J, Hawkins D, et al. Ciprofloxacin and amoxicillin as continuation treatment of febrile neutropenia in pediatric cancer patients. Med Pediatr Oncol 2003;40:93.

Parsons SK, Mayer DK, Alexander SW, et al. Growth factor practice patterns among pediatric oncologists: results of a 1998 pediatric oncology group survey. Economic Evaluation Working Group. The Pediatric Oncology Group. J Pediatr Hematol Oncol 2000;22:227.

Patterson TF, Kirkpatrick WR, White M, et al. Invasive aspergillosis: disease spectrum, treatment practices, and outcomes. Medicine (Baltimore) 2000;79:250.

Petrilli AS, Dantas LS, Campos MC, et al. Oral ciprofloxacin vs. intravenous ceftriaxone administered in an outpatient setting for fever and neutropenia in low-risk pediatric oncology patients: randomized prospective trial. Med Pediatr Oncol 2000;34:87.

Pizzo PA. Management of fever in patients with cancer and treatment-induced neutropenia. N Engl J Med 1993;328:1323.

Pizzo PA, Hathorn JW, Hiemenz J, et al. A randomized trial comparing ceftazidime alone with combination antibiotic therapy in cancer patients with fever and neutropenia. N Engl J Med 1986;315:552.

Pizzo PA, Ladisch S, Robichaud K. Treatment of gram-positive septicemia in cancer patients. Cancer 1980;45:206.

Pizzo PA, Robichaud KJ, Gill FA. Duration of empirical antibiotic therapy in granulocytopenic cancer patients. Am J Med 1979;67:194.

Pizzo PA, Robichaud KJ, Gill FA, Witebsky FG. Empiric antibiotic and antifungal therapy of cancer patients with prolonged fever and granulocytopenia. Am J Med 1982a;72:101.

Pizzo PA, Robichaud KJ, Wesley R, Commers JR. Fever in the pediatric and young adult patient with cancer: a prospective study of 1,001 episodes. Medicine 1982b;61:153.

Postovsky S, Ben Arush MW, Kassis E, et al. Pharmacokinetic analysis of gentamicin thrice and single daily dosage in pediatric cancer patients. Pediatr Hematol Oncol 1997;14:547.

Prentice HG, Hann IM, Herbrecht R, et al. A randomized comparison of liposomal versus conventional amphotericin B for the treatment of pyrexia of unknown origin in neutropenic patients. Br J Haematol 1997;98:711.

Rackoff WR, Ge J, Sather HN, et al. Central venous catheter use and the risk of infection in children with acute lymphoblastic leukemia: a report from the Children's Cancer Group. J Pediatr Hematol Oncol 1999;21:260.

Rackoff WR, Gonin R, Robinson C, et al. Predicting the risk of bacteremia in children with fever and neutropenia. J Clin Oncol 1996;14:919.

Reed EC, Bowden RA, Dandliker PS, et al. Treatment of cytomegalovirus pneumonia with ganciclovir and intravenous cytomegalovirus immunoglobulin in patients with bone marrow transplants. Ann Intern Med 1989;109:783.

Roilides E, Lyman C, Panagopoulou P, et al. Immunomodulation in fungal infections. Infect Dis Clin North Am 2003;17:193-219.

Roilides E, Walsh TJ, Pizzo PA, Rubin M. Granulocyte colony–stimulating factor enhances the phagocytic and bactericidal activity of normal and defective human neutrophils. J Infect Dis 1991;163:579.

Rotstein C, Bow EJ, Laverdiere M, et al. Randomized placebo-controlled trial of fluconazole prophylaxis for neutropenic cancer patients: benefit based on purpose and intensity of cytotoxic therapy. Clin Infect Dis 1999;28:331.

Rubin LG, Tucci V, Cercenado E, et al. Vancomycin-resistant *Enterococcus faecium* in hospitalized children. Infect Control Hosp Epidemiol 1992;13:700.

Rubin M, Hathorn JW, Marshall D, et al. Gram-positive infections and the use of vancomycin in 550 episodes of fever and neutropenia. Ann Intern Med 1988;108:30.

Salzman MB, Rubin LG. Intravenous catheter-related infections. Adv Pediatr Infect Dis 1995;10:337.

Sanders J, Powers N, Moore R. Ceftazidime monotherapy for empiric treatment of febrile, neutropenic patients: A meta-analysis. J Infect Dis 1992;164:907.

Saral R, Burns WH, Laskin OL, et al. Acyclovir prophylaxis of herpes simplex virus infections: a randomized, double-blind, controlled trial in bone-marrow-transplant recipients. N Engl J Med 1981;305:63.

Sarlis NJ, Chanock SJ, Nieman LK. Cortisolemic indices predict severe infections in Cushing syndrome due to ectopic production of adrenocorticotropin. J Clin Endocrinol Metab 2000;85:42.

Schlatter M, Snyder K, Freyer D. Successful nonoperative management of typhlitis in pediatric oncology patients. J Pediatr Surg 2002;37:1151.

Schmidt GM, Horak DA, Niland JC, et al. A randomized, controlled trial of prophylactic ganciclovir for cytomegalovirus pulmonary infection in recipients of allogeneic bone marrow transplants. N Engl J Med 1991;324:1005.

Schutze GE, Mason EO Jr, Wald ER, et al. Pneumococcal infections in children after transplantation. Clin Infect Dis 2001;33:16.

Segal BH, Holland SM. Primary phagocytic disorders of childhood. Pediatr Clin North Am 2000;47:1311.

Shamberger RC, Weinstein HJ, Delorey MJ, Levey RH. The medical and surgical management of typhlitis in children with acute nonlymphocytic (myelogenous) leukemia. Cancer 1986;57:603.

Shaul DB, Scheer B, Rokhsar S, et al. Risk factors for early intervention of central venous catheters in pediatric patients. J Am Coll Surg 1998;186:654.

Sidi V, Roilides E, Bibashi E, et al. Comparison of efficacy and safety of teicoplanin and vancomycin in children with antineoplastic therapy–associated febrile neutropenia and gram-positive bacteremia. J Chemother 2000;12:326.

Skibber JM, Matter GJ, Pizzo PA, Lotze MT. Right lower quadrant pain in young patients with leukemia: a surgical perspective. Ann Surg 1987;206:711.

Slavin MA, Osborne B, Adams R, et al. Efficacy and safety of fluconazole prophylaxis for fungal infections after marrow transplantation—a prospective, randomized, double-blind study. J Infect Dis 1995;171:1545.

Sloas MM, Flynn PM, Kaste SC, Patrick CC. Typhlitis in children with cancer: a 30-year experience. Clin Infect Dis 1993;17:484.

Soker M, Colpan L, Ece A, et al. Serum levels of IL-1 beta, sIL-2R, IL-6, IL-8, and TNF-alpha in febrile children with cancer and neutropenia. Med Oncol 2001;18:51.

Sommers LM, Hawkins DS. Meningitis in pediatric cancer patients: a review of forty cases from a single institution. Pediatr Infect Dis J 1999;18:902.

Sotiropoulos SV, Jackson MA, Woods GM, et al. Alpha-streptococcal septicemia in leukemic children treated with continuous or large dosage intermittent cytosine arabinoside. Pediatr Infect Dis J 1989;8:755.

Stroncek DF, Leonard K, Eiber G, et al. Alloimmunization after granulocyte transfusions. Transfusion 1996;36:1009.

Talcott JA, Finberg RW. Fever and neutropenia—how to use a new treatment strategy. N Engl J Med 1999;341:362.

Talcott JA, Finberg R, Mayer RJ, Goldman L. The medical course of cancer patients with fever and neutropenia: clinical identification of a low-risk subgroup at presentation. Arch Intern Med 1988;148:2561.

Talcott JA, Whalen A, Clark J, et al. Home antibiotic therapy for low-risk cancer patients with fever and neutropenia: a pilot study of thirty patients based on a validated prediction rule. J Clin Oncol 1994;12:107.

Taylor JG, Choi E, Foster CB, Chanock SJ. Using genetic variation to study human disease. Trends in Mol Med 2001;7:507.

Wade JC, Schimpff SC, Newman KA, Wiernik PH. Staphylococcus epidermidis: an increasing cause of infection in patients with granulocytopenia. Ann Intern Med 1982;97:503.

Wald A, Leisenring W, Van Burik JA, et al. Epidemiology of Aspergillus infections in a large cohort of patients undergoing bone marrow transplantation. J Infect Dis 1997;175:1459.

Walsh FW, Rolfe MW, Rumbak MJ. The initial pulmonary evaluation of the immunocompromised patient. Chest Surg Clin North Am 1999a;9:19.

Walsh TJ, Chanock SJ. Diagnosis of invasive fungal infections: advances in nonculture systems. Curr Clin Top Infect Dis 1998;18:101.

Walsh TJ, Finberg RW, Arndt C, et al. Liposomal amphotericin B for empirical therapy in patients with persistent fever and neutropenia. N Engl J Med 1999b;340:764.

Walsh TJ, Goodman JL, Pappas P, et al. Safety, tolerance, and pharmacokinetics of high-dose liposomal amphotericin B (Ambisome) in patients infected with Aspergillus species and other filamentous fungi: maximum tolerated dose study. Antimicrob Agents Chemother 2001;45:3487.

Walsh TJ, Lutsar I, Driscoll T, et al. Voriconazole in the treatment of aspergillosis, scedosporiosis, and other invasive fungal infections in children. Pediatr Infect Dis J 2002a;21:240.

Walsh TJ, Pappas P, Winston DJ, et al. Voriconazole compared with liposomal amphotericin B for empirical antifungal therapy in patients with neutropenia and persistent fever. N Engl J Med 2002b;346:225.

Walsh TJ, Seibel NL, Arndt C, et al. Amphotericin B lipid complex in pediatric patients with invasive fungal infections. Pediatr Infect Dis J 1999c;18:702.

Wehl G, Allerberger F, Heitger A, et al. Trends in infection morbidity in a pediatric oncology ward, 1986-1995. Med Pediatr Oncol 1999;32:336.

Whimbey E, Champlin RE, Englund JA, et al. Combination therapy with aerosolized ribavirin and intravenous immunoglobulin for respiratory syncytial virus disease in adult bone marrow transplant recipients. Bone Marrow Transplant 1995;16:393.

Wiley JM, Smith N, Leventhal BG, et al. Invasive fungal disease in pediatric acute leukemia patients with fever and neutropenia during induction chemotherapy: a multivariate analysis of risk factors. J Clin Oncol 1990;8:280.

Wilimas JA, Hudson M, Rao B, et al. Late vascular occlusion of central lines in pediatric malignancies. Pediatrics 1998;101:E7.

Wingard JR. Infections due to resistant Candida species in patients with cancer who are receiving chemotherapy. Clin Infect Dis. 1994;19:49.

Wingard JR, Merz WG, Rinaldi MG, et al. Increase in Candida krusei infection among patients with bone marrow transplantation and neutropenia treated prophylactically with fluconazole. N Engl J Med 1991;325:1274.

Winkelstein JA, Marino MC, Johnston RB Jr, et al. Chronic granulomatous disease: report on a national registry of 368 patients. Medicine 2000;79:155.

Winston DJ, Chandrasekar PH, Lazarus HM, et al. Fluconazole prophylaxis of fungal infection in patients with acute leukemia: results of a randomized, placebo-controlled, double-blind, multicenter trial. Ann Intern Med 1993;118:495.

Winston DJ, Hathorn JW, Schuster MG, et al. A multicenter, randomized trial of fluconazole versus amphotericin B for empiric antifungal therapy of febrile neutropenic patients with cancer. Am J Med 2000;108:282.

Wolk J, Stuart M, Stockman J, et al. Neutropenia, fever, and infection in children with acute lymphocytic leukemia. Am J Dis Child 1977;131:157.

Wong-Beringer A, Jacobs RA, Guglielmo BJ. Lipid formulations of amphotericin B: clinical efficacy and toxicities. Clin Infect Dis 1998;27:603.

Wood DJ, Corbitt G. Viral infections in childhood leukemia. J Infect Dis 1985;152:266.

Yu VL, Muder RR, Poorsattar A. Significance of isolation of *Aspergillus* from the respiratory tract in diagnosis of invasive pulmonary aspergillosis: results from a 3-year prospective study. Am J Med 1986;81:249.

Zaman MM, Landman D, Burney S, et al. Treatment of experimental endocarditis due to multidrug-resistant *Enterococcus faecium* with clinafloxacin and penicillin. J Antimicrob Chemother 1996;37:127.

Zeidler C, Welte K. Kostmann syndrome and severe congenital neutropenia. Semin Hematol 2002;39:82.

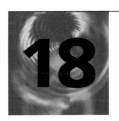

18 KAWASAKI SYNDROME

ANNE H. ROWLEY

Kawasaki syndrome, formerly termed *mucocutaneous lymph node syndrome*, is an acute vasculitis of young children that results in coronary artery aneurysm formation in 20% of untreated patients; sudden death may result from myocardial infarction, myocarditis, or aneurysm rupture. It was described first in the Japanese-language medical literature in 1967, when Tomisaku Kawasaki reported his experience with 50 children who presented with symptoms distinct from those of other known febrile childhood illnesses (Kawasaki, 1967). He originally thought that the syndrome represented a benign childhood illness, because symptoms resolved spontaneously after 1 to 3 weeks. However, it soon became apparent that a small subset of children with the illness abruptly died, usually when their clinical condition appeared improved. Kawasaki's original report was followed by that of Melish and colleagues in 1976, who reported the same illness in 16 children in Hawaii (Melish et al., 1976). Melish and Kawasaki independently developed the same diagnostic criteria that are still used today to diagnose classic Kawasaki syndrome. It is now recognized that Kawasaki syndrome occurs worldwide in children of all ethnic groups, although Asian children appear to be at highest risk. About 1 in 200 Japanese children develops Kawasaki syndrome by the age of 5 years. Since Dr. Kawasaki's description of the clinical features of the illness, about 170,000 cases have been diagnosed in Japan. In the United States, Japan, and other developed nations, Kawasaki syndrome has replaced acute rheumatic fever as the most common cause of acquired heart disease in childhood (Taubert et al., 1994). The etiology of the illness remains unknown, but clinical and epidemiologic data indicate an infectious cause. Intravenous gammaglobulin (IVIG) and aspirin therapy are highly effective in reducing the prevalence of coronary artery abnormalities from 20% in untreated patients to 5% in those who receive these therapies (Newburger et al., 1991), although the mechanism of action is unknown.

ETIOLOGY

Despite intense investigation over the last 40 years, the etiology of Kawasaki syndrome remains a mystery, although an infectious cause appears most likely. The clinical features—a self-limited, generally nonrecurring illness with fever, rash, enanthem, exanthem, conjunctival injection, and cervical adenitis—are consistent with an infectious cause. Epidemiologic features of the illness, including well-defined epidemics with periodicity, winter-spring predominance in temperate climates, and a geographic wavelike spread of illness during epidemics, are also compatible with an infectious etiology. However, conventional bacterial and viral cultures and serologic investigations have failed to yield a causative agent (Bell et al., 1981; Dean et al., 1982). A variety of viral and bacterial agents have been proposed as being related to Kawasaki syndrome over the years, but none has been confirmed with additional research. The marked cytokine activation that occurs in acute Kawasaki syndrome has led some to propose a superantigen as the cause of the illness. Some investigators have reported selective expansion of T cells expressing T-cell receptor variable regions Vβ2 and/or Vβ8 in acute Kawasaki syndrome (Abe et al., 1992; Curtis et al., 1995), suggesting the presence of a circulating superantigen, but other studies have not confirmed this finding (Mancia et al., 1998; Melish et al., 1994; Pietra et al., 1994). An initial report suggesting a relationship between colonization of mucosal surfaces with toxic shock syndrome toxin-1–producing *Staphylococcus aureus* and Kawasaki syndrome (Leung et al., 1993) has not been confirmed in subsequent studies (Melish et al., 1994; Terai et al., 1995). Comparison of pathologic findings in toxic shock syndrome and those in Kawasaki syndrome does not support the hypothesis that these illnesses are different expressions of the same disease (Larkin et al., 1982). Still, a possible superantigen etiology of Kawasaki syndrome remains an area of intense investigation. Recent data, however, suggest that immunologic findings in Kawasaki syndrome fit best with stimulation of the immune system by a conventional antigen (Choi et al., 1997; Rowley et al., 2001). Unfortunately, the nature of any superantigens or conventional antigens involved in the pathogenesis of Kawasaki syndrome remains unknown. It is clear that identification of the etiology of the illness is critical to further advances in the field. A diagnostic test and more specific therapy based on the pathogenesis of the illness are urgently needed. Additionally, prevention of Kawasaki syndrome is not likely to be feasible without knowledge regarding the etiologic agent.

A particularly attractive hypothesis regarding etiology is that Kawasaki syndrome is caused by a ubiquitous infectious agent that leads to clinically apparent disease in certain genetically predisposed individuals. The rarity of the illness in the first few months of life suggests protection by maternal antibody, and the virtual absence of the disease in adults suggests widespread immunity. The paucity of evidence of person-to-person transmission of Kawasaki syndrome is compatible with this hypothesis, because most individuals would develop asymptomatic infection and only a restricted number would develop clinical illness. In view of the marked predisposition of Asian children to develop Kawasaki syndrome, genetic factors are clearly involved and potentially influence the ability of the infectious etiologic agent(s) to cause disease. The genetic factors responsible for increased susceptibility to Kawasaki syndrome remain unknown; no consistent human leukocyte antigen association appears to exist.

Newer molecular biologic methods are now being applied to the study of the etiology and genetics of Kawasaki syndrome and, it is hoped, will result in identification of the causative agent(s) and understanding of the basis for increased susceptibility in Asian children in the near future.

PATHOLOGY AND PATHOGENESIS

Kawasaki syndrome is characterized by inflammatory lesions in many organs and tissues, particularly medium-sized arteries such as the coronary arteries. Although the likely infectious trigger of the marked inflammatory immune response remains unknown, the pathologic findings have been well-described and are virtually identical in all patients with the illness, varying only in the severity of the lesions. In addition to vascular tissue, the following organ systems typically demonstrate inflammatory lesions: cardiovascular system (myocarditis, pericarditis, and less commonly endocarditis); respiratory system (bronchitis and interstitial pneumonia); digestive system (stomatitis, sialoduct adenitis, enteritis, hepatitis, cholangitis, pancreatitis, and pancreatic ductitis); urinary system (focal interstitial nephritis, cystitis, and prostatitis); nervous system (aseptic meningitis and neuritis); and hematopoietic system (lymphadenitis and splenitis) (Amano et al., 1980). In the first month after onset of illness, the inflammatory lesions are quite severe. They begin to subside in the second month after onset, and then subside more rapidly in the third month (Amano et al., 1980).

Inflammatory cell infiltrates in the acute phase are initially neutrophils, but these are rapidly replaced by lymphocytes, which are largely CD8+ T cells, macrophages, and plasma cells (Brown et al., 2001). Notably, IgA plasma cells are prominent in the inflammatory infiltrate in vascular tissue and nonvascular tissues such as kidney and pancreas (Rowley et al., 1997; Rowley et al., 2000). Examination of the clonality of the IgA antibodies produced in the vascular wall demonstrated an oligoclonal or antigen-driven response (Rowley et al., 2001), indicating that either microbial or, possibly, human antigens are being targeted in the vascular wall by the IgA antibodies. Edema and necrosis are apparent in the arterial wall even in the earliest stages of the disease. Endothelial cell changes and inflammation in the adventitial layer appear first; the most severely involved vessels also demonstrate inflammation, edema, and necrosis of smooth muscle cells in the media. Fibrinoid necrosis is mostly absent. Splitting and fragmentation of the internal and external elastic laminae can occur, weakening the structural integrity of the vascular wall. Eventually the layers of the wall become indistinguishable. Such vessels may "balloon" and undergo aneurysmal dilatation, occasionally resulting in sudden death from aneurysm rupture. Myocardial inflammation can be severe and involve the atrioventricular conduction pathway, resulting in fatal arrhythmias or death from intractable congestive heart failure. At 1 to 3 months following the onset of illness, the inflammatory cell infiltrate resolves and fibrous connective tissue begins to form in the vessel wall. The intima proliferates and becomes thickened. Over time, the lumen of the vessel may narrow, because of either thrombosis or stenosis from intimal thickening. Significantly reduced blood flow through the abnormal vessel may lead to myocardial infarction or sudden death. In some cases, calcification of the vessel occurs. Thrombus in the lumen may become organized and recanalized. Inflammatory changes in nonvascular tissues appear to resolve without sequelae.

It is now recognized that before Kawasaki's report of the clinical features of the illness, Kawasaki syndrome was identified only on postmortem examination by pathologists, who termed the illness *infantile periarteritis nodosa*. Careful study indicates that infantile periarteritis nodosa and fatal Kawasaki syndrome are pathologically indistinguishable (Amano et al., 1980; Landing and Larson, 1977) and represent the same clinical entity.

The presence of IgA plasma cell infiltration in targeted tissues in acute Kawasaki syndrome suggests stimulation of the immune system at a mucosal site such as the respiratory or gastrointestinal tract. Pathologic examination of the upper respiratory tract of patients with fatal acute Kawasaki syndrome reveals marked infiltration of IgA plasma cells around large bronchi, similar to findings in children with fatal acute respiratory viral infection (Rowley et al., 2000). This suggests a respiratory portal of entry for the Kawasaki syndrome pathogen. Epidemiologic study of outbreaks of Kawasaki syndrome (Bell et al., 1981) have demonstrated a higher incidence of a preceding respiratory illness in Kawasaki patients when compared with controls. The winter-spring predominance of Kawasaki syndrome also supports a respiratory pathogen, as these are the seasons in which respiratory illnesses of childhood are most common.

There is remarkable systemic immune activation in acute Kawasaki syndrome. Elevations of interleukin (IL)-1, tumor necrosis factor (TNF)-α, interferon-γ, IL-4, IL-6, IL-8, IL-10, and a variety of other cytokines have been noted in the peripheral blood (Hirao et al., 1997; Lin et al., 1992). A decreased level of serum IgG is characteristic of acute Kawasaki syndrome and appears to be correlated with the severity of coronary disease (Newburger et al., 1991). In the subacute phase of illness (day 10 to 21 after the onset), elevations in serum IgG, IgM, IgA, and IgE have been reported (Kusakawa and Heiner, 1976; Lin and Hwang, 1987). IgG and IgA immune complexes can be detected in the peripheral blood in the subacute phase, but their presence does not appear to correlate with the development of coronary artery disease, and immune complexes are not deposited in tissues in Kawasaki syndrome. There is a reduction in total CD8+ T cells in the peripheral blood in acute Kawasaki syndrome, without significant changes in the numbers of CD4+ T cells, giving rise to an elevated CD4-CD8 ratio (Leung et al., 1982; Terai et al., 1987). Examination of CD45RO+ T-cells (activated and memory T cells) in the peripheral blood in acute Kawasaki syndrome indicates an expansion of the CD8+, but not the CD4+ T-cell compartment (Pietra et al., 1994). Clonal expansion of CD8+ T cells in the peripheral blood in acute Kawasaki syndrome has also been documented, suggesting that the CD8+ T cells are targeting specific antigens (Choi et al., 1997). The decrease in overall numbers of CD8+ T cells in the peripheral blood in acute Kawasaki syndrome is in marked distinction to their presence in fourfold to fivefold greater numbers than CD4+ T cells in the coronary artery aneurysm wall (Brown et al., 2001). These studies strongly suggest that an antigen-driven immune response involving CD8+ T lymphocytes occurs in acute Kawasaki syndrome. CD8+ T cells may be selectively removed from the circulation into the major target tissue in the disease, the coronary artery. The presence of an expanded CD45RO+ CD8+ T-cell compartment and clonal expansion of CD8+ T cells in the peripheral blood is consistent with an antigen-driven immune response, targeting antigens in the vascular wall and other sites.

The CD8+ T-cell infiltrate in the arterial wall in acute Kawasaki syndrome suggests antigen processing of an intracellular pathogen, such as a virus, by major histocompatibility complex class I molecules. Clonal expansion of CD8+ T cells and IgA plasma cells fits the hypothesis that Kawasaki syndrome results from an antigen-driven immune response to a mucosal, potentially viral, pathogen.

EPIDEMIOLOGY

Kawasaki syndrome occurs primarily in young children, with 80% of patients under the age of 4 years. The illness is rare under the age of 3 months, but severe coronary artery disease can occur in infants less than 3 months of age who develop Kawasaki syndrome. Older children are also much less commonly affected than those 6 months to 8 years of age, but the disease may be more severe and the diagnosis delayed in children over 8 years (Momenah et al., 1998; Stockheim et al., 2000). Boys are 1.4 to 1.6 times more likely to be affected than girls. Kawasaki syndrome occurs worldwide and in children of all ethnic groups, although Asians are at highest risk.

In Japan, the incidence rate in the year 2000 was 134 per 100,000 children <5 years of age. Thus, approximately 1 in 200 Japanese children develops Kawasaki syndrome by the age of 5. In young infants, aged 3 to 11 months, the incidence rate is higher, up to 240 children per 100,000. Japan experienced epidemics of Kawasaki syndrome in 1979, 1982, and 1986. No clear nationwide epidemic has been observed since 1986, although incidence rates have been increasing over the past 10 years (Yanagawa et al., 2001). During epidemics, an increased number of cases have been noted in the winter and spring (Yanagawa et al., 1996). A wavelike spread of illness has been observed during epidemics, similar to that observed in outbreaks of infectious diseases such as measles and influenza (Yanagawa et al., 1986). The recurrence rate of Kawasaki syndrome in Japan is about 3%. A study of Kawasaki syndrome in Japanese families revealed that the overall rate of occurrence of a second case in a household within 1 year after onset of the first case was significantly higher than the rate of occurrence in the general population of age-matched children. More than half of the second cases occurred within 10 days of the index case, and in three of four sets of twins who both developed Kawasaki syndrome the illness began on the same date (Fujita et al., 1989). These findings suggest common exposure to an infectious agent in genetically predisposed individuals.

In the United States, incidence rates are approximately tenfold less than in Japan, but attack rates approaching those seen in Japan have been observed during epidemics (Bell et al., 1981). Incidence rates in U.S. children of Japanese ethnicity are similar to those in Japanese children in Japan. The incidence rate in blacks lies between the rates in whites and Asians. Multiple epidemics of illness have been reported in the United States: Hawaii in 1978 (Dean et al., 1982); Rochester, New York and eastern and central Massachusetts in 1979 to 1980 (Bell et al., 1981); Maryland in 1983 (Lin et al., 1985); and 10 areas of the United States in 1984 to 1985 (Centers for Disease Control, 1985). The peak age of illness in the United States appears to be 18 to 24 months of age, in contrast to the peak age in Japan of 6 to 11 months. The recurrence rate is about 1%. In the United States, Kawasaki syndrome occurs more commonly in children of middle and upper socioeconomic status. Patients with Kawasaki syndrome also have a higher incidence of an antecedent, primarily respiratory illness than controls matched for age, sex, and race (Bell et al., 1981). An association between rug shampooing and the illness has been reported in some outbreaks but not in others. Similarly, proximity to a body of water has been implicated as a risk factor in some reports but not in others, and the significance of both observations is unclear.

Epidemiology from countries other than Japan and the United States generally reveal that other Asian nations experience high incidence rates, and countries with primarily white populations experience rates closer to those seen in the United States. Both Korea and Finland have reported epidemics of Kawasaki syndrome (Lee, 1987; Salo et al., 1986).

CLINICAL MANIFESTATIONS

The classic form of Kawasaki syndrome is a distinctive clinical illness. Because a diagnostic test for the disorder does not yet exist, diagnosis is based upon the presence of prolonged fever with four of five principal manifestations of illness (Box 18-1; plate 46); these are the clinical criteria developed by Dr. Kawasaki.

Fever

Fever generally begins abruptly and is high spiking (often to 40° C or higher) and remittent,

---

BOX 18-1

DIAGNOSTIC CRITERIA FOR KAWASAKI SYNDROME

Fever, daily for more than 5 days, high spiking and intermittent, with four of the five following clinical features:

- Bulbar conjunctival injection, generally nonpurulent
- Changes in the oral mucosa, consisting of:
  - Red, fissured lips
  - Redness of the mouth
  - Strawberry tongue
- Changes in the hands and feet, consisting of:
  - Redness of the palms and soles
  - Swelling of the hands and feet
  - Peripheral desquamation in the subacute stage of illness
- Rash, erythematous and polymorphous but nonvesicular:
  - Maculopapular
  - Erythema multiforme–like
  - Scarlatiniform
- Cervical lymphadenopathy, greater than 1.5 cm in diameter

---

with two to four peaks per day. The duration of fever is generally 1 to 2 weeks in the absence of treatment but may extend for 3 to 5 weeks. The first day of fever is considered to be the first day of illness, although one or more other clinical features may have developed the day before the fever begins. In patients treated with high dose aspirin and IVIG, fever generally resolves dramatically within 24 to 48 hours.

Conjunctival Injection

Discrete vascular injection of the bulbar conjunctiva is characteristic; palpebral conjunctiva are generally less affected. Decreased redness close to the iris (limbal sparing) is commonly observed. Conjunctival injection occurs in the first week of illness. Exudate is not characteristic, and ulcerations and edema of the conjunctiva and cornea do not occur, distinguishing the illness from Stevens-Johnson syndrome. Mild acute iridocyclitis or anterior uveitis may be present on slit-lamp examination, and photophobia may be associated.

Oral Mucosal Changes

Changes in the mouth and lips are characterized by erythema, dryness, fissuring, peeling, and bleeding of the lips; erythema of the oral and pharyngeal mucosa; and strawberry tongue with prominent papillae and erythema. Oral ulcerations, Koplik's spots, and pharyngeal exudates are not observed. These changes occur in the first week of illness.

Findings in the Hands and Feet

Changes in the hands and feet are quite distinctive and include erythema confined to the palms and soles. The erythema is often striking, with an abrupt change to normal-appearing skin at or just above the palms and soles. The hands and feet can be edematous or firmly indurated, and patients frequently refuse to walk or to hold objects in their hands because of discomfort. In the subacute phase of illness, from day 10 to day 20 of illness, a characteristic desquamation begins at the fingertips just under the nailbed, and is often followed by desquamation of the toes. Extensive desquamation of the entire palm and sole in sheets can develop. It is important to recognize that peeling occurs after resolution of the acute phase; diagnosis should be made prior to the onset of peeling so that therapy can be instituted within the first 10 days of illness, preferably within the first week of illness. Transverse grooves across the fingernails and toenails (Beau's lines) can develop 1 to 2 months after the onset of illness and grow out with the nail.

Rash

The rash of Kawasaki syndrome is erythematous and nonvesicular but is otherwise polymorphic. Most common is a diffuse maculopapular rash that begins on the trunk and extremities. Although this rash may resemble a measles rash, it differs in distribution and does not progress from the face and behind the ears to the trunk, as does the measles rash. An erythema multiforme–type rash with raised, deeply erythematous pruritic plaques is also common, as is a scarlatiniform erythroderma. Fine pustules over the extensor surfaces are occasionally seen. Often, accentuation of the rash in the groin is observed. Erythema and desquamation in the groin are quite common and observed in both diapered and toilet-trained children. This occurs earlier than periungual desquamation and may be present in the acute febrile phase.

Lymph Nodes

The final diagnostic criterion, cervical lymphadenopathy, is observed in 50% of patients, whereas the other features are each present in approximately 90% of patients with Kawasaki syndrome. When present, lymphadenopathy is usually unilateral with considerable firm induration and may result in torticollis. The node is nonpurulent and may be erythematous. Although cervical adenopathy is the least common diagnostic feature, it may be the most prominent (Stamos et al., 1994); patients with acute febrile cervical adenitis unresponsive to antibiotic therapy may have unrecognized Kawasaki syndrome.

Incomplete (Atypical) Kawasaki Syndrome

Not all patients with Kawasaki syndrome have fever with four of the five other clinical manifestations, which are required to fulfill classic diagnostic criteria. Children may have fever and fewer than four of the clinical features and yet develop significant coronary artery disease (Rowley et al., 1987). The clinical illness in these patients has been termed *atypical* or *incomplete* Kawasaki disease. *Incomplete* is a more descriptive term, as these patients do not show complete clinical symptoms of Kawasaki syndrome. The term *atypical* Kawasaki disease should not be misconstrued to imply that these patients have clinical features not generally associated with the illness. Patients with incomplete Kawasaki syndrome have been identified worldwide, and the existence of such cases creates a diagnostic dilemma for the clinician. Recognition of such cases can be quite difficult, and fatal outcomes have occurred. Autopsy findings are identical in classic and incomplete cases (Fujiwara et al., 1986). Incomplete Kawasaki syndrome appears particularly common in young infants (Burns et al., 1986; Rosenfeld et al., 1995), who are unfortunately at greatest risk of developing coronary artery abnormalities. The laboratory profile of incomplete cases is similar to that of classic cases. Kawasaki syndrome should be considered in the differential diagnosis of prolonged fever in infants. The existence of incomplete Kawasaki syndrome emphasizes the need to identify the etiologic agent of the illness so that a diagnostic test can be developed.

Associated Features

Just as the pathologic features of Kawasaki syndrome indicate inflammatory lesions in a large number of tissues, so, too, do the clinical associated features of the illness attest to its multisystem nature (Box 18-2). Genitourinary, musculoskeletal, gastrointestinal, respiratory, and neurologic signs and symptoms can be present; however, cardiovascular involvement is the most important associated feature and is discussed separately below. Sterile pyuria resulting from urethritis occurs in 50% to 90% of patients. Arthritis can occur in the first week of illness, involving multiple joints and associated with synovial fluid counts of 100,000 to 300,000/mm^3, or it can occur in the subacute phase, with less intense inflammation in joint fluid and involving large weight-bearing joints. Arthritis occurs in 30% of untreated patients, but appears to be much

---

BOX 18-2

ASSOCIATED FEATURES OF KAWASAKI SYNDROME

Cardiovascular Features
- Coronary artery aneurysms
- Myocarditis
- Pericarditis
- Less commonly: endocarditis, systemic artery aneurysms

Neurologic Features
- Extreme irritability in infants
- Aseptic meningitis
- Less commonly: facial palsy

Gastrointestinal Features
- Diarrhea
- Abdominal pain
- Hepatitis
- Gallbladder hydrops
- Less commonly: obstructive jaundice, pancreatitis

Genitourinary Features
- Urethritis and pyuria
- Hydrocele

Musculoskeletal Features
- Arthritis and arthralgia

Respiratory Features
- Interstitial pneumonitis, radiographically but not clinically apparent

Other Findings
- Anterior uveitis

less common in IVIG-treated patients. Arthrocentesis may result in significant clinical improvement in those patients with arthritis despite IVIG therapy. Abdominal pain, diarrhea, and nausea are common, as are mild elevations of the transaminases. Hydrops of the gallbladder may occur; this complication resolves spontaneously without surgical intervention. Obstructive jaundice and pancreatitis have rarely been reported. Respiratory symptoms are mild, but chest radiographs indicate the presence of mild interstitial pneumonitis in 15% of patients. Extreme irritability, particularly in infants, can be present, as can lethargy. Aseptic meningitis is observed in about 40% of patients and is characterized by a median cell count of 20/mm^3 in the cerebrospinal fluid (CSF), with 90% polymorphonuclear cells and normal CSF glucose and protein levels. Otitis media is often noted.

An interesting feature of Kawasaki syndrome is erythema and induration at the site of a recent vaccination with Calmette-Guérin bacillus (BCG) for tuberculosis (Takayama et al., 1982). Since BCG is rarely given in the United States, this finding is rarely present in U.S. patients. In contrast, this feature is commonly seen in Japan, where the vaccine is routinely administered to children, and generally occurs when Kawasaki syndrome develops 6 months to 1 year following immunization. In one series, this complication was observed in 36% of 295 patients with acute Kawasaki syndrome. This finding has been incorporated into diagnostic guidelines for Kawasaki syndrome outlined by the Japan Research Committee on Kawasaki disease. The cause of this reaction is unknown.

Clinical Phases of Kawasaki Syndrome

The course of Kawasaki syndrome can be divided into three clinical phases. The acute febrile phase, generally lasting 1 to 2 weeks, is characterized by fever, conjunctival injection, oral mucosal changes, erythema and swelling of the hands and feet, rash, cervical adenopathy, aseptic meningitis, and diarrhea. Myocarditis is common and a pericardial effusion may be present. Coronary arteritis may be present, but aneurysms are not yet visible by echocardiography.

The subacute phase begins when fever, rash, and lymphadenopathy resolve at about 1 to 2 weeks after the onset of fever, but irritability,

anorexia, conjunctival injection, and oral mucosal changes may persist. Desquamation of the fingers and toes and thrombocytosis are seen during this stage, which generally lasts until 4 weeks after the onset of fever. Coronary artery aneurysms usually develop during this time, and the risk for sudden death is highest during this stage.

The convalescent stage begins when all clinical signs of the illness have disappeared and continues until the sedimentation rate normalizes, usually at 6 to 8 weeks after the onset.

Cardiovascular Manifestations

About 20% of untreated Kawasaki syndrome patients develop coronary artery abnormalities, including diffuse dilatation and aneurysm formation. Coronary dilatation is first detected at a mean of 10 days after onset of illness, and the peak frequency of coronary dilatation or aneurysms occurs within 4 weeks of onset (Hirose et al., 1981). Saccular and fusiform aneurysms usually develop between 18 and 25 days after the onset. The fatality rate is dependent on prompt recognition of cases and institution of appropriate therapy. Initial reports of 2% fatality rates from Japan in the 1970s has dropped dramatically to less than 0.1% because of improved recognition and therapy. Fatality rates as high as 6% in Auckland and 3.7% in the British Isles have been reported (Dhillon et al., 1993; Gentles et al., 1990). Death generally occurs when the patient's symptoms appear improved, at 2 to 12 weeks after the onset. The most common cause of death is myocardial infarction secondary to thrombosis of a coronary artery aneurysm. Rupture of a large coronary aneurysm is the next most common cause of death in the subacute stage. Deaths occurring in patients without an apparent myocardial infarction or aneurysm rupture may result from arrhythmias secondary to myocarditis affecting atrioventricular conduction pathways, or from intractable congestive heart failure. Deaths during or following the convalescent stage are usually the result of myocardial infarction secondary to thrombosis or stenosis of a coronary artery aneurysm.

Myocarditis occurs in more than 50% of children with acute Kawasaki syndrome. Pericarditis with pericardial effusion is present in about 25% of cases. Valvular disease is present in about 1% of patients and occasionally has required valve replacement (Akagi et al.,

1990). Systemic artery aneurysms occur in 2% of patients, generally in those who also have coronary artery aneurysms. The most commonly affected arteries are the renal, paraovarian or paratesticular, mesenteric, pancreatic, iliac, hepatic, splenic, and axillary arteries (Naoe et al., 1991).

A rare but serious complication of Kawasaki syndrome is the development of severe peripheral ischemia with resultant gangrene (Tomita et al., 1992). Patients with this complication are generally less than 7 months of age and non-Asian. Most of these infants have giant coronary artery aneurysms, the most serious coronary artery complication of Kawasaki syndrome, and some have peripheral aneurysms, particularly axillary aneurysms. Pathogenetic mechanisms giving rise to this complication likely include small vessel arteritis with thrombosis or vasospasm. Unfortunately, most of these patients experience autoamputation of fingers or require amputation of distal extremities. Although optimal therapy is unknown, salicylates and IVIG should be administered, and prostaglandin E_1, sympathetic nerve block, and thrombotic or anticoagulant therapy have shown some success.

DIAGNOSIS

Kawasaki syndrome should be considered in the differential diagnosis of patients with fever and any of the clinical symptoms of illness described above. A diagnosis of Kawasaki syndrome is considered secure when fever with four of the five principal clinical criteria are present in a patient without another explanation for the illness or in a patient with fever and fewer than four of the other clinical features and coronary artery aneurysms. If all clinical features of Kawasaki syndrome are present, it is not necessary to wait for the fifth day of fever to make the diagnosis.

Laboratory features of Kawasaki syndrome are nonspecific but quite characteristic. Patients generally have an elevated white blood cell count, or a normal white blood cell count with a predominance of neutrophils and immature forms on peripheral blood smear. Anemia is common, and its severity correlates with the severity of coronary artery disease (Asai, 1983). A low platelet count at presentation, although uncommon, is a risk factor for more severe coronary artery disease (Asai, 1983). Elevations of the platelet count to as high as 800,000/mm³

to 1,200,000/mm³ are characteristic but do not occur until the subacute phase of illness and are therefore not useful for timely diagnosis of Kawasaki syndrome. Elevations in acute phase reactants such as the erythrocyte sedimentation rate and C-reactive protein levels are almost universally observed and generally persist for several weeks. Thus, Kawasaki syndrome is unlikely in a febrile patient in whom acute phase reactants normalize in a matter of days. Mild elevations in the serum transaminases are often seen; hyperbilirubinemia is less common. Low serum albumin is another risk factor for more severe coronary disease (Asai, 1983). Cerebrospinal fluid pleocytosis with neutrophil predominance and normal glucose and protein levels may be present. Sterile pyuria is characteristic, but may be intermittent.

The differential diagnosis of Kawasaki syndrome includes measles, scarlet fever, staphylococcal scalded skin syndrome, Stevens-Johnson syndrome and other drug reactions, Rocky Mountain spotted fever, toxic shock syndrome, leptospirosis, and juvenile rheumatoid arthritis.

Identification of Kawasaki syndrome in areas where measles remains epidemic is difficult. Important differences between measles and Kawasaki syndrome include exudative conjunctivitis, Koplik's spots, and severe cough in measles. The measles rash generally starts on the face behind the ears, becomes confluent as it fades, and leaves a distinctive brownish hue, whereas the rash in patients with Kawasaki syndrome is most prominent on the trunk and extremities and generally fades abruptly without residua. Perineal accentuation of the rash is typical of Kawasaki syndrome but not measles. Swelling of the hands and feet occurs in both illnesses. The white blood cell count and sedimentation rate in patients with uncomplicated measles are low, whereas both are generally high in patients with Kawasaki syndrome. When the two diseases are difficult to distinguish, a measles IgM titer will be useful.

Kawasaki syndrome also demonstrates clinical similarities to staphylococcal and streptococcal diseases. Toxic shock syndrome can be differentiated from Kawasaki syndrome in that hypotension and renal involvement are rare in Kawasaki syndrome but common in toxic shock syndrome. Elevations of creatinine phosphokinase are also common in toxic shock syndrome but not in Kawasaki syndrome. Scarlet fever can be easily diagnosed by the presence of group A streptococci on throat culture. A common clinical problem is differentiating scarlet fever from Kawasaki syndrome in children who are carriers of group A streptococci. Up to 20% to 25% of children may be carriers of group A streptococci; thus, many children with Kawasaki syndrome will have positive throat cultures for group A streptococci. Because scarlet fever patients respond rapidly to appropriate treatment, antibiotic therapy for 24 to 48 hours with clinical reassessment generally clarifies the diagnosis.

Experienced clinicians can usually distinguish drug reactions from Kawasaki syndrome based on the nature of the rash and features such as periorbital edema (common in drug reactions but not in Kawasaki syndrome) and oral ulcers, which are common in Stevens-Johnson syndrome but not in Kawasaki syndrome. The sedimentation rate is usually less elevated in patients with drug reactions, in contrast to the very high sedimentation rates characteristic of Kawasaki syndrome.

Systemic onset juvenile rheumatoid arthritis may resemble Kawasaki syndrome. The presence of hepatosplenomegaly and lymphadenopathy suggests juvenile rheumatoid arthritis, as does the presence of an evanescent, salmon-colored rash. Rarely, a patient with systemic onset juvenile rheumatoid arthritis will be treated for Kawasaki syndrome with IVIG and aspirin therapy. Symptoms will often flare after high-dose aspirin is reduced to a low dose. Persistent or relapsing symptoms may make this diagnosis clear over time.

TREATMENT

As soon as possible after diagnosis, patients should receive treatment with a single dose of 2 g/kg of IVIG over 10 to 12 hours with 80 to 100 mg/kg/day of aspirin given orally every 6 hours. Treatment of patients with Kawasaki syndrome with this regimen within the first 10 days of illness reduces the prevalence of coronary artery abnormalities from between 20% and 25% in patients treated with aspirin alone to 4% in those treated with IVIG and aspirin (Newburger et al., 1991). Although this regimen does provide a substantial fluid and protein load, it does not increase the risk of congestive heart failure, and in fact improves cardiac function when administered over 10 to 12 hours (Newburger et al., 1989). IVIG not only reduces the prevalence of coronary disease

but also results in rapid resolution of fever and acute phase reactants. Some data suggest that patients who develop coronary disease despite IVIG and aspirin therapy have less severe dilatation and more prompt resolution of abnormalities than those who never received IVIG therapy. Aspirin is given for its anti-inflammatory and antithrombotic effects. Children with acute Kawasaki syndrome manifest decreased absorption and increased clearance of aspirin (Koren et al., 1988), and aspirin toxicity is distinctly unusual. More often, aspirin levels are subtherapeutic, but measurement of aspirin levels are generally not needed, as they do not appear to correlate with clinical response. Somewhat lower doses of aspirin (30 to 50 mg/kg/day) are used for patients with acute Kawasaki syndrome in Japan. To date, there is no conclusive evidence favoring any one aspirin dosage. Aspirin is generally continued at high doses (80 to 100 mg/kg/day) until the 14th illness day, at which time it is reduced to 3 to 5 mg/kg given as a single daily dose.

All patients with Kawasaki syndrome should be admitted to the hospital for administration of therapy and observation until fever has resolved. Cardiovascular function should be carefully monitored. Patients should have a baseline echocardiogram performed at presentation. If fever rapidly resolves following treatment and the patient remains afebrile for 24 hours, the patient may be discharged. Persistent fever is a risk factor for more severe coronary disease; patients with fever that has not resolved by 48 hours after the IVIG infusion is complete and those in whom fever recurs following an afebrile period are at particular risk and should be closely monitored. In patients who respond to therapy, a repeat echocardiogram is performed at 2 to 3 weeks after the onset of illness and again at 6 to 8 weeks after the onset. If all of these studies are normal, additional echocardiograms are not necessary. The peak time for coronary abnormalities to be diagnosed by echocardiography is at about 3 to 4 weeks after onset. Patients without evidence of coronary abnormalities should continue to receive low-dose aspirin therapy (3 to 5 mg/kg/day) in the first 2 months after the onset. It can be discontinued if there is no evidence of coronary artery dilatation and the sedimentation rate has normalized (usually 6 to 8 weeks after the onset of fever).

Limited data exist to guide therapy of patients who present after the tenth day of illness. If patients are still febrile, IVIG and aspirin therapy should be administered, as it is likely to result in prompt clinical improvement. Patients who present 1 or more weeks after fever has subsided are less likely to respond to IVIG; no evidence suggests any beneficial effect after active inflammation has subsided. Such patients should be treated with low-dose aspirin therapy until data demonstrate normal coronary arteries and resolution of acute phase reactants 2 months after the onset of illness.

The mechanism of action of IVIG in acute Kawasaki syndrome is unknown. Potential mechanisms include neutralization of a toxin, nonspecific immune modulation, and provision of specific antibody against the causative agent. The mechanism of action will be difficult to determine until the etiology of the illness is identified.

Unfortunately, not all patients with acute Kawasaki syndrome respond to initial treatment with IVIG and aspirin. Patients who remain febrile 48 to 72 hours after initial therapy, so-called nonresponders, should be re-treated with a second 2-g/kg infusion of IVIG. Re-treatment should also be considered for patients who respond to initial therapy but then have recurrence of fever following an afebrile period. Both of these patient groups are at high risk of developing coronary artery abnormalities. Uncontrolled data suggest that most nonresponders will improve following a second IVIG infusion (Han et al., 2000). However, some patients still remain febrile, and controversy exists regarding the optimal treatment of these patients. Some investigators advocate steroid therapy (Wright et al., 1996), but the efficacy of such treatment is unknown. Steroid therapy, if prescribed, should be reserved for those patients who fail to respond to two doses of IVIG. It is important to remember that Kawasaki syndrome resolves spontaneously, usually at about 3 to 6 weeks after the onset of illness. Persistence of fever with or without other symptoms after 2 to 3 months should suggest another diagnosis.

Myocardial infarction occurs most often in patients with giant coronary artery aneurysms 8 mm or larger. It may occur as early as 1 to 2 months after the onset of illness, if acute coronary thrombosis develops. Prompt fibrinolytic therapy with streptokinase, urokinase, or tissue plasminogen activator, performed at a tertiary care center by a team of cardiologists and intensivists, can be lifesaving.

LONG-TERM MANAGEMENT

The routine administration of live parenteral viral vaccines (MMR, varicella) should be delayed for 11 months following IVIG treatment for Kawasaki syndrome because the presence of specific antiviral antibodies may interfere with the immune responses to the vaccine. If significant exposure to varicella occurs in an unvaccinated patient receiving long-term aspirin therapy for Kawasaki syndrome, temporary discontinuation of aspirin can be considered. Similarly, aspirin therapy can be interrupted if the patient develops an illness suspected to be varicella or influenza, to reduce the risk of Reye's syndrome. In patients at particularly high risk for myocardial infarction, the use of an alternative antiplatelet agent should be considered. To reduce the risk of Reye's syndrome in patients on long-term aspirin therapy, administration of influenza vaccine is recommended.

Long-term management of coronary artery disease resulting from Kawasaki syndrome is based on risk stratification (Dajani et al., 1994).

Patients With No Coronary Artery Changes on Echocardiography at Any Stage of the Illness

No antiplatelet therapy is needed after the initial 6 to 8 weeks following the onset of illness. No restriction on physical activity is needed after 6 to 8 weeks. Pediatric cardiology follow-up and diagnostic testing are not indicated beyond the first year.

Patients With Transient Coronary Artery Ectasia That Disappears During the Acute Illness

No antiplatelet therapy or restriction on physical activity is needed after 6 to 8 weeks following the onset of illness. Pediatric cardiology follow-up and diagnostic testing are not essential beyond the first year, but some cardiologists prefer to follow these patients at 3- to 5-year intervals.

Patients With a Small to Medium Solitary Coronary Artery Aneurysm

Long-term antiplatelet therapy with aspirin (3 to 5 mg/kg once daily) should be administered, at least until abnormalities resolve. Physical activity of infants and children in the first decade is permitted without restriction after 6 to 8 weeks following the onset of illness. Stress testing with myocardial perfusion scan may be performed every other year in the second decade to guide recommendations for physical activity. Participation in competitive contact athletics with endurance training is discouraged. Annual follow-up with a pediatric cardiologist is recommended, with echocardiographic evaluation. Coronary angiography may be indicated if a stress test or perfusion imaging study suggests myocardial ischemia or if cardiac ultrasound suggests significant stenosis.

Patients With Giant Coronary Artery Aneurysms 8 mm or Larger

Indefinite therapy with aspirin (3 to 5 mg/kg once daily), with or without adjunctive therapy with warfarin sodium (Coumadin) anticoagulation, is warranted. Close follow-up by a pediatric cardiologist is essential. Diagnostic testing is likely to include yearly or more frequent echocardiograms; cardiac catheterization if indicated; and annual stress testing with evaluation of myocardial perfusion in patients in the second decade of life, or pharmacologic stress testing with myocardial perfusion scan in younger patients in whom obstruction is demonstrated by angiography. Physical activity is regulated on the basis of stress test results and the level of anticoagulation. Patients with obstructive lesions or signs of ischemia may need evaluation for possible surgical intervention. In 168 patients who underwent coronary bypass surgery in Japan following Kawasaki syndrome, the patency rate at 85 months after surgery was 77% for arterial grafts compared with 46% for vein grafts (Kitamura et al., 1994). Recent reports document successful treatment of coronary obstruction with catheter intervention rather than bypass surgery in patients with significant localized stenosis confined to a single vessel, although high-pressure balloon inflation has been associated with neoaneurysm formation (Akagi et al., 2000). In patients with distal aneurysms or severe myocardial dysfunction, heart transplantation has been performed (Checchia et al., 1997).

PROGNOSIS

The fate of coronary aneurysms over time has been well-described (Kato et al., 1982). At 1 to 3 months after the onset of Kawasaki syndrome, 15% of patients in this study had angiographic evidence of coronary artery aneurysms. Repeat angiography 5 to 18 months later in those with aneurysms showed resolution of the abnormality in about 50% of patients. Of those with persistent aneurysms, half had smaller aneurysms than previously, with or without stenosis, one third had resolution of the aneurysms but had developed obstruction or stenosis of the coronary arteries, and the remainder had fine irregularities of the vessel walls without stenosis. Stenosis, which occurs as a result of intimal proliferation as the vessel heals, often leads to significant coronary obstruction and myocardial ischemia. A longer-term follow-up study (Kato et al., 1996) indicated that 10 to 21 years after acute Kawasaki syndrome, additional patients with persistent aneurysms had developed stenosis of the vessel. Myocardial infarction occurred in 39% of patients with persistent aneurysms with stenosis, or 1.9% of all the Kawasaki syndrome patients in this series. Bypass surgery was performed in 1.2% of all patients, or 25% of those with persistent aneurysms with stenosis. Mortality in this group of 594 patients was 0.8%.

Although smaller aneurysms may resolve by echocardiography, intravascular ultrasound studies indicate that such vessels generally have a significantly thickened intima-media complex and are thus not normal (Sigamura et al., 1994; Suzuki et al., 1996). These vessels have lower distensibility and reduced vasodilatory response than normal vessels (Kurisu et al., 1987; Sigamura et al, 1992). So-called giant aneurysms, in which the lumen diameter is ≥8 mm, rarely resolve and most often result in complications such as myocardial ischemia. In the long-term follow-up study discussed above, 26 of 594 patients (4.4%) developed giant coronary artery aneurysms. In 12 of the 26 (46%), stenosis or complete obstruction occurred over time. Of the 12, 8 (67%) experienced a myocardial infarction, with a 50% mortality rate.

Myocardial infarction in children has a different clinical presentation than in adults. A review of 195 cases of myocardial infarction due to Kawasaki syndrome indicated that the chief symptoms were shock, unrest, vomiting, and abdominal pain; chest pain was most common in older children (Kato et al., 1986). In a recent U.S. case of myocardial infarction secondary to unrecognized Kawasaki syndrome, a 3-year-old patient was brought repeatedly to a local emergency room because of abdominal pain. Two sequential investigations for intussusception were performed before it was recognized that the patient's chest radiograph showed an enlarged heart, the ECG showed changes characteristic of myocardial infarction, and echocardiography revealed giant coronary aneurysms.

There is no direct evidence at present to indicate that a prior history of Kawasaki syndrome is a risk factor for the development of early atherosclerosis, but studies to address this question are in progress.

Noncardiovascular complications of Kawasaki syndrome are apparently entirely self-limited, are present for less than 3 months following the onset, and are not associated with chronic or progressive disability or recurrent attacks. Children who recover from Kawasaki syndrome have normal immune function and are not at higher risk of developing other infectious diseases.

Recurrence of Kawasaki syndrome is uncommon, with 1% 3% of patients developing a second episode. Recurrences may occur in the same year as the first attack, or many years later.

PREVENTION

Prevention of Kawasaki syndrome will not be possible until the etiology of the disorder is identified.

BIBLIOGRAPHY

Abe J, Kotzin BL, Jujo K, et al. Selective expansion of T cells expressing T-cell receptor variable regions Vβ2 and Vβ8 in Kawasaki disease. Proc Natl Acad Sci 1992;89:4066-4070.

American Heart Association. AHA Scientific Statement: Diagnostic Guidelines for Kawasaki Disease. Circulation 2001;103:335-336.

Akagi T, Kato H, Inoue O, et al. Valvular heart disease in Kawasaki syndrome: incidence and natural history. Am Heart J 1990;120:366-372.

Akagi T, Ogawa S, Ino T, et al. Catheter interventional treatment in Kawasaki disease: a report from the Japanese Pediatric Interventional Cardiology Investigation Group. J Pediatr 2000;137:181-186.

Amano S, Hazama F, Hamashima Y. Pathology of Kawasaki disease. I. Pathology and morphogenesis of the vascular changes. Jpn Circ J 1979;43:633-643.

Amano S, Hazama F, Hamashima Y. Pathology of Kawasaki disease. II. Distribution and incidence of the vascular lesions. Jpn Circ J 1979;43:741-748.

Amano S, Hazama F, Kubagawa H, et al. General pathology of Kawasaki disease. Acta Pathol Jpn 1980;30:681-694.

Asai T. Evaluation method for the degree of seriousness in Kawasaki disease. Acta Pediatr Jpn 1983;25:170-175 (overseas edition).

Bell DM, Brink EW, Nitzkin JL, et al. Kawasaki Syndrome: description of two outbreaks in the United States. N Engl J Med 1981;304:1568-1575.

Brown TJ, Crawford SE, Cornwall M, et al. CD8+ T cells and macrophages infiltrate coronary artery aneurysms in acute Kawasaki disease. J Infect Dis 2001;184:940-943.

Burns JC, Wiggins JW, Toews WH, et al. Clinical spectrum of Kawasaki disease in infants younger than 6 months of age. J Pediatr 1986;109:759-763.

Centers for Disease Control. Multiple outbreaks of Kawasaki syndrome—United States. MMWR Morb Mortal Wkly Rep 1985;34:33-35.

Checchia PA, Pahl E, Shaddy RE et al. Cardiac transplantation for Kawasaki disease. Pediatrics 1997;100:695-699.

Choi IH, Chwae YJ, Shim WP, et al. Clonal expansion of CD8+ T cells in Kawasaki Disease. J Immunol 1997;159:481-486.

Curtis N, Zheng R, Lamb JR, Levin M. Evidence for a superantigen mediated process in Kawasaki disease. Arch Dis Child 1995;72:308-311.

Dajani AS, Taubert KA, Takahashi M, et al. Guidelines for long-term management of patients with Kawasaki disease. Circulation 1994;89:916-930.

Dean AG, Melish ME, Hicks R. An epidemic of Kawasaki syndrome in Hawaii. J Pediatr 1982;100:552-557.

Dhillon R, Newton L, Rudd PT, et al. Management of Kawasaki disease in the British Isles. Arch Dis Child 1993;69:631-638.

Fujita Y, Nakamura Y, Sakata K et al. Kawasaki Disease in Families. Pediatrics 1989;84:666-669.

Fujiwara H, Fujiwara T, Kao T, et al. Pathology of Kawasaki disease in the healed stage. Relationships between typical and atypical cases of Kawasaki disease. Acta Pathol Jpn 1986;36:857-867.

Gentles TL, Clarkson PM, Trenholme AA, et al. Kawasaki disease in Auckland, 1979-1988. NZ Med J 1990;103:389-391.

Han RK, Silverman ED, Newman A, et al. Management and outcome of persistent or recurrent fever after initial intravenous gammaglobulin therapy in acute Kawasaki Disease. Arch Pediatr Adolesc Med 2000;154:694-699.

Hirao J, Hibi S, Andoh T, et al. High levels of circulating interleukin-4 and interleukin-10 in Kawasaki disease. Int Arch Allergy Immunol 1997;112:152-156.

Hirose O, Misawa H, Kijima Y, et al. Two-dimensional echocardiography of coronary artery in Kawasaki disease (MCLS): detection , changes in acute phase, and follow-up observation of the aneurysm. J Cardiography 1981;11:89-104 (in Japanese with English abstract).

Kato H, Ichinose E, Kawasaki T. Myocardial infarction in Kawasaki disease: clinical analyses in 195 cases. J Pediatr 1986;108:923-927.

Kato H, Ichinose E, Yoshoka F, et al. Fate of coronary aneurysms in Kawasaki disease: serial coronary angiography and long-term follow-up study. Am J Cardiol 1982;49:1758-1766.

Kato H, Sugimura T, Akagi T, et al. Long-term consequences of Kawasaki disease. Circulation 1996;94:1279-1285.

Kawasaki T. Acute febrile mucocutaneous syndrome with lymphoid involvement with specific desquamation of the fingers and toes in children [Japanese]. Jpn J Allergy 1967; 16:178-222.

Kitamura S, Kameda Y, Seki T, et al. Long-term outcome of myocardial revascularization in patients with Kawasaki coronary artery disease. J Thorac Cardiovasc Surg 1994;107:663-674.

Koren G, Schaffer F, Silverman E, et al. Determinants of low serum concentrations of salicylates in patients with Kawasaki disease. J Pediatr 1988;112:663-667.

Kurisu Y, Azumi T, Sugahara T, et al. Variation in coronary arterial dimension (distensible abnormality) after disappearing aneurysm in Kawasaki disease. Am Heart J 1987;114:532-538.

Kusakawa S, Heiner DC. Elevated levels of immunoglobulin E in the acute febrile mucocutaneous lymph node syndrome. Pediatr Res 1976;10:108-111.

Landing BH, Larson EJ. Are infantile periarteritis nodosa with coronary artery involvement and fatal mucocutaneous lymph node syndrome the same: comparison of 20 patients from North America with patients from Hawaii and Japan. Pediatrics 1977;59:651-662.

Larkin SM, Williams DN, Osterholm MT, et al. Toxic shock syndrome: clinical, laboratory, and pathologic findings in nine fatal cases. Ann Intern Med 1982;96:858-864.

Lee DB. Epidemiologic study of Kawasaki disease in Korea. Prog Clin Biol Res 1987;250:55-60.

Leung DYM, Meissner HC, Fulton DR, et al. Toxic shock syndrome toxin-secreting *Staphylococcus aureus* in Kawasaki syndrome. Lancet 1993;342:1385-1388.

Leung DYM, Siegel RL, Grady S, et al. Immunoregulatory abnormalities in mucocutaneous lymph node syndrome. Clin Immunol Immunopathol 1982;23:100-112.

Lin CY, Hwang B. Serial immunologic studies in patients with mucocutaneous lymph node syndrome (Kawasaki disease). Ann Allergy 1987;59:291-297.

Lin CY, Lin CC, Hwang B, et al. Serial changes of serum interleukin-6, interleukin-8, and tumor necrosis factor alpha among patients with Kawasaki disease. J Pediatr 1992;121:924-926.

Lin FYC, Bailowitz A, Koslowe P, et al. Kawasaki syndrome. A case-control study during an outbreak in Maryland. Am J Dis Child 1985;139:277-279.

Mancia L, Wahlstrom J, Schiller B, et al. Characterization of the T-cell receptor V-β repertoire in Kawasaki disease. Scand J Immunol 1998;48:443-449.

Melish ME, Hicks RM, Larson EJ. Mucocutaneous lymph node syndrome in the United States. Am J Dis Child 1976;130:599-607.

Melish ME, Parsonett J, Marchette N. Kawasaki syndrome (KS) is not caused by toxic shock syndrome toxin-1 (TSST-1)+ staphylococci. Pediatr Res 1994;35:187A.

Momenah T, Sanatani S, Potts J, et al. Kawasaki disease in the older child. Pediatrics 1998;102:e7.

Naoe S, Shibuya K, Takahashi K, et al. Pathological observations concerning the cardiovascular lesions in Kawasaki disease. Cardiol Young 1991;1:212-220.

Newburger JW, Sanders SP, Burns JC, et al. Left ventricular contractility and function in Kawasaki syndrome. Effect of intravenous gammaglobulin. Circulation 1989;79:1237-1246.

Newburger JW, Takahashi M, Beiser AS, et al. A single intravenous infusion of gamma globulin as compared with four infusions in the treatment of acute Kawasaki syndrome. N Engl J Med 1991;324:1633-1639.

Pietra BA, de Inocencio J, Giannini EH, Hirsch R. TCR Vβ family repertoire and T cell activation markers in Kawasaki disease. J Immunol 1994;153:1881-1888.

Rosenfeld EA, Corydon KE, Shulman ST. Kawasaki disease in infants less than one year of age. J Pediatr 1995;126:524-529.

Rowley AH, Eckerley CA, Jack H-M, et al. IgA plasma cells in vascular tissue of patients with Kawasaki syndrome. J Immunol 1997;159:5946-5955.

Rowley AH, Gonzalez-Crussi F, Gidding S, et al. Incomplete Kawasaki disease with coronary artery involvement. J Pediatr 1987;110:409-413.

Rowley AH, Shulman ST, Mask CA, et al. IgA plasma cell infiltration of proximal respiratory tract, pancreas, kidney, and coronary artery in acute Kawasaki disease. J Infect Dis 2000;182:1183-1191.

Rowley AH, Shulman ST, Spike BT, et al. Oligoclonal IgA response in the vascular wall in acute Kawasaki disease. J Immunol 2001;166:1334-1343.

Salo E, Pelkonen P, Pettay O. Outbreak of Kawasaki syndrome in Finland. Acta Pediatr Scand 1986;75:75-80.

Sigamura T, Kato H, Inoue O, et al. Intravascular ultrasound of coronary arteries in children. Assessment of the wall morphology and the lumen after Kawasaki disease. Circulation 1994;89:258-265.

Sigamura T, Kato H, Inoue O, et al. Vasodilatory response of the coronary arteries after Kawasaki disease: evaluation by intracoronary injection of isosorbide dinitrate. J Pediatr 1992;121:684-688.

Stamos JK, Corydon K, Donaldson J, et al. Lymphadenitis as the dominant manifestation of Kawasaki disease. Pediatrics 1994;93:525-528.

Stockheim JA, Innocentini N, Shulman ST. Kawasaki disease in older children and adolescents. J Pediatr 2000;137:250-252.

Suzuki A, Yamagishi M, Kimura K, et al. Functional behavior and morphology of the coronary artery wall in patients with Kawasaki disease assessed by intravascular ultrasound. J Am Coll Cardiol 1996;27:291-296.

Takayama J, Yanase Y, Kawasaki T. A study on erythematous change at the site of the BCG inoculation. Acta Paediatr Jpn 1982;86:567-572.

Taubert KA, Rowley AH, Shulman ST. Seven-year national survey of Kawasaki disease and acute rheumatic fever. Pediatr Infect Dis J 1994;13:704-708.

Terai M, Kohno Y, Niwa K, et al. Imbalance among T-cell subsets in patients with coronary arterial aneurysms in Kawasaki disease. Am J Cardiol 1987;60:555-559.

Terai M, Miwa K, Williams T, et al. The absence of evidence of Staphylococcal toxin involvement in the pathogenesis of Kawasaki disease. J Infect Dis 1995;172:558-561.

Tomita S, Chung K, Mas M, et al. Peripheral gangrene associated with Kawasaki disease. Clin Infect Dis 1992;14:121-126.

Wright DA, Newburger JW, Baker A, et al. Treatment of immune globulin-resistant Kawasaki disease with pulsed doses of corticosteroids. J Pediatr 1996;128:146-149.

Yanagawa H, Nakamura Y, Kawasaki T, et al. Nationwide epidemic of Kawasaki disease in Japan during winter of 1985-1986. Lancet 1986;2:1138-1139.

Yanagawa H, Nakamura Y, Yashiro M, et al. Update of the epidemiology of Kawasaki disease in Japan from the results of the 1993-1994 nationwide survey. J Epidemiol 1996;6:148-157.

Yanagawa H, Nakamura Y, Yashiro M, et al. Incidence survey of Kawasaki disease in 1997 and 1998 in Japan. Pediatrics 2001;107:e33.

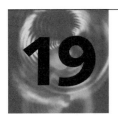

19 MALARIA

JOHANNA P. DAILY

Malaria remains a major health problem for children in tropical areas of the world. Despite the discovery of the causative agent of malaria in the 1880s, many features of its biology and pathogenesis are unknown and it remains a very potent threat. The underlying mechanism of age-related disease severity and why some children suffer severe disease while others do not are not understood. This parasite has coevolved with humans for centuries and over this time has developed survival and transmission strategies to allow maintenance in the human population. For example, the parasite antigens expressed on the surface of red blood cells have been found to undergo variation to evade host immune responses (Borst et al., 1995; Contamin et al., 1996). While antimalarial agents remain the mainstay of prevention and treatment, the development of drug resistance to the various classes of compounds, particularly in *Plasmodium falciparum*, has occurred. Furthermore, adjunctive therapeutics to further decrease mortality in cases of severe malaria have had only limited success. These events and the lack of new agents may actually have increased the global impact of malaria.

The diagnosis of malaria is commonly considered in patients who live and are cared for in malaria endemic areas, although it is an unusual cause of illness in children returning from the tropics. The signs and symptoms of malaria are very nonspecific, and infection can occur despite proper antimalarial prophylaxis. For this reason a high suspicion of this diagnosis must be maintained when treating children returning from endemic areas.

ETIOLOGY

Malaria is a disease caused by a protozoan parasite that has an asexual life cycle that takes place in the human host liver cells and erythrocytes and a sexual stage that occurs in the anopheline mosquito. The infection is transmitted during the blood meal of a female *Anopheles*, and malarial sporozoites are incidentally discharged into the bloodstream of the human host. Within minutes, these sporozoites find their way to the liver. Asexual development takes place as the parasite moves through the trophozoite and schizont stages, which have distinctive morphology. Merozoites are released from hepatocytes into the circulation 1 to 3 weeks later, although disease caused by *Plasmodium vivax* strains may occasionally emerge after months. The merozoites quickly invade erythrocytes and continue the asexual life cycle, with each schizont producing 8 to 32 merozoites. There is a febrile response to each release of merozoites, resulting in the classic periodic fever pattern in established infection; the burden of infection can rise rapidly through this process. A small percentage of these intraerythrocytic forms develop into transmissible forms, male and female gametocytes. Gametocytes are incidentally acquired during an anopheline blood meal and undergo sexual stage replication within the midgut of the mosquito. Sporozoites are formed and then inoculated into another human host to continue the transmission cycle. Four primary species of *Plasmodium* infect humans, each with different patterns of endemicity, virulence, incubation period, and morphology. They include *P. vivax, Plasmodium ovale, P. falciparum*, which have an asexual stage life cycle of 48 hours, and *Plasmodium malariae*, which has a 72-hour asexual life cycle. *P. falciparum* and *P. vivax* cause the vast majority of infections worldwide. In addition, the majority of severe disease and death is related to infection with *P. falciparum*, and subsequent discussion of severe disease will refer to disease caused by this species. In rare instances, malaria can be transmitted without traveling to an endemic area, such as in cases of airport malaria or extremely rare occurrence of transfusion-related malaria (Layton et al., 1995; Mungai et al., 2001; Van den Ende et al., 1998).

EPIDEMIOLOGY

There are an estimated 300 to 500 million cases of malaria each year, with 1.5 to 2.7 million deaths annually (World Health Organization, 1997). The vast majority of these *P. falciparum*–related deaths occur in children in Africa (Murphy and Breman, 2001; Olliaro et al., 1996). This disease is endemic in areas that contain 40% of the world's population and include Africa, Latin America, the Caribbean, India, Southeast Asia, the Eastern Mediterranean, the Western Pacific, and parts of Europe (World Health Organization, 1997). Transmission of *P. vivax* malaria, however, also occurs in temperate areas of China and Russia and parts of Korea (Siegel, 1998). Many factors including rainfall, season, altitude, local vegetation, temperature, and personal protective measures modulate transmission risk. Although in many areas there is transmission of more than one species, certain species may predominate, and this information will assist in determining causative species (Table 19-1). For example, *P. falciparum* is the predominant species in Africa and is found in Asia and South America, whereas *P. vivax* is rare in Africa and is found commonly in Asia and Latin America. Large urban centers in Asia generally are free of malaria, whereas transmission in cities in Africa is common.

Knowledge of these details of transmission and patient exposure is important when planning prophylaxis or determining if a child is at risk for infection. It is often overlooked that two species—*P. vivax* and *P. ovale*—can remain latent in the liver for years, resulting in illness long after the exposure. In addition, *P. malariae*, which causes a very rare form of malaria, can remain at a subpatent level for years before causing illness.

Drug Resistance

P. ovale and *P. malariae* remain chloroquine sensitive. *P. vivax* infections are generally chloroquine sensitive, although there are rare case reports of resistance to chloroquine in, for example, areas in Papua New Guinea, Indonesia, and Columbia (Baird et al., 1997; Rieckmann et al., 1989; Soto et al., 2001; Whitby, 1997). *P. falciparum* has become chloroquine resistant in most geographic areas except in the Dominican Republic, Haiti, Central America west of the former Panama Canal Zone, parts of China, Peru, Argentina, and some countries in North Africa (for instance, Egypt). In addition, resistance of *P. falciparum* to both chloroquine and sulfadoxine-pyrimethamine (SP; Fansidar) is widespread in Thailand, Myanmar, Cambodia, the Amazon River basin area of South America, and, increasingly, parts of East Africa. *P. falciparum* resistance to mefloquine has been confirmed on the borders of Thailand with Myanmar and Cambodia, in the western provinces of Cambodia, and in the eastern states of Myanmar (Figure 19-1) (Centers for Disease Control and Prevention, 2001). Updates on malaria epidemiology and drug

TABLE 19-1	Epidemiology of *Plasmodium* Species by Geographic Location			
Region	*Plasmodium falciparum*	*Plasmodium vivax*	*Plasmodium malariae*	*Plasmodium ovale*
Africa	Very high	Rare, except in Northeast	Low	Moderate in West
Southeast Asia	Moderate to high	Moderate to high	Low	Low (Philippines and Indonesia)
South Asia	Low to moderate	Moderate to high	Rare	None
South America	Moderate	Moderate to high	Low	None
Central America	Low	Low to moderate	Rare	None
Southwest Asia	Rare	Low	Rare	None
Oceania	High	Moderate to high	Low	Low

Modified from Baird and Hoffman: Med Clin North Am 1999;83:923-944.

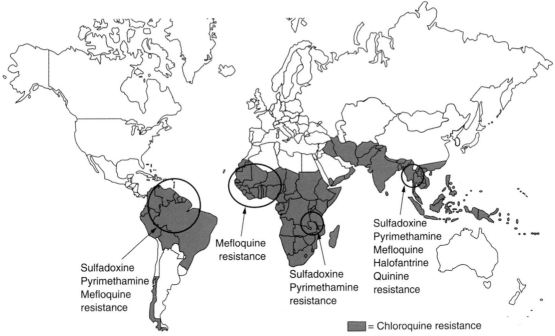

Fig. 19-1 Epidemiology of antimalarial drug resistance. (Modified from Centers for Disease Control and Prevention, National Center for Infectious Diseases, Atlanta, Ga.)

resistance prevalence can be found at the World Health Organization's Web site (http://www.who.int/ith/) and in the Centers for Disease Control and Prevention (CDC) "Yellow Book" (http://www.cdc.gov/ncidod/guidelines/guide-lines_topic_travel.htm) (Centers for Disease Control and Prevention, 2001).

PATHOGENESIS

Disease is secondary to parasite biology including invasion leading to erythrocyte loss, attachment to microvasculature, glucose metabolism, and host response (Chen et al., 2000). Multiple genetic host factors protect from severe disease, and in addition there may be variation in the virulence of parasites strains (Aitman et al., 2000; Gupta et al., 1994; Hill et al., 1991; Hill et al., 1992; May et al., 2001; McGuire et al., 1994). *P. vivax* and *P. ovale* can rarely cause severe symptoms. Severe morbidity and mortality in general are secondary to *P. falciparum* infection in young children or nonimmune adults. The vast majority of immune adult patients with *P. falciparum* infection are asymptomatic or have mild symptoms. Newborns of immune mothers appear to be protected from severe disease until approximately 6 months of

age, although the mechanism of this protection remains unknown (McGuinness et al., 1998; Riley et al., 2000). After this time period, young children are at risk for severe disease, particularly severe anemia and cerebral malaria, which are related to age and transmission intensity. For example, severe anemia is more common in infants (>6 months) and young children (<3 years), whereas cerebral malaria affects slightly older children (Allen et al., 1996; Greenwood, 1997b; Snow et al., 1997). The fatality rate of severe malarial anemia is generally less than that of cerebral malaria, in which the mortality rates approach 20% (Bondi, 1992; Imbert et al., 1997; Molyneux et al., 1989; Newton et al., 1991; Waller et al., 1995). Overlap of these two clinical syndromes is common. *P. falciparum* has particular biologic properties that are postulated to confer this deadly potential. First, this parasite, unlike the other species, can invade a wider range of ages of red blood cells. This results in a higher burden of parasites compared with other species, and, in general, parasitemias >2% are secondary to infection with *P. falciparum*. Second, *P. falciparum* late-stage trophozoites and schizonts can adhere to microvasculature and sequester out of the circulation (Fujioka and Aikawa, 1996). This is thought to provide the parasite a mechanism to avoid clearance by the spleen. Sequestration likely plays a role in the minority of patients who go on to develop cerebral malaria and, in addition, may play a role in other clinical manifestations. For example, cytoadherence to the pulmonary microvasculature has been associated with respiratory involvement (Corbett et al., 1989). Finally, it has been postulated that *P. falciparum* schizonts release a malaria "toxin" at the time of schizont rupture; this results in cytokine response, which contributes to the clinical illness. Studies are underway to determine if antibodies to this parasite phospholipid are protective against severe disease (Naik et al., 2000).

Loss of erythrocytes due to parasitization is an obvious contributor to anemia, although in many studies the degree of anemia does not correlate with the degree of parasitemia (Menendez et al., 2000; Molyneux et al., 1989; Phillips et al., 1986; Price et al., 2001). In fact, there are multiple mechanisms that result in malaria-induced anemia, including extravascular hemolysis or erythrophagocytosis of both parasitized and nonparasitized erythrocytes, bone-marrow suppression, and dyserythropoiesis (Menendez et al., 2000). Patients from endemic areas often have concomitant processes that contribute to anemia, such as malnutrition, iron or folate deficiency, hemoglobinopathies, sickle-cell disease, human immunodeficiency virus (HIV) infection, or helminthic infections. Evaluation for these conditions should be undertaken if the hematocrit does not normalize after antimalarial therapy.

The pathophysiology of coma in cerebral malaria remains unknown, and it is possible that there are distinct and varied mechanisms that result in a comatose state. The striking feature of this syndrome is that the vast majority of patients awake within 2 to 3 days, without neurologic sequela. Children often have raised intracranial pressure presumably secondary to increase in cerebral blood volume (Newton et al., 1991). Seizures, hyperthermia, anemia, and sequestration of parasitized and unparasitized red cells are thought to contribute to this phenomenon (Newton and Warrell, 1998). Gross and microscopic brain pathology reveal multiple visible petechial hemorrhages in the gray matter, with intact endothelium and occasional inflammatory cells (Brown et al., 2001;

MacPherson et al., 1985; Silamut et al., 1999; Turner et al., 1994). The sequestration of infected red cells via parasite proteins expressed on red-cell surface with cerebral microvascular endothelial ligands is thought to be a critical component of coma. Sequestered parasites likely compromise the local blood flow of the microcirculatory system. Seizures are frequent, prolonged, and repeated and are believed to contribute to the comatose state. Together, production of tumor necrosis factor (TNF), hypoglycemia, release of nitric oxide and free radicals, seizures, and microvasculature obstruction contribute to the encephalopathy (Clark et al., 1992). Computed tomography performed in a small series of children with cerebral malaria revealed that some of the children exhibited diffuse brain swelling or swelling with widespread areas of low density. In follow-up, this latter group developed cerebral atrophy and infarction associated with clinical neurologic sequela (Newton et al., 1994).

CLINICAL MANIFESTATIONS

Malaria can manifest in children with a wide range of symptoms. There is nothing specific in the history or examination to suggest this diagnosis, and therefore a high index of suspicion should be maintained when treating any sick child who has been exposed to an endemic area. For example, cough, vomiting, and diarrhea are common symptoms associated with malaria (Hendrickse et al., 1971; O'Dempsey et al., 1983). Clinical diagnosis is unreliable, and blood smears or alternative diagnostic tests must be performed (Hendrickse et al., 1971). Lack of fever periodicity is common and does not rule out the diagnosis of malaria. The classic fever pattern generally does not occur during the acute phase of infection and often does not occur in *P. falciparum* infection. Periodicity may develop after a week of infection with *P. vivax*, *P. ovale*, and *P. malariae*. A majority of children do not present with severe disease. Instead, young children exhibit fever, gastrointestinal symptoms such as diarrhea, irritability, and respiratory symptoms. Pallor and splenomegaly may be more specific indicators of malaria, but there are no clinical signs that provide sufficient specificity (Redd et al., 1996).

It is important to recognize severe disease so that proper supportive measures can be arranged, and specific principles are kept in mind (Box 19-1). The category of severe disease includes patients whose presenting signs include severe anemia, coma from which the patient cannot be aroused, pulmonary edema, circulatory failure, disseminated intravascular coagulation, acidosis, renal failure, and repeated generalized convulsions (Warrell et al., 1990). Non–P. *falciparum* malaria can cause marked symptoms but rarely causes severe malaria or death. P. *vivax*–induced hypersplenism can result in splenic rupture, however. Aside from the species of organism causing the malaria, host factors also modulate disease severity, and, of greatest importance, the age of patients from endemic areas modulates the manifestations of the disease (Baird, 1998). Nonimmune children of all ages are at risk for severe malaria secondary to P. *falciparum*.

Severe Malarial Disease

Indicators of life-threatening malaria include impaired consciousness, particularly if associated with extensor posturing; respiratory distress; jaundice; and laboratory markers including hypoglycemia, hyperlactemia (plasma lactate level >5 mmol/L), and presence of late-stage forms on the blood smear (Marsh et al., 1995; Silamut and White, 1993; Waller et al., 1995). Respiratory distress with acidosis and hyperlactemia has been found to be a very important indicator of prognosis and may suggest total tissue hypoxia (English et al., 1996b; Krishna et al., 1994; Marsh et al., 1996; Taylor et al., 1993). Signs of malarial hyperpneic syndrome include alar flaring, chest recession (intercostal or subcostal), use of accessory muscles for respiration or abnormally deep breathing (Marsh et al., 1995). Metabolic acidosis

generally improves rapidly with antimalarial treatment and with oral or intravenous fluids (Taylor et al., 1993).

Anemia

Malaria-related anemia is defined as reduction in the red blood cell count below normal for age in the presence of malaria parasitemia of any density in an endemic area. Severe anemia is defined as hemoglobin <5 g/dl or hematocrit <15%, with parasitemia of >10,000 parasites/ul (Warrell et al., 1990).

Cerebral Malaria

Cerebral malaria should be considered if the patient is unarousable, if parasitemia of any density is present, if alternative diagnoses such as hypoglycemia and meningitis have been ruled out, and if the state of unconsciousness lasts more than 30 minutes after seizures have stopped (Warrell et al., 1990). Cerebral malaria may develop rapidly in children, as reported in a study from East Africa in which patients were febrile less than 2 days and the mean time of occurrence of unconsciousness was only 7.8 hours prior to presentation (Greenwood et al., 1987; Molyneux et al., 1989). The manifestations of neurologic involvement are extremely diverse, ranging from diffuse cortical involvement to specific brainstem dysfunction. Clinical findings include posturing, absence of corneal reflexes, pupillary changes, gaze abnormalities, and abnormal respiratory patterns, including Kussmaul's and Cheyne-Stokes respirations and periodic apnea (Molyneux et al., 1989; Schmutzhard and Gerstenbrand, 1984; Waller et al., 1995). Patients with cerebral malaria

---

BOX 19-1

APPROACH TO CHILD WITH SEVERE MALARIA

- Perform lumbar puncture and measure glucose levels if there are seizures or mental status changes.
- Consider secondary processes related to other diseases such as typhoid, pneumonia, or bacteremia.
- Rarely, peripheral smear is negative for malaria; treat presumptively, and continue to obtain smears.
- Initiate parenteral antimalarial therapy and continue until patient's condition improves and therapy can be administered orally.
- Monitor glucose during quinine or quinidine infusion.
- Replete intravascular space if metabolic acidosis and respiratory distress occur.
- Consider exchange transfusion with high parasitemia.
- Examine patient carefully for subtle signs of seizure, and treat appropriately.

often have retinal hemorrhages, retinal whitening, retinal vessels with patches of whitening, and papilledema; occasionally these are detected before the onset of coma (Lewallen, 1999; Lewallen, 2000; Looareesuwan et al., 1983).

Despite the depth of coma and temporary neurologic abnormalities during the hospital course, very few patients have gross long-term neurologic sequelae. A wide range of abnormalities, though, can persist after discharge as a result of the acute illness, including residual seizures, hemiparesis, generalized hypotonia, generalized spasticity of limbs, cerebeller ataxia, persistent extrapyramidal tremor, aphasia, blindness, cerebral palsy, behavior disturbances, and psychosis (Brewster et al., 1990; Carme et al., 1993; Molyneux et al., 1989; Musoke, 1966; Schmutzhard and Gerstenbrand, 1984). Risk factors for persistent deficits include protracted convulsions, prolonged coma, and severe anemia (Brewster et al., 1990; Crawley et al., 1996). Many patients recover fully over time, although in a proportion of them a neurologic deficit remains. Long-term follow-up studies are not available on the prevalence of subtle neurologic defects after an episode of cerebral malaria.

Seizures

Seizures are a very common presenting sign, and persistence of seizures is associated with increased morbidity and mortality (Bondi, 1992). Fever is an important factor, but often the mechanism of these seizures is directly related to the *P. falciparum* infection specifically, and frequently they occur when the temperature is below 38° C. A study in children from Thailand found that *P. vivax* infection is much less likely to result in seizure than is *P. falciparum* infection (Crawley et al., 1996; Waruiru et al., 1996; Wattanagoon et al., 1994). Seizures can also occur with minimal clinical signs, and close neurologic evaluation should be performed frequently to detect them (Crawley, 1996). Subtle signs may include nystagmus and salivation, and ongoing seizure activity may contribute to hypoventilation and acid-base disturbances (Crawley et al., 1996; White, 1971).

Hypoglycemia

Not uncommonly, children with severe malaria present with hypoglycemia (Taylor et al., 1988; White et al., 1987). In addition, rapid infusions

of quinine can precipitate hypoglycemia, as quinine is a potent insulin secretagogue (Okitlonda et al., 1987; White et al., 1983). Presenting hypoglycemia and, in particular, persistent hypoglycemia correlate with heightened mortality (Jaffar et al., 1997; Musoke, 1966; Taylor et al., 1988). Intensive care unit–management of this condition is a critical component of the treatment of the seriously ill child with *P. falciparum* infection.

Renal Manifestations

Dehydration with hyponatremia, reduction in creatinine clearance, and hypokalemia and hyperkalemia have been reported in children during acute falciparum infection (Sowunmi, 1996). Renal failure secondary to *P. falciparum* infection is a very rare occurrence in children. Notably, the nephrotic syndrome and chronic glomerulonephritis have been specifically associated with *P. malariae* infections.

Respiratory Manifestations

Respiratory signs and symptoms are not uncommon in acute *P. falciparum* malaria. The spectrum includes clinical features that overlap with pneumonia (O'Dempsey et al., 1993). In one study of 200 children admitted to a hospital in Kenya with the diagnosis of acute severe respiratory infection, 45% were ultimately given the diagnosis of malaria alone and had normal chest x-ray films (English et al., 1996a). Rare complications in severe malaria include adult respiratory distress syndrome and noncardiogenic pulmonary edema, although these are more likely to occur in adults. It is important to keep in mind that children who display signs of respiratory distress are often intravascularly depleted. If the patient is severely anemic, blood transfusion can be safely given (English et al., 1996b).

Malaria in Pregnancy and Congenital Malaria

Malaria infection during pregnancy can have severe effects on the outcome. These complications include low birth weight, intrauterine growth retardation, and heightened infant mortality (Steketee et al., 2001). Primigravid and nonimmune patients are at greatest risk. Malaria prophylaxis has been shown in some studies to decrease these complications (Nyirjesy et al., 1993). Congenital malaria is rare and has been found to occur in up to 0.3% of immune mothers and up to 7.4% of nonimmune mothers, although higher rates have been reported elsewhere (Covell, 1950; McGregor, 1984; Akindele et al, 1993). In a review of cases occurring in the United States, the mean age of onset of symptoms in a series of 46 infants was 5.5 weeks. All these children had fever and the majority had hepatosplenomegaly, anemia, and thrombocytopenia (Hulbert, 1992). Manifestations of illness, however, can occur as early as 48 hours after delivery.

DIAGNOSIS

Delay in diagnosis can result in poor outcome and has resulted in disastrous consequences among young children with imported malaria (Moore et al., 1994). Microscopy performed by an experienced operator is very sensitive, rapid, and inexpensive and remains the gold standard (Dorsey et al., 2000; Kain et al., 1998). Thin and thick smears can be examined with Giemsa, Wright's, or Field's staining. Giemsa stain provides the greatest detail and will allow the detection of Schüffner's dots, whereas the application of Field's stain is much more rapid. Thick smears are more sensitive for detecting the presence of parasites, and thin smears can provide more details for species determination. Table 19-2 outlines morphologic clues for determination of species. An adequate amount of time must be spent to analyze multiple forms and to determine if there is a mixed infection. If an experienced microscopist is not available there are a number of rapid diagnostic devices available. In general, limitations of these alternative tests include low sensitivity with low parasitemia, inability to differentiate between species, and positive results despite cure. Improved tests to overcome these issues are being developed. The QBC test (Becton, Dickinson and Company, Franklin Lakes, New Jersey) was one of the first rapid tests developed using acridine orange dye, which allows species determination, although sensitivity with low parasitemia is less than that of microscopy (Baird et al., 1992; Rickman et al., 1989). Other rapid tests include ICT Malaria Pf (ICT Diagnostics, Sydney, Australia); ICT Malaria P.f/P.v (ICT Diagnostics); and PATH Falciparum Malaria IC Strip (Program for Appropriate Technology, Seattle, Washington) (Jelinek et al., 2001; Mills et al., 1999). OptiMAL and ICpLDH (Flow, Inc, Portland, Oregon) detect parasite lactate dehydrogenase enzyme and can distinguish *P. falciparum* from the other species. Rapid, inexpensive poly-merase chain reaction assay, which is often the most sensitive technology, is being developed for detection of malaria (Schindler et al., 2001). It is important to know the limitation of the test being used, and it is imperative to repeat the test if the result is negative in order to enhance sensitivity.

DIFFERENTIAL DIAGNOSIS

Malaria has nonspecific symptoms and clinical findings, and a differential diagnosis must take into consideration other common illnesses to which the patient may have been exposed, such as influenza, viral hepatitis, typhoid, diarrheal illness, respiratory infection, bacteremia, meningitis, tuberculosis, HIV infection, and other parasitic infections. Because of immunity, many patients are parasitemic without disease, and the simple presence of parasites in a patient with fever can be misleading; therefore, one should always consider the differential diagnosis (Rougemont et al., 1991).

TREATMENT

Once the diagnosis is arrived at, determining the severity of illness is critical to allow prompt therapy and supportive measures. The epidemiology of drug-resistant parasites to which the patients has been exposed will direct the appropriate antimalarial therapy (Figure 19-1, Table 19-3.) Prognosis is improved with early initiation of chemotherapy, which should be administered parentally in cases of severe disease (Warrell, 1999).

Chloroquine is inexpensive and well tolerated and requires a short oral treatment course. It is available for intravenous or intramuscular administration for severe disease, but administration by these routes should be undertaken with caution, as it can lead to hypotension (Table 19-3). Persistence of parasites after 4 to 5 days of treatment suggests drug resistance.

Quinine remains the mainstay of initial therapy for severely ill children in areas where parasites are quinine susceptible. An initial loading of quinine (20 mg quinine dihydrochloride/kg infused over 4 hours) has been shown to improve outcomes and is safe (Mehta et al., 1994; van der Torn et al., 1998; White et al., 1983a). Hypoglycemia can accompany this method of administration, and glucose levels should be monitored during the infusion. Side effects include gastrointestinal upset, tinnitus,

TABLE 19-2 Morphologic Features of *Plasmodium* Species

Species	MORPHOLOGIC FEATURES				
	Only early trophozoites (rings) seen in blood smear	Schüffner's dots	Other diagnostic characteristics	Hypnozoite form	Drug resistance
Plasmodium falciparum	Yes	No	Double chromatin dot common Multiply infected erythrocytes common Infects young and old red blood cells Parasitemia may exceed 2% Accolé form	No	Chloroquine resistance: parts of Africa, Latin America, Asia, Southeast Asia, Oceania Sulfadoxine-pyrimethamine resistance in parts of Amazon River basin, Southeast Asia, Southern and Eastern Africa Multiple drug resistance at Myanmar-Thailand border
Plasmodium vivax	No, all stages seen	Yes	Rarely double chromatin dot Occasionally multiply infected erythrocytes Infects young red blood cells Parasitemia <2%	Yes	Chloroquine sensitive Rare reports of resistance in Columbia, New Guinea, Indonesia, Myanmar, India, Irian Jaya, and the Solomon Islands
Plasmodium ovale	No, all stages seen	Yes	No multiply infected erythrocytes Infects young red blood cells Red cells become oval with tufted ends Parasitemia <2%	Yes	Chloroquine sensitive
Plasmodium malariae	No, all stages seen	No	No multiply infected erythrocytes Infects old red blood cells Parasitemia <2% Band form	No, but can persist in blood for years without symptoms	Chloroquine sensitive

TABLE 19-3	Antimalarial Agents Used for Treatment	
Antimalarial agent	Treatment	Comments
Chloroquine phosphate (Aralen)	10 mg base/kg (not to exceed 600 mg base), 5 mg base/kg (not to exceed 300 mg base) 6 h later, then 5 mg base/kg at 24 and 48 h	Although side effects are rare, nausea and vomiting, headache, dizziness, blurred vision, and pruritus have been reported, particularly in black-skinned patients. May worsen the symptoms of psoriasis.
Quinine dihydrochloride	20 mg/kg loading dose IV in 5% dextrose over 4 h, followed by 10 mg/kg over 2-4 hq8h (max 1800 mg/d) until oral therapy can be started; complete treatment with second agent such as doxycycline, sulfadoxine-pyrimethamine, clindamycin	Can cause hypotension if infused too quickly. Can induce hypoglycemia
Quinidine gluconate	10 mg base/kg loading dose (max 600 mg) in normal saline over 1-2 hours, followed infused by 0.02 mg/kg/min continuous infusion until oral therapy can be started; complete treatment with second agent such as doxycycline, sulfadoxine-pyrimethamine, clindamycin	Monitor for QT prolongation and hypotension.
Quinine sulfate	25 mg/kg/day PO divided into 3 doses for 3-7 days; complete treatment with second agent such as doxycycline, sulfadoxine-pyrimethamine, clindamycin	In general, poorly tolerated; may cause tinnitus, nausea, deafness.
Sulfadioxone (500 mg)-pyrimethamine (25 mg) (Fansidar)	<1 yr, ¼ tab PO qd 1-3 yr, ½ tab single dose 4-8 yr, 1 tab single dose 9-14 yr, 2 tabs single dose >14 yr 3 tabs single dose	Contraindicated in patients with sulfa allergy and in those less than 2 months of age; can cause gastrointestinal upset and headache.
Mefloquine (Lariam)	15 mg/kg PO followed in 8-12 h by 10 mg/kg	Not recommended for persons with epilepsy and other seizure disorders, severe psychiatric disorders, or cardiac conduction abnormalities.
Atovaquone and proguanil (Malarone) Adult formulation: 250 mg/100 mg	11-20 kg: 1 adult tab PO qd × 3 days 21—30 kg: 2 adult tabs PO qd as single dose × 3 days 31—40 kg: 3 adult tabs PO as single dose × 3 days > 40 kg: 4 adult tabs as single dose × 3 days	Not indicated in patients <11 kg; contraindicated in patients with severe renal impairment (creatinine clearance <30 ml/min); rare reports of elevated liver function tests.
Doxycycline (Vibramycin, Monodox)	In combination with quinine Children over 8: 2 mg/kg PO qd × 7 days, not to exceed 100 mg bid	Contraindicated in children <8 years of age; can cause photosensitivity.
Clindamycin	20-40 mg/kg day PO in 3 divided doses × 5 days (single dose not to exceed 900 mg) in combination with quinine	Can cause gastrointestinal upset.
Halofantrine (Halfan)	8 mg/kg q6h × 3 doses PO, repeat in 7 days	Avoid use in patients taking mefloquine prophylactically and those with baseline QT abnormalities.

and high-tone deafness. Severely ill patients should be monitored closely. Quinine treatment should be combined with a second agent such as doxycycline (not for use in children under 8 years of age), clindamycin, or SP. Change to oral therapy can occur once the patient no longer has severe disease and is taking medications orally. Quinidine can be used if quinine is not available. Prolongation of the QT interval is more marked than with use of quinine and therefore cardiac monitoring is necessary. In addition, hypotension can occur with rapid infusion.

SP is often used in areas with chloroquine-resistant organisms, as it is also inexpensive and requires only a single dose. It is no longer recommended for prophylaxis because of adverse cutaneous reactions. Unfortunately drug resistance has been increasing in parts of Africa, Southeast Asia, and Brazil. Patients with G6PD deficiency are at risk for hemolysis with this drug. In general SP is contraindicated for use in the first 1 to 2 months of life because of the potential for kernicterus.

Mefloquine is an expensive alternative if the patient is from an area with chloroquine- and SP-resistant organisms. Doses effective for treatment can result in significant gastrointestinal side effects, particularly in children (Luxemburger et al., 1996). It should not be used with quinine or quinidine. There is no parenteral formulation.

Halofantrine is an option for treatment of drug resistant parasites. The limitations include expense, cross-resistance to mefloquine, and concentration-related effect on QT interval. This drug is contraindicated in patients taking mefloquine.

Drug resistance, particularly at the Thailand-Myanmar border has resulted in the development of new compounds including artemisinin (quinghaosu) derivatives such as water-soluble artesunate and oil-soluble artemether. This class of compounds results in the fastest time to clearance of the parasite but no clear improvement in outcomes compared with quinine (Murphy et al., 1996; van Hensbroek et al., 1996). Clinical experience with these compounds in areas where parasites are highly drug resistant has been extensive (Price et al., 1999b). To improve on the significant mortality rate of 10% to 30% in severe malaria patients treated with standard anti-malarial agents, combination therapy has been used. The addition of arsenate to quinine showed no benefit over quinine alone in adult patients with acute falciparum malaria (Newton et al., 2001). A combination of arte-sunate and SP has been shown to be safe and to result in faster elimination of fever and clearance of parasites in a study of uncomplicated malaria in Gambian children (Doherty et al., 1999). The use of artemisinin is indicated in areas where parasites are quinine resistance or where there is evidence of recurrent quinine-induced hypoglycemia or quinine-induced intravascular hemolysis (Warrell, 1997). Atovaquone treatment results in unacceptably high relapse rates and rapid development of resistance (Looareesuwan et al., 1996). In combination with proguanil it has shown excellent efficacy for treatment and prophylaxis (Lell et al., 1998; Looareesuwan et al., 1999). This is a very good option, particularly for areas of high drug resistance (Sabchareon et al., 1988). Other options for patients with highly drug-resistant parasites include artesunate with mefloquine (Price et al., 1999a). To counter the continual emergence of antimalarial drug–resistant organisms, the strategy of combination therapy is being evaluated for the future (Brockman et al., 2000).

Adjunct Therapy

Exchange transfusion is often used as an adjunct to parental antimalarial therapy when a patient's level of parasitemia exceeds 10% and severe manifestations are present (Miller et al., 1989). Iron has been shown in some studies to facilitate faster hematologic recovery in children after acute falciparum malaria. Folic acid supplementation, however, may affect efficacy of SP therapy and is not routinely recommended (van Hensbroek et al., 1995).

Pure anemia without any associated symptoms that predict poor prognosis, such as respiratory distress or high lactate levels, suggests a good prognosis. Transfusion has been suggested for children with hemoglobin <5.0 g/dl and heart failure or those with hemoglobin <3 g/dl without clinical complication (Lackritz et al., 1992). In some studies malarial anemia is not associated with mortality (Allen et al., 1996; Marsh et al., 1995; Waller et al., 1995). In locales where blood for transfusions is in short supply or there are risks of transfusion-associated infections, this lack of association between strict anemia and mortality supports the practice of restricting blood transfusion to those children who have complications such as acidosis in addition to severe anemia (Lackritz et al., 1992; Newton et al., 1992).

Improved outcome in patients with acidosis may be accomplished by intravascular repletion with blood or volume (English et al., 1996c). Sustained lactic acidosis has been shown to be correlated with mortality, and, in a Gambian study, elevated plasma lactate concentration between 4 and 24 hours following initiation of treatment was the best single predictor of fatal outcomes (Krishna et al., 1994).

Hypoglycemia should be evaluated in any patient with altered consciousness or seizures, and repeat fingersticks should be carried out until this resolves. Intravenous infusion of 50% dextrose (1ml/kg) for severe hypoglycemia can be used. If glucose measurement is not possible in a timely manner, empiric dextrose should be considered in a parasitemic, unconscious patient.

Despite availability of effective drugs, even in children who are brought promptly to health-care centers, the mortality rate from severe malaria remains high. To improve the outcome of cerebral malaria (CM), other treatments have been attempted to inhibit the process that results in severe disease. For example, dexamethasone was studied in severely ill patients as adjunctive therapy to antimalarial agents. These trials found that dexamethasone did not improve outcome and may have had detrimental effect on duration of coma and secondary infection (Warrell et al., 1982; Hoffman et al., 1988). TNF inhibitors have been used but did not improve survival, and there were excessive neurologic sequelae noted at the 6-month follow-up (van Hensbroek et al., 1996).

PREVENTIVE MEASURES

It is important to determine risk of infection, and this can be done by referring to updated Web sites such as those maintained by the Centers for Disease Control and Prevention (http://www.cdc.gov/travel) and the Virtual Naval Hospital (http://www.vnh.org/Malaria/Malaria.html). There is no vaccine presently available, although they are under development (Alonso et al., 1994; Bojang et al., 2001; D'Alessandro et al., 1995a). If transmission of malaria is a risk, then minimizing contact with its vectors is part of prevention. Reduction of contact with or exposure to anopheline mosquitoes will reduce transmission. Anopheline mosquitoes feed particularly between dusk and dawn. Use of bed nets has been shown to reduce death rates by up to 38% in areas of the Gambia and in other study sites (D'Alessandro et al., 1995b; Greenwood, 1997a; Habluetzel et al., 1997). Screening rooms and wearing clothing that covers the skin reduce infection (Nevill et al., 1996). Insect spray containing permethrin can be used on clothes and mosquito nets in living and sleeping areas during evening and nighttime hours. Use of N,N-diethylmetatoluamide (DEET) is recommended, but care must be taken to avoid getting DEET on children's hands to reduce its inoculation into their eyes or mouth. DEET should not be used on abraded skin. Chemoprophylaxis is an important adjunct to reducing risk of transmission (Table 19-4). It is important to know if the patient has had any previous difficulties with a chemoprophylactic regimen and if they are visiting an area with drug-resistant organisms. Prophylaxis, except for atovaquone-proguanil or doxycycline, should start 1 to 2 weeks before travel. This allows enough time that a therapeutic drug level can be attained and any unacceptable side effects or intolerances can be detected before the patient embarks on the trip. Chemoprophylaxis should continue during travel in the malarious areas and after leaving the malarious areas. It is critical that patients continue to take the prophylactic medications upon return to prevent infection. After travel, 4 weeks of treatment are required for chloroquine, mefloquine, and doxycycline, and 7 days of treatment are required for atovaquone-proguanil. Note that sulfa is contraindicated in children less than 2 months of age and that doxycycline should not be used before the age of 8 years. Malarone is not indicated for infants less than 11 kg. If a child is too young or unable to swallow whole tablets the pharmacist can grind the tablet and store the proper dose in gelatin capsules. In addition, Mefloquine, chloroquine, and Malarone taste very bitter. These medicines can be put into something sweet, such as applesauce, chocolate syrup, or jelly.

TABLE 19-4 Antimalarial Agents Used for Prophylaxis		
Antimalarial agent	*Dosing regimen*	
Chloroquine phosphate (Aralen)	5 mg/kg base not to exceed 300 mg base PO once per week while in endemic area	Start 1-2 weeks, once per week, before visiting endemic area, and continue once per week for 4 weeks after leaving area
Hydroxychloroquine (Plaquenil) For regions with chloroquine-sensitive organisms	5mg/kg base PO once per week while in endemic area, up to maximum dose of 310 mg base	Start 1-2 weeks, once per week, before visiting endemic area, and continue once per week for 4 weeks after leaving area
Mefloquine (Lariam)	≤15 kg: 5.0 mg/kg base once per week while in endemic areas 15-19 kg: ¼ tablet once per week 20-30 kg: ½ tablet once per week 31-45 kg: ¾ tablet once per week ≥45 kg: 1 tablet once per week	Start 1-2 weeks, once per week, before visiting endemic area, OR alternatively can administer once per day for 3 days before travel and continue once per week for 4 weeks after leaving area
Atovaquone and proguanil (Malarone) Pediatric formulation:62.5mg/25mg	Not indicated for children <11 kg 11-20 kg: 1 pediatric tablet every day while in endemic area 21-30 kg: 2 pediatric tablets every day 31-40 kg: 3 pediatric tablets every day 40 kg: 1 adult formulation tablet (250 mg atovaquone and 100mg proguanil)	Start 1-2 days before visiting endemic area, and continue every day for 7 days after leaving area
Doxycycline (Vibramycin)	Not indicated for children <8 yr ≥8 yr: 2 mg/kg PO every day while in endemic areas, not to exceed 100 mg day	Start 1-2 days, once per day, before visiting endemic area, and continue once per day for 4 weeks after leaving area
Primaquine phosphate 15 mg base tablet	To eradicate hypnozoite stage in *P. vivax* and *P. ovale* <2 yr: ¼ tablet every day 2-5 yr: ½ tablet every day 6-12 yr: 1 tablet every day 12 yr: 2 tablets every day for 14 days after leaving malarious area	Contraindicated in patients with G6PD deficiency.

Modified from Centers for Disease Control and Prevention: U.S. Department of Health and Human Services, Public Health Service 2001.

Bibliography

Aitman TJ, Cooper LD, Norsworthy PJ, et al. Malaria susceptibility and CD36 mutation. Nature 2000;405:1015-1016.

Akindele JA, Sowunmi A, Abohweyere AE. Congenital malaria in a hyperendemic area: a preliminary study. Ann Trop Paediatr 1993;13:273-276.

Allen SJ, O'Donnell A, Alexander ND, et al. Severe malaria in children in Papua New Guinea. QJM 1996;89:779-788.

Alonso PL, Smith T, Schellenberg JR, et al. Randomised trial of efficacy of SPf66 vaccine against *Plasmodium falciparum* malaria in children in southern Tanzania. Lancet 1994;344:1175-1181.

Baird JK. Age-dependent characteristics of protection v. susceptibility to *Plasmodium falciparum*. Ann Trop Med Parasitol 1998;92:367-390.

Baird JK, Hoffman S. Prevention of malaria in travelers. Med Clin North Am 1999;83:923-944.

Baird JK, Purnomo, Jones TR. Diagnosis of malaria in the field by fluorescence microscopy of QBC capillary tubes. Trans R Soc Trop Med Hyg 1992;86:3-5.

Baird JK, Wiady I, Fryauff DJ, et al. In vivo resistance to chloroquine by *Plasmodium vivax* and *Plasmodium falciparum* at Nabire, Irian Jaya, Indonesia. Am J Trop Med Hyg 1997;56:627-631.

Bojang KA, PJ Milligan, M Pinder, et al. Efficacy of RTS,S/AS02 malaria vaccine against *Plasmodium falciparum* infection in semi-immune adult men in the Gambia: a randomised trial. Lancet 2001;358:1927-1934.

Bondi FS. The incidence and outcome of neurological abnormalities in childhood cerebral malaria: a long-term follow-up of 62 survivors. Trans R Soc Trop Med Hyg 1992;86:17-19.

Borst P, Bitter W, McCulloch R, et al. Antigenic variation in malaria. Cell 1995;82:1-4.

Brewster DR, Kwiatkowski D, White NJ. Neurological sequelae of cerebral malaria in children. Lancet 1990;336:1039-1043.

Brockman A, Price RN, van Vugt M, et al. *Plasmodium falciparum* antimalarial drug susceptibility on the northwestern border of Thailand during five years of extensive use of artesunate-mefloquine. Trans R Soc Trop Med Hyg 2000;94:537-544.

Brown H, Rogerson S, Taylor T, et al. Blood-brain barrier function in cerebral malaria in Malawian children. Am J Trop Med Hyg 2001;64:207-213.

Carme B, Bouquety JC, Plassart H. Mortality and sequelae due to cerebral malaria in African children in Brazzaville, Congo. Am J Trop Med Hyg 1993;48:216-221.

Centers for Disease Control and Prevention. Health Information for the International Traveler 2001-2002. Atlanta, Ga: U.S. Department of Health and Human Services, Public Health Service, 2001.

Chen Q, Schlichtherle M, Wahlgren M. Molecular aspects of severe malaria. Clin Microbiol Rev 2000;13:439-450.

Clark IA, Rockett KA, Cowden WB. Possible central role of nitric oxide in conditions clinically similar to cerebral malaria. Lancet 1992;340:894-896.

Contamin H, Fandeur T, Rogier C, et al. Different genetic characteristics of *Plasmodium falciparum* isolates collected during successive clinical malaria episodes in Senegalese children. Am J Trop Med Hyg 1996;54:632-643.

Corbett CE, Duarte MI, Lancellotti CL, et al. Cytoadherence in human falciparum malaria as a cause of respiratory distress. J Trop Med Hyg 1989;92:112-120.

Covell G. Congenital malaria. Trop Dis Bull 1950:1147-1167.

Crawley J, English M, Waruiru C, et al. Abnormal respiratory patterns in childhood cerebral malaria. Trans R Soc Trop Med Hyg 1998;92:305-308.

Crawley J, Smith S, Kirkham F, et al. Seizures and status epilepticus in childhood cerebral malaria. QJM 1996;89:591-597.

D'Alessandro U, Leach A, Drakeley CJ, et al. Efficacy trial of malaria vaccine SPf66 in Gambian infants. Lancet 1995a;346:462-467.

D'Alessandro U, Olaleye BO, McGuire W, et al. Mortality and morbidity from malaria in Gambian children after introduction of an impregnated bednet programme. Lancet 1995b;345:479-483.

Doherty JF, Sadiq AD, Bayo L, et al. A randomized safety and tolerability trial of artesunate plus sulfadoxine-pyrimethamine versus sulfadoxine-pyrimethamine alone for the treatment of uncomplicated malaria in Gambian children. Trans R Soc Trop Med Hyg 1999;93:543-546.

Dorsey G, Gandhi M, Oyugi JH, et al. Difficulties in the prevention, diagnosis, and treatment of imported malaria. Arch Intern Med 2000;160:2505-2510.

English M, Punt J, Mwangi I, et al. Clinical overlap between malaria and severe pneumonia in Africa children in hospital. Trans R Soc Trop Med Hyg 1996a; 90:658-662.

English M, Waruiru C, Amukoye E, et al. Deep breathing in children with severe malaria: indicator of metabolic acidosis and poor outcome. Am J Trop Med Hyg 1996b;55:521-524.

English M, Waruiru C, Marsh K. Transfusion for respiratory distress in life-threatening childhood malaria. Am J Trop Med Hyg 1996c;55:525-530.

Forney JR, Magill AJ, Wongsrichanalai CJ, et al. Malaria rapid diagnostic devices: performance characteristics of the ParaSight F device determined in a multisite field study. J Clin Microbiol 2001;39:2884-2890.

Fujioka H, Aikawa M. The molecular basis of pathogenesis of cerebral malaria. Microb Pathog 1996;20:63-72.

Funk M, Schlagenhauf P, Tschopp A, et al. MalaQuick versus ParaSight F as a diagnostic aid in traveler's malaria. Trans R Soc Trop Med Hyg 1999;93:268-272.

Greenwood BM: What's new in malaria control? Ann Trop Med Parasitol 1997a;91:523-531.

Greenwood BM: The epidemiology of malaria. Ann Trop Med Parasitol 1997b;91:763-769.

Greenwood BM, Bradley AK, Greenwood AM, et al. Mortality and morbidity from malaria among children in a rural area of the Gambia, West Africa. Trans R Soc Trop Med Hyg 1987;81:478-486.

Gupta S, Hill AV, Kwiatkowski D, et al. Parasite virulence and disease patterns in *Plasmodium falciparum* malaria. Proc Natl Acad Sci USA 1994;91:3715-3719.

Habluetzel A, Diallo DA, Esposito F, et al. Do insecticide-treated curtains reduce all-cause child mortality in Burkina Faso? Trop Med Int Health 1997;2:855-862.

Hendrickse RG, Hasan AH, Olumide LO, et al. Malaria in early childhood. An investigation of five hundred seriously ill children in whom a "clinical" diagnosis of malaria was made on admission to the children's emergency room at University College Hospital, Ibadan. Ann Trop Med Parasitol 1971;65:1-20.

Hill AV: Malaria resistance genes: a natural selection. Trans R Soc Trop Med Hyg 1992;86:225-226,232.

Hill AV, Allsopp CE, Kwiatkowski D, et al. Common West African HLA antigens are associated with protection from severe malaria [see comments]. Nature 1991;352:595-600.

Hoffman SL, Rustama D, Punjabi NH, et al. High-dose dexamethasone in quinine-treated patients with cerebral malaria: a double-blind, placebo-controlled trial. J Infect Dis 1988;158:325-331.

Hulbert TV: Congenital malaria in the United States: report of a case and review. Clin Infect Dis 1992;14:922-926.

Humar A, Ohrt C, Harrington MA, et al. Parasight F test compared with the polymerase chain reaction and microscopy for the diagnosis of *Plasmodium falciparum* malaria in travelers. Am J Trop Med Hyg 1997;56:44-48.

Imbert P, Sartelet I, Rogier C, et al. Severe malaria among children in a low seasonal transmission area, Dakar,

Senegal: influence of age on clinical presentation. Trans R Soc Trop Med Hyg 1997;91:22-24.

Jaffar S, Van Hensbroek MB, Palmer A, et al. Predictors of a fatal outcome following childhood cerebral malaria. Am J Trop Med Hyg 1997;57:20-24.

Jelinek T, Grobusch MP, Harms G. Evaluation of a dipstick test for the rapid diagnosis of imported malaria among patients presenting within the network TropNetEurop. Scand J Infect Dis 2001;33:752-754.

Kain KC, Harrington MA, Tennyson S, et al. Imported malaria: prospective analysis of problems in diagnosis and management. Clin Infect Dis 1998;27:142-149.

Krishna S, Waller DW, ter Kuile F, et al. Lactic acidosis and hypoglycaemia in children with severe malaria: pathophysiological and prognostic significance. Trans R Soc Trop Med Hyg 1994;88:67-73.

Lackritz EM, Campbell CC, Ruebush TK II, et al. Effect of blood transfusion on survival among children in a Kenyan hospital. Lancet 1992;340:524-528.

Layton M, Parise ME, Campbell CC, et al. Mosquito-transmitted malaria in New York City, 1993. Lancet 1995;346:729-731.

Lell B, Luckner D, Ndjave M, et al. Randomised placebo-controlled study of atovaquone plus proguanil for malaria prophylaxis in children. Lancet 1998;351:709-713.

Lewallen S, Harding SP, Ajewole J, et al. A review of the spectrum of clinical ocular fundus findings in *P. falciparum* malaria in African children with a proposed classification and grading system. Trans R Soc Trop Med Hyg 1999; 93:619-622.

Lewallen S, White VA, Whitten RO, et al. Clinical-histopathological correlation of the abnormal retinal vessels in cerebral malaria. Arch Ophthalmol 2000;118: 924-928.

Looareesuwan S, Viravan C, Webster HK, et al. Clinical studies of atovaquone, alone or in combination with other antimalarial drugs, for treatment of acute uncomplicated malaria in Thailand. Am J Trop Med Hyg 1996;54:62-66.

Looareesuwan S, Chulay JD, Canfield CJ, et al. Malarone (atovaquone and proguanil hydrochloride): a review of its clinical development for treatment of malaria. Malarone Clinical Trials Study Group. Am J Trop Med Hyg 1999;60:533-441.

Looareesuwan S, Warrell DA, White NJ, et al. Retinal hemorrhage, a common sign of prognostic significance in cerebral malaria. Am J Trop Med Hyg 1983;32:911-915.

Luxemburger C, Price RN, Nosten F, et al. Mefloquine in infants and young children. Ann Trop Paediatr 1996;16:281-286.

Mabeza GF, Moyo VM, Thuma PE, et al. Predictors of severity of illness on presentation in children with cerebral malaria. Ann Trop Med Parasitol 1995;89:221-228.

MacPherson GG, Warrell MJ, White NJ, et al. Human cerebral malaria. A quantitative ultrastructural analysis of parasitized erythrocyte sequestration. Am J Pathol 1985;119:385-401.

Marsh K, English M, Crawley J, Peshu N. The pathogenesis of severe malaria in African children. Ann Trop Med Parasitol 1996;90:395-402.

Marsh K, Forster D, Waruiru C, et al. Indicators of life-threatening malaria in African children. N Engl J Med 1995;332:1399-1404.

May J, Lell B, Luty AJ, et al. HLA-DQB1*0501-restricted Th1 type immune responses to *Plasmodium falciparum* liver stage antigen 1 protect against malaria anemia and reinfections. J Infect Dis 2001;183:168-172.

McGregor IA. Epidemiology, malaria and pregnancy. Am J Trop Med Hyg 1984;33:517-525.

McGuinness D, Koram K, Bennett S, et al. Clinical case definitions for malaria: clinical malaria associated with very low parasite densities in African infants. Trans R Soc Trop Med Hyg 1998;92:527-531.

McGuire W, Hill AV, Allsopp CE, et al. Variation in the TNF-alpha promoter region associated with susceptibility to cerebral malaria. Nature 1994;371:508-510.

Mehta SR, Lazar AI, Kasthuri AS. Experience on loading dose—quinine therapy in cerebral malaria. J Assoc Physicians India 1994;42:376-378.

Menendez C, Fleming AF, Alonso PL. Malaria-related anaemia. Parasitol Today2000;16:469-476.

Miller KD, Greenberg AE, Campbell CC. Treatment of severe malaria in the United States with a continuous infusion of quinidine gluconate and exchange transfusion. N Engl J Med 1989;321:65-70.

Mills CD, Burgess DC, Taylor HJ, et al. Evaluation of a rapid and inexpensive dipstick assay for the diagnosis of *Plasmodium falciparum* malaria. Bull World Health Org 1999;77:553-559.

Molyneux ME, Taylor TE, Wirima JJ, Borgstein A. Clinical features and prognostic indicators in paediatric cerebral malaria: a study of 131 comatose Malawian children [see comments]. QJM 1989;71:441-459.

Moore TA, Tomayko JF Jr, Wierman AM, et al. Imported malaria in the 1990s. A report of 59 cases from Houston, Texas. Arch Fam Med 1994;3:130-136.

Mungai M, Tegtmeier G, Chamberland M, et al. Transfusion-transmitted malaria in the United States from 1963 through 1999. N Engl J Med 2001;344:1973-1978.

Murphy S, English M, Waruiru C, et al. An open randomized trial of artemether versus quinine in the treatment of cerebral malaria in African children. Trans R Soc Trop Med Hyg 1996;90:298-301.

Murphy SC, Breman JG. Gaps in the childhood malaria burden in Africa: cerebral malaria, neurological sequelae, anemia, respiratory distress, hypoglycemia, and complications of pregnancy. Am J Trop Med Hyg 2001;64:57-67.

Musoke LK. Neurological manifestations of malaria in children. East Afr Med J 1966;43:561-564.

Naik RS, Branch OH, Woods AS, et al. Glycosyl-phosphatidylinositol anchors of *Plasmodium falciparum*: molecular characterization and naturally elicited antibody response that may provide immunity to malaria pathogenesis. J Exp Med 2000;192:1563-1576.

Nevill CG, Some ES, Mung'ala VO, et al. Insecticide-treated bednets reduce mortality and severe morbidity from malaria among children on the Kenyan coast. Trop Med Int Health 1996;1:139-146.

Newton CR, Warrell DA. Neurological manifestations of falciparum malaria. Ann Neurol 1998;43:695-702.

Newton CR, Kirkham FJ, Winstanley PA, et al. Intracranial pressure in African children with cerebral malaria. Lancet 1991;337:573-576.

Newton CR, Marsh K, Peshu N, et al. Blood transfusions for severe anaemia in African children. Lancet 1992;340:917-918.

Newton CR, Peshu N, Kendall B, et al. Brain swelling and ischaemia in Kenyans with cerebral malaria. Arch Dis Child 1994;70:281-287.

Newton PN, Chierakul W, Ruangveerayuth R, et al. A comparison of artesunate alone with combined artesunate and quinine in the parenteral treatment of acute falciparum malaria. Trans R Soc Trop Med Hyg 2001;95:519-523.

Nyirjesy P, Kavasya T, Axelrod P, Fischer PR. Malaria during pregnancy: neonatal morbidity and mortality and the efficacy of chloroquine chemoprophylaxis. Clin Infect Dis 1993;16:127-132.

O'Dempsey TJ, McArdle TF, Laurence BE, et al. Overlap in the clinical features of pneumonia and malaria in African children. Trans R Soc Trop Med Hyg 1993;87:662-665.

Okitolonda W, Delacollette C, Malengreau M, et al. High incidence of hypoglycaemia in African patients treated with intravenous quinine for severe malaria. Br Med J (Clin Res Ed) 1987;295:716-718.

Olliaro P, Cattani J, Wirth D. Malaria, the submerged disease. JAMA 1996;275:230-233.

Phillips RE, Looareesuwan S, Warrell DA, et al. The importance of anaemia in cerebral and uncomplicated falciparum malaria: role of complications, dyserythropoiesis and iron sequestration. Q J Med 1986;58:305-323.

Price RN, Simpson JA, Nosten F, et al. Factors contributing to anemia after uncomplicated falciparum malaria. Am J Trop Med Hyg 2001;65:614-622.

Price RN, Simpson JA, Teja-Isavatharm P, et al. Pharmacokinetics of mefloquine combined with artesunate in children with acute falciparum malaria. Antimicrob Agents Chemother 1999a;43:341-346.

Price RN, van Vugt M, Phaipun L, et al. Adverse effects in patients with acute falciparum malaria treated with artemisinin derivatives. Am J Trop Med Hyg 1999b;60:547-555.

Redd SC, Kazembe PN, Luby SP, et al. Clinical algorithm for treatment of Plasmodium falciparum malaria in children. Lancet 1996;347:223-237.

Rickman LS, Long GW, Oberst R, et al. Rapid diagnosis of malaria by acridine orange staining of centrifuged parasites. Lancet 1989;1:68-71.

Rieckmann KH, Davis DR, Hutton DC. Plasmodium vivax resistance to chloroquine? Lancet 1989;2:1183-1184.

Riley EM, Wagner GE, Ofori MF, et al. Lack of association between maternal antibody and protection of African infants from malaria infection. Infect Immun 2000;68:5856-5863.

Rougemont A, Breslow N, Brenner E, et al. Epidemiological basis for clinical diagnosis of childhood malaria in endemic zone in West Africa. Lancet 1991;338:1292-1295.

Sabchareon A, Attanath P, Phanuaksook P, et al. Efficacy and pharmacokinetics of atovaquone and proguanil in children with multidrug-resistant Plasmodium falciparum malaria. Trans R Soc Trop Med Hyg 1998;92:201-206.

Schindler HC, Montenegro L, Montenegro R, et al. Development and optimization of polymerase chain reaction–based malaria diagnostic methods and their comparison with quantitative buffy coat assay. Am J Trop Med Hyg 2001;65:355-361.

Schmutzhard E, Gerstenbrand F. Cerebral malaria in Tanzania. Its epidemiology, clinical symptoms and neurological long term sequelae in the light of 66 cases. Trans R Soc Trop Med Hyg 1984;78:351-353.

Siegel D. An unusual case of Plasmodium vivax infection from Korea with delayed presentation. Mil Med 1998;163:244-245.

Silamut K, Phu NH, Whitty C, et al. A quantitative analysis of the microvascular sequestration of malaria parasites in the human brain. Am J Pathol 1999;155:395-410.

Silamut K, White NJ. Relation of the stage of parasite development in the peripheral blood to prognosis in severe falciparum malaria. Trans R Soc Trop Med Hyg 1993;87:436-443.

Snow RW, Omumbo JA, Lowe B, et al. Relation between severe malaria morbidity in children and level of Plasmodium falciparum transmission in Africa. Lancet 1997;349:1650-1654.

Soto J, Toledo J, Gutierrez P, et al. Plasmodium vivax clinically resistant to chloroquine in Colombia. Am J Trop Med Hyg 2001;65:90-93.

Sowunmi A. Renal function in acute falciparum malaria. Arch Dis Child 1996;74:293-298.

Steketee RW, Nahlen BL, Parise ME. The burden of malaria in pregnancy in malaria-endemic areas. Am J Trop Med Hyg 2001;64:28-35.

Taylor TE, Borgstein A, Molyneux ME. Acid-base status in paediatric Plasmodium falciparum malaria. Q J Med 1993;86:99-109.

Taylor TE, Molyneux ME, Wirima JJ, et al. Blood glucose levels in Malawian children before and during the administration of intravenous quinine for severe falciparum malaria. N Engl J Med 1988;319:1040-1047.

Turner GD, Morrison H, Jones M, et al. An immunohistochemical study of the pathology of fatal malaria. Evidence for widespread endothelial activation and a potential role for intercellular adhesion molecule-1 in cerebral sequestration. Am J Pathol 1994;145:1057-1069.

Van den Ende J, Lynen L, Elsen P, et al. A cluster of airport malaria in Belgium in 1995. Acta Clin Belg 1998;53:259-263.

van der Torn M, Thuma PE, Mabeza GF, et al. Loading dose of quinine in African children with cerebral malaria. Trans R Soc Trop Med Hyg 1998;92:325-331.

van Hensbroek MB, Morris-Jones S, Meisner S, et al. Iron, but not folic acid, combined with effective antimalarial therapy promotes haematological recovery in African children after acute falciparum malaria. Trans R Soc Trop Med Hyg 1995;89:672-676.

van Hensbroek MB, Onyiorah E, Jaffar S, et al. A trial of artemether or quinine in children with cerebral malaria. N Engl J Med 1996;335:69-75.

Waller D, Krishna S, Crawley J, et al. Clinical features and outcome of severe malaria in Gambian children. Clin Infect Dis 1995;21:577-587.

Warrell DA. Cerebral malaria: clinical features, pathophysiology and treatment. Ann Trop Med Parasitol 1997;91:875-884.

Warrell DA. Management of severe malaria. Parassitologia 1999;41:287-294.

Warrell DA, Looareesuwan S, Warrell MJ, et al. Dexamethasone proves deleterious in cerebral malaria. A double-blind trial in 100 comatose patients. N Engl J Med 1982;306:313-319.

Warrell DA, Molyneux ME, Beales PF. Severe and complicated malaria, ed 2. Trans R Soc Trop Med Hyg 1990;84(suppl 2):1-65.

Waruiru CM, Newton CR, Forster D, et al. Epileptic seizures and malaria in Kenyan children. Trans R Soc Trop Med Hyg 1996;90:152-155.

Wattanagoon Y, Srivilairit S, Looareesuwan S, et al. Convulsions in childhood malaria. Trans R Soc Trop Med Hyg 1994;88:426-428.

Whitby M. Drug resistant *Plasmodium vivax* malaria. J Antimicrob Chemother 1997;40:749-752.

White JC: Epileptic nystagmus. Epilepsia 1971;12:157-164.

White NJ, Looareesuwan S, Warrell DA, et al. Quinine loading dose in cerebral malaria. Am J Trop Med Hyg 1983a;32:1-5.

White NJ, Miller KD, Marsh K, et al. Hypoglycaemia in African children with severe malaria. Lancet 1987;1:708-711.

White NJ, Warrell DA, Chanthavanich P, et al. Severe hypoglycemia and hyperinsulinemia in falciparum malaria. N Engl J Med 1983b;309: 61-66.

World Health Organization: World malaria situation in 1994. Part I. Population at risk. Wkly Epidemiol Rec 1997;72:269-274.

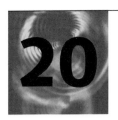

20 MEASLES (RUBEOLA)

Samuel L. Katz

Measles is an acute, highly contagious viral disease characterized by fever, coryza, conjunctivitis, cough, and a specific enanthem (Koplik's spots) followed by a generalized maculopapular eruption, which usually appears on the fourth day of the disease. The rash and accompanying illness reach a climax on approximately the sixth day, followed by subsidence in a few days and, in most cases, complete recovery. Serious complications involving the gastrointestinal and respiratory tracts and central nervous system (CNS) occur in 5% to 15% of patients in developed countries. In other parts of the world, however, the high mortality and morbidity associated with measles present serious problems. The widespread use of live attenuated measles virus vaccine has been followed by a sharp decline in the incidence of the disease in the Americas, as well as in other nations in which immunization has been established as a cornerstone of child health practices.

Prior to availability of measles virus vaccine the World Health Organization (WHO) estimated there were annually 8 million deaths due to measles throughout the world. With widespread availability of vaccine this number had decreased by 2002 to approximately 700,000 deaths, still an unacceptable number for a disease that is fully preventable through vaccination. The major mortality persists in areas of sub-Saharan Africa and the Asian subcontinent. With the success of the global smallpox eradication program in 1980 and the anticipated achievements early in the twenty-first century of the global polio eradication effort, major attention has been focused on the possible control and elimination of measles, the third major disease target. A measles initiative has been organized by the American Red Cross, joined by the United Nations Foundation, the Centers for Disease Control and Prevention (CDC), the United Nations Children's Fund (UNICEF), WHO, the Pan American Health Organization (PAHO), and many national Red Cross and Red Crescent Societies and other nongovernmental organizations, initially to reduce measles mortality in Africa and eventually throughout the remainder of the world. In its first year of operation large campaigns were conducted in Tanzania, Uganda, Benin, Mali, Burkina Faso, Togo, Cameroon, and Ghana. More than 20 million infants and children were vaccinated, with the resultant prevention of an estimated 140,000 deaths. In the last decade of the twenty-first century global coverage with single dose measles vaccine varied from 74% to 82%, but individual national rates in many of the most severely afflicted countries were less than 50%.

ETIOLOGY

Although measles had been demonstrated to be a transmissible infection of viral etiology early in the twentieth century, it was not until 1954 that Enders and Peebles reported the successful isolation of measles virus in human and rhesus monkey kidney cell cultures. The characteristic cytopathic changes in tissue culture included (1) formation of multinucleated giant cells, (2) vacuolization in the syncytial cytoplasm, and (3) presence of eosinophilic intranuclear and intracytoplasmic inclusion bodies. Measles virus has been adapted to a number of tissue cultures, both primary as well as a variety of human and simian cell lines and chick embryo cells. The cytopathic effects in tissue culture have provided a basis for virus isolation procedures, for assay of infectivity, and for determination of neutralizing antibody. The property of hemagglutination of simian erythrocytes by infected tissue culture fluids has been utilized as the basis for a convenient serologic test.

Measles is the sole human member of the genus Morbillivirus, family Paramyxoviridae. Other viruses of that genus are the causative agents of canine distemper; rinderpest of cattle; peste des petits ruminants (sheep and goats); and four morbilliviruses of dolphins, seals, and porpoises.

Measles virions are spherical, pleomorphic, lipid-enveloped particles, ranging from 100 to 250 nm in diameter, with a helical nucleocapsid. They are morphologically identical to the other paramyxoviruses. Two transmembrane glycoproteins, H (hemagglutinin) and F (fusion), project from the surface of the virus envelope, a lipid bilayer derived from the plasma membrane of infected cells. The M (matrix) protein is in the inner surface of the membrane. The helical nucleocapsid within the envelope contains the nucleoprotein (N) bound to the genomic RNA, along with the phosphoprotein (P) and the large polymerase protein (L). The genome is linear, single stranded, of negative polarity, and nonsegmented and contains approximately 16,000 nucleotides. It has been fully sequenced, and there is a surprising degree of stability and homogeneity among various strains and isolates, but with some minor changes in the N and H genes (Rota et al., 1998). These observations coincide with the apparent clinical and immunologic stability of measles over the centuries of observation and nearly five decades of laboratory investigations. Naniche et al. (1993) identified a member of the regulators of complement activation, CD46, as the cell receptor for measles virus permitting binding of virus to the host cell. It is a 57- to 67-kd protein expressed on nearly all human cell types except erythrocytes. A monoclonal antibody to CD46 inhibits measles virus binding, syncytium formation, and subsequent viral replication. Later it was demonstrated that the CD150 signaling lymphocyte activation molecule (SLAM) may also be utilized for binding and cell entry by measles virions (Tatsuo et al., 2000; Duke and Mgone, 2003).

Measles virus is temperature sensitive and is also inactivated by ultraviolet light, ether, trypsin, and β-propiolactone. Formalin destroys infectivity, but it does not alter complement-fixing activity. The virus in the presence of protein is well preserved at low temperature, surviving storage at −15° to −70° C for 5 years and at 4° C for 5 months. In the lyophilized state with a protein stabilizer it is preserved at 4° C for 18 months.

PATHOLOGY

Because measles is a generalized infection, the pathologic lesions are widespread (Degen, 1937). The virus initiates infection in the upper respiratory tract epithelium and spreads to the local lymph nodes in macrophages. Following replication in the lymph nodes, virus is released to the bloodstream, from which it disseminates to the reticuloendothelial system where another round of replication produces a secondary viremia with distribution of virus to multiple tissue sites with generalized infection of vascular endothelium and the epithelium of the respiratory and gastrointestinal tracts. During the prodromal period there is hyperplasia of the lymphoid tissue in the tonsils, adenoids, lymph nodes, spleen, and appendix. Large (100 μm) multinucleated giant cells can be demonstrated in these tissues and in the pharyngeal and bronchial mucosa.

Suringa et al. (1970) found that Koplik's spots and the skin lesions of measles share the following histologic features: foci of syncytial epithelial giant cells with pale-staining cytoplasm, intercellular and intracellular edema, and parakeratosis and dyskeratosis. Many of the giant cell nuclei contain pink-staining inclusion bodies. Electron microscopy reveals aggregates of "viral" microtubules within the nuclei and cytoplasm of syncytial giant cells. These tubules are indistinguishable from those seen in tissue cultures infected with measles virus.

The lungs show evidence of a peribronchiolar inflammatory reaction with a mononuclear cell infiltrate in the interstitial tissues. The large giant cells are occasionally identified there.

The brain and spinal cord in measles encephalomyelitis show gross evidence of edema, congestion, and scattered petechial hemorrhages. Microscopically, the early stage is characterized by perivascular hemorrhages and lymphocytic cell infiltration. Later there is evidence of demyelination throughout the CNS. Histologically, these lesions are very similar to those encountered in postvaccinal encephalitis.

CLINICAL MANIFESTATIONS

The clinical course of a typical case of measles is illustrated in Figure 20-1. After an incubation period of 10 to 11 days the illness is ushered in by fever and malaise. Within 24 hours there is onset of coryza, conjunctivitis, and cough. These symptoms gradually increase in severity, reaching a peak with the appearance of the eruption on the fourth day. Approximately 2 days before the development of the rash, Koplik's spots appear on the buccal mucous membranes opposite the molars. Over a 3-day period these lesions increase in number and spread to involve the entire mucous membrane. Koplik's spots disappear by the end of the second day of the rash. The coryza and conjunctivitis clear considerably by the third day of the rash. The duration of the exanthem rarely exceeds 5 to 6 days.

Fever

The temperature curve illustrated in Figure 20-1 is the one most commonly observed. There is a stepwise increase until the fifth or sixth day of illness at the height of the eruption. Occasionally, however, the temperature curve may be biphasic: an initial elevation for the first 24 to 48 hours followed by a normal period for 1 day and then a rapid rise when the rash is in full bloom. In some cases the temperature may reach its peak by the end of the first day and remain elevated at levels of 39.4° to 40.6° C (103° to 105° F) for the remaining prodromal and early rash period. In uncomplicated measles the temperature falls by crisis or rapid lysis between the second and third days after the onset of the exanthem.

Coryza

The coryza of measles is indistinguishable from that of a severe common cold. The early sneez-

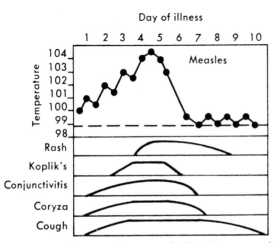

Fig. 20-1 Schematic diagram of clinical course of typical case of measles. The rash appears 3 to 4 days after onset of fever, conjunctivitis, coryza, and cough. Koplik's spots usually develop 2 days before the rash.

ing is followed by nasal congestion and a mucopurulent discharge that becomes most profuse at the height of the eruption. It clears very rapidly after the patient becomes afebrile.

Conjunctivitis and Keratitis

A transverse marginal line of conjunctival injection across the lower lids may be observed in the early prodromal period. Subsequently, it is obscured by an extensive conjunctival inflammation associated with edema of the lids and the caruncles. There is increased lacrimation, and complaints of photophobia. In severe cases, Koplik's spots may be observed on the caruncle. The conjunctivitis, like the coryza, disappears shortly after the fever has subsided. Among children with malnutrition accompanied by vitamin A deficiency, a more severe conjunctivitis with accompanying keratitis and corneal ulcerations may leave damage sufficient to impair vision permanently.

Cough

The cough is caused by the inflammatory reaction of the respiratory tract. Like the other catarrhal manifestations, it increases in frequency and intensity, reaching its climax at the height of the eruption. However, it persists much longer, gradually subsiding over the next several weeks.

Koplik's Spots

Approximately 2 days before the rash appears, the pathognomonic Koplik's spots may be detected. These lesions were described by Koplik (1896) as small irregular spots of bright red color; in the center of each red spot is seen a minute bluish-white speck. There may initially be only a few such spots, but they rapidly increase in number. The combination of a bluish-white speck with a rose-red background on the buccal and labial mucous membrane is pathognomonic of measles. Sometimes the bluish-white speck is so small and delicately colored that only in a very direct and strong daylight is it possible to bring out the above effect.

Koplik's spots increase so that by the end of the first day of rash they usually involve the entire buccal and labial mucosa. The rose-red areas coalesce to form a diffuse erythematous background that is peppered with many pinpoint blue-white elevations. At this stage, Koplik's spots resemble grains of salt sprinkled on a red background (Plate 47). By the end of the second day of the rash the spots begin to slough, and by the third day of rash the mucous membranes look perfectly normal.

Rash

As indicated in Figure 20-1, the rash of unmodified measles first makes its appearance 3 to 4 days after the onset of catarrhal symptoms. Occasionally the prodromal period may be as short as 1 or as long as 7 days.

The exanthem begins as an erythematous maculopapular eruption (Figure 20-2). It appears first at the hairline and involves the forehead, the area behind the earlobes, and the upper part of the neck. It then spreads downward to involve the face, neck, upper extremities, and trunk. It continues downward until it reaches the feet by the third day. The earlier sites contain many more lesions than those that are affected later. Consequently, the lesions on the face and neck tend to become confluent, whereas those more peripheral on the extremities tend to remain discrete (Figure 20-3).

The rash begins to fade by the third day in order of appearance. Therefore, although the face and upper trunk may be clear by the fourth day, an eruption may still be apparent on the lower extremities. The early erythematous lesions blanch on pressure. After 3 or 4 days they assume a brownish appearance. This staining of the skin, which is probably the result of capillary hemorrhages, does not fade on pressure. With the disappearance of the rash, a fine branny desquamation may be noted over the sites of most extensive involvement. In contrast to the extensive peeling seen in scarlet fever, the skin of the hands and feet does not desquamate. Morley (1962) observed extensive desquamation, however, after severe measles in West African children who were protein deficient.

Other Manifestations

Anorexia and malaise are usually present during the febrile period. Gastroenteritis with both vomiting and diarrhea is commonly present and in malnourished children may be especially severe, often accompanied by painful stomatitis (Makhene and Diaz, 1993). Generalized lymphadenopathy is noted in moderate to severe cases. Like rubella, measles may be associated with enlarged postauricular, cervical, axillary, inguinal, and occipital lymph nodes. Occasionally a transient prodromal rash may be observed. This eruption may be scarlatiniform or morbilliform and usually disappears within 24 hours. Laryngotracheitis, sometimes of severity sufficient to require intubation in patients under 2

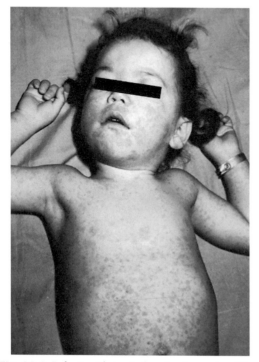

Fig. 20-2 Infant with typical rash of measles. Note confluent maculopapular lesions on face.

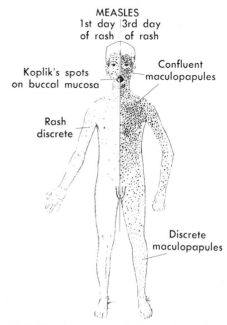

Fig. 20-3 Development and distribution of measles rash.

years of age (Fortenberry et al., 1992), bronchitis, bronchiolitis, and pneumonitis caused by the primary viral infection are present in various degrees in most patients.

Convalescence

The illness reaches its climax between the second and third days of the rash. At this time, the temperature is at its peak, Koplik's spots have covered the entire buccal mucous membrane and are beginning to slough, the eyes are puffy and red, the coryza is profuse, and the cough is most distressing. The child looks "measly" and feels miserable. Within the next 24 to 36 hours the temperature falls by crisis or rapid lysis, the coryza and conjunctivitis clear, and the cough decreases in severity. Within a few days the child feels normal. Fever persisting beyond the third day of rash is usually caused by a complication. The convalescent period of measles is of short duration, although cough often persists for weeks.

ATYPICAL MEASLES IN CHILDREN PREVIOUSLY IMMUNIZED WITH INACTIVATED MEASLES VIRUS VACCINE

A severe, atypical form of measles was first reported by Rauh and Schmidt in 1965, by Nader et al. in 1968, and by Fulginiti et al. in 1967 in children who had received inactivated measles virus vaccine 2 to 4 years previously. The following clinical manifestations have been observed: fever, pneumonitis, pneumonia with pulmonary consolidation and pleural effusion, and an unusual rash. The eruption has been urticarial, maculopapular, petechial, purpuric, and occasionally vesicular with a predilection for the extremities. Edema of the hands and feet, myalgia, and severe hyperesthesia of the skin also have been observed. The appearance and distribution of the exanthem resemble Rocky Mountain spotted fever.

Patients with atypical measles had extraordinarily high measles hemagglutination-inhibition (HI) antibody titers (1:25,000 to 1:200,000). These levels are sixfold or more higher than those observed following typical measles infection.

It has been estimated that 600,000 to 900,000 children were immunized with inactivated measles vaccine between the time of licensure in 1963 and 1967, when it was withdrawn from use. Consequently, this disease now is seen exclusively in adults (Cherry et al.,

1990). It was appropriate for Martin et al. (1979) and Hall and Hall (1979) to describe this problem in detail in the adult medical literature.

This syndrome was thought initially to result from failure of inactivated vaccine to induce antibody to the F protein of the virus (Annunziato et al., 1982). However, further studies suggested that it was more of a hypersensitivity reaction, with the vaccine having primed for a measles-specific but nonprotective Th2 response, resulting in immune complex deposition, complement activation, and an eosinophilia with elevated IgE (Polack et al.,1999; Polack et al., 2002).

SEVERE HEMORRHAGIC MEASLES

Severe hemorrhagic measles (black measles) is a rare form of the illness. It may begin with sudden onset of fever (40.6° to 41.1° C; 105° to 106° F), convulsions, delirium, or stupor that may progress to coma. This is followed by marked respiratory distress and an extensive confluent hemorrhagic eruption of the skin and mucous membranes. Bleeding from the mouth, nose, and bowel may be severe and uncontrollable. This type of measles is often fatal, probably because it involves disseminated intravascular coagulation.

Hemorrhagic measles should not be confused with the purpuric rash that may occur in fair-skinned children with severe ordinary measles. This latter eruption is not associated with excessive toxicity, and the illness pursues a more favorable course.

MODIFIED MEASLES

Modified measles most commonly develops in children who have been passively immunized with immune globulin (IG) after exposure to the disease. Occasionally it may also occur in infants whose maternal transplacental antibodies persist. The incubation period may be prolonged to 14 to 20 days. The illness itself is an abbreviated, milder version of ordinary measles.

The usual prodromal period of 3 to 4 days may be decreased to 1 or 2 days, or it may even be absent. The fever is generally low grade, or the temperature may be normal. The coryza, conjunctivitis, and cough are usually minimal and may even be absent. Koplik's spots may not be present; if they do appear, they are few in number and disappear within a day. The rash is generally sparse, discrete, and in some cases so mild that it may be missed.

Modification of measles converts a severe 6- to 9-day illness to one that is very mild and of much shorter duration. In contrast to the unmodified disease, it is rarely followed by complications. Nevertheless, the patient with modified illness is a potential source of infection to susceptible contacts.

DIAGNOSIS
Confirmatory Clinical Factors

The development of a generalized maculopapular eruption preceded by a 3- to 4-day period of fever, cough, coryza, and conjunctivitis associated with the pathognomonic Koplik's spots points to a clear-cut diagnosis of measles. During the prevaccine era, confirmatory laboratory procedures were usually unnecessary, and parents as well as health personnel made the diagnosis with ease.

Identification of Causative Agent

Measles virus may be isolated from the blood, urine, or nasopharyngeal secretions during the febrile period of the illness. However, doing so involves costly, arduous, and technically demanding cell culture procedures that are infrequently available or used for purposes other than investigation. A sensitive and specific polymerase chain reaction assay with reverse transcription (RT-nested PCR) has been employed successfully by Matsuzono et al. (1994).

Serologic Tests

A significant titer of antibodies may be detected in serum collected 2 weeks after the onset of illness. IgM antibodies first appear within 1 to 3 days after onset of rash. Peak titers are reached after 2 to 4 weeks. IgG neutralizing and HI antibodies rise later but may be detected for years thereafter. The pattern of development and persistence of measles HI antibody is illustrated in Figure 20-4. A fourfold or greater increase in antibody titer during convalescence is strongly indicative of measles infection. The enzyme immunoassay (EIA), because of its increased sensitivity and rapidity and its relative simplicity, is the test currently used most often to assay measles-specific antibodies. A single determination of IgM antibody to measles in an acute-phase serum specimen confirms the diagnosis. Helfand et al. (1996, 1997) have demonstrated the reliability of an antibody-capture IgM EIA for detection of measles-specific IgM in capillary blood and in oral fluids obtained from a cotton-fiber pad rubbed between the cheek and gum of infants. Their results correlated well (91% with positive results, 95% with negative results) when compared with serum specimens from the same infants. The most sensitive assay for measles antibodies is a plaque reduction neutralization test, which has detected antiviral activity at levels below those obtained by enzyme-linked immunosorbent assay, hemagglutination inhibition, or complement fixation. It has been used in evaluating persistence of transplacental antibodies in infants and duration of immunity in vaccine recipients who have become seronegative by the usual, more convenient methods of measurement (Albrecht et al., 1977).

Other Laboratory Findings

Uncomplicated measles typically is associated with leukopenia. A characteristic multinucleated giant cell has been identified in sputum and nasal secretions of patients during the prodromal period and in urinary sediment throughout the course of the disease (Scheifele and Forbes, 1972; Tompkins and Macaulay, 1955).

DIFFERENTIAL DIAGNOSIS

Differential diagnosis of measles is discussed in Chapter 20.

COMPLICATIONS

The measles virus is responsible for an inflammatory reaction that extends from the nasopharynx down the respiratory tract to the bronchi. Nasopharyngitis and tracheobronchitis with cough are therefore both manifestations of the natural disease. The more common complications are usually caused by (1) an extension of the inflammation caused by the virus, (2) an invasion of damaged tissues by bacteria, or (3) a combination of both. The sites of involvement of complications of measles include the middle ear, the respiratory tract, the gastrointestinal tract, the CNS, the eyes, and the skin.

Otitis Media

Infection of the middle ear is one of the most common complications of measles. Early in the course of illness the tympanic membranes may

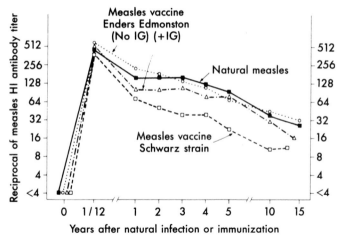

Fig. 20-4 Measles hemagglutination-inhibition (HI) antibody response and persistence. Fifteen-year follow-up. (From Krugman S: J Pediatr 1977;90:1.)

on examination reveal redness, bulging, and obliteration of the light reflex and landmarks. Particularly in infants, the first sign of otitis media may be a purulent discharge from a perforated tympanic membrane. Complicating otitis media is usually responsible for persistence of pyrexia beyond the normal course.

The incidence of otitis media as a complication of measles is affected by factors related to the disease, the host, and the environment. Severe measles is more likely to be complicated than are mild forms. Susceptibility is increased in infants as compared with older children and in patients of any age with a history of previous ear infections. In the 1990 U.S. outbreak, nearly 7% of reported cases of measles were complicated by otitis media (Centers for Disease Control, 1991).

Mastoiditis

Mastoiditis formerly was a common sequela of otitis media. Prompt antibacterial therapy has virtually eliminated this complication.

Pneumonia

Pulmonary complications are as frequent as otitis media but of greater severity. The pneumonia may result from (1) an extension of the viral infection, (2) a superimposed bacterial infection, or (3) a combination of both. It is manifested clinically as bronchiolitis (in infants), bronchopneumonia, or lobar pneumonia. The presence of a pneumonic complication should be suspected when any child with measles develops respiratory distress associated with persistence or recrudescence of fever. Examination of the chest may reveal dullness to percussion, suppression of breath sounds, bronchial breathing, and localized or generalized rales. A chest x-ray should clarify the diagnosis.

In some adults and especially in immunocompromised individuals of any age lacking normal cellular immune functions, a persisting giant cell pneumonia may occur as a result of chronic replication of measles virus in the bronchi and lungs. This has usually been a fatal complication, sometimes occurring without any measles rash (Enders et al., 1959).

Obstructive Laryngitis and Laryngotracheitis

Transient mild laryngitis and tracheitis are both part of the normal course of measles. Occasionally, however, the inflammatory process progresses and causes airway obstruction. The increased hoarseness, barking cough, and inspiratory stridor associated with suprasternal retractions indicate the development of this complication. These symptoms usually subside when the rash begins to fade. The development of increasing restlessness, dyspnea, and tachycardia points to increasing obstruction, which may necessitate intubation and maintenance of airway support until the subsidence of the acute inflammation.

Gastroenteritis

Measles virus replicates in the gastrointestinal tract and often results in diarrhea, which may be severe. With the painful glossitis, seen most often among malnourished children with measles, the combination of reduced oral intake and increased intestinal fluid losses results in dehydration. Gastroenteritis is second only to pneumonia as a cause of death related to measles complications.

Cervical Adenitis

Generalized lymphadenopathy is associated with most cases of measles and represents the lymphoid hyperplasia caused by the virus. Bacterial cervical adenitis may occur as an extension of pharyngitis secondary to upper respiratory flora.

Acute Encephalomyelitis

Acute encephalomyelitis is a serious, potentially crippling or fatal complication that occurs in approximately 0.1% of measles cases. It begins most commonly between the second and sixth days after onset of the rash. However, rarely it develops during the preeruptive period.

Fever, headache, vomiting, drowsiness, convulsions, coma, or personality changes may usher in this complication. Frequently, there are signs of meningeal irritation, such as a stiff neck and Brudzinski's and Kernig's signs. The cerebrospinal fluid (CSF) shows a modest pleocytosis with a predominance of lymphocytes. The protein level is generally elevated; the glucose level is either normal or elevated. In rare instances the CSF may be normal.

The course of encephalomyelitis is quite variable. It may be very mild, clearing completely within several days, or it may be rapidly progressive and fulminating, terminating fatally within 24 hours. Between these two extremes are many variations. In general, approximately 60% of patients recover completely; 15% die; and 25% subsequently show manifestations of brain damage such as mental retardation, recurrent seizures, severe behavior disorders, nerve deafness, hemiplegia, and paraplegia. The course is unpredictable. It is not unusual for a child to be in a coma for several weeks and subsequently to recover completely without sequelae.

Other CNS complications of measles include cerebellar ataxia, retrobulbar neuritis, and hemiplegia caused by infarctions in the distribution of major arteries (Tyler, 1957). Although the pathogenesis of measles encephalomyelitis remains uncertain, it does not seem to involve viral replication in the CNS; rather, it more closely resembles the neuropathologic findings of experimental allergic encephalomyelitis, suggesting an autoimmune-mediated process (Johnson et al., 1984).

Subacute Sclerosing Panencephalitis

The rare condition of subacute sclerosing panencephalitis (SSPE) is a late complication of measles, with onset 5 to 10 years later and with an incidence of approximately 1 per 100,000 cases. It has clinical and pathologic features that are characteristic of a "slow virus" infection. The syndrome, first described by Dawson in 1934 and then by van Bogaert in 1945, has also been called *subacute inclusion-body encephalitis*.

The early clinical manifestations are characterized by insidious and progressive behavioral and intellectual deterioration, possibly initially manifested by declining school performance. These symptoms are associated with awkwardness, stumbling, and falling. Later, the course may be characterized by involuntary myoclonic seizures and increasing mental deterioration followed by death within a 6-month period. The confirmatory laboratory findings include (1) an electroencephalogram with paroxysmal spiking at regular intervals and depressed activity between spikes; (2) elevation of the CSF globulin, predominantly the IgG fraction; (3) an exceptionally high serum measles antibody titer; and (4) detectable oligoclonal measles antibody in the CSF.

The early neuropathologic features of SSPE include perivascular round cell infiltration, neuronal degeneration, and intranuclear and intracytoplasmic inclusion bodies. Later, extensive gliosis and demyelination occur. A defective structurally incomplete variant of the virus is responsible. Further confirmation of the role of measles virus in SSPE has been provided by electron microscopic demonstration of paramyxovirus nucleocapsids in the inclusion bodies, immunofluorescence with specific measles antiserum of affected cells, and recovery in the laboratory by cocultivation techniques of infectious measles–like virus from brain biopsy or autopsy specimens.

There is a spectrum of gene defects in virus recovered from brains of SSPE patients, but most frequently the virus demonstrates absent or defective synthesis of M protein. By a method combining in situ reverse transcriptase (RT)–PCR amplification with labeled-probe hybridization (in situ RT-PCR-LPH) Isaacson et al. (1996)

have detected measles virus RNA in neurons, astrocytes, oligodendrocytes, and vascular endothelial cells of SSPE patients, suggesting a far wider spread of the virus in the brain than had been appreciated by previous neuropathologic and virus culture studies. Since the advent of measles immunization programs, SSPE has disappeared from countries with high rates of vaccination. However, it persists in those nations where measles vaccines are not yet widely used (Bonthius et at., 2000).

Subacute Measles Encephalitis

In addition to acute measles encephalitis and SSPE, a third CNS syndrome has been described: subacute measles encephalitis (SME). SME occurs primarily in immunodeficient patients, most commonly children undergoing treatment for acute leukemia, but also, more recently, patients infected with human immunodeficiency virus (HIV). Whereas patients with SSPE have a latency period of years between measles and the onset of the syndrome, patients with SME have usually had measles within the past 6 months. Focal or generalized seizures, altered level of consciousness, and a variety of other CNS dysfunctions are observed. The mortality rate is 85%, with death occurring a few weeks to several months after onset. Mustafa et al. (1993) reviewed the past literature and reported two additional SME patients studied during the outbreaks of measles in Dallas from 1989 to 1991. Confirmatory findings include the characteristic intranuclear or intracytoplasmic inclusions on neurohistologic staining, paramyxovirus nucleocapsids on electron microscopy, measles virus RNA detected through PCR, and isolation of measles virus from affected brain cells.

Other Complications

Purpura, thrombocytopenic and nonthrombocytopenic, rarely may complicate measles. The deleterious effect of measles on pregnancy and on tuberculosis was clearly demonstrated in the southern Greenland epidemic (Christensen et al., 1953). Of 26 pregnant women with measles, half either aborted or gave birth to premature infants; there were no congenital malformations. There apparently were a reactivation of previously arrested cases, a striking increase of new cases of tuberculosis, and an increased mortality rate with this disease.

A positive tuberculin test may temporarily revert to negative during the course of measles. This anergy may persist for as long as 6 weeks. In the majority of cases the tuberculin test becomes positive again within 2 weeks.

Pneumomediastinal and subcutaneous emphysema may occur in rare instances. Bloch and Vardy (1968) described four cases that occurred during an epidemic in a small town in the northern Negev in Israel.

Corneal ulceration is a potentially serious complication that fortunately is uncommon. However, nearly all patients have a mild superficial keratoconjunctivitis.

Among children with nutritional deficiencies, particularly of vitamin A, the combination of infection and epithelial cell vulnerability has resulted in a more extensive involvement frequently ending in blindness (Morley, 1962).

Appendicitis may develop, as a result of lymphoid hyperplasia in the appendix, that may be so extensive it obliterates the lumen. In most instances perforation occurs before the complication is recognized.

In those areas of the world (sub-Saharan Africa and India) where measles remains a severe and often-fatal disease, the following complications are frequently observed: severe diarrhea and dehydration, kwashiorkor, pyogenic infections of the skin, cancrum oris, and septicemia. Of deaths attributable to measles, 98% occur in developing countries, where case fatality rates are 1% to 5% ordinarily but may in some settings reach 10% to 30%.

Among children infected with HIV, measles has an enhanced severity, with a higher incidence of pneumonia, hospitalization, and death (Kaplan et al., 1992; Krasinski and Borkowsky, 1989) (see also Chapter 1). Because those regions where measles remains endemic and epidemic are also those where HIV rates are highest among infants and children, this coinfection may influence not only the individual response to the disease but also impair the programs for disease control and eradication of measles (Moss et al., 1999; Permar et al., 2001).

An association between either intrapartum exposure to measles virus (Ekbom et al., 1996) or childhood receipt of measles vaccine (Thompson et al., 1995) and inflammatory bowel disease has been suggested but questioned by a number of critical reviewers (Patriarca and Beeler, 1995). Somewhat similarly, allegations of a causative relationship among inflammatory bowel disease, measles, mumps, and rubella (MMR) vaccine, and autism have been promulgated for several years (Wakefield, 1999; Wakefield et al., 1998) but refuted by expert review groups (Institute of Medicine Immunization Safety Reviews, 2001).

PROGNOSIS

The prognosis for patients with measles has improved significantly during the past three decades. Many of the serious bacterial complications are successfully treated with antimicrobial therapy. In general, the prognosis is better in older children than in infants. A preexisting tuberculous infection may be aggravated. The majority of deaths result from severe bronchopneumonia or encephalitis. In 1989 and 1990 in outbreaks in the United States the reported case fatality rates were from 3 to 4 per 1,000 (Centers for Disease Control, 1991).

Modified measles, which is rarely complicated, has an excellent prognosis.

IMMUNITY
Active Immunity

One attack of measles is generally followed by permanent immunity. Most so-called recurrent attacks reflect errors in diagnosis. The available evidence suggests that in most cases lasting immunity also follows an attack of modified measles. Contemporary studies indicate that comparable lasting immunity will follow immunization with live attenuated measles virus vaccine. Markowitz et al. (1990a) conducted an extensive review of the literature on duration and quality of measles vaccine–induced immunity 27 years after licensure of vaccine. Although a number of issues remain unresolved, waning immunity has been demonstrated in only a very small proportion of vaccinees (Anders et al., 1996; Edmunson et al., 1990).

A number of studies have explored the causes of the suppression of cell-mediated immune responses observed during and following measles for weeks or months. These same alterations to a lesser degree have been detected after live measles virus vaccination (Hussey et al., 1996). Reported factors include a downregulation of interleukin (IL)-12 production by infected monocyte-macrophages and a suppression of Th1 type cytokines, including IL-4, which inhibits CD4 and CD8 cell-mediated

responses. The effects on the monocyte-macrophages resulted from binding of measles virus to the cells (Karp et al., 1996) with or without the initiation of productive virus infection. This binding occurs at the CD46 receptor on the cell membrane, suggesting an interaction with the complement system, since C3b binds to the same site. The persisting cellular immunosuppression induced by measles is responsible for greatly enhanced susceptibility to a variety of bacterial and fungal opportunistic infections during the days and weeks after the initial virus infection. There is a continuing general proliferative unresponsiveness of T cells and a perturbation of cytokine elaboration (Schneider-Schaulies et al., 2002). A complex series of interactions initiated by infected antigen presenting cells produces this T-cell and cytokine imbalance. These alterations remain the subject of intensive laboratory investigation.

Passive Immunity

Neutralizing antibodies for measles virus are present in convalescent-phase serum and in pooled adult serum. These antibodies are contained in the IG fraction that has been used for passive immunization. Passively acquired measles antibody is detected in cord blood and is usually not measurable after the infant reaches 12 months of age.

Studies by Albrecht et al. (1977) revealed the presence of passively acquired measles-neutralizing antibody in serum specimens obtained from 12-month-old infants who had no detectable HI antibody. In those populations where measles vaccines have been widely used since the mid-1960s, most pregnant women have vaccine-induced antibodies rather than those resulting from the natural infection. Because these are of lower titer, they are catabolized earlier in the first year of life by their infants, who then may lack detectable antibody by 9 to 12 months of age (Markowitz et al., 1996).

EPIDEMIOLOGIC FACTORS

Patients with measles harbor the virus in their nasopharyngeal secretions during the acute stage of the disease. Epidemiologic evidence suggests that the patients are contagious for at least 7 days after the onset of the first symptom. Contacts may acquire the infection (1) directly, by being sprayed with droplets emanating from a cough or sneeze; or (2) by airborne spread. The most common mode of spread is by direct contact. Indirect contact within a house or a hospital ward is also possible but is an unlikely mode of transmission. In crowded settings such as classrooms, residential institutions, day-care centers, and homes, the spread is mostly via large respiratory droplets. Air-borne spread by viruses persisting in fine droplets for several hours in physicians' waiting rooms has also been demonstrated.

Measles virus is present in the nasopharynx during the first day of rash and during the preceding catarrhal period of the disease. The larger quantities of virus present during the pre-rash catarrhal period are undoubtedly most responsible for spread of the disease.

During the prevaccine era (before 1963) the age incidence varied with the particular environment. In general, measles was a disease of childhood. In congested urban areas the highest incidence occurred in the infant and preschool age-groups. In rural and less crowded urban areas the highest incidence was in children 5 to 10 years of age. In epidemics that occurred in isolated communities, children of all ages were equally affected. In developing countries, measles is most common in infants 1 to 2 years of age and is often seen in those less than 9 months old. Because of this early occurrence among small infants, for whom morbidity and mortality are often very marked, a number of programs were initiated to evaluate the immunogenicity, safety, and efficacy of several higher-titered live virus measles vaccines administered early (Aaby et al., 1988; Markowitz et al., 1990b; Tidjani et al., 1989; Whittle et al., 1988a; Whittle et al., 1988b).

Vaccines containing 100 times more virus than usual were administered to 4- to 6-month-old infants in an attempt to overcome maternal transplacental immunity and "close the window of susceptibility" that exists between catabolism of maternal antibody and ability to immunize successfully with conventional titer attenuated live measles virus vaccines. The success of these studies in a number of nations (Senegal, Guinea-Bissau, Gambia, Haiti, Togo, Sudan, Mexico, and Peru) led to a 1989 WHO recommendation that high-titered vaccines (10^5 infectious units rather than the usual $10^{3\ to\ 4}$ per dose) be administered at 6 months of age, instead of waiting until 9 months with conventional vaccines, in those areas where measles

below age 9 months caused significant mortality (World Health Organization, 1990). In the subsequent 3 years, surveillance revealed that, despite the successful prevention of measles, there was an unexplained increase in deaths from other infections especially in female recipients (Aaby et al., 1993; Aaby et al., 1996). This was an inconsistent finding among the study populations, but its occurrence in Senegal, Guinea-Bissau, and Haiti was of sufficient concern to call a halt to further use of high-titered vaccines (World Health Organization, 1992). It is uncertain whether the phenomenon was due to the previously described persisting immune suppression caused by measles viruses, with resultant susceptibility to other infections. The lack of autopsy data or microbiology precludes exploration of this hypothesis. The female gender bias is similarly unexplained.

The disease is extremely rare in infants less than 3 to 4 months of age because of passively acquired maternal antibodies. If the mother, however, has never had measles, the newborn infant is susceptible.

Seasonal incidence in the temperate zones was essentially that of a winter-spring disease, with the peak occurring during March and April. In heavily populated areas, epidemics usually occurred at intervals of 2 to 3 years during the prevaccine era. This periodicity was in part caused by the accumulation of a new group of susceptible children during this interval. The extensive use of live attenuated measles virus vaccine since licensure in 1963 has had a profound effect on the incidence of measles (Figure 20-5).

Following the initiation in 1966 of major federal funding for measles vaccine programs, a precipitous drop in the reported cases of disease resulted. By 1981 a reduction of greater than 99% from levels seen in prevaccine years had occurred. In 1983 an all-time low was reached, with fewer than 1,500 cases, in contrast to the half million or more reported annually before 1963. In 1989 and 1990 a striking increase in measles cases was observed, especially among inner-city, poor, unimmunized preschool children (see inset of Figure 20-5). This resulted in great part from a failure to reach these infants and children with recommended health care measures, including basic immunizations (Katz, 1991). With enhanced efforts to immunize children and with the introduction of second doses

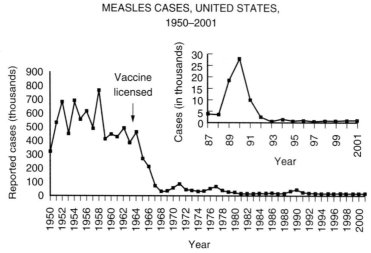

Fig. 20-5 Number of reported cases of measles in the United States, 1950 to 2001. (From National Immunization Program, Centers for Disease Control and Prevention, Atlanta, Ga.)

of vaccine, measles was reduced to fewer than 1,000 reported cases annually in the years 1993 through 1997 (Katz, 1998), fewer than 100 in 2000 and 2001 and only 37 in 2002 (MMWR). Using genomic analysis as a technique for molecular epidemiology, it has been demonstrated that measles virus isolates in the United States have been of international origin, with no indigenous U.S. strain or transmission of virus since 1993 (Watson et al., 1998). Most importations since then have originated in Western Europe and Eastern Asia.

Geographic distribution is worldwide. Modern air transportation can carry an infected individual to all parts of the world within the incubation period. Through the leadership of PAHO, an effort directed toward measles control and elimination has been initiated and has progressed rapidly in much of Latin America and the Caribbean countries (de Quadros et al., 1996). The English-speaking Caribbean countries have reported no cases of measles since 1991 despite careful surveillance and laboratory investigation of suspect patients with febrile rash illnesses (Pan American Health Organization, 1996a).

Measles is one of the most highly contagious diseases. The secondary attack rate after an intimate household exposure is greater than 90%. Reductions in intimacy and duration of exposure in a school, bus, or hospital ward are followed by a lower attack rate in susceptible persons—less than 25%.

TREATMENT

Measles is a self-limited disease. No specific antiviral agent is available, and the course of uncomplicated infection is not altered by antibiotics. Treatment is chiefly supportive.

Studies in Africa by Barclay et al. (1987) and by Hussey and Klein (1990) have demonstrated the striking beneficial effects of giving vitamin A to poorly nourished children with severe measles. In a randomized, double-blind trial of hospitalized children (median age, 10 months), Hussey and Klein found that those who received 400,000 IU of vitamin A within 5 days of onset of rash had less croup, recovered more rapidly from pneumonia and diarrhea, spent fewer days in the hospital, and had a much lower mortality rate than those given a placebo. Only 2 of 92 patients died among the vitamin A recipients; 10 of 97 placebo patients died. The WHO has recommended vitamin A supplementation for all children in regions where vitamin A deficiency exists or where the measles mortality rate is 1% or higher. To take advantage of the 9-month health visit at which measles vaccine is administered in the Expanded Programme on Immunization (EPI), it is recommended that vitamin A be given at that time (Ross and Cutts, 1997).

Supportive Therapy

Bed rest is advisable and not difficult to enforce during the febrile period. The diet should be either liquid or soft as tolerated. When the child becomes afebrile and the anorexia subsides, regular indoor activity and diet may be resumed.

The measles cough is difficult to control but some suppressants may help. The coryza is unaffected by treatment and runs a self-limited course. The skin around the nares, however, can be protected with petrolatum.

The conjunctivitis usually requires no medication. The eyelids should be cleansed with warm water to remove any secretions or crusts. The cornea should be examined for possible ulceration. Corneal complications should be treated by an ophthalmologist. If photophobia is present, bright lights should be avoided.

Infants with very high fever and children with headache should be treated with appropriate doses of antipyretic drugs.

Prevention of Bacterial Complications

Antibiotics should not be routinely administered to children with measles for the purpose of preventing bacterial complications. These agents not only may fail to achieve this goal but also may have the adverse effect of encouraging overgrowth by antibiotic-resistant bacteria or fungi that later may be responsible for complicating secondary infections (pneumonia, otitis, mastoiditis, sinusitis). This was demonstrated clearly by Weinstein (1955) in his studies of measles and its complications in the prevaccine era. Consequently, each case of measles should be carefully evaluated before antimicrobial agents are prescribed. The following factors pertaining to the host, the environment, and the disease may influence the decision to administer or withhold these drugs.

Host factors. Age and past experience influence the development of complications. Infants are more prone to develop complications than are older children. Children with a past history of recurrent otitis media may be particularly susceptible to another episode.

Environmental factors. Patients at home are less likely than those in hospital wards to acquire a secondary infection.

Disease factors. A mild case of measles is usually uncomplicated and need not be treated. A severe case, however, more likely will be complicated by otitis media or pneumonia.

Treatment of Complications

Otitis media. The pathogenesis and the treatment of otitis media that arises as a com-

plication of measles are no different from those following other respiratory virus infections. For a complete discussion, see Chapter 24.

Pneumonia. Bacterial pneumonia may be caused by *Streptococcus pneumoniae*, hemolytic streptococci, *Staphylococcus* species, or *Haemophilus influenzae*. These infections are discussed in Chapters 14, 29, 34, 35.

Bronchiolitis. The treatment of infants who develop complicating bronchiolitis is difficult. The details are discussed in Chapter 29.

Obstructive laryngitis and laryngotracheitis. The development of a severe measles croup requires emergency treatment. The child should be hospitalized and placed in an intensive care unit. Treatment of this complication is discussed in detail in Chapter 29.

Encephalitis. Treatment is primarily symptomatic. There is no measles-specific antiviral drug currently available. Most patients require the detailed monitoring and supportive interventions available in a critical care unit. These may include stabilization of circulatory function, maintenance of respiration and ventilation, anticonvulsant therapy, lowering of increased intracranial pressure, and management of fluid and electrolyte balance (Chapter 43).

The use of corticosteroids remains controversial. The very favorable clinical experience reported by Applebaum and Abler in 1956 with 17 treated cases and by Allen in 1957 with 10 treated cases appeared impressive. Although the number of cases was small (27), the reported incidence of 26 complete recoveries was striking. On the other hand, in 1959 Meade reported comparable results without corticosteroid therapy. He cited a personal observation of more than fifty patients, many with respiratory paralysis and status epilepticus, who recovered without sequelae. The evidence for the efficacy of corticosteroids in the treatment of measles encephalitis is not convincing.

An important aspect of the treatment of encephalitis is the supportive medical and nursing care necessary to tide over a comatose child for a period of days and sometimes weeks. This includes careful attention to hydration and nutrition and the prevention and treatment of intercurrent infections.

PREVENTIVE MEASURES
Immune Globulin

Measles can be modified or prevented by human IG, which induces passive immunity of variable duration. The dose for prevention is 0.25 ml/kg of body weight given within 6 days of exposure.

With the increasing use of human IG preparations for a variety of conditions, especially intravenous IG (IGIV), measles and measles vaccine virus infections are inadvertently modified or prevented in a number of scenarios, depending on the product used and the dose administered (Halsey, 1995). Although the Food and Drug Administration has established a minimum concentration of measles antibody for IG preparations, there is no such standard for IGIV. Because of the resultant uncertainty regarding duration of protection from such globulin administration, measles vaccine should be given to recipients promptly after a known exposure in hopes of providing active protection if the exogenous antibody has been catabolized to an extent unlikely to prevent illness.

MEASLES VIRUS VACCINES

Within a decade of the first report of successful isolation and replication of measles virus in cell culture systems (Enders and Peebles, 1954), an attenuated live measles virus vaccine was licensed in the United States (Enders et al., 1960) and subsequently in a number of other nations (Markowitz and Katz, 1994). With rare exceptions (Japan, China, Russia) these products are all descendants of the prototype Edmonston virus. Widespread administration of these vaccines in developed nations and through the EPI of the WHO has resulted in a marked decrease in both morbidity and mortality resulting from measles. Previously in the United States, 500,000 to 800,000 cases were reported annually, but this was gross underreporting, because nearly an entire birth cohort (3.5 to 4.0 million children) was infected each year. From a global perspective the WHO estimates that before initiation of the EPI in 1977 there were 8 million deaths annually from measles; by 2001 there were fewer than 1 million. After a brief resurgence of measles in the United States, mainly among unimmunized inner-city children 1989 through 1991 (Hutchin et al., 1996; Katz, 1991), increased efforts to immunize all children shortly after their first birthday and to administer second doses at elementary or middle school entry have resulted in elimination of endemic disease since 1993. In the years 1999, 2000, and 2001, total measles cases in the United States hovered

around 100 annually. With optimism regarding the possibility of measles elimination (following the examples of the eradication of smallpox and of current progress in the global polio eradication program), participants at a July 1996 meeting sponsored by PAHO, the CDC, and WHO agreed that progress to date in measles control justified the establishment of a target date of 2010 for global measles eradication (Pan American Health Organization, 1996b). Currently the EPI schedule calls for administration of measles vaccine at age 9 months. In the United States, vaccine is given between 12 and 15 months of age and a second dose before school entry. In the United States, measles vaccine is ordinarily administered as a combination covering measles, mumps, and rubella. EPI uses monovalent measles vaccine without mumps or rubella.

Measles vaccine is produced in cell cultures of chick embryo fibroblasts and is stabilized with human albumin, sorbitol, and hydrolyzed gelatin to yield a final concentration of at least 1,000 tissue culture infectious doses of virus. There is also a small amount of neomycin in the final solution. The only measles vaccine currently licensed in the United States is Moraten (an Enders-Edmonston descendant) (Merck and Company, Inc). Although the complete genome of measles virus has been sequenced (Kobune et al., 1995), and it is therefore possible to differentiate vaccine strain from circulating wild virus, the molecular basis for attenuation or virulence has not been identified. Past epidemiologic history and current laboratory observations confirm the overall antigenic stability of the virus, but there are sufficient variations in the F and H gene products to permit the discrimination of vaccine from wild strains (Chibo et al., 2002). Immunologically, it is reassuring to note that sera from vaccine recipients are capable in vitro of neutralizing wild viruses isolated more than 40 years ago. Likewise, sera from individuals infected many years ago neutralize current measles virus isolates.

In the United States, two committees are mainly responsible for recommendations governing the use of measles virus vaccines. The Advisory Committee on Immunization Practices of the U.S. Public Health Service publishes its recommendations as supplements to the Morbidity and Mortality Weekly Report, and the Committee on Infectious Diseases (the "Redbook Committee") of the American

Academy of Pediatrics publishes its recommendations in the journal *Pediatrics* and in its Redbook publication, which is issued approximately every 3 years, most recently its 26th edition in 2003.

In susceptible children, measles vaccine produces febrile response (≥39.4° C) in 5% to 15% of recipients 7 to 12 days after vaccination and rash in approximately 5% 7 to 10 days after vaccine administration. More than 95% of susceptible recipients show seroconversion with a measles-specific antibody response first detectable 12 to 15 days after vaccination and achieving peak titers 21 to 28 days thereafter. Serum antibodies are of the IgM, IgG, and IgA isotypes, and there is also detectable measles-specific secretory IgA at the respiratory mucosal surfaces. In general, these antibodies are enduring but may fall to undetectable levels in a variable number of recipients over lengthy periods of observation. Reexposure to vaccine results in a rapid anamnestic response, indicating persistence of effective immune memory. Undoubtedly, a significant aspect of this memory resides in T-cell function, an essential component of the measles immune response. Concern regarding secondary vaccine failures (that is, those individuals who initially responded to vaccine but subsequently lost their immunity) has challenged full resolution over the years. Recent observations suggest that, if they occur, they are extremely unusual, probably occurring in less than 0.2% (Anders et al., 1996; Guris et al., 1996; Watson et al., 1996b).

As noted, fever and rash are the most common reactions observed after primary immunization of susceptible children. From an exhaustive review by a committee of the Institute of Medicine (Stratton et al., 1994) available evidence pointed to febrile seizures, thrombocytopenia, and anaphylaxis as the only adverse events for which sufficient evidence existed to establish a causal relationship. Anaphylaxis has been reported in less than 1 per 1 million doses of MMR vaccine in the United States. Although children may have febrile seizures after MMR vaccination, especially those with a prior history of seizures, there is no evidence for the production of a residual seizure disorder or chronic neurologic disability. Suspected encephalopathies follow a nonrandom distribution between days 5 and 14 after vaccine administration. If measles vaccine is the cause, the frequency may be 1 to 10 per million, significantly fewer than the 1 per 1,000 rate observed following natural measles. Thrombocytopenia, which may be an unusual complication of natural measles, has also been reported after monovalent measles vaccine at an estimated rate of 1 per 75,000 doses. This may be a more frequent complication for patients who have previously had an immune thrombocytopenic purpura and is reported to occur more frequently with MMR vaccines.

Because vaccine is derived from chick embryo cell cultures, there has been a concern regarding its administration to children with egg allergy. James et al. (1995) studied 54 children with severe allergies to egg, 26 of whom had anaphylaxis after ingestion of eggs. None of the 54 had either an immediate or a delayed adverse reaction on receipt of a standard dose of MMR subcutaneously.

Because the vaccine is a live, replicating virus, its administration to immunocompromised patients has received careful scrutiny. In early studies with the first (less attenuated) Edmonston vaccine, two children under chemotherapy for acute leukemia developed giant cell pneumonia after vaccination (Mitus et al., 1962). After subsequent further attenuation of the vaccine virus and extensive experience over three decades, only six severely immunocompromised patients have been reported who suffered fatal complications attributable to vaccine virus. This occurs in a background denominator of more than 300 million doses administered. In the current era of HIV and acquired immunodeficiency syndrome, increased attention has been focused on the possible risks associated with measles immunization of HIV-infected children. Because wild measles has resulted in such a high mortality rate among these patients (Kaplan et al., 1992), the hypothetical risk of vaccine-induced disease has been an acceptable one, so until 1996 MMR was recommended for asymptomatic HIV-infected persons and considered for symptomatic ones. The publication in 1996 (Centers for Disease Control and Prevention, 1996) of a single, highly unique exception initiated a reconsideration of this policy. One year after receipt of his second dose of MMR, given to fulfill a college prematriculation requirement, a young man developed a progressive illness with pneumonia, shown later to be giant cell pneumonia resulting from measles virus, which was identified as vaccine strain by its sequence analysis. As a result, recommendations were reformulated, advising the withholding of measles vaccine from HIV-infected individuals with severe immunosuppression (for children age 1 to 5 years, CD4 counts of less than 200 or percentages less than 15). Among those infants and children who have received measles vaccine, there has been a spectrum of response with lower antibody titers, fewer seroconversions, and shortened persistence of detectable antibodies (Palumbo et al., 1992; Walter et al., 1994).

Despite the impressive success of current vaccines in controlling measles and eliminating transmission in some countries, the challenge of immunizing infants at an even younger age (when transplacentally acquired maternal antibody aborts the infection with attenuated virus) has stimulated attempts to develop other forms of vaccine that would immunize successfully despite circulating measles-specific antibody. These have included the use of recombinant vaccinia virus or canarypox virus expressing measles F and H proteins, immune-stimulating complexes containing these same proteins (Hsu et al., 1996), and chimeras of measles and other viruses. In attempts to avoid the needle-syringe route of vaccination and in hopes of bypassing residual maternal measles antibody, a number of studies have explored aerosol nebulization of vaccine (Cutts et al., 1997). Another approach involves the inhalation of powdered vaccine. These studies continue at varied stages of development while the WHO and EPI programs press forward with injectable vaccine at age 9 months. When administered at 9 months of age to infants in Bangladesh, 95% seroconversion has been achieved (Schnorr et al., 2001), with 70% at age 6 months. As an indicator of the immune modulation produced by vaccine, these children had increased 1L-12 production for 6 to 24 weeks after vaccination. A number of studies suggest that cellular immunity with memory may be induced at 6 months by measles vaccine even in the absence of a detectable antibody response, reflecting a differential in immunologic maturation of infancy (Gans et al., 2001).

Other modifications of current measles vaccine include the incorporation of live attenuated varicella vaccine in a tetravalent preparation (measles-mumps-rubella-varicella vaccine [MMRV]), which has been immunogenic and safe in initial studies (Watson et al., 1996a; also see Chapter 41).

Global elimination of measles is an enormous challenge, given the marked communicability of the infection, the susceptibility of infants once maternal antibody has been catabolized, the need to immunize close to 100% of susceptible individuals, and the lack of public health infrastructure in those countries where it remains endemic (Katz and Gellin, 1994).

ISOLATION AND QUARANTINE

In general, isolation and quarantine procedures are of limited value in the prophylaxis of measles. Exposure usually occurs before the diagnosis is obvious. Attempts to isolate siblings from one another are useless. The availability of IG and live attenuated measles virus vaccine for household and other susceptible contacts has obviated the need for quarantine.

Isolation of Patient

Epidemiologic evidence has indicated that measles is no longer contagious after the fourth day of rash. Consequently, children may return to school or other group activities after this time.

Quarantine of Contact

The susceptible contact is a potential source of infection from the eighth day after exposure to as long as the twenty-first day if IG has been administered. Consequently, if quarantine were to be instituted, a child would have to be isolated for almost 2 weeks. Experience has shown that quarantine rarely affects the course of an epidemic. On the contrary, it usually disrupts household and school activities unnecessarily. Once the outbreak has occurred, it is best to continue normal school and group activities and to rely chiefly on IG and live attenuated measles virus vaccine as prophylactic agents. Vaccine administered to a susceptible individual within 72 hours of contact has great likelihood of protection.

Bibliography

Aaby P, Jensen TG, Hansen HL, et al. Trial of high-dose Edmonston-Zagreb measles vaccine in Guinea-Bissau: protective efficacy. Lancet 1988;2:809-811.

Aaby P, Knudsen K, Whittle H, et al. Child mortality after Edmonston-Zagreb measles vaccination in Guinea-Bissau increased female mortality rate. J Pediatr 1993;122:904-908.

Aaby P, Samb B, Simondon F, et al. Five-year follow-up of morbidity and mortality among recipients of high-titer measles vaccines in Senegal. Vaccine 1996;14:226-229.

Albrecht P, Ennis FA, Saltzmann EJ, Krugman S. Persistence of maternal antibody in infants beyond 12 months: mechanism of measles vaccine failure. J Pediatr 1977;91:715.

Allen JE. Treatment of measles encephalitis with adrenal steroids. Pediatrics 1957;20:87.

Anders JF, Jacobson RM, Poland GA, et al. Secondary failure rates of measles vaccines: a metaanalysis of published studies. Pediatr Infect Dis J 1996;15:62-66.

Annunziato D, Kaplan MH, Hall WW, et al. Atypical measles syndrome: pathologic and serologic findings. Pediatrics 1982;70:203-209.

Applebaum E, Abler C. Treatment of measles encephalitis with corticotropin. Am J Dis Child 1956;92:47.

Barclay AJG, Foster A, Sommer A. Vitamin A supplements and mortality related to measles: a randomized clinical trial. Br Med J 1987;294:294-296.

Bellini WJ, Rota PA. Genetic diversity of wild-type measles viruses: implications for global measles elimination programs. Emerg Infect Dis 1998:4:1-7.

Bloch A, Vardy P. Pneumomediastinum and subcutaneous emphysema in measles. Clin Pediatr 1968;7:7.

Bonthius DJ, Stanek N, Grose C. Subacute sclerosing panencephalitis, a measles complication in an internationally adopted child. Emerg Infect Dis 2000;6:377-382.

Centers for Disease Control and Prevention. Measles pneumonitis following M-M-R vaccination of a patient with HIV infection, 1993. MMWR Morb Mortal Wkly Rep 1996;45:603-606.

Cherry JD, Cohen LM, Panosian CB. Diarrhea, fever, hypoxia, and rash in a house officer. Rev Infect Dis 1990;12:1044-1051.

Chibo D, Riddell M, Catton M, Birch C. Novel measles virus genotype, East Timor and Australia. Emerg Infect Dis 2002;8:735-737.

Christensen PO, Schmidt H, Bang HO, et al. An epidemic of measles in Southern Greenland in 1951. Acta Med Scand 1953;144:430,450.

Cutts FT, Clements JC, Bennett J. Alternative routes of measles immunization: a review. Biologicals 1997;25:323-338.

Cutts FT, Henao-Restrepo AM, Olive JM. Measles elimination: progress and challenges. Vaccine 1999;17(suppl 3): S47-S52.

Dawson JR Jr. Cellular inclusions in cerebral lesions of epidemic encephalitis. Arch Neurol Psychiatr 1934;31:685.

Degen JA Jr. Visceral pathology in measles: a clinicopathological study of 100 fatal cases. Am J Med Sci 1937;194:104.

de Quadros C, Olive J, Hersh B, et al. Measles elimination in the Americas: evolving strategies. JAMA 1996;275:224-229.

Duke T, Mgone CS. Measles: not just another viral exanthem. Lancet 2003;361:763-773.

Edmunson MB, Addiss DG, McPherson JT, et al. Mild measles and secondary vaccine failure during a sustained outbreak in a highly vaccinated population. JAMA 1990;263:2467-2471.

Ekbom A, Daszak P, Kraaz W, et al. Crohn's disease after in utero measles virus exposure. Lancet 1996;348:515-517.

Enders JF, Katz SL, Milovanovic MJ, Holloway A. Studies on an attenuated measles virus vaccine. I. Development and preparation of the vaccine: techniques for assay of effects of vaccination. N Engl J Med 1960;263:153.

Enders JF, McCarthy K, Mitus A, Cheatham WJ. Isolation of measles virus at autopsy in cases of giant-cell pneumonia without rash. N Engl J Med 1959; 261:875.

Enders JF, Peebles TC. Propagation in tissue cultures of cytopathogenic agents from patients with measles. Proc Soc Exp Biol Med 1954;86:277.

Fortenberry J, Mariscalco M, Louis P, et al. Severe laryngotracheobronchitis complicating measles. Am J Dis Child 1992;146:1040-1043.

Fulginiti VA, Eller JJ, Downie AW, Kempe CH. Altered reactivity to measles virus: atypical measles in children previously immunized with inactivated measles virus vaccine. JAMA 1967;202:1075.

Gans H, Yasukawa L, Rinti M et al. Immune responses to measles and mumps vaccination of infants at 6, 9 and 12 months. J Infect Dis 2001;184:817-826.

Guris D, McCready J, Watson JC, et al. Measles vaccine effectiveness and duration of vaccine-induced immunity in the absence of boosting from exposure to measles virus. Pediatr Infect Dis J 1996;15:1082-1086.

Hall WJ, Hall CB. Atypical measles in adolescents: evaluation of clinical and pulmonary function. Ann Intern Med 1979;90:882.

Halsey N. Dose-adjusted timing of measles vaccine after administration of Ig. Rep Pediatr Infect Dis 1995;5: 21-22.

Harp CL. Measles, immunosuppression, interleukin-12 complement receptors. Immunol Rev 1999;168: 91-101.

Helfand R, Kebede S, Alexander J, et al. Comparative detection of measles-specific IgM in oral fluid and serum from children by an antibody-capture IgM EIA. J Infect Dis 1996;173:1470-1474.

Helfand RF, Heath JL, Anderson LJ, et al. Diagnosis of measles virus with an IgM capture EIA: the optimal timing of specimen collection after rash onset. J Infect Dis 1997;175:195-199.

Hsu S, Schadeck E, Delmas A, et al. Linkage of a fusion peptide to a CTL epitope from the nucleoprotein of measles virus enables incorporation into ISCOMs and induction of CTL responses following intranasal immunization. Vaccine 1996;14:1159-1166.

Hussey G, Goddard E, Hughes J, et al. The effect of Edmonston-Zagreb and Schwarz measles vaccines on immune responses in infants. J Infect Dis 1996;173:1320-1326.

Hussey GD, Klein M. A randomized controlled trial of vitamin A in children with severe measles. N Engl J Med 1990;323:160-164.

Hutchin S, Markowitz L, Atkinson W, et al. Measles outbreaks in the United States, 1987 through 1990. Pediatr Infect Dis J 1996;15:31-38.

Institute of Medicine Immunization Safety Reviews. Measles-Mumps-Rubella Vaccine and Autism. Washington, D.C.: National Academy Press, 2001.

Isaacson S, Asher D, Godec M, et al. Widespread, restricted low-level measles virus infection of brain in a case of subacute sclerosing panencephalitis. Acta Neuropathol 1996;91:135-139.

James J, Burks A, Roberson P, et al. Safe administration of the measles vaccine to children allergic to eggs. N Engl J Med 1995;332:1262-1266.

Johnson RT, Griffin DE, Hirsch RL, et al. Measles encephalomyelitis: clinical and immunologic studies. N Engl J Med 1984;310:137-141.

Kaplan LJ, Daum RS, Smaron M, McCarthy CA. Severe measles in immunocompromised patients. JAMA 1992; 267:1237-1241.

Karp C, Wysocka M, Wahl L, et al. Mechanism of suppression of cell-mediated immunity by measles virus. Science 1996;273:228-231.

Katz SL. Measles in the United States: 1989 and 1990. In Arnoff SC (ed). Advances in Pediatric Infectious Diseases, vol 6. St. Louis: Mosby, 1991.

Katz SL. Commentary: the disappearance of indigenous measles in the United States. Pediatr Infect Dis J 1998;17:366-367.

Katz SL, Gellin BG. Measles vaccine: do we need new vaccines or new programs? Science 1994;265:1391-1392.

Kobune F, Funatu M, Takahashi H, et al. Characterization of measles viruses isolated after measles vaccination. Vaccine 1995;13:370-372.

Koplik H. The diagnosis of the invasion of measles from a study of the exanthema as it appears on the buccal mucous membrane. Arch Pediatr 1896;13:918.

Krasinski K, Borkowsky W. Measles and measles immunity in children infected with human immunodeficiency virus. JAMA 1989;261:2512-2516.

Makhene M, Diaz P. Clinical presentations and complications of suspected measles in hospitalized children. Pediatric Infect Dis J 1993;12:836-840.

Markowitz L, Albrecht P, Rhodes P, et al. Changing levels of measles antibody titers in women and children in the United States: impact on response to vaccination. Pediatrics 1996;97:53-58.

Markowitz LE, Katz SL. Measles vaccine. In Plotkin SA, Mortimer EA Jr (eds). Vaccines. Philadelphia: Saunders, 1994.

Markowitz LE, Preblud SR, Fine PEM, et al. Duration of live measles vaccine–induced immunity. Pediatr Infect Dis 1990a;9:101-110.

Markowitz LE, Sepulveda J, Diaz-Ortega JL, et al. Immunization of six-month-old infants with different doses of Edmonston-Zagreb and Schwarz measles vaccines. N Engl J Med 1990b;322:580-587.

Martin DB, Werher LB, Nieburg PI, et al. Atypical measles in adolescents and young adults. Ann Intern Med 1979;90:977.

Matsuzono Y, Narita M, Ishiguro N, et al. Detection of measles virus from clinical samples using the polymerase chain reaction. Arch Pediatr Adolesc Med 1994;148: 289-293.

Meade RH III. Common viral infections in childhood: a discussion of measles, German measles, mumps, chickenpox, vaccinia, and smallpox. Med Clin North Am 1959;43:1355.

Mitus A, Holloway A, Evans AE, Enders JF. Attenuated measles vaccine in children with acute leukemia. Am J Dis Child 1962;103:243-248.

Morley DC. Measles in Nigeria. Am J Dis Child 1962;103:230.

Morris DL, Montgomery SM, Thompson NP, et al. Measles vaccination and inflammatory bowel disease: a national British cohort study. Am J Gastroenterol 2000;95:3507-3512.

Moss WJ, Cutts F, Griffin DE. Implications of the Human Immunodeficiency Virus epidemic for control and eradication of measles. Clin Infect Dis 1999;29:100-112.

Mustafa M, Weitman S, Winick N, et al. Subacute measles encephalitis in the young immunocompromised host: report of two cases diagnosed by polymerase chain reaction and treated with ribavirin and review of the literature. Clin Infect Dis 1993;16:654-660.

Nader PR, Horwitz MS, Rousseau J. Atypical exanthem following exposure to natural measles: 11 cases in children previously inoculated with killed vaccine. J Pediatr 1968;72:22.

Naniche D, Varior G, Cervoni F, et al. Human membrane cofactor protein (CD46) acts as a cellular receptor for measles virus. J Virol 1993;67:6025-6032.

Pan American Health Organization. Record five years measles-free! EPI Newsletter 1996a;18:1-3.

Pan American Health Organization. Global measles eradication: target 2010? EPI Newsletter 1996b;18(4):1-3.

Palumbo P, Hoyt L, Demasio K, et al. Population-based study of measles and measles immunization in human immunodeficiency virus–infected children. Pediatr Infect Dis J 1992;11:1008-1014.

Patriarca PA, Beeler JA. Measles vaccination and inflammatory bowel disease. Lancet 1995;345:1062-1063.

Permar SR, Moss WJ, Ryan JJ, et al. Prolonged measles virus shedding in Human Immunodeficiency Virus–infected children, detected by reverse transcriptase-polymerase chain reaction. J Infect Dis 2001;183: 532-538.

Polack FP, Auwaerter PG, Lee SH, et al. Production of atypical measles in rhesus macaques: evidence for disease mediated by immune complex formation and eosinophils in the presence of fusion-inhibiting antibody. Nat Med 1999;5:629-634.

Polack FP, Hoffman SJ, Moss WJ, Griffin DE. Altered synthesis of Interleukin-12 and type 1 and type 2 cytokines in rhesus macaques during measles and atypical measles. J Infect Dis 2002;185:13-19.

Rauh LW, Schmidt R. Measles immunization with killed virus vaccine. Am J Dis Child 1965;109:232.

Ross DA, Cutts FT. Vindication of policy of vitamin A with measles vaccination. Lancet 1997;350:81-82.

Rota JS, Rota PA, Redd SB, et al. Genetic analysis of measles viruses isolated in the United States. J Infect Dis 1998;177:204-208.

Scheifele DW, Forbes CE. Prolonged giant cell excretion in severe African measles. Pediatrics 1972;50:867.

Schneider-Schaulies S, Bieback K, Avota E, et al. Regulation of gene-expression in lymphocytes and antigen-presenting cells by measles virus: consequences for immunomodulation. J Mol Med 2002;80:73-85.

Schnorr J-J, Cutts FT, Wheeler JG, et al. Immune modulation after measles vaccination of 6-9 months old Bangladeshi infants. Vaccine 2001;19:1503-1510.

Seng R, Samb B, Simondon F, et al. Increased long-term mortality associated with rash after early measles vaccination in rural Senegal. Pediatr Infect Dis J 1999;18: 48-52.

Stratton K, Howe C, Johnson R (eds). Adverse Events Associated with Childhood Vaccines: Evidence Bearing on Causality. Washington, D.C.: National Academy Press, 1994.

Suringa DWR, Bank LJ, Ackerman AB. Role of measles virus in skin lesions and Koplik's spots. N Engl J Med 1970;283:1139.

Tatsuo H, Ono N, Tanaka K, Yanagi Y. SLAM (CDw 150) is a cellular receptor for measles virus. Nature 2000;406:893-897.

Thompson N, Montgomery S, Pounder R, et al. Is measles vaccination a risk factor for inflammatory bowel disease? Lancet 1995;345:1071-1074.

Tidjani O, Grunitsky G, Guerin N, et al. Serological effects of Edmonston-Zagreb, Schwarz, and AIK-C measles vaccine strains given at 4-5 or 8-10 months. Lancet 1989;2:1357-1360.

Tompkins V, Macaulay JC. A characteristic cell in nasal secretions during prodromal measles. JAMA 1955;157:711.

Tyler HR. Neurological complications of rubeola (measles). Medicine 1957;25:147-167.

van Bogaert L. Une leuco-encephalite sclerosante subaigu. J Neurol Neurosurg Psychiatry 1945;8:101.

Wakefield AJ. MMR vaccination and autism. Lancet 1999;354:949-951.Wakefield AJ, Murch SH, Anthony A, et al. Ileal-lymphoid-nodular hyperplasia, non-specific colitis, and pervasive development disorder in children. Lancet 1998;351:632-641.

Walter EB, Katz SL, Bellini WJ. Measles immunity in HIV-infected children. Pediatr AIDS HIV Infect 1994;5:300-304.

Watson B, Laufer D, Kuter B, et al. Safety and immunogenicity of a combined live attenuated measles, mumps, rubella, and varicella vaccine (MMRV) in healthy children. J Infect Dis 1996a;173:731-734.

Watson J, Pearson J, Markowitz L, et al. An evaluation of measles revaccination among school-entry-aged children. Pediatr 1996b;97:613-618.

Watson JC, Redd SC, Rhodes PH, Hadler SC. The interruption of indigenous measles in the United States during 1993. Pediatr Infect Dis J 1998;17:363-366.

Weinstein L. Failure of chemotherapy to prevent the bacterial complications of measles. N Engl J Med 1955;253:679.

Whittle HC, Hanlon P, O'Neill K, et al. Trial of high-dose Edmonson-Zagreb measles vaccine in the Gambia: antibody response and side effects. Lancet 1988a;2:811-814.

Whittle HC, Mann G, Eccles M, et al. Effects of dose and strain of vaccine on success of measles vaccination of infants aged 4-5 months. Lancet 1988b;1:963-966.

World Health Organization, Expanded Programme on Immunization, Global Advisory Group. Measles immunization before 9 months of age (part 1). Wkly Epidemiol Rec 1990;65:5-12.

World Health Organization, Expanded Programme on Immunization. Safety of high titer measles vaccines. Wkly Epidemiol Rec 1992;67:357-361.

21 MENINGITIS

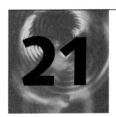

Xavier Sáez-Llorens and George H. McCracken, Jr.

Bacterial meningitis is a potentially fatal acute infectious disease caused by a variety of microorganisms. Current case fatality rates associated with this entity can be as low as 2% in infants and children and as high as 30% in neonates. Deafness or other long-term neurologic sequelae are present in up to one third of survivors. Antimicrobial agents have had a profound effect on the clinical course and prognosis of meningitis. Sophisticated medical intensive care technology and the availability of newer, extraordinarily active β-lactam antibiotics, however, have resulted in only a slight improvement in outcome from this disease.

In the last decade there has been an increasing recognition that further improvements in the treatment of bacterial meningitis can result only from a better understanding of the pathophysiologic events that occur after activation of the host's inflammatory pathways by either the bacteria or their products (Leib and Tauber, 1999; Sáez-Llorens et al., 1990; Sande et al., 1989) and of the molecular mechanisms involved in the genesis of brain damage (Braun and Tuomanen, 1999; Pfister et al., 1994).

With the advent of effective conjugated vaccines against *Haemophilus influenzae* type b organisms, the incidence of bacterial meningitis caused by these organisms has declined more than 98%. Enthusiasm has been neutralized, however, by the worldwide spread of pneumococcal strains exhibiting resistance to multiple, commonly used, antimicrobial agents and the continued widespread epidemics of meningococcal disease in many areas of the developing world. The recent introduction of conjugated vaccines against seven of the most prevalent *Streptococcus pneumoniae* strains causing invasive disease in children will reduce the burden of pneumococcal meningitis worldwide.

Postlicensure data on these conjugated vaccines indicate a greater than 85% reduction in invasive pneumococcal disease in the population of Kaiser Permanente in Northern California. Current research is focusing at developing more immunogenic meningococcal vaccines against the various bacterial groups involved in endemic and epidemic disease.

ETIOLOGY

A wide range of pathogenic and nonpathogenic bacteria have been incriminated as causative agents of purulent meningitis. The most commonly implicated organisms are listed for the various pediatric age-groups.

Newborn infants
- Group B streptococci (*Streptococcus agalactiae*)
- *Escherichia coli* K1 and other gram-negative enteric bacilli
- *Listeria monocytogenes*
- Enterococci

Infants and children
- *S. pneumoniae*
- *Neisseria meningitidis*
- *H. influenzae* type b (rare in areas with routine *Haemophilus* vaccination)

Children older than 5 years
- *S. pneumoniae*
- *N. meningitidis*

In immunocompromised hosts and in patients undergoing neurosurgical procedures, meningitis can be caused by a variety of different bacteria, such as *Staphylococcus* species, gram-negative enteric bacilli, or *Pseudomonas aeruginosa*.

In the neonatal period, group B streptococci are the most common organisms causing bacterial meningitis in many developed countries. Most cases of meningitis are caused by subtype III strains, and the disease usually occurs after the first week of life. Coliform bacilli are the second most common meningeal pathogens, particularly strains of *E. coli* possessing K1 antigen. In many developing countries *E. coli* and other gram-negative enteric bacilli, such as species of *Klebsiella*, *Enterobacter*, and *Salmonella*, are the leading cause of meningitis in newborns. *L. monocytogenes* can be recovered in 1% to 10% of all cases of bacterial meningitis in this age-group. As with group B streptococcal infections, meningeal infection caused by *L. monocytogenes* usually occurs after the first week of life. *Listeria* serotype IVb has been implicated in most cases.

In infants and children, *N. meningitidis*, *S. pneumoniae*, and *H. influenzae* type b (unvaccinated cases) are responsible for the vast majority of bacterial meningitis cases. Young infants 1 to 3 months of age, however, are in a special category because pathogens found both in neonates and in older infants and children can cause meningitis.

Encapsulated strains of *H. influenzae* are classified by capsular polysaccharide types a through f; however, more than 95% of invasive diseases are caused by type b strains. With the routine use of conjugated vaccines against the type b strain in many countries, disease caused by this organism has almost disappeared. The capsule of the type b strain (polyribosyl ribitol phosphate [PRP]) is believed to play an important role in the ability of these pathogens to evade immunologic recognition by the host, whereas the lipopolysaccharide or endotoxin component of the bacterial outer cell membrane constitutes the main virulence factor (Syrogiannopoulos et al., 1988).

Although more than 90 serotypes of pneumococci have been identified on the basis of their capsular polysaccharides, only relatively few have commonly been associated with invasive disease and with meningitis. Almost all penicillin-resistant pneumococcal strains causing meningitis belong to serotypes 6, 14, 19, and 23. The capsule of these organisms aids the bacteria to resist phagocytosis, whereas the teichoic acid polymers of the pneumococcal cell wall are important in determining virulence and eliciting the host's inflammatory responses (Tuomanen et al., 1985).

Meningococci have been divided into serogroups on the basis of antigenic differences in their capsular polysaccharides (A, B, C, D, X, Y, Z, W-135, and 29-E). Groups B, C, Y, and W-135 are the predominant serogroups associated with severe clinical disease in the United States and in other developed countries, whereas the group A strain accounts for epidemic disease in many other countries, especially sub-Saharan Africa. Group B strains are the most common isolates in Latin America (Riedo et al., 1995). Meningococcal serotypes are defined on the basis of antigenic differences in the class 2 and 3 outer membrane proteins (OMPs), whereas differences in the class 1 OMPs determine subtypes. There are currently more than 20 serotypes and at least 10 class 1 subtypes. As with the pathogenesis of *H. influenzae* disease, the presence of the meningococcal capsule is important in avoiding the host's clearance mechanisms, whereas its endotoxin contributes to virulence.

PATHOGENESIS

Meningitis most commonly follows invasion of the bloodstream by organisms that have colonized mucosal areas. In the neonatal period pathogens are acquired primarily, although not exclusively, during birth by contact and aspiration of intestinal and genital tract secretions at the time of delivery. Neonates with longer nursery stays can also be exposed to multiple nosocomial pathogens. Colonization of babies with potential meningeal organisms can result in bacteremia and subsequent cerebrospinal fluid (CSF) invasion in a small percentage of cases, especially in very low–birth-weight infants.

In infants and children meningitis usually develops after hematogenous dissemination with encapsulated bacteria that have colonized the nasopharynx. It is believed that mild upper respiratory viral infections commonly precede bloodstream bacterial invasion (Feldman, 1966). Consequently, organisms penetrate vulnerable sites of the blood-brain barrier (e.g., choroid plexus and cerebral capillaries) and reach the subarachnoid space.

In some cases meningitis may also develop by direct extension from a paranasal sinus or from the middle ear to the mastoid and finally to the meninges. Severe head trauma with a skull fracture and/or CSF rhinorrhea may lead to meningitis, usually caused by *S. pneumoniae*. Direct inoculation of bacteria into the CSF may occur, with congenital dural defects (dermal sinus or meningomyelocele), neurosurgical procedures (CSF derivation shunts), penetrating wounds, or extension from a suppurative parameningeal focus.

Infants with underlying illnesses such as malignancy, sickle cell disease, agammaglobulinemia, complement deficiency, and acquired immunodeficiency syndrome (AIDS) are predisposed to develop meningitis by both common and uncommon bacterial pathogens.

PATHOPHYSIOLOGY

The intense inflammation within the subarachnoid space as reflected in lumbar CSF and the resulting neurologic damage are not the direct result of the pathogenic bacteria but instead of activation of the host's inflammatory pathways by either the microorganisms or their products (Sáez-Llorens et al., 1990).

Once the meningeal pathogens have entered the central nervous system (CNS), they replicate rapidly and liberate active cell wall or membrane-associated components (i.e., lipoteichoic acid and peptidoglycan fragments of gram-positive organisms and endotoxin of gram-negative bacteria). Effective antimicrobial treatment causes rapid lysis of bacteria, which results in an initial enhanced release of these active bacterial products into CSF. These potent inflammatory substances are capable of stimulating macrophage-equivalent brain cells (e.g., astrocytes, microglia) and/or cerebral capillary endothelia to produce cytokines such as tumor necrosis factor (TNF), interleukin-1 (IL-1), and other inflammatory mediators such as IL-6, IL-8, platelet-activating factor, nitric oxide, arachidonic acid metabolites (e.g., prostaglandin and prostacycline), and macrophage-derived proteins. The presence of these mediators in the CSF of infants and children with bacterial meningitis has been documented by many investigators. The cytokines activate adhesion-promoting receptors on cerebral vascular endothelial cells and leukocytes, resulting in attraction of neutrophils to these sites. Subsequently, leukocytes penetrate the intercellular junctions of the capillary endothelium and release proteolytic products and toxic oxygen radicals. These events result in injury to the vascular endothelium and alteration of blood-brain barrier permeability. Depending on the potency and duration of the inflammatory stimuli, the alterations in permeability result in penetration of low-molecular-weight serum proteins into CSF and in vasogenic edema. Additionally, large numbers of leukocytes enter the subarachnoid space and release toxic substances that contribute to the production of cytotoxic edema. As a result of the high protein and cell content, the increased CSF viscosity contributes to generation of interstitial edema. All these inflammatory events, if not modulated promptly and effectively, eventually cause alteration of CSF dynamics (brain edema, intracranial hypertension), of brain metabolism, and of cerebrovascular autoregulation (decreased cerebral blood flow). Current research focuses on delineating the mechanisms involved in neuronal injury, possibly through the participation of potential mediators such as reactive oxygen and nitrogen substances, excitatory amino acids, metalloproteinases, and cellular apoptosis mediated by caspases. Induction of all these molecular pathways can eventually result in irreversible focal or diffuse brain damage (Braun and Tuomanen, 1999; Pfister et al., 1994).

PATHOLOGY

The gross appearance of the brain in a patient with meningitis is striking. The entire surface and base can be covered by a layer of thick purulent fibrinous exudate. As a result of generalized vasculitis, thrombosis of vessels and/or sinuses and necrosis of vessel walls can occur, causing compromise of perfusion and cerebral edema.

Histologically, the lesion begins with hyperemia and hemorrhages, followed by a purulent inflammatory reaction in the arachnoid and pia mater. The inflammatory exudate consists of masses of polymorphonuclear leukocytes, fibrin, bacterial clumps, and red blood cells.

As the infection extends to the ventricles, thick pus or adhesions may occlude the various foramina or aqueducts and cause obstructive hydrocephalus. Communicating hydrocephalus results because CSF reabsorption by the arachnoid villi can be impaired because of occlusion of the sagittal or lateral sinuses, high concentrations of CSF protein, or obstruction within the basilar cisterns. The exudate can involve the intracranial portion of the optic nerve, with subsequent neuritis and possible blindness. Involvement of the cochlear aqueduct and/or the internal auditory canal with development of acute suppurative labyrinthitis is considered responsible for the early deafness that commonly occurs in bacterial meningitis.

EPIDEMIOLOGIC FACTORS

The incidence of neonatal meningitis varies greatly among different institutions and geographic areas, with approximate rates of 2 to 10 cases per 10,000 live births (Klein et al., 1986). More than two thirds of all cases of neonatal meningitis in developed countries currently are caused by group B streptococci, viridans streptococci, and gram-negative enteric bacilli. *L. monocytogenes* is encountered occasionally and usually is associated with maternal infection that was acquired from contaminated milk products. In developing countries gram-negative enteric bacilli are the predominant organisms causing bacterial meningitis in newborns; nonetheless, group B streptococci and *L. monocytogenes* have been increasingly isolated in recent years (Moreno et al., 1994). Vertical transmission is the principal mode of acquisition, but nosocomial transmission is also important, especially in low–birth-weight preterm infants who require long-term intensive care management. Viridans streptococci, enterococci, staphylococci, and nontypable *H. influenzae* strains can also be implicated. Although virtually all newborn infants are colonized by many of the organisms with which they have contact, sepsis occurs in less than 1% of them. Approximately one fourth of infants with septicemia develop meningitis.

H. influenzae type b meningitis is primarily a disease of infancy. The highest incidence occurs in the first year of life, with most of the cases occurring in children 3 months to 3 years of age. It occurs uncommonly in infants less than 3 months and in children greater than 5 years of age. During the first few months most infants are protected by passively acquired maternal antibodies. Children naturally develop immunity to *H. influenzae* after the third year of life, and concentrations of PRP antibodies reach adult levels by 7 years of age (Dajani et al., 1979). Routine immunization of infants and children with the conjugated *Haemophilus* vaccines against this organism has resulted in the virtual disappearance of *Haemophilus* meningitis in developed countries (Adams et al., 1993; Peltola et al., 1992). For example, in Dallas County, Texas, the annual incidence of *Haemophilus* disease in children younger than 5 years was reduced from 158 cases per 100,000 person-years in 1983 to 9 cases per 100,000 in 1991 (Murphy et al., 1993). There was only one case of *Haemophilus* meningitis at Children's Medical Center of Dallas between 1998 and 2003.

Meningococcal and pneumococcal meningitis have their highest incidence in the first year of life and rarely occur in infants younger than 3 months of age. Unlike *H. influenzae* infections, these two microorganisms can cause systemic infection at any age in both children and adults.

Although poor living conditions increase the risk of developing meningitis, other factors such as crowding in day-care facilities contribute to the incidence of disease. The increased incidence in certain ethnic groups (American Indians, Eskimos, and blacks) and in families, however, and the observation that siblings of patients with meningitis can have deficient antibody synthesis against *H. influenzae*, have suggested that there is also a genetic predisposition to infection.

All types of meningitis occur sporadically; only meningococcal infections occur in epidemic form. Meningococci are transmitted from person to person by nasopharyngeal secretions from a patient or carrier, and transmission usually requires close contact. Major epidemics have occurred in South America, Finland, Mongolia, and sub-Saharan Africa. Outbreaks among military recruits have been observed in training camps and bases during periods of national mobilization and, recently, in U.S. college freshmen living in dormitories.

The risk of acquiring a secondary case of meningococcal or *Haemophilus* disease after household exposure to primary infection is greatly increased compared with that in the normal population. The risk for acquiring *Haemophilus* disease is greatest for unvaccinated infants and children less than 4 years of age, whereas for meningococcal disease the incidence of secondary cases is increased for family members regardless of age. Pneumococcal disease can also occur in families.

CLINICAL MANIFESTATIONS

Clinical findings of acute bacterial meningitis depend principally on the patient's age. Classic manifestations observed in older children and adults are rarely present in infants. In general, the younger the patient, the more subtle and atypical are the symptoms.

Classic Meningitis of Children and Adults

Classic meningitis usually begins with fever, chills, vomiting, photophobia, and severe headache. Occasionally, the first sign of illness is a convulsion that can recur during evolution of the disease. Irritability, delirium, drowsiness, lethargy, and coma can also develop.

As the CSF inflammatory response intensifies in bacterial meningitis, the most consistent physical finding is the presence of nuchal rigidity associated with Brudzinski's and Kernig's signs. Brudzinski's sign is elicited by rapid flexion of the neck of the supine patient, followed involuntarily by brisk flexion of the knees in the presence of meningeal irritation. Kernig's sign is present if there is marked resistance to extension of the leg when the patient is in the supine position with the thigh flexed at the hip and the leg flexed at the knee. As the disease progresses, the neck stiffness increases, causing the head to draw backward. Because of the spasm of the back muscles, the patient assumes a position of opisthotonos.

The signs and symptoms just described are common to all types of meningitis. There are other manifestations, however, peculiar to specific infections. Petechial and purpuric eruptions are usually indicative of meningococcemia, although they may be present with *H. influenzae* meningitis. Rashes very rarely occur with pneumococcal infections. The rapid development of multiple hemorrhagic eruptions in association with a shocklike state is almost pathognomonic of meningococcemia (Waterhouse-Friderichsen syndrome). Joint involvement suggests meningococcal or *H. influenzae* infection and can occur early (suppurative arthritis) or late (reactive arthritis) in the illness.

The presence of a chronically draining ear or a history of head trauma with or without skull fracture is most likely associated with pneumococcal meningitis.

Meningitis in Infancy

Infants 3 months to 1 year of age seldom develop the classic picture of meningitis. Fever, vomiting, marked irritability, convulsions, somnolence, and abnormal cry usually characterize the illness. A significant physical finding is a tense, bulging fontanelle, which usually occurs late during the course of illness. Nuchal rigidity may be absent, and Brudzinski's and Kernig's signs are difficult to elicit in this age-group.

Because the highest incidence of meningitis occurs between 6 and 12 months of age, any unexplained, persistent febrile illness in an infant should prompt suspicion of CNS involvement.

Neonatal Meningitis

Meningitis in newborn and premature infants is extremely difficult to recognize. Clinical manifestations are vague and nonspecific. In general, if the diagnosis of sepsis is entertained, the presence of meningitis should be ruled out. Fever is frequently absent. Refusal of feedings, vomiting, excessive irritability or drowsiness, irregular respirations, and jaundice are commonly associated with sepsis and meningitis. At later stages, the fontanelle may be full, tense, or bulging in approximately one third of cases.

DIAGNOSIS

Diagnosis of acute bacterial meningitis cannot be made on the basis of symptoms and signs alone. Classic meningeal findings are frequently minimal or absent or can result from meningismus or from tuberculous or aseptic meningitis. Definitive diagnosis is dependent on CSF examination and culture.

Indications for Lumbar Puncture

A properly performed lumbar puncture is a relatively innocuous procedure. Nevertheless, because of its invasiveness, it should not be done indiscriminately. Whenever the physician suspects meningitis, a lumbar puncture should be performed. Early diagnosis followed by appropriate medical management can have a favorable effect on the outcome; consequently, it is preferable to perform a lumbar puncture that yields normal CSF than to miss an early diagnosis of bacterial meningitis. In neonates, the procedure should be considered when sepsis is suspected, because meningitis accompanies sepsis in 20% to 25% of cases. It may be necessary to postpone the lumbar puncture for hours or several days in some infants with significant cardiopulmonary instability that could be a result of elevated intracranial pressure.

In many instances, particularly in infants, fever and convulsions may be the only initial signs of meningitis. It is hazardous to attribute seizures to uncomplicated febrile convulsions. In children older than 1 year of age clinical acumen may enable the skilled physician to differentiate those children with uncomplicated febrile seizures from those who have meningitis. Nevertheless, it is prudent to perform a lumbar puncture in any infant or child with a febrile convulsion when meningitis cannot be excluded from the diagnosis.

When focal neurologic signs, especially pupillary signs or cardiovascular instability, are present, whether accompanied by papilledema or not, the use of cranial computed tomography (CT) or magnetic resonance imaging (MRI) should be considered before the lumbar puncture to exclude a brain abscess or generalized cerebral edema and to avoid the danger of herniation. If such a procedure will significantly delay treatment, however, antibiotic therapy should be started before the lumbar puncture. The subsequent lumbar puncture, when clinically indicated, is conducted under manometric guidance, using a small-gauge needle, with slow removal of the smallest volume of CSF necessary for the diagnostic tests.

CSF Findings

Examination of the CSF of a patient with acute bacterial meningitis characteristically reveals the following: (1) a cloudy appearance, (2) an increased white blood cell count with a polymorphonuclear leukocyte predominance, (3) a low glucose concentration in relation to the serum glucose concentration, (4) an elevated protein concentration, (5) a smear and culture positive for the causative microorganism, and (6) a high manometric pressure. The CSF findings in patients with bacterial meningitis are shown in Table 21-1.

Cell count. Normal white blood cell count values depend on the patient's age. During the neonatal period CSF from uninfected infants contains less than 11 leukocytes/mm³, with an average ±1 standard deviation of 7.3 ± 14.0 cells/mm³ (Ahmed et al., 1996). As many as two thirds of those cells can be polymorphonuclear leukocytes. In very low–birth-weight infants the normal range of values is greater (Rodriguez

et al., 1990). By 1 month of age, counts in the range of 0 to 6 cells/mm³ are noted, and there is rarely more than 1 polymorphonuclear cell/mm³.

In patients with acute bacterial meningitis the cell count can be extremely variable, but it is usually in the range of 1,000 to 5,000 leukocytes/mm³. In rare instances, particularly very early in the illness, the cell count may be normal despite a positive CSF culture. In these cases, a lumbar puncture repeated several hours later usually shows characteristic leukocyte values. Although predominance of polymorphonuclear leukocytes is the rule, some patients with bacterial meningitis show a monocytic pattern, particularly patients with *L. monocytogenes* meningitis.

Glucose. In most patients with bacterial meningitis the CSF glucose concentration is low as a result of increased utilization from metabolic demands. A CSF glucose concentration that is less than half the simultaneously obtained blood glucose concentration usually is considered abnormal. A CSF glucose concentration of less than 20 mg/dl is associated with a higher incidence of hearing impairment. The rapid return of the glucose concentration to near normal is generally a good early index of a favorable response to therapy.

Protein. Protein concentrations usually are elevated in patients with bacterial meningitis. Values less than 40 mg/dl are considered normal in infants and children, and those greater than 100 mg/dl suggest bacterial disease is present. Protein concentrations of more than 100 to 120 mg/dl commonly are observed in healthy, uninfected newborn infants, especially premature babies.

Smears. The probability of visualizing bacteria on a gram-stained CSF preparation is

---

TABLE 21-1 **Normal and Characteristic Abnormal CSF Findings in Pediatric Age-Groups With or Without Bacterial Meningitis***

| Finding | NEONATES[†] | | INFANTS AND CHILDREN | |
	Normal	Abnormal	Normal	Abnormal
Leukocyte count (cells/µl)	<30	>100	<10	>1000
Polymorphonuclear (%)	<60	>80	≤10	>60-80
Protein (mg/dl)	<170	>200	<40	>100
CSF/blood glucose ratio	>0.6	<0.5	>0.5	<0.4
Manometric pressure (mm H₂O)	<60	>100	<90	>150

*Patients with aseptic meningitis can have CSF findings that are indeterminate or fit in the abnormal category.
†Normal values may be different in very low–birth-weight infants (Rodriguez et al., 1990).

dependent on the number of organisms present. In general, a properly prepared smear examined by an experienced person is positive in as many as 80% of cases. The sensitivity is low, however, when *L. monocytogenes* is the cause of meningitis because usually a small number of organisms ($\leq 10^3$ colony-forming units/ml) is present in CSF. Because of the possibility of misidentification, antibiotic therapy should not be tailored for a specific organism on the basis of the stained smear; instead, the results of the culture are the best guide for selecting specific therapy.

CSF cultures. Culture should be performed routinely on all spinal fluid specimens, even those that are clear on gross inspection and show no increase in the leukocyte count. The yield of positive CSF cultures falls from 70% to 85% to below 50% in patients previously treated with antibiotics (particularly in meningococcal infection), although often there is insignificant change in the CSF inflammatory indices.

CSF pressure. The mean opening lumbar CSF pressure is generally elevated in patients with bacterial meningitis. Normal values usually do not exceed 50 to 60 mm H_2O in newborns and 80 to 90 mm H_2O in infants and children (Minns et al., 1989). At the time of diagnosis opening pressures greater than 150 to 200 mm H_2O are commonly found in infants and children with bacterial meningitis.

Rapid Diagnostic Tests

Antigen detection by latex particle agglutination was once a routine part of the diagnosis of bacterial meningitis. Identification of the capsular polysaccharides of meningococci, pneumococci, group B streptococci, and *H. influenzae* type b in CSF is possible in many cases. These tests are not meant to replace the CSF culture but are a useful adjunct to the CSF examination and immediate diagnosis, especially in previously treated patients. False-negative and rare false-positive test results can occur. A positive antigen test result is usually meaningful, but a negative test result is unreliable for excluding a diagnosis of bacterial meningitis. The sensitivity of the rapid antigen tests for meningeal pathogens is highest for *H. influenzae* type b. Many authorities have questioned the value of these rapid tests in an era of a virtual disappearance of *H. influenzae* invasive infections.

In patients who have received effective antimicrobial therapy before the first lumbar puncture the CSF findings likely will be modified but still indicative of bacterial meningitis. On the second day of treatment the leukocyte count can be higher than at the time of diagnosis. Thereafter it decreases, and there can be a predominance of lymphocytes by the fifth day or later. Gram-stained smear and culture may be negative in pretreated patients, but antigen detection tests can still be useful. The CSF glucose and protein concentrations generally will remain abnormal for several days despite effective treatment.

DIFFERENTIAL DIAGNOSIS

Acute bacterial meningitis can simulate other inflammatory diseases that involve the meninges either directly or indirectly. Typical cases do not usually pose a diagnostic dilemma. In some instances, however, the spinal fluid findings in patients with bacterial disease do not conform to the typical picture, and confusion can occur in distinguishing viral or mycobacterial meningitis from meningitis caused by the usual bacterial agents.

Aseptic Meningitis

In children with aseptic or proved viral meningitis the spinal fluid characteristically shows an increase in lymphocytes and a normal or only slightly decreased glucose concentration, with a slightly elevated protein concentration. Early in the disease the CSF can reveal a large number of polymorphonuclear cells, but a repeat lumbar tap 24 to 48 hours later can demonstrate the typical lymphocyte predominance in CSF in many patients. Amplification of genetic material using polymerase chain reaction provides a specific diagnosis within hours, especially for enteroviruses and herpesvirus. This rapid procedure provides invaluable information to aid in treatment decisions.

Tuberculous Meningitis

Tuberculous meningitis can be clinically indistinguishable from acute bacterial meningitis. The diagnosis is established by (1) an increase in number of CSF leukocytes, usually from 50 to 500 cells/mm^3, with a predominance of lymphocytes, a low glucose, very elevated protein concentrations, and a culture negative for the usual pathogenic organisms but subsequently positive for tubercle bacilli; (2) a positive tuberculin skin test; (3) chest roentgenograms showing evidence of a tuberculous lesion; and (4) a positive history of contact with an active case of tuberculosis.

Brain Abscess

Brain abscess can result from head trauma, chronic otitis media and sinusitis, or septic embolization in children with cyanotic congenital heart disease. The symptoms are usually not as acute as those of meningitis, and focal neurologic signs can be present. If a lumbar puncture is performed because this diagnosis is not considered, the results of the spinal fluid examination are highly variable and can either be normal or show an increase in leukocytes, a normal glucose value, and a slightly elevated protein concentration. The culture of the CSF specimen is usually sterile. Cranial computed tomography or magnetic resonance imaging with contrast confirm the diagnosis and are useful in documenting success of therapy. Rupture of the abscess into the subarachnoid space or ventricles will result in purulent meningitis with a positive CSF culture. Abscess is frequently associated with *Citrobacter diversus* meningitis of the neonate.

Brain Tumor

The findings in patients with a brain tumor are similar to those occurring with brain abscess except that the course is more insidious, fever is usually absent, and the patient is usually not acutely ill.

Meningismus

Meningismus is characterized by symptoms and signs of meningeal irritation and normal results from spinal fluid examination and culture. It is usually associated with pneumonia, acute otitis media, acute tonsillopharyngitis, or other infectious disease.

Lead Encephalopathy

Lead encephalopathy in infants and children can simulate meningitis. The spinal fluid has a normal glucose concentration, an increased protein concentration, and normal or slightly elevated lymphocyte count. Helpful diagnostic aids include (1) a blood smear showing basophilic stippling, (2) roentgenographic evidence of a line of increased density at the metaphyseal ends of the long bones in growing children, (3) coproporphyrinuria, and (4) an increased blood lead value.

COMPLICATIONS

Complications of acute bacterial meningitis can develop early in the course of illness, either before diagnosis or several days after starting treatment.

Systemic Circulatory Manifestations

Systemic circulatory manifestations usually occur during the first hospital day of acute bacterial meningitis. Peripheral circulatory collapse is one of the most dramatic and most serious complications of meningitis. It most frequently is associated with meningococcemia but can accompany other types of infection. Profound shock usually develops early in the course of the illness and, if untreated, progresses rapidly to a fatal outcome. Disseminated intravascular coagulation can be an associated finding. Gangrene of the distal extremities can occur in patients with fulminant hemorrhagic meningococcal meningitis. It has been recognized that in some patients antibiotic therapy can initially aggravate these systemic phenomena, probably as a result of release of cell wall or membrane active components such as endotoxin from rapidly lysed microorganisms.

It has been commonly believed that many patients with bacterial meningitis have inappropriate antidiuretic hormone (SIADH) secretion requiring fluid restriction in the initial management of patients with neuroinfection. Experimental and clinical investigations conducted in the last decade have suggested, however, that the elevated antidiuretic hormone serum concentration is an appropriate host response to unrecognized hypovolemia and that a more liberal use of parenteral fluids can be beneficial (Moller et al., 2001; Powell et al., 1990; Singhi et al., 1995; Tureen et al., 1992). In addition, systemic blood pressure must be maintained at levels sufficient to prevent compromise of cerebral perfusion.

Neurologic Complications

Focal neurologic findings such as hemiparesis, quadriparesis, facial palsy, and visual field defects occur early or late in approximately 10% to 15% of patients with meningitis and may correlate with persistent abnormal neurologic examinations on long-term follow-up assessments. Presence of focal signs can be associated with cortical necrosis, occlusive vasculitis, or thrombosis of the cortical veins. Extension of the meningeal inflammatory process can involve the second, third, sixth, seventh, and eighth cranial nerves that course through the subarachnoid space. Inflammation of the cochlear aqueduct and the auditory nerve can lead to reversible or permanent deafness in 5% to 20% of cases. Hydrocephalus of either the communicating or obstructive type is occasionally seen in patients in whom treatment has been either suboptimal or delayed, occurring more often in younger infants. Brain abscesses can rarely complicate the course of meningitis, particularly in newborn infants infected with *C. diversus* or *Proteus* species.

Seizures

Seizures occur before or in the first several days after admission to the hospital in as many as one third of patients with meningitis. Although most of these episodes are generalized, focal seizures are more likely to presage an adverse neurologic outcome. In addition, seizures that are difficult to control or that persist beyond the fourth hospital day and seizures that occur for the first time late in the patient's hospital course have a greater likelihood of being associated with neurologic sequelae.

Subdural Collections of Fluid

Subdural effusions are not generally associated with signs and symptoms, commonly resolve spontaneously, are present in more than one third of patients with meningitis, and usually are not associated with permanent neurologic abnormalities (Snedeker et al., 1990). These collections are less frequently present with meningococcal than with *H. influenzae* or pneumococcal meningitis. Subdural effusions occur principally in infants less than 2 years of age. Indications for performing needle puncture of a subdural effusion include a clinical suspicion that empyema is present (prolonged fever and irritability, stiff neck coupled with CSF leukocytosis), a rapidly enlarging head circumference in a child without hydrocephalus, focal neurologic findings, and/or evidence of increased intracranial pressure.

Arthritis

Joint involvement may be present initially or may develop during the course of bacterial meningitis. Early occurrence suggests direct invasion of the joint by the microorganism, usually *H. influenzae* type b, whereas arthritis that develops after the fourth day of therapy is believed to be an immune complex–mediated event that usually involves several joints and is most frequently seen with meningococcal infections.

Other Complications

Buccal or preseptal cellulitis, pneumonia, and pericarditis can also be present in patients with bacterial meningitis, particularly complicating invasive *H. influenzae* infections in infants.

PROGNOSIS

The prognosis in individual patients with bacterial meningitis is predicated on many factors, including (1) age of patient, (2) duration and type of illness before effective antibiotic therapy is instituted, (3) type of causative microorganism, (4) number of bacteria or the quantity of active bacterial products in CSF at the time of diagnosis, (5) intensity of the host's inflammatory response, and (6) time needed to sterilize CSF cultures.

As a rule, the younger the patient, the poorer the prognosis. The highest mortality and morbidity rates occur in the neonatal period. Infections caused by group B streptococci, gram-negative enteric bacilli, and pneumococci are associated with poorer outcome from disease than those caused by *H. influenzae* and meningococci. Delay in starting antimicrobial therapy in some patients or in sterilizing CSF cultures has been recognized to increase the rate of adverse outcome. The amount of bacteria or their products correlates with an increased host production of inflammatory mediators such as TNF, IL-1, and prostaglandins. The greater the host's inflammatory response in the subarachnoid space to the microorganism and its products, the greater the likelihood of permanent sequelae.

With prompt and adequate antimicrobial and supportive therapy, the chances for survival today are excellent, especially in infants and children, for whom case fatality rates have been reduced to less than 10%. Long-term sequelae, however, have not been dramatically reduced, despite the advent of extraordinarily active β-lactam antibiotics and highly sophisticated intensive care management. The incidence rate of residual abnormalities in postmeningitic children is approximately 15% (with a range of

10% to 30%). Infants and children who survive bacterial meningitis are more apt to have seizures, hearing deficits, learning and/or behavioral problems, and lower intelligence compared with their siblings who did not have meningitis. Several studies conducted during the last decade have demonstrated that residual neurologic and audiologic abnormalities are reduced in patients who received early dexamethasone therapy (see the following discussion).

TREATMENT

Optimal management of infants and children with bacterial meningitis requires appropriate antimicrobial therapy, fluid and electrolyte adjustments, control of cardiovascular stability and intracranial pressure, and anticonvulsant therapy. The role of corticosteroids has been extensively studied in animal models of meningitis and in patients with bacterial meningitis, and evidence strongly suggests that dexamethasone given before parenteral antimicrobial therapy is beneficial in rapid modulation of the meningeal inflammatory response and in improving long-term outcome in infants and children (Kanra et al., 1995; McIntyre et al., 1997; Odio et al., 1991; Schaad et al., 1993), particularly in those with meningitis caused by *H. influenzae* and penicillin-susceptible pneumococcal strains.

Antimicrobial Therapy

Optimal antibiotic therapy entails the selection of appropriate agents that are effective against the likely pathogens and are able to attain adequate bactericidal activity in CSF. The initial empiric regimen chosen for treatment should be broad enough to cover the potential organisms for the age-group involved (see Table 21-4). Recommended dosages are listed in Tables 21-2 and 21-5.

Newborn infants. In the neonatal period the organisms most often responsible for meningitis are group B *Streptococcus* (GBS), *E. coli* and other gram-negative enteric bacilli, *L. monocytogenes*, and enterococci. The initial empiric regimen used conventionally has been ampicillin and an aminoglycoside. Because of the emergence of aminoglycoside-resistant gram-negative enteric bacilli in some neonatal units, the concern about possible adverse auditory and renal effects, and the relatively low bactericidal activity of aminoglycosides in the CSF, many centers in the United States and other developed and developing countries are now using ampicillin and cefotaxime for initial, empiric treatment of neonatal meningitis. Although cefotaxime is effective for treatment of bacterial meningitis, there is concern that the routine use of a

---

TABLE 21-2   Daily Dosages of Recommended Antimicrobial Agents for Treatment of Bacterial Meningitis in Pediatric Age-Groups[*]

Drugs	NEONATES[†]		Infants and children
	0-7 Days	8-28 Days	
Amikacin[‡]	15-20 div q12	20-30 div q8	20-30 div q8
Ampicillin	100-150 div q12	150-200 div q8 or 6	200-300 div q6
Cefepime	—	—	150 div q8
Cefotaxime[§]	100 div q12	150-200 div q8 or 6	200-225 div q8
Ceftazidime	60 div q12	90 div q8	150 div q8
Ceftriaxone	—	—	100 once daily
Chloramphenicol[‡]	25 once daily	50 div q12	75-100 div q6
Gentamicin[‡]	5 div q12	7.5 div q8	7.5 div q8
Meropenem	—	—	120 div q8
Nafcillin/oxacillin	100-150 div q12	150-200 div q8 or 6	200 div q6
Penicillin G	150,000 div q12	200,000 div q8 or 6	250,000 div q6 or 4
Tobramycin[‡]	5 div q12	6 div q8	6 div q8
Vancomycin[‡]	30 div q12	45 div q8	60 div q6

[*]Dosages are expressed in milligrams per kilogram of body weight per day and divided *(div)* for administration every *(q)* 12, 8, 6, or 4 hours. Penicillin is expressed in units per kilogram.
[†]Daily dosages may be different for very low–birth-weight infants (Prober et al., 1990).
[‡]Serum concentrations should be monitored and dosages adjusted accordingly.
[§]Cefotaxime has been used at dosages up to 360 mg/kg/day for resistant pneumococci.

cephalosporin in neonatal intensive care units will lead to rapid emergence of resistant organisms, especially among *Enterobacter, Proteus, Serratia,* and *Citrobacter* species. By contrast, the use of cefotaxime is advantageous from the standpoint of achieving high CSF bactericidal activity against most coliforms and of avoiding the necessity to monitor serum concentrations of the aminoglycoside to attain safe and therapeutic concentrations. Ceftriaxone, although equivalent in activity to cefotaxime, is not recommended for use in the neonatal period because of the potential displacement of bilirubin from albumin-binding sites and its profound inhibitory effect on growth of the bacterial flora of the intestinal tract. We continue to recommend ampicillin and an aminoglycoside for initial empiric treatment of suspected neonatal sepsis. When the CSF examination is indicative of meningitis, cefotaxime can be substituted for the aminoglycoside. Once the specific pathogen is identified and results of susceptibilities are known, antimicrobial therapy can be modified accordingly. In newborns with meningitis caused by susceptible gram-negative enteric organisms, cefotaxime can be used safely and effectively, either alone or combined with an aminoglycoside. For meningitis caused by group B streptococci or *L. monocytogenes,* ampicillin alone is usually satisfactory after an initial 48 to 72 hours of combined therapy with an aminoglycoside. For disease caused by a rare tolerant strain (inhibited but not killed by achievable CSF concentrations of ampicillin) of GBS or by an *Enterococcus* species, combination therapy with ampicillin and an aminoglycoside is indicated. The duration of therapy for neonatal meningitis depends on the clinical response and duration of positive CSF cultures after therapy is initiated. Usually, treatment for 10 to 14 days is satisfactory for disease caused by GBS and *L. monocytogenes,* and a minimum of 2 weeks of treatment after CSF cultures are sterile is required for gram-negative enteric meningitis. Enterococcus meningitis is usually treated for 2 to 3 weeks. Because of the unpredictable clinical course of illness and the unreliability of the clinical examination in assessing response to therapy in neonates, we believe that the CSF should be examined and cultured at completion of therapy to determine whether additional treatment is required. Additionally, we recommend a cranial CT scan or MRI be performed during treatment to be certain that intracranial complications have not occurred.

Infants 1 to 3 months old. Infants 1 to 3 months old are arbitrarily considered as a special category because of the broad array of possible causative agents implicated in meningitis. These agents include the pathogens encountered in neonates and those that usually cause disease in older infants, namely *H. influenzae* type b, *S. pneumoniae,* and *N. meningitidis.* Ampicillin and cefotaxime or ampicillin and ceftriaxone constitute a suitable initial empiric regimen, because in some patients *Listeria* or enterococci (resistant to the cephalosporin) can be the causative agent. Addition of vancomycin to the third-generation cephalosporin is advised when *S. pneumoniae* is suspected on the basis of a CSF smear in areas where penicillin and cephalosporin-resistant pneumococcal strains have been encountered.

Infants and children. Therapy with ampicillin and chloramphenicol was effective for many years. Currently, however, cefotaxime and ceftriaxone are widely recommended for treatment of meningitis in infants and children because of their extraordinary in vitro activity against the common meningeal pathogens, their excellent safety record, and their ability to promptly sterilize CSF cultures. Chloramphenicol is rarely used today in developed countries because of its unpredictable metabolism in young infants; its pharmacologic interaction when administered concomitantly with phenobarbital, phenytoin, rifampin, or acetaminophen; and the requirement for monitoring its serum concentrations to avoid toxic or subtherapeutic values.

Another reason for using third-generation cephalosporins in the management of meningitis is the fact that currently 20% to 30% or more of *S. pneumoniae* strains in many countries are resistant to penicillin. This figure is even higher in some European and Latin American countries. As many as two thirds of these strains have intermediate resistance (minimum inhibitory concentration [MIC] 0.1 to 1.0 mg/ml), and the rest are considered highly resistant (MIC >1.0 mg/ml). These strains are also resistant to chloramphenicol and to third-generation cephalosporins. Although many of the infections caused by intermedially resistant strains can be successfully treated with either cefotaxime or ceftriaxone (especially at high dosages), we recommend the addition of vancomycin to the initial empiric regimen to ensure eradication of these strains from CSF. Of concern is the recent in vitro demonstration and in vivo isolation of pneumococcal strains exhibiting vancomycin tolerance; the clinical significance of this finding is uncertain. To face potential antimicrobial failures in patients infected by multiresistant meningeal pathogens in the near future, evaluation of new fluoroquinolones (e.g., gatifloxacin, moxifloxacin) is currently under clinical assessment. Strains of *N. meningitidis* with partial resistance to penicillin have also been encountered in the United States and some other parts of the world. To date, however, no penicillin failures have been reported for these isolates.

We recommend strongly that a repeat lumbar puncture be performed at 24 to 48 hours after admission if a resistant pneumococcus has been isolated from the initial CSF culture and if the patient has not shown clear clinical improvement. Modification of the antimicrobial regimen should be made according to bacteriologic and clinical findings. Treatment for 4 to 7 days is satisfactory for most infants and children with uncomplicated meningococcal meningitis, for 7 to 10 days for *Haemophilus* disease, and for 10 days or longer for pneumococcal meningitis. Performing a lumbar puncture on completion of therapy in a child with uncomplicated meningitis is not recommended, because the information obtained is not useful in predicting which patient will develop bacteriologic relapse (Schaad et al., 1981).

Steroid Therapy

Several prospective, double-blind, placebo-controlled studies evaluating the role of steroids in infants and children with bacterial meningitis have been published. In most trials dexamethasone therapy has been associated with improvement in meningeal inflammatory indices, with reduction in CSF cytokine concentrations, and with fewer audiologic and/or neurologic sequelae when compared with placebo recipients. Dexamethasone treatment was not associated with delayed sterilization of CSF cultures or with a higher incidence of recurrent disease. A few children developed gastrointestinal bleeding while receiving the steroid. Superior outcome versus that in placebo recipients was seen when dexamethasone was given early (i.e., before the first parenteral antibiotic dose) as opposed to late (i.e., after several hours or more of antimicrobial treatment) (Table 21-3). Animal studies have confirmed the critical importance of timing to achieve optimal beneficial effects with dexamethasone therapy. Initial studies used a dexamethasone dosage of 0.15 mg/kg every 6 hours for a total of 4 days. From more recent reports it appears that similar beneficial results can be obtained by using a dosage of 0.4 mg/kg every 12 hours for 2 days (Schaad et al., 1993; Syrogiannopoulos et al., 1994).

TABLE 21-3 Long-Term Sequelae Observed in Children With Meningitis Given in 6 Randomized, Double-Blind, Placebo-Controlled Studies of Dexamethasone Therapy: Outcome in Relation to Timing of the First Steroid Dose

Author	Number of patients	Antibiotic	Steroid administration in relation to antibiotic	TOTAL SEQUELAE (%)		
				Placebo	Dexamethasone	P-value
Early Dexamethasone Therapy[*]						
Odio	101	Cefotaxime	15-20 min before	38	14	0.007
Schaad	115	Ceftriaxone	10 min before	16	5	0.066
Kanra	56	Ampicillin Sulbactam	15 min before	27	7	0.062
Late Dexamethasone Therapy[†]						
Lebel	95	Ceftriaxone	2-3 hours after	20	6	0.065
Wald	143	Ceftriaxone	≤4 hours after	14	9	0.434
King	101	Ceftriaxone	>10 hours after	14	15	1.00

[*]Sequelae in the early group: steroid—9%; placebo—26%. $P = 0.0003$; odds ratio (OR) 0.27 (95% confidence intervals (CI): 0.13-0.57).

[†]Sequelae in the late group: steroid—10%; placebo—16%. $P = 0.14$; OR 0.058 (95% CI: 0.29-1.17).

Although most of the meningitis cases in these prospective studies were caused by *H. influenzae*, data suggest that the salutary effects associated with dexamethasone therapy apply also to pneumococcal meningitis (Kanra et al., 1995; Kennedy et al., 1991; McIntyre et al., 1997). Concern, however, has been raised regarding the use of steroids in patients with infection caused by resistant pneumococcal strains because of the decreased penetration of antibiotics when dexamethasone is used (Cabellos et al., 2000; Paris et al., 1994). Clinical data, however, suggest that dexamethasone does not interfere with eradication of resistant pneumococci achieved by combined treatment with a third-generation cephalosporin and vancomycin. Based on currently available data, we believe that the advantages of dexamethasone therapy, especially when given before the first parenterally administered antibiotic dose, outweigh the possible disadvantages and that its use should be strongly recommended for therapy of bacterial meningitis in infants and children. In a recently conducted large clinical trial in adults with bacterial meningitis employing excellent methodological design and early dexamethasone administration, treatment with steroids was associated with a reduction in mortality and a more favorable outcome, especially for disease caused by *S. pneumoniae* (74% vs 48% for dexamethasone and placebo, respectively) (Degan et al, 2002). Some physicians, however, do not recommend adjunctive steroid therapy (Kaplan, 1995), especially now that *H. influenzae* meningitis has disappeared in the United States. Its usefulness in infants younger than 6 weeks has not been established.

SUPPORTIVE THERAPY

Adequate oxygenation, prevention of hypoglycemia and hyponatremia, anticonvulsant therapy, and measures designed to decrease intracranial hypertension and to prevent fluctuation in cerebral blood flow are a crucial part of the management of patients with bacterial meningitis.

Infants and children with alteration of consciousness, pupillary changes, and/or cardiovascular instability should have intracranial pressure monitored. Among measures to reduce abnormal pressures are elevation of the head of the bed to approximately 30 degrees, avoidance of vigorous suctioning and chest physiotherapy, maintenance of normal serum osmolarity, fluid

restriction in documented cases of SIADH (dehydration and hypotension should be avoided), and use of mannitol to decrease cerebral edema. An unconfirmed report (Kilpi et al., 1995) suggested that glycerol, another hyperosmolar agent given orally, significantly improved the outcome in infants and children as compared with placebo recipients. Further placebo-controlled, blinded studies are required before glycerol can be recommended as an adjunctive measure.

Optimal cerebral perfusion can be maintained by controlling fever to reduce the brain's metabolic demands, by maintaining arterial blood pressures within normal limits, and by hyperventilation to reduce arterial carbon dioxide tension (P_{CO_2}) to a range of 25 to 30 mm Hg (Ross and Scheld, 1989). The use of hyperventilation, however, has been questioned by some authorities who believe that it should not be used in children with bacterial meningitis and evidence of cerebral edema on CT scan, because intracranial pressure would be decreased at the expense of a reduction in cerebral blood flow, possibly approaching ischemic thresholds (Ashwal et al., 1994).

PREVENTION
Vaccination

Immunization is the most effective means of preventing bacterial meningitis in children. Before vaccination, 60% to 70% of all *H. influenzae* meningitis cases occurred in infants younger than 18 months old. The conjugated *Haemophilus* vaccines are considerably more immunogenic than the polysaccharide vaccine, and studies in Finland and in the United States have demonstrated immunogenicity and protection after initiation of a two- to three-dose vaccine regimen at 2 to 3 months of age (Black et al., 1991; Madore et al., 1990; Makela et al., 1990; Santosham et al., 1991). Vaccination beginning at this age was approved for routine use in the United States in late 1990; depending on the vaccine used, a three- or four-dose regimen is recommended. Routine use of these conjugated vaccines has been associated with disappearance of invasive diseases caused by *H. influenzae* type b organisms in developed areas of the world (Adams et al., 1993; Peltola et al., 1992) and in some developing countries (Diaz et al., 2001; Peltola, 2000).

A polyvalent meningococcal vaccine, containing the purified polysaccharide capsules of groups A, C, Y, and W-135 organisms, is available but is not recommended for general use in infants and young children. The vaccine is recommended for children older than 2 years of age who are at high risk of infection, such as those with asplenia and those with terminal complement deficiencies, and recently for college freshmen living in some U.S. dormitories. Several European countries have recently adopted routine vaccination against group C meningococcal disease with a new conjugated vaccine. Cuba and Norway have also manufactured OMP vaccines against the group B meningococcus. Field trials performed in several parts of the world showed a modest estimated efficacy, with the lowest protection observed in young children (Riedo et al., 1995). It is possible, but unproved, that these vaccines can provide the potential for control of epidemic disease caused by this organism. More immunogenic vaccines directed against multiple meningococcal serotypes are clearly needed to prevent these infections in infants and young children. Ongoing experimental and clinical research of meningococcal vaccine candidates is encouraging.

Recently, a new conjugate vaccine, directed against the seven most prevalent pneumococcal strains causing invasive disease in United States, has been approved for routine use in infants, starting at 2 months of age. Three doses of this vaccine, given at 2, 4, and 6 months of age, were associated with a significant reduction in invasive pneumococcal infections (Black et al., 2001). Thus an important decline of pneumococcal meningitis cases is expected to occur in the near future. The former pneumococcal polysaccharide vaccine is composed of purified capsular polysaccharide antigen from 23 pneumococcal serotypes. It is recommended for children older than 2 years of age who are at increased risk of developing pneumococcal disease, including those with asplenia, especially patients with sickle-cell hemoglobinopathies, with HIV infection and immunosuppression, with nephrotic syndrome, and with recurrent meningitis after head trauma. These children should receive one or two doses of the conjugate vaccine followed 2 or more months later with the polysaccharide vaccine. Investigators are evaluating promising protein-conjugated polysaccharide pneumococcal vaccines, which have incorporated 9 to 11 serotypes that most commonly infect young children.

Chemoprophylaxis

Intrapartum ampicillin or penicillin given to high-risk women with prenatal vaginal or rectal group B streptococcal colonization has been associated with reduced rates of neonatal colonization and of early-onset group B streptococcal sepsis (Baltimore et al., 2001a; Gotoff, 1984). Risk factors include preterm labor at less than 37 weeks gestation, premature rupture of membranes beyond 12 to 18 hours, intrapartum fever, multiple births, maternal group B streptococcal urinary tract infection, and previous delivery of a sibling with invasive GBS disease. Penicillin-allergic women may be given intravenous clindamycin. As expected, the incidence of late-onset neonatal GBS meningitis has not been affected by intrapartum prophylaxis.

In infants and children, rifampin prophylaxis for *Haemophilus* disease is recommended for all household contacts, irrespective of age, when at least one unvaccinated contact is younger than 4 years of age. The dosage is 20 mg/kg daily given for 4 days. The index case should receive rifampin at or near completion of therapy for the *H. influenzae* infection. Treatment of meningitis with a third-generation cephalosporin effectively eliminates nasopharyngeal carriage of *H. influenzae organisms*, making prophylaxis in the index case unwarranted (Goldwater, 1995). Management of day-care and extended home-care groups must be individualized. The efficacy of rifampin prophylaxis in day-care attendees is unproved, and the difficulties in delivering prophylaxis to many individuals in such centers can be considerable. Accordingly, prophylaxis is recommended only after two cases of *Haemophilus* disease have occurred among attendees within 2 months in a day-care or home-care setting, provided that many of these children have not been fully vaccinated.

Household and day-care contacts of an index case of meningococcal disease should be given rifampin prophylaxis in a dosage of 10 mg/kg given every 12 hours for four doses or in the same regimen as recommended for *Haemophilus* prophylaxis. Ceftriaxone given in a single intramuscular dose (125 mg for children younger than 12 years; 250 mg for those older than 12 years and adults) has been demonstrated to be more effective than oral rifampin in eliminating meningococcal group A nasopharyngeal carriage, thereby allowing its

TABLE 21-4 Recommended Empiric Selection of Antibiotics for Previously Healthy Children With Suspected Bacterial Meningitis According to Age and Epidemiologic Situation

Patient group	Likely pathogens	Empiric antibiotics
Neonate		
Vertical acquisition	*Streptococcus agalactiae, Escherichia coli, Klebsiella pneumoniae,* enterococci, *Listeria monocytogenes*	Ampicillin + cefotaxime
Nosocomial infection	Staphylococci[*], gram-negative enteric bacilli, *Pseudomonas aeruginosa*	Nafcillin/oxacillin or vancomycin + ceftazidime[‡]
Age 1-3 months	Same as for vertical acquisition, plus *Streptococcus pneumoniae, Neisseria meningitidis,* and *Haemophilus influenzae*	Ampicillin + cefotaxime or ceftriaxone
Age 3 months to 5 years	*S. pneumoniae, N. meningitidis,* and *H. influenzae*[†]	Cefotaxime or ceftriaxone
Age more than 5 years	*S. pneumoniae* and *N. meningitidis*	Cefotaxime or ceftriaxone
Children in areas with moderate or greater prevalence of resistant *S. pneumoniae*	Multiresistant pneumococci	Cefotaxime or ceftriaxone + Vancomycin

[*]Methicillin-susceptible or methicillin-resistant *Staphylococcus aureus* or *Staphylococcus epidermidis.*
[†]This pathogen is almost disappearing in children fully immunized with *H. influenzae* type b (Hib) vaccine.
[‡]With or without the addition of an aminoglycoside.

TABLE 21-5 Recommendations for Pathogen-Specific Antimicrobial Therapy of Children With Bacterial Meningitis

Bacteria	Antibiotic of choice	Other useful antibiotics
Neisseria meningitidis	Penicillin G or ampicillin	Cefotaxime or ceftriaxone
Haemophilus influenzae	Cefotaxime or ceftriaxone	Ampicillin, chloramphenicol[*]
Streptococcus pneumoniae		
Penicillin-susceptible (MIC <0.1 μg/ml)	Penicillin G, ampicillin	Cefotaxime or ceftriaxone
Penicillin-intermediate (MIC = 0.1-1.0 μg/ml)	Cefotaxime or ceftriaxone	Cefepime or meropenem
Penicillin-resistant (MIC >1.0 μg/ml)	Cefotaxime or ceftriaxone[†] plus vancomycin[‡]	Cefepime or meropenem
Cephalosporin-resistant (MIC >0.5 μg/ml)	Cefotaxime or ceftriaxone plus vancomycin	Meropenem? New fluoroquinolones?
Listeria monocytogenes	Ampicillin + gentamicin	Trimethoprim-sulfamethoxazole
Streptococcus agalactiae	Penicillin G ± gentamicin	Ampicillin + gentamicin
Enterococcus species	Ampicillin + aminoglycoside	Vancomycin
Enterobacteriaceae	Cefotaxime or ceftriaxone	Cefepime or meropenem
Pseudomonas aeruginosa	Ceftazidime + aminoglycoside	Cefepime or Meropenem

[*]In areas with economic constraints.
[†]Higher dosages are advised.
[‡]Vancomycin is administered until results of cefotaxime susceptibility is known.

use when oral rifampin cannot be taken (e.g., during pregnancy) or when compliance with the oral regimen is unlikely (Schwartz et al., 1988). Ciprofloxacin or azythromycin given as a single, oral dose of 500 mg to adults is also effective in eradicating meningococcal carriage.

BIBLIOGRAPHY

Adams WG, Deaver KA, Cochi SL, et al. Decline of childhood *Haemophilus influenzae* type b disease in the Hib vaccine era. JAMA 1993;269:221.

Ahmed A, Hickey SM, Ehrett S, et al. Cerebrospinal fluid values in the term neonate. Pediatr Infect Dis J 1996; 15:298.

Ahmed A, Jafri H, Lutsar I, et al. Pharmacodynamics of vancomycin for the treatment of experimental penicillin- and cephalosporin-resistant pneumococcal meningitis. Antimicrob Agents Chemother 1999;43:876

Appelbaum PC, Scragg JN, Bowen AJ, et al. *Streptococcus pneumoniae* resistant to penicillin and chloramphenicol. Lancet 1977;2:995.

Arditi M, Ables L, Yogev R. Cerebrospinal fluid endotoxin levels in children with H. influenzae meningitis before and after administration of intravenous ceftriaxone. J Infect Dis 1989;160:1005.

Arditi M, Mason EO, Bradley JS, et al. Three-year multicenter surveillance of pneumococcal meningitis in children: clinical characteristics and outcome related to penicillin susceptibility and dexamethasone use. Pediatrics 1998;102:1087

Ashwal S, Perkin RM, Thompson JR, et al. Bacterial meningitis in children: current concepts of neurologic management. Curr Probl Pediatr 1994;267:84.

Auslander MC, Meskan ME. The pattern and stability of post meningitic hearing loss in children. Laryngoscope 1988; 98:940.

Baker CJ. Prevention of neonatal group B streptococcal disease. Pediatr Infect Dis 1983;2:1.

Baker CJ, Paoletti LC, Rench MA, et al. Use of capsular polysaccharide-tetanus toxoid conjugate vaccine for type II group B Streptococcus in healthy women. J Infect Dis 2000;182:1129

Baltimore RS, Huie SM, Meek JI, et al. Early-onset neonatal sepsis in the era of group B streptococcal prevention. Pediatrics 2001a;108:1094

Baltimore RS, Jenson HB. Meningococcal vaccine: new recommendations for immunization of college freshmen. Curr Opin Pediatr 2001b;13:47

Black SB, Shinefield H, Fireman B, et al. Efficacy in infancy of oligosaccharide conjugate *Haemophilus influenzae* type b (HbOC) vaccine in a United States population of 61,080 children. Pediatr Infect Dis 1991;10:97.

Black SB, Shinefield H, Fireman B, et al. Efficacy, safety, and immunogenicity of heptavalent pneumococcal conjugate vaccine in children. Pediatr Infect Dis J 2000;19: 187.

Braun JS, Tuomanen EI. Molecular mechanisms of brain damage in bacterial meningitis. Adv Pediatr Infect Dis 1999;14:49

Burnes LE, Hodgman JE, Cass AB. Fatal circulatory collapse in premature infants receiving chloramphenicol. N Engl J Med 1959;261:1318.

Cabellos C, Martinez-Lacasa J, Tubau F, et al. J Antimicrob Chemother 2000;45:315.

Converse GM, Gwaltney JM Jr, Strassburg DA, et al. Alteration of cerebrospinal fluid findings by partial treatment of bacterial meningitis. J Pediatr 1973;83:220.

Dajani AS, Asmar Bl, Thirumoorthi MC. Systemic *Haemophilus influenzae* disease: an overview. J Pediatr 1979;94:355.

De Kleijn ED, de Groot R, Lafeber AB, et al. Prevention of meningococcal serogroup B infections in children: a protein-based vaccine induces immunologic memory. J Infect Dis 2001;184:98

Del Rio M, Chrane D, Shelton S, et al. Ceftriaxone versus ampicillin and chloramphenicol for treatment of bacterial meningitis in children. Lancet 1983;1:1241.

Diaz JM, Catalan L, Urrutia MT, et al. Trends of etiology of acute bacterial meningitis in Chilean children from 1989 to 1998. Impact of the anti-*H. influenzae* type b vaccine. Rev Med Chil 2001;129:719

Drean J, van de Beek D, and the European doxamethasone in adulthood bacterial meningitis study investigators. NEJM 2002; 347:1549-1556.

Dodge PR, Swartz MN. Bacterial meningitis. A review of selected aspects. N Engl J Med 1965;272:725.

Feldman HA. Meningococcal disease. JAMA 1966;196: 105.

Feldman WE. Concentrations of bacteria in cerebrospinal fluid of patients with bacterial meningitis. J Pediatr 1976;88:549.

Feldman WE. Relation of concentrations of bacteria and bacterial antigen in cerebrospinal fluid to prognosis in patients with bacterial meningitis. N Engl J Med 1977; 296:433.

Fishman RA. Brain edema. N Engl J Med 1975;193:706.

Fraser DW, Darby CP, Koehler RE, et al. Risk factors in bacterial meningitis. J Infect Dis 1973;127:271.

Galaid El, Cherubin CE, Marr JS, et al. Meningococcal disease in New York City, 1973 to 1978 recognition CR groups Y and W-135 as frequent pathogens. JAMA 1980;211:2167.

Gartner JC, Michaels RM. Meningitis from a pneumococcus moderately resistant to penicillin. JAMA 1979;241: 1707.

Ginsburg CM, McCracken GH Jr, Rae S, et al. *Haemophilus influenzae* type b disease: incidence in a day care center. JAMA 1977;12:604.

Girgis NL, Farid Z, Makhail IA, et al. Dexamethasone treatment for bacterial meningitis in children and adults. Pediatr Infect Dis J 1989;8:848.

Goldwater PN. Effect of cefotaxime or ceftriaxone treatment on nasopharyngeal *Haemophilus influenzae* type b colonization in children. Antimicrob Agents Chemother 1995;39:2150.

Gotoff SP. Chemoprophylaxis of early onset group B streptococcal disease. Pediatr Infect Dis J 1984;3:401.

Graham DR, Band JD. *Citrobacter diversus* brain abscess and meningitis in neonates. JAMA 1981;245:1923.

Istre GR, Tarpay M, Anderson M, et al. Invasive disease due to *Streptococcus pneumoniae* in an area with a high rate of relative penicillin resistance. J Infect Dis 1987; 156:732.

Jacobs MR, Koornhof HJ, Robins-Browne RM, et al. Emergence of multiply resistant pneumococci. N Engl J Med 1978;299:735.

Jacobs RF, His S, Wilson CB, et al. Apparent meningococcemia: clinical features of disease due to *Haemophilus influenzae* and *Neisseria meningitidis*. Pediatrics 1983; 72:469.

Kanra GY, Ozen H, Secmeer G, et al. Beneficial effects of dexamethasone in children with pneumococcal meningitis. Pediatr Infect Dis J 1995;14:490.

Kaplan SL. Adjunctive therapy in meningitis. Adv Pediatr Infect Dis 1995;10:167.

Kaplan SL. Clinical manifestations, diagnosis, and prognostic factors of bacterial meningitis. Infect Dis Clin North Am 1999;13:579.

Kaplan SL, Goddard J, Van Kleeck M, et al. Ataxia and deafness in children due to bacterial meningitis. Pediatrics 1981;68:8.

Kennedy WA, Hoyt MJ, McCracken GH Jr. The role of corticosteroid therapy in children with pneumococcal meningitis. Am J Dis Child 1991;145:1374.

Kessler SL, Dajani AS. *Listeria meningitis* in infants and children. Pediatr Infect Dis 1990;9:61.

Kilpi T, Peltola H, Jauhiainen T, et al. Oral glycerol and intravenous dexamethasone in preventing neurologic and audiologic sequelae of childhood bacterial meningitis. Pediatr Infect Dis J 1995;14:270.

King SM, Law B, Langley JM, et al. Dexamethasone therapy for bacterial meningitis: better never than late? Can J Infect Dis 1994;5:219.

Klein JO, Feigin RD, McCracken GH Jr. Report of the task force on diagnosis and management of meningitis. Pediatrics 1986;78:959.

Lebel MH, Freij BJ, Syrogiannopoulos GA, et al. Dexamethasone therapy for bacterial meningitis; results of two double-blind, placebo-controlled trials. N Engl J Med 1988;319:964.

Lebel MH, Hoyt MJ, McCracken GH Jr. Comparative efficacy of ceftriaxone and cefuroxime for treatment of bacterial meningitis. J Pediatr 1989;114:1049.

Leedom MJ, Inler D, Mathies AW, et al. The problems of sulfadiazine-resistant meningococci. Antimicrob Agents Chemother 1966;6:281.

Leib SL, Tauber MG. Pathogenesis of bacterial meningitis. Infect Dis Clin North Am 1999;13:527

Leib SL, Leppert D, Clements J, Tauber MG. Matrix metalloproteinases contribute to brain damage in experimental pneumococcal meningitis. Infect Immun 2000; 68:615

Lingappa JR, Rosenstein N, Zell ER, et al. Surveillance for meningococcal disease and strategies for use of conjugate meningococcal vaccines in the United States. Vaccine 2001;19:4566

Linnan MJ, Mascola L, Lou XD, et al. Epidemic listeriosis associated with Mexican-style cheese. N Engl J Med 1988;319:823.

Madore DV, Johnson CL, Phipps DC, et al. Safety and immunologic response to *Haemophilus influenzae* type b oligosaccharide-CRM 197 conjugate vaccine in 1- to 6-month-old infants. Pediatrics 1990;85:331.

Makela PH, Eskola J, Peltola HO, et al. Clinical experience with *Haemophilus influenzae* type b conjugate vaccines. Pediatrics 1990;85:651.

McCracken GH Jr. Neonatal septicemia and meningitis. Hosp Pract 1976;11:89.

McCracken GH Jr. New developments in the management of children with bacterial meningitis. Pediatr Infect Dis 1984;3:532.

McCracken GH Jr, Lebel MH. Dexamethasone therapy for bacterial meningitis in infants and children. Am J Dis Child 1989;143:287.

McIntyre PB, Berkey CS, King SM, et al. JAMA 1997;278:925.

Mertsola J, Ramilo O, Mustafa MM, et al. Release of endotoxin after antibiotic treatment of gram negative bacterial meningitis. Pediatr Infect Dis 1989;8:904.

Minns RA, Engleman KIM, Stirling H. Cerebrospinal fluid pressure in pyogenic meningitis. Arch Dis Child 1989;64:814.

Mitchell L, Tuomanen EI. Vancomycin-tolerant *Streptococcus pneumoniae* and its clinical significance. Pediatr Infect Dis J 2001;20:531

Moller K, Larsen FS, Bie P, Skinhoj P. The syndrome of inappropriate secretion of antidiuretic hormone and fluid restriction in meningitis—how strong is the evidence? Scand J Infect Dis 2001;33:13

Moreno MT, Vargas S, Poveda R, Sáez-Llorens X. Neonatal sepsis and meningitis in a developing Latin American country. Pediatr Infect Dis J 1994;13:516.

Murphy TV, White KS, Pastor P, et al. Declining incidence of *Haemophilus influenzae* type b disease since introduction of vaccination. JAMA 1993;269:246.

Mustafa MM, Ramilo O, Sáez-Llorens X, et al. Cerebrospinal fluid prostaglandins, interleukin-1β and tumor necrosis factor in bacterial meningitis: clinical and laboratory correlations in placebo and dexamethasone-treated patients. Am J Dis Child 1990;144:883.

Nelson JD. How preventable is bacterial meningitis? N Engl J Med 1982;307:1265.

Nelson JD. Cerebrospinal fluid shunt infections. Pediatr Infect Dis 1984;3:530.

Novak R, Henriques B, Charpentier E, et al. Emergence of vancomycin tolerance in *Streptococcus pneumoniae*. Nature 1999;399:590

Odio CM, Faingezicht I, Paris M, et al. The beneficial effects of early dexamethasone administration on infants and children with bacterial meningitis. N Engl J Med 1991;324:1525.

Paredes A, Taber LH, Yow MD, et al. Prolonged pneumococcal meningitis due to an organism with increased resistance to penicillin. Pediatrics 1976;58:378.

Paris MM, Hickey SM, Uscher MI, et al. Effect of dexamethasone on therapy of experimental penicillin- and cephalosporin-resistant pneumococcal meningitis. Antimicrob Agents Chemother 1994;38:1320.

Peltola H, Kilpi T, Anttila M. Rapid disappearance of *Haemophilus influenzae* type b meningitis after routine childhood immunization with conjugated vaccines. Lancet 1992;340:592.

Peltola H. Worldwide *H. influenzae* type b disease at the beginning of the 21st century: global analysis of the disease burden 25 years after the use of the polysaccharide vaccine and a decade after the advent of conjugates. Clin Microbiol Rev 2000;13:302

Pfister HW, Fontana A, Tauber MG, et al. Mechanisms of brain injury in bacterial meningitis: workshop summary. Clin Infect Dis 1994;19:463.

Portnoy JM, Olsen LC. Normal cerebrospinal fluid values in children: another look. Pediatrics 1985;75:484.

Powell KR, Sugarman LI, Eskenazi AE, et al. Normalization of plasma arginine vasopressin concentrations when children with meningitis are given maintenance plus replacement fluid therapy. J Pediatr 1990;117:515.

Prober CG, Stevenson DK, Benitz WE. The use of antibiotics in neonates weighing less than 1200 grams. Pediatr Infect Dis 1990;9:111.

Ramilo O, Sáez-Llorens X, Mertsola J, et al. Tumor necrosis factor α/cachectin and interleukin-1β initiate meningeal inflammation. J Exp Med 1990;172:497.

Rapkin RH. Repeat lumbar punctures in the diagnosis of meningitis. Pediatrics 1974;54:34.

Rennels MB, Edwards KM, Keyserling HL, et al. Safety and immunogenicity of four doses of Neisseria meningitides group C vaccine conjugated to CRM197 in United States infants. Pediatr Infect Dis J 2001;20:153

Riedo FX, Plikaytis BD, Broome CV. Epidemiology and prevention of meningococcal disease. Pediatr Infect Dis J 1995;14:643.

Rodriguez AF, Kaplan SL, Mason EO Jr. Cerebrospinal fluid values in the very low birth weight infant. J Pediatr 1990;116:971.

Ross KL, Scheld WM. The management of fulminant meningitis in the intensive care unit. Infect Dis Clin North Am 1989;3:137.

Sáez-Llorens X, McCoig C, Feris JM, et al. Quinolone treatment for pediatric bacterial meningitis : a comparative study of trovafloxacin and ceftriaxone with or without vancomycin. Pediatr Infect Dis J 2002;21:14

Sáez-Llorens X, McCracken GJ Jr. Antimicrobial and anti-inflammatory treatment of bacterial meningitis. Infect Dis Clin North Am 1999;13:619

Sáez-Llorens X, O'Ryan M. Cefepime in the empiric treatment of meningitis in children. Pediatr Infect Dis J 2001;20:356

Sáez-Llorens X, Ramilo O, Mustafa MM, et al. Molecular pathophysiology of bacterial meningitis: current concepts and therapeutic implications. J Pediatr 1990;116:671.

Sande MA, Tauber MG, Scheld M, et al. Pathophysiology of bacterial meningitis: summary of the workshop. Pediatr Infect Dis 1989;8:929.

Santosham M, Wolff M, Reid R, et al. The efficacy in Navajo infants of a conjugate vaccine consisting of Haemophilus influenzae type b polysaccharide and Neisseria meningitidis outer-membrane protein complex. N Engl J Med 1991;324:1767-1772.

Schaad UB, Lips U, Gnehm HE, et al. Dexamethasone therapy for bacterial meningitis in children. Lancet 1993;342:457.

Schaad UB, Nelson JD, McCracken GH Jr. Recrudescence and relapse in bacterial meningitis of childhood. Pediatrics 1981;67:188.

Scheld WM, Fletcher DD, Fink FN, et al. Response to therapy in an experimental rabbit model of meningitis due to Listeria monocytogenes. J Infect Dis 1979;140:287.

Schwartz B, Al-Ruwais A, As Ashi J, et al. Comparative efficacy of ceftriaxone and rifampicin in eradicating pharyngeal carriage of group A Neisseria meningitidis. Lancet 1988;1:1239.

Sell SH. Long term sequelae of bacterial meningitis in children. Pediatr Infect Dis 1983;2:90.

Shapiro ED. Prophylaxis for contacts of patients with meningococcal or Haemophilus influenzae type b disease. Pediatr Infect Dis 1982;1:132.

Shinefield HR, Black S, Ray P, et al. Safety and immunogenicity of heptavalent pneumococcal CRM197 conjugate vaccine in infants and toddlers. Pediatr Infect Dis J 1999;18:757

Siegel JD, Shannon KM, DePasse BM. Recurrent infection associated with penicillin-tolerant group B streptococci: a report of two cases. J Pediatr 1981;99:920.

Singhi SC, Singhi PD, Srinivas B, et al. Fluid restriction does not improve the outcome of acute meningitis. Pediatr Infect Dis J 1995;14:495.

Snedecker JD, Kaplan SL, Dodge PR, et al. Subdural effusion and its relationship with neurologic sequelae of bacterial meningitis in infancy: a prospective study. Pediatrics 1990;S6:163.

Syrogiannopoulos GA, Hansen EJ, Erwin AL, et al. Haemophilus influenzae type b lipopolysaccharide induces meningeal inflammation. J Infect Dis 1988;157:237.

Syrogiannopoulos GA, Lourida AN, Theodoridou MC, et al. Dexamethasone therapy for bacterial meningitis in children: 2 versus 4 day regimen. J Infect Dis 1994;169:853.

Tarafdar K, Rao S, Recco RA, Zaman MM. Lack of sensitivity of the latex agglutination test to detect bacterial antigen in the cerebrospinal fluid of patients with culture-negative meningitis. Clin Infect Dis 2001;33:406

Tauber MC. Brain edema, intracranial pressure, and cerebral blood flow in bacterial meningitis. Pediatr Infect Dis 1989;8:915.

Tauber MG, Sehibl AM, Hackbarth CJ, et al. Antibiotic therapy, endotoxin concentration in cerebrospinal fluid, and brain edema in experimental Escherichia coli meningitis in rabbits. J Infect Dis 1987;156:456.

Tikhomirov E. Meningococcal meningitis: global situation and control measures. World Health Stat Q 1987;40:98.

Toews WH, Bass JW. Skin manifestations of meningococcal infection. Am J Dis Child 1974;127:173.

Tuomanen E. Molecular mechanisms of inflammation in experimental pneumococcal meningitis. Pediatr Infect Dis 1987;6:1146.

Tuomanen E, Liu H, Hengstler B, et al. The induction of meningeal inflammation by components of the pneumococcal cell wall. J Infect Dis 1985;151:859.

Tureen JH, Dworkin RJ, Kennedy SL, et al. Loss of cerebrovascular autoregulation in experimental meningitis in rabbits. J Clin Invest 1990;85:577.

Tureen JM, Tauber MG, Sande MA. Effect of hydration status on cerebral blood flow and cerebrospinal fluid lactic acidosis in rabbits with experimental meningitis. J Clin Invest 1992; 89:947.

Waage A, Halstensen A, Espevik T. Association between tumor necrosis factor in serum and fatal outcome in patients with meningococcal disease. Lancet 1987;1:355.

Wald ER, Kaplan SL, Mason EO, et al. Dexamethasone therapy for children with bacterial meningitis. Pediatrics 1995;95:21.

Ward JI, Fraser DW, Baroff LJ, et al. Haemophilus influenzae meningitis a national study of secondary spread in household contacts. N Engl J Med 1979;301:122.

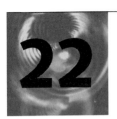

22 MUMPS

Mumps (epidemic parotitis) is an acute contagious disease caused by a paramyxovirus that has a predilection for glandular and nervous tissue. Mumps is characterized most commonly by enlargement of the salivary glands, particularly the parotid glands. One or more of the following manifestations of mumps may be associated with or may occur without parotitis: meningoencephalitis, orchitis, pancreatitis, and other glandular involvement. Inapparent infection occurs in a significant percentage of persons (30% to 40%).

ETIOLOGY

Mumps is caused by a virus belonging to the parainfluenza subgroup of the paramyxoviruses. It ranges in size from 100 to 600 nm and is composed of RNA and five proteins. A capsid and an envelope with glycoprotein projections surround the RNA. There are two envelope glycoproteins: a hemagglutinin-neuraminidase and a cell fusion protein. The envelope also contains a matrix protein. Internally there are two proteins: a nucleocapsid protein and an RNA polymerase protein. The virus is infective for monkeys and chick embryos and produces cytopathic effects in a variety of tissue cultures, such as primary monkey kidney, human embryonic kidney, and human diploid fibroblasts. Infectivity is lost as a result of heating at 55° to 60°C for 20 minutes and after exposure to formalin or to ultraviolet light. Infectivity is maintained for years at temperatures of −20° to −70°C. Mumps virus has an antigenic relationship to other members of the myxovirus group, including Newcastle disease virus and the parainfluenza viruses. Although only one antigenic type has been identified by neutralization assays, minor antigenic differences and differences in neurovirulence have been identified by molecular analyses (Swierkosz, 1999). Using polymerase chain reaction (PCR) it is possible to distinguish geographic differences between mumps viruses (Jin et al., 1999).

PATHOLOGY

The mumps-infected parotid gland is rarely available for pathologic examination. The interstitial tissue shows edema and infiltration with lymphocytes. With accumulation of necrotic debris and polymorphonuclear leukocytes in the lumina, the cells of the ducts degenerate. Inclusion bodies are not seen. Mumps orchitis is characterized by edema and a perivascular lymphocytic infiltrate that progress to involve the interstitial tissue. There are focal hemorrhage and destruction of germinal epithelium, producing plugging of the tubules by epithelial debris, fibrin, and polymorphonuclear leukocytes.

PATHOGENESIS

The current concept of the pathogenesis of mumps stems from experience gained from a variety of epidemiologic, immunologic, clinical, and experimental studies. Virus probably enters through the respiratory tract. Proliferation takes place in either the parotid gland or the superficial epithelium of the respiratory tract. This is followed by viremia, with subsequent localization of virus in glandular or nervous tissue. The parotid gland is most often involved. Mumps virus has been isolated from human saliva, blood, urine, and cerebrospinal fluid (CSF) during the acute phase of the illness. The salivary glands, brain, and spinal cord of experimentally infected monkeys also have yielded virus. The concept of mumps as a generalized infection is well documented.

391

CLINICAL MANIFESTATIONS

For a long time the terms *mumps* and *epidemic parotitis* were used interchangeably. Mumps was recognized as primarily an infection of the salivary glands. The isolation of the virus and the development of serologic specific tests, however, have contributed to a better understanding of the pathogenesis and a clarification of the clinical picture of the disease.

Infection with mumps virus usually develops after an incubation period of 16 to 18 days. In approximately 30% to 40% of the patients the resulting infection is inapparent. The remaining 60% to 70% of the patients develop an illness of variable severity, with symptoms that depend on the site or sites of infection. In the majority of instances clinical mumps is characterized only by parotitis, either unilateral or bilateral. Additional relatively common manifestations include submaxillary and sublingual gland infection, orchitis, and meningoencephalitis. Pancreatitis, oophoritis, thyroiditis, and other glandular infections are relatively rare. These various manifestations of mumps may precede, accompany, follow, or occur without parotitis.

Salivary Gland Involvement

The classic illness is ushered in by fever, headache, anorexia, and malaise. Within 24 hours the child complains of an "earache" localized near the lobe of the ear and aggravated by chewing movements of the jaw. The following day the enlarged parotid gland is noticeable and rapidly progresses to its maximum size within 1 to 3 days. The fever usually subsides after a variable period of 1 to 6 days, with the temperature returning to normal before the glandular swelling disappears.

The normal parotid gland is not palpable. It is horseshoe shaped, with the concave portion adjacent to the lobe of the ear (Figure 22-1). An imaginary line bisecting the long axis of the ear and passing through the ear lobe divides the gland into two relatively equal parts. These anatomic relationships are not altered by the enlarging parotid gland. As the swelling progresses, the lobe of the ear is displaced upward and outward. During the phase of rapid parotid enlargement, the pain and tenderness may be severe. These symptoms subside after the swelling has reached its peak. The enlarged parotid gland gradually decreases in size over a period of 3 to 7 days. Thus the swelling may be present for possibly 6 to 10 days. Usually one parotid gland enlarges first, and within a few days the other enlarges. Occasionally, both sides swell simultaneously. Approximately 25% of all patients have unilateral parotitis.

The submaxillary swelling, when present, may be seen and palpated beneath the

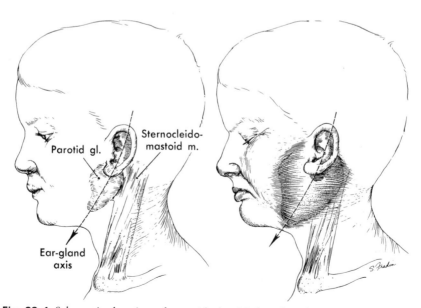

Fig. 22-1 Schematic drawing of parotid gland infected with mumps, *right*, compared with normal gland, *left*. An enlarged cervical lymph node is usually posterior to the imaginary line.

mandible just anterior to the angle of the jaw and directly beneath the anterior portion of the masseter muscle (Figure 22-2). During the early stages the edema surrounding the submaxillary gland may spread over the mandible onto the cheek and downward toward the neck. When submaxillary mumps occurs without parotitis, it is clinically indistinguishable from cervical adenitis.

Sublingual mumps is usually bilateral and begins as a swelling in the submental region and on the floor of the mouth. Of the three salivary glands, the sublinguals are the least commonly involved.

The clinical picture of mumps just described is the classic one. The disease, however, is extremely variable. Occasionally, the appearance of local glandular swelling and tenderness may be the only manifestation of infection. Fever and constitutional symptoms may be absent.

Frequently, the orifices of the ducts show inflammatory changes. The openings of Stensen's (parotid) and Wharton's (submaxillary) ducts may be reddened and edematous. Patients with extensive salivary gland involvement may develop edema in the presternal area. It has been postulated that this is caused by an obstruction of the lymphatic vessels by the enlarged salivary glands.

Epididymo-Orchitis

Epididymo-orchitis is the second most common manifestation of mumps infection in the adult male. It usually follows parotitis, but it may precede it or occur as an isolated manifestation of mumps. Epididymitis invariably is associated with the orchitis. Unilateral involvement occurs in 20% to 30% of males who develop the disease after puberty. The incidence of bilateral orchitis is low—approximately 2%. Under epidemic conditions the incidence of orchitis may be higher. In 1959 Philip et al. described an epidemic of 363 cases of mumps in a "virgin" population on St. Lawrence Island in the Bering Sea. The incidence of orchitis in males more than 10 years of age was approximately 35%; bilateral orchitis occurred in approximately 12%. Orchitis develops within the first 2 weeks of infection, most commonly during the first week. In rare instances it may be delayed to the third week. Mumps orchitis may occur in the absence of salivary gland involvement.

Orchitis begins abruptly with fever, chills, headache, nausea, vomiting, and lower abdominal pain. The systemic reaction usually parallels the extent of gonadal involvement. The temperature may vary from normal to over 40°C (104°F). The duration of fever rarely exceeds 1 week. It persists for 3 days or less in approximately 20% of cases, 4 days or less in 50%, and 5 days or less in 80%. The temperature falls by crisis in approximately half the cases and by lysis in the remainder.

With the appearance of the fever, the testis begins to swell rapidly and becomes very painful and tender. It may increase in size very

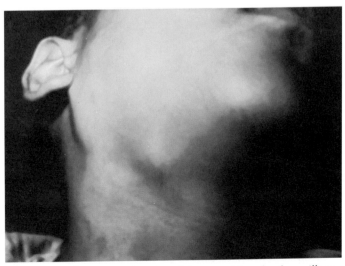

Fig. 22-2 Patient with mumps showing right parotid and submaxillary swelling. Note displacement of ear and characteristic location of both glands.

slightly or to as much as four times that of the normal gland. As the fever subsides, the pain and swelling disappear. The tenderness, however, persists for a longer period. As the testis decreases in size, a change of consistency is noted—loss of turgor. In approximately half of the cases this is subsequently followed by atrophy. However, at least half of the involved glands do return to normal. One of the most important concerns of men with mumps orchitis is the fear that sexual impotence and sterility will follow, but this sequela is rare. Most orchitis is unilateral. Even with bilateral involvement, it would be rare to have complete atrophy of both glands. The extensive experience with mumps orchitis in World Wars I and II failed to demonstrate that impotence and sterility are frequent consequences of this infection.

Meningoencephalitis

Central nervous system (CNS) involvement is another common manifestation of mumps. Symptomatic disease has been estimated to occur in approximately 10% of all cases. In a study by Bang and Bang (1944) 62% of 371 patients with mumps parotitis had cells in the CSF. Of this group 106 (28%) had CNS symptoms. Mumps meningoencephalitis usually follows the parotitis by 3 to 10 days. However, it may precede or even occur in the absence of salivary gland involvement (Figure 22-3).

The illness is characterized by fever, headache, nausea, vomiting, nuchal rigidity, change in sensorium, and, only rarely, convulsions. Brudzinski's and Kernig's signs can be elicited. The CSF shows pleocytosis, with a predominance of lymphocytes, normal glucose content, and elevated protein level. Although the glucose content is usually normal, cases with hypoglycorrhachia have been reported (Wilfert, 1969). The temperature usually falls by lysis over a period of 3 to 10 days. As the fever subsides, the symptoms clear, and recovery is usually uneventful. The infection follows the course of benign aseptic meningitis (see Chapter 38) and usually has no sequelae.

Pancreatitis

Pancreatitis is a severe but uncommon manifestation of mumps infection. There is a sudden onset of severe epigastric pain and tenderness associated with fever, chills, extreme weakness,

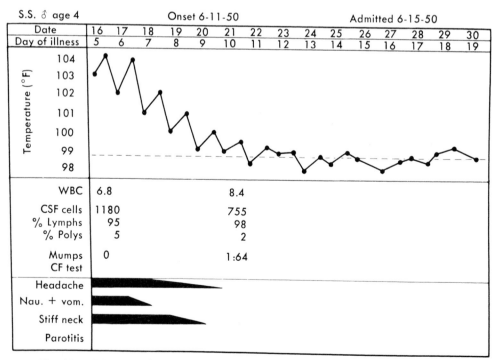

Fig. 22-3 Diagram of clinical course of mumps meningoencephalitis without salivary gland involvement. Pleocytosis with predominance of lymphocytes was found. The diagnosis was established by the development of complement-fixing antibody between the fifth and tenth days of illness.

prostration, nausea, and repeated bouts of vomiting. The symptoms gradually subside over a period of 3 to 7 days, and the patient usually recovers completely.

Other Clinical Manifestations

The development of fever, nausea, vomiting, and lower abdominal pain in the female with mumps points to oophoritis. When the right ovary is involved, the signs and symptoms may be indistinguishable from those of acute appendicitis. Many other glands may be involved in the infection. Thyroiditis, mastitis, dacryoadenitis, and bartholinitis are rare manifestations of mumps. In general, except for the symptoms caused by the local swelling, the course is essentially the same as for any other mumps infection.

DIAGNOSIS
Confirmatory Clinical Factors

The following factors should point to mumps as a diagnostic possibility: (1) a history of exposure to mumps 2 to 3 weeks before onset of illness, (2) a compatible clinical picture of parotitis or other glandular involvement, and (3) signs of aseptic meningitis.

In the classic case of so-called epidemic parotitis, confirmatory laboratory procedures are usually unnecessary. In the absence of parotitis or in the presence of recurrent parotitis, however, use of the following specific diagnostic aids may be necessary.

Isolation of Causative Agent

Mumps virus can be recovered from the saliva, mouth washings, or urine during the acute phase of parotitis and from the CSF early in the course of meningoencephalitis. Shedding of virus in the urine may persist for as long as 2 weeks after disease onset. Mumps virus is readily isolated after inoculation of appropriate clinical specimens into a variety of host systems such as rhesus monkey kidney cells and human embryonic lung fibroblasts. Rapid identification of the agent may be accomplished by use of cells grown in shell vials with fluorescein-labeled monoclonal antibodies to identify the virus. Both virus isolation and PCR are useful for diagnosis of mumps (Jin et al., 1999; Swierkosz, 1999).

Serologic Tests

A number of serologic tests are used to demonstrate the development of specific mumps antibody: complement fixation (CF), hemagglutination-inhibition (HI), enzyme-linked immunosorbent assay (ELISA), and virus neutralization. The CF and ELISA tests are the most practical and most reliable of these diagnostic procedures.

The formation of mumps CF antibody after infection is shown in Figure 22-4. The antibody becomes detectable in the blood by the end of the first week, and by the end of the second week a fourfold or greater rise in antibody titer can be demonstrated. When a diagnosis of mumps is suspected, acute and convalescent sera should be tested simultaneously. A fourfold or greater rise in the level of antibody confirms the diagnosis. This test is particularly useful for the diagnosis of mumps meningoencephalitis without parotitis, as is illustrated in Figure 22-3.

Ancillary Laboratory Findings

The serum amylase level is elevated in both mumps parotitis and pancreatitis. The levels seem to parallel the parotid swelling. The values reach a peak during the first week, gradually returning to normal by the second and third weeks. Serum amylase determinations are abnormal in approximately 70% of cases of mumps parotitis. The finding of normal serum amylase levels may aid in the identification of obscure swellings about the jaw that resemble parotid involvement. The white blood cell count may be normal or slightly elevated. Usually there is a slight predominance of lymphocytes, but at times the reverse is true.

DIFFERENTIAL DIAGNOSIS
Parotitis

Mumps parotitis may be simulated by various conditions affecting the parotid glands or neighboring lymph nodes. Anterior cervical or preauricular adenitis involvement of the lymph nodes, with surrounding edema, may simulate mumps parotitis. The parotid gland can usually be identified by its characteristic location, consistency, and outline. Its anatomic relationship to the ear is illustrated in Figure 22-1. A line bisecting the long axis and lobe of the ear passes through the center of the gland. It has a brawny consistency with a well-defined posterior border and ill-defined anterior and inferior borders. In contrast, an enlarged lymph node has a well-defined, discrete border, is firm, and does not have the characteristic anatomic relationship to the ear. The appearance of the

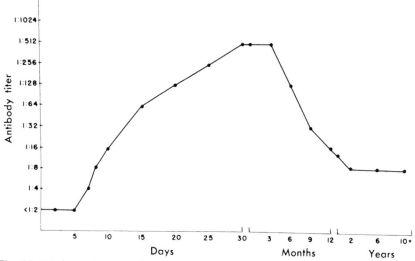

Fig. 22-4 Schematic curve illustrating development of mumps complement-fixing antibody. A significant rise in the level of antibody can be demonstrated in the serum by the end of the second week of illness. The acute and convalescent serum specimens should be tested simultaneously.

opening of Stensen's duct does not help very much. An elevated serum amylase level would point to parotid involvement. A mumps antibody test clarifies the diagnosis.

Suppurative parotitis. In suppurative parotitis the skin over the gland is usually red and hot, and the gland is exquisitely tender. Pus may be expressed from Stensen's duct by massaging the gland. An increase in the number of polymorphonuclear leukocytes is usually present. Although aerobic bacteria such as *Staphylococcus aureus* are the most common cause of acute suppurative parotitis, occasionally anaerobic bacteria (*Bacteroides, Fusobacterium,* and *Peptostreptococcus*) may be responsible (Brook and Finegold, 1978).

Recurrent parotitis. Recurrent parotitis, a condition of unknown and probably varied causes, is characterized by frequent recurrent swellings of the parotid gland. Infection and hypersensitivity to certain drugs such as iodides and phenothiazines may have a role in the causation of this disease. Roentgenographic studies of the duct system reveal evidence of sialectasia in some cases. The individual attack may be clinically indistinguishable from mumps parotitis. The submaxillary and sublingual glands, which are frequently associated with mumps parotitis, are not involved in recurrent parotitis. The history of previous attacks and a negative or unchanging CF test clarifies the diagnosis.

Calculus. A calculus that obstructs Stensen's duct causes a swelling of the parotid gland that is usually intermittent.

Coxsackie virus infection. In 1957 Howlett et al. described a syndrome of parotitis and herpangina caused by Coxsackie virus.

Parainfluenza 3 virus infection. In 1970 Zollar and Mufson reported on two children in whom acute parotitis was associated with detection of parainfluenza 3 virus and a significant rise in the level of homologous antibody.

Mixed tumors, hemangiomas, and lymphangiomas of the parotid. Mixed tumors, hemangiomas, and lymphangiomas of the parotid are responsible for chronic enlargement of the gland and are confused with mumps only during the early stages.

Sjögren's syndrome. In Sjögren's syndrome there is chronic bilateral parotid and lacrimal gland enlargement, usually associated with dryness of the mouth and absence of tears. It is a chronic condition associated with autoimmunity and development of lymphoma.

Uveoparotid fever. Uveoparotid fever is a manifestation of sarcoidosis, which may be confused with mumps.

Human immunodeficiency virus infection. Bilateral parotid swelling may accompany human immunodeficiency virus (HIV) infection in children, but this condition is chronic, lasting for months to years. Parotitis in HIV-infected children is often associated with pulmonary lymphoid interstitial hyperplasia.

Meningoencephalitis

Mumps meningoencephalitis without parotitis is clinically indistinguishable from aseptic meningitis caused by Coxsackie virus, ECHO virus, lymphocytic choriomeningitis virus, and a variety of other agents (see Chapter 43). The specific mumps antibody test or virus isolation usually establishes the diagnosis.

COMPLICATIONS
Deafness

Deafness is a very rare but serious complication of mumps. There is usually a sudden onset of vertigo, tinnitus, ataxia, and vomiting followed by permanent deafness. In most cases it is unilateral. The cause has been ascribed to neuritis of the auditory nerve.

Other Neurologic Complications

Other neurologic complications, also very rare, include facial neuritis, myelitis, and postinfectious encephalitis. The latter, like measles encephalitis, may be fatal or complicated by serious sequelae. This type of encephalitis occurs very infrequently.

Myocarditis

Myocarditis as a complication of mumps has occasionally been observed (Chaudary and Jaski, 1989; Brown and Richmond, 1980). Electrocardiographic findings indicate that the incidence may be 15%. The development of dyspnea, tachycardia, or bradycardia during the first 2 weeks of illness associated with T-wave changes and prolongation of the PR interval should suggest this diagnosis. The myocarditis is usually followed by an uneventful recovery. More rarely, pericarditis also may occur. Molecular diagnostic methods have implicated mumps virus in endocardial fibroelastosis (Ni et al., 1997). These investigators suggested that fibroelastosis might be a long-term complication of mumps myocarditis.

Arthritis

Arthritis also has been described as a rare complication of mumps. It usually appears as migrating polyarthritis involving the larger and smaller joints and clears spontaneously (Harel et al., 1990).

Diabetes Mellitus

It has been suggested that some cases of diabetes mellitus may be associated with a previous mumps virus infection. The relationship of mumps virus to diabetes mellitus has been studied epidemiologically and experimentally for many years without clear resolution of the possible role of the virus in the pathogenesis of this disease (Banatvala et al., 1985; Sultz et al., 1975).

Hepatitis

Hepatitis has been reported as a rare complication of mumps. From the available descriptions, however, it is difficult to determine whether it is truly a complication or possibly a coincident development of viral hepatitis.

Hematologic Complications

Unusual hematologic complications have included thrombocytopenia and hemolytic anemia. They have been severe but self-limited (Graham et al., 1974).

PROGNOSIS

In general, the prognosis of mumps is excellent. Fatalities are very rare. Meningoencephalitis is usually benign and is rarely followed by sequelae. In spite of high incidence of testicular atrophy following orchitis, sterility is extremely rare. In a small percentage of cases permanent deafness may complicate the disease.

IMMUNITY

One attack usually confers lifelong immunity. Mumps may recur, and the rate (4%) cited for second attacks probably reflects some errors in diagnosis. Clinical reinfections with mumps have been reported on occasion (Gut et al., 1995). Acute cervical adenitis and recurrent parotitis are likely to be erroneously diagnosed as mumps. A survey of 100 patients referred to a communicable disease hospital with a diagnosis of mumps revealed that 5% of the group had cervical adenitis. Permanent immunity is conferred by an attack of any type of mumps infection, including unilateral parotitis, meningoencephalitis without parotitis, or orchitis without parotitis. Indeed, even clinically inapparent infections also confer a lasting immunity. Infants born of mothers who have had mumps have passive immunity that lasts for several months.

A number of tests are available to measure the immune status of a person. These include

HI, CF, ELISA, and virus neutralization. Note in Figure 22-4 that the titer of mumps complement-fixing antibody persists at a low level for many months or years after infection. In a small percentage of cases the antibody level may fall below the detectable range. However, a positive CF test usually indicates past infection.

Several studies have correlated the results of serologic tests with patients who have past histories of a clinical case of mumps. Analysis of the data indicates that 30% to 40% of all susceptible persons exposed to mumps develop the infection in an inapparent form. Henle et al. confirmed these conclusions experimentally in 1948 (Figure 22-5). Of a group of 15 susceptible subjects who were deliberately exposed to mumps, four developed parotitis, two developed submaxillary swelling, and one developed orchitis. The remaining eight subjects developed an inapparent infection as indicated by the isolation of virus and the rise in mumps complement-fixing antibody.

EPIDEMIOLOGIC FACTORS

During the prevaccine era mumps was an endemic disease in most urban populations. In institutions in which crowding favored virus transmission, epidemics occurred frequently. Most cases of mumps occurred in the 5- to 10-year age group, with approximately 85% of the infections among children less than 15 years of age. It was uncommon in infancy. The age group affected by mumps was older than those groups affected by measles, varicella, and pertussis. Consequently, there were epidemics among adolescents in boarding schools and among adults in the armed forces. The disease has occurred in persons of all ages, ranging from 1 day to 99 years.

Live attenuated mumps virus vaccine was introduced in the United States in 1967; there were 185,691 reported cases of mumps in 1968. After routine use of the vaccine was recommended in 1977, there was a progressive decline in the number of cases. The number of

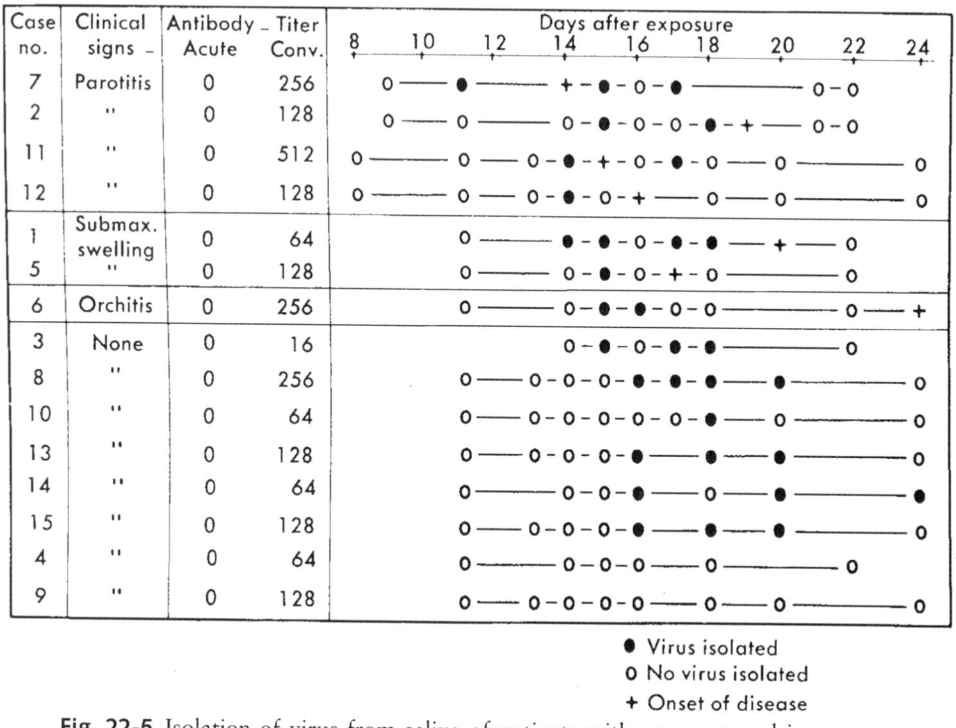

Fig. 22-5 Isolation of virus from saliva of patients with apparent and inapparent mumps infection. Virus was detected from 1 to 6 days before onset of salivary gland involvement. Virus was also readily isolated from six to eight patients with inapparent infection. Significant antibody levels developed in all 15 patients who were studied. (Reproduced from Henle G, Henle W, Wendell KK, et al: J Exp Med 1948;88:223. Copyright Rockefeller University Press.)

reported cases in 1995 was 906, a 99% decrease from 1968 (Centers for Disease Control and Prevention, 1998).

The source of infection may be saliva or other virus-containing secretions of an infected person. Transmission of mumps occurs by direct contact or by droplet infection. The available epidemiologic evidence suggests that the period of infectivity is from several days before the onset of symptoms to the subsidence of the salivary gland swelling. In the average case this represents a period of approximately 7 to 10 days.

The study of experimentally induced mumps infection by Henle et al. (1948) (Figure 22-5) has contributed significant data clarifying the period of infectivity. In the patients who developed parotitis 14 to 19 days after exposure, mumps virus was isolated from the saliva as many as 1 to 4 days before onset of parotitis. One patient who developed only submaxillary swelling on the twentieth day yielded mumps virus from the saliva 6 days before. It is of interest that six of the patients with inapparent infection secreted mumps virus in the saliva between the fifteenth and twenty-fourth days after exposure. This is a striking example of how an inapparent case of mumps can be the potential source for the spread of mumps infection.

Outbreaks of mumps have also on occasion been reported in highly immunized populations (Hersh, et al., 1991) underscoring the need for extremely high rates of immunization with two doses of vaccine to prevent disease.

Based on experience with other live attenuated vaccines, it is likely that live attenuated mumps virus vaccine could abort an epidemic in progress. The high incidence of inapparent cases and the infectivity of patients before onset of parotitis both combine to limit the effectiveness of quarantine or isolation. In the past the patient was isolated until the swelling of the salivary gland had subsided. In our opinion, too much time and effort should not be wasted on outmoded rigid isolation and quarantine procedures.

TREATMENT

Mumps is a self-limited infection, the course of which is not altered by use of any of the antimicrobial drugs. Treatment is symptomatic, and supportive measures are used. Acetaminophen will usually control the pain caused by glandular swelling. Warm applications seem to help some patients; others prefer cold. Topical ointments are useless. Parenteral administration of fluids is indicated for the support of patients with persistent vomiting associated with pancreatitis or meningoencephalitis.

PREVENTIVE MEASURES
Passive Protection

Passive immunization is not effective against mumps. During an epidemic of mumps in Alaska, Reed et al. (1967) evaluated the effect of mumps immune globulin (IG). The attack rate of mumps was 46% among 56 susceptible individuals who received globulin; it was 45% among 185 susceptible persons who did not receive globulin. Under the conditions of this study there was no evidence that the mumps IG prevented orchitis or meningoencephalitis.

Active Immunization[*]

Mumps virus vaccine is prepared in chick-embryo cell culture; it was introduced into the United States in December 1967. The vaccine produces a subclinical, noncommunicable infection with very few side effects. Mumps vaccine is available both in monovalent (mumps only) form and in combinations: mumps-rubella and measles-mumps-rubella (MMR) vaccines. The Urabe strain of mumps vaccine, which was associated with the side effect of aseptic meningitis (Brown, et al., 1996) was not used in the United States.

The vaccine is approximately 95% efficacious in preventing mumps disease, and vaccine-induced antibody is protective and long lasting, although of considerably lower titer than antibody resulting from natural infection. Estimates of clinical vaccine efficacy ranging from 75% to 95% have been calculated from data collected in outbreak settings using different epidemiologic study designs.

Susceptible children, adolescents, and adults should be vaccinated against mumps, unless vaccination is contraindicated. MMR vaccine is the vaccine of choice for routine administration and should be used in all situations in which recipients are also likely to be susceptible to measles and/or rubella. Persons should be considered susceptible to mumps unless they have documentation of (1)

---

[*]Abstracted from MMWR Morb Mortal Wkly Rep 1989;38:388-392, 397-400.

physician-diagnosed mumps, (2) adequate immunization with live mumps virus vaccine on or after their first birthday, or (3) laboratory evidence of immunity. Because live mumps vaccine was not used routinely before 1977 and because the peak age-specific incidence was in 5 to 9 year olds before the vaccine was introduced, most persons born before 1957 are likely to have been infected naturally between 1957 and 1977. Therefore they generally may be considered to be immune, even if they may not have had clinically recognizable mumps disease. However, this cutoff date for susceptibility is arbitrary. Persons who are unsure of their mumps disease history and/or mumps vaccination history should be vaccinated. Testing for susceptibility before vaccination, especially among adolescents and young adults, is not necessary.

Reports of illnesses after mumps vaccination have mainly been episodes of parotitis and low-grade fever. Allergic reactions including rash, pruritus, and purpura have been temporally associated with mumps vaccination but are uncommon and usually mild and of brief duration. The reported occurrence of encephalitis within 30 days of receipt of a mumps-containing vaccine (0.4 per million doses) is not greater than the observed background incidence rate of CNS dysfunction in the normal population. Other manifestations of CNS involvement, such as febrile seizures and deafness, have also been infrequently reported. Complete recovery is usual. Although mumps vaccine virus has been shown to infect the placenta and fetus, there is no evidence that it causes congenital malformations in humans. However, because of the theoretic risk of fetal damage, it is prudent to avoid giving live virus vaccine to pregnant women. Because live mumps vaccine is produced in chick-embryo cell culture, persons with a history of anaphylactic reactions (hives, swelling of the mouth and throat, difficulty breathing, hypotension, or shock) after egg ingestion should be vaccinated only with caution using published protocols.

Passively acquired antibody can interfere with the response to live attenuated virus vaccines. Therefore mumps vaccine should be given at least 2 weeks before the administration of IG or deferred until approximately 3 months after the administration of IG. In theory, replication of the mumps vaccine virus may be potentiated in patients with immune deficiency diseases and by the suppressed immune responses that occur with leukemia, lymphoma, or generalized malignancy or with therapy with corticosteroids, alkylating drugs, antimetabolites, or radiation. In general, patients with such conditions should not be given live mumps virus vaccine. Because vaccinated persons do not transmit mumps vaccine virus, the risk of mumps exposure for those patients may be reduced by vaccinating their close susceptible contacts. An exception to these general recommendations is in children infected with HIV; all asymptomatic HIV-infected children should receive MMR at 15 months of age. Patients with leukemia in remission whose chemotherapy has been terminated for at least 3 months may also receive live mumps virus vaccine.

BIBLIOGRAPHY

Banatvala JE, Bryant J, Schernthaner G, et al. Coxsackie B, mumps, rubella, and cytomegalovirus specific IgM responses in patients with juvenile-onset insulin-dependent diabetes mellitus in Britain, Austria, and Australia. Lancet 1985;1:1409.

Bang HO, Bang J. Involvement of the central nervous system in mumps. Bull Hyg 1944;19:503.

Brook I, Finegold SM. Acute suppurative parotitis caused by anaerobic bacteria: report of two cases. Pediatrics 1978;62:1019.

Brown EG, Dimock K, Wright KE. The Urabe AM9 mumps vaccine is a mixture of viruses differing at amino acid 335 of the hemagglutinin-neuraminidase gene with one form associated with disease. J Infect Dis 1996;174:619.

Brown NJ, Richmond SJ. Fatal mumps myocarditis in an 8-month-old child. Br Med J 1980;281:356.

Centers for Disease Control and Prevention. Measles, mumps, and rubella–vaccine use and strategies for elimination of measles, rubella, and congenital rubella syndrome and control of mumps. MMWR Morb Mortal Wkly Rep 1998;47:1.

Chaudary S, Jaski BE. Fulminant mumps myocarditis. Ann Intern Med 1989;110:569.

Graham DY, Brown CH, Benrey J, Butel JS. Thrombocytopenia: a complication of mumps. JAMA 1974;227:1162.

Gut JP, Lablache C, Behr S, et al. Symptomatic mumps virus reinfections. J Med Virol 1995;45:17.

Harel L, Amir J, Reish O, et al. Mumps arthritis in children. Pediatr Infect Dis J 1990;9:928.

Henle G, Henle W, Wendell KK, Rosenberg P. Isolation of mumps virus from human beings with induced apparent or inapparent infections. J Exp Med 1948;88:223.

Hersh BS, Fine PE, et al. Mumps outbreak a highly vaccinated population. J Pediatr 1991;119:187-193.

Howlett JG, Somlo F, Kalz F. A new syndrome of parotitis with herpangina caused by the Coxsackie virus. CMAJ 1957;77:5.

Jin L, Beard S, Brown DW. Genetic heterogeneity of mumps virus in the United Kingdom: identification of two new genotypes. J Infect Dis 1999;180:829.

Ni J, Bowles NE, Kim YH, et al. Viral infection of the myocardium in endocardial fibroelastosis. Molecular evidence for the role of mumps virus as an etiologic agent. Circulation 1997;95:133.

Philip RN, Reinhard KR, Lackmann DB. Observations on a mumps epidemic in a "virgin" population. Am J Hyg 1959;69:91.

Reed D, Brown G, Merrick R, et al. A mumps epidemic on St. George Island, Alaska. JAMA 1967;199:113.

Sultz HA, Hart BA, Zielezny M. Is mumps virus an etiologic factor in juvenile diabetes mellitus? J Pediatr 1975;86:654.

Swierkosz EM. Mumps. In Murray PR (ed). Manual of Clinical Microbiology. Washington D.C.: ASM Press, 1999.

Wilfert CM. Mumps meningoencephalitis with low cerebrospinal fluid glucose, prolonged pleocytosis and elevation of protein. N Engl J Med 1969;280:855.

Zollar LM, Mufson MA. Acute parotitis associated with parainfluenza 3 virus infection. Am J Dis Child 1970;119:147.

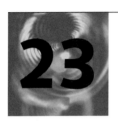

23 OSTEOMYELITIS AND SUPPURATIVE ARTHRITIS

KATHLEEN MCKENNA VOZZELLI AND LAURA GUTMAN

Suppurative skeletal infections are relatively uncommon in childhood, but when they occur, they are most likely to afflict young children. More than half of all cases occur in children under 5 years of age. This is a time of rapid skeletal growth, so damage to the growth plate or to joints has the potential for lifelong consequences. Skeletal infections are often difficult to recognize or localize early in the course of illness, and many are difficult to manage medically and surgically. Because prompt medical and surgical intervention probably decreases the likelihood of permanent sequelae, physicians who care for children should be aware of the earliest signs and symptoms of suppurative skeletal infections and be aggressive about establishing the diagnosis.

PATHOGENESIS AND EPIDEMIOLOGY

The majority of bone and joint infections are hematogenous in origin. However, infection less commonly can follow penetrating injuries or various medical and surgical maneuvers (e.g., arthroscopy, prosthetic joint surgery, intraarticular steroid injection, and various orthopedic surgeries). Impaired host defenses can also increase the risk of skeletal infection.

Significant blunt trauma is a preceding event in approximately one third of cases of osteomyelitis. Animal models of experimental osteomyelitis involve inflicting trauma to the bone of an animal that is bacteremic. The unique anatomy of the ends of long bones explains the predilection for localization of blood-borne bacteria. In the metaphysis are tiny vascular loops in which blood flow is sluggish. Rupture of some of these vessels as a result of trauma provides a favorable environment for multiplication of bacteria.

In the newborn and young infant there are blood vessels connecting the metaphysis and epiphysis, so it is common for pus from the metaphysis to rupture into the joint space. However, in the latter part of the first year of life the physis (growth plate) forms, there are no transphyseal blood vessels, and purulent infection of the joint occurs only rarely when the synovial attachment allows perforation of the periosteum to occur within the joint space. Bone is not distensible, so pus under pressure, prevented from decompressing into the joint, moves laterally through cortical vascular channels and accumulates under the loosely attached periosteum. After growth ceases, once again blood vessels connect the metaphysis and epiphysis.

Preceding trauma is less common in patients with suppurative arthritis, and the pathogenesis of hematogenous arthritis is poorly understood. The synovium is rich in blood vessels, and insignificant, unremembered trauma may play a role in pathogenesis. Possibly, synovial membrane receptors for bacteria play a role in localization. For example, in the era before universal vaccination for *Haemophilus influenzae*, type B accounted for only approximately 10% of cases of osteomyelitis in the first 2 years of life, but it was the pathogen in 45% of cases of arthritis in that age group.

Both conditions are most common in young children (Table 23-1); this is particularly true of arthritis, in which one half of all cases occur in the first 2 years of life and three fourths of all cases by 5 years of age. The figures for osteomyelitis in those two age groups are approximately one third and one half, respectively.

Skeletal infections consistently occur more commonly in boys than in girls in all reported series. The male-to-female ratio is approximately 2:1 in most series. If trauma is truly an important risk factor, it may be that the lifestyle of boys predisposes to traumatic events.

TABLE 23-1	Frequency of Disease by Age Group*				
		AGE-GROUPS (YR)			
Disease	*Number of cases*	*<2*	*2-5*	*6-10*	*11-15*
Osteomyelitis					
Number	399	127	101	108	63
Percent	100	32	25	27	16
Arthritis					
Number	682	362	172	102	46
Percent	100	53	25	15	1

*Based on J Nelson's series of cases.

Apparently there is no particular predilection for arthritis or osteomyelitis based on race. In most series the racial distribution of cases reflects the local population.

CLINICAL FINDINGS

The earliest signs and symptoms of skeletal infection are often subtle. This is particularly true of the neonate, who characteristically is not ill. In a report summarizing 83 cases of neonatal osteomyelitis from the literature, 52% had no fever, and only 8% were described as appearing septic or toxic. In infants, only pseudoparalysis of an extremity or apparent pain on movement of the affected extremity may be present.

In older infants and children the majority have fever and localized signs. Redness and swelling of skin and soft tissue overlying the site of infection usually are seen earlier in patients with arthritis than in those with osteomyelitis. The exception is with hip involvement, in which these signs are usually absent because of the deep location of that joint. In other joints, the bulging infected synovium is relatively near the surface, whereas the metaphyses are located deeper under the soft tissues. Local swelling and redness in a patient with osteomyelitis mean that the infection has spread out of the metaphysis into the subperiosteal space and that there is a secondary soft-tissue inflammatory response. Nonspecific systemic signs of infection such as nausea, vomiting, diarrhea, and headache are not prominent features of skeletal infections even though many of the patients have bacteremia. If those signs are present, disseminated infection syndrome with multiple foci of disease should be suspected; this is most likely to occur with *Staphylococcus aureus* or group B streptococci.

Long bones are principally involved in osteomyelitis (Table 23-2). The femur and tibia are equally affected and together constitute almost half of all cases. The bones of the upper extremities account for one fourth of all cases. Flat bones are less commonly affected.

Joints of the lower extremity constitute three quarters of all cases of arthritis. The elbow, wrist and shoulder joints are involved in approximately 20% of all cases, and small joints uncommonly are affected.

A single locus usually is involved in bone or joint infection. Multifocal osteomyelitis and polyarticular arthritis occur in fewer than 10% of cases (Tables 23-3 and 23-4). An exception is gonococcal infection, which is polyarticular in more than half of the cases.

DIAGNOSIS

The differential diagnosis of bone and joint infections includes trauma, cellulitis, pyomyositis, malignancy, and collagen vascular diseases. It is not unusual for patients with leukemia or neuroblastoma to present with fever and focal signs suggesting bone or joint infection. A biopsy establishes the diagnosis. History and roentgenographic findings help in distinguishing trauma from infection. Pyomyositis is rare outside central Africa and parts of Southeast Asia. Sonography and magnetic resonance imaging (MRI) are very helpful in identifying pyomyositis. In most cases the differential diagnosis between cellulitis and similar soft-tissue findings secondary to bone and joint infection becomes obvious during physical examination. When there is doubt, three-phase radionuclide scanning can be helpful. Various collagen vascular diseases may mimic arthritis if the patient has a single joint involved. In most cases, multiple joint involvement, disease in other organ

TABLE 23-2 Infected Bones in 372 Patients With Monosteal Disease and 27 Patients With Polysteal Disease*

Bone	Monosteal	Polysteal
Femur	93	12
Tibia	89	18
Humerus	50	8
Fibula	16	10
Phalanx	18	5
Calcaneus	18	0
Radius	13	4
Ischium	14	1
Metatarsus	8	0
Ulna	7	3
Ilium	7	0
Vertebra	7	2
Sacrum	3	0
Skull	3	0
Talus	3	1
Clavicle	2	2
Rib	2	1
Scapula	2	1
Carpal bone	2	0
Cuneiform	2	0
Pubis	3	1
Sternum	3	0
Metacarpus	2	0
One case each: maxilla, mandible, cuboid, bone of pyriform aperture, acetabulum	6	0

TABLE 23-3 Distribution of Affected Joints in Patients With Septic Arthritis

Joint	DALLAS SERIES (646 JOINTS, 591 PATIENTS)		FIVE OTHER SERIES (377 JOINTS, 357 PATIENTS)	
	Total joints	Percentage	Total joints	Percentage
Knee	258	40	144	38
Hip	146	23	121	32
Elbow	89	14	21	6
Ankle	85	13	52	14
Wrist	27	4	3	1
Shoulder	28	4	11	3
Hand/foot	8	1	15	4
Other	5	1	10	2

Modified from Fink CW, Nelson JD: Clin Rheum Dis 1986;12:423-435.

systems, failure to respond to antibiotic therapy, and the chronic or remittent nature of the process leads to the correct diagnosis.

Results from routine laboratory tests such as the white blood cell count and differential, erythrocyte sedimentation rate, and C-reactive protein are nonspecific and may not be helpful in differentiating skeletal infections from other conditions.

The radiologic assessment of infectious diseases of bones and joints has enjoyed rapid advances over the past decade and continues to

TABLE 23-4	Monarticular and Polyarticular Involvement in Septic Arthritis			
	DALLAS SERIES (591 JOINTS)		**OTHER SERIES (307 JOINTS)**	
Joints	*Number of patients*	*Percentage*	*Number of patients*	*Percentage*
Monarticular	552	93.4	295	96
Two joints	26	4.4	8	2.6
Three joints	10	1.7	3	1
Four joints	3	0.5	1	0.3

Modified from Fink CW, Nelson JD: Clin Rheum Dis 1986;12:423-435.

be the subject of much research. The application of various radiologic techniques (plain roentgeongrams, sonography, radionuclide imaging, indium-label leukocytes, MRI) has specific uses for specific clinical settings. It is recommended that for the diagnosis of complicated cases of suspected bone and joint infections, advice be sought from an experienced radiologist regarding appropriate use of these modalities. Plain roentgenograms are useful in selected cases. Distention of the joint space is often visible in the knee and shoulder but seldom is detected in other joints. Distortion of the deep soft tissues around the metaphyses is a very useful radiographic sign when it is present because it is seen only in two other conditions: crush injuries and pyomyositis. Destructive changes in bone are not seen until at least 10 to 14 days after onset of infection (Figure 23-1).

Radionuclide imaging with technetium radiophosphate or gallium bone scintigraphy is useful in selected cases, but there are limitations in sensitivity, specificity, and predictive values (Figure 23-2). Imaging is not so successful in cases of acute suppurative arthritis. When three-phase technetium phosphate scans were interpreted "blindly" by radiologists, only 13% of scans of children with proved arthritis were

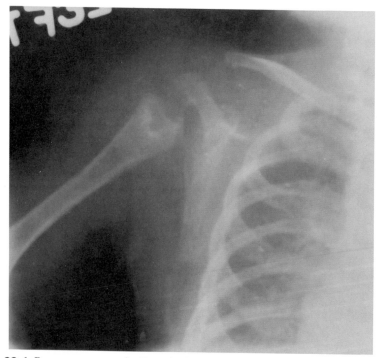

Fig. 23-1 Roentgenogram of a 7-week-old infant with osteomyelitis of the head of the humerus, showing destruction of areas of metaphysis and epiphysis. Pyarthrosis was also present initially.

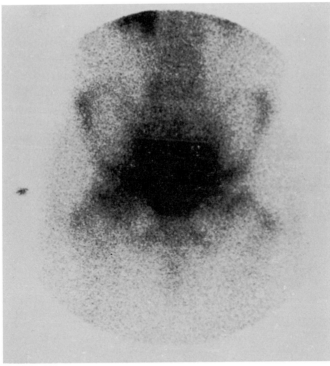

Right   Left

Fig. 23-2 Image intensified technetium pyrophosphate bone scan of the hips and pelvis of a 10-year-old boy with 1 day of point tenderness over the head of the right femur and blood cultures positive for *Staphylococcus aureus*. Roentgenographic areas of the radiolucency never appeared.

interpreted correctly, and arthritis was incorrectly identified in 32% of children with no evidence of suppurative arthritis. When the radiologists were provided clinical data about each case, the sensitivity rose to 70% and the specificity was 68%; positive predictive value was 62%, and negative predictive value was 70%. Technetium scans may be uninterpretable in neonates. When a scan is ordered for patients at any age, detailed clinical information should be provided to the radiologist to optimize the interpretation. A negative scan should not rule out bone or joint disease if the clinical findings suggest osteomyelitis or arthritis. Radionuclide imaging is not necessary in most cases, but it can be useful when there is doubt about the diagnosis or the localization.

Radioactive indium-labeled leukocytes have been used successfully for localizing infection, but the technique is not generally available. Gallium scanning is more sensitive and specific than technetium scanning for determining osteomyelitis, but it is slower and involves more radiation.

Application of MRI to musculoskeletal disorders has emerged as a major tool for diagnostically challenging situations. Suppurative arthritis, cellulitis, and osteomyelitis can be differentiated. Generally, the sensitivity for MRI in diagnosing osteomyelitis is high, with values ranging from 82% to 100%. Specificity, however, is lower because of abnormalities that can produce similar alterations in signal intensity. These may include tumors, stress fractures, surgical scarring, and reactive changes in the bone marrow as a result of adjacent soft-tissue inflammation.

Ultrasonography has been used to detect fluid in the hip joint. The most recent development in radionuclide scanning for detection of focal infection is the use of indium-labeled intravenous gamma globulin. Successful localization of skeletal infection was achieved in 12 or 13 cases.

The ultimate diagnostic tool for skeletal infections is the aspirating needle, and the procedure should be done unless there are unusual circumstances that contraindicate its use. Most joint spaces are easy to enter, but the hip can pose technical problems.

Sonographic guidance can facilitate aspiration. If no fluid is obtained, a small amount of air or contrast material is injected and a roentgenogram obtained to confirm the needle tip was in the joint cavity. In cases of osteomyelitis, a steel needle is needed to penetrate the cortex into the metaphysis. If pus is encountered in the subperiosteal space, going further is unnecessary. Aspiration of joint or bone pus not only serves to confirm the diagnosis of infection, but also provides the best specimen for bacteriologic culture.

MICROBIOLOGY

A microbial cause is revealed in approximately two thirds of cases of suppurative arthritis (Table 23-5) and three fourths of cases of osteomyelitis (Table 23-6). Some negative cultures are explained by prior antibiotic therapy and some by the inhibitory effect of pus on microorganisms, but it is possible that some cases that are treated as bacterial arthritis are actually reactive arthritis.

In patients with osteomyelitis, *S. aureus* is the most common infecting organism in all age groups, including the newborn. Group B streptococci and coliform bacteria are also prominent pathogens in the neonate. Group A streptococci are next in frequency but constitute less than 10% of all cases. Prior to widespread immunization for *H. influenzae* type b, this organism had accounted for 7% of all cases in children 5 year of age or younger. *Pseudomonas aeruginosa* cases are almost exclusively related to puncture wounds of the foot. After 5 years of age virtually all cases of

---

TABLE 23-5 Causative Agents Found in Patients With Suppurative Arthritis

Organism	DALLAS SERIES (591 JOINTS)		OTHER SERIES (343 JOINTS)	
	Number of patients	Percentage found	Number of patients	Percentage found
Staphylococcus aureus	97	17	139	41
Haemophilus influenzae	149	25	41	12
Others	144	25	67	19
Unknown	201	33	96	28

Modified from Fink CW, Nelson JD: Clin Rheum Dis 1986;12:423-435.

TABLE 23-6 Causative Agents of Osteomyelitis by Ages of Patients

Organism	Number of cases	AGE-GROUPS (YR)		
		<2	2-5	5
Staphylococcus aureus	200	27*	56	64
Streptococci†	44	16	13	6
Haemophilus influenzae type b	16	11	2	0
Pseudomonas aeruginosa	11	2	2	4
Staphylococcus epidermidis	10	6	1	0
Gram-negative enteric bacilli	10	4	4	0.6
S. aureus and group A Streptococcus	2	0.8	0	0
Mycobacterium tuberculosis	1	0	1	0
Moraxella kingae	1	0.8	0	0
Brucella abortus	1	0	1	0
Unknown	103	34	20	23
TOTAL	399	127	101	171

*Percent of cases in age-group.
†Twenty-nine *Streptococcus pyogenes*, eight *Streptococcus agalactiae*, six *Streptococcus pneumoniae*, one not specified.

osteomyelitis are caused by gram-positive cocci except for the *P. aeruginosa* cases.

In young patients with suppurative arthritis, *H. influenzae* type b previously outranked *S. aureus* in frequency. The control of *H. influenzae* type b through immunization has decreased the incidence of suppurative arthritis and osteomyelitis attributable to this organism to near zero in the United States. After 5 years of age, *S. aureus* predominates.

In both conditions occasional cases caused by fungal infections or tuberculosis are encountered, and some viral infections are associated with arthritis.

SPECIAL CONSIDERATIONS
Newborn Infants

The indolent nature of skeletal infections in neonates is noteworthy. Because of the lack of fever and other systemic signs of illness in approximately one half of the neonates, the pain with movement of an extremity is often mistakenly attributed to trauma.

In the series of 83 neonates with osteomyelitis collected from three reports in the literature there was abnormal delivery in 33%, and a preceding infection in 46%. Unlike older patients in whom a single bone is involved in more than 90% of cases, polyosteal disease was present in 40% of neonates. Infection of the adjacent joint occurred in 70% of cases. The bacteria involved were *S. aureus* in 53%, streptococci (mostly group B) in 23%, gram-negative enteric bacilli in 13%, and unknown organisms in 11%. Calcaneal osteomyelitis has occurred as a complication of heel puncture.

In 23 neonates with suppurative arthritis the pathogens were staphylococci in 9; streptococci in 5; coliform bacilli in 3; *Candida albicans* in 3; and *P. aeruginosa*, *H. influenzae* type b, and *Neisseria gonorrhoeae* in 1 each. *Candida* infections occur in neonates with vascular catheters in place who have received prior broad-spectrum antibiotic therapy.

Group B streptococcal infections differ in several respects from other infections. The age of onset is later, and the infants have had no preceding infections. Possibly because of trauma during delivery, a single bone is involved, typically the proximal right humerus. Spread to the contiguous joint is less common with group B streptococcal infection than with staphylococcal or coliform infection.

Sickle Cell Anemia

Skeletal infections in patients with sickle cell anemia often are caused by uncommon pathogens, and distinguishing between episodes of aseptic infarction and infection is exceedingly difficult. With infarction there is fever, pain, swelling, redness, leukocytosis and an increase in the acute phase reactants just as in infection, and the progress of roentgenographic changes is the same. However, infarction episodes are far more common than skeletal infections. Gallium and technetium scanning do not discriminate between infection and infarction, probably because infarction also occurs in the presence of infection. If the usual supportive measures for bone infarct episodes do not lead to improvement, osteomyelitis should be suspected and an aspirate of bone taken for culture.

In a series of 14 episodes of osteoarticular infection in 13 sicklemic patients there were eight cases of osteomyelitis and six cases of arthritis. The causative bacteria in osteomyelitis were *Salmonella* species (four cases) and one case each with *Escherichia coli*, *Enterobacter aerogenes*, *H. influenzae* type b, and *S. aureus*. In contrast, the pathogens in arthritis were *Streptococcus pneumoniae* in five cases and *H. influenzae* type b in one case. (Pneumococci are very uncommon causes of arthritis in nonsicklemic patients.) More recent data from a retrospective study performed in 2000 reveal similar epidemiologic patterns.

Hemophilia

Hemarthrosis apparently predisposes to joint infections. It has been calculated that there is a threefold to twelvefold increased risk of suppurative arthritis in persons with hemophilia in comparison with the general population. In a review of 139 children with hemophilia, four (2.9%) developed joint infection during a 6-year period. Just as with sickle cell disease, pneumococcus is the most common pathogen.

The Immunocompromised Host

In addition to infection with common pathogens, children with congenital, acquired, or iatrogenic immune deficiency may be subject to infections with unusual organisms. Bone and joint infections as a result of fungal organisms, gram-negative bacteria, atypical mycobacteria, and tuberculosis, among others, have been described in higher rates in the immunocompromised population. Patients with chronic granulomatous disease are particularly susceptible to *Aspergillus* osteomyelitis. Atypical mycobacteria, tuberculous bacteria, and *Bartonella henselae,* the organism responsible for cat-scratch disease, are more common in the HIV-infected population.

Transient Synovitis of the Hip

The syndrome of transient synovitis is the most common cause of hip pain in children. The cause is unknown.

A review of 497 cases during a 30-year period provides useful information, but it is biased toward the more severe cases because all the children were hospitalized. Many children with mild cases are not hospitalized.

The syndrome typically occurs in children 4 to 10 years of age and is twice as common in boys as in girls. Approximately half of the patients have a preceding upper respiratory infection. Body temperature, leukocyte count, and erythrocyte sedimentation rate are normal or slightly elevated. The most prominent symptoms are thigh pain and a limp or a failure to bear weight. Physical examination reveals limitation of internal rotation.

Radiographs of the hip are normal in most children, but a small percentage show a mild increase in joint space size or blurring of deep muscle planes. Of 41 patients who had technetium scans, 22 showed increased uptake of isotope consistent with synovitis. Aspirated joint fluid is serous or serosanguineous.

In mild cases managed on an outpatient basis, symptoms last only a few days. In the 497 hospitalized patients treated with bed rest, with or without Buck's traction, symptoms lasted less than 1 week in 67% and less than 1 month in an additional 21%. The outcome is excellent in almost all cases. Because an occasional case of Legg-Calvé-Perthes disease mimics toxic synovitis initially, it is recommended that the children be examined once or twice over the ensuing 6 months.

Reactive Arthritis

Reactive arthritis is defined as inflammation of one or more joints related to infection at a site distant from the affected joints; no infectious agent can be found within the joint. Reiter's syndrome is the best known type of reactive arthritis, but the condition is associated with several types of gastrointestinal infection, group A streptococcal infections,

and certain viral infections. Reactive arthritis occurs 3 to 10 days after onset of meningococcal or *Haemophilus* meningitis in 3.5% of patients.

Results of cell counts and differential counts of synovial fluid are similar in patients with bacterial and reactive arthritis. Some patients with culture-negative arthritis who are treated with antibiotics for presumed bacterial infections probably actually have reactive arthritis.

Large concentrations of tumor necrosis factor (TNF)–α and interleukin-1β (IL-1β) are present in synovial fluid in cases of suppurative arthritis but not in cases of reactive arthritis. In a study performed on 75 synovial fluid samples taken from patients with various forms of arthritis, elevated levels of TNF-α were present in nearly 100% of samples that were culture-positive for bacterial arthritis. IL-1β and IL-6 showed poorer sensitivity. These tests may prove to be of value as additional research is performed and as the assays become widely available. Treatment of reactive arthritis is with antiinflammatory drugs.

Acute or Subacute Epiphyseal Osteomyelitis

Acute or subacute epiphyseal osteomyelitis is a little known condition that affects the proximal tibia or distal femoral epiphysis. Presenting signs mimicking those of arthritis. Roentgenographic changes in the epiphysis are not seen in the acute form; it is likely that some patients are treated with antibiotics for arthritis and the diagnosis of epiphyseal osteomyelitis is never made because follow-up radiographs are never obtained. *S. aureus* sometimes is grown from the synovial fluid, but in most cases the cultures are sterile. The condition responds coincident with administration of antistaphylococcal antibiotics.

Infection Secondary to Trauma

The most common forms of traumatic skeletal infection follow puncture wounds of the feet or compound fractures. A great variety of bacteria are involved, and polymicrobial infections are common. Wound cultures fail to predict bone culture results in most patients.

When puncture wounds occur through the soles of sneakers, *P. aeruginosa* osteochondritis often ensues because these organisms can exist in the foam layer of the shoe. Performing thorough surgical débridement is essential for treating this disease. Even prolonged courses of antipseudomonal therapy fail to eradicate the infection in the absence of surgical débridement. When meticulous surgery is performed, a regimen of postoperative antibiotics for only 7 days is effective therapy.

Suppurative Bursitis

Infections of bursae are rare in children. Ten cases were diagnosed in three Denver hospitals during a 25-year period. Eight involved the prepatellar bursa, and there was one each in the olecranon and subacromial bursa. Blunt trauma was a predisposing event in six cases; however, in young infants suppurative bursitis apparently is hematogenous in origin. Most cases are manifested by swelling and fluctuance but normal range of motion of the adjacent joint. S. aureus and group A streptococci are the usual pathogens.

Chronic Recurrent Multifocal Osteomyelitis

Originally reported as *subacute and chronic symmetrical osteomyelitis,* this condition has since been termed *chronic recurrent multifocal osteomyelitis (CRMO).*

The disease affects children and young adults. It commonly begins between 8 and 12 years of age and affects females twice as often as males. As its name implies, several sites are involved during each episode, and the condition remits and relapses for several years before stopping spontaneously. The metaphyses of long bones are involved, but other bones rarely infected in bacterial osteomyelitis are frequently involved, namely the clavicle and spine. Biopsy studies of the lesions reveal acute and chronic inflammation, with necrosis and granulation tissue. Sclerosis and hyperostosis are progressive.

Patients with CRMO commonly have chronic inflammatory skin conditions such as palmoplantar pustulosis, psoriasis, and Sweet's syndrome. There is also a subset of patients with CRMO and associated synovitis, acne, pustulosis, hyperostosis and osteitis, giving rise to the acronym SAPHO. CRMO is considered a noninfectious inflammatory condition that may affect other organ systems such as the lung. There have also been case reports of associations between CRMO and inflammatory bowel disease, Wegener's granulomatosis, Takayasu arteritis, and pyoderma gangrenosum. However, in one case *Mycoplasma hominis* was cultured from a bone biopsy specimen, and the disease apparently was improved by therapy with clindamycin and later tetracycline.

TREATMENT

Optimal treatment of skeletal infections requires collaborative efforts of the pediatrician or family physician, the orthopedic surgeon, and the physiatrist.

Initial Antibiotic Therapy

Initial empiric antibiotic therapy is based on knowledge of likely bacterial pathogens at various ages, the results of the gram stain of aspirated material, and special considerations. In the newborn an antistaphylococcal penicillin such as methicillin or nafcillin and a broad-spectrum cephalosporin such as cefotaxime provide coverage for methicillin-sensitive S. aureus, group B streptococci, and coliform bacilli. An aminoglycoside could be used in place of the cephalosporin, but aminoglycosides have somewhat reduced activity with decreased oxygen tension and pH, and these conditions are present in tissue infections. If the neonate is a small premature infant who has been in the neonatal intensive care unit for a long period of time or who has a central vascular catheter, the possibility of the presence of nosocomial, multiple antibiotic–resistant gram-negative bacteria, methicillin-resistant staphylococci, or fungi must be considered.

In infants and children up to approximately 4 to 5 years of age, the principle pathogens are S. aureus and streptococci. Several antibiotics are useful for treating these types of infection. Cephalosporins such as cefuroxime, cefotaxime, or ceftriaxone commonly are used. Beyond 5 years of age, unless there are special circumstances, almost all cases of skeletal infection are caused by gram-positive cocci, so an antistaphylococcal antibiotic such as nafcillin can be used.

Some clinical situations dictate special considerations about empiric antibiotic selection. In sicklemic patients with osteomyelitis, coliform bacteria are common pathogens, so a broad-spectrum cephalosporin such as cefotaxime or ceftriaxone should be used in addition to an antistaphylococcal drug. Arthritis in patients with sickle cell disease is unlikely to be caused by coliform bacteria, so use of the usual antibiotics would be appropriate. Clindamycin is a useful alternative drug for patients who are expected to have a *Staphylococcus* infection. In addition to good antistaphylococcal activity, clindamycin has broad activity against anaerobes, so it is useful for treatment of infections secondary to penetrating injuries or compound fractures.

In instances of *Pseudomonas* osteomyelitis, which often results from a puncture wound of the foot through tennis shoes, ceftazidime or piperacillin plus an aminoglycoside provide appropriate care. Ciprofloxacin has been successfully used as a transition to oral therapy in adolescent patients with calcaneal puncture-wound–associated osteomyelitis. An integral aspect of management is surgical débridement of the lesions.

In cases of suspected or culture-proved methicillin-resistant *S. aureus* (MRSA) infection, vancomycin is the treatment of choice. Two newer antibiotics, linezolid and quinpristin-dalfopristin are both active against MRSA. Data concerning these drugs for the treatment of bone and joint infections are scarce. A study evaluating the efficacy of linezolid for treatment of osteomyelitis in an animal model did not show promise. There are case reports in the literature of successful treatment of MRSA osteomyelitis with linezolid in human subjects. The high oral bioavailability of linezolid would make this drug an attractive treatment option if further data prove its efficacy.

The fluoroquinolones have been used widely in the therapy of chronic osteomyelitis in adults with good results. Their use in children remains controversial because of the development of arthropathy in juvenile animals, although to date there have been no reports of drug-associated human arthropathy. Because there are often treatment alternatives available, the use of quinolones should be dictated by antimicrobial susceptibility patterns. They may have a role in the treatment of bone and joint infections caused by *Salmonella*, *Pseudomonas*, and drug-resistant gram-negative pathogens in immunocompromised hosts.

For immunocompromised patients the potential pathogens are legion. Combination therapy usually is initiated. Use of several combinations of two to three drugs would be rational. Currently, vancomycin with ceftazidime or ticarcillin-clavulanate is used in many places, especially in neutropenic patients.

Subsequent Antibiotic Therapy

When the pathogen has been identified, appropriate adjustments in antibiotics are made when necessary. If a pathogen is not identified and the patient is improving, therapy is usually continued with the antibiotic selected initially; however, consideration should be given to the possibility of a noninfectious inflammatory condition. Similarly, if a pathogen is not identified and the patient is not improving, consideration is given to performing reaspiration or biopsy and to the possibility of a noninfectious condition.

In recent years it has become common practice to change the route of administration of antibiotics from parenteral to oral once the patient's condition has stabilized, after approximately 1 week of parenteral therapy and after it has been shown that serum concentrations of antimicrobial agents following oral dosing are expected to be efficacious for the particular isolate.

The oral regimen decreases the risk of nosocomial infections related to prolonged intravenous therapy, may be more comfortable for the patient, and permits treatment outside the hospital if compliance with the regimen can be ensured. However, the improved availability of home parenteral therapy with home monitoring and assistance has also made the completion of a parenteral regimen very accessible. Because of issues of compliance and clinical experiences with treatment failures due to noncompliance, some centers prefer that the entire course of therapy be delivered parenterally.

Duration of Antibiotic Therapy

Prolonged courses of antibiotic therapy have traditionally been recommended, but there has been a trend toward shorter courses.

The Centers for Disease Control and Prevention guidelines recommend 7 days of therapy for gonococcal tenosynovitis. As mentioned previously, 7 postoperative days of treatment is adequate for *Pseudomonas* osteochondritis or arthritis, if surgically débrided. Immunocompromised patients generally require prolonged courses of therapy, as do patients with fungal or tuberculous disease.

For the typical case of staphylococcal, streptococcal, or *Haemophilus* infection, treatment is continued for a minimum of 4 weeks provided that the signs of inflammation have disappeared. Duration of antibiotic therapy should be individualized, and if the clinical response has been slow, a course of 4 to 6 weeks is commonly used.

As mentioned above, there has been a trend toward shorter courses of therapy, most notably more rapid transitions to oral antibiotics. As part of a prospective study performed by the Finnish Study Group, 50 children with sensitive *S. aureus* osteomyelitis were treated with short-course antibiotic therapy. The patients received 3 to 4 days of either clindamycin or a first-generation cephalosporin parenterally, followed by a 3-week course of oral therapy. Less than half received adjunctive surgical intervention. All 50 children were well without relapse or sequelae 1 year later. Retrospective data from Scotland indicate that the average duration of parenteral therapy for osteomyelitis prescribed by local physicians is 1 day, followed by a mean of 4 weeks or oral therapy.

If inflammatory markers such as the white blood cell count, C-reactive protein, and erythrocyte sedimentation rate are elevated upon presentation, subsequent serial measurements can be helpful during therapy to gauge resolution of inflammation. In comparative studies, C-reactive protein has been proved to be the most useful marker, as it is often elevated early in infection and decreases rapidly in a healing infection.

Surgical Therapy

No randomized, prospective study has compared two or more surgical procedures in patients with skeletal infections. The measures used derive from training and experience. For example, after arthrotomy some surgeons leave drains and some do not. Of those who use drains, some use collapsible drains and some use rigid ones. Of those who use rigid drains, some use suction and some do not. None of these approaches has been evaluated in a controlled manner.

Hip joint infection is a surgical emergency because of the threat to the blood supply to the head of the femur. When a penetrating injury has occurred and the presence of a foreign body is likely, surgical intervention is indicated. In other situations the need for surgery is individualized.

For joints other than the hip, daily percutaneous needle aspirations of synovial fluid are done. Generally one or two subsequent aspirations suffice. If fluid is still accumulating after 4 to 5 days, arthrotomy is performed. At the time of surgery the joint is flushed with sterile saline solution. Antibiotics are not instilled because they are irritating to synovial tissue, and adequate amounts of antibiotic are achieved in joint fluid with systemic administration.

If frank pus is obtained from a subperiosteal or metaphyseal aspiration, the patient may benefit from surgery for drainage through a cortical window. In one series, incision and drainage were done in 36% of cases of arthritis and 69% of cases of osteomyelitis.

Infected weight-bearing limbs should be protected from the trauma of weight bearing during the initial course of therapy. Good attention to nutrition is essential for satisfactory healing.

Physical Medicine

The major role of physical medicine is a preventive one. If a child is allowed to lie in bed with an extremity in flexion, limitation of extension can develop in a few days. The affected extremity should be kept in extension with sand bags, splints, or, if necessary, casts. Casts are indicated when there is a potential for pathologic fracture.

After 2 or 3 days, when pain is easing, passive range-of-motion exercises are started and then continued until the child resumes normal activity.

In neglected cases with flexion contractures, prolonged physical therapy is required.

PROGNOSIS

Because children are in a dynamic state of growth, sequelae of skeletal infections may not become apparent for months or years, so long-term follow-up is important. In a series of 40 neonates with osteomyelitis treated from 1970 to 1979, 10 had severe sequelae and 6 had moderate sequelae. Major problems related to retarded growth of an affected bone. Growth disturbance was evident in 20 of 36 nonoperated foci and in 4 of 19 operated foci.

Relapses and chronic infections are uncommon. A group of 50 infants and children with osteomyelitis was followed for an average of 36 months (range 12 to 56 months) after treatment. At diagnosis 32 were classified as acute, 15 as subacute (symptoms for longer than 7 days), and 3 as chronic. Relapses occurred in only two patients, one of whom was originally classified as acute and the other as chronic. In another series, 8 of 60 patients did not respond to antibiotics within 48 hours and required surgical drainage. Of the remaining 52 patients, 35 patients were treated with parenteral antibiotics for an average of 21 days, and 17 were treated parenterally for 8 days, followed by 4 weeks of oral antibiotics. Chronic infection ensued in one of the operatively treated patients and in two of the remaining 52.

In 49 patients with suppurative arthritis of weight-bearing joints followed for an average of 4.3 years (range 18 months to 12 years) after treatment, 13 patients (27%) had sequelae, and in eight (16%) ambulation was impaired. Residual damage was more common with hip involvement (40% of cases) and ankle involvement (33%) than knee joint disease (10%). Sequelae were equally common after *S. aureus* and *H. influenzae* infection. Evaluation at the time of hospital discharge correctly identified only 4 of the 13 children with sequelae, and four others who were normal at follow-up had been thought to have permanent damage at discharge. Children with sequelae tended to have been sick longer before diagnosis, and in them drainage of pus was delayed.

Thirty-seven children with hip joint infection treated at the Mayo Clinic from 1943 through 1973 had long-term (mean 8.3 years) follow-up evaluation. Nineteen had satisfactory results, and 18 had unsatisfactory results. "Unsatisfactory" was defined as more than 2.5 cm limb length discrepancy (seven patients), persisting pain (five patients), limitation of movement (seven patients), or need for secondary surgical procedures (nine patients). Duration of symptoms was the most important prognostic factor. There were no sequelae among the nine patients treated within 4 days of onset of symptoms. Of 11 patients with symptoms persisting for more than 1 week, only two had satisfactory results. Associated metaphyseal osteomyelitis was another bad prognostic sign: only 2 of 14 had a satisfactory result.

Even with appropriate medical and surgical therapy, there is potential for permanent disabling sequelae in patients with skeletal infections. Prompt recognition and vigorous medical, surgical, and physical therapy offer the best hope for a satisfactory outcome.

SUGGESTED READINGS

Blyth MJG, Kincaid R, Craigen MAC, et al. The changing epidemiology of acute and subacute haemotogenous osteomyelitis in children. J Bone Joint Surg Br 2001; 83m-B:99-102.

Boutin RD, Brossman J, Sartoris DJ, et al. Update on imaging of orthopedic infections. Orthop Clin N Am 1998;29:41-66.

Bousvaros A, Marcon M, Treem W. Chronic recurrent multifocal osteomyelitis associated with inflammatory bowel disease in children. Dig Dis Sci 1999;44:2500-2507.

Bowerman SG, Green NG, Mencio GA. Decline of bone and joint infections attributable to *Haemophilus influenzae* type B. Clin Orthop 1997;341:128-133.

Centers for Disease Control and Prevention. 1998 Guidelines for Sexually Transmitted Diseases. MMWR Recomm Rep 1998;47:63-64.

Chambers JB, Forsythe DA, Bertrand SL, et al. Retrospective review of osteoarticular infection in a pediatric sickle cell age group. J Pediatr Orthop 2000;20:682-685.

Dagan O, Barak Y, Metzger A. Pyoderma gangrenosum and sterile multifocal osteomyelitis preceding the appearance of Takayasu arteritis. Pediatr Dermatol 1995;12:39-42.

Howard AW, Viskontas D, Sabbagh C. Reduction in osteomyelitis and septic arthritis related to *Haemophilus influenzae* type B vaccination. J Pediatr Orthop 1999;19:705-709.

Jeng GW, Wang CR, Liu ST. Measurement of synovial TNF-α in diagnosing emergency patients with bacterial arthritis. Am J Emerg Med 1997;15:626-629.

Marshall GS, Mudido P, Rabalais GP, et al. Organism isolation and serum bacterial titers in oral antibiotic therapy for pediatric osteomyelitis. South Med J 1996;89:68-70.

Melzer M, Goldsmith D, Gransden W. Successful treatment of vertebral osteomyelitis with linezolid in a patient receiving hemodialysis and with persistent methicillin-resistant *Staphylococcus aureus* and vancomycin-resistant *Enterococcus* bacteremias. Clin Infect Dis 2000;31:208-209.

Patel R, Piper KE, Rouse MS, et al. Linezolid therapy for *Staphylococcus aureus* experimental osteomyelitis. Antimicrob Agents Chemother 2000:3438-3440.

Pelkonen P, Pyoppy S, Jasskilainen J, et al. Chronic osteomyelitis-like disease with negative bacterial cultures. Am J Dis Child 1998;142:1167-1173.

Peltola H, Unkila-Kallio L, Kallio M, the Finnish Study Group. Simplified treatment of acute staphylococcal osteomyelitis of childhood. Pediatrics 1997;99:846-850.

Puffinbarger WR, Guiel CR, Hendon WA, et al. Osteomyelitis of the calcaneus in children. J Pediatr Orthop 1996;16:224-230.

Rissing JP. Antimicrobial therapy for chronic osteomyelitis in adults: role of the quinolones. Clin Infect Dis 1997;25:1327-1333.

Roine I, Faingezicht I, Arguedas A, et al. Serial C-reactive protein to monitor recovery from acute hematogenous osteomyelitis in children. Pediatr Infect Dis J 1995;14:40-44.

Schaad UB. Pediatric use of quinolones. Pediatr Infect Dis J 1999;18:469-470.

Sundaram M, McDonald D, Engel E, et al. Chronic recurrent multifocal osteomyelitis: an evolving clinical and radiological spectrum. Skeletal Radiol 1996;25: 333-336.

Unkila-Kallio L, Kallio MJ, Eskola J, et al. Serum C-reactive protein, erythrocyte sedimentation rate, and white blood cell count in acute hematogenous osteomyelitis of children. Pediatrics 1994;93:59-62.

Vassilopoulos D, Chalasani P, Jurado RL, et al. Musculoskeletal infections in patients with human immunodeficiency virus infection. Medicine 1997;76: 284-294.

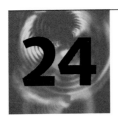

24 OTITIS MEDIA

JEROME O. KLEIN

Acute otitis media and middle ear effusion are among the most common illnesses of childhood. After every episode of acute otitis media, fluid persists in the middle ear for varying periods of time, usually weeks to months. The signs of acute infection resolve with appropriate antibiotic therapy, but the middle ear effusion, now sterile (in episodes of bacterial infection), persists. Conductive hearing loss usually accompanies middle ear effusion, although the extent of the loss varies from child to child. Because of the frequency of acute otitis media and accompanying hearing loss, pediatricians have been concerned that children who suffer from persistent or recurrent middle ear disease might also suffer from delay or impairment of speech, language, or cognitive abilities.

EPIDEMIOLOGY

Otitis media is a disease of infants and young children. The peak age-specific attack rate occurs between 6 and 18 months of age. By 3 years of age, most children have had at least one episode of acute otitis media, and up to one half have had recurrent acute otitis media (three or more episodes). Few children have first episodes of acute otitis media after 3 years of age (Teele et al., 1989). Among the variables associated with acute otitis media are the following host factors: sex (males have more middle ear disease than females); race (there is an extraordinary incidence of infection in some racial groups such as American Indians, Alaskan and Canadian Eskimos, and African and Australian aboriginal children); age at first episode (the earlier in life the first episode occurs, the more likely the child is to have recurrent disease); and sibling or parent history of severe or recurrent acute otitis media (suggesting a genetic basis for the disease).

Environmental factors that influence the incidence of acute otitis media include allergy to antigens and pollutants (including atmospheric conditions and air pollution) (Kim et al., 1996); exposure to smoke (Etzel et al., 1992); breast-feeding (infants who are breast-fed for as little as 3 months have less disease in the first year of life than children who are not breast-fed); season (the incidence of otitis media parallels the seasonal variations of respiratory tract infections); frequent exposure to infectious agents such as occurs in day-care centers (Wald et al., 1988); poverty and associated crowded living conditions and poor sanitation; and access to medical care. Parents with children who have problems with otitis media should be made aware of these risk factors. Although little can be done about most of the host factors, the incidence of otitis media may be reduced by encouraging breast-feeding and discouraging smoking in the household and attendance of the child in large group day care.

ETIOLOGY

The microbiology of otitis media has been documented by appropriate culture of middle ear fluids obtained by needle aspiration (Bluestone and Klein, 2001) (Table 24-1). The findings of bacteriologic studies performed in the United States and Scandinavia are remarkably consistent: *Streptococcus pneumoniae* is the most frequent agent in all age groups; *Haemophilus influenzae* is the next most frequent pathogen in all age groups; *Moraxella catarrhalis* is isolated from middle ear fluids with increasing frequency; *Streptococcus pyogenes* has been a significant pathogen in some studies from Scandinavia but not in studies done in the United States; and *Staphylococcus aureus*, gram-negative enteric bacilli, and anaerobic bacteria are infrequent causes of otitis media (Table 24-1).

TABLE 24-1 Bacterial Pathogens Isolated From Middle Ear Fluids in Children With Acute Otitis Media, 1985-1992[*]

Pathogen	Mean (%)	Range (%)
Streptococcus pneumoniae	38	27-52
Haemophilus influenzae	27	16-52
Moraxella catarrhalis	10	2-15
Streptococcus pyogenes	3	0-11
Staphylococcus aureus	2	0-16
None or nonpathogens	28	12-35

From Bluestone CD, Klein JO: Otitis Media in Infants and Children, ed 3. Philadelphia: Saunders, 2000;79.[*]Data from 12 reports from United States, Columbia, and Finland.

Because *S. pneumoniae* is the most important cause of otitis media, investigators have carefully studied the types responsible for infection of the middle ear. The results indicate that relatively few types are responsible for most disease. In recent studies (Eskola et al., 2001) the most common serotypes were 19F, 23F, 11, 15, 6A, and 19A. All are included in the currently available 23-type polysaccharide pneumococcal vaccine; 6B, 14, 19F, and 23F are included in the valent conjugate pneumococcal vaccine. Otitis media caused by *H. influenzae* is associated with nontypeable strains in the vast majority of patients. At one time *H. influenzae* was believed to be of limited importance to otitis media in school-age children and adolescents, but several studies indicate that this organism is a significant cause of otitis media in all age groups (Grönroos et al., 1964; Herberts et al., 1971; Howie et al., 1970; Schwartz et al., 1977).

Gram-negative enteric bacilli are responsible for approximately 20% of cases of otitis media in young infants (to 6 weeks of age), but these organisms are rarely present in the middle ear effusion of older children. Other than the greater prevalence of otitis media caused by gram-negative bacilli and the presence of other organisms responsible for neonatal sepsis such as group B streptococci and *S. aureus*, the bacteriology of otitis in the infant up to 6 weeks of age is similar to that in older children (Table 24-2) (Berman et al., 1978; Bland, 1972; Shurin et al., 1978; Tetzlaff et al., 1977).

Studies in Cleveland (Shurin et al., 1983) and Pittsburgh (Kovatch et al., 1983) indicate a significant increase in isolation of *M. catarrhalis*. During 1980 and 1981, *M. catarrhalis* was iso-

TABLE 24-2 Bacterial Pathogens Isolated From 169 Infants With Otitis Media During the First 6 Weeks of Life[*]

Pathogen	Percent of infants with microorganism
Respiratory bacteria	
Streptococcus pneumoniae	18.3
Haemophilus influenzae	12.4
S. pneumoniae and H. influenzae	3.0
Staphylococcus aureus	7.7
Streptococci, groups A and B	3.0
Moraxella catarrhalis	5.3
Enteric bacteria	
Escherichia coli	5.9
Klebsiella-Enterobacter	5.3
Pseudomonas aeruginosa	1.8
Miscellaneous	5.3
None or nonpathogens	32.0

[*]Reports from Honolulu, Hawaii (Bland, 1972); Dallas, Texas (Tetzlaff et al., 1977); Denver, Colorado (Berman et al., 1978); and Huntsville, Alabama and Boston, Massachusetts (Shurin et al., 1978).

lated from 27% and 19% of children with acute otitis media, respectively. Approximately three fourths of the isolates produced β-lactamase and were therefore resistant to ampicillin. Other bacteria responsible for occasional cases of acute otitis media include group A *Streptococcus, S. aureus,* anaerobic bacteria, and, in developing countries, *Mycobacterium tuberculosis, Clostridium tetani,* and *Corynebacterium diphtheriae.*

Use of polymerase chain reaction (PCR) assay for bacterial and viral genome sequences adds an additional technique for identifying the role of microorganisms in middle ear fluids. Post and colleagues (1995) identified DNA of *S. pneumoniae, H. influenzae,* and *M. catarrhalis* in 97 middle ear fluids of patients with otitis media with effusion; 30% were both culture and PCR positive, but an additional 48% were PCR positive and culture negative for these bacterial species.

Epidemiologic data suggest that viral infection is associated with acute otitis media (Henderson et al., 1982). Respiratory syncytial virus (RSV), influenza virus, rhinoviruses, and enteroviruses with or without concurrent bacterial pathogens (Arola et al., 1990; Chonmaitree et al., 1986) have been isolated from middle ear fluids from some children. In addition, there is evidence of viral infection obtained by enzyme-linked immunosorbent assay (ELISA) techniques that identify viral antigens in middle ear fluids in children with acute otitis media (Klein et al., 1982). Ruuskanen et al. (1991) summarized eight studies published between 1982 and 1990 using immunoassay or isolation; virus was

identified in middle ear fluids in 17% of samples. Pitkaranta and colleagues (1998) found evidence of rhinovirus RNA in 22% of patients with acute otitis media and 19% of patients with otitis media with effusion; evidence of RSV infection was found in 18% and 8%; and coronavirus in 7% and 3% of the fluids from acute and chronic infections.

Only one report of isolation of a mycoplasma *(Mycoplasma pneumoniae)* from middle ear fluid of a child with acute otitis media has been reported (Sobeslavsky et al., 1965). *Chlamydia trachomatis* infection results in a mild but prolonged pneumonitis in infants and may be accompanied by otitis media. *C. trachomatis* has been isolated from middle ear fluids of such infants (Tipple et al., 1979). *Chlamydia pneumoniae* has been isolated uncommonly from the middle ear fluids of children with acute otitis media but more frequently from children with otitis media with effusion (Storgaard et al., 1997).

PATHOGENESIS

The pathogenesis of otitis media must be approached with the understanding that the disease involves a system having contiguous parts, including the nares, nasopharynx, eustachian tube, middle ear, and mastoid antrum and air cells (Figure 24-1). The middle ear resembles a flattened box, which is approximately 15 mm from top to bottom, 10 mm wide, and only 2 to 6 mm deep. The lateral wall includes the tympanic membrane, and the medial wall includes the oval and round windows. The mastoid air cells lie behind, and the

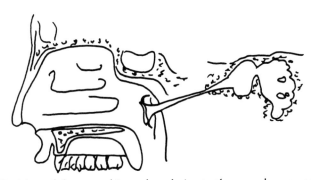

Fig. 24-1 Position of the eustachian tube relative to the nasopharynx and the middle ear. The eustachian tube is a double-horned organ with the proximal two thirds lying in cartilage and the distal one third in bone. The segments are connected by the narrow isthmus, the site most vulnerable to obstruction. Thus the system consists of the nares, nasopharynx, eustachian tube, middle ear, and mastoid air cells.

orifice of the eustachian tube is in the superior portion of the front wall.

The eustachian tube connects the middle ear with the posterior nasopharynx, and its lateral one third lies in bone and is open. The medial two thirds are in cartilage, and the walls are in apposition except during swallowing or yawning. In the young infant the eustachian tube is both shorter and proportionately wider than in the older child; the cartilaginous and osseous portions of the tube form a relatively straight line. In an older child the angle of the tube is more acute. These anatomic differences may predispose some infants to early and repeated illness.

The eustachian tube has at least three important physiologic functions with respect to the middle ear: protection of the ear from nasopharyngeal secretions, drainage into the nasopharynx of secretions produced within the middle ear, and ventilation of the middle ear to equalize air pressure within the box with pressure in the external ear canal. When one or more of these functions is compromised, the result may be obstruction of the tube, accumulation of secretions in the middle ear, and, if pyogenic organisms are present, development of suppurative otitis media. Dysfunction of the eustachian tube because of anatomic or physiologic factors apparently is the most important feature of the pathogenesis of infection of the middle ear.

The most likely sequence of events in most episodes of acute otitis media includes an antecedent event (usually caused by an upper respiratory viral infection) that results in congestion of the respiratory mucosa; congestion of the mucosa in the eustachian tube results in obstruction of the narrowest portion of the tube, the isthmus; the obstruction results in negative pressure in the middle ear and then development of middle ear effusion; the secretions of the mucosa of the middle ear, which usually drain through the eustachian tube, now have no egress and accumulate in the middle ear; if pathogenic bacteria that colonize the nasopharynx are present in the middle ear after obstruction of the tube has taken place, the organisms multiply, resulting in an acute suppurative infection.

CLINICAL MANIFESTATIONS

Otalgia (ear pain), otorrhea (ear drainage), hearing impairment affecting one or both ears, and fever suggest infection of the middle ear. However, many children with otitis media do not have these signs. Infants may manifest only general signs of distress, including irritability, bouts of crying, diarrhea, and feeding problems. Less commonly, the patient may exhibit conjunctivitis or complain of vertigo or tinnitus. Swelling about the ear may be a sign of mastoiditis. Acute otitis media is defined by the presence of middle ear effusion accompanied by a sign or symptom of acute illness.

Hyperemia of the tympanic membrane caused by injection of blood vessels is an early sign of otitis media. However, redness of the tympanic membrane may be caused by inflammation elsewhere in the system, because the mucous membrane is continuous from the nares and eustachian tube and lines the walls of the middle ear cleft. Thus a "red ear" alone does not establish the diagnosis of otitis media.

Fluid in the middle ear persists for variable periods of time after onset of the acute episode. At the conclusion of a 10- to 14-day course of antimicrobial therapy, one half to two thirds of children still have fluid in the middle ear. The fluid in the middle ear persists in approximately 40% of children at 1 month, 20% at 2 months, and 10% at 3 months after onset of acute otitis.

DIAGNOSIS
Clinical

For optimal assessment of the tympanic membrane and its mobility, a pneumatic otoscope should be used. The otoscopic examination should include observation of the following conditions of the tympanic membrane:

- *Position*—Normal is slightly convex; bulging indicates increased pressure from positive air pressure or fluid; a retracted drum indicates negative pressure with or without effusion.
- *Appearance and color*—The normal color is pearly gray and translucent; congestion of the mucous membrane is indicated by a pink appearance of the membrane; a blue discoloration suggests blood in the middle ear, sometimes associated with basal skull fracture; acute suppurative otitis usually is reflected in a bright red or red-yellow membrane.
- *Integrity*—The four quadrants of the membrane should be inspected for perforation, retraction pockets, or cholesteatoma.

- *Mobility*—The normal tympanic membrane moves inward with positive pressure and outward with negative pressure (Figure 24-2). The motion observed is proportional to the pressure applied by gently squeezing and then releasing the rubber bulb attachment on the head of the otoscope. Normal mobility of the tympanic membrane is indicated when positive and then negative pressure is applied and the membrane moves rapidly inward and outward like a sail in a brisk wind. Either presence of fluid in the middle ear or high negative middle ear pressure dampens tympanic membrane mobility.

Tympanometry uses an electroacoustic impedance bridge to record compliance of the tympanic membrane and middle ear pressure. Many instruments are available for use in pediatric practice. After a small probe is inserted into the external canal by means of a snug-fitting cuff, a tone of fixed characteristics is delivered by an oscillator-amplifier through the probe. A microphone measures the compliance of the tympanic membrane while a pump manometer varies the external canal pressure. The tone is delivered at a given intensity as the air pressure in the canal is varied over a positive and negative range. The recording that results—the tympanogram—reflects the dynamics of the middle ear system, including the tympanic membrane, middle ear, mastoid air cells, and eustachian tube. The technique is reliable, simple, and readily carried out by nonprofessional personnel. However, there are technical problems in applications of presently available instruments to young children, particularly those less than 7 months of age. Tympanometry is of particular value in diagnosis of ambiguous cases of otitis media, in screening for ear disease, and in training of students and young physicians.

Acoustic reflectometry uses principles of reflected energy from the middle ear space to provide information about the presence or absence of middle ear effusion. A microphone located in the probe tip measures the level of transmitted and reflected sound. Acoustic energy is reflected back toward the probe tip from the ear canal and eardrum. The more sound reflected, the greater is the likelihood of the presence of an effusion. In contrast to tympanometry, a seal of the probe is not required, and the reading of reflected sound is almost instantaneous. A hand-held, lightweight portable instrument is available for clinical use (EarCheck, MDI Instruments, Chesree, New Jersey) and there is a similar device for home use.

Radiography

Roentgenographic evaluation of the temporal bone is indicated when complications or sequelae of otitis media are suspect or present. Plain radiographs are of limited value in the diagnosis of mastoiditis or cholesteatoma; computed tomography (CT) and magnetic resonance imaging (MRI) are more precise and should be obtained if a suppurative intratemporal or intracranial complication is suspected.

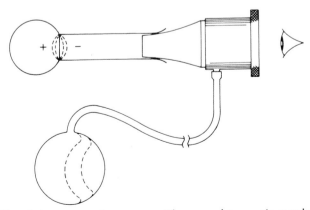

Fig. 24-2 Use of the pneumatic otoscope. The normal tympanic membrane moves inward with positive pressure in the ear canal and outward with negative pressure. The presence of effusion or negative pressure dampens movement of the tympanic membrane.

Microbiology

The results of bacterial cultures of the nasopharynx and oropharynx correlate poorly with those of middle ear fluids. The results are sensitive but not specific for the middle ear pathogen. Thus cultures of the upper respiratory tract are of limited value in specific bacteriologic diagnosis of otitis media. If the child is in a toxic state or has localized infection elsewhere, culture of blood and/or the focus of infection should be performed.

Needle aspiration of a middle ear effusion provides immediate and specific information about the bacteriology of the infection. Although the consistent results of investigations of the bacteriology of acute otitis media provide a guide to the most likely pathogens, *S. pneumoniae* and *H. influenzae,* needle aspiration should be considered in selected children. These children include those who are critically ill at first visit and those who fail to respond adequately to initial therapy and remain in a toxic state and febrile 48 to 72 hours after onset of therapy. Also included are patients with altered host defenses who may be infected with an unusual agent, such as those with malignancy or immunosuppressive disease, newborn infants, and those with chronic otitis media. When spontaneous perforation occurs, the exudate in the ear canal is contaminated with flora from the canal. Culture should be obtained, after cleansing the canal with alcohol, by needle aspiration of fluid emerging from the area of perforation or preferably from within the middle ear.

COMPLICATIONS AND SEQUELAE

Suppurative complications of acute infection of the middle ear are now uncommon in areas where children have access to medical care. Contiguous spread of infection, however, may be responsible for mastoiditis, petrositis, labyrinthitis, brain abscess, and meningitis.

Of more concern, at present, is impairment of hearing associated with fluid in the middle ear. Audiograms of children with middle ear effusion usually indicate a mild to moderate conductive hearing loss. The median loss is approximately 25 dB (Fria et al., 1985), which is the equivalent of putting plugs in the ears. The hearing loss is conductive and due to the presence of fluid in the middle ear and is less influenced by the quality of fluid (serous, mucoid, or purulent) than by its volume (partially or completely filling the middle ear

space). The conductive hearing impairment is usually reversed with resolution of the middle ear effusion. High negative pressure in the middle ear or atelectasis, both in the absence of middle ear effusion, may also result in conductive hearing loss.

Sensorineural hearing loss is uncommonly associated with otitis media. Permanent sensorineural loss has been described, presumably as a result of the spread of microorganisms or products of inflammation through the round window membrane or because of a suppurative complication of acute otitis media such as labyrinthitis. Permanent hearing loss also may result from irreversible inflammatory changes, including adhesive otitis media and ossicular discontinuity.

The significance of hearing loss associated with acute infection or persistent middle ear effusion is uncertain. Retrospective studies suggest that chronic middle ear disease with effusion occurring during the first few years of life has adverse effects on development of speech and language, hearing, intelligence, and performance in school (Holm and Kunze, 1969; Kaplan et al., 1973; Lewis, 1976; Needleman, 1977; Teele et al., 1990; Zinkus et al., 1978).

Longitudinal studies indicate that children who have had recurrent episodes of otitis media or persistent middle ear effusion perform less well on tests of speech, language, and cognitive abilities than do their disease-free peers. These data suggest that delay or impairment of development may be an important sequela of otitis media. Boston children observed for ear disease from birth were evaluated at age 7 years by Teele et al. (1990). Estimated time with middle ear effusion during the first 3 years of life was associated significantly with lower scores on tests of cognitive abilities (full-scale, performance, and verbal intelligence quotients), speech and language (articulation and use of morphologic markers), and school performance (lower scores in mathematics and reading).

TREATMENT
Acute Otitis Media

The preferred antimicrobial agent for the patient with otitis media must be active against *S. pneumoniae, H. influenzae,* and *M. catarrhalis.* Group A streptococci and *S. aureus* are infrequent causes of acute otitis media and need not be considered in initial therapeutic decisions. Gram-negative enteric bacilli must be considered when otitis media occurs in the newborn infant, in the patient with a depressed immune response, and in the patient with suppurative complications of chronic otitis media.

Surveys of susceptibilities of *S. pneumoniae* in the United States identify increasing rates of multidrug resistance beginning in the mid 1980s. A survey of 51 medical centers in 1996 and 1997 by Thornsberry and colleagues (1999) found that 36% of strains were nonsusceptible to penicillin; about one half of these were highly resistant, suggesting possible clinical failure. The prevalence of resistance varied by region, with rates highest in the South East and South Central States and lowest in New England and the Midwest. Most of the penicillin-resistant strains were also resistant to cephalosporins and include variable patterns of resistance to macrolides and sulfonamides. The basis for resistance to penicillins and cephalosporins is alteration of the penicillin-binding proteins with less affinity for the drug. The resistance is indicated by increments in the amount of drug required to inhibit the organism—the minimum inhibitory concentration (MIC). Penicillin-susceptible organisms have MICs <0.1 ug/ml; intermediate strains are defined as having MICs of 0.1 to 1.0 ug/ml; and resistant strains have MICs ≥2 ug/ml. Risk factors for multidrug resistant pneumococci

include use of an antimicrobial agent in the preceding 28 days, hospitalization, and out-of-home day care. No clinical features distinguish infection with resistant organisms from infection with susceptible organisms, and there does not appear to be increased virulence with disease caused by resistant strains.

Almost all resistance of *H. influenzae* to susceptible penicillins (including penicillins G and V, ampicillin and amoxicillin, and carbenicillin and ticarcillin) is based on production of β-lactamase; the enzyme cleaves the β-lactam ring of susceptible penicillins, rendering the drug inactive against the organism. The vast majority of *M. catarrhalis* strains are β-lactamase producers. The proportion of β-lactamase–producing strains of *H. influenzae* isolated from middle ear fluids in the United States in recent years is approximately 40% (Jacobs et al., 1999).

The U.S. Food and Drug Administration has approved 17 products for treatment of acute otitis media (Table 24-3) and an eighteenth ototopical agent, ofloxacin otic, for management of acute otorrhea in children who have tympanostomy tubes in place. Amoxicillin remains the drug of choice because it continues to be effective, safe, and relatively inexpensive (Dowell et al., 1999). Doubling the dosage schedule from 40 mg/kg/day to 80 mg/kg/day in 2 doses increases the concentration of the drug

TABLE 24-3 **Antimicrobial Agents for Acute Otitis Media and Dosage Schedules**

Drug (trade name)	No. doses × day	Dosage (kg/day)
Amoxicillin (Amoxil)	2-3/day × 10	40-80 mg
Amoxicillin-clavulanate (Augmentin)	2/day × 10	40-80 mg
Azithromycin (Zithromax)	1/day × 1	30 mg
	1/day × 3	10 mg
	1/day × 1	10 mg
	Followed by 1/day × 2-5	5 mg
Clarithromycin (Biaxin)	2/day × 10	15 mg
Erythromycin-sulfisoxazole (Pediazole)	4/day × 10	50-150 mg
Ceftriaxone (Rocephin)	1 IM × 1-3	50 mg
Ceftibuten (Cedax)	1/day × 10	9 mg
Loracarbef (Lorabid)	2/day × 10	30 mg
Cefprozil (Cefzil)	2/day × 10	30 mg
Cefpodoxime (Vantin)	2/day × 5	10 mg
Cefuroxime axetil (Ceftin)	2/day × 10	30 mg
Cefaclor (Ceclor)	3/day × 10	40 mg
Cefdinir (Omnicef)	1/day × 10	14 mg
	2/day × 5 or 10	7 mg
Cefixime (Suprax)	1/day × 10	8 mg
Trimethoprim-sulfamethoxazole (Bactrim, Septra)	2/day × 10	8-40 mg
Trimethoprim (Primsol)	2/day × 10	10 mg

in the middle ear fluid (Seikel et al., 1997) and is recommended in communities with increased rates of penicillin-nonsusceptible strains (more than 25%). Although most experts agree on the continued use of amoxicillin as the drug of choice for initial treatment of acute otitis media, there is less consensus on the appropriate drug to use when amoxicillin fails. A Centers for Disease Control and Prevention consensus report suggested amoxicillin clavulanate (80 to 90 mg/kg/day in 2 doses), cefuroxime axetil, and intramuscular ceftriaxone (Dowell et al., 1999). A macrolide (erythromycin plus sulfisoxazole, azithromycin, or clarithromycin) is the preferred drug for acute otitis media for children who are allergic to β-lactam antibiotics; trimethoprim sulfamethoxazole is now less useful for otitis media because of high rates of resistance.

Nasal and oral decongestants, administered either alone or in combination with an antihistamine, are currently among the most popular medications for the treatment of acute otitis media with effusion. The common concept is that these drugs reduce congestion of the respiratory mucosa and relieve the obstruction of the eustachian tube that results from inflammation caused by respiratory infection. The results of clinical trials, however, indicate no significant evidence of efficacy of any of these preparations used alone or in combination for relief of signs of disease or decrease in time that fluid remains in the middle ear after acute infection (Collip, 1961; Fraser et al., 1977; Olson et al., 1978).

Chronic Otitis Media With Effusion

Appropriate management of the child with chronic otitis media remains controversial. The difficulty of arriving at a consensus for management of otitis media with effusion is reflected in an extensive review published by the Agency for Health Care Policy and Research of the U.S. Department of Health and Human Services (Stool et al., 1994b). The major goal of management of persistent middle ear effusion is to achieve and maintain an aerated middle ear that is free of fluid and has a normal mucosa. Current therapies of otitis media with effusion include courses of antimicrobial agents, with or without steroids, myringotomy, adenoidectomy, and use of tympanostomy (ventilating) tubes.

Another 10-day course of a broad-spectrum antimicrobial agent that has activity against β-lactamase–producing organisms should be considered before surgical intervention. Bacterial pathogens are found in approximately one quarter of patients with otitis media with effusion, and a metaanalysis of blinded studies (Stool et al., 1994a) identified resolution of the effusion in 14% of cases after the additional course of antimicrobial agent. Steroid therapy alone or with an antibiotic has been demonstrated to be effective in some children with otitis media with effusion. Berman (1995) recommended a regimen of prednisone, 1 mg/kg/day given orally in 2 doses for 7 days, with an antibiotic for 14 to 21 days.

Before the introduction of antimicrobial agents, myringotomy was the major method of managing suppurative otitis media. Currently, use of myringotomy is limited to the relief of intractable ear pain, hastening resolution of mastoid infection, and drainage of persistent middle ear effusion that is unresponsive to medical therapy. The procedure is of limited value in otitis media with effusion, because the incision heals quickly and before the middle ear mucosa has normalized.

Enlarged adenoids may obstruct the orifice of the eustachian tube in the posterior portion of the nasopharynx and interfere with adequate ventilation and drainage of the middle ear. Recent studies of the use of adenoidectomy in children with prolonged effusions in the middle ear identify a beneficial effect in reducing time spent with effusion in selected children (Gates et al., 1987; Paradise et al., 1990).

Tympanostomy tubes, resembling small collar buttons placed in the tympanic membrane, provide drainage of middle ear fluid and ventilate the middle ear. The effect in children who have impaired hearing because of the presence of fluid is restoration of normal hearing. Placement of the tube treats the effect rather than the cause of the persistent effusion. The criteria for placement of ventilating tubes, management of tubes once they are placed, and long-term benefits, if any, are uncertain. The indications for placement of tympanostomy tubes include persistent middle ear effusions that are unresponsive to adequate medical treatment, persistent tympanic membrane retraction pockets with impending cholesteatoma, and persistent negative pressure with significant hearing loss (Bluestone and Shurin, 1974). Follow-up management of children with tympanostomy tubes requires close liaison between the primary care provider and the otolaryngologist. Guidelines for following such children were presented by the American Academy of Pediatrics (American Academy of Pediatrics, 2002).

PREVENTION
Advising Parents

Parents of children who have severe and recurrent otitis media or risk factors for middle ear infections should be advised of measures that may reduce the incidence of infection, such as breast-feeding; enrolling children in small rather than large, group day-care centers; and reducing exposure to tobacco smoke.

Chemoprophylaxis

Chemoprophylaxis has been successful in reducing the number of new symptomatic episodes of acute otitis media in children who have a history of recurrent infections. The results of 15 reports of controlled clinical trials of modified courses of antimicrobial agents compared with those in which placebo or historic controls were used were reviewed recently (Klein, 1994). The majority of studies used a sulfonamide or a broad-spectrum penicillin. All of the reports indicated benefit to the enrollees in reduction of new episodes when they were compared with controls. The interested reader should review selected original studies (Biedel, 1978; Liston et al., 1983; Maynard et al., 1972; Perrin et al., 1974; Principi et al., 1989; Schuller, 1983; Schwartz et al., 1982). The data are persuasive that children who are prone to recurrent episodes of acute infection of the middle ear are benefited by the following program:

1. Enrollment criteria—children who have had three documented episodes of acute otitis media in 6 months or four episodes in 12 months
2. Drugs and dosage—amoxicillin or sulfisoxazole offers the advantages of demonstrated efficacy, safety, and low cost; the drugs can be administered once a day in one half the therapeutic dosage (sulfisoxazole, 50 mg/kg of body weight; amoxicillin, 20 mg/kg)
3. Duration—approximately 6 months, usually during the winter and spring seasons when respiratory tract infections are most frequent
4. Observation—children should be examined at approximately 1-month intervals when free of acute signs to determine if middle ear effusion is present; management of

prolonged middle ear effusion should be considered separately from prevention of recurrences of acute infection.

Chemoprophylaxis should be used selectively because a modified dosage schedule of antibiotic used continuously may result in colonization with bacteria resistant to the agent used. Breakthrough episodes should be treated with an alternative antibiotic likely to be effective against resistant strains (see discussion of treatment).

Bacterial Vaccines

A conjugate vaccine combining the polysaccharides of the pneumococcus with a protein carrier, a diphtheria toxin mutant (CRM_{197}), was approved by the Food and Drug Administration in February 2000. The vaccine contains polysaccharides for the serotypes 4, 6B, 9V, 14, 18C, 19F, and 23 F. The vaccine is immunogenic in children as young as 2 months (Black et al., 2000; Fireman et al., 2003). Protective titers were achieved after doses administered at ages 2, 4, and 6 months but waned during the following 6 months, necessitating a booster between ages 12 and 15 months.

The vaccine was effective in preventing vaccine-type invasive disease (97.4% in fully immunized infants) and pneumonia (35% decrease for radiographically identifiable disease) (Black et al., 2000). In contrast, only a 7% reduction in episodes of acute otitis media occurred. A 25% reduction in surgical procedures for placement of tympanostomy tubes occurred in the cohort of children who received the conjugate pneumococcal vaccine, suggested that the vaccine was most effective for infants who were susceptible to recurrent infections (and would be candidates for the surgical procedure).

Bacteriologic efficacy of the conjugate pneumococcal vaccine was evaluated in studies of Finnish children (Eskola et al., 2001). The reduction of episodes of acute otitis media (7%) was similar to that in California children. The microbiologic data identified a 57% decrease in episodes due to vaccine serotype pneumococcal otitis media, a 51% decrease in acute otitis media due to cross-reactive pneumococcal serotypes, and a 34% decrease for culture-confirmed pneumococcal acute otitis media (irrespective of the serotype). Of concern were a 33% increase in episodes of acute otitis media due to serotypes not in the vaccine and an 11% increase in disease caused by *H. influenzae*. Thus, the efficacy of the conjugate pneumococcal vaccine for prevention of new episodes of pneumococcal otitis media was more modest than the efficacy of the vaccine for invasive pneumococcal disease.

Each pneumococcal antigen in the currently available 23-type polysaccharide vaccine produces an independent antibody response in children beginning at 2 years of age and in adults. Antibody develops in about 2 weeks, and the polysaccharide vaccine should be considered in conjunction with the conjugate vaccine for children older than 2 years of age who are still suffering recurrent episodes of acute otitis media.

Because the vast majority of *H. influenzae* strains responsible for otitis media are nontypeable and current vaccines are prepared from type b capsular polysaccharide, prospects for a vaccine against nontypeable strains lie in the future.

Viral Vaccines

Influenza virus vaccine resulted in a reduction of cases of influenza A as well as a 36% decline in otitis media in children attending a day-care center (Clements et al., 1995). A similar reduction (30%) in episodes of febrile otitis media was reported in children after administration of a live attenuated cold-adapted intranasal influenza vaccine (Belshe et al., 1998). The intranasal vaccine was approved by the Food and Drug Administration in December 2002 but only for healthy subjects 5 to 49 years old; use of the vaccine for infants and toddlers is expected at a later time. Use of available influenza virus vaccines should be part of the strategy for reducing the incidence of acute otitis media for children with recurrent and severe disease.

RSV is the viral pathogen most closely associated with acute otitis media. Immunoprophylaxis against RSV is available with use of high-titered RSV immune globulin (Simoes et al., 1996) and with a high-titered RSV monoclonal antibody, palivizumab (Impact-RSV Study Group, 1998). The RSV immune globulin, but not the monoclonal antibody, was effective in reducing the number of episodes of acute otitis media.

BIBLIOGRAPHY

American Academy of Pediatrics. Follow-up management of children with tympanostomy tubes. Pediatrics 2002;109:328-329.

Arola M, Ruuskanen O, Ziegler T, et al. Clinical role of respiratory virus infection in acute otitis media. Pediatrics 1990;86:848-855.

Belshe RB, Mendelman PM, Treanor J, et al. The efficacy of live, attenuated, cold-adapted, trivalent, intranasal influenza virus vaccine in children. N Engl J Med 1998;338:1459-1461.

Berman S. Otitis media in children. N Engl J Med 1995;332:1560-1565.

Berman SA, Balkany TJ, Simmons MA. Otitis media in infants less than 12 weeks of age: differing bacteriology among inpatients and outpatients. J Pediatr 1978;93:453-454.

Biedel CW. Modification of recurrent otitis media by short-term sulfonamide therapy. Am J Dis Child 1978;132:681-683.

Black S, Shinefield H, Fireman B, et al. Efficacy, safety and immunogenicity of heptavalent pneumococcal conjugate vaccine in children. Pediatr Infect Dis J 2000;19:187-195.

Bland RD. Otitis media in the first six weeks of life: diagnosis, bacteriology, and management. Pediatrics 1972;49:187.

Bluestone CD, Klein JO. Otitis Media in Infants and Children, ed 3. Philadelphia: Saunders, 2001.

Bluestone CD, Shurin PA. Middle ear disease in children. Pathogenesis, diagnosis, and management. Pediatr Clin North Am 1974;21:379.

Chonmaitree T, Howie VM, Truant AL. Presence of respiratory viruses in middle ear fluids and nasal wash specimens from children with acute otitis media. Pediatrics 1986;77:698.

Clements DA, Langdon L, Bland C, Walter E. Influenza A vaccine decreases the incidence of otitis media in 6 to 30 month old children in day care. Arch Pediatr Adolesc Med 1995;149:1113-1117.

Collip PJ. Evaluation of nose drops for otitis media in children. Northwest Med 1961;60:999.

Dowell SF, Butler JC, Giebink GS, et al. Acute otitis media: management and surveillance in an era of pneumococcal resistance—a report from the Drug-Resistant *Streptococcus pneumoniae* Therapeutic Working Group. Pediatr Infect Dis J 1999;18:1-9.

Eskola J, Kilpi T, Palmu A, et al. Efficacy of a pneumococcal conjugate vaccine against acute otitis media. N Engl J Med 2001;344:403-409.

Etzel RA, Pattishall EN, Haley NJ, et al. Passive smoking and middle ear effusion among children in day care. Pediatrics 1992;90:228-232.

Fireman B, Black SB, Shinefield HR, et al. Impact of the pneumococcal conjugate vaccine on otitis media. Pediatr Infect Dis 2003;22:10-16.

Fraser JG, Mehta M, Fraser PM. The medical treatment of secretory otitis media: a clinical trial of three commonly used regimens. J Laryngol Otol 1977;91:757.

Fria TJ, Cantekin EI, Eichler JA. Hearing acuity of children with otitis media with effusion. Arch Otolaryngol 1985;111:10-16.

Gates GA, Avery CA, Prihoda TJ, Cooper JC. Effectiveness of adenoidectomy and tympanostomy tubes in the treatment of chronic otitis media with effusion. N Engl J Med 1987;317:1444-1451.

Grönroos JA, et al. The etiology of acute middle ear infection. Acta Otolaryngol 1964;58:149.

Henderson FW, Collier AM, Sanyal MA, et al. A longitudinal study of respiratory viruses and bacteria in the etiology of acute otitis media with effusion. N Engl J Med 1982; 306:1377-1383.

Herberts G, Jeppsson PH, Nylen O. Acute otitis media. Pract Otorhinolaryngol 1971;33:191.

Holm VA, Kunze LH. Effect of chronic otitis media on language and speech development. Pediatrics 1969;43:833.

Howie V, Ploussard J, Lester R. Otitis media: a clinical and bacteriologic correlation. Pediatrics 1970;45:29.

Impact-RSV Study Group. Palivizumab, a humanized respiratory syncytial virus monoclonal antibody, reduces hospitalization from respiratory syncytial virus infection in high-risk infants. Pediatrics 1998;102:531-537.

Jacobs MR, Bajaksouzian S, Zilles A, et al. Susceptibilities of *Streptococcus pneumoniae* and *Haemophilus influenzae* to 10 oral antimicrobial agents based on pharmacodynamic parameters: 1997 U.S. surveillance study. Antimicrob Agents Chemother 1999;43:1901-1908.

Kaplan GJ, et al. Long-term effects of otitis media. A ten-year cohort study of Alaskan Eskimo children. Pediatrics 1973;52:577.

Kim PE, Musher DM, Glezen WP, et al. Association of invasive pneumococcal diseases with season, atmospheric condition, air pollution, and the isolation of respiratory viruses. Clin Infect Dis 1996;22:100-106.

Klein BS, Dollette FR, Yolken RH. The role of respiratory syncytial virus and other viral pathogens in acute otitis media. J Pediatr 1982;101:16-20.

Klein JO. Preventing recurrent otitis: what role for antibiotics? Contemp Pediatr 1994;11:44-60.

Kovatch AJ, Wald ER, Michaels RH. β-Lactamase–producing *Branhamella catarrhalis* causing otitis media in children. J Pediatr 1983;102:261-264.

Lewis N. Otitis media and linguistic incompetence. Arch Otolaryngol 1976;102:387.

Liston TE, Foshee WS, Pierson WD. Sulfisoxazole chemoprophylaxis for frequent otitis media. Pediatrics 1983;71:524-530.

Maynard JE, Fleshman JK, Tschopp CF. Otitis media in Alaskan Eskimo children. JAMA 1972;219:597-599.

Needleman H. Effects of hearing loss from early recurrent otitis media on speech and language development. In Jaffee B (ed). Hearing Loss in Children. Baltimore: University Park Press, 1977.

Olson AL, Klein SW, Charney E, et al. Prevention and therapy of serous otitis media by oral decongestant: a double-blind study in pediatric practice. Pediatrics 1978;61:679.

Paradise JL, Bluestone CD, Rogers KD, et al. Efficacy of adenoidectomy for recurrent otitis media in children previously treated with tympanostomy-tube placement: results of parallel randomized and non-randomized trials. JAMA 1990;263:2066-2073.

Perrin JM, et al. Sulfisoxazole as chemoprophylaxis for recurrent otitis media. A double-blind crossover study in pediatric practice. N Engl J Med 1974;291:664.

Pitkaranta A, Virolainen A, Jero J, et al. Detection of rhinovirus, respiratory syncytial virus and coronavirus infections in acute otitis media by reverse transcriptase polymerase chain reaction. Pediatrics 1998;102:291-299.

Post JC, Preston RA, Aul JJ, et al. Molecular analysis of bacterial pathogens in otitis media with effusion. JAMA 1995;273:1598-1604.

Principi N, Marchisio P, Massironi E, et al. Prophylaxis of recurrent acute otitis media and middle-ear effusion: comparison of amoxicillin with sulfamethoxazole and trimethoprim. Am J Dis Child 1989;143:1414-1418.

Ruuskanen O, Arola M, Heikkinen T, et al. Viruses in acute otitis media: increasing evidence for clinical significance. Pediatr Infect Dis J 1991;10:425.

Schuller DE. Prophylaxis of otitis media in asthmatic children. Pediatr Infect Dis 1983;2:280-283.

Schwartz R, Rodriguez J, Khan WN, Ross S. Acute purulent otitis media in children older than 5 years: incidence of *Haemophilus* as a causative organism. JAMA 1977;238:1032.

Schwartz RH, Puglise J, Rodriguez WJ. Sulfamethoxazole prophylaxis in the otitis media–prone child. Arch Dis Child 1982;57:590-593.

Seikel K, Shelton S, McCracken GH Jr. Middle ear fluid concentrations of amoxicillin after large dosages in children with acute otitis media. Pediatr Infect Dis J 1997;16:710-711.

Shurin PA, et al. Bacterial etiology of otitis media during the first six weeks of life. J Pediatr 1978;92:893.

Shurin PA, Marchant CD, Kim CH, et al. Emergence of beta-lactamase-producing strains of *Branhamella catarrhalis* as important agents of acute otitis media. Pediatr Infect Dis 1983;2:34-38.

Simoes EA, Groothuis JR, Tristram DA, et al. Respiratory syncytial virus–enriched globulin for the prevention of acute otitis media in high risk children. J Pediatr 1996;129:214-219.

Sobeslavsky O, et al. The etiological role of *Mycoplasma pneumoniae* in otitis media in children. Pediatrics 1965;35:652.

Stool SE, Berg AO, Berman S, et al. Otitis media with effusion in young children. Clinical practice guideline. Number 12. AHCPR Publication No 94-0622. Rockville, Md: Agency for Health Care Policy and Research, Public Health Service, U.S. Department of Health and Human Services, July 1994a, p 52.

Stool SE, Berg AO, Carney CJ, et al. Managing otitis media with effusion in young children. Quick reference guide for clinicians. AHCPR Publication No 94-0623. Rockville, Md: Agency for Health Care Policy and Research, Public Health Service, U.S. Department of Health and Human Services, July 1994b.

Storgaard M, Ostergaard L, Jensen JS, et al. *Chlamydia pneumoniae* in children with otitis media. Clin Infect Dis 1997;25:1090-1093.

Teele DW, Klein JO, Chase C, et al. Otitis media in infancy and intellectual ability, school achievement, speech, and language at age 7 years. J Infect Dis 1990;162:685-694.

Teele DW, Klein JO, Rosner B, Greater Boston Otitis Media Study Group. Epidemiology of otitis media during the first seven years of life in children in greater Boston: a prospective, cohort study. J Infect Dis 1989;160:83-94.

Tetzlaff TR, Ashworth C, Nelson ND. Otitis media in children less than 12 weeks of age. Pediatrics 1977;59:827-832.

Thornsberry C, Olivie PT, Holley HP Jr, Sahm DF. Survey of susceptibilities of *Streptococcus pneumoniae*, *Haemophilus influenzae* and *Moraxella catarrhalis* isolates to 26 antimicrobial agents: a prospective U.S. study. Antimicrob Agents Chemother 1999; 43:2612-2623.

Tipple MA, Beem MO, Saxon EM. Clinical characteristics of afebrile pneumonia associated with *Chlamydia trachomatis* infections in infants less than 6 months of age. Pediatrics 1979;63:192.

Wald ER, Dashefshy B, Byers C, et al. Frequency and severity of infections in day care. J Pediatr 1988;112:540-544.

Welby PL, Keller DS, Cromien JL, et al. Resistance to penicillin and non-β-lactam antibiotics of *Streptococcus pneumoniae* at a children's hospital. Pediatr Infect Dis J 1994;13:281-287.

Zinkus PW, Gottlieb MI, Schapiro M. Developmental and psychoeducational sequelae of chronic otitis media. Am J Dis Child 1978;132:1100.

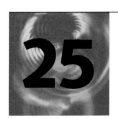

25 PARVOVIRUS INFECTIONS

STUART P. ADLER AND WILLIAM C. KOCH

The Parvoviridae families of viruses are the smallest known DNA-containing viruses. Their genomes contain sufficient DNA to encode only a few proteins. Within the Parvoviridae family is the genus Parvovirus. These viruses differ from other Parvoviridae because they replicate their DNAs without assistance from a helper virus. Parvoviruses infect many mammalian species, but cross-infection between species does not occur. For example, the canine parvovirus does not infect humans and the human parvovirus does not infect dogs. Similarly each mammalian parvovirus causes a different illness in its mammalian host so that parvovirus disease in dogs is very different from that in humans. Parvoviruses were known to cause illness in small mammals long before it was discovered that a parvovirus infected humans. The human parvovirus, also called *human parvovirus B19* or *erythrovirus B19,* is the only known parvovirus to infect humans, but this single virus causes a wide spectrum of both acute and chronic human diseases.

Cossart et al. (1975) discovered B19 in human sera. They were testing sera for hepatitis B surface antigen and found several sera (one of which was encoded B19) that had small spherical viral particles with many disrupted fragments and empty shells. They showed that this virus was not hepatitis B virus and that 40% of adults had IgG antibodies to the new viral antigen (Cossart et al., 1975; Paver and Clarke, 1976). The virus subsequently was characterized by genetic and biochemical analysis as being a parvovirus. (Summers et al., 1983). Initially B19 was not associated with any specific disease. However, the availability of serologic tests for B19 infection allowed testing of sera from patients, and this eventually led to the discovery of human disease caused by this virus.

CLINICAL MANIFESTATIONS

Since its discovery in 1975, B19 has been associated with a number of diverse clinical syndromes. Knowledge of the molecular aspects of B19 infection shed light on the relationships among these seemingly disparate syndromes. The major syndromes associated with B19 infection are listed in Table 25-1. Asymptomatic infection with B19 also occurs commonly in both children and adults. In studies of large outbreaks, asymptomatic infection is reported in approximately 20% of serologically proved cases (Chorba et al., 1986; Plummer et al., 1985).

Erythema Infectiosum (Fifth Disease)

Erythema infectiosum (EI) is the most common manifestation of infection with parvovirus B19. This is a benign exanthematous illness of childhood, also known as *fifth disease* because it was the fifth in a numeric classification scheme of common childhood exanthems. This scheme included: (1) measles, (2) scarlet fever, (3) rubella, (4) Filatov-Dukes disease (a variant of scarlet fever that is no longer recognized), (5) EI, and (6) roseola (Thurn, 1988). Although the numbering scheme is no longer used, the designation of fifth disease for EI has persisted. Anderson first proposed B19 as the cause of EI in 1983, and subsequent studies confirmed this association (Anderson et al., 1983; Anderson et al., 1984; Plummer et al., 1985).

EI begins with a mild prodromal phase consisting of low-grade fever, headache, malaise, and upper respiratory symptoms. This prodrome may be so mild as to go unnoticed. The hallmark of the illness is the characteristic rash. The rash usually occurs in three phases but these are not always distinguishable. The initial stage consists of an erythematous facial flushing described as a "slapped-cheek" appearance.

TABLE 25-1	Clinical Manifestations of Parvovirus B19 Infection
Diseases	*Patients*
Diseases Associated with Acute Infection	
Erythema infectiosum (fifth disease)	Normal children
Polyarthropathy	Normal adolescents and adults
Transient aplastic crisis	Patients with transient aplastic crisis
Papular-purpuric gloves and socks syndrome	Normal adolescents and adults
Diseases Associated with Chronic Infection	
Persistent anemia	Immunodeficient or immunocompromised children and adults
Nonimmune hydrops fetalis	Intrauterine infection
Congenital anemia	Intrauterine infection
Chronic arthropathy	Rare patients with B19-induced joint disease
Virus-associated hemophagocytosis	Normal or immunocompromised patients
Vasculitis or purpura	Normal adults and children
Myocarditis	Intrauterine infection and normal adults and children

In the second stage the rash spreads quickly or concurrently to the trunk and proximal extremities as a diffuse macular erythema. Central clearing of macular lesions occurs promptly, giving the rash a lacy, reticulated appearance. Palms and soles are usually spared and the rash tends to be more prominent on the extensor surfaces. Affected children at this point are afebrile and feel well. Adolescents and adult patients often complain of pruritus or arthralgias concurrent with the rash. The rash resolves spontaneously usually within 3 weeks but typically may recur in response to a variety of environmental stimuli such as sunlight, heat, exercise, and stress. Lymphadenopathy is not a consistent feature. Atypical rashes not recognizable as classic EI have also been associated with acute B19 infections, including morbilliform, vesiculopustular, desquamative, petechial, and purpuric rashes (Török, 1997).

Transient Aplastic Crisis (Erythroid Aplasia)

This was the first clinical syndrome to be definitively linked to B19 infection. An infectious etiology was suspected for the aplastic crisis of sickle-cell disease because it usually occurred only once in a given patient, had a well-defined incubation and duration of illness, and occurred in clusters within families and communities. Attempts, however, to link it to infection with a single agent had repeatedly failed. In 1981, Pattison and colleagues reported six positive tests for B19 (seroconversion or antigenemia) among 600 admissions to a London hospital. All six were children with sickle-cell anemia and aplastic crisis. This association was later confirmed by retrospective studies on the population with sickle-cell disease in Jamaica (Serjeant et al., 1981).

In contrast to children with EI, patients with an aplastic crisis are ill at presentation with fever, malaise, and signs and symptoms of profound anemia (pallor, tachypnea, tachycardia, and so on). Rash is rarely present in these patients (Brown, 1997; Saarinen et al., 1986). The acute infection causes a transient arrest of erythropoiesis with a profound reticulocytopenia leading to a sudden and often life-threatening fall in serum hemoglobin. Children with sickle hemoglobinopathies may also develop a concurrent vaso-occlusive pain crisis, which further complicates the diagnosis.

Although transient aplastic crises are most common with sickle-cell anemia and B19 is the primary cause of the aplastic crisis of sickle-cell anemia, any patient with increased red-cell turnover and accelerated erythropoiesis can experience an aplastic crisis due to B19. B19-induced aplastic crises have occurred in many hematologic disorders including hemoglobinopathies (e.g., thalassemia, sickle-C hemoglobin, etc.), red-cell membrane defects (hereditary spherocytosis, stomatocytosis), enzyme deficiencies (e.g., pyruvate kinase deficiency, glucose-6-phosphate dehydrogenase deficiency, etc.), antibody-mediated red-cell destruction (e.g., autoimmune hemolytic anemia), and decreased red-cell production (iron deficiency, blood loss, etc.) (Brown, 1997).

B19, however, is not a cause of transient erythroblastopenia of childhood, another condition of transient red-cell hypoplasia that usually occurs in younger, hematologically normal children and follows a more indolent course (Brown and Young, 1995).

Neutropenia and thrombocytopenia also occur during an aplastic crisis, but the incidence varies. In a French study of 24 episodes of aplastic crisis (mostly hereditary spherocytosis), 35% to 40% of patients were either leukopenic or thrombocytopenic compared with 10% to 15% in a large American study (mainly sickle-cell disease) (Lefrere et al., 1986; Saarinen et al., 1986). These transient declines in leukocyte count and/or platelets follow a similar time course as the reticulocytopenia, although they are not as severe and the counts return to normal without sequelae. The preservation of leukocytes and platelets in sickle-cell anemia compared with other hereditary hemolytic anemias is presumably due to the functional asplenia associated with sickle-cell disease (Young, 1988). Varying degrees of neutropenia and thrombocytopenia occur after natural B19 infection in hematologically normal patients as well (Anderson et al., 1985). Some cases of idiopathic thrombocytopenic purpura (ITP) and neutropenia in childhood have been associated with acute B19 infection (Lefrere et al., 1989; Saunders et al., 1986). These few reports aside, larger studies have not confirmed B19 as a common cause of either ITP or chronic neutropenia (Brown and Young, 1995).

A typical transient aplastic crisis may be the first manifestation of an underlying hemolytic condition in certain patients who are hemodynamically well compensated and undiagnosed. This is especially well documented in patients with hereditary spherocytosis (Lefrere et al., 1986). The diagnosis of a typical transient aplastic crisis in an otherwise well patient should prompt a thorough hematologic investigation to exclude underlying hemolytic conditions.

Arthropathy

Up to 80% of adolescents and adults have joint symptoms associated with a B19 infection, whereas joint symptoms are uncommon in children (Ager et al., 1966). Arthritis/arthralgia may either be associated with EI or be the only manifestation of infection. Females are more frequently affected than males (Ager et al., 1966; Anderson et al., 1984).

The joint symptoms of B19 infection usually are a symmetric peripheral polyarthropathy with a sudden onset (Brown, 1997). The joints most often affected are the hands, wrists, knees, and ankles but the larger joints also can be involved (White et al., 1985). The joint symptoms have a wide range of severity from mild morning stiffness to frank arthritis with erythema, warmth, tenderness, and swelling. Like the rash of EI, the arthropathy has been presumed to be immunologically mediated because the onset of joint symptoms coincides with the development of specific antibodies. Rheumatoid factor may also be transiently positive, leading to some diagnostic confusion with rheumatoid arthritis (RA) in adult patients (Naides and Field, 1988). Fortunately, there is no joint destruction and in the majority of patients joint symptoms resolve within 2 to 4 weeks. For some patients joint discomfort may last for months or, in rare individuals, years. The role of B19 in these more chronic arthropathies is not clear. In patients with symptoms for over 1 year, B19 IgM antibody is usually undetectable, and some patients have evidence of chronic viral infection. Viral DNA has been detected in the bone marrow of four patients with chronic B19 arthropathy (Foto et al., 1993). The viral and host factors involved in disease expression in these patients remain unknown.

The arthritis associated with B19 infection may persist long enough to satisfy clinical diagnostic criteria for RA or juvenile RA (JRA). This has led some to suggest that B19 may be the etiologic agent of these conditions. This speculation has been supported by the detection of B19 DNA in synovial tissue from patients with RA and reports of increased seropositivity among patients with these conditions (Dijkmans et al., 1988; Saal, et al., 1992). The recent finding of DNA from other viruses in addition to B19 in synovial tissue from patients with arthritis, as well as the finding of B19 DNA in synovium from persons without arthritis, suggests that this may be a nonspecific effect of inflammation (Soderlund et al., 1997; Stahl et al., 2000). A recent review of the accumulated evidence on this topic has concluded that B19 is unlikely to be etiologic in these rheumatic diseases but may be one of several viral triggers (Kerr, 2000).

Infection in the Immunocompromised or Immunodeficient Host

Patients with impaired humoral immunity are at risk for developing chronic and recurrent infections with parvovirus B19. Persistent anemia, sometimes profound, with reticulocytopenia is the most common manifestation of such infections, which may also be accompanied by neutropenia, thrombocytopenia, or complete marrow suppression. Chronic infections with B19 occur in children with cancer receiving cytotoxic chemotherapy (Koch et al., 1990; Van Horn et al., 1986); children with congenital immunodeficiency states (Kurtzman et al., 1987); children and adults with acquired immunodeficiency syndrome (AIDS) (Frickhofen et al., 1990; Naides et al., 1993); transplant recipients (Weiland et al., 1989); and even patients with more subtle and specific defects in IgG class-switching who are able to produce measurable antibodies to B19 but are unable to generate adequate neutralizing antibodies (Kurtzman et al., 1989a; Kurtzman et al., 1989b).

B19 has also been associated with the viral-associated hemophagocytic syndrome (VAHS) (Koch et al., 1990; Muir et al., 1992). This condition of histiocytic infiltration of bone marrow and associated cytopenias usually occurs in immunocompromised patients. B19 is one of several viruses that have been implicated as causing VAHS. Thus VAHS is generally considered a nonspecific response to a variety of viral insults rather than a specific manifestation of a single pathogen.

Intrauterine Infection

Maternal infection with B19 during pregnancy may cause nonimmune fetal hydrops, intrauterine fetal demise, and stillbirth (Anand et al., 1987). The primary pathogenetic mechanism is a viral-induced red-cell aplasia occurring when the fetal erythroid fraction is rapidly expanding. This leads to fetal anemia, hypoxemia, congestive heart failure, fetal hydrops, and fetal death (Brown, 1997). Fetal myocarditis also occurs and may contribute to fetal congestive heart failure and hydrops (Respondek et al., 1997; von Kaisenberg et al., 2001; von Kaisenberg and Jonat, 2001). Viral DNA is found in infected abortuses, but fetal production of viral-specific IgM is often absent despite documented fetal infection, especially in the first half of pregnancy (Anand, et al., 1987; Morey et al., 1991).

The fetus seems to be at highest risk during the second trimester (<20 weeks), but fetal losses have occurred in every stage of gestation. Fortunately, the incidence of fetal demise is low and the majority of infants infected in utero will be delivered normally at term (Hall and the Public Health Laboratory Service, 1990).

Human parvovirus B19 causes about 27% of the cases of nonimmune fetal hydrops (von Kaisenberg and Jonat, 2001). The fetal loss rate attributable to B19, however, has been estimated at between 0% and 9% in prospective studies (Gratacos et al., 1995; Hall and the Public Health Laboratory Service, 1990; Harger et al., 1998; Rodis et al., 1990). Based on the presence of B19-specific IgM in cord blood or viral DNA in fetal samples, however, the rate of intrauterine infection ranges from 25% to 50% (Gratacos, et al., 1995; Hall and the Public Health Laboratory Service, 1990; Koch et al., 1998). In most fetuses with evidence of intrauterine infection and mild hydrops seen via ultrasound, the condition resolves spontaneously and the infants are delivered normally at term (Brown, 1997; Harger et al., 1998; Morey et al., 1991). For fetuses with severe intrauterine anemia and/or hydrops only one third will experience spontaneous resolution, but empiric evidence indicates that intrauterine transfusion significantly improves this survival rate (Rodis et al., 1998; von Kaisenberg and Jonat, 2001).

Some infants infected in utero develop a chronic or recurrent asymptomatic postnatal infection with B19, the long-term consequences of which are not known (Koch et al., 1993; Koch et al., 1998). There is one report of three cases of infants born with severe central nervous system abnormalities after confirmed maternal infection during pregnancy (Török, 2001). Several cases of congenital anemia after intrauterine B19 infections have also been reported (Brown et al., 1994b). Also reported are three children with Diamond-Blackfan anemia (congenital red-cell aplasia) who had B19 DNA in their bone marrow (Heegard et al., 1996). There are a few reports of congenital malformations in B19-infected fetuses but there are no reports to date of live-born infants with malformations after intrauterine B19 infection (Hartwig, et al., 1989). The incidence of birth defects in the children of mothers with a B19 infection during pregnancy has been no higher than that in children of noninfected mothers

(Kinney et al., 1988). Thus B19 is unlikely to be a significant cause of birth defects.

Papular-Purpuric "Gloves and Socks" Syndrome

Papular-purpuric "gloves and socks" syndrome (PPGSS) is a distinctive self-limited dermatosis first described in the dermatologic literature in 1990 (Smith et al., 1997). The syndrome is characterized by fever, pruritus, and painful edema and erythema localized to the distal extremities in a glove and sock distribution, followed by acral petechiae and oral lesions. Resolution of all symptoms usually occurs in 1 to 2 weeks. A search for serologic evidence of viral infection led to discovery of an association with acute B19 infection in many of these patients based on demonstration of specific IgM or seroconversion. This association has been further confirmed with subsequent reports and demonstration of B19 DNA in skin biopsy samples and sera from these patients (Grilli 1999; Smith et al., 1997). Initially described in adults, a number of children have now been described with this condition (Saulsbury, 1998). There appears to be sufficient evidence to suggest that PPGSS is a rare but distinctive manifestation of primary infection with parvovirus B19, primarily in young adults but also affecting children. Other diagnoses to consider on presentation include other infectious agents such as enteroviral and rickettsial infections and allergic reactions.

Vasculitis and Purpura

There are reports of confirmed acute B19 infections associated with nonthrombocytopenic purpura and vasculitis, including several cases clinically diagnosed as Henoch-Schönlein purpura (HSP), an acute leukocytoclastic vasculitis of unknown etiology in children. Chronic B19 infection has also been associated with a necrotizing vasculitis including cases of polyarteritis nodosa and Wegener's granulomatosis (Finkel et al., 1994). These patients had no underlying hematologic disorder and were generally not anemic at diagnosis. The pathogenesis is unknown but suggests an endothelial cell infection as occurs with other viruses, such as rubella. Parvovirus B19 capsid antigens and DNA were found in a skin biopsy from a patient with EI, and this observation lends support to a role for B19 in these vascular disorders (Schwarz et al., 1994). In a controlled

study of 27 children with HSP, B19 was not a common cause (Ferguson et al., 1996). Only three of 27 children had B19 IgM, indicating a recent infection. The question of whether B19 is a causative agent in these conditions remains unresolved.

Myocarditis

The anemia associated with B19 infection is due to a specific viral tropism for progenitor erythroid cells, specifically P antigen that is found on these cells (Brown, 1998). However, clinical and laboratory evidence has been accumulated to suggest that B19 has a wider tropism than only erythroblasts (Heegaard and Hornsleth, 1995). Direct infection of myocardial cells following fetal B19 infection of extramedullary erythroid progenitor cells has been demonstrated by in situ DNA hybridization or electron microscopy (Morey et al., 1992; Naides and Weiner, 1989; Respondek et al., 1997). This is not surprising, because fetal myocardial cells contain P antigen (Heegaard and Hornsleth, 1995).

B19 infection of the heart is probable because case reports have described eight fetuses, five children, and four adults with myocarditis associated with a concurrent B19 infection (Brandenburg et al., 1996; Chia and Jackson, 1996; Enders et al., 1998; Heegaard et al., 1998; Malm et al., 1993; Moore et al., 1993; Morey et al., 1992; Naides and Weiner, 1989; Orth et al., 1997; Respondek et al., 1997). One case occurred post transplantation (Heegaard et al., 1998). In five of these cases B19 DNA was identified in cardiac tissue by polymerase chain reaction (PCR) assay (Heegaard et al., 1998; Porter et al., 1988; Saint-Martin et al., 1990).

A retrospective study of endomyocardial tissue from 360 children with suspected myocarditis, 200 children with suspected post-transplant cardiac rejection, and 250 control biopsies identified parvoviral genomes in myocardial tissue of nine additional children (six in heart tissue obtained after transplantation, three in heart tissue from normal children with myocarditis) (Schowengerdt et al., 1997). For the nine children with B19-associated myocarditis, some had cardiac arrest, some had dilated cardiomyopathy, and some recovered, but no detailed clinical or serologic data were given (Schowengerdt et al., 1997). One report describes the progression to persistent myocarditis in a child with an early and persistently active B19 infection.

Although B19 DNA occurs in myocardial tissue no one has convincingly demonstrated viral replication in myocardial tissue. B19 is mildly cardiotropic and acute lymphocytic myocarditis probably results from the cellular response to either myocardial tissue or the virus infecting the heart tissue. We found elevated levels of interleukin (IL)-6, IL-8, TNF, and IFN-γ in the acute phase of the disease in both children who recovered, and persistently high levels in one patient who developed persistent myocarditis (Nigro et al., 2000). The levels of these cytokines correlated with the course of acute lymphocytic myocarditis and were not associated with B19 infection without clinical myocarditis (Nigro et al., 2000). If elevated cytokine levels are associated with myocarditis not associated with B19 is unknown.

Even though B19-associated myocarditis appears to occur infrequently, there is sufficient evidence to consider B19 as a cause of lymphocytic myocarditis. In patients with this disease clinicians should search for evidence of a concurrent B19 infection. Additional prospective studies starting from infancy are needed to determine the true incidence of cardiac involvement associated with B19 infections and the long-term consequences of B19-associated cardiac disease.

PATHOGENESIS

Because of its small genome, parvovirus B19, like other autonomously replicating parvoviruses, requires a mitotically active host cell for its own replication (Hauswirth, 1984). B19 can propagate only in human erythroid progenitor cells from bone marrow (Ozawa et al., 1987), fetal liver (Yaegashi et al., 1989), peripheral blood (Schwarz et al., 1992), umbilical cord blood (Sosa et al., 1992), and a few leukemic cell lines (Shimomura et al., 1992). The cellular receptor for B19 is globoside, a neutral glycosphingolipid found primarily on erythroid cells where it is known as the *P blood group antigen* (Brown et al., 1993). This receptor is necessary but not sufficient for B19 infection (Weigel-Kelley et al., 2001). Bone marrow from patients who lack the P antigen (p phenotype) cannot be infected in vitro with B19, and individuals without this antigen on their red cells are naturally immune to B19 infection (Brown et al., 1994b). The tissue distribution of the cellular receptor explains the predominance of hematologic effects in B19 infection. P antigen is also found on vascular endothelial cells, megakaryocytes, placenta, fetal liver, and fetal myocardial cells, a tissue distribution that may have implications for the pathogenesis of other B19 syndromes (Brown et al., 1993).

The primary target of B19 infection is the erythroid progenitor cell in the marrow near the pronormoblast stage (Ozawa et al., 1987). The virus lytically infects these cells leading to an arrest of erythropoiesis (Young, 1988). Susceptibility to infection appears to increase with increasing differentiation, and the pluripotent stem cells are spared (Takahashi et al., 1990). Infected bone marrow cultures are characterized by the presence of giant pronormoblasts or so-called lantern cells (Brown and Young, 1995). These are large, early erythroid cells recognized by their cytoplasmic vacuolization, immature chromatin, and large eosinophilic nuclear inclusion bodies. These cells are also found in bone marrow of clinically infected patients (Kurtzman et al., 1987; Van Horn et al., 1986).

The viral suppression of erythropoiesis by B19 is demonstrated in vitro by its effect on colony assays of erythroid cells. Addition of virus to erythroid colony assays results in near complete inhibition of erythroid colony-forming units (CFU-E) and variable inhibition of erythroid blast-forming units (BFU-E) (Mortimer et al., 1983a). This suppressive effect can be reversed by the addition of convalescent serum containing IgG antibodies to B19. The virus has no effect on the myeloid cell lines (CFU-GM) but causes inhibition of megakaryocytopoiesis in vitro without viral replication or cell lysis (Srivastava et al., 1990). Infection of such cells that are nonpermissive for replication leads to accumulation of a viral nonstructural protein, NS1, that may itself be toxic to the cell (Ozawa et al., 1988).

For patients with a transient aplastic crisis, this pathophysiologic process makes the clinical presentation understandable. Individuals with conditions of chronic hemolysis and increased red-cell turnover are very sensitive to any perturbations in erythropoiesis. Infection with B19 leads to a transient arrest in red-cell production and a resultant precipitous fall in serum hemoglobin and hematocrit, usually requiring transfusion. The reticulocyte count falls to near zero, reflecting the lysis of infected erythroblasts. Viral-specific IgM appears within 1 to 2 days of the peak of viremia followed by IgG antibodies to B19, and the infection is controlled. Control of the infection and the relative resistance of the pluripotent stem cells to infection contribute to marrow recovery with a reactive reticulocytosis and rise in serum hemoglobin (Takahashi et al., 1990).

Normal volunteers infected with B19 develop a mild biphasic illness rather than an aplastic crisis (Anderson et al., 1985). Seven to 11 days after inoculation, such volunteers develop viremia with fever, malaise, and mild upper respiratory symptoms. Their reticulocyte counts drop to undetectable levels but, with a normal red-cell half-life of 120 days, this results in only a mild, clinically insignificant dip in serum hemoglobin concentration. Their symptoms resolve spontaneously and the reticulocyte counts return to normal with the appearance of specific antibodies. Some volunteers develop a generalized rash 17 to 18 days after inoculation and arthralgias coincident with the appearance of specific antibodies. Thus, some manifestations of B19 infection are a direct result of lytic viral infection (transient aplastic crisis, fetal hydrops), whereas others (EI, arthropathy) are postinfectious phenomena related to the immune response and possibly immune complex development (Anderson, 1990). Skin biopsies from patients with EI have shown only edema and perivascular mononuclear infiltrates. In one skin biopsy, viral capsid proteins and DNA were identified in epidermal cells suggesting B19 may have a more direct effect in the production of exanthema (Schwarz et al., 1994).

Like other parvoviruses, B19 infects the placenta and the fetus causing fetal viremia after a primary maternal infection (Jordan and DeLoia, 1999). The fetus is at risk for serious disease because of both its hematologic status and immature immune status (Anderson, 1990). The fetus has a rapidly expanding red-cell mass, a relatively short red-cell half-life, and impaired humoral immunity. Intrauterine infection may lead to a profound fetal anemia, and this, with or without myocarditis, may lead to cardiac failure. Fetal hydrops ensues, and fetal mortality is high. There may also be a direct effect of the virus on the fetal heart as evidenced by the presence of B19 DNA in myocardial tissue from abortuses and sup-

ported by the tissue distribution of the P antigen (Brown et al., 1993; Porter et al., 1988).

IMMUNITY

In the normal host, infection with parvovirus B19 induces a brisk IgM and IgG response. Experimental infection of human volunteers has elucidated the course of the immune response (Anderson et al., 1985). Viremia occurs between 7 and 11 days after inoculation with a peak at 8 to 9 days. IgM antibody to B19 appears 10 to 14 days after infection (generally 1 to 2 days after the peak of viremia) and remains detectable for 6 to 8 weeks but may persist for several months. IgG antibody follows within a few days and persists for life, serving as a marker of prior infection and immunity. The early antibody responses are directed against the major capsid protein, VP2, but as the immune response matures, reactivity to the minor capsid protein VP1 predominates (Kurtzman et al., 1989b). The immune response to VP1 appears to be crucial for the development of protective immunity: VP1 must be present in recombinant capsids to elicit a neutralizing antibody response in animals (Kajigaya et al., 1991). Some patients with persistent B19 infections have antibody to VP2 but lack antibodies to VP1 (Kurtzman et al., 1989b).

Less is known about the IgA responses to B19 infection. In patients with typical EI, serum IgA appears to parallel IgG response but to a lesser degree, peaking in 1 to 2 weeks and gradually declining over 6 to 12 months (Erdman et al., 1991). No information is available on the secretory IgA response.

Humoral responses appear to control B19 infection. Recovery from infection correlates with the appearance of circulating viral-specific antibody; administration of commercial immunoglobulins appears to cure or ameliorate persistent B19 infections in immunodeficient patients (Frickhofen et al., 1990; Koch et al., 1990; Kurtzman et al., 1989a). Cellular responses to B19 have also been detected, although their importance in the control of this infection is unknown.

DIAGNOSIS

The diagnosis of EI (fifth disease) is usually based on the clinical recognition of the typical exanthem, benign course, and exclusion of other similar conditions. A presumptive diagnosis of a

B19-induced transient aplastic crisis in a known sickle-cell patient (or other condition of chronic hemolysis) is based on an acute febrile illness, severe fall in serum hemoglobin, and an absolute reticulocytopenia.

Specific laboratory diagnosis depends on identification of B19 antibodies, viral antigens, or viral DNA. In the immunologically normal patient, determination of anti-B19 IgM is the best marker of recent or acute infection on a single serum sample. IgM antibodies develop rapidly after infection and are generally detectable for 6 to 8 weeks (Anderson et al., 1986). IgG antibodies become detectable a few days after IgM and persist for years and probably life. Seroconversion from IgG-negative to IgG-positive on paired sera also confirms a recent infection. Anti-B19 IgG, however, primarily serves as a marker of past infection or immunity. Patients with EI or acute B19 arthropathy are almost always IgM-positive, so a diagnosis can usually be made from a single serum sample. Patients with B19-induced aplastic crisis may present before antibodies are detectable; however, IgM will be detectable within 1 to 2 days of presentation and IgG will follow within days (Saarinen et al., 1986).

Recombinant cell lines that express B19 capsid proteins provide a reliable source of antigen (Cohen and Bates, 1995; Koch, 1995).

In immunocompromised or immunodeficient patients, serologic diagnosis is unreliable because humoral responses are impaired, and methods to detect viral particles or viral DNA are necessary to make the diagnosis of a B19 infection. As noted, the virus cannot be isolated on routine cell cultures so viral culture is not useful. Detection of viral DNA by DNA hybridization techniques or by PCR are useful methods in these patients (Clewley, 1985; Clewley, 1989; Koch and Adler, 1990). Both techniques can be applied to a variety of clinical specimens including serum, amniotic fluid, fresh tissues, bone marrow, and paraffin-embedded tissues.

Histologic examination is also helpful in diagnosing B19 infection in certain situations. Examination of bone marrow aspirates in anemic patients often reveals giant pronormoblasts or lantern cells against a background of general erythroid hypoplasia. However, the absence of such cells does not exclude B19 infection (Brown et al., 1994b; Heegaard et al., 1996). Electron microscopy may reveal viral particles in serum of some infected patients and cord blood or tissues of hydropic infants (Caul et al., 1988; Cossart et al., 1975).

DIFFERENTIAL DIAGNOSIS

The differential diagnosis of EI includes rubella, measles, enteroviral infections, scarlet fever, and drug reactions. Rubella is the most similar condition to exclude. Measles and scarlet fever should be clinically distinguishable by the significant fever and typical coryzal prodrome of measles and the fever and pharyngitis of scarlet fever. A suggestive rash and joint symptoms in older children and adolescents should prompt consideration of other rheumatologic disorders such as juvenile chronic arthritis and systemic lupus erythematosus.

Whereas B19 is by far the most common cause of the transient aplastic crisis in sickle-cell anemia patients, infection with other pathogens, especially systemic bacterial infections, may cause relative degrees of erythroid hypoplasia and subsequent worsening of the chronic anemia (Serjeant et al., 1981). The degree of suppression of hematopoiesis, however, is much less dramatic, the fall in the reticulocyte count is not as extreme, and usually other signs of infection are present, such as pneumonia, abscess, or osteomyelitis.

COMPLICATIONS

EI is often accompanied by arthralgias or arthritis in adolescents and adults, which may persist after resolution of the rash. Joint symptoms occur in 60% to 80% of adults with EI, whereas the incidence in children (<9 years of age) is less than 10% (Ager et al., 1966). Prior to the discovery of B19, neurologic complications of encephalitis and aseptic meningitis were rarely described after EI; subsequently, reports have appeared describing B19-associated meningitis, encephalitis, hepatitis, and a peripheral neuropathy (Barah et al., 2001; Koduri and Naides, 1995; Sokal et al., 1998; Török, 1997). The majority resolved without sequelae.

EPIDEMIOLOGY AND TRANSMISSION

B19 is a highly contagious infection. In the U.S. 60% or more of white adults are seropositive (i.e., have IgG antibodies to B19 in their sera). This indicates a previous infection usually acquired in childhood. Among blacks the rate of seropositivity is lower, about 30%.

Transmission of B19 from person to person is probably by droplets from oral or nasal secretions. This is suggested by the rapid transmission among those in close physical contact such as schoolmates or family members and by the fact that in a study of healthy volunteers, virus was found in blood and nasopharyngeal secretions for several days beginning a day or two before symptoms appeared (Anderson et al., 1985). In the volunteer study no virus was detected in urine or stool.

Given the highly contagious nature of B19 infections and that transmission requires close contact, most outbreaks occur in elementary schools. Seronegative adult school personnel are at high risk for acquiring the infection from students (Adler et al., 1993). Some outbreaks in schools may be epidemic with many children and staff acquiring the infection and developing symptoms of EI. At other times the infection is often endemic, with transmission occurring slowly and with only a few manifesting symptoms.

Other settings where B19 transmission is facilitated include the hospital and the family. B19 can readily be transmitted from infected patients to hospital workers (Bell et al., 1989). Therefore, patients with erythrocyte aplasia should be presumed to have a B19 infection until proved otherwise. These patients should receive respiratory and contact isolation while hospitalized. The family is another setting in which transmission is rapid, although no intervention is generally necessary to interrupt transmission here.

Outbreaks of B19 also occur in day-care centers, although transmission here is less common than among school-age children. B19 has also been transmitted via infusion of coagulation factors, although this is uncommon (Mortimer et al., 1983b). B19 transmission has not been reported but is theoretically possible after routine erythrocyte transfusions or organ transplantation.

B19 AND PREGNANCY

The risk for fetal death from a maternal B19 infection or exposure is relatively low. Approximately half of women between 20 and 40 years of age will be seropositive; for seronegative women the maternal B19 infection rate ranges from 30% for exposures by the woman's own children to between 10% and 18% for other exposures, and the expected

fetal morbidity and mortality risk is maximally 2%. Thus the overall risk of fetal death following exposure varies from a high of only 0.3% ($\frac{1}{2} \times \frac{3}{10} \times \frac{1}{50} = \frac{3}{1,000}$) to a low of 0.1% ($\frac{1}{2} \times \frac{1}{10} \times \frac{1}{50} = \frac{1}{1,000}$). Because of these low risks, removing pregnant day-care workers or schoolteachers from their workplaces even during out-breaks in the school is unnecessary.

Because EI may be seasonal—occurring in the spring in temperate climates—exposure of pregnant women to B19 is most likely March through July; however, sporadic cases of exposure and infection may occur year around. Pregnant women who suspect exposure to EI should be questioned in detail about their exposure. The single greatest risk for a pregnant woman comes from children living in her own household, where 30% of susceptible pregnant women will become infected. On the other hand, brief contact not involving touching the potential source carries less risk.

The symptoms and signs of adult B19 infection are nonspecific. One study found that 67% of the 52 IgM-positive, parvovirus-infected women reported at least one of the following symptoms: malaise (52%), arthralgia (46%), rash (38%), coryza (23%), and fever ≥38.0° C (19%) (Harger et al., 1998). Pregnant women expressing such symptoms, especially malaise with symmetric arthralgias in the hands, wrists, knees, or feet, should be tested for B19 infection. Also to be tested are women with signs of a rapidly enlarging uterus (fundal height exceeding dates by more than 3 centimeters), an elevated serum alpha-fetoprotein, preterm labor, or decreased fetal movement and women with ultrasonic evidence of fetal hydrops, ascites, pleural or pericardial effusion, skin thickening, polyhydramnios, or placentomegaly. Serum should be tested for IgG and IgM antibodies against parvovirus B19. Serum should be drawn at least 10 days after the exposure to allow time for IgG and IgM antibodies to develop. Fetal morbidity rarely occurs within 2 weeks of exposure, so immediate serologic testing should be reserved for a woman or fetus already displaying symptoms or signs of actual B19 infection.

If a pregnant women seroconverts or her serum contains IgM antibodies to B19 and the gestational age of the fetus exceeds 20 weeks, an initial negative ultrasound should be repeated each week for 12 weeks to detect the onset of hydrops fetalis. The average interval between maternal B19 exposure or infection and fetal death or hydrops fetalis is 6 weeks, with a range of 1 to 19 weeks (Adler et al., 2001). Electronic fetal monitoring is not effective in detecting hydrops fetalis or in predicting the outcome of pregnancy in B19-IgM–positive women. Contraction stress tests and "nonstress" tests are not accurate predictors of fetal well-being in cases of fetal anemia and/or hydrops fetalis, whereas ultrasound scans provide specific information about fetal status in these cases. Similarly, fetal assessment with estriol measurements or other biochemical markers have no documented role in cases of hydrops fetalis.

If hydrops fetalis is detected before 18 weeks, there is no effective intervention available currently. Other causes of fetal hydrops such as chromosomal disorders and anatomic abnormalities should be sought. The fetus should be scanned again by ultrasound at 18 weeks and, if it is still viable, consideration given to percutaneous umbilical blood sampling (PUBS), also termed cordocentesis. At 18 weeks the umbilical vein diameter is about 4 mm, the minimum size required for successful PUBS. Fetal blood should be obtained for measurement of hematocrit, Kleihauer-Betke test, reticulocyte count, platelet count, leukocyte count, determination of presence of antiparvovirus B19-IgM, karyotype, and perhaps tests for B19-DNA by PCR. The hematocrit must be determined immediately and, if fetal anemia is present, an intrauterine intravascular fetal transfusion performed with the same needle puncture. If anemia is not confirmed, another cause of hydrops fetalis other than B19 should be considered in lieu of fetal transfusion.

If the fetus is already between 18 and 32 weeks of gestation at the diagnosis of hydrops fetalis, fetal transfusion should be considered. If the fetus is ≥32 weeks when hydrops is discovered, immediate delivery with neonatal exchange transfusion is usually the safest management.

THERAPY

The only specific therapy currently available is intravenous immunoglobulin. Since most B19 infections are self-limited, therapy mainly has been used in immunocompromised patients and fetuses with prolonged anemia for which red blood cell transfusions may also be necessary.

PREVENTION

Specific preventive measures are not available. Respiratory and contact isolation of all hospitalized patients with suspected B19 infection is recommended. To reduce the risk of infection to seronegative pregnant school personnel during major school outbreaks, furloughing or transfer of such personnel to jobs without child contact is an option, but is of unproved benefit.

BIBLIOGRAPHY

Adler SP, Harger JH, Koch WC. Infections due to human parvovirus B19 during pregnancy. In Faro S, Soper D (eds). Infectious Diseases in Women. Philadelphia: Saunders, 2001.

Adler SP, Manganello A-M, Koch WC, et al. Risk of human parvovirus B19 infections among school and hospital employees during endemic periods. J Infect Dis 1993;168:361-368.

Ager EA, Chin TDY, Poland JD. Epidemic erythema infectiosum. N Engl J Med 1966;275:1326-1331.

Anand A, Gray ES, Brown T, et al. Human parvovirus infection in pregnancy and hydrops fetalis. N Engl J Med 1987; 316:183-186.

Anderson LJ. Human parvoviruses. J Infect Dis 1990;161:603-608.

Anderson LJ, Tsou C, Parker RA, et al. Detection of antibodies and antigens of human parvovirus B19 by enzyme-linked immunosorbent assay. J Clin Microbiol 1986;24:522.

Anderson MJ, Higgins PG, Davis LR, et al. Experimental parvoviral infection in humans. J Infect Dis 1985;152:257-265.

Anderson MJ, Jones SE, Fisher-Hoch SP, et al. Human parvovirus, the cause of erythema infectiosum (fifth disease)? (letter) Lancet 1983;1:1378.

Anderson MJ, Lewis E, Kidd IM, et al. An outbreak of erythema infectiosum associated with human parvovirus infection. Epidemiol Infect 1984;93:83.

Barah F, Vallely PJ, Chiswick ML, et al. Association of human parvovirus B19 infection with acute meningoencephalitis. Lancet 2001;358:729-730.

Bell LM, Naides SJ, Stoffman P, et al. Human parvovirus B19 infection among hospital staff members after contact with infected patients. N Engl J Med 1989;321:485.

Brandenburg H, Los FJ, Cohen-Overbeek TE. A case of early intrauterine parvovirus B19 infection. Prenat Diagn 1996;16:75-77.

Brown KE. Human parvovirus B19 epidemiology and clinical manifestations. In Anderson LJ, Young NS (eds). Human Parvovirus B19. Monographs in Virology, vol 20. Basel: Karger, 1997

Brown KE. Human parvovirus B19 infections in infants and children. Adv Pediatr Infect Dis 1998;13:101-126

Brown KE, Anderson SM, Young NS. Erythrocyte P antigen: cellular receptor for B19 parvovirus. Science 1993;262:114-117.

Brown KE, Green SW, de Mayolo JA, et al. Congenital anemia after transplacental B19 parvovirus infection. Lancet 1994a;343:895-896.

Brown KE, Hibbs JR, Gallinella G, et al. Resistance to parvovirus B19 infection due to lack of virus receptor (erythrocyte P antigen). N Engl J Med 1994b;330:1192-1196.

Brown KE, Young NS. Parvovirus B19 infection and hematopoiesis. Blood Rev 1995;9:176-182.

Caul EO, Usher MJ, Burton PA. Intrauterine infection with human parvovirus B19: a light and electron microscopy study. J Med Virol 1988;24:55-66.

Chia JKS, Jackson B. Myopericarditis due to parvovirus B19 in an adult. Clin Infect Dis 1996;23:200-201.

Chorba T, Coccia P, Holman RC, et al. The role of parvovirus B19 in aplastic crisis and erythema infectiosum (fifth disease). J Infect Dis 1986;154:383-393.

Clewley JP. Detection of human parvovirus using a molecularly cloned probe. J Med Virol 1985;15:173.

Clewley JP. Polymerase chain reaction assay of parvovirus B19 DNA in clinical specimens. J Clin Microbiol 1989;27:2647.

Cohen BJ, Bates CM. Evaluation of 4 commercial test kits for parvovirus B19-specific IgM. J Virol Methods 1995;55:11-25.

Cossart YE, Cant B, Field AM, et al. Parvovirus-like particles in human sera. Lancet 1975;1:72.

Dijkmans BA, van Elsacker-Niele AM, Salimans MMM, et al. Human parvovirus B19 DNA in synovial fluid. Arthritis Rheum 1988;31:279-281.

Enders G, Dötsch J, Bauer J, et al. Life-threatening parvovirus B19-associated myocarditis and cardiac transplantation as possible therapy: two case reports. Clin Infect Dis 1998;26:355-358.

Erdman DD, Usher MJ, Tsou C, et al. Human parvovirus B19 specific IgG, IgA, and IgM antibodies and serum DNA in serum specimens from persons with erythema infectiosum. J Med Virol 1991;35:110-115.

Ferguson PJ, Saulsbury FT, Dowell SF, et al. Prevalence of human parvovirus B19 infection in children with Henoch-Schönlein purpura. Arthritis Rheum 1996;39:880-881.

Finkel TH, Török TJ, Ferguson PJ, et al. Chronic parvovirus B19 infection and systemic necrotising vasculitis: opportunistic infection or aetiological agent? Lancet 1994;343:1255-1258.

Foto F, Saag KG, Scharosch LL, et al. Parvovirus B19-specific DNA in bone marrow from arthropathy patients: evidence for B19 virus persistence. J Infect Dis 1993;167:744-748.

Frickhofen N, Abkowitz JL, Safford M, et al. Persistent B19 parvovirus infection in patients infected with human immunodeficiency virus type 1 (HIV-1): a treatable cause of anemia in AIDS. Ann Intern Med 1990;113:926-933.

Gratacos E, Torres P-J, Vidal J, et al. The incidence of human parvovirus B19 infection during pregnancy and its impact on perinatal outcome. J Infect Dis 1995;171:1360-1363.

Grilli R, Izquierdo MJ, Farina MC, et al. Papular-purpuric "gloves and socks" syndrome: polymerase chain reaction demonstration of parvovirus B19 DNA in cutaneous lesions and sera. J Am Acad Dermatol 1999;41:793-796.

Hall SM, the Public Health Laboratory Service Working Party on Fifth Disease. Prospective study of human parvovirus (B19) infection in pregnancy. Br Med J 1990;300:1166-1170.

Harger JH, Adler SP, Koch WC, et al. Prospective evaluation of 618 pregnant women exposed to parvovirus B19: risks and symptoms. Obstet Gynecol 1998;91:413-420.

Hartwig NG, Vermeij-Keers C, Van Elsacker-Niele AMW, et al. Embryonic malformations in a case of intrauterine parvovirus B19 infection. Teratology 1989;39:295-302.

Hauswirth WW. Autonomous parvovirus DNA structure and replication. In Berns KI (ed). The Parvoviruses. London: Plenum Press, 1984.

Heegaard ED, Eiskjaer H, Baandrup U, et al. Parvovirus B19 infection associated with myocarditis following adult cardiac transplantation. Scand J Infect Dis 1998;30:607-610.

Heegard ED, Hasle H, Clausen N, et al. Parvovirus B19 infection and Diamond-Blackfan anaemia. Acta Pediatr 1996;85:299-302.

Heegaard ED, Hornsleth A. Parvovirus: the expanding spectrum of disease. Acta Paediatr 1995;84:109-117.

Jordan JA, DeLoia JA: Globoside expression within the human placenta. Placenta 1999;20:103-108.

Kajigaya S, Fujii H, Field A, et al. Self-assembled B19 parvovirus capsids, produced in a baculovirus system, are antigenically and immunologically similar to native virions. Proc Natl Acad Sci USA 1991;88:4646-4650.

Kerr JR. Pathogenesis of human parvovirus B19 in rheumatic disease. Ann Rheum Dis 2000;59: 672-683.

Kinney JS, Anderson LJ, Farrar J, et al. Risk of adverse outcomes of pregnancy after intrauterine infection with human parvovirus B19 infection. J Infect Dis 1988;157:663-667.

Koch WC. A synthetic parvovirus B19 capsid protein can replace viral antigen in antibody-capture enzyme immunoassays. J Virol Methods 1995;55:67-82.

Koch WC, Adler SP. Detection of human parvovirus B19 DNA by using the polymerase chain reaction. J Clin Microbiol 1990;28:65-69.

Koch WC, Adler SP, Harger J. Intrauterine parvovirus B19 infection may cause an asymptomatic or recurrent postnatal infection. Pediatr Infect Dis J 1993;12:747-750.

Koch WC, Harger JH, Barnstein B, Adler SP. Serologic and virologic evidence for frequent intrauterine transmission of human parvovirus B19 with a primary maternal infection during pregnancy. Pediatr Infect Dis J 1998;17: 489-494.

Koch WC, Massey G, Russell CE, et al. Manifestations and treatment of human parvovirus B19 infection in immunocompromised patients. J Pediatr 1990;116: 355-359.

Koduri PR, Naides SJ. Aseptic meningitis caused by parvovirus B19. Clin Infect Dis 1995;21:1053.

Kurtzman G, Frickhofen N, Kimball J, et al. Pure red-cell aplasia of ten years' duration due to persistent parvovirus B19 infection and its cure with immunoglobulin therapy. N Engl J Med 1989a;321:519-523.

Kurtzman GJ, Cohen BJ, Field AM, et al. Immune response to B19 parvovirus and antibody defect in persistent viral infection. J Clin Invest 1989b;84:1114-1123.

Kurtzman GJ, Ozawa K, Cohen B, et al. Chronic bone marrow failure due to persistent B19 parvovirus infection. N Engl J Med 1987;317:287-294.

Lefrere J-J, Courouce A-M, Bertrand Y, et al. Human parvovirus and aplastic crisis in chronic hemolytic anemias: a study of 24 observations. Am J Hematol 1986;23:271-275.

Lefrere J-J, Courouce A-M, Kaplan C. Parvovirus and idiopathic thrombocytopenic purpura (letter). Lancet 1989;i:279.

Malm C, Fridell E, Jansson K. Heart failure after parvovirus B19 infection. Lancet 1993;341:1408-1409.

Moore L, Chambers HM, Foreman AR, Khong TY. A report of human parvovirus B19 infection in hydrops fetalis. First Australian case confirmed by serology and immunohistology. Med J Aust 1993;159:344-345.

Morey AL, Nicolini U, Welch CR, et al. Parvovirus B19 infection and transient fetal hydrops (letter). Lancet 1991;337:496.

Morey AL, Porter HJ, Keeling JW, Fleming KA. Non-isotopic in situ hybridisation and immunophenotyping of infected cells in investigation of human fetal parvovirus infection. J Clin Pathol 1992;45:673-678.

Mortimer PP, Humphries RK, Moore JG, et al. A human parvovirus-like virus inhibits haematopoietic colony formation in vitro. Nature 1983a;302:426-429.

Mortimer PP, Luban NLC, Kelleher JF, et al. Transmission of serum parvovirus-like virus by clotting-factor concentrates. Lancet 1983b;2:482.

Muir K, Todd WTA, Watson WH, et al. Viral-associated haemophagocytosis with parvovirus B19-related pancytopenia. Lancet 1992;339:1139-1140.

Naides SJ, Field EH. Transient rheumatoid factor positivity in acute human parvovirus B19 infection. Arch Intern Med 1988;148:2587-2589.

Naides SJ, Howard EJ, Swack NS, et al. Parvovirus B19 infection in human immunodeficiency virus type 1–infected persons failing or intolerant to zidovudine therapy. J Infect Dis 1993;168:101-105.

Naides SJ, Weiner CP. Antenatal diagnosis and palliative treatment of non-immune hydrops fetalis secondary to fetal parvovirus B19 infection. Prenat Diagn 1989;9:105-114.

Nigro G, Bastianon V, Colloridi V, et al. Human parvovirus B19 infection in infancy associated with acute and chronic lymphocytic myocarditis and high cytokine levels: report of 3 cases and review. Clin Infect Dis 2000;31:65-69.

Orth T, Herr W, Spahn T, et al. Human parvovirus B19 infection associated with severe acute perimyocarditis in a 34-year-old man. Eur Heart J 1997;18:524-525.

Ozawa K, Ayub J, Kajigaya S, et al. The gene encoding the nonstructural protein of B19 (human) parvovirus may be lethal in transfected cells. J Virol 1988;62:2884-2889.

Ozawa K, Kurtzman G, Young N. Productive infection by B19 parvovirus of human erythroid bone marrow cells in vitro. Blood 1987;70:384-391.

Pattison JR, Jones SE, Hodgson J. Parvovirus infections and hypoplastic crisis in sickle-cell anaemia (letter). Lancet 1981;1:664.

Paver WK, Clarke SKR. Comparison of human fecal and serum parvo-like viruses. J Clin Microbiol 1976;4:67.

Plummer FA, Hammond GW, Forward K, et al. An erythema infectiosum-like illness caused by human parvovirus infection. N Engl J Med 1985;313:74-79.

Porter HJ, Quantrill AM, Fleming KA. B19 parvovirus infection of myocardial cells (letter). Lancet 1988;1:535.

Respondek M, Bratosiewicz J, Pertynski T, et al. Parvovirus particles in a fetal heart with myocarditis: ultrastructural and immunohistochemical study. Arch Immunol Ther Exp (Warsz) 1997;45:465-470.

Rodis JF, Borgida AF, Wilson M, et al. Management of parvovirus infection in pregnancy and outcomes of hydrops: a survey of members of the society of perinatal obstetricians. Am J Obstet Gynecol 1998;179:985-988.

Rodis FJ, Quinn DL, Gary GW, et al. Management and outcomes of pregnancies complicated by human B19 parvovirus infection: a prospective study. Am J Obstet Gynecol 1990;163:1168-1171.

Saal JG, Stendle M, Einsele H, et al. Persistence of B19 parvovirus in synovial membranes of patients with rheumatoid arthritis. Rheumatology 1992;12:147-151.

Saarinen UM, Chorba TL, Tattersall P, et al. Human parvovirus B19–induced epidemic acute red cell aplasia in patients with hereditary hemolytic anemia. Blood 1986;67:1411-1417.

Saint-Martin J, Choulot JJ, Bonnaud E, et al. Myocarditis caused by parvovirus. J Pediatr 1990;116:1007-1008.

Saulsbury FT. Petechial gloves and socks syndrome caused by parvovirus B19. Pediatr Dermatol 1998;15:35-37.

Saunders PWG, Reid MM, Cohen BJ. Human parvovirus induced cytopenias: a report of five cases. Br J Haematol 1986; 407-410.

Schowengerdt KO, Ni J, Denfield SW, et al. Association of parvovirus B19 genome in children with myocarditis and cardiac allograft rejection. Diagnosis using the polymerase chain reaction. Circulation 1997;96:3549-3554.

Schwarz TF, Serke S, Hottentrager B, et al. Replication of parvovirus B19 in hematopoietic progenitor cells generated in vitro from normal human peripheral blood. J Virol 1992;66:1273-1276.

Schwarz TF, Wiersbitzky S, Pambor M. Case report: detection of parvovirus B19 in skin biopsy of a patient with erythema infectiosum. J Med Virol 1994;43:171-174.

Serjeant GR, Topley JM, Mason K, et al. Outbreak of aplastic crises in sickle cell anaemia associated with parvovirus-like agent. Lancet 1981;2:595-597.

Shimomura S, Komatsu N, Frickhofen N, et al. First continuous propagation of B19 parvovirus in a cell line. Blood 1992;79:18-24.

Smith PT, Landry ML, Carey H, et al. Papular-purpuric gloves and socks syndrome associated with acute parvovirus B19 infection: case report and review. Clin Infect Dis 1997;27:164-168.

Soderlund M, von Essen R, Haapasaari J, et al. Persistence of parvovirus B19 DNA in synovial membranes of young patients with and without chronic arthropathy. Lancet 1997;349:1063-1065.

Sokal EM, Melchior M, Cornu C, et al. Acute parvovirus B19 infection associated with fulminant hepatitis of favourable prognosis in young children. Lancet 1998;352:1739-1741.

Sosa CE, Mahoney JB, Luinstra KE, et al. Replication and cytopathology of human parvovirus B19 in human umbilical cord blood erythroid progenitor cells. J Med Virol 1992;36:125-130.

Srivastava A, Bruno E, Briddell R, et al. Parvovirus B19-induced perturbation of human megakaryocytopoiesis in vitro. Blood 1990;76:1997-2004.

Stahl HD, Hubner B, Seidl B, et al. Detection of multiple viral DNA species in synovial tissue and fluid of patients with early arthritis. Ann Rheum Dis 2000;59:342-346.

Summers J, Jones SE, Anderson MJ. Characterization of the genome of the agent of erythrocyte aplasia permits its classification as a human parvovirus. J Gen Virol 1983;64:2527.

Takahashi T, Ozawa K, Takahashi K, et al. Susceptibility of human erythropoietic cells to B19 parvovirus in vitro increases with differentiation. Blood 1990;75: 603-610.

Thurn J. Human parvovirus B19: historical and clinical review. Rev Infect Dis 1988;10:1005-1011.

Török T. Human parvovirus B19. In Remington JS, Klein JO (eds). Infectious Diseases of the Fetus and Newborn Infant, ed 5. Philadelphia: Saunders, 2001.

Török TJ. Unusual clinical manifestations reported in patients with parvovirus B19 infection. In Anderson LJ, Young NS (eds). Human Parvovirus B19, vol 20. Monographs in Virology. Basel: Karger, 1997.

Van Horn DK, Mortimer PP, Young N, et al. Human parvovirus–associated red cell aplasia in the absence of underlying hemolytic anemia. Am J Pediatr Hematol Oncol 1986;8:235-329.

von Kaisenberg CS, Bender G, Scheewe J, et al. A case of fetal parvovirus B19 myocarditis, terminal cardiac heart failure, and perinatal heart transplantation. Fetal Diagn Ther 2001; 16:427-432.

von Kaisenberg CS, Jonat W. Fetal parvovirus B19 infection. Ultrasound Obstet Gynecol 2001; 18:280-288.

Weigel-Kelley KA, Yoder MC, Srivastava A. Recombinant human parvovirus B19 vectors: erythrocyte P antigen is necessary but not sufficient for successful transduction of human hematopoietic cells. J Virol 2001;75:4110-4116.

Weiland HT, Salimans MMM, Fibbe WE, et al. Prolonged parvovirus B19 infection with severe anaemia in a bone marrow transplant recipient (letter). Br J Haematol 1989;71:300.

White DG, Woolf AD, Mortimer PP, et al. Human parvovirus arthropathy. Lancet 1985;1:419-421.

Yaegashi N, Shiraishi H, Takeshita T, et al. Propagation of human parvovirus B19 in primary culture of erythroid lineage cells derived from fetal liver. J Virol 1989;63:2422-2426.

Young N. Hematologic and hematopoietic consequences of B19 parvovirus infection. Semin Hematol 1988;25: 159-172.

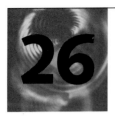

26 PERTUSSIS (WHOOPING COUGH)

EDWARD A. MORTIMER, JR.[†] AND JAMES D. CHERRY

Pertussis is a devastating contagious disease of childhood, particularly infancy, that is now well controlled in the United States and other developed countries by immunization. However, at the turn of the century in the United States approximately 5 of every 1,000 infants born alive died of the disease before their fifth birthdays (Mortimer and Jones, 1979). Today, fewer than 10 deaths are reported annually in the United States. Thus the disease remains well controlled in the developed world, although local outbreaks continue to occur. In contrast, in the developing world as recently as the early 1980s, according to the Expanded Programme on Immunization (EPI) in 1992, the rate of childhood pertussis deaths exceeded 7 per 1,000 births. Morbidity and mortality, however, have declined, and it is a remarkable tribute to the efforts of the EPI that by 1992 (in less than 10 years) this rate was reduced by 60% (World Health Organization, 1996).

In the past decade, several other developments related to the control of pertussis have occurred. In the United States there is further confirmation of adolescents and adults with atypical pertussis as an important reservoir of the disease. The polymerase chain reaction (PCR) assay has been confirmed as a useful method for identification of the organism in respiratory secretions, although it is not yet widely available for routine use. Acellular pertussis DTP preparations (DTaP vaccines) have replaced whole-cell DTP vaccines in the United States and are now licensed and used in many developed countries. DTaP vaccines are being considered for use as boosters in adolescents and adults.

The first description of the disease did not appear until the sixteenth century, which is rather curious for an epidemic disorder with such a characteristic clinical picture. An explanatory hypothesis for this curiosity is that pertussis was a disease new to humans at that time. Recent studies suggest that *Bordetella bronchiseptica*, a pathogen of several lower mammals, is the likely evolutionary progenitor of *Bordetella pertussis*—the causative organism of epidemic pertussis (Cotter and Miller, 2001). *B. pertussis* was first recovered by Bordet and Gengou in 1906, and in the mid 1940s effective vaccines became available. Current whole-cell vaccines are essentially the same as those in use 50 years ago. Over the last 25 years, biotechnological advances have allowed the development of DTaP vaccines that are less reactogenic than their DTP vaccine predecessors (Hewlett and Cherry, 1997).

ETIOLOGY

Epidemic pertussis is caused by *B. pertussis*. Similar nonepidemic illness is caused by *Bordetella parapertussis*, and rarely *B. bronchiseptica* can cause a pertussis-like cough illness. *B. pertussis* is a fastidious gram-negative, aerobic pleomorphic bacillus. It can be recovered from the surface of ciliated epithelial cells of the respiratory tract. Specimens for culture can be obtained by nasopharyngeal swab (calcium alginate or Dacron), nasopharyngeal aspiration, or nasal wash. Specimens should be directly plated on special medium (Regan-Lowe or Bordet-Gengou agar) and inoculated in modified Stainer-Scholte broth. In situations when direct plating cannot be carried out, the use of Regan-Lowe transport medium is recommended. The highest isolation rates occur when specimens are obtained early in the illness and the laboratory personnel are experienced in isolating the organism.

Antigens and Biologically Active Components

Among the many bacteria that affect humans, *B. pertussis* has been one of the more difficult to study in terms of its biologic anatomy. Indeed, only in the last 25 years or so has it been possible to dissect the organism and relate its various components to disease pathogenesis and immunity in man, although as yet imperfectly. Previously, various physiologic effects and attributes of the organism, recognized in the laboratory and to some extent in humans, could not be assigned to identifiable components. Recent advances in genetic and molecular techniques (the entire genome of *B. pertussis* has been sequenced) have led to a greatly increased understanding of *Bordetella* pathogenesis and what identified antigens and biologically active components can do (Cotter and Miller, 2001). However, because there is no natural-host animal model system for *B. pertussis*, the actual events in human infection can only be speculated. A brief review of the constituents of the organism and their probable or possible roles in disease pathogenesis and immunity are outlined in Table 26-1 and presented later. All known virulence factors, with the exception of tracheal cytotoxin (TCT), are regulated by a single genetic locus *bvg*AS (Cotter and Miller, 2001). A component of *B. pertussis* assigned considerable importance in the pathogenesis and immunology of pertussis has been variously designated *pertussis toxin* (PT), *lymphocytosis-promoting factor* (LPF), and *pertussigen,* with the first term used most commonly (Table 26-1). PT is a classic bacterial toxin with an enzymatically active A subunit and a B oligomer-binding protein. PT is associated with the production of lymphocytosis in humans and experimental animals. It is also the histamine-sensitizing factor, the effect of which has been long recognized in experimental animals, although this effect does not occur in humans. PT also stimulates the release of insulin

in humans and animals; in animals, but not in humans, significant hypoglycemia results. PT has a variety of other actions, including (1) mitogenicity for some human and animal cells, and (2) hemagglutination (Wardlaw and Parton, 1988). It is likely that PT plays an important role in the pathogenesis of pertussis. It appears to facilitate attachment of the organism to respiratory ciliated cells, and it may be an important contributor to respiratory mucosal damage. The finding in the mid-1970s that PT was a classic bacterial toxin, like diphtheria toxin, led to the idea that pertussis was a single-toxin disease and that pertussis could be controlled in a manner similar to diphtheria with a toxoid vaccine (Cherry, 1992). However, it is clear today that pertussis is not a single PT toxin disease and its major clinical manifestation, paroxysmal cough, is not caused by PT. This statement is supported by the fact that *B. parapertussis* causes a cough illness similar to that caused by *B. pertussis,* but *B. parapertussis* does not express PT. Antibodies to PT develop in humans after infection or immunization, and antibodies to PT are important in clinical immunity to pertussis.

Filamentous hemagglutinin (FHA) is a cell wall component of all *Bordetella* species, and animal model studies suggest that it participates in the attachment of the organism to ciliated respiratory epithelial cells. It is nontoxic to cells and with infection or immunization it elicits a vigorous antibody response.

It was noted over 50 years ago that antibody to *B. pertussis* caused agglutination of the organism. It is now known that the most important antigens (agglutinogens) in agglutination are two fimbrial serotypes (fimbriae 2 and 3). Fimbriae also participate in the attachment of *B. pertussis* to ciliated respiratory epithelial cells.

TABLE 26-1 Putative Roles of Constituents of *Bordetella pertussis* in Humans

Constituent	Pathogenesis	Immunity
Pertussis toxin (PT)	Attachment; cell damage; causes lymphocytosis	Important
Filamentous hemaglutinin (FHA)	Minor attachment factor	Possibly important
Fimbriae 2 and 3	Attachment	Important
Pertactin	Attachment	Most important
Adenylate cyclase toxin	Cell damage	Probably not important
Dermonecrotic toxin	Possible cell damage	None
Tracheal cytotoxin (TCT)	Cell damage	None
Lipopolysaccharide (LPS); endotoxin	Attachment	Probably important
Tracheal colonization factor (TCF)	Attachment	Probably important

Another important antigen of *B. pertussis* is pertactin, a 69-kDa outer-membrane protein (Shahin et al., 1990). It functions as an adhesin in infection, and recent studies suggest that antibody to pertactin is most important in human protection (Cherry et al., 1998a; Storsaeter et al., 1998).

Adenylate cyclase toxin is a cellular enzyme that disrupts host cell metabolism and very likely participates in ciliary cell destruction. It is also immunogenic, but there is no evidence to date that antibodies to this enzyme play a role in clinical immunity.

Another identified component of the organism is TCT, which very likely plays a role in cell damage. A relatively small molecule, TCT is not immunogenic. A heat-labile toxin, sometimes known as dermonecrotic toxin, is also produced. It is lethal to animals when given systemically and produces dermonecrosis on local injection. It appears to play no role in clinical immunity, and whether or how it participates in the pathogenesis of the disease is unknown. Like other gram-negative bacteria, *B. pertussis* produces a lipopolysaccharide (LPS, endotoxin). Compared with the endotoxins of enteric bacilli, the toxicity of this lipopolysaccharide is weak, being one tenth to one hundredth as potent. It is immunogenic, and it is an attachment factor. It is a major cause of local reactions and fever following immunization with whole-cell component DTP vaccines.

Recently described is tracheal colonization factor (TCF), which may also be an important attachment factor.

EPIDEMIOLOGY

Pertussis is highly contagious, transmitted primarily by intimate respiratory contact. Nearly all nonimmune, exposed household contacts acquire the disease, and approximately 50% of susceptible individuals exposed in school settings develop pertussis. Because there is minimal transplacental immunity, young infants, in whom the disease is most dangerous, are usually fully susceptible.

In the absence of immunization it is likely that no individuals escape *B. pertussis* infection during life. However, as with many notifiable infections, pertussis is considerably underreported. Indeed, a well-conducted study indicated that as few as one quarter of all cases are actually reported (Sutter and Cochi, 1992). The reasons for lack of notification are multiple and

probably include failure to suspect and diagnose the disease (particularly when the manifestations are atypical or mild); the difficulty in laboratory confirmation; and, unfortunately, the failure of some physicians to appreciate the importance of reporting. Curiously, the disease is more often reported in girls than in boys, and mortality rates are higher in girls. An explanation for this phenomenon is not evident; it may be, given that almost every unimmunized child acquires *B. pertussis* infection, that the disease is inexplicably more severe and therefore more recognizable, and thus reported, in girls. In the past, pertussis was both endemic and epidemic; major increases in incidence occurred every 2 to 5 years (usually 3). Widespread immunization has not altered this cyclic pattern, although incidence rates, both endemic and peak, are strikingly lower (Cherry, 1984).

Seasonal influences on the incidence of pertussis in the United States are difficult to interpret. There is no unanimity among descriptions of the seasonal epidemiology of pertussis before widespread use of the vaccine. Some reports indicated higher incidence in the summer when young infants probably were in more contact with one another. Others stated that the peak incidence was in late winter and early spring, and some alleged no seasonal variation. However, examination of tabulated deaths from pertussis by month for the 5 years 1936 through 1940, allowing a 4- to 8-week lag between onset and date of death, provides support for the assertion that the incidence of pertussis was highest during the first half of the calendar year, at least in younger children, the group most likely to succumb from the disease. Closer examination of these mortality data shows that this seasonal variation was accounted for by the 2 years (1937 and 1938) when deaths were the highest (70% greater than the other 3 years). Recorded deaths for the 3 years with fewer deaths show no month-to-month variation. This suggests that in colder, temperate zones such as the United States pertussis was endemic year-round before the advent of widespread immunization and that epidemics were more apt to occur in the winter and spring. Remarkably, the seasonal epidemiology of pertussis is presently very different. For the years 1980 through 1989, pertussis was two or three times more frequent in the late summer or autumn, with a curious disparity between northern and southern states (Farizo et al.,

1992). In southern states the peak occurred in midsummer; in northern states peak months were July to October. In Cincinnati in the years 1989 through 1993, cases of pertussis were far more frequent in the latter half of the year (Christie et al., 1994). No explanation is available for the past and current seasonality of pertussis or for the apparent shift.

There have also been remarkable changes in the age distribution of pertussis from the pre-vaccine era to the present, but these changes very likely are explained by widespread immunization beginning in the 1950s. Before World War II approximately half of all reported cases occurred in elementary school–age children, who served as the major reservoir of the disease. Less than 20% of cases occurred in infants under 1 year of age, but 50% to 70% of all deaths occurred in this age group. Fewer than 1% of reported cases occurred in individuals older than 14 years (Dauer, 1943). The present age distribution of pertussis in the United States has changed markedly, very likely as a consequence of several interrelated factors. The first is widespread immunization against the disease. A second factor is the requirement for immunization before school entry in the United States. In some states this requirement includes day-care and preschool classes, but in all states immunization requirements are mandated for entry into elementary school. A factor of indeterminable impact is possible enhanced recognition and reporting of pertussis as a result of augmented interest in the disease and better diagnostic methods. Finally, it is increasingly recognized that pertussis occurs in adolescents and adults, ranging from mild atypical cases to the full-blown syndrome (Cherry, 1995; Cherry, 1999a; Deen et al., 1995; Izurieta et al., 1996; Mortimer, 1990). It is likely that *B. pertussis* infections in adolescents and adults have always been common because of waning immunity from both past infections and immunization (Cherry, 1999a; Cherry, 1999b). These infections are recognized today because of attention generated by a number of recent studies and the availability of better laboratory methods for diagnosis. It is also important to note that infections may occur in hospital personnel, even as outbreaks (Cherry, 1995). It is logical to assume that these adult infections, whether mild or severe, represent important sources of continuing transmission of *B. pertussis*. Table 26-2 compares the age distributions of pertussis for 1979 through 1981 and 1992 through 1994 in the United States. Because there is firm evidence that partially immune adolescents and adults with pertussis often exhibit mild symptoms, these data probably underestimate the true incidence of infection in older persons. In 1998, 7,405 cases were reported and 30% of these were in patients older than 14 years of age (Centers for Disease Control and Prevention, 1998). Whatever the reasons, the striking reductions in pertussis morbidity and mortality in the United States have been associated with clear-cut changes in the age distribution of reported cases. These changes have important implications for the control of the disease.

Determining the effects of race on pertussis epidemiology is complicated by a number of factors. In the late 1930s overall pertussis mortality rates for blacks strikingly exceeded those for whites (Dauer, 1943). This was in part a result of the fact that disease incidence rates for blacks compared with whites were considerably higher in infants and very young children, who are at greatest risk of death. Additionally, age-specific mortality rates for blacks were higher in all age groups. These differences in morbidity and mortality are undoubtedly explained in large part by socioeconomic status. Curiously, overall mortality rates from

| TABLE 26-2 | Age Distribution of Reported Pertussis Cases in the United States, 1979-1981 and 1992-1994 |

Year	Total cases	PERCENT BY AGE GROUP IN YEARS				
		<1	1-4	5-14	15-19	>19
1979-1981	4,601	56	26	12	2	4
1992-1994	14,829	41	20	21	6	12

From Centers for Disease Control and Prevention from annual summaries published in the *Morbidity and Mortality Weekly Report* for the respective years.

pertussis were always higher in rural areas in the United States; it is likely that this is in part explained by very high mortality rates in blacks in the rural South. These differences persisted through the first decade or two of the pertussis vaccine era, probably for similar reasons and because of lower rates of immunization in blacks. It is therefore unlikely that any differences in morbidity and mortality by race are related to the genetics of race (Dauer, 1943).

PATHOLOGY

The pathologic findings in patients with pertussis are primarily bronchopulmonary; changes in other organs are of anoxic origin stemming from bronchopulmonary damage. The key changes are bronchial and bronchiolar, with ciliary damage and destruction, edema, and the accumulation of mucoid secretions. Secondary findings are bronchiolar obstruction; atelectasis; areas of bronchopneumonia; and, occasionally, spotty emphysematous changes. Pneumothorax occurs but is uncommon, and secondary bacterial pneumonia such as lobar pneumonia is uncommon except as a complication of assisted ventilation. Mortality from pertussis relates directly to the severity of pulmonary involvement (Lapin, 1943). Other manifestations occur mainly in the brain and are of two varieties. The first consists of edema and other changes characteristic of anoxia. Hemorrhages constitute the other type of cerebral changes. They may be moderately extensive but usually are small or petechial.

PATHOGENESIS

Knowledge of the actions of the various components of B. pertussis permits the development of a hypothesis about the series of pathologic events that occur in the course of whooping cough. Because the likelihood of infection varies directly with the intimacy and duration of contact, it is probable that large numbers of organisms are required to infect the respiratory tract. Attachment of organisms to respiratory cilia is facilitated by pertactin, fimbriae 2 and 3, PT, LPS, TCF, and possibly FHA. After attachment it is necessary for the organism to evade host defenses; major roles in this process are presumably played by PT and adenylate cyclase. It is logical that TCT and dermonecrotic toxin participate. Cell damage is a consequence of the actions of PT and adenylate cyclase. It is probable that TCT and dermonecrotic toxins also contribute (Cotter and Miller, 2001; Wardlaw and Parton, 1988). Similarly, there is no evidence that the rather weak endotoxin of B. pertussis contributes to disease manifestations (Wardlaw and Parton, 1988). An obvious contribution of PT is the characteristic lymphocytosis of pertussis. There is no evidence that PT induces histamine stimulation during the illness, nor does the insulin-stimulating activity exert any clinically recognizable effect in humans. B. pertussis is noninvasive; accordingly, all the manifestations of pertussis except lymphocytosis may be explained by the unique effects on respiratory endothelium with disruption of function or cell death (Wardlaw and Parton, 1988). As a consequence of ciliary destruction or dysfunction, the normal toilet of the pulmonary tree is compromised. The processes that remove foreign material, cell debris, and secretions are impaired, resulting in the accumulation of viscid mucoid material. Retained secretions obstruct smaller bronchi and bronchioles, with consequent atelectasis and occasional emphysema. Nonspecific bronchopneumonia occurs frequently. The thick ropy secretions that accumulate are very difficult to expel, resulting in episodes of repetitious, paroxysmal coughing, often followed by vomiting. The mechanism of vomiting is probably the accumulation of this viscid material in the pharynx. The characteristic whoop follows a protracted spasm that has nearly emptied the bronchopulmonary tree of air and represents an attempt to inspire through vocal cords that may be partially narrowed because of secretions and consequent spasm. Indeed, it may well be that in some instances inspiration is possible only when some relaxation of vocal cords occurs as a result of severe anoxia. The mechanism of the encephalopathy that sometimes occurs in the course of pertussis, often with permanent brain damage or death, was the subject of considerable debate in the past. A hypothesis often voiced was that one or another toxic product of B. pertussis was responsible. No such toxin has been identified; currently, there is general consensus that encephalopathy during the course of pertussis is explained by anoxia engendered by the episodes of paroxysmal coughing and, in some instances, by cerebral hemorrhages of varying extent that result from the combination of increased intracranial pressure during paroxysms and the vascular effects of anoxia. In those children who die of pertussis there are three apparent mechanisms of death that often act in concert. Severe bronchopulmonary disease with bronchopneumonia is of major importance. Often associated with it is the central nervous system damage described earlier. In the past, and perhaps in the developing world today, inanition secondary to repeated emesis following spasms of coughing was undoubtedly a major factor in mortality from whooping cough in infants and children. Additionally, in the past in the United States and presently in the developing world, other underlying disorders such as low birth weight; malnutrition; gastrointestinal infections; and other debilitating conditions, including measles and severe respiratory illnesses, strongly compromise survival of infants and children with whooping cough.

CLINICAL MANIFESTATIONS

The clinical presentation of *B. pertussis* infection depends on a number of factors, such as age, previous immunization or infection, the presence of passively required antibody, degree of exposure, host genetic and acquired traits, and perhaps the genotype of the infecting organism. The incubation period for the majority of cases is 7 to 10 days and most cases occur between 6 and 20 days after exposure. The initial symptoms are nonspecific. Throughout the course of the disease, fever is absent or low. There may be mild coryza-like symptoms, plus a mild, dry cough. The cough progresses in frequency and severity, and, approximately 2 weeks after onset, spells of paroxysmal coughing are recognized. The paroxysms progress in severity and frequency; ultimately, dozens of such spells may occur daily. As the paroxysms increase, the characteristic whoop occurs, often followed by vomiting. With severe paroxysms, cyanosis often occurs, the eyes roll back, and the child may appear semiconscious. When a paroxysm terminates, it appears that the respiratory tract has been nearly emptied of air; the characteristic whoop is produced by the initial attempt to inspire through the glottis, which is narrowed by spasm caused by the irritative effects of the secretions and the cough. The vomiting apparently is a consequence of thick mucoid secretions in the pharynx. Frequently, a series of paroxysms may occur in immediate succession. Severe paroxysms are very frightening to the child and to all observers. After an

episode the child appears exhausted. In full-blown pertussis, paroxysms with whooping usually persist at least 2 weeks and may continue for 6 weeks. The paroxysms frequently are precipitated by a variety of events, such as feeding, crying, or even hearing another person cough; in the past, when several children with pertussis were in the same hospital room, a paroxysm in one child would precipitate episodes in others. In convalescence the cough gradually disappears over a month or more, although minor exacerbations may occur with exertion or in the course of an intercurrent respiratory infection. The two major and potentially lethal complications of pertussis, bronchopneumonia and encephalopathy, are most apt to occur at the height of the paroxysmal stage. In patients with severe whooping cough it may be difficult to maintain adequate intake of fluid and nourishment because of the vicious cycle of feeding inducing paroxysms and vomiting. In the past, when the incidence of whooping cough was high, particularly in infants, some nurses in contagious disease hospitals were highly valued for their skill and patience in feeding and refeeding infants with severe whooping cough.

In addition to typical pertussis, which is described above, mild nonclassic illness due to *B. pertussis* infection is common. As might be expected, it occurs in previously vaccinated children, but also frequently occurs in primary infections in nonvaccinated children. In mild illness paroxysms still occur but the total duration of disease is shortened. In one study involving 2,592 culture-positive previously unvaccinated children, it was found that 17% had cough illness duration of 3 weeks or less (Heininger et al., 1997).

B. pertussis infection in neonates is particularly severe and often not recognized as pertussis. Illness often presents as apnea, and typical coughing is not observed. However, the infants have repetitive expiration of air without inspiration. This leads to hypoxia, apnea, and often seizures. Marked leukocytosis with lymphocytosis is particularly notable in neonates and correlates with severe disease.

Adults with *B. pertussis* infections are noted to have prolonged afebrile cough illnesses that are most often not recognized as pertussis and are thought to be bronchitis or allergic conditions (Cherry, 1999a). However, most have paroxysmal cough with significant posttussive phlegm. Choking sensation is described and posttussive vomiting is common. Some adults experience unique sweating episodes and others fainting in association with coughing.

Illness caused by *B. parapertussis* is similar to that caused by *B. pertussis* but is most often less severe and of shortened duration (Heininger et al., 1994). Leukocytosis with lymphocytosis does not occur in *B. parapertussis* infection.

DIAGNOSIS

The clinical picture of full-blown pertussis is so characteristic that the disease is readily suspected and recognized by physicians, other health-care personnel, and grandparents who have had prior experience with its manifestations, particularly if a paroxysm is observed. The presence of pertussis in the community or a history of exposure provides strongly supportive evidence; however, the source of infection may be an individual with a mild, atypical illness, particularly a household member who in the past had been infected or vaccinated and whose immunity had waned. Also strongly supportive of the diagnosis is absolute lymphocytosis, which is usually present at the beginning of the paroxysmal stage and persists for 3 or 4 weeks (Figure 26-1). However, in infants and in

partially immune persons with antibodies to PT, lymphocytosis does not occur.

Proof of the diagnosis of pertussis is achieved by recovery of the organism on culture (Onorato and Wassilak, 1987). The organism is most readily recovered during the catarrhal stage but disappears within 2 or 3 weeks after the onset of paroxysms (Figure 26-1). The best source of material for culture is nasopharyngeal mucus obtained by nasopharyngeal swab, nasopharyngeal aspiration, or nasal wash. Use of cough plates, often the practice in the past, is less frequently successful.

Isolation of *B. pertussis* depends on careful transport and efficient processing of the materials obtained for culture and is particularly enhanced if the clinical microbiologist is experienced with the organism. If the specimen cannot be processed soon after it is obtained it should be placed in Regan-Lowe transport medium. While direct plating is preferable, specimens in transport medium will have a good yield even if shipped by post. In the laboratory, the specimen should be inoculated onto Bordet-Gengou or Regan-Lowe agar and into modified Stainer-Scholte broth. There are other satisfactory laboratory culture media and methods.

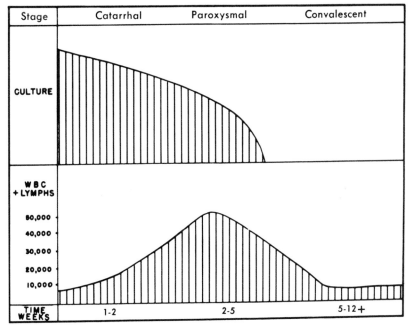

Fig. 26-1 Diagnostic laboratory findings in pertussis. *Bordetella pertussis* may be recovered, usually during catarrhal and early paroxysmal stages (first 4 weeks of illness). The white blood cell count usually is elevated during the paroxysmal stage (second to fifth weeks). Lymphocytes predominate.

In addition to a specific pattern of biochemical reactions, serologic identification of *B. pertussis* will confirm the isolation. A slide agglutination test can be performed with a standard inoculum of organisms and specific antiserum, which is available commercially (Onorato and Wassilak, 1987). Direct fluorescent antibody (DFA) staining has been used to identify *B. pertussis* from direct smears of nasopharyngeal swabs and for identification of organisms growing on Bordet-Gengou plates. The DFA examination of nasopharyngeal swab material is often unreliable except in experienced hands. However, in patients who have received antibiotics, the DFA may be positive when cultures are negative. In recent years a new approach to the diagnosis of pertussis is the polymerase chain reaction (PCR) (Ewanowich et al., 1993; He et al., 1994; Schlapfer et al., 1995). By PCR assay one or more characteristic nucleic acid sequences of specific genes of *B. pertussis* can be identified in respiratory secretions. Requiring relatively few organisms in the specimen, PCR is very sensitive and highly specific. Initially developed as a research tool, it probably will become more widely available. However, a major problem with PCR in the diagnosis of pertussis is the risk of false positive results because of contaminated specimens. Contamination can occur in the doctor's office from the air if another patient has pertussis. Contamination can also occur in the laboratory if PCR is not performed in a separate area.

In the past, assessment of antibodies in the serum was usually accomplished by measuring agglutinins, but today few laboratories in the United States are prepared to perform tests for *B. pertussis* agglutinin titers.

Specific tests for antibodies to PT and FHA have been developed, and enzyme-linked immunosorbent assays (ELISAs) for IgG and IgA antibodies correlate well with infection and are of considerable use in recognizing culture-negative pertussis, including mild or asymptomatic infections (Granstrom et al., 1988; Steketee et al., 1988). Many commercial laboratories now perform ELISA for *B. pertussis* antibodies. With satisfactory standardization, a 100% (twofold) or greater increase in antibody to PT IgG or IgA between acute-phase and convalescent-phase serum specimens is indicative of infection. IgG and IgA antibodies to FHA are also often used in documenting pertussis. However, other *Bordetella* species and perhaps other microorganisms can elicit false positive results.

Most instances of the whooping cough syndrome in infants and children represent true pertussis, particularly during outbreaks, although on rare occasions other disorders may be associated with prolonged cough and result in confusion. Illness due to *B. parapertussis* cannot be clinically differentiated from that caused by *B. pertussis,* although it is normally less severe and of a shortened duration (Heininger et al., 1997). *Mycoplasma pneumoniae* and *Chlamydia pneumoniae* both cause pneumonia with prolonged periods of coughing. However, the illnesses usually are associated with significant fever, and the cough, although repetitive, is not paroxysmal. Pneumonia due to *Chlamydia trachomatis* in young infants is associated with a staccato cough without the distress of a pertussis paroxysm. In the past, several studies suggested that adenoviruses could cause pertussis-like illness. However, it is likely that cases in these studies had both *B. pertussis* and adenoviral infections. Confusion occasionally arises in the case of some children with bronchiolitis or protracted bronchopneumonia. Previously unrecognized cystic fibrosis may cause confusion, as may respiratory foreign bodies. In the past, tuberculosis with hilar nodes pressing on the trachea or bronchi occasionally resulted in similar symptoms. Ordinarily, however, there is little confusion, but other conditions should be suspected when confirmatory or supportive evidence such as a positive culture, lymphocytosis, and epidemiologic linkage to a proved case or to an outbreak is lacking.

More important than misclassifying other conditions as pertussis at the present time is the problem of failure to diagnose pertussis in cases that are mild or atypical. Such mild illnesses may lack characteristics that distinguish them from a wide variety of other, more common respiratory disorders, and thus pertussis is not suspected. Mild cases in older siblings or parents in a household are often recognized retrospectively when an infant, as yet unimmunized, develops full-blown whooping cough. In individuals with mild disease the diagnosis, even if suspected early, is not easily made. The organism may be more difficult to recover on culture, either because of the lack of copious respiratory secretions or because the number of organisms is small. Additionally, lymphocytosis may be inhibited by residual antibody to PT. Nonetheless, such individuals appear to constitute a major reservoir for pertussis and a source of infection for others.

COMPLICATIONS

There are three major complications of pertussis: respiratory problems, effects on the central nervous system, and malnutrition. Respiratory complications usually consist of varying degrees of atelectasis and nonspecific bronchopneumonia. Localized emphysema may occur, but pneumothorax is rare. True lobar pneumonia is uncommon. In the past, 90% of deaths caused by pertussis resulted from pulmonary complications; this proportion is no doubt reduced considerably at present by modern measures of intensive care, including mechanical ventilation and, perhaps, antimicrobial therapy.

Central nervous system complications occur rarely in the course of pertussis, particularly during the paroxysmal stage, and they may be severe (Litvak et al., 1948). They apparently are secondary to anoxia and cerebral hemorrhages that are usually petechial but may be larger. The clinical findings are those of nonspecific encephalopathy, usually including repeated convulsions and obtunding. Visual disturbances and paralyses may occur. Central nervous system complications are most frequent in young infants. Estimates of the risk of encephalopathy associated with whooping cough are quite imprecise because they are based on hospitalized cases and do not include in the denominator the much larger numbers of children with pertussis who do not require hospitalization. However, from two populations in which it was possible to estimate the total number of cases of pertussis, the apparent risks of severe encephalopathy were 1:11,000 and 1:12,500 (Litvak et al., 1948; Miller et al., 1985). Undoubtedly, the risk is markedly age dependent; it is probably negligible in older children and much higher in young infants. Permanent sequelae—seizure disorders, developmental retardation, and pareses—frequently ensue. There is also evidence, mostly but not all anecdotal, that milder forms of encephalopathy, insufficiently severe to warrant hospitalization, occur and may be associated with more subtle neurologic disturbances, including developmental disorders. In the past in the United States, malnutrition secondary to repeated vomiting and sometimes progressing to inanition was a major problem, particularly in infants. It remains a serious complication in developing countries, where it is often superimposed on, or concomitant with, other debilitating factors. The combination of large populations of unimmunized children with consequently high rates of pertussis and high case-fatality rates explains the excessive mortality from whooping cough in these countries. Minor complications of pertussis include otitis media and hemorrhagic phenomena such as epistaxis, petechiae, and subconjunctival bleeding. In infants and children young enough to have lower incisors, ulceration of the frenum may occur because of protrusion of the tongue during coughing spells. Occasionally, a hernia may become manifest because of increased abdominal pressure during coughing spells, and, rarely, prolapse of the rectum occurs. Apnea is a significant problem in neonates and young infants, and sudden death occurs. Rib fractures are not uncommon in severe adult cases.

PROGNOSIS

In the United States the mortality rate has declined remarkably since the turn of the century. At that time approximately 1 of every 200 children born alive died of pertussis before the fifth birthday; in the last decade this risk has been reduced to no more than 1 in 500,000. This decline cannot be attributed solely to the advent of pertussis vaccines; indeed, by the late 1930s, before pertussis vaccine was available, the mortality rate from pertussis in young children had declined approximately 80% from 1900 (Mortimer and Jones, 1979). This remarkable decline by 1940 must be attributed to a decrease in the case-fatality rate because nearly every child experienced pertussis, a highly contagious disease. Undoubtedly, many factors contributed to this decline in the case-fatality rates. Possible factors include the diminished frequency of diarrheal diseases of infancy as a result of pasteurization of milk; better nutrition; improved socioeconomic status; and smaller family size, resulting both in decreased exposure of high-risk young infants and in better supportive care of ill infants. With the advent of increasingly widespread immunization against pertussis beginning in the late 1940s, there was a striking acceleration in the decline of mortality from pertussis. A similar decrease was observed in Britain a few years later when pertussis immunization was instituted. Although the vaccine-induced near-elimination of pertussis is clearly the major factor in this accelerated decline, case-fatality rates have undoubtedly also decreased as a result of better supportive care, including respiratory assistance; better nutrition; and, perhaps, the availability of antibiotics (Mortimer and Jones, 1979).

TREATMENT

The treatment of pertussis is largely supportive. In most instances this protracted disease, although fatiguing or exhausting and very unpleasant, can be managed at home. Most patients who require hospitalization are young infants. For children managed at home, maintenance of adequate nutrition and hydration is ordinarily easily achieved. Providing high humidity is probably of no value. Cough suppressants, if used at all, should be used in low doses to avoid interference with expulsion of secretions (Bass, 1985).

For those children who must be hospitalized, usually infants, symptomatic management depends on disease manifestations and their severity. The infant or child with severe pertussis must be constantly monitored so that immediate help can be provided for severe paroxysms. A means of suction should be at hand. In patients unable to handle their own secretions, removal of mucoid material is facilitated by placing the child in a head-down position (45 to 60 degrees) to take advantage of gravity. Suction of the oropharynx with a catheter large enough to permit flow of tenacious secretions is required during paroxysms. In a severely ill child, assisted ventilation and oxygen may be needed. The child's state of hydration must be monitored and maintained at an adequate level. Caloric intake also requires observation, although, during the most severe phase of the disease, optimal intake may not be possible.

Specific therapy is less than satisfactory. *B. pertussis* is susceptible to a number of antibiotics in vitro, but the only agent with extensive evidence of clinical efficacy is erythromycin. Erythromycin may be expected to eradicate *B. pertussis* from the upper respiratory tract; for this reason all children with pertussis should receive 14 days of this antibiotic 50 mg/kg daily in four divided doses to minimize transmission.

The dose for adults is 2 g/day given every 6 hours Unfortunately, erythromycin has been shown to exert only a minimal effect on the clinical course of full-blown pertussis. Clearly, it will prevent or modify the course of the disease when given promptly to exposed persons or during the incubation period before the onset of symptoms (DeSerres et al., 1995). There is also some evidence that, when given early in the catarrhal stage, it will ameliorate symptoms or shorten the course of the disease. Unfortunately, the potential value of erythromycin is sorely compromised because exposure usually is not recognized and because the symptoms of those with early pertussis in the catarrhal stage are indistinguishable from those with a common respiratory infection. Nonetheless, in a household with a case of recognized pertussis, all family members with or without symptoms should receive a full course of erythromycin promptly in the stated dosage in an effort to prevent further disease and subsequent spread. Trimethoprim-sulfamethoxazole can be used in children allergic to erythromycin. On the basis of in vitro sensitivity testing it is likely that the newer macrolide antibiotics (clarithromycin and azithromycin) are effective, but few clinical trials are available to date. Because adults tolerate the full dose of erythromycin poorly, it is probably better when an antibiotic is being administered for prophylaxis to use azithromycin (Cherry, 1995).

IMMUNITY

Immunity to pertussis had once been considered lifelong after a first attack (Mortimer, 1990), but in recent years improved diagnostic methods, enhanced surveillance, careful historical review, and seasonal epidemiologic studies have shown this belief to be false (Cherry, 1999a; Cherry, 1999b; Cherry et al., 1995; Schmitt-Grohé et al., 1995). Immunity following immunization with most present-day DTP vaccines is good but relatively short lived. Similarly, immunity following infection is also good but relatively short lived. A population study of IgA antibodies (which are a marker for past infection and not immunization) noted similar values in two groups of young adults; most in one group had been vaccinated during early childhood, whereas in the other group few had been vaccinated (Cherry et al., l995). These data coupled with findings in a number of adult pertussis studies indicate that recurrent infections with *B. pertussis* are frequent in both previously vaccinated and unvaccinated persons (Cherry, 1999a). In general, infections in persons who were previously vaccinated are less severe, and it is probable that most reinfections in persons who had pertussis in childhood are also modified.

It is repeatedly stated that the nature of immunity in pertussis is not known and that there are no serologic correlates of immunity. Although there is clearly much more to learn, both old and new data indicate that specific serum antibodies protect against infection (Cherry and Olin, 1999; Cherry et al, 1998a; Storsaeter et al., 1998). It was demonstrated 40 to 50 years ago that high levels of agglutinating serum antibodies were protective. We now know that agglutinating antibodies are a composite response to four *B. pertussis* antigens: fimbriae 2 and 3, pertactin, and LPS. In two recent studies it was found that antibody to pertactin was most important in protection and that additional antibodies to fimbriae and PT augmented this protection.

PREVENTION

Active immunization is the mainstay of pertussis control worldwide because treatment of pertussis is far from satisfactory, transmission occurs from early or unrecognized infections, and passive immunization has not been proved to be effective and is not available (Cherry, 1984; American Academy of Pediatrics, 2000; Mortimer and Jones, 1979). Beginning approximately in 1910, a few years after identification and isolation of the organism, various attempts were made to develop vaccines for primary immunization. For many years these hit-or-miss efforts were largely unsuccessful. Most preparations consisted of killed, whole organisms, although around 1940 attempts were made to immunize with cell-free filtrates of cultures of the organism. By the early 1940s clinically effective whole-cell preparations were produced, and by 1945 they were licensed and marketed. In the United States, pertussis vaccine was standardized by federal regulation in 1954, and in 1964 an international standard was established. Current whole-cell pertussis vaccines are relatively unchanged since that time, except for technical refinements such as better control of the number of organisms required for an immunizing dose.

Today acellular pertussis vaccines (DTaP) are replacing whole-cell vaccines (DTP) in many countries throughout the world, but at present and for a number of years in the future DTP vaccines will continue to be used because they are cheaper and have been proven to be efficacious.

White-cell Vaccines

Today's killed, whole-cell pertussis vaccines are combined with diphtheria and tetanus toxoids and adsorbed onto an aluminum salt, forming the familiar diphtheria and tetanus toxoids and pertussis vaccine (DTP).

Whole-cell pertussis vaccines, widely used in the industrialized world during the past four decades, have achieved a remarkable record of success. For the 10 years 1983 through 1992, an average of less than six deaths from pertussis were reported annually in the United States. Additionally, during the years 1985 through 1994 an average of about 4,100 cases were reported annually, compared with more than 220,000 four decades ago. Acknowledging that the disease is vastly underreported, even if recognized, this is a remarkable achievement (Sutter and Cochi, 1992).

For many years it has been recognized that DTP is undesirably reactive (Mortimer and Jones, 1979). Most of the reactivity is attributable to the pertussis component (Cody et al., 1981). Local reactions include pain at the site of injection in approximately half of all recipients; redness and swelling are observed in approximately 40%. Systemic reactions include fever of 38° C or more in nearly half of recipients; more than half display irritability. Drowsiness is noted in approximately one third and anorexia in approximately 20%. These systemic symptoms are largely limited to the first 48 hours after injection; fever is most apt to occur between 6 and 12 hours after receipt of the vaccine. Rare but disturbing events that occur after DTP injection include so-called hypotensive-hyporesponsive episodes. These episodes usually occur within a few hours of the injection and always within 12 hours. Duration is usually a matter of minutes or 1 or 2 hours, but rarely episodes have lasted longer (up to 36 hours). The best estimate of their frequency is 1 per 1,750 doses, but with a wide confidence interval. These episodes are frightening to observe because the child appears cold, clammy, and bluish and responds poorly. Nonetheless, spontaneous recovery occurs, and death has not been observed. The mechanism is unclear; similar episodes have been observed following administration of diphtheria and tetanus toxoids (DT) (Pollock and Morris, 1983).

As would be expected, febrile convulsions occur occasionally after DTP injection but appear to be without sequelae (Baraff et al., 1988; Barlow et al., 2001; Cody et al., 1981; Shields et al., 1988). The best estimate of their frequency is 1 per 1,750 doses, with a wide confidence interval and variation with age. Occasionally, convulsions after DTP injection occur in the absence of fever; rarely, more complex or protracted seizures may occur with or without fever. It is likely that most, if not all, of these more worrisome convulsive episodes represent the precipitation of overt manifestations of preexisting central nervous system disorders by the systemic effects of DTP. Persistent, inconsolable crying has also been observed after the child is given DTP or, less often, DT. These episodes are without sequelae and probably are caused by pain at the site of injection (Cody et al., 1981). For nearly 60 years, beginning with the original hit-or-miss experimental vaccines, there have been dozens of anecdotal reports suggesting that, on occasion, within 1 or 2 days after injection, pertussis vaccine produces acute, severe encephalopathy, sometimes with permanent brain damage or death (Cherry et al., 1988). Because the disease itself was known to produce encephalopathy and because other vaccines such as those for rabies and smallpox were recognized to cause severe neurologic sequelae, these rare events were accepted as an unfortunate price to pay for the control of a serious disease. As widespread use of the vaccine reduced the threat of the disease markedly, these events became magnified in importance, not only in the United States but also in other industrialized nations, including the United Kingdom, Japan, and Sweden. Widespread publicity about these occurrences caused near boycotts of pertussis vaccine in the United Kingdom and Japan, with reappearance of major outbreaks of the disease (Cherry, 1984; Kanai, 1980; Noble, 1987). In the United States, similar publicity about these alleged injuries exerted only a minor effect on vaccine use, but widespread litigation ensued, resulting in major price increases because of insurance costs. These problems prompted systematic efforts to assess the causative role of pertussis vaccine in severe neurologic disease, both in the United States and in the United Kingdom, with the latter nation being particularly suited to

such studies because of the organization of its health-care system.

In the British National Childhood Encephalopathy Study, over a 3-year period during which approximately 2,100,000 doses of DTP were administered, 1,182 hospitalized children age 3 months to 3 years with acute neurologic disorders without obvious causes were studied (Alderslade et al., 1981; Miller et al., 1981). For each of these children, two age-matched controls were selected, and for all case and control children it was determined whether a vaccine had been administered in the prior 28 days and, if so, when. The results of this study were analyzed and reanalyzed by multiple investigators subsequent to the initial publication and subsequent to a 10-year follow-up publication (Bellman et al., 1983; Bowie, 1990; Cherry, 1989; Cherry, 1990; Howson and Fineberg, 1992; Institute of Medicine, 1991; MacRae, 1988; Madge et al., 1993; Miller et al., 1985; Miller et al., 1993; Stephenson, 1988; Stratton et al., 1994). Although this study was the most extensive and rigorously controlled study of the possible association between pertussis immunization and neurologic events in vaccines ever carried out, the original analyses of the results were flawed (Cherry, 1989; Cherry, 1990; MacRae, 1988; Stephenson, 1988). A major problem was the misclassification of complex febrile convulsing as acute encephalopathy (Stephenson, 1988.) This study demonstrated a statistical association between pertussis immunization and neurologic illness. Children who had received DTP immunization within 3 to 7 days were 2 to 5 times more likely to have neurologic disease than children not immunized during the same time intervals. However, since both cases and controls had an equal rate of immunization during the month preceding the index date it is more appropriate to interpret the results as representing not cause and effect but a redistribution of events during the time period (Cherry, 1989; Cherry, 1990). The vaccine calls attention to or brings out an event that is to occur; it moves its appearance forward in time. The 10-year follow-up analysis noted that children hospitalized with neurologic events originally studied were more likely than controls (well children) to have died or to have educational, behavioral, neurologic, or physical dysfunction 10 years after their original illness (Madge et al., 1993; Miller et al., 1993). However, outcomes in children whose original illness followed DTP immunization were similar to those in children who had not been recently immunized. These findings are reassuring and what would be expected. They do not support a causative association between DTP immunization and brain damage

In the United States the most common severe neurologic illness noted in temporal association with DTP vaccination was the first seizure of what turned out to be severe epilepsy (Cherry, 1990). Four additional extensive epidemiologic studies found no causative role of DTP vaccine in infantile epilepsy. In addition there is no causative relationship between DTP and other disorders such as hyperactivity; learning problems; infantile autism; behavior problems; transverse myelitis; or other overt, subtle, or slowly progressive neurologic conditions (Butler et al., 1982; Cherry, 1990; Golden, 1990). Sudden infant death syndrome (SIDS) has also been noted to follow DTP immunization. This is not surprising, because routine immunization was carried out at the peak age occurrence of SIDS. However, excellent control studies have found no causative association between DTP and SIDS (Cherry et al., 1988; Griffin et al., 1998; Hoffman et al., 1987).

Acellular Vaccines

The development of acellular pertussis vaccines was made possible by technical advances beginning in the 1970s. These advances enabled dissection of the organism, isolation of its various components, and determination (as yet incomplete) of their roles in disease pathogenesis and clinical immunity. The obvious, practical purpose of these efforts was to develop a less reactive vaccine, free of components thought to be irrelevant to clinical immunity. This endeavor was stimulated by increasing concern about serious sequelae attributed to whole-cell vaccines, a concern that turned out to be erroneous on the basis of subsequent information. Nonetheless, whole-cell vaccines are relatively crude compared, for example, with tetanus toxoid, and undoubtedly contain components that may be unpleasantly reactive and irrelevant or of minor importance to immunity. Understandable misinterpretation of the effects of this reactivity resulted in, or contributed to, rejection of vaccine acceptance in the 1970s, with consequent recrudescence of epidemic pertussis in Japan, the United Kingdom, and

Sweden, as well as major concern and litigation in the United States.

On the basis of antibody responses the first acellular pertussis vaccines (DTaP) for clinical use were licensed and used in Japan in 1981 for children age 2 years and older. Infants were excluded because of the assumption that immunization of older children would inhibit transmission to infants; this assumption proved to be false, but nevertheless epidemic pertussis in Japan has been controlled for the past two decades (Kimura and Kuno-Sakai, 1990). Six products, containing two to five antigens, were licensed in Japan. A four-antigen acellular preparation combined with diphtheria and tetanus toxoids that was shown in an uncontrolled study to be clinically protective in Japan (Mortimer et al., 1990) and demonstrated to be less reactive and satisfactorily immunogenic in U.S. children was licensed in the United States in 1991 for the fourth and fifth doses of DTP. Following a controlled efficiency trial in Sweden, a second two-component DTaP was licensed for the same doses in 1992. Because clinical efficacy of these DTaP vaccines had not been demonstrated in infants, whole-cell DTP was continued for the first three doses.

The first prospective controlled trial in infants of two acellular pertussis vaccines was performed in Sweden from 1984 to 1987 (Ad Hoc Group for the Study of Pertussis Vaccines, 1988). Although this trial was well controlled it had several unusual aspects, which detracted from its usefulness. It enrolled only infants who were older than 6 months of age; they received only two doses of vaccine; and there was no whole-cell vaccine control. As mentioned previously, the data for one of the two study vaccines allowed its licensure in the United States for booster doses. At this time it was decided that more extensive efficacy trials in infants with many candidate vaccines should be carried out. Therefore, many phase II reactogenicity and immunogenicity studies were performed with some 14 different candidate vaccines. Subsequently, eight different vaccines were evaluated in eight different efficacy trials in the 1990s.

DTaP vaccines vary from one another by the number of *B. pertussis* antigens that they contain and the concentration of these antigens. They also vary in the amount of diphtheria toxoid and aluminum adjuvant that they contain, the method by which PT is toxoided, and the preservative that they contain. However, a unifying factor of all DTaP vaccines is that they contain virtually no LPS. This fact is responsible for their overall decreased reactogenicity when compared with DTP vaccines.

In one carefully controlled study the reactogenicity of 13 candidate DTaP vaccines was compared with that of a DTP vaccine after doses given at 2, 4, and 6 months of age (Decker et al., 1995). Local redness, swelling, and pain and fever, fussiness, drowsiness, and anorexia were all significantly less common in DTaP recipients than in DTP recipients, as was the use of antipyretic agents. Local redness, swelling, and fever increased in frequency from the first to the third dose whereas the complaint of drowsiness decreased. In other studies it has been noted that the frequency and severity of local erythema and induration increase considerably with fourth and fifth doses of DTaP vaccines. Particularly disconcerting has been the observation of extensive swelling of the thigh with booster doses with some DTaP vaccines. This event was most common in vaccines with a high diphtheria toxoid content.

Less common, more severe DTP-vaccine–related events (persistent crying, seizures, and hypotonic-hyporesponsive episodes) were evaluated in DTaP vaccinees in five large trials. All three events were extremely uncommon and markedly less common than following DTP vaccines (Greco et al., 1996; Gustafsson et al., 1996; Liese et al., 1997; Trollfors et al., 1995; Uberall et al., 1997).

During preparation for the extensive infant efficacy trials that were performed in the early 1990s, it was noted from analysis of the original Swedish trial that case definitions had a marked effect on calculated efficacy. Therefore, in an effort to make the results of different trials comparable, a WHO committee put forward a primary case definition in 1991 (World Health Organization, 1991). This definition required ≥21 days of paroxysmal cough and laboratory confirmation of B. pertussis infection. Although this definition is specific it is not sensitive. A vaccine that lessens the severity of disease but does not prevent disease will have inflated efficacy. In general this definition tends to make the efficacy of all vaccines appear similar (Cherry, 1997). Fortunately in the more rigorous of the efficacy trials carried out in the 1990s the investigators also evaluated less severe illness and in these studies a more accurate picture of vaccine efficacy is available (Greco et al., 1996; Gustafsson et al., 1996; Stehr et al., 1998; Trollfors et al., 1995).

The reported efficacy of DTaP vaccines can also be markedly influenced by other aspects of study design and procedure in addition to case definition (Cherry, 1997; Cherry and Olin, 1999; Cherry et al., 1998b). In general, double-blind trials with both placebo and DTP controls are best. However, observer bias can significantly affect the results of all studies, even those with double blinding. In general, studies with frequent investigator monitoring will identify more mild cases than will studies with infrequent monitoring or in which only parent reporting is used. Studies in which serology as well as culture is used for case identification also will identify more mild cases. In general, household contact studies, unless they are nested within a prospective cohort trial, are particularly subject to observer bias. Finally, it has been demonstrated in the past that case-control studies significantly inflate vaccine efficacy data (Fine, 1997).

From 1984 to 1997 nine trials were carried out in four countries with eight DTaP vaccines and two aP vaccines. When consideration is given to all the possible confounding factors presented previously, the following can be stated:

- The most efficacious vaccine was a multi-component vaccine that contained PT, FHA, pertactin, and fimbriae 2 and 3 (five-component vaccine).
- Three- and four-component vaccines (PT, FHA, and pertactin, with or without fimbriae 2) are more efficacious than monocomponent (PT) or two-component (PT and FHA) vaccines.
- Two-component vaccines (PT and FHA) are more efficacious than PT toxoids.
- One U.S. DTP vaccine in use in the early 1990s was found to have very poor efficacy.
- Only one DTaP vaccine (the five-component product) had an efficacy that was comparable to a good DTP vaccine.

In addition to the use of DTaP vaccines in Japan, where they have been used exclusively since 1981, DTaP vaccines are the only vaccines available in the United States and are used extensively in Europe and Canada (Heininger, 2001). Vaccination schedules with DTaP vaccines vary from country to country. For example, in the United States the traditional schedule of 2, 4, 6, and 12 to 15 months and 4 to 6 years is recommended. In contrast in Denmark, Norway, and Sweden, DTaP vaccines are administered at 3, 5, and 12 months. In Germany DTaP vaccines are administered at 2, 3, 4, and 12 months and at 11 years.

Although few data are available to support the various schedules, some aspects are relatively clear. For example, the high concentrations of PT and pertactin in one three-component vaccine used in the United States should allow an alternative schedule, such as 2, 4, and 6 months and 4 to 6 years or 2, 4, and 12 to 15 months and 4 to 6 years. Finally, because adolescents and adults play an important role in the continued circulation of *B. pertussis*, future schedules should include adolescent and adult booster doses.

BIBLIOGRAPHY

Ad Hoc Group for the Study of Pertussis Vaccines. Placebo-controlled trial of two acellular pertussis vaccines in Sweden: protective efficacy and adverse events. Lancet 1988;1:955-960.

Alderslade R, Bellman MH, Rawson NSB, et al. The National Childhood Encephalopathy Study. In Whooping Cough: Reports from the Committee on Safety and the Joint Committee on Vaccination and Immunization. London: Department of Health and Social Security, Her Majesty's Stationary Office, 1981.

American Academy of Pediatrics. Pertussis. In Peter G (ed): 1994 Red Book: Report of the Committee on Infectious Diseases, ed 23. Elk Grove Village, Ill: American Academy of Pediatrics, 1994.

American Academy of Pediatrics, Committee on Infectious Diseases. The relationship between pertussis vaccine and central nervous system sequelae: continuing assessment. Pediatrics 1996;97:279-281.

American Academy of Pediatrics. Active immunization: pertussis. In Pickering LK (ed): 2000 Red Book: Report of the Committee on Infectious Diseases, ed 25. Elk Grove Village, Ill: American Academy of Pediatrics, 2000.

Baraff LJ, Shields WD, Beckwith L, et al. Infants and children with convulsions and hypotonic-hyporesponsive episodes following diphtheria-tetanus-pertussis immunization: follow-up evaluation. Pediatrics 1988;81:789-794.

Barlow WE, Davis RL, Glasser JW, et al. The risk of seizure after receipt of whole-cell pertussis or measles, mumps, and rubella vaccine. New Engl J Med 2001;345:656-661.

Bass JW. Pertussis: current status of prevention and treatment. Pediatr Infect Dis J 1985;4:614-619.

Bellman MH, Ross EM, Miller DL. Infantile spasms and pertussis immunization. Lancet 1983;1:1031-1034.

Bowie C. Viewpoint: lessons from the pertussis vaccine court trial. Lancet 1990;335:397-399.

Butler NR, Haslum M, Golding J, Stewart-Brown S. Recent findings from the 1970 child health and education study: preliminary communication. J R Soc Med 1982;75:781-784.

Centers for Disease Control and Prevention. Summary of notifiable diseases, United States, 1994. MMWR Morb Mortal Wkly Rep 1994;43:3-80.

Centers for Disease Control and Prevention. Summary of notifiable diseases, United States, 1998. MMWR Morb Mortal Wkly Rep 1998;47:12.

Cherry JD. The epidemiology of pertussis and pertussis vaccine in the United Kingdom and the United States: a comparative study. In Lockhart JD (ed). Current Problems in Pediatrics. Chicago: Year Book, 1984.

Cherry JD. Pertussis and the vaccine controversy. In Root RK, Griffiss JM, Warren KS, et al (eds). Immunization. New York: Churchill Livingstone, 1989.

Cherry JD. "Pertussis vaccine encephalopathy": it is time to recognize it as the myth it is. JAMA 1990;263:1679-1680.

Cherry JD. Pertussis: the trials and tribulations of old and new pertussis vaccines. Vaccine 1992;10:1033-1038.

Cherry JD. Nosocomial infections in the nineties. Infect Control Hosp Epidemiol 1995;16:553-555.

Cherry JD: Comparative efficacy of acellular pertussis vaccines: an analysis of recent trials. Pediatr Infect Dis J 1997;16:990-996.

Cherry JD. Epidemiological, clinical, and laboratory aspects of pertussis in adults. Clin Infect Dis 1999a;28(suppl 2):S112-S117.

Cherry JD. Pertussis in the preantibiotic and prevaccine era, with emphasis on adult pertussis. Clin Infect Dis 1999b;28(suppl 2):S107-S111.

Cherry JD, Beer T, Chartrand SA, et al. Comparison of antibody values to *Bordetella pertussis* antigens in young German and American men. Clin Infect Dis 1995;20:1271-1274.

Cherry JD, Brunell PA, Golden GS, Karzon DT. Report of the Task Force on Pertussis and Pertussis Immunization—1988. Pediatrics 1988;81(suppl):939-984.

Cherry JD, Gombein J, Heininger U, et al. A search for serologic correlates of immunity to *Bordetella pertussis* cough illnesses. Vaccine 1998a;16:1901-1906.

Cherry JD, Heininger U, Stehr K, et al. The effect of investigator compliance (observer bias) on calculated efficacy in a pertussis vaccine trial. Pediatrics 1998b;102:909-912.

Cherry JD, Olin P. Commentaries: the science and fiction of pertussis vaccines. Pediatrics, 1999;104:1381-1384.

Christie CDC, Marx ML, Marchant CD, Reising SF. The 1993 epidemic of pertussis in Cincinnati: resurgence of disease in a highly immunized population of children. New Engl J Med 1994;331:16-21.

Cody CL, Baraff LJ, Cherry JD, et al. Nature and rates of adverse reactions associated with DTP and DT immunizations in infants and children. Pediatrics 1981;68:650-660.

Cotter PA, Miller JF: *Bordetella*. In Groisrnan EA (ed). Principles of Bacterial Pathogenesis. San Diego: Academic Press, 2001.

Dauer CC. Reported whooping cough morbidity and mortality in the United States. Public Health Rep 1943;58:661-676.

Decker MD, Edwards KM (eds). Report of the nationwide multicenter acellular pertussis vaccine trial. Pediatrics 1995;96(suppl):547-603.

Decker MD, Edwards KM, Steinhoff MC, et al. Comparison of 13 acellular pertussis vaccines: adverse reactions. Pediatrics 1995;96:557-566.

Deen JL, Mink CM, Cherry JD, et al. Household contact study of *Bordetella pertussis* infections. Clin Infect Dis 1995;21:1211-2119.

DeSerres G, Boulianne N, Duval B. Field effectiveness of erythromycin prophylaxis to prevent pertussis within families. Pediatr Infect Dis J 1995;14:969-975.

DeSerres G, Boulianne N, Duval B, et al. Effectiveness of a whole-cell pertussis vaccine in child-care centers and schools. Pediatr Infect Dis J 1996;15:519-524.

Edwards KM, Decker MD. Acellular pertussis vaccines for infants. New Engl J Med 1996;344:391-392.

Expanded Programme on Immunization. EPI for the 1990s. Geneva: World Health Organization, 1992.

Ewanowich CA, Chui LW-L, Paranchych MG, et al. Major outbreak of pertussis in northern Alberta, Canada: analysis of discrepant direct fluorescent-antibody and culture results by using polymerase chain reaction methodology. J Clin Microbiol 1993;31:1715-1725.

Farizo KM, Cochi SL, Zell ER, et al. Epidemiological features of pertussis in the United States, 1980-1989. Clin Infect Dis 1992;14:708-719.

Fine PEM. Implications of different study designs for the evaluation of acellular pertussis. Dev Biol Stand 1997;89:123-133.

Golden GS. Pertussis vaccine and injury to the brain. J Pediatr 1990;116:854-861.

Granstrom G, Wretlind B, Salenstedt C-R, Granstrom M. Evaluation of serologic assays for diagnosis of whooping cough. J Clin Microbiol 1988;26:1818-1823.

Granstrom M, Olinder-Neilsen AM, Holmblad P, et al. Specific immunoglobulin for treatment of whooping cough. Lancet 1991;338:1230-1233.

Greco D, Salmaso S, Mastrantonio P, et al. A controlled trial of two acellular vaccines and one whole-cell vaccine against pertussis. N Engl J Med 1996;334:341-348.

Griffin MR, Ray WA, Livengood JR, et al. Risk of sudden infant death syndrome after immunization with the diphtheria-tetanus-pertussis vaccine. N Engl J Med 1988;319:618-623.

Gustafsson L, Hallander HO, Olin P, et al. A controlled trial of a two-component acellular, a five-component acellular, and a whole-cell pertussis vaccine. N Engl J Med 1996;334:349-355.

He Q, Mertsola J, Soini H, Vijanen MK. Sensitive and specific polymerase chain reaction assays for detection of *Bordetella pertussis* in nasopharyngeal specimens. J Pediatr 1994;124:421-426.

Heininger U. Recent progress in clinical and basic pertussis research. Eur J Pediatr 2001;160:203-213.

Heininger U, Klich K, Stehr K, et al. Clinical findings in *Bordetella pertussis* infections: results of a prospective multicenter surveillance study. Pediatrics 1997;100. Available at: http://www.pediatrics.org/cgi/content/full/100/6/el0.

Heininger U, Stehr K, Schimtt-Grohe S, et al. Clinical characteristics of illness caused by *Bordetella parapertussis* compared with illnesses caused by *Bordetella pertussis*. Pediatr Infect Dis J 1994;13:306-309.

Hewlett EL, Cherry JD. New and improved vaccines against pertussis. In Levine MM, Woodrow GC, Kaper JB, Cobon GS (eds). New Generation Vaccines. New York: Marcel Dekker, 1997.

Hoffman HJ, Hunter JC, Damus K, et al. Diphtheria-tetanus-pertussis immunization and sudden infant death: results of the National Institute of Child Health and Human Development Cooperative Epidemiological Study of Sudden Infant Death Syndrome Risk Factors. Pediatrics 1987;79:598-611.

Howson CP, Fineberg HV. Adverse events following pertussis and rubella vaccines: summary of a report of the Institute of Medicine. JAMA 1992;267:392-396.

Institute of Medicine. Committee report: adverse effects of pertussis and rubella vaccines. Washington, D.C.: National Academy Press, 1991.

Izurieta HS, Kenyon TA, Strebel PM, et al. Risk factors for pertussis in young infants during an outbreak in Chicago in 1993. Clin Infect Dis 1996;22:503-507.

Kanai K. Japan's experience in pertussis epidemiology and vaccination in the past thirty years. Jpn J Sci Biol 1980;33:107-143.

Kimura M, Kuno-Sakai H. Developments in pertussis immunization in Japan. Lancet 1990;336:30-32.

Lapin LH. Whooping Cough. Springfield, Ill: Charles C Thomas, 1943.

Liese JG, Meschievitz CK, Harzer E, et al. Efficacy of a two-component acellular pertussis vaccine in infants. Pediatr Infect Dis J 1997;16:1038-1044.

Litvak AM, Gibel H, Rosenthal SE, Rosenblatt P. Cerebral complications in pertussis. J Pediatr 1948;32:357-379.

MacRae KD. Epidemiology, encephalopathy, and pertussis vaccine. In FEMS Symposium Pertussis: Proceedings of the Conference Organized by the Society of Microbiology and Epidemiology of the GDR, Berlin, 1988.

Madge N, Diamond J, Miler D, et al. The national childhood encephalopathy study: a 10-year follow-up. Dev Med Child Neurol 1993;68(suppl):1-119.

Marchant CD, Loughlin AM, Lett SM, et al. Pertussis in Massachusetts, 1981-1991: incidence, serologic diagnosis, and vaccine effectiveness. New Engl J Med 1994;169:1297-1305.

Marwick C. Acellular pertussis vaccine is licensed for infants. JAMA 1996;276:516-517.

Miller D, Madge N, Diamond J, et al. Pertussis immunization and serious acute neurological illness in children. Br Med J 1993;307:1171-1176.

Miller D, Wadsworth J, Diamond J, Ross E. Pertussis vaccine and whooping cough as risk factors for acute neurological illness and death in young children. Dev Biol Stand 1985;61:389-394.

Miller DL, Ross EM, Alderslade R, et al. Pertussis immunisation and serious acute neurological illness in children. Br Med J 1981;282:1595-1599.

Mortimer EA Jr. Perspective: pertussis and its prevention—a family affair. J Infect Dis 1990;161:473-479.

Mortimer EA Jr, Jones PK. An evaluation of pertussis vaccine. Rev Infect Dis 1979;1:927-932.

Mortimer EA Jr, Kimura M, Cherry JD, et al. Protective efficacy of the Takeda acellular pertussis vaccine combined with diphtheria and tetanus toxoids following household exposure of Japanese children. Am J Dis Child 1990;144:899-904.

Nennig ME, Shinefield HR, Edwards KM, et al. Prevalence and incidence of adult pertussis in an urban population. JAMA 1996;275:1672-1674.

Noble GR, Bernier RH, Esber EC, et al. Acellular and whole-cell pertussis vaccine in Japan: report of a visit by U.S. scientists. JAMA 1987;257:1351-1356.

Olin P. Defining surrogate serologic tests with respect to predicting vaccine efficacy: pertussis vaccination. Ann New York Acad Sci 1995;754:273-277.

Onorato IM, Wassilak SG, Meade G. Efficacy of whole-cell pertussis vaccine in preschool children in the United States. JAMA 1992;267:2745-2749.

Onorato IM, Wassilak SGF. Laboratory diagnosis of pertussis: the state of the art. Pediatr Infect Dis J 1987;6:145-151.

Poland GA. Acellular pertussis vaccines: new vaccines for an old disease. Lancet 1996;347:209-210.

Pollock TM, Morris J. A 7-year survey of disorders attributed to vaccination in North West Thames region. Lancet 1983;1:753-757.

Public Health Laboratory Service. Efficacy of whooping-cough vaccines used in the United Kingdom before 1968. Br Med J 1973;1:259-262.

Schlapfer G, Cherry JD, Heininger V, et al. Polymerase chain reaction identification of *Bordetella pertussis* infections in vaccinees and family members in a pertussis vaccine efficacy trial in Germany. Pediatr Infect Dis J 1995;14:209-214.

Schmitt-Grohe S, Cherry JD, Heininger U, et al. Pertussis in German adults. Clin Infect Dis 1995;21:860-866.

Shahin RD, Brennan MJ, Li ZM, et al. Characterization of the protective capacity and immunogenicity of the 69-kD outer membrane protein of *Bordetella pertussis*. J Exp Med 1990;171:63-73.

Shields WD, Nielsen C, Buch D, et al. Relationship of pertussis immunization to the onset of neurologic disorders: a retrospective epidemiologic study. J Pediatr 1988;113:801-805.

Stehr K, Cherry JD, Heininger U, et al. A comparative efficacy trial in Germany in infants who received either the Lederle/Takeda acellular pertussis component DTP (DTaP) vaccine, the Lederle whole-cell component DTP vaccine or DT vaccine. Pediatrics 1998;101:1-11.

Steketee RW, Burstyn DG, Wassilak SGF, et al. A comparison of laboratory and clinical methods for diagnosing pertussis in an outbreak in a facility for the developmentally disabled. J Infect Dis 1988;157:441-449.

Stephenson JBP. A neurologist looks at neurological disease temporally related to DTP immunization. Tokai J Exp Clin Med 1988;13:157-164.

Storsaeter J, Hallander HG, Gustafsson L, et al. Levels of anti-pertussis antibodies related to protection after household exposure to *Bordetella pertussis*. Vaccine 1998;16:1907-1916.

Stratton KR, Howe CJ, Johnston RB (eds). DPT vaccine and chronic nervous system dysfunction: a new analysis. Washington, D.C.: National Academy Press, 1994.

Sutter RW, Cochi SL. Pertussis hospitalizations and mortality, 1985-1988: evaluation of the completeness of national reporting. JAMA 1992;267:386-391.

Trollfors B, Taranger J, Lagergard T, et al. A placebo-controlled trial of a pertussis-toxoid vaccine. N Engl J Med 1995;333:1045-1050.

Uberall MA, Stehr K, Cherry JD, et al. Severe adverse events in a comparative efficacy trial in Germany in infants receiving either the Lederle/Takeda acellular pertussis component DTP (DTaP) vaccine, the Lederle whole-cell component DTP (DTP) or DT vaccine. Dev Biol Stand 1997;89:83-89.

Wardlaw AC, Parton R (eds). Pathogenesis and Immunity in Pertussis. New York: John Wiley & Sons, 1988.

World Health Organization. Meeting on Case Definition of Pertussis, Geneva, 1991.

World Health Organization, Global Programme for Vaccines and Immunization. State of the World's Vaccines and Immunization. Geneva: World Health Organization, 1996.

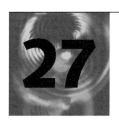

27 PSEUDOMONAS AERUGINOSA AND CYSTIC FIBROSIS

EMILY DIMANGO AND ALICE PRINCE

PSEUDOMONAS AERUGINOSA

Pseudomonas aeruginosa is a ubiquitous organism that thrives in aqueous environments such as ponds, puddles, sinks, and shower heads, as well as in hospital settings, contaminating respiratory therapy equipment, disinfectants, and moist surfaces in general. Although it is infrequently a cause of infection in normal hosts, it is a highly successful opportunistic pathogen and is a major cause of nosocomial infection, as well as infections in immunocompromised hosts, burn patients, and patients with cystic fibrosis (CF) (Baltch et al., 1994).

MICROBIOLOGY

P. aeruginosa is a gram-negative bacillus that does not ferment lactose but oxidizes glucose and xylose. Although usually considered an aerobic pathogen, *P. aeruginosa* can grow anaerobically using nitrate as an inorganic electron acceptor. It has few nutritional requirements and has diverse metabolic capabilities. These bacteria are usually characterized biochemically as indophenol oxidase-positive, citrate-positive, and L-arginine dehydrolase–positive organisms. In addition, *P. aeruginosa* often produces the fluorescent pigments pyoverdin and pyochelin siderophores, which scavenge iron, as well as pyocyanin, which together give the organism its characteristic blue-green hue. The genome of the prototypic *P. aeruginosa*, strain PAO1, has been sequenced (http://pseudomonas.bit.uq.edu.au) and is relatively large for a prokaryote (5,570 protein-encoding genes), encompassing numerous metabolic genes as well as pathogenicity islands that encode clusters of virulence factors, accounting for its success as an opportunistic pathogen.

PATHOGENESIS

P. aeruginosa thrives under conditions that are adverse to many other bacteria. In response to specific environmental signals, groups of virulence factors are coordinately expressed that enable the organism to survive and replicate under conditions inimical to many other bacteria. Many *P. aeruginosa* gene products, including pili, flagella, and lipopolysaccharide (LPS) interact with host cell targets and activate inflammatory responses (Prince, 2000). Several secreted exoproducts including proteases, phospholipases, exotoxin A, and exoenzyme S are directly toxic to tissues and mediate local damage to the host. The specific roles of many *P. aeruginosa* virulence factors have been studied in animal models of infection that are relevant to disseminated infections in neutropenic hosts or pulmonary infection, as in CF. Despite the prodigious abilities of *P. aeruginosa* to cause infection as an opportunist, the normal host is quite resistant to infection by the organism unless there is a loss of the epithelial barrier, iatrogenic neutropenia, or defective airway clearance mechanisms.

Most environmental strains of *P. aeruginosa* express flagella, which enable the organism to swim toward specific carbon sources (chemotaxis) and mediate binding to mucin (Ramphal et al., 1996). Organisms entrapped in mucin can be removed from the airways by normal mucociliary clearance mechanisms. Flagella are also major virulence factors, facilitating the dissemination of organisms both in the respiratory tract (Feldman et al., 1998) and in burns. These structures may be glycosylated and are highly immunogenic, stimulating epithelial cells to produce chemokines such as interleukin (IL)-8 (Feldman et al., 1998) or mucin (McNamara et al., 2001) and thus initiate a host inflammatory response. *P. aeruginosa* also express pili, antigenically diverse organelles that mediate attachment to epithelial surfaces via recognition of asialoglycolipids (Saiman and Prince,

1993). Piliated *P. aeruginosa* organisms activate the expression of numerous genes in the airway epithelium (Ichikawa et al., 2000), including IL-8, a neutrophil chemokine that is important in the inflammation typical of airway diseases such as chronic bronchitis and CF (DiMango et al., 1995). Other superficial components of *P. aeruginosa* also activate inflammation. LPS stimulates mucin expression (Li et al., 1997), and the combined effects of these multiple bacterial-host interactions results in the florid polymorphonuclear leukocyte response characteristic of *P. aeruginosa* infection.

Once these bacteria have colonized the host, they express a number of secreted virulence factors and can initiate an invasive infection. Following pilin-mediated attachment, several toxins are injected into the host cells via type III mediated secretion pathways. These toxins, such as exoenzymes S and T, interact with host cytoskeletal components, disrupting epithelial tight junctions and enabling the organisms to invade locally and destroy tissues (Pederson et al., 1999). Other potent toxins, such as exotoxin A—an ADP-ribosylating enzyme—destroy tissue, as do secreted proteases such as elastase, alkaline protease, and phospholipases, which are toxic to leukocytes, as well (Baltch and Smith, 1994). As a gram-negative organism, *P. aeruginosa* produces and sheds LPS, a major immunostimulant for macrophages, T cells, and endothelial cells. *P. aeruginosa* endotoxin causes sepsis with severe and often fatal systemic consequences (Kurahashi et al., 1999). Strains of *P. aeruginosa* isolated from sites of chronic infection, such as the lung of a patient with CF, have specific mutations in LPS genes (Ernst et al., 1999) and make modified, "rough" LPS that lacks the O-side chains associated with classic serotyping schemes.

The expression of many of these virulence factors is coordinately regulated through bacterial expression of small diffusible molecules or "quorum sensing systems" (Parsek and Greenberg, 2000). An acyl homoserine lactone is expressed by the organism and diffuses out of the cell. When present in sufficient quantity, it diffuses back into the bacteria, where it acts in concert with transcriptional activators to induce the expression of groups of genes important in pathogenesis. This quorum sensing system also enables bacterial colonies to produce extracellular polysaccharides to form biofilms (Costerton, 2001). Although biofilms are often associated with the bacteria that cause infections in the presence of intravascular catheters and foreign bodies, *P. aeruginosa* growing within the airways can also be considered to be a biofilm. Organisms growing in a biofilm have a highly structured colonial morphology and differential rates of growth and are especially difficult to eradicate either with conventional antibiotic therapy or by phagocytosis.

P. aeruginosa organisms are formidable pathogens because of their ability to express such diverse virulence factors, as well as their genetic and metabolic flexibility. They readily adapt to specific environments, effectively thwarting immune responses by cleaving antibody or by altering surface components to prevent phagocytosis and clearance. For example, a selected group of virulence genes are actively expressed within the context of CF airway infection (Storey et al., 1998) as opposed to other conditions. The selection of mutants with excessive amounts of alginate expression, the mucoid organisms pathognomonic for *P. aeruginosa* infection in CF, is another example of the ability of this species to adapt to specific environments (Deretic et al., 1994). Alginate production and the failure to express flagella and pili, which often accompanies this mucoid phenotype, prevents effective opsonization and polymorphonuclear leukocytic ingestion of these organisms.

P. aeruginosa infection occurs when these ubiquitous organisms gain access to a usually sterile site through a breach in the normal host defenses. This breach could be a lower airway infection in a patient with CF who is unable to clear inhaled organisms and mounts an inappropriately excessive proinflammatory response to these bacteria; infection of a burn wound, where the epithelial barrier has been lost; or sepsis in a profoundly neutropenic patient who lacks normal polymorphonuclear leukocyte function. Although antimicrobial resistance per se is not a virulence factor, the intrinsic and acquired resistance of *P. aeruginosa* to many commonly used antimicrobial agents enables them to flourish in a hospital setting and predisposes hospitalized patients to *P. aeruginosa* infection.

EPIDEMIOLOGY

P. aeruginosa causes diverse clinical syndromes depending on the host that is infected. These can range from folliculitis associated with bathing in hot tubs to septic shock in bone marrow–transplant patients. There has been extensive epidemiologic analysis of *P. aeruginosa*, especially as relevant to nosocomial outbreaks of infection, which are frequent (Foca et al., 2000; Gales et al., 2001; Toltzis et al., 2001). Outbreaks have been associated with diverse sources of *P. aeruginosa* contamination including intravenous solutions, multiple-dose vials of drugs, and artificial fingernails that have been colonized by medical personnel (Foca et al., 2000). The analysis of nosocomial *P. aeruginosa* infection due to multiply antibiotic resistant organisms in relationship to the widespread use of specific antimicrobial agents has also been studied in detail (Gales et al., 2001). There is a great deal of epidemiologic data to follow the acquisition and phenotypic changes of the organisms in chronic pulmonary infections in CF. Historically, *P. aeruginosa* strains were serotyped on the basis of LPS O-side chain antigenicity. However, mutation and alterations in LPS phenotype in different environments have led to the development of much more accurate molecular typing schemes, including the analysis of DNA restriction fragment polymorphisms and polymerase chain reaction (PCR)–based ribotyping by pulsed field gel electrophoresis (Foca et al., 2000; Toltzis et al., 2001).

Clinical Syndromes

Skin and soft-tissue infection. P. aeruginosa is a cause of folliculitis, typically associated with hot tubs (Baltch and Smith, 1994). Inadequate chlorination leads to the overgrowth of the organisms and ability to invade microabrasions in the skin. Often these infections are minor, and they clear without specific antimicrobial therapy. *P. aeruginosa* is also associated with more significant soft-tissue infections and osteochondritis. As a contaminant of the moist environment within soft-soled sneakers, *P. aeruginosa* can be introduced into the soft tissues through puncture wounds that pierce the sole of the shoe (Jacobs et al., 1989). These infections do not respond to the usual empiric antistaphylococcal treatment, and deeper aspirates or biopsies can reveal *P. aeruginosa*.

In immunocompromised hosts, *P. aeruginosa* is associated with much more severe skin and soft-tissue infection. Ecthyma gangrenosum lesions are embolic sites of *P. aeruginosa* infection, typically with a necrotic center (Baltch and Smith, 1994). Although *P. aeruginosa* has been a much-feared complication of burns wounds, recent techniques to rapidly re-epithelialize the burn wound have led to a significant decrease in *P. aeruginosa* infection at these sites.

P. aeruginosa is a relatively common cause of superficial ocular infection, often associated with keratitis and trauma in patients with contact lenses. It has also been reported to be a cause of endophthalmitis in immunocompromised CF patients following lung transplantation. Combined topical, intravenous, and intravitreous therapy in severe cases may be used.

Otitis externa. P. aeruginosa is frequently a cause of "swimmer's ear" or otitis externa. This may be the result of retained fluids in the externa auditory canal that become contaminated with *P. aeruginosa* organisms. Small abrasions in the canal are sufficient to establish a nidus of infection and initiate a local inflammatory response. Topical therapy is adequate, and several otic preparations of anti-*Pseudomonas* drugs are available (Klein, 2001). Otitis externa in immunocompromised patients or those with diabetes is a much more serious entity, often referred to as *maliganant otitis externa* due to *P. aeruginosa*. This condition requires aggressive parenteral therapy.

Pulmonary infection. P. aeruginosa is the major cause of infection and lung disease in patients with CF, as described in detail later in the chapter. *P. aeruginosa* is a cause of nosocomial pulmonary infection, particularly in patients with damaged airways and loss of normal mucociliary clearance mechanisms, such as patients in intensive care units who have been intubated (Lynch, 2001). These ubiquitous organisms are inhaled but not cleared, a result of mechanical and immunologic defects in these patients. Interactions among the bacteria, their many virulence factors, and the host epithelium and immune cells initiate a polymorphonuclear leukocyte response and more damage to the airways. It is often difficult to differentiate airway infection from invasive *P. aeruginosa* infection in these patients. Because of the severity of the inflammatory response, endobronchial infection is usually treated aggressively. The *P. aeruginosa* pulmonary disease associated with CF is discussed later in this chapter.

Urinary tract infection. Although *P. aeruginosa* is not often the initial cause of urinary tract infection (UTI) in normal hosts, it is a frequent nosocomial pathogen, causing infection in patients with indwelling urinary catheters because of its ability to form biofilms and causing recurrent infection in patients who have been treated with antimicrobial agents that lack anti-*Pseudomonas* properties. Effective treatment of *P. aeruginosa* UTI can be achieved through the use of oral agents, and the fluoroquinolones are widely used (Drago et al., 2001).

Sepsis. *P. aeruginosa* is a major cause of bloodstream infection in immunocompromised hosts. In a hospital setting it colonizes these patients and, because of its elaboration of virulence factors, can invade the bloodstream from a nidus on a mucosal surface, from the urinary tract, or from the gut, especially in the setting of mucositis associated with chemotherapy. Although the LPS of *P. aeruginosa* does not appear to be any more "toxic" than that of other gram-negative rods, the resistance of the organism to many antimicrobial agents is likely to be important in the poor outcome associated with *P. aeruginosa* sepsis. Many of these patients are on antimicrobial agents while febrile and neutropenic, and *P. aeruginosa* is selected out by its ability to develop resistance to these drugs (Collins et al., 2001; El Amari et al., 2001; Grisaru-Soen et al., 2000). The antimicrobial susceptibility of bloodstream isolates of *P. aeruginosa* depends on the antibiotics given previously (El Amari et al., 2001), as well as the underlying condition of the patient (Grisaru-Soen et al., 2000). The incidence of *P. aeruginosa* bacteremia does not appear to be increasing; however, it is still associated with significant mortality, because of both its intrinsic resistance and the nature of the patients at risk for this infection (Grisaru-Soen et al., 2000).

Therapy. Antimicrobial therapy of *P. aeruginosa* infection is complicated by the intrinsic resistance of the species to many classes of antibiotics as well as the ability of the organism to either induce or acquire the genes associated with resistance to even the "anti-*Pseudomonas*" antimicrobial agents (Hancock, 1998). In a setting in which there are large numbers of organisms, as in the CF lung, mutants can be selected that are resistant to an entire class of antibiotics. Similarly, in an oncology patient previously exposed to multiple classes of antibacterial agents, mutants can be selected

that are associated with invasive infection when the patient becomes neutropenic (Collins et al., 2001). For these reasons, most serious infections due to *P. aeruginosa* are treated with combinations of antibiotics with different targets of action.

Antimicrobial Resistance. The failure of many classes of antimicrobial agents to accumulate within *P. aeruginosa* is due to the presence of several efflux systems that enable the organisms to actively pump antibiotics including tetracyclines, fluoroquinolones, chloramphenicol, macrolides, trimethoprim, and β-lactams, and β-lactamase inhibitors out of the cell (Li et al., 1995). The *mexAB* operon is a prototype of this system. It consists of three components: an inner membrane exporter, an outer membrane channel, and a membrane fusion protein that forms a link between the inner and outer membranes. Genomic analysis indicates that at least 20 homologues of this system are present in *P. aeruginosa*. Antibiotics must get across the bacterial cell wall through selectively permeable porins (Wong and Hancock, 2000). The drugs then gain access to specific targets, such as the penicillin binding proteins for the β-lactam compounds, or get through the cytoplasmic membrane to interact with intracellular targets, such as the ribosome (for aminoglycosides) or topoisomerases (for the fluoroquinolones). These efflux systems enable the bacteria not only to limit the amount of drug that gets through the porins, but also to selectively pump out drugs that would get across the cytoplasmic membrane.

Enzyme Production. *P. aeruginosa* organisms express many enzymes that inactivate antimicrobial agents. Of these, the β-lactamases, which destroy the activity of the penicillins, cephalosporins, and related compounds, are of considerable clinical importance. The limited permeability of the *P. aeruginosa* porins, combined with the expression of both constitutive and inducible β-lactamases in the cell periplasm, provides an efficient means to inactivate many β-lactam antibiotics. *P. aeruginosa* express an inducible chromosomal cephalosporinase, which is relatively resistant to the β-lactamase inhibitors clavulanate and tazobactam, compounds that have more activity against plasmid-mediated penicillinases. *P. aeruginosa* can acquire transposons or plasmids encoding penicillinases (clavulanate- and tazobactam-susceptible); the acquisition of extended spectrum β-lactamases, enzymes that can degrade ceftazidime, cefepime, and other "anti-*Pseudomonas*" cephalosporins, has been described in many hospitals. Thus, *P. aeruginosa* has both constitutive and inducible β-lactam production, which can have major clinical relevance depending on the general use of antibiotics in a given hospital.

P. aeruginosa can also acquire genes encoding aminoglycoside-modifying enzymes, enabling them to become resistant to clinically achievable levels of the aminoglycosides. Plasmid-encoded or transposon-associated enzymes that can acetylate, phosphorylate, or adenylylate specific sites on aminoglycosides can be associated with clinically significant aminoglycoside resistance. The prevalence of these genes varies widely among hospitals. In airway infections in CF, aminoglycoside resistance often can be overcome by administering high doses of aminoglycosides by aerosol (MacLeod et al., 2000).

Therapy

For uncomplicated infections in a normal host (puncture wound–associated osteomyelitis or severe folliculitis) a single drug such as a fluoroquinolone (ciprofloxacin) for oral therapy is usually sufficient. Piperacillin and tazobactam, ceftazidime, or cefepime would be appropriate parenteral therapy if the organism is susceptible. Many clinicians would add an aminoglycoside for more severe infections, although this class of drugs has significant nephrotoxicity. Aminoglycosides can be given in once-daily dosing (Fishman and Kaye, 2000) (Table 27-1).

UTIs are readily treated with many of the anti-*Pseudomonas* antibiotics, because high concentrations are achieved in the urine of patients with normal renal function. A single drug, usually a fluoroquinolone such as ciprofloxacin, can be used even in patients with abnormalities of the urinary tract. Because of biofilm formation, foreign bodies must be removed, and patients with stones or anatomic abnormalities frequently have recurrent infection.

Immunocompromised Hosts. Treatment of systemic *P. aeruginosa* infection in immunocompromised hosts invariably includes two anti-*P. aeruginosa* agents. Synergistic combinations of drugs, especially in neutropenic hosts, are associated with more favorable outcomes. Clinicians are also concerned about the antimicrobial susceptibility of this organism and the frequent development of resistance. *P. aeruginosa* has been associated with high mortality in neutropenic patients, and empiric therapy in the febrile neutropenic host should include antimicrobial agents with anti-*P. aeruginosa* activity and should take into consideration local resistance patterns. Imipenem and meropenem are often useful against organisms with induced chromosomal β-lactamase activity, and therapeutic levels for treatment of meningitis can be achieved (Odio et al., 1999). *P. aeruginosa* resistance to all currently available antibiotics is found; therefore, susceptibility testing is important to guide therapy.

CYSTIC FIBROSIS

CF is the most common autosomal recessive disorder in whites, affecting approximately 22,000 persons in the United States (Cystic Fibrosis Foundation Patient Registry, 2001),

---

TABLE 27-1	Activity of Common Antimicrobial Agents Against *Pseudomonas aeruginosa* 3817 Cystic Fibrosis Isolates 1997-2001		
Antibiotic	*MIC 50 (μg/ml)*	*MIC 90 (μg/ml)*	*MIC range (μg/ml)*
Piperacillin + tazobactam	8	64	8->512
Cefepime	64	>64	2-64
Ceftazidime	2	32	2-128
Imipenem	1	>8	1->64
Meropenem	8	64	0.25->64
Aztreonam	4	16	4-64
Tobramycin	1	4	1-16
Amikacin	8	32	8-64
Ciprofloxacin	0.25	1	0.25-4

MIC, Minimum inhibitory concentration.

with a carrier rate of 1 in 25 (Fitzsimmons, 1993). The primary cause of morbidity and mortality in patients with CF is persistent bacterial infection of the airways, with subsequent bronchiectasis, fibrosis, and obstructive lung disease. Chronic respiratory infection with resultant respiratory failure accounts for over 90% of fatalities in this disease (Abman et al., 1991; Konstan and Berger, 1993). The disorder was first recognized in 1938 by Dorothy Anderson, who described a syndrome in children that resulted in pancreatic insufficiency, malnutrition, and chronic respiratory infections. At that time 70% of babies with CF died within the first year of life. Data from the Cystic Fibrosis Foundation Patients Registry of 2000 show median survival of 32.2 years among CF patients in the United States, largely as a result of the development of effective antibiotics and improved nutritional status (Cystic Fibrosis Foundation Patient Registry, 2001).

The disease is caused by a mutation in a single gene on the long arm of chromosome 7 that encodes the CF transmembrane conductance regulator (CFTR) (Collins, 1992). CFTR has multiple functions involving fluid and electrolyte balance across epithelial cells. It acts as a chloride channel activated by adenosine triphosphate (ATP).

PATHOGENESIS

Lung infection in CF is primarily endobronchial and chronic with superimposed acute exacerbations. Localized infections at nonrespiratory sites or systemic infections are rare. The spectrum of bacteria, viruses, and fungi associated with CF respiratory infection is comparatively restricted (Gilligan, 1991; Govan and Deretic, 1996; Karem et al., 1990). The microbial pathogens most commonly isolated include *Staphylococcus aureus*, *Haemophilus influenzae*, and particularly *P. aeruginosa*, which infects more than 80% of CF patients by the age of 18 years (Cystic Fibrosis Foundation Patient Registry, 2001).

The earliest observed morphologic lesions are mucous obstruction of small airways and inflammation of the bronchiolar walls (Konstan et al., 1993). Concomitant with the persistent infection is chronic neutrophil-dominated airway inflammation, which contributes greatly to lung damage (McElvaney et al., 1992; Rosenfeld et al., 2001). Bronchoalveolar lavage studies

demonstrate neutrophil-rich inflammation in airway lining fluid of infants with CF in the first year of life (Armstrong et al., 1995; Wotjczak et al., 2001). Mediators released by these inflammatory cells overwhelm the normal antiinflammatory defense screen of the epithelial surface and contribute directly to lung damage (Birrer et al., 1994). Several abnormalities in the lungs of patients with CF have been proposed as possible explanations for the chronic infection seen in this disease. As a consequence of the viscid nature of airway secretions in CF, mucociliary clearance of bacteria from the lungs is impaired (Konstan et al., 1993). Bacteria are loosely enmeshed in the viscous endobronchial mucous layer, which contains large amounts of cellular debris. Epithelial defensins, naturally occurring bactericidal peptides that serve as one of the first local lines of defense against inhaled organisms, do not function effectively in the lungs of patients with CF, contributing to the inability to clear inspired organisms (Smith et al., 1996). In patients with CF, these bacteria grow endobronchially into biofilms—structured communities of bacteria encased in a self-produced polymeric matrix—in the airway (Costerton et al., 2000; Hoiby et al., 2001). *P. aeruginosa* uses extracellular quorum sensing signals (chemical signals that cue cell-density–dependent gene expression) to coordinate biofilm formation (Singh et al., 2000). Bacteria growing in such biofilms are relatively resistant to antibiotics and to phagocytosis by airway macrophages.

As the organisms persist within the lung in the CF patient, mutants adapted for this milieu are selected. Strains of *P. aeruginosa* isolated from chronically infected individuals acquire mutations in genes regulating alginate synthesis, lose flagellar expression, and downregulate expression of most of the classical virulence determinants—all features consistent with the mucoid phenotype that overproduces alginate (Govan and Deretic, 1996). Recovery of this unusual mucoid phenotype of *P. aeruginosa* is a somewhat unique feature of CF. The *P. aeruginosa* strains that infect the airways of CF patients are not necessarily unique, but rather the environment of the lung in CF facilitates selection of the mucoid phenotype.

ETIOLOGIC AGENTS

The sequence of events leading from the defective CFTR protein to bacterial colonization and inflammation of the airway is not yet well understood. Several factors may contribute to the selection of *P. aeruginosa* specifically. It is this pathogen that is most closely associated with decline of lung function and clinical deterioration (Kosorok et al., 2001). There are an increased number of *Pseudomonas* receptors available on CF epithelial cells, compared with normal epithelial cells, as a direct result of a sialylation defect in CF (Barasch et al., 1991; Poschet et al., 2001; Saiman and Prince, 1993). CFTR mutations are associated with undersialylation of glycolipids and glycoproteins on the apical membranes of epithelial cells. These asialylated glycoconjugates provide receptors for the major *P. aeruginosa* adhesin, pilin. Pilin-mediated attachment to these receptors directly stimulates epithelial cytokine expression and the ensuing inflammatory response (DiMango et al., 1995).

Pulmonary infection in CF is primarily restricted to the airways rather than the lung parenchyma and typically occurs in an age-related sequence. *S. aureus* colonization occurs in young infants; *H. influenzae* appears in early childhood, with *P. aeruginosa* following, although infants with *P. aeruginosa* infection are being recognized with increasing frequency (Armstrong et al., 1995; Gilligan, 1991; Govan and Deretic, 1996). Other organisms found include *Burkholderia cepacia* and other glucose nonfermenters, such as *Stenotrophomonas mal-tophilia* and *Alcaligenes* species (Cystic Fibrosis Foundation Patient Registry, 2001) (Box 27-1 and Table 27-2).

S. aureus was the first organism recognized to cause chronic lung infections in young patients with CF and was the leading cause of mortality in the preantibiotic era. It continues to be an important pulmonary pathogen, especially in patients with CF who are under 10 years of age. Methicillin-resistant *S. aureus* has been isolated with increasing frequency from the lungs of patients with CF, although it does not appear to be associated with worse outcome (Miall et al., 2001). Although intermittent infection may occur for a period of time early in the disease process, once chronic infection with *P. aeruginosa* is established, organisms are rarely, if ever, eradicated, and infection with mucoid *P. aeruginosa* heralds the onset of progressive decline in pulmonary function (Bedard et al., 1993; Kosorok et al., 2001). There is some evidence that it may be possible to prevent or delay the onset of chronic infection in some patients with CF by eliminating cross-infection and by early aggressive antibiotic treatment beginning with the first positive sputum culture and continuing through subsequent intermittent colonization (Hoiby, 2000; Valerius et al., 1991).

The immune response to the organism, initiated by the antibody response and dominated

---

BOX 27-1

RESPIRATORY MICROBIOLOGY RESULTS IN PATIENTS WITH CYSTIC FIBROSIS

Type of Culture	Percent of Patients
Sputum	69.2
Throat	29.4
Bronchoscopy	1.4
TOTAL	16,993
	(91% of all patients seen in clinic)

Organisms Cultured	
Pseudomonas aeruginosa	60.1
Staphylococcus aureus	36.4
Haemophilus influenzae—any strain	15
Aspergillus species	6.0
Burkholderia cepacia	3.5
Stenotrophomonas maltophilia	3.4

Data from Cystic Fibrosis Foundation Patient Registry, 1995.

TABLE 27-2 Concurrent Infections	
Infection type	Number of cystic fibrosis patients affected (1995)
Pseudomonas aeruginosa	10,185
Burkholderia cepacia	333
Staphylococcus aureus	3,389
Methicillin-resistant S. aureus	12
Stenotrophomonas maltophilia	343
Other pseudomonads	252
Haemophilus influenzae	1,156
Klebsiella species	111
Alcaligenes species	47
Other gram-negative organisms	747
Aspergillus species	777

Data from Cystic Fibrosis Foundation Patient Registry, 1995.

by polymorphonuclear neutrophil leukocytes and their proteolytic and oxidative products, makes a significant contribution to the tissue damage seen in the lungs of patients with CF. Patients with CF who have high levels of circulating immune complexes have poorer lung function than those with lower levels (Wheeler et al., 1984). Besides immune complex–mediated damage to the lung, there are very high levels of elastase and protease of phagocytic cell origin in the lungs of CF patients infected with P. aeruginosa. These proteases contribute to lung damage and airway inflammation by stimulating secretion of inflammatory cytokines (McElvaney et al., 1992; Sagel et al., 2001).

During the early 1980s B. cepacia emerged as a pathogen of importance in patients with CF. Although a variable clinical course has been reported with the acquisition of B. cepacia in patients who have CF, this organism has been associated with significant mortality at CF centers in the United States and Canada, often in the setting of epidemic spread within institutions (LiPuma, 1998; Millar-Jones et al., 1992). Ribotyping, a method of strain identification based on analysis of bacterial genomic restriction fragment length polymorphisms (RFLPs), proved person-to-person transmission of B. cepacia in the setting of an educational camp (LiPuma et al., 1988). There is also evidence that transmission may be strain dependent, with some strains being more virulent and more likely to cause epidemics (Govan et al., 1993, Mahenthiralingam et al., 2001).

Factors that lead to colonization by B. cepacia are just beginning to be understood. The risk for B. cepacia colonization is increased by the severity of underlying pulmonary disease, the existence of a sibling with CF who has also been colonized, increasing age, and hospitalization in the previous 6 months (Millar-Jones et al., 1992; Tablan et al., 1987). The characteristic multidrug resistance of B. cepacia to anti–P. aeruginosa agents makes antimicrobial therapy difficult, and aggressive therapy seldom results in significant clinical improvement or even reduction in the numbers of bacteria cultured from sputum (Pitt et al., 1996). Recent studies report that triple antibiotic combinations are more likely than double and single antibiotic combinations to be bactericidal against B. cepacia in vitro and that multiple combination bactericidal testing is useful for assisting with decisions regarding appropriate combination therapy for patients infected with this organism (Aaron et al., 2000). Infection with B. cepacia usually follows one of three clinical courses. In some CF patients, long-term colonization occurs without adversely affecting lung function. In others, chronic infection associated with slowly declining lung function is seen. Finally, in about 20% of patients, acute fulminant lung infection with necrotizing pneumonia, fever, bacteremia, elevated erythrocyte sedimentation rate, and leukocytosis leads to death in weeks to months. The 2000 CF Registry reported the overall prevalence of the organism to be less than that seen in specific centers, with an overall mean isolation rate of 3.2% (Fitzsimmons and Brooks, 1994). The implications of *B. cepacia* infection and the ultimate success of lung transplantation remain an area of controversy (Chaparro et al., 2001).

OTHER PATHOGENS

In addition to the bacterial agents mentioned in the preceding section, there are several microorganisms that seem to have a high predilection for the lung of CF patients. CF patients are frequently colonized with *Aspergillus* species. The high rate of colonization in CF patients is due to the propensity of *Aspergillus* to grow in thick secretions in diseased lungs. Colonization may lead to chronic antigenic stimulation, which can lead to sensitization in a susceptible host, resulting in allergic bronchopulmonary aspergillosis (ABPA), variously reported to occur in 1% to 15% of patients with CF (Mroueh and Spock, 1994). Wheezing, episodic pulmonary infiltrates, and bronchiectasis occurring most commonly in the upper lobes characterize the clinical course. The diagnosis of ABPA in patients with CF is difficult because the signs and symptoms of each disease mimic those of the other. Positive results of skin-prick testing, elevated total serum IgE, *Aspergillus* in respiratory secretions, eosinophilia, and the presence of *Aspergillus* serum precipitins are used as diagnostic criteria for ABPA. Recent data report that in addition to traditional treatment with glucocorticoids or other more active drugs, such as variconazole, itraconazole treatment of ABPA is safe, allows for a reduction of steroid dosing, and is associated with fewer acute episodes of ABPA (Nepomuceno et al., 1999).

Nontuberculous mycobacteria (NTM), particularly *Mycobacterium avium* complex, has also been isolated with increased frequency from the sputum of patients with CF, with an overall prevalence of 13% (Olivier, 1996). Distinguishing airway colonization by NTM from pathogenic NTM infection that contributes to the progression of the underlying CF lung disease can be particularly difficult. Initial therapy for patients from whom this organism is recovered usually involves intensive bronchial hygiene, including antibacterial antibiotics, in an attempt to rid the lung of this colonizer. Patients sometimes require directed therapy for the NTM, particularly if there is convincing evidence that the organism is contributing to clinical deterioration. Ongoing screening for NTM in patients with CF will contribute to understanding the relevance of these pathogens with regard to deterioration in clinical status.

Later in the course of CF lung disease, multiple resistant gram-negative organisms including *S. maltophilia* and *Alcaligenes* species are recovered from the lung (Beringer and Appleman, 2000; Valdezate et al., 2001). Multicenter surveillance studies are needed to more clearly establish the pathogenicity of these organisms in CF.

CLINICAL MANIFESTATIONS

The major clinical manifestations of CF are due to the progressive lung disease. Pancreatic insufficiency is adequately treated with pancreatic enzyme supplements and replacement of the fat-soluble vitamins A, D, E, and K (Ramsey et al., 1992). The inability to eradicate bacterial pathogens from the airways results in chronic pulmonary symptoms. Patients have cough with expectoration of thick, purulent sputum and progressive deterioration in pulmonary function (Karem et al., 1990). Acute episodes of clinical infectious exacerbations are superimposed on chronic pulmonary symptoms. Because of wide variation in the severity of underlying manifestations, it is often difficult to define a pulmonary exacerbation on clinical criteria alone. An exacerbation is heralded by a quantitative change in ongoing respiratory symptoms (e.g., an increase in frequency and intensity of cough or in the quantity and purulence of sputum) or a greater than 10% decline in the forced expiratory volume in 1 second (FEV1). The acute and chronic symptoms are largely the result of the vigorous inflammatory response to endobronchial infection. Increased airway disease is manifest by tachypnea and increased work of breathing (retractions, use of accessory respiratory muscles, and wheezing). Systemic manifestations of pulmonary exacerbation include malaise, myalgia, anorexia, weight loss, and occasionally low-grade fever (Karem et al., 1990).

Decline in pulmonary function is the most accurate and objective indicator of a pulmonary exacerbation. Unfortunately, most patients younger than 5 years cannot perform pulmonary function tests reproducibly, making the diagnosis of an exacerbation more difficult. The appearance of a new pulmonary infiltrate on the chest radiograph may be helpful; however, most pulmonary exacerbations, especially in patients with advanced disease, are not associated with significant radiographic changes.

Sputum culture can identify the bacterial pathogens colonizing lower airway secretions; oropharyngeal culture (a suggested alternative in the nonexpectorating patient) is a relatively insensitive measure of lower airway pathogens (Ramsey et al., 1991). A study comparing oropharyngeal cultures with bronchoalveolar cultures showed that oropharyngeal cultures yielding *P. aeruginosa* or *S. aureus* are highly predictive, but cultures lacking these organisms do not rule out their presence in the lower airways. The use of selective media and quantitative culturing methods to identify infecting organisms in sputum may also be useful, particularly when mucoid strains of *P. aeruginosa* obscure the growth of more fastidious organisms such as *H. influenzae* (Bauernfeind et al., 1987).

Other laboratory studies that may be helpful in defining a pulmonary exacerbation include white blood cell count with differential and acute phase reactants, such as erythrocyte sedimentation rate and C-reactive protein. Bacteremia is seen rarely in patients with CF, except in a subpopulation of patients with *B. cepacia*. It is hypothesized that the low incidence of bacteremia is due to the relatively low virulence of the infecting organism; intense antibody response; and endobronchial, rather than parenchymal, location of the infectious process. In addition to pulmonary disease, almost all patients with CF have chronic sinusitis, often associated with nasal polyps (Ramsey et al., 1992). This is likely to be the result of the CFTR defect affecting the lining cells of the sinuses. Etiologic agents include the usual sinus pathogens plus the organisms that colonize the lower airways in this population. In addition to causing acute and chronic disease, sinuses may serve as a reservoir for antibiotic-resistant organisms in patients undergoing lung transplantation (Flume et al., 1994).

Nonpulmonary symptoms of CF that can mimic infection include immune complex–mediated manifestations such as vasculitic skin rashes and arthritis. In addition to pancreatic insufficiency, gastrointestinal manifestations include severe constipation, intestinal obstruction, and unrecognized or unusual presentations of acute appendicitis.

TREATMENT

Current therapy for lung disease in CF requires a multidisciplinary approach consisting of outpatient and inpatient care. Outpatient therapy includes postural drainage and chest percussion performed daily to help mobilize the inspissated secretions, along with administration of oral or inhaled antibiotics, bronchodilators, and recombinant human DNase (Webb, 1995). Optimizing nutritional status has been shown to have a positive impact on pulmonary function and should be aggressively addressed; sometimes necessitating gastrostomy feedings (Ramsey et al., 1992). Intravenous antibiotic therapy is often necessary for infectious exacerbations and is frequently performed as outpatient therapy, particularly in older children and adults; hospitalization is required for severe exacerbations or complications such as hemoptysis, pneumothorax, respiratory failure, pulmonary hypertension, or cor pulmonale.

Effective antibiotics administered to CF patients are thought to act by decreasing the sputum bacterial density and hence the ensuing inflammatory response. Antibiotics are typically directed against the major pathogens isolated from the sputum, with attention to antibiotic sensitivity (Table 27-3).

One important consideration in the treatment of patients with CF is antibiotic dosing. These patients have increased total body clearance of β-lactams and aminoglycosides as a result of an increased rate of elimination by the kidney (de Groot and Smith, 1987). As a result, CF patients often require higher doses of antibiotics to achieve therapeutic levels. Because sputum concentration is dependent on the peak serum concentration, patients with CF require larger doses of most antibiotics.

During the last two decades, chronic *P. aeruginosa* lung infection has emerged as the most difficult therapeutic problem in patients with CF. There is no universal agreement on how or when to treat this infection, and, regardless of the regimen used, *P. aeruginosa* is seldom permanently eradicated. Infections are typically treated with two antipseudomonal antibiotics: an aminoglycoside in addition to a second drug, usually a β-lactam antibiotic. Synergistic antibiotic testing is typically performed for multiply resistant bacteria. The intravenous administration of antibiotics is the currently accepted treatment for pulmonary exacerbations of CF in patients infected with *P. aeruginosa*. After 14 days of administration of intravenous antibiotics, the FEV1 typically increases approximately 20%, and the density

TABLE 27-3	Intravenous Treatment of Pathogens Associated with Pulmonary Exacerbations of Cystic Fibrosis*		
Organism	Drug	Dose (mg/kg)	Interval
Staphylococcus aureus	Nafcillin	25-50	q6h
	Cephalothin	25-50	q6h
	Vancomycin	15	q6h
	Linezolid	600	q12h[†]
Haemophilus influenzae	Ticarcillin/clavulanate	100/3.3	q6h
Pseudomonas aeruginosa[‡]	Piperacillin/tazobactam	100/12.5	q6h
		9	qd
	Tobramycin	3	q8h
	Amikacin	5-7.5	q8h
	Ceftazidime	50-75	q8h
	Ciprofloxacin	15	q12h
	Aztreonam	50	q6h
	Piperacillin	100	q6h
	Imipenem	15-25	q6h

*Treatment often depends on sputum sensitivity testing.
†Adult dosing *not* per kg
‡Use two agents simultaneously; aminoglycoside + β-lactam or quinolone.

of *P. aeruginosa* in sputum decreases substantially (Redding et al., 1982).

Some physicians treat patients only when there is evidence of clinical deterioration, whereas others treat at regular intervals regardless of symptoms. A single study of Danish patients with CF followed between 1971 and 1980 showed that patients treated every 3 months with anti-*Pseudomonas* antibiotics had improved 5-year survival (82% in the regularly treated group versus 54% in the as-needed group) and improved pulmonary function compared with those patients treated only during an exacerbation.

Another approach is the institution of early and aggressive anti-*Pseudomonas* treatment with oral or inhaled antibiotics as soon as organisms are recovered from sputum (Valerius et al., 1991). The use of direct aerosol delivery of aminoglycosides such as tobramycin to the lower airways has been shown to result in improved lung function, decreased density of *P. aeruginosa* in sputum, and decreased use of systemic antibiotics (Ramsey et al., 1999). Administration of tobramycin solution for inhalation (TOBI) at a dose of 300 mg by nebulizer twice daily during alternating months is now common practice for patients with CF who have moderate to severe lung disease and are infected with *P. aeruginosa* (Ramsey et al., 1999).

Treatment for allergic ABPA usually includes administration of corticosteroids, with more recent addition of itraconazole, an oral antifungal azole that may obviate the need for steroids (Nepomuceno et al., 1999).

RECENT ADVANCES

Although life expectancy for CF patients has increased dramatically over the past two decades, mainly through the development of better anti-*Pseudomonas* drugs and improved nutrition, airway obstruction resulting from chronic infection remains the main cause of mortality (Figure 27-1). Extracellular DNA released by disintegrating inflammatory cells, particularly polymorphonuclear leukocytes, is present in infected sputum of patients with CF in very high concentrations and likely contributes to the increased viscosity of the sputum (Shak et al., 1990). Aerosolized recombinant human DNase, an enzyme that cleaves high–molecular-weight DNA, has been shown to result in improvement of mean FEV1 to 10% to 15% over baseline in some patients and to reduce the frequency of infectious exacerbations requiring antibiotics (Fuchs et al., 1994).

Bilateral lung transplantation for CF was first performed in 1983. Ion transport in the lung is corrected after transplantation; however, because transport abnormalities associated with CF persist in the native proximal

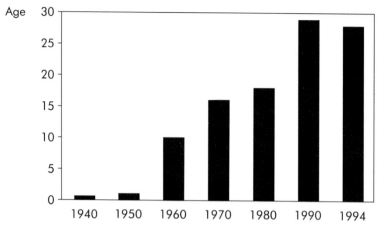

Fig. 27-1 Median survival age in patients with cystic fibrosis.

airways and sinuses, it has been suggested that the presence of airway pathogens before lung transplantation may place patients with CF at a higher risk for infectious complications after transplant (Flume et al., 1994). However, 5-year survival in lung-transplant patients with CF who are not infected with *B. cepacia* is the same as that for patients undergoing transplant because of other diseases (Flume et al., 1994). Pretransplant infection with *B. cepacia* portends worsened posttransplant survival for many patients (Chaparro et al., 2001).

With the knowledge that the clinical manifestations of CF are predominantly a result of abnormalities on the epithelial surface of the airways, combined with the discovery of the CFTR gene, there is a major research effort to develop methods to deliver the normal CFTR gene to respiratory epithelial cells. Different vectors—including recombinant viruses, liposomes, and other vector systems—are presently being investigated.

It is presently unclear how many epithelial cells need to be corrected or which cells are the proper targets. Although effective transfer of the gene to epithelial cells has been achieved, the transfer is not long lived, and many of the vectors themselves result in airway inflammation. Current work involves modification of the vectors and potential alteration of the host immune response to these vectors. Although human gene therapy is still in its infancy, hope remains that it may lead to a cure of the respiratory manifestations of CF.

Approaches to the prevention of *P. aeruginosa* colonization in patients with CF have included the development of anti-*Pseudomonas*

vaccines for use in uncolonized patients, but none are currently available. CF patients should receive routine childhood immunizations (including *H. influenzae* type B vaccine). In addition, patients and their families should receive influenza vaccine annually because of the high morbidity associated with infection. There is no indication for routine administration of pneumococcal vaccine.

Ongoing studies involve use of macrolide antibiotics as antiinflammatory agents in the treatment of lung disease in CF. Low-dose macrolide therapy has dramatically increased survival in patients with diffuse panbronchiolitis, a disease with many similarities to CF (Jaffe and Bush, 2001). Studies to determine efficacy of these agents in CF are currently under way.

BIBLIOGRAPHY

Aaron SD, Ferris W, Henry DA, et al. Multiple combination bactericidal antibiotic testing for patients with cystic fibrosis infected with Burkholderia cepacia. Am J Respir Crit Care Med 2000;161:1206-1212.

Abman SH, Ogle JW, Harbeck RJ, et al. Early bacteriologic, immunologic, and clinical courses of young infants with cystic fibrosis identified by neonatal screening. J Pediatr 1991;119:211-217.

Anderson DH. Cystic fibrosis of the pancreas and its relation to celiac disease: a clinical and pathologic study. Am J Dis Child 1938;56:344-399.

Armstrong DSK, Grimwood R, Carzmo JB, et al. Lower respiratory infection and inflammation in infants with newly diagnosed cystic fibrosis. Br Med J 1995;310:1571-1572.

Baltch AL, Smith RP (eds). *Pseudomonas aeruginosa* Infections and Treatment. New York: Marcel Dekker, 1994.

Barasch J, Kiss B, Prince A, et al. Defective acidification of intracellular organelles in cystic fibrosis. Nature 1991;52:70-73.

Bauernfeind A, Rotter K, Weisslein-Pfister CH. Selective procedure to isolate *H. influenzae* from sputa with large quantities of *P. aeruginosa*. Infection 1987;15:278-280.

Bedard M, McClure D, Schiller NL, et al. Release of IL-8, IL-6, and colony stimulating factor by upper airway epithelial cells: implications for cystic fibrosis. Am J Respir Cell Mol Biol 1993; 9:455-462.

Beringer PM, Appleman MD. Unusual respiratory bacterial flora in cystic fibrosis: microbiologic and clinical features. Curr Opin Pulm Med 2000;6:545-550.

Birrer P, McElvaney NG, Ruderberg A, et al. Protease-antiprotease imbalance in the lungs of children with cystic fibrosis. Am J Respir Crit Care Med 1994;150: 207-213.

Chaparro C, Maurer J, Gutierrez C, et al. Infection with *Burkholderia cepacia* in cystic fibrosis: outcome following lung transplantation. Am J Respir Crit Care Med 2001;163:43-48.

Collins BA, Leather HL, Wingard JR, et al. Evolution, incidence, and susceptibility of bacterial bloodstream isolates from 519 bone marrow transplant patients. Clin Infect Dis 2001;33:947-953.

Collins FA. Cystic fibrosis: molecular biology and therapeutic implications. Science 1992;256:774-777.

Costerton JW. Cystic fibrosis pathogenesis and the role of biofilms in persistent infection. Trends Microbiol 2001;9:50-52.

Costerton JW, Stewart PS, Greenberg, EP. Bacterial biofilms: a common cause of persistent infections. Science 2000;284:1318-1332.

Cystic Fibrosis Foundation Patient Registry, 2000. Annual Data Report. Bethesda, Md: Cystic Fibrosis Foundation, 2001.

de Groot R, Smith AL. Antibiotic pharmacokinetics in cystic fibrosis: differences and clinical significance. Clin Pharmacokinet 1987;13:228-253.

Deretic V, Schurr MJ, Boucher JC, et al. Conversion of *Pseudomonas aeruginosa* to mucoidy in cystic fibrosis: environmental stress and regulation of bacterial virulence by alternative sigma factors. J Bacteriol 1994;176:2773-2780.

DiMango E, Zar HJ, Prince AS, et al. Diverse *Pseudomonas aeruginosa* gene products stimulate respiratory epithelial cells to produce interleukin-8. J Clin Invest 1995;96:2204-2210.

Drago L, de Vecchi E, Mombelli B, et al. Activity of levofloxacin and ciprofloxacin against urinary pathogens. J Antimicrob Chemother 2001;48:37-45.

El Amari EB, Chamot E, Auckenthaler R, et al. Influence of previous exposure to antibiotic therapy on the susceptibility pattern of *Pseudomonas aeruginosa* bacteremic isolates. Clin Infect Dis 2001;33:1859-1864.

Ernst RK, Yi EC, Guo L, et al. Specific lipopolysaccharide found in cystic fibrosis airway *Pseudomonas aeruginosa*. Science. 1999;286:1561-1565.

Feldman M, Bryan R, Prince AS, et al. Role of flagella in pathogenesis of *Pseudomonas aeruginosa* pulmonary infection. Infect Immun 1998;66:43-51.

Fishman DN, Kaye KM. Once-daily dosing of aminoglycoside antibiotics. Infect Dis Clin North Am 2000;14:475-487.

Fitzsimmons SC. The changing epidemiology of cystic fibrosis. J Pediatr 1993;122:1-9.

Fitzsimmons SC, Brooks M. Annual Cystic Fibrosis Patient Registry Report. Bethesda, Md: Cystic Fibrosis Foundation, 1994.

Flume PA, Egan TM, Paradowski LJ, et al. Infectious complications of lung transplantation. Am J Respir Crit Care Med 1994; 149:1601-1607.

Foca M, Jakob K, Whittier S, et al. Endemic *Pseudomonas aeruginosa* infection in a neonatal intensive care unit. N Engl J Med 2000;343:695-700.

Fuchs HJ, Borowitz DS, Christiansen DH, et al. Effect of aerosolized recombinant human DNase on exacerbations of respiratory symptoms and on pulmonary function in patients with cystic fibrosis. N Engl J Med 1994;331: 637-642.

Gales AC, Jones RN, Turnidge J, et al. Characterization of *Pseudomonas aeruginosa* isolates: occurrence rates, antimicrobial susceptibility patterns, and molecular typing in the global SENTRY Antimicrobial Surveillance Program, 1997-1999. Clin Infect Dis 2001;32(suppl 2):S146-S155.

Gilligan PH. Microbiology of airway disease in patients with cystic fibrosis. Clin Microbiol Rev 1991;4:35.

Govan JF, Brown PH, Maddison J, et al. Evidence for transmission of *Pseudomonas cepacia* by social contact in cystic fibrosis. Lancet 1993;342:15-19.

Govan JRW, Deretic V. Microbial pathogenesis in cystic fibrosis: mucoid *Pseudomonas aeruginosa* and *Burkholderia cepacia*. Microbiol Rev 1996;60:539-574.

Grisaru-Soen G, Lerner-Geva L, Keller N, et al. *Pseudomonas aeruginosa* bacteremia in children: analysis of trends in prevalence, antibiotic resistance and prognostic factors. Pediatr Infect Dis J 2000;19:959-963

Hancock RE. Resistance mechanisms in *P. aeruginosa* and other non-fermentative gram negative bacteria. Clin Infect Dis 1998;27(suppl):S93-S99.

Hoiby N. Prospects for the prevention and control of Pseudomonal infection in children with cystic fibrosis. Paediatr Drugs 2000;2:451-463.

Hoiby N, Krogh JH, Moser C. *Pseudomonas aeruginosa* and the in vitro and in vivo biofilm mode of growth. Microbes Infect 2001;3:23-35.

Ichikawa JK, Norris A, Bangera MG, et al. Interaction of *P. aeruginosa* with epithelial cells: identification of differentially regulated genes by expression microarray analysis of human cDNAs. Proc Natl Acad Sci USA 2000;97:9659-9664.

Jacobs RF, McCarthy RE, Elser JM. *Pseudomonas* osteochondritis complicating puncture wounds of the feet in children: a 10 year evaluation. J Infect Dis 1989;160:657-661.

Jaffe A, Bush A. Anti-inflammatory effects of macrolides in lung disease. Pediatr Pulmonol 2001;31:464-473.

Karem E, Corey M, Gold R. Pulmonary function and clinical course in patients with cystic fibrosis after pulmonary colonization with *Pseudomonas aeruginosa*. J Pediatr 1990;116:714.

Klein JO. In vitro and in vivo antimicrobial activity of topical ofloxacin and other ototopical agents. Pediatr Infect Dis J 2001;20:102-103,120-122.

Konstan MW, Berger M. Infection and inflammation of the lung in cystic fibrosis. In Davis PB (ed). Cystic Fibrosis. New York: Marcel Dekker, 1993.

Kosorok MR, Zeng L, West SE, et al. Acceleration of lung disease in children with cystic fibrosis after *Pseudomonas aeruginosa* acquisition. Pediatr Pulmonol 2001;32:277-287.

Kurahashi K, Kajikawa O, Sawa T, et al. Pathogenesis of septic shock in *Pseudomonas aeruginosa* pneumonia. J Clin Invest 1999;104:743.

Li J-D, Dohrman AF, Gallup M, et al. Transcriptional activation of mucin by *Pseudomonas aeruginosa* lipopolysaccharide in the pathogenesis of cystic fibrosis lung disease. Proc Natl Acad Sci USA 1997.

Li X, Nikaido H, Poole K. Role of MexA-MexB-OprM in antibiotic efflux in *Pseudomonas aeruginosa*. Antimicrob Agents Chemother 1995;39:1948-1953.

LiPuma J. *Burkholderia cepacia*: management issues and new insights. Clin Chest Med 1998;19:473-486.

LiPuma JL, Mortensen JE, Dasen SE, et al. Ribotype analysis of *Pseudomonas cepacia* from cystic fibrosis treatment centers. J Pediatr 1988;113:859-862.

Lynch JP. Hospital-acquired pneumonia: risk factors, microbiology, and treatment. Chest 2001; 119(suppl 2):373S-384S.

MacLeod DL, Nelson LE, Shawar RM, et al. Aminoglycoside-resistance mechanisms for cystic fibrosis *Pseudomonas aeruginosa* isolates are unchanged by long-term, intermittent, inhaled tobramycin treatment. J Infect Dis 2000;181:1180.

Mahenthiralingam E, Vandamme P, Campbell ME, et al. Infection with *Burkholderia cepacia* complex genomovars in patients with cystic fibrosis: virulent transmissible strains of genomovar III can replace *Burkholderia multivorans*. Clin Infect Dis 2001;33:1469-1475.

McElvaney NGH, Nakamura B, Birrer CA, et al. Modulation of airway inflammation in cystic fibrosis. J Clin Invest 1992;90:1296-1301.

McNamara N, Khong A, McKemy D, et al. ATP transduces signals from ASGM1, a glycolipid that functions as a bacterial receptor. Proc Natl Acad Sci USA 2001;98:9086-9091.

Miall LS, McGinley NT, Brownlee KG, et al. Methicillin resistant *Staphylococcus aureus* infection in cystic fibrosis. Arch Dis Child 2001;84:160-162.

Millar-Jones L, Paull A, Saurnelers Z, et al. Transmission of *Pseudomonas cepacia* among cystic fibrosis patients. Lancet 1992;340:491

Mroueh S, Spock A. Allergic bronchopulmonary aspergillosis in patients with cystic fibrosis. Chest 1994;105:32-36.

Nepomuceno IB, Esrig S, Moss R. Allergic bronchopulmonary aspergillosis in cystic fibrosis: role of atopy and response to itraconazole. Chest 1999;115:364-370.

Odio CM, Puig JR, Feris JM, et al. Prospective, randomized, investigator-blinded study of the efficacy and safety of meropenem vs. cefotaxime therapy in bacterial meningitis in children. Meropenem Meningitis Study Group. Pediatr Infect Dis J 1999;18:581-590.

Olivier KN, Yankaskas JR, Knowles MR. Nontuberculous mycobacterial pulmonary disease in cystic fibrosis. Semin Respir Infect 1996;11:272-284.

Parsek MR, Greenberg EP. Acyl-homoserine lactone quorum sensing in gram-negative bacteria: a signaling mechanism involved in associations with higher organisms. Proc Nat Acad Sci USA 2000;97:8789.

Pederson KJ, Vallis AJ, Aktories K, et al. The amino-terminal domain of *Pseudomonas aeruginosa* ExoS disrupts actin filaments via small-molecular-weight GTP-binding proteins. Mol Microbiol 1999;32:393.

Pitt TL, Kaufmann P, Patel BS, et al. Type characterization and antibiotic susceptibility of *Burkholderia cepacia* isolates from patients with cystic fibrosis in the United Kingdom and the Republic of Ireland. J Med Microbiol 1996;44:203-210.

Poschet JF, Boucher JC, Tatterson L, et al. Molecular basis for defective glycosylation and *Pseudomonas* pathogenesis in cystic fibrosis lung. Proc Natl Acad Sci USA 2001;98:13972-13977.

Prince A. Bacterial induction of cytokine secretion in pathogenesis of airway inflammation. In Virulence Mechanisms of Bacterial Pathogens. Washington, D.C.: ASM Press, 2000.

Ramphal R, Arora SK, Ritchings SW. Recognition of mucin by the adhesin-flagellar system of *Pseudomonas aeruginosa*. Am J Respir Crit Care Med 1996;154:S170-S174.

Ramsey B, Richardson M. Impact of sinusitis in cystic fibrosis. J Allergy Clin Immunol 1992;90:547-552.

Ramsey BW, Farrel PM, Pencharz P. Nutritional assessment and management in cystic fibrosis: a consensus report. Am J Clin Nutr 1992;55:108-116.

Ramsey BW, Pepe MS, Quan JM, et al. Intermittent administration of inhaled tobramycin in patients with cystic fibrosis. N Engl J Med 1999;340:23-30.

Ramsey BW, Wentz KR, Smith AL, et al. Predictive value of oropharyngeal cultures for identifying lower airway bacteria in cystic fibrosis patients. Am Rev Respir Dis 1991;144:331-337.

Redding GJ, Restuccia R, Cotton EK. Serial changes in pulmonary functions in children hospitalized with cystic fibrosis. Am Rev Respir Dis 1982;126:31-36.

Rosenfeld M, Gibson RL, McNamara S, et al. Pediatr Pulmonol 2001;32:356-366.

Sagel SD, Kapsner R, Osberg I, et al. Airway inflammation in children with cystic fibrosis and healthy children assessed by sputum induction. Am J Respir Crit Care Med 2001;164:1425-1431.

Saiman L, Prince AS. *P. aeruginosa* pili bind asialoGM1 which is increased on the surface of cystic fibrosis epithelial cells. J Clin Invest 1993;92:1875-1880.

Shak I, Capon DJ, Hellmiss R, et al. Recombinant human DNase reduces the viscosity of CF sputum. Proc Natl Acad Sci USA 1990;87:9188-9192.

Singh PK, Schaefer AL, Parsek MR, et al. Quorum-sensing signals indicate that cystic fibrosis lungs are infected with bacterial biofilms. Nature 2000;407:762-764.

Smith JJ, Travis SM, Greenberg EP. Cystic fibrosis airway epithelia fail to kill bacteria because of abnormal airway surface fluid. Cell 1996;85:229-236.

Storey DG, Ujack EE, Rabin HR, et al. *Pseudomonas aeruginosa* lasR transcription correlates with the transcription of lasA, lasB, and toxA in chronic lung infections associated with cystic fibrosis. Infect Immun 1998;66:2521-2528.

Tablan OC, Martone WJ, Doershuk CF, et al. Colonization of the respiratory tract with *Pseudomonas cepacia* in cystic fibrosis: risk factors and outcomes. Chest 1987;91:527-532.

Toltzis P, Dul MJ, Hoyen C, et al. Molecular epidemiology of antibiotic-resistant gram-negative bacilli in a neonatal intensive care unit during a nonoutbreak period. Pediatrics 2001;108:1143-148.

Valdezate S, Vindel A, Maiz L, et al. Persistence and variability of *Stenotrophomonas maltophilia* in cystic fibrosis patients, Madrid, 1991-1998. Emerg Infect Dis 2001;7:113-122.

Valerius NH, Koch C, Hoiby N. Prevention of chronic *P. aeruginosa* colonization in cystic fibrosis by early treatment. Lancet 1991;338:725-726.

Webb AK. The treatment of pulmonary infection in cystic fibrosis. Scand J Infect Dis 1995;96:24-27.

Wheeler WB, Williams M, Matthews WJ, et al. Progression of cystic fibrosis lung disease as a function of serum immunoglobulin G levels: a 5-year longitudinal study. J Bacteriol 1984;104:695-699.

Wong KKY, Hancock REW. Insertion mutagenesis and membrane topology model of the *Pseudomonas aerugi-nosa* outer membrane protein OprM. J Bacteriol 2000;182:2402.

Wojtczak HA, Kerby GS, Wagener JS, et al. Beclometha-sone diproprionate reduced airway inflammation in young children with cystic fibrosis: a pilot study. Pediatr Pulmonol 2001;32:293-302.

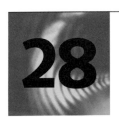

28

RABIES (HYDROPHOBIA, RAGE, LYSSA)

STANLEY A. PLOTKIN

Rabies is a viral infection that terminates in a fatal encephalomyelitis; rabies is acquired usually from the bite or scratch of a mammal suffering from the disease. Because of its inexorable course it has been called *the incurable wound*, and its history is full of romance, ranging from the sinister stories of vampirism to the triumph of Louis Pasteur.

Although relatively rare in the United States, where the principal risk now comes from bats, rabies is an important disease in Southeast Asia, where it continues to kill thousands each year.

Pasteur pioneered the development of rabies vaccine in 1885, when, without knowing that the virus was a filterable agent, he managed to transmit it to animals and to chemically attenuate the agent by desiccation. His successful human trials, though based on insufficient animal experimentation, launched the field of vaccine development (Pasteur coined the word *vaccination*) and resulted in the worldwide establishment of Pasteur Institutes to produce rabies vaccine.

ETIOLOGY

The rabies virus is classified within the lyssavirus family of rhabdoviruses and shares homology with at least six other viruses (such as Mokola and Duvenhage) that are considerably rarer as causes of disease in man, and about which relatively little is known. Moreover, although rabies virus is classified as lyssavirus type 1, and all rabies viruses belong to that type, the virus varies genetically, and strains coming from different animals and from different geographic areas can be distinguished, facilitating epidemiologic investigation. For example, the fact that human rabies cases of occult origin had been acquired from bats was established by molecular epidemiologic studies, as was the documentation that spread of rac-coon rabies to the northeastern United States had been the result of importation of animals for hunting purposes.

Physical and Chemical Properties

Rabies virus is bullet shaped and has a symmetric structure giving it the appearance of a beehive. The virus measures 75 nm in diameter and 160 to 180 nm in length (Wunner et al., 1988). The negative single-stranded genome is nonsegmented RNA approximately 12,000 nucleotides long. The genome has been cloned and sequenced. The glycoprotein of the spikes on the surface of the virus is encoded by the G gene. This is the attachment protein and is the antigen that elicits neutralizing antibodies. The virulence of the virus is dramatically altered by single amino acid substitutions in the glycoprotein. Monoclonal antibodies against the glycoprotein or the nucleoprotein distinguish strains of virus and, together with sequencing, have served to clarify the epidemiology of rabies (Smith, 1989).

Rabies virus survives storage at 4° C for weeks and in the frozen state for much longer periods in the absence of carbon dioxide; therefore in dry-ice cabinets it must be stored in sealed glass ampules. It keeps for years in the dried state at 4° C. Rabies virus is killed by temperatures of 56° C in 1 hour and of 60° C in 5 minutes. It is quickly inactivated by sunlight and ultraviolet light. The virus is resistant to phenol and thimerosal (Merthiolate). It is inactivated by ß-propiolactone, ether, formalin, mercury bichloride, and nitric acid.

Host Range

Rabies virus has an extensive host range; all warm-blooded animals are susceptible. Rabies virus was the first virus transmitted experimentally to a laboratory animal, the rabbit.

Rabies virus has also been propagated in chick and duck embryos, in tissue cultures of mouse, in hamster kidneys, in continuous cell lines of African green monkey kidney origin (Vero), and in human diploid cell lines. For immunization of animals, only inactivated virus vaccines prepared from these substrates are used in the United States.

Newer techniques of rabies virus cultivation permitted the development of safer and more immunogenic vaccines for humans, starting in 1957 with a vaccine propagated in duck embryos. Subsequently, cell culture vaccines were developed, and in the 1970s a concentrated, purified rabies virus vaccine was prepared from the supernatants of human diploid cell cultures, thereby eliminating the risks of injecting animal proteins, including those originating in the central nervous system (CNS). Currently, several different cell substrates are used to make rabies vaccine, including Vero cells, chick embryo fibroblasts, and duck embryo fibroblasts.

Immunologic Properties

Both neutralizing antibodies (which attach to the viral glycoprotein) and complement-fixing antibodies are formed late in the course of rabies infection, and they may also develop as a result of vaccination. The level of 0.5 IU of neutralizing antibody is associated with protection against illness. Cell-to-cell spread of virus is prevented by neutralizing antibody in vitro. Postexposure administration of antibody may prevent virus from reaching the CNS.

A measurable cytotoxic T-cell response is generated after vaccination, but the role in pathogenesis or protection is unknown. In vitro the cellular response contributes to clearance of virus from cells, and this can be enhanced by antibody.

PATHOLOGY

Introduction of virus by virtually any route usually gives rise to infection, but intracerebral inoculation with virus from canines almost invariably produces fatal encephalomyelitis. In infected animals, rabies virus is widely distributed. The salivary glands of infected dogs have yielded high titers of virus; lesser quantities have been detected in the lacrimal glands, pancreas, kidney, adrenal glands, and breast tissue. In humans, rabies virus has been recovered from various parts of the CNS, including the olfactory bulbs, horn of Ammon, frontal and occipital cortices, and medulla. It has also been recovered from cervical and abdominal sympathetic ganglia, salivary glands, adrenal glands, myocardium, walls of both small and large intestines, mesenteric lymph nodes, tonsillar and pharyngeal tissues, and lungs.

The principal changes produced by rabies virus are found throughout the CNS, consisting mainly of neuronal necrosis, which is most pronounced in the thalamus, hypothalamus, substantia nigra, pons, and medulla. The cranial nerve nuclei are severely damaged, and mononuclear cell infiltration is likely to be greater there than elsewhere. The spinal cord shows neuronal changes, especially in the posterior horns. The most distinctive feature of the pathologic changes is the presence of Negri bodies, which are pathognomonic of rabies, although not always present. These specific inclusion bodies are found in the cytoplasm of nerve cells. They consist of acidophilic structures approximately 2 to 10 μm in diameter, are sharply demarcated, and are usually round or oval; they occur most abundantly in the hippocampus (horn of Ammon), basal ganglia, pons, and medulla.

Changes similar to those in the brain may be found in the sympathetic ganglia and dorsal root ganglia of the spinal cord. The salivary glands may show degenerative changes of the acinar cells and neurons; Negri bodies may be found in the latter.

PATHOGENESIS

The attack rate in persons bitten by rabid animals is hard to estimate; it depends on the extent and location of the bites and the dose of virus entering the wound. Lacerations of the head and neck are followed by higher attack rates than are those of the feet and ankles. The amount of virus reaching the nerves is influenced by several additional factors: (1) lack of virus in saliva of 50% of rabid dogs; (2) protection afforded by clothing so that little or no virus enters the wound; and (3) removal or inactivation of virus by soap and water, benzalkonium (Zephiran), and other agents.

Overall, the risk of rabies after human exposures to the bites of rabid animals appears to range from 15% to 40%, with wolf bites to the head exemplifying the high end of the range. The virus usually enters the body through a saliva-contaminated bite or scratch. Rabies has rarely been acquired by inhalation, by contamination of mucosal surfaces, and by transplantation of infected corneas. Replication of virus appears to occur initially in nonneural cells such as myocytes, where it may continue at low levels for weeks. Eventually, virus attaches to receptors on nerve cells, like the nicotinic acetylcholine receptor. After entry, the virus is occult to the immune system until late in the course of infection.

Available evidence indicates that rabies virus multiplies initially in the muscle at the inoculation site, reaches neuromuscular junctions, and travels through the axoplasm of peripheral nerves to dorsal root ganglia and the CNS. After multiplication in neurons centrally, the virus travels peripherally along nerve pathways to invade many distal tissues and organs. Up to this point, little inflammatory response or measurable host response can be demonstrated. See the discussion of diagnosis, later in this chapter.

CLINICAL MANIFESTATIONS IN ANIMALS AND HUMANS

The term *street virus* is used to designate strains of wild viruses freshly isolated from animals. Such strains are characterized by incubation periods that usually vary from 10 days to several months. However, much longer incubation periods may be observed. Rabies viruses produce either prolonged excitation and viciousness (furious type) or depression and paralysis with early onset (dumb type) or, as occurs in most infected dogs, some manifestations of both types. Street virus rabies is almost always associated with the presence of Negri bodies. The term *fixed virus* refers to laboratory strains transferred in series from brain to brain, usually in the rabbit, characterized by a short and constant incubation period of 4 to 6 days, absence of Negri bodies, and diminished ability to spread centrifugally. The Pasteur strain of fixed virus has been maintained in rabbits since its original isolation in 1882 and is the strain generally used for nerve tissue vaccines.

In the United States human rabies is rare; the average annual incidence of human rabies declined from 40 cases per year during the 1940s to 0 to 2 cases per year in the 1980s. Some of the cases are imported; monoclonal serotyping of rabies isolates from four human cases of rabies occurring in the United States in the 1980s revealed viruses similar to those in the country of origin of the patient. The important feature was long incubation periods with probable acquisition of infection before entry into the United States (Smith et al., 1991). However, in 1995 alone there were four indigenous cases linked to bat exposures, and the difficulty of ascertaining those exposures became evident.

The incubation period in humans is usually 1 to 2 months, but wide ranges from 7 days to 6 years have been observed. The incubation period appears to be shorter in children. Multiple severe lacerations, the introduction of large doses of virus, and bites on the head and neck are associated with short incubation periods.

The illness may begin, as do other kinds of encephalitis, with prodromal symptoms of malaise, fever, headache, anorexia, nausea, sore throat, drowsiness, irritability, and restlessness (Bhatt et al., 1974; Hemachuda, 1994). The patient may complain of hyperesthesia, paresthesia, or anesthesia in the area of the bite and along the course of the involved peripheral nerves.

Progression of the infection occurs in two forms: furious or paralytic. The former is associated with increased anxiety and hyperexcitability accompanied by mounting fever. Delirium, involuntary twitching movements, and generalized convulsions are often seen. Manic behavior may alternate with periods of lethargy. Violent spasmodic contractions of the muscles of the mouth, pharynx, or larynx when the patient attempts to drink or merely at the sight of water are the striking characteristics that gave rabies its common name—*hydrophobia*. These painful spasms may be set off by relatively mild stimuli such as noise, light touch, or air currents. The patient may drool profusely from the mouth to avoid swallowing, which is associated with painful spasm.

Within a few days the patient's condition worsens, the pulse rate increases, respirations become more labored or irregular, and the temperature rises steadily. Periods of responsiveness become less frequent, and muscular spasms may give way to paralysis. Peripheral vascular collapse, coma, and death quickly follow. The disease runs its entire course usually in no more than 5 to 6 days and ends fatally.

In 5% to 20% of patients, particularly those bitten by insectivorous or frugivorous bats, the clinical picture of rabies is that of an ascending, symmetric, flaccid paralysis without hyperexcitability; spasmodic muscle contractions may also be manifest until coma develops. This picture resembles that of Guillain-Barré syndrome so that, in the absence of known history of rabies virus exposure, such patients may go through the entire course of illness with no suspicion of the diagnosis of rabies until the characteristic findings are observed at autopsy (Baer, 1975).

The cerebrospinal fluid (CSF) is usually normal: the pressure is normal or slightly increased, the fluid is clear, and in most cases the number of cells is not increased. In patients with pleocytosis the CSF cell count rarely exceeds 100, and the cells are mostly mononuclear leukocytes. There may be a slight increase in the level of protein.

The peripheral white blood cell count shows an increase in the number of leukocytes, which may reach 20,000 to 30,000, with a predominance of polymorphonuclear leukocytes. Abnormal urinary findings may include albumin, casts, reducing substances, and acetone.

■ **Case 1**   An 11-year-old boy was bitten on the forehead by a dog 32 days before onset of the disease; the wound was cauterized, but no antirabies vaccine was given. The patient's illness began with headache, drowsiness, anorexia, and malaise that progressed in 2 days to delirium accompanied by fever and vomiting.

Delirium associated with visual hallucinations and delusions of persecution were the outstanding and persistently recurring features. He was often manic and struck and bit attendants. Except for transient difficulty in swallowing and slurring of speech on the fourth and fifth days, there was a striking absence of localizing neurologic signs. The CSF was normal. The temperature was sustained between 38.9° and 40.3° C (102° and 104.5° F) for 1 week. On the tenth day, irregular respirations were observed, with periods of apnea lasting as long as 45 seconds. He died on the twelfth day from respiratory and circulatory failure. Postmortem touch preparations of the hippocampus showed typical Negri bodies, and rabies virus was isolated from various parts of the brain and other tissues.

DIAGNOSIS

Confirmation of rabies in a biting animal is often the first and crucial step toward the prevention of rabies in humans. All nondomesticated animals and bats should be considered rabid; their heads or, if small, their entire carcasses should be preserved at 0° to 4° C and submitted to rabies diagnostic laboratories, where rabies virus is sought in brain tissue by fluorescent rabies antibody staining for viral antigen, virus isolation in mice inoculated intracerebrally, and more recently by polymerase chain reaction (PCR) detection of viral nucleic acid. Negri bodies may be absent, and diagnosis should not depend on their presence.

In a typical human case, rabies is easily recognized. The characteristic history is that of an animal bite followed in several weeks or months by the onset of overwhelming encephalitis; the CNS signs include excitement, anxiety, manic behavior, and delirium associated with spasmodic concentrations of muscles used in swallowing and speech. Clinical laboratory findings are generally of little help. In humans the premortem diagnosis is made best by demonstration of antigen in a skin biopsy. Corneal impressions have been difficult to obtain and unreliable for detection of antigen. During the first week of illness, virus can be isolated occasionally from saliva, CSF, and urine and consistently from the brain. Virus can be demonstrated by immunofluorescence, by identification of Negri bodies, or by inoculation of brain tissue into mice and cell cultures. The presence of IgM antibody in blood and CSF indicates acute infection. PCR improves the sensitivity and specificity of diagnosis.

Table 28-1 summarizes the results of a diagnostic study (Noah et al., 1998), which shows that reverse transcriptase (RT)–PCR of saliva and brain biopsy is the most accurate method of diagnosis in terms of sensitivity, specificity, and early positivity.

Tetanus may be confused with rabies. Excitement accompanied by spasms of the laryngeal and pharyngeal muscles is not so common in patients with tetanus and is virtually constant in patients with rabies. Tetanus is characterized by trismus and spasmodic contractions of the muscles of the body. Other intoxications, including porphyria, should also be considered. Paralytic cases of rabies pose more of a diagnostic problem and may be confused with poliomyelitis, Japanese encephalitis, Guillain-Barré syndrome, or encephalomyelitis after nerve tissue rabies vaccine.

PROGNOSIS

Rabies was considered 100% lethal until recent years. A small number of cases have now been reported in which survival from rabies infection appears probable, at least in part because of vaccination during the incubation period. However, these cases are rare, and the prognosis in unvaccinated persons is still uniformly fatal.

■ **Case 2**   *Probable human rabies with survival.* On October 10, 1970, in Lima, Ohio, a 6-year-old boy was bitten on his left thumb by a bat while he was asleep. The bat

TABLE 28-1	Antemortem Diagnostic Test Results for 20 Human Patients With Rabies in the United States, 1980-1996		
Test	Number of patients positive for rabies virus/total number tested (%)		Earliest positive (day of illness)
RT-PCR of saliva for rabies virus RNA	10/10	(100)	5
Brain biopsy for rabies virus antigen	3/3	(100)	8
Nuchal skin biopsy for rabies virus antigen	10/15*	(67)	5
Virus isolation from saliva	9/15†	(60)	5
Antibody to rabies virus in serum	10/18	(56)	5‡
Rabies virus antigen in touch impression from cornea	2/8	(25)	14
Antibody to rabies virus in CSF	2/13	(15)	15§

Data from Noah DL, Drenzek CL, Smith JS, et al: Ann Intern Med 1998;128:922-930.
RT-PCR, Reverse transcriptase polymerase chain reaction; CSF, cerebrospinal fluid.
*Two patients had earlier skin biopsies that were negative for rabies virus but became positive on subsequent biopsy.
†One patient had an earlier test that was negative for rabies virus.
‡Latest negative 24 days, median to positive 10 days.
§Latest negative 24 days.

was captured by the boy's father and was submitted to the Ohio Health Department, where rabies was confirmed on examination of the brain by fluorescent antibody (FA) technique. On October 14 a 14-day course of treatment with duck embryo vaccine (DEV) was begun on the boy.

The boy showed no symptoms until October 30, when he complained of neck pain, and during the next several days he became lethargic and showed malaise and anorexia. His condition worsened, and on November 4 he entered a local hospital with a temperature of 40° C (104° F). During the next 10 days the boy's temperature dropped but he became more lethargic. On November 13 stiffness of the neck developed and the CSF yielded 125 white blood cells. During the next several days the boy's condition deteriorated; he showed total aphasia, weakness of left arm, bilateral Babinski's signs, and coma. A tracheostomy was done because of respiratory difficulty, tachypnea, and increased pharyngeal secretions. The patient was in and out of coma for a week and then gradually began to improve. In December his condition continued to improve, and he was able to walk with assistance and speak in short sentences. As of October 1971 the patient was reported to be normal.

Efforts to establish the diagnosis included biopsy of the brain, which was negative for rabies virus by culture, and FA tests. There were no detectable serum antibodies to St. Louis encephalitis, eastern or western

equine encephalomyelitis, or leptospirosis. Serum complement–fixing antibody titer to California virus was 1/8 on October 13, 1970, and biweekly determinations through December 3 remained the same. Serum-neutralizing antibody titers against rabies were 1/300 on November 13, rose to 1/37,000 on November 27, and remained between 1/39,000 and 1/47,000 during December and January. The question arose whether the 14-day course of treatment with DEV could be responsible for these high antibody titers. It can be stated that rabies antibody titers after a 14-day course of treatment with DEV rarely exceed 1:500 and, therefore, that titers of the magnitude seen in this patient strongly support the diagnosis of rabies. Indeed, the only aspect of this patient's course not compatible with rabies infection is recovery. The clinical management of this patient included the continuous monitoring of cardiac and pulmonary functions, the prevention of hypoxia by prophylactic tracheostomy, and intensive pulmonary assistance. These measures may have contributed to the arrest of clinical illness and to eventual recovery.

TRANSMISSION AND EPIDEMIOLOGY

Rabies virus is primarily excreted through the salivary glands, but bats do excrete virus in their guano and any innervated tissue in an infected animal can contain the virus. Thus, implantation of saliva by bites or by saliva-contaminated claws is the main route of transmission. Inhalation of bat guano or aerosols created in the laboratory are also risks. Transplantation of corneas, and in principle other tissues, is also a risk, and donation from patients dying of undiagnosed encephalitis should not be accepted.

Geographic distribution of rabies includes most of the world. The mammalian host range is so large that areas free of rabies are primarily island nations. The British Isles, Australia, New Zealand, and the Hawaiian Islands are rabies free through eradication efforts and quarantine to eliminate enzootic cycles. Rabies occurs in any climate and in any season but is most common in Asia and Africa. Thailand and Ethiopia are the countries with the highest infection rates.

The sources of the vast majority of rabies exposures in the high-incidence parts of the world are domesticated dogs and cats. In theory, population control and vaccination of these animals could sharply reduce rabies in humans, but in practice poverty and social customs prevent those measures.

Rabies in domestic animals in the United States has decreased in recent years. In 1946 there were more than 8,000 cases of rabies in dogs, compared with fewer than 1,000 cases in all domestic animals in 2000 (Figure 28-1). Rabid domestic animals comprise <10% of all rabid animals but are responsible for the majority of exposures requiring treatment. Rabid cats are the most commonly reported rabid domestic species in the United States.

In 1999 there were over 7,000 confirmed cases of wildlife rabies in 53 states and territories, of which only 8.5% occurred in domestic animals (Table 28-2) (Krebs and Rupprecht, 2000). These data originate in state and federal laboratories of the United States but reflect the worldwide epizootic in wildlife hosts, extending from the Arctic Circle to the tropics in the Eastern and Western hemispheres. Wild animals currently constitute the most important source of infection for domestic animals in the United States. Skunks and raccoons are the main sources of rabies for domestic animals and the main source of exposure in humans. The recent epidemiology of rabies in the United States has been strongly influenced by the spread of raccoon rabies throughout the Northeast. Introduced into Virginia by the transfer of raccoons from the South for hunting purposes, the epizootic has spread north to New York and to New England, resulting in

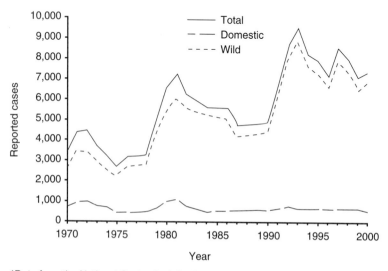

Rabies. Reported Wild and Domestic Animal Cases by Year*—
United States and Puerto Rico, 1970-2000

*Data from the National Center for Infectious Diseases.

Fig. 28-1 Rabies in wild and domestic animals, by year, in the United States and Puerto Rico, 1970 to 2000. (From Centers for Disease Control and Prevention: MMWR Morb Mortal Wkly Rep 2002;49:59.)

TABLE 28-2	Cases of Animal Rabies in the United States, 2000	
	Number	*Percent*
Wild Animals		
Raccoons	2,778	38
Skunks	2,223	10
Bats	1,240	17
Foxes	453	6.2
Rodents/Lagomorphs	52	0.7
Other	109	1.5
TOTAL	6,855	93
Domestic Animals		
Cats	249	3.4
Dogs	114	1.6
Cattle	83	1.1
Horses or mules	52	0.14
Sheep or goats	10	0.14
Other	1	0.01
TOTAL	509	6.9

Data from Krebs et al: J Am Vet Med Assoc 2000; 217:1799-1811.

with great success using baits containing live viruses—either vaccinia-rabies recombinants or attenuated strains of rabies virus.

In the Americas, canine rabies is still important in Mexico and other parts of Central and South America, and bats (including vampire bats) are important vectors throughout the hemisphere. Although only insectivorous bats are found in the United States, they have recently been implicated in the majority of the rare human cases, presumably because their bites may go undetected in a sleeping individual. Silver-haired and Eastern pipistrelle bats are the species usually incriminated.

The incidence of rabies is high in Asian and African children because of the increased chance of exposure resulting from their friendliness toward animals and their inability to defend themselves against attack. Also, because of their small size, children are more often bitten on the head and face, and thus are more susceptible to disease. Additional factors leading to a higher risk in children include provocative behavior and failure to recognize the signs of rabies in dogs.

Winkler (1968) pointed out the possibility of airborne respiratory infection acquired in caves inhabited by large numbers of infected bats. Although transmission by inhalation is probably very rare, it must be considered in patients with compatible clinical illnesses who have a history of visits to bat-infested caves. Spelunkers may be listed among those with

numerous human exposures. In Canada the fox is the principal species affected by rabies. Transmission from one domestic species to another rarely occurs in North America (Figure 28-2) (Krebs et al., 2000).

In Europe the fox is the main source of human exposure. Recently, vaccination of wild foxes has been practiced in Western Europe

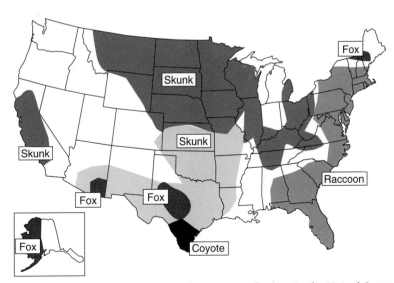

Fig. 28-2 Distribution of major terrestrial reservoirs of rabies in the United States.

"high-risk" vocations or avocations for whom preexposure prophylaxis is justified.

Human-to-human transmission of rabies by bite is extremely rare. However, iatrogenic transmission has been reported (Houff et al., 1979), resulting from a corneal transplant to a healthy recipient from a donor who had died of a CNS illness with progressive ascending paralysis similar to Guillain-Barré syndrome. One month after the transplant procedure, the recipient developed an acute fatal meningoencephalitis that was recognized as rabies only at autopsy. Studies of the donor's and the recipient's eyes then demonstrated the presence of rabies virus in both.

PREVENTIVE MEASURES

The prevention of rabies depends on the elimination of virus before it invades nerve cells. This can be done prophylactically through immunization before exposure and therapeutically through immunization after exposure because of the long interval between contamination of a wound and invasion of the nerve cell (Plotkin, 2000).

The general treatment of the bite and the question of whether or not to immunize those persons bitten or scratched by animals suspected of being rabid is no longer a difficult decision, now that better tolerated vaccines are available. The decision to immunize must be made immediately after exposure because the likelihood that any prophylactic measure will contribute to the prevention of rabies dimin-

ishes rapidly as the interval between exposure and treatment increases.

Although a case of rabies may occasionally develop in persons who receive antirabies treatment, evidence from laboratory and field experience in many parts of the world indicates that postexposure prophylaxis is highly effective when local cleansing, antiserum, and vaccine are appropriately used (Wilde et al., 1996).

Attack rates in persons bitten by rabid animals and the effect of specific prophylactic measures are shown in Table 28-3. Sabeti et al. (1964) described the results of treatment of individuals bitten in Iran by wolves proved rabid. The evidence is clear that use of the combination of hyperimmune serum and vaccine was superior to vaccine alone, especially in cases of head bites, which are associated with shorter incubation periods and higher attack rates than those in cases in which the head and neck are not involved.

In 1964 Veeraraghaven et al. (Johnson, 1965) compared the attack rates in persons bitten by proved rabid animals in India from 1946 to 1962, when a total of 581 persons exposed in this manner were given a complete course of antirabies vaccine; of them, 49 (8.4%) died. In contrast, of 153 persons who were not vaccinated, 77 (50%) died (Table 28-1). Hattwick and Gregg (1975) and Baer (1975) give a lower estimate of between 15% and 40% for rabies after proven exposure. However, the Indian patients were exposed mostly to rabid dogs, whereas American patients are exposed to a

TABLE 28-3	**Attack Rates in Human Beings Bitten by Animals Proved to Be Rabid: Effects of Specific Preventive Measures**				
	PERSONS BITTEN				
Authors	*Number*	*Bitten on head?*	*Number of rabies deaths*	*Mortality (%)*	*Type of prophylaxis*
Sabeti	96	Yes	38	40	Vaccine alone
et al., 1964[*]	71	No	6	8.4	
TOTAL	167		44	26	
	50	Yes	3	6	Serum and vaccine
	24	No	0	0	
TOTAL	74		3	4	
Veeraraghavan	153	[†]	77	50	No vaccine
et al., 1964[*]	581	[†]	49	8.4	Vaccine

[*]Cited by Johnson HN: In Horsfall FL Jr, Tamm I (eds): Philadelphia: Lippincott, 1965.
[†]No data.

variety of animals, which may account for the difference.

In recent years, cell culture vaccines have been developed to replace the original nerve tissue vaccines pioneered by Pasteur in 1885, although, unfortunately, even today the majority of human vaccinations in the developing world are performed using vaccines produced in the brains of animals.

Cell culture vaccines are highly immunogenic, free of serious reactions, and effective in postexposure prophylaxis (Aoki et al., 1992), as described previously. They have also been reliable in stimulating high antibody titers when administered in a three-dose schedule to high-risk individuals before exposure (Plotkin and Wiktor, 1979).

The standard rabies cell culture vaccine is prepared from cultures of human diploid cells and has been tested extensively. However, to reduce the cost of vaccination, other cell culture vaccines have been developed, particularly ones prepared in Vero African green monkey kidney cell lines, chick embryo cells, and duck embryo cells. All cell culture vaccines appear to be equally effective. The two vaccines currently available in the United States are made in human diploid cells (Aventis Pasteur) and chick embryo cells (Chiron Behring).

RABIES-IMMUNIZING PRODUCTS

The following information is *based on* the recommendations of the Immunization Practices Advisory Committee (Centers for Disease Control and Prevention, 1999). Because of space limitations, the following information may be incomplete for certain purposes, and medical personnel intending to use vaccination for rabies prevention are urged to consult the entire original document for complete information.

There are two types of rabies-immunizing products.

Rabies vaccines induce an active immune response that includes the production of neutralizing antibodies. This antibody response requires approximately 7 to 10 days to develop and usually persists for more than 2 years.

Rabies immune globulins (RIGs) provide rapid, passive immune protection that persists for only a short time (half-life of approximately 21 days). In almost all postexposure prophylaxis regimens, both products should be used concurrently.

Vaccines

Three inactivated rabies vaccines are currently licensed for preexposure and postexposure prophylaxis in the United States.

Rabies vaccine: human diploid cell. In the human diploid cell vaccine (HDCV), the PM rabies strain is inactivated with ß-propiolactone and is supplied in a form for intramuscular (IM) administration (Imovax Rabies Vaccine, Aventis Pasteur, Swiftwater, Pennsylvania).

Rabies vaccine adsorbed. Rabies vaccine adsorbed (RVA) (Michigan Department of Public Health) was licensed in 1988; it was developed by the Biologics Products Program of the Michigan Department of Public Health and is distributed by GlaxoSmithKline, Philadelphia, Pennsylvania. The vaccine is prepared from the Kissling strain of Challenge Virus Standard (CVS) rabies virus adapted to fetal rhesus lung diploid cell culture. However, RVA is currently unavailable.

Rabies vaccine: primary chick embryo fibroblasts. Recently licensed by Chiron Corporation (Emeryville, California), primary chick embryo vaccine (PCEV) consists of the inactivated Flury LEP virus prepared for IM use (Briggs et al., 2000).

All products are rehydrated to form a 1.0-ml dose.

No intradermal preparation is currently available in the United States. However, in many developing countries vials for IM administration are used for multiple intradermal vaccination using volumes of 0.1 to 0.2 ml depending on the antigenic concentration of the vaccine. Although this practice has been successful and reduces substantially the cost of vaccination, it is no longer officially accepted practice in the Unites States, although extensively used in the Far East.

Rabies immune globulins. RIGs licensed for use in the United States include human rabies immune globulin (HRIG; Hyperab, Cutter Biologicals [a division of Miles, Inc.]) and Imogam Rabies (Aventis Pasteur, distributed by Connaught Laboratories, Inc.) is an antirabies gamma globulin concentrated by cold ethanol fractionation from plasma of hyperimmunized human donors. Rabies-neutralizing antibody content, standardized to contain 150 IU per ml, is supplied in 2-ml (300 IU) and 10-ml (1,500 IU) vials for pediatric and adult use, respectively.

Outside of the United States, equine RIGs (ERIGs) are available and are used in a dose of 40 IU/kg.

PREEXPOSURE VACCINATION

Any one of the cell culture vaccines can be used to immunize those who are likely to come into contact with rabid animals. In developed countries, groups such as veterinarians, spelunkers, and laboratory workers are candidates (Table 28-4) (Centers for Disease Control and Prevention, 1999). Some have suggested that in developing countries where rabies is enzootic, consideration should be given to routine vaccination of children (Lange et al., 1997). Travelers to countries where rabies is common might also consider vaccination if contact with animals is likely.

The regimen for preexposure vaccination is three doses at 0, 7, and 21 to 28 days. A booster is usually administered at 1 year. Subsequent boosters depend on serologic surveillance and the extent of continued exposure.

POSTEXPOSURE PROPHYLAXIS: RATIONALE FOR TREATMENT

Physicians should evaluate each possible exposure to rabies and if necessary consult with local or state public health officials regarding the need for rabies prophylaxis (Table 28-5) (Centers for Disease Control and Prevention, 1999). In the United States the following factors should be considered before specific antirabies treatment is initiated.

TABLE 28-4	Rabies Preexposure Prophylaxis Guide—United States, 1999		
Risk category	Nature of risk	Typical populations	Preexposure recommendations
Continuous	Virus present continuously, often in high concentrations. Specific exposure likely to go unrecognized. Bite, nonbite or aerosol exposure.	Rabies research laboratory workers* Rabies-biologics production workers	Primary course. Serologic testing every 6 months; booster vaccination if antibody titer is below acceptable level.†
Frequent	Exposure usually episodic with source recognized, but exposure also might be unrecognized. Bite, nonbite, or aerosol exposure.	Rabies diagnostic lab workers.* Spelunkers, veterinarians and staff, and animal-control and wildlife workers in rabies-enzootic areas.	Primary course. Serologic testing every 2 years; booster vaccination if antibody titer is below acceptable level.†
Infrequent (greater than population at large)	Exposure nearly always episodic with source recognized. Bite or nonbite exposure.	Veterinarians and animal-control and wildlife workers in areas with low rabies rates. Veterinary students. Travelers visiting areas where rabies is enzootic and immediate access to appropriate medical care including biologic agents is limited.	Primary course. No serologic testing or booster vaccination.
Rare (population at large)	Exposure always episodic with source recognized. Bite or nonbite exposure.	U.S. population at large, including persons in rabies-epizootic areas.	No vaccination necessary.

*Judgment of relative risk and extra monitoring of vaccination status of laboratory workers is responsibility of the laboratory supervisor.
†Minimum acceptable antibody level is complete virus neutralization at a 1:5 serum dilution by the rapid fluorescent focus inhibition test. A booster dose should be administered if the titer falls below this level.

TABLE 28-5	Rabies Postexposure Prophylaxis Guide—United States, 1999	
Animal type	*Evaluation and disposition of animal*	*Postexposure prophylaxis recommendations*
Dogs, cats, and ferrets	Healthy and available for 10 days observation	Persons should not begin prophylaxis unless animal develops clinical signs of rabies
	Rabid or suspected rabid	Immediately vaccinate*
	Unknown (e.g., escaped)	Consult public health officials
Skunks, raccoons, foxes, and most other carnivores; bats	Regarded as rabid unless assumption proved negative by laboratory tests†	Consider immediate vaccination
Livestock, small rodents, lagomorphs (rabbits and hares), large rodents (woodchucks and beavers), and other mammals	Consider individually	Consult public health officials; bites of squirrels, hamsters, guinea pigs, gerbils, chipmunks, rats, mice, other small rodents, rabbits, and hares almost never require antirabies postexposure prophylaxis

*During the 10-day observation period, begin postexposure prophylaxis at the first sign of rabies in a dog, cat, or ferret that has bitten someone. If the animal exhibits clinical signs of rabies, it should be killed immediately and tested.
†The animal should be killed and tested as soon as possible. Holding for observation is not recommended. Discontinue vaccine if immunofluorescence test results of the animal are negative.

Type of Exposure

Rabies is transmitted only when the virus is introduced into open cuts or wounds in skin or mucous membranes. If there has been no exposure (as described in this section), postexposure treatment is not necessary. The likelihood of rabies infection varies with the nature and extent of exposure. Two categories of exposure (bite and nonbite) should be considered.

Bites and scratches. Any penetration of the skin by teeth constitutes a bite exposure. Bites to the face and hands carry the highest risk, but the site of the bite should not influence the decision to begin treatment. Scratches, abrasions, open wounds, or mucous membranes contaminated with saliva or other potentially infectious material (such as brain tissue) from a rabid animal also constitute serious exposures.

Although occasional reports of transmission by nonbite exposure suggest that such exposures constitute sufficient reason to initiate postexposure prophylaxis under some circumstances, nonbite exposures rarely cause rabies. The nonbite exposures associated with the highest risk appear to be exposures to large amounts of aerosolized rabies virus, transplantation of organs (e.g., corneas) from donors who died of rabies, and scratches from rabid animals.

Other contact by itself—such as petting a rabid animal or contact with the blood, urine, or feces of a rabid animal—does not constitute an exposure and is not an indication for prophylaxis. However, see the section on bats below.

Animal Rabies Epidemiology and Evaluation of Involved Species

Wild animals. All bites by wild carnivores and bats must be considered possible exposures to the disease. Postexposure prophylaxis should be initiated when patients are exposed to wild carnivores unless (1) the exposure occurred in a region known to be free of terrestrial rabies and the results of immunofluorescence antibody testing is available within 48 hours, or (2) the animal is tested and shown not to be rabid. If treatment has been initiated and subsequent immunofluorescence testing shows that the exposing animal was not rabid, treatment can be discontinued.

Signs of rabies among carnivorous wild animals cannot be interpreted reliably; therefore any such animal that bites or scratches a person should be killed at once (without unnecessary damage to the head) and the brain submitted for rabies testing. If the results of testing are negative by immunofluorescence, the saliva can be assumed to contain no virus, and the person bitten does not require treatment.

If the biting animal is a particularly rare or valuable specimen and the risk of rabies small, public health authorities may choose to administer postexposure treatment to the bite victim in lieu of killing the animal for rabies testing. Such animals should be quarantined for 30 days.

Rodents (such as squirrels, hamsters, guinea pigs, gerbils, chipmunks, rats, and mice) and lagomorphs (including rabbits and hares) are almost never found to be infected with rabies and have not been known to cause rabies among humans in the United States. However, woodchucks can be rabies infected, and from 1971 through 1988 woodchucks accounted for 70% of the 179 cases of rabies among rodents reported to the Centers for Disease Control and Prevention (CDC). In all cases involving rodents, the state or local health department should be consulted before a decision is made to initiate postexposure antirabies prophylaxis. Exotic pets (including ferrets) and domestic animals crossbred with wild animals are considered wild animals by the National Association of State Public Health Veterinarians and the Conference of State and Territorial Epidemiologists because they may be highly susceptible to rabies and could transmit the disease. These animals should be killed and tested rather than confined and observed when they bite humans.

Domestic animals. In areas where canine rabies is not enzootic (including virtually all of the United States and its territories), a healthy domestic dog or cat that bites a person should be confined and observed for 10 days. Any illness in the animal during confinement or before release should be evaluated by a veterinarian and reported immediately to the local health department. If signs suggestive of rabies develop, the animal should be humanely killed and its head removed and shipped, under refrigeration, for examination by a qualified laboratory. Any stray or unwanted dog or cat that bites a person should be killed immediately and the head submitted as described for rabies examination.

In most developing countries of Asia, Africa, and Central and South America, dogs are the major vector of rabies; exposures to dogs in such countries represent a special threat.

Travelers to these countries should be aware that about 50% of the rabies cases among humans in the United States result from exposure to dogs outside the United States. Although dogs are the main reservoir of rabies in these countries, the epizootiology of the disease among animals differs sufficiently by region or country to warrant the evaluation of all animal bites. Exposures to stray dogs in canine rabies-enzootic areas outside the United States carry a high risk; authorities therefore recommend that postexposure rabies treatment be initiated immediately after such exposures. Treatment can be discontinued if the dog or cat can be caught and remains healthy during the 10-day observation period, but often the animal cannot be identified.

Bats. The importance of occult exposure to rabid bats in the United States has become evident recently (Krebs et al., 2000) More than half of the viruses isolated from human rabies cases since 1980 have been identified as being of bat origin, although in many of these there was no history of bat bite. The mandibles of bats are sufficiently small that bites may be difficult to detect, and the animal may attack sleeping persons. Therefore it is now advised that exposures of sleeping persons, particularly children, to bats be taken more seriously, even if no evidence of bite is found. Thus, in situations in which a bat is found to be present and bite exposure is possible, postexposure prophylaxis should be given unless capture and testing of the bat excludes rabies infection. Obviously this recommendation must be applied with discretion, and it underlines the need for consultation with experts in many instances of putative exposure to rabies.

Circumstances of biting incident and vaccination status of exposing animal. An unprovoked attack by a domestic animal is more likely than a provoked attack to indicate that the animal is rabid. Bites inflicted on a person attempting to feed or handle an apparently healthy animal should generally be regarded as provoked. However, in countries where canine rabies is enzootic this rule should be ignored and all bites should be considered as unprovoked.

A fully vaccinated dog or cat is unlikely to become infected with rabies, although rare cases have been reported. In a nationwide study of rabies among dogs and cats in 1988, only one dog and two cats that were vaccinated contracted rabies. All three of these animals had received only single doses of vaccine; no documented vaccine failures occurred among dogs or cats that had received two vaccinations.

POSTEXPOSURE PROPHYLAXIS: LOCAL TREATMENT OF WOUNDS AND VACCINATION

The essential components of rabies postexposure prophylaxis are local wound treatment and the administration, in most instances, of both HRIG and vaccine (Table 28-6) (Centers for Disease Control and Prevention, 1999). Persons who have been bitten by animals suspected or proved rabid should begin treatment within 24 hours. However, there have been instances when the decision to begin treatment was not made until many months after the exposure because of a delay in recognition that an exposure had occurred, and awareness

that incubation periods of >1 year have been reported. In 1977 the World Health Organization recommended a regimen of RIG and 6 doses of HDCV over a 90-day period. This recommendation was based on studies in Germany and Iran. When used this way, the vaccine was found to be safe and effective in protecting persons bitten by animals proved rabid, and it induced an excellent antibody response in all recipients. Studies conducted in the United States by the CDC have shown that a regimen of one dose of HRIG and five doses of HDCV over a 28-day period was safe and induced an excellent antibody response in all recipients.

With use of the new rabies vaccines of culture origin (Wiktor et al., 1977), there now have been several convincing studies of efficacy in postexposure rabies prophylaxis. Bahmanyar

---

TABLE 28-6	Rabies Postexposure Prophylaxis Schedule—United States, 1999	
Vaccination status	*Treatment*	*Regimen**
Not previously vaccinated	Wound cleansing	All postexposure treatment should begin with immediate thorough cleansing of all wounds with soap and water. If available, a virucidal agent should be used to irrigate the wounds.
	RIG	Administer 20 IU/kg body weight. If anatomically feasible, the full dose should be infiltrated around the wound(s) and any remaining volume should be administered IM at an anatomic site distant from vaccine administration. Also, RIG should not be administered in the same syringe as vaccine. Because RIG might partially suppress active production of antibody, no more than the recommended dose should be given.
	Vaccine	HDCV, RVA, or PCEC 1.0 mL, IM (deltoid area[†]), once each on days 0[‡], 3, 7, 14, and 28.
Previously vaccinated[¶]	Wound cleansing	All postexposure treatment should begin with immediate thorough cleansing of all wounds with soap and water. If available, a virucidal agent such as a povidone-iodine solution should be used to irrigate the wounds.
	RIG	RIG should not be administered.
	Vaccine	HDCV, RVA, or PCEC 1.0 mL, IM (deltoid area[†]), one each on days 0[‡] and 3.

Data from Centers for Disease Control and Prevention: MMWR Recomm Rep 1999; RR2:48.
RIG, Rabies immune globulin; *IM,* intramuscular; *HDCV,* human diploid cell vaccine; *RVA,* rabies vaccine adsorbed; *PCEC,* purified chick embryo cell vaccine.
*These regimens are applicable for all age groups, including children.
[†]The deltoid area is the only acceptable site of vaccination for adults and older children. For younger children, the outer aspect of the thigh may be used. Vaccine should never be administered in the gluteal area.
[‡]Day 0 is the day the first dose is administered.
[¶]Any person with a history of preexposure vaccination with HDCV, RVA, or PCEC; prior postexposure prophylaxis with HDCV, RVA, or PCEC; or previous vaccination with any other type of rabies vaccine and documented history of antibody response to the prior vaccination.

et al. (1976) described the successful protection of eight groups, totaling 45 persons, who were severely bitten in Iran by six dogs and two wolves that were proved rabid. A total of only six doses of vaccine, plus an initial injection of antirabies serum prepared in mules, was administered to each patient. None developed rabies despite deep wounds of the extremities and in some cases the face and head. In Germany all of 31 persons bitten by animals that were proved rabid were protected from rabies by a similar vaccine schedule (Kuwert et al., 1976). Extensive United States experience has also shown protection (Anderson et al., 1984; Centers for Disease Control and Prevention, 1999).

Immediate and thorough washing of all bite wounds and scratches with soap and water is an important measure for preventing rabies. Caustic compounds should not be used, but alcohol, povidone-iodine, and quaternary ammonium compounds may be used if available.

HRIG is administered only once (i.e., at the beginning of antirabies prophylaxis) to provide immediate antibodies until the patient responds to vaccine by actively producing antibodies. If HRIG was not given when vaccination was begun, it can be given through the seventh day after administration of the first dose of vaccine. Beyond the seventh day, HRIG is not indicated, because an antibody response to cell culture vaccine is presumed to have occurred. The recommended dose of HRIG is 20 IU/kg. This formula is applicable for all age groups, including children. If anatomically feasible, all the dose of HRIG should be thoroughly infiltrated in the area around the wound. If that is not possible, the rest should be administered intramuscularly in the gluteal area. HRIG should never be administered in the same syringe or into the same anatomic site as vaccine. Because HRIG may partially suppress active production of antibody, no more than the recommended dose should be given. The above recommendations also apply to ERIG, which is given in a dose of 40 IU/kg.

Rabies vaccine is administered in conjunction with HRIG at the beginning of postexposure therapy. A regimen of five doses of 1 ml each of HDCV or PCEV should be given intramuscularly. The first dose of vaccine in the five-dose course should be given as soon as possible after exposure. Additional doses should be given on days 3, 7, 14, and 28 after the first vaccination. For adults the vaccine should always be administered IM in the deltoid area. For children the anterolateral aspect of the thigh is also acceptable. The gluteal area should never be used for rabies vaccine injections, because administration in this area results in lower neutralizing antibody titers.

Patients who are HIV infected, particularly those with CD4+ cell counts less than 300/ml^3, may need increased doses, and definitely need monitoring for development of rabies antibodies.

BIBLIOGRAPHY

Anderson LJ, Nicholson KG, Rauxe RV, et al. Human rabies in the United States, 1960 to 1979; epidemiology, diagnosis, and prevention. Ann Intern Med 1984;100:728-735.

Aoki FY, Rubin ME, Fast MV. Rabies-neutralizing antibody in serum of children compared to adults following postexposure prophylaxis. Biologicals 1992;20:283-287.

Baer GM (ed). The Natural History of Rabies. New York: Academic Press, 1975.

Bahmanyar M, Fayaz A, Nour-Salehi S, et al. Successful protection of humans exposed to rabies infection: postexposure treatment with the new human diploid cell rabies vaccine and antirabies serum. JAMA 1976;236:2751.

Bhatt DP, et al. Human rabies: diagnosis, complications, and management. Am J Dis Child 1974;127:862.

Briggs DJ, Dreesen DW, Nicolay U, et al. Purified chick embryo cell culture rabies vaccine: interchangeability with human diploid cell culture rabies vaccine and comparison of one versus two-dose post-exposure booster regimen for previously immunized persons. Vaccine 2000;19:1055-1060.

Centers for Disease Control and Prevention. Human rabies prevention—United States, 1999. Recommendations of the Advisory Committee on Immunization Practices (ACIP). MMWR Morb Mortal Wkly Rep 1999;48:1-21.

Hattwick MA, Gregg MB. The disease in man. In Baer GM (ed). The Natural History of Rabies. New York: Academic Press, 1975.

Hemachuda T. Human rabies: clinical aspects, pathogenesis, and potential therapy. Curr Top Microbiol Immunol 1994;187:121-143.

Houff SA, Burton RC, Wilson RW, et al. Human-to-human transmission of rabies virus by corneal transplant. N Engl J Med 1979;300:603.

Johnson HN. Rabies virus. In Horsfall JL Jr, Tamm I (eds). Viral and Rickettsial Infections of Man, ed 4. Philadelphia: JB Lippincott, 1965.

Krebs JW, Rupprecht CE. Rabies surveillance in the United States during 1999. J Am Vet Med Assoc 2000;217:1799-1811.

Krebs JW, Smith JS, Rupprecht CE, et al. Mammalian reservoirs and epidemiology of rabies diagnosed in human beings in the United States, 1981-1998. Ann NY Acad Sci 2000;916:345-353.

Kuwert EK, Marcus I, Hoher PG. Neutralizing and omplement-fixing antibody responses in preexposure and postexposure vaccinees to a rabies vaccine produced in human diploid cells. J Biol Stand 1976;4(4): 249.

Lang J, Hoa DQ, Gioi NV, et al. Randomized feasibility trial of pre-exposure rabies vaccination with DTP-IPV in infants. Lancet 1997;349:1663-1665.

Noah DL, Drenzek CL, Smith JS, et al. Epidemiology of human rabies in the United States, 1980 to 1996. Ann Intern Med 1998;128:922-930.

Plotkin S, Wiktor TJ. Rabies vaccination. Ann Rev Med 1979;29:583.

Plotkin SA. Rabies. Clin Infect Dis 2000;30:4-12.

Sabeti A, Bahmanyar M, Ghodssi M, et al. Traitement des mordus par loups enragés en Iran. Ann Inst Pasteur 1964;106:303.

Smith JS. Rabies virus epitopic variation: use in ecologic studies. Adv Virus Res 1989;36:215-253.

Smith JS, Rupprecht CE, Fishbein DB, et al. Unexplained rabies in three immigrants in the United States: a virologic investigation. N Engl J Med 1991;324: 205-211.

Wiktor TJ, Plotkin SA, Koprowski H. Development and clinical trials of the new human rabies vaccine of tissue culture (human diploid cell) origin. Dev Biol Stand 1977;40:3.

Wilde H, Sirikawin S, Sabchoaren A, et al. Failures of postexposure treatment of rabies in children. Clin Infect Dis 1996;22:228-232.

Winkler WG. Airborne rabies virus infection. Bull Wildl Dis Assoc 1968;4:37.

Wunner WH, Larson JK, Dietzschold B, et al. The molecular biology of rabies viruses. Rev Infect Dis 1988;10(suppl 4):771-784.

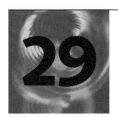

29 RESPIRATORY INFECTIONS

Margaret Burroughs, Maria-Arantxa Horga, Matthew T. Murrell, and Anne Moscona

Respiratory tract infections cause many of the most significant childhood diseases in both developed and underdeveloped areas of the world. This chapter is organized around the major forms of respiratory disease. Within each of these sections, pathogens that are primarily responsible for the clinical entity are discussed in detail. The major clinical syndromes and pathogens are summarized in Table 29-1.

CROUP (LARYNGOTRACHEOBRONCHITIS)
Etiology

Most cases of croup are caused by human parainfluenza virus (HPIV) types 1, 2, and 3. Other viral causes of croup include adenovirus, influenza A and B, rhinoviruses, respiratory syncytial virus (RSV), measles, and enteroviruses. Much less frequent are bacterial causes such as *Haemophilus influenzae*, group A hemolytic streptococci, *Corynebacterium diphtheriae*, *Streptococcus pneumoniae*, *Staphylococcus aureus*, and *Mycoplasma pneumoniae*.

The rest of this section deals specifically with the parainfluenza viruses (PIVs), because they represent the major cause of croup; other causes are discussed briefly at the end of this section and in detail in the relevant sections of the chapter.

HPIV types 1, 2, and 3. The HPIVs, taken together, are the most important cause of croup. HPIV type 3 alone is responsible for approximately 11% of pediatric respiratory hospitalizations (Chanock, 1990; Murphy, 1988) and is an important cause of croup as well as bronchiolitis and pneumonia in young infants. HPIV types 1 and 2 tend to infect older children and adolescents. Infection with HPIV in immunocompromised children such as liver-transplant recipients has been associated with a range of disease, from mild upper respiratory symptoms to requirement of mechanical ventilation and

death, especially in young children, in those whose infections occur soon after transplant, and in those whose immunosuppression has been augmented (Apalsch et al., 1995).

Classification and Structure. The HPIVs types 1 through 4 are members of the paramyxovirus family of nonsegmented, negative-strand RNA viruses. The molecular organization of the HPIV genome and the general structural features of the virus follow the pattern observed for all paramyxoviruses. The envelope of the HPIVs contains two viral glycoproteins, the receptor binding protein hemagglutinin-neuraminidase (HN) and the fusion protein (F). In addition, the virion possesses a non-glycosylated membrane-associated matrix protein (M), and a core comprised of a helical nucleocapsid containing the RNA genome and three viral proteins, the nucleocapsid protein (NP), the phosphoprotein (P) and a subunit of the RNA polymerase (L). Infection of cells by HPIV-3 is initiated by attachment of the virus to the host cell through interaction of the HN glycoprotein with a neuraminic acid–containing molecule on the host cell surface. During infection, the two virus-encoded glycoproteins, F and HN, are inserted into the plasma membrane of infected cells. The virion envelope is formed by budding from the surface of the infected cell and consists of the cell membrane–derived lipid bilayer containing the F and HN glycoproteins. Penetration and uncoating of the virus occur by fusion of the viral envelope with the plasma membrane of the cell, resulting in the release of the viral nucleocapsid into the cytoplasm. A characteristic feature of paramyxovirus infection is the induction of cell fusion at neutral pH.

HN is the receptor binding protein of HPIV-3, and has both hemagglutinating and neuraminidase activities. The hemagglutinating activity is responsible for attachment of virus to

TABLE 29-1   Acute Respiratory Tract Disease—Clinical Syndromes and Causative Agents

	CAUSATIVE AGENTS		
Clinical syndrome	Viruses	Bacteria	Other agents
Common cold; coldlike illness	Respiratory syncytial virus Parainfluenza Nonpolio virus Enteroviruses Adenoviruses Coronaviruses	*Mycoplasma pneumoniae*	
Febrile nasopharyngitis (in infants)		*Streptococcus*, group A pneumococci	
Acute tonsillopharyngitis with exudate or membrane	Adenoviruses Epstein-Barr	*Streptococcus*, group A *Corynebacterium diphtheriae*	
With vesicles or ulcers	Herpes simplex Group A coxsackie		
Acute laryngitis; laryngotracheobronchitis (croup)	Parainfluenza Influenza Adenoviruses Rhinoviruses Respiratory syncytial virus Measles	*C. diphtheriae*	
Acute epiglottitis		*Haemophilus influenzae* type b	
Bronchiolitis	Respiratory syncytial virus Parainfluenza Adenoviruses Influenza		
Pneumonia	Respiratory syncytial virus Parainfluenza Measles Adenoviruses Influenza Cytomegalovirus Varicella-zoster Hantavirus	*M. pneumoniae* Ureaplasma urealyticum *Staphylococcus* Pneumococci Hemolytic streptococci *H. influenzae* Enterobacteriaceae *Pseudomonas aeruginosa* *Klebsiella pneumoniae* Anaerobes Mycobacteria *Nocardia* *Legionella* *Chlamydia* Others	*Pneumocystis carinii* *Coxiella burnettii* (Q fever) *Toxoplasma gondii* Fungi (e.g., *Candida,* *Aspergillus,* *Coccidioides,* *Histoplasma,* *Blastomyces,* *Cryptococcus*)
Influenza-like illness	Influenza Parainfluenza Adenoviruses Lymphocytic choriomeningitis		
Acute sinusitis	Parainfluenza Adenoviruses	Pneumococci *H. influenzae* *Moraxella catarrhalis* *Streptococcus pyogenes* Anaerobes	

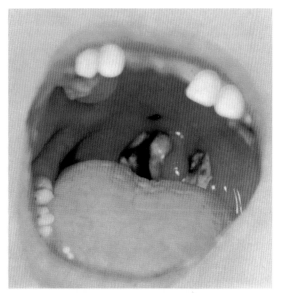

Plate 1 Tonsillar diphtheria. (Courtesy Franklin H. Top, MD; Professor and Head of the Department of Hygiene and Preventive Medicine, State University of Iowa, College of Medicine, Iowa City, Iowa; and Parke, Davis & Company's *Therapeutic Notes.*)

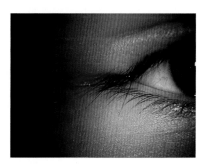

Plate 3 Chalazion (with inflammation) on right upper lid.

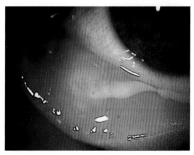

Plate 4 Chalazion on right lower lid, with inward discharge.

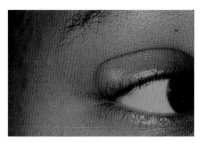

Plate 2 Chalazion on right upper lid.

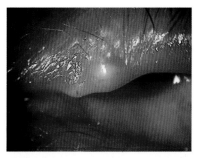

Plate 5 Folliculitis.

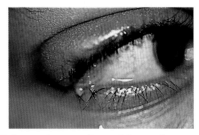

Plate 6 Pyogenic granuloma. Note red mass prolapsing from behind the right upper lid.

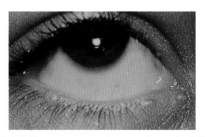

Plate 9 Molluscum contagiosum along the left inferior lid.

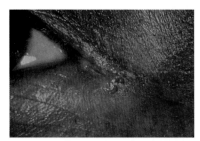

Plate 7 *Moraxella* angular blepharitis affecting only the left lateral canthus.

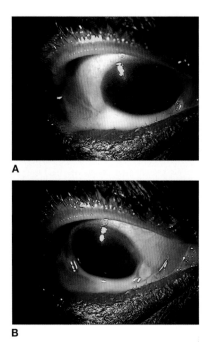

A

B

Plate 10 Bacterial conjunctivitis with mucous discharge.

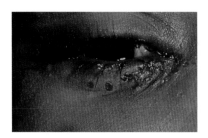

Plate 8 Primary herpes simplex virus blepharitis.

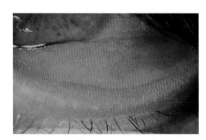

Plate 11 Hyperpurulent gonococcal conjunctivitis.

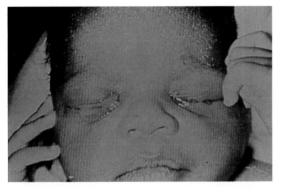

Plate 12 *Neisseria* ophthalmia neonatorum with purulent discharge.

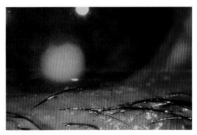

Plate 15 Early corneal ulcer secondary to trichiasis.

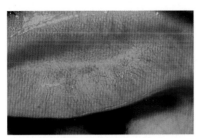

Plate 13 Everted right upper lid showing conjunctival chlamydial linear scarring (Arlt's line).

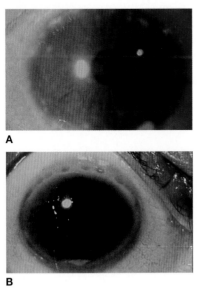

A

B

Plate 14 A, Perilimbal infiltrates. Note the clear space between the infiltrates and the limbus-sclera. **B,** Herbert's pits along superior limbus.

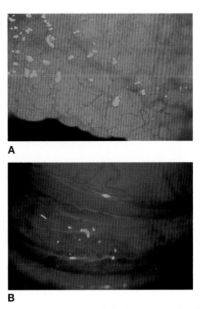

A

B

Plate 16 A, Conjunctival follicles. Note the clear, avascular centers. **B,** Conjunctival follicles with fluorescein stain.

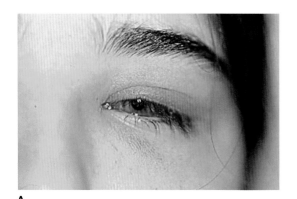

A

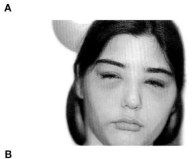

B

Plate 17 Hemorrhagic conjunctivitis with characteristic subconjunctival hemorrhages and lid swelling.

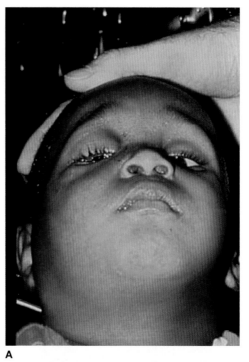

A

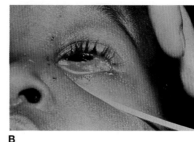

B

Plate 18 Parinaud's oculoglandular syndrome. Note the swollen right upper lid, right preauricular lymphadenopathy, and right cervical adenopathy.

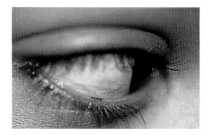

Plate 19 Raised nodular conjunctival phlycten.

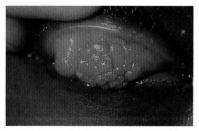

Plate 20 Upper lid eversion showing giant papillae seen in vernal conjunctivitis or contact lens overwear.

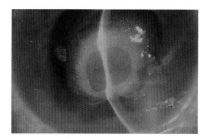

Plate 23 Typical *Pseudomonas* ulcer in a contact lens wearer.

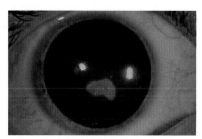

Plate 21 Corneal abrasion, highlighted by fluorescein stain. Note the lack of any white infiltrate in the surrounding cornea.

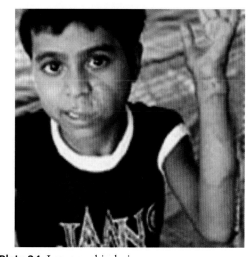

Plate 24 Leprosy skin lesions.

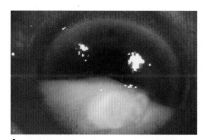

A

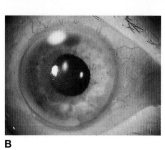

B

Plate 22 Corneal ulcer and hypopyon in anterior chamber.

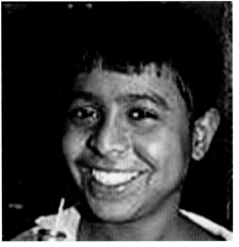

Plate 25 Child from Plate 24 with healed, treated skin lesions.

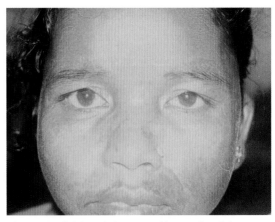

Plate 27 Child with leprosy affecting her lids. Note the superior lid retraction.

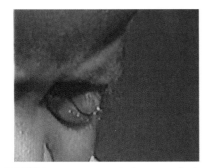

Plate 26 White cornea seen in keratomalacia.

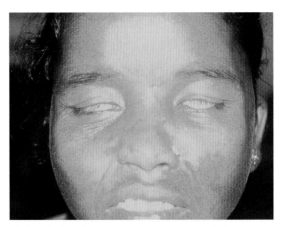

Plate 28 Child with leprosy attempting lid closure. Lagophthalmos is evident. Inferior white sclera is seen between the palpebra because the eyes are in up-gaze, owing to a normal Bell's effect.

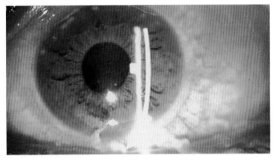

Plate 29 Staphylococcal hypersensitivity perilimbal infiltrates. Note the clear zone between infiltrates and the limbus.

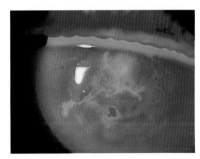

Plate 32 HSV dendrites stained with fluorescein.

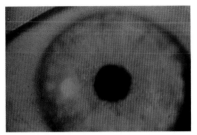

Plate 30 HSV dendrites stained with rose bengal.

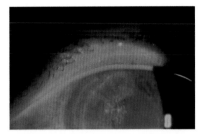

Plate 33 HSV dendrites stained with fluorescein.

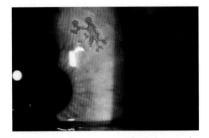

Plate 31 HSV dendrites stained with rose bengal.

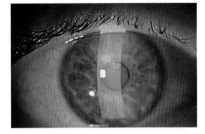

Plate 34 Small HSV dendrites stained with fluorescein.

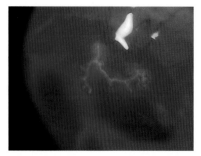

Plate 35 HSV dendrites stained with fluorescein.

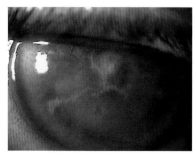

Plate 36 HSV dendrites stained with fluorescein, with surrounding corneal stroma infiltrate.

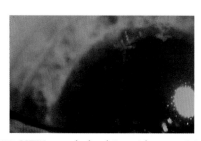

Plate 37 HZV pseudodendrite without staining.

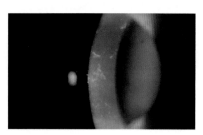

Plate 38 HZV pseudodendrite with rose bengal staining.

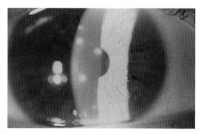

Plate 39 EBV nummular keratitis.

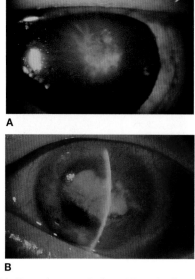

A

B

Plate 40 Fungal stromal ulcer. Note feathery edges.

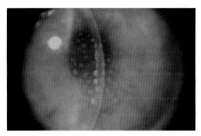

Plate 41 Granulomatous uveitis with "mutton fat" keratitic precipitates—clumps of white blood cells on the endothelium inside surface of cornea.

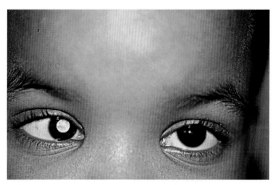

Plate 43 White pupil or leukokoria of the right eye.

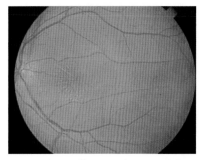

Plate 42 Macular stellate exudates and disc edema characteristic of neuroretinitis.

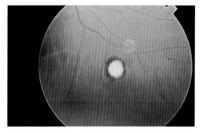

Plate 44 Old, inactive, chorioretinal toxoplasmosis scar without satellite lesions or overlying vitritis.

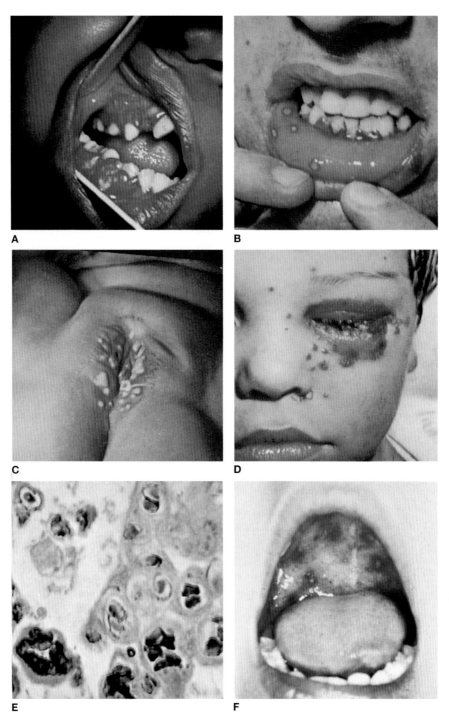

Plate 45 Herpes simplex infections. **A**, Primary herpetic gingivostomatitis in a child. **B**, Same disease in a young adult. **C**, Primary HSV1 vulvovaginitis in an infant. **D**, Primary herpetic keratoconjunctivitis. **E**, Biopsy of herpetic vesicle. Eosinophilic intranuclear inclusions and giant cells (×800). **F**, Ulcerative lesions on palate and tongue in hand-foot-and-mouth syndrome caused by Coxsackie A-16 virus. (A-E from Blank H, Rake G. Viral and rickettsial diseases of the skin, eye, and mucous membranes of man. Boston: Little, Brown, 1995. F courtesy James D. Cherry, MD.)

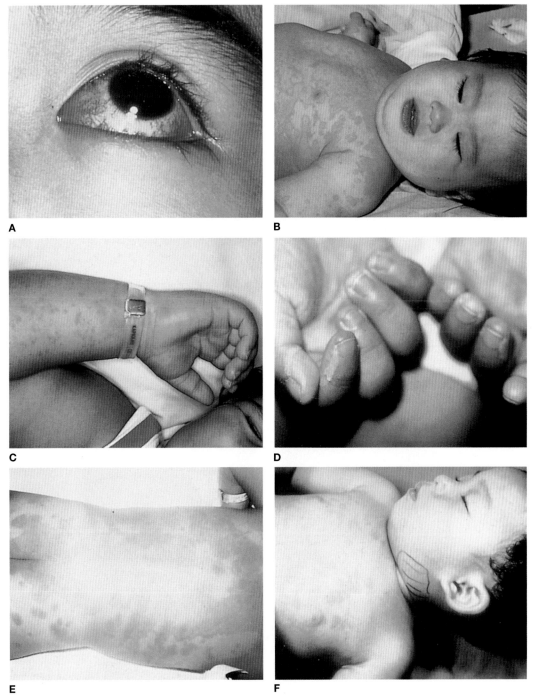

Plate 46 Some clinical signs of Kawasaki syndrome. **A,** Discrete vascular injection of the bulbar conjunctiva. **B,** Generalized lip erythema with mild edema, cracking, and bleeding fissures. **C,** Diffuse red-purple discoloration of the palm(s). **D,** Desquamation beginning at the fingertips just below the nailbeds. **E,** Diffuse erythematous, nonvesicular and nonbullous, polymorphic rash. **F,** Unilaterally enlarged cervical lymph node.

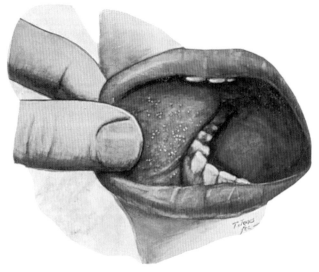

Plate 47 Koplik's spots. (From Zahorsky J, Zahorsky TS. Synopsis of pediatrics, St. Louis: Mosby, 1953.)

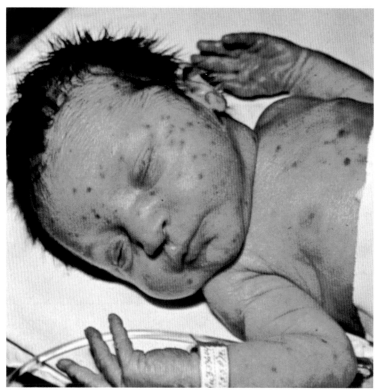

Plate 48 A 3-day-old infant with generalized macular lesions characteristic of neonatal purpura resulting from congenital rubella. His jaundice is caused by rubella hepatitis. (Courtesy Dr. Kenneth Schiffer, Albert Einstein College of Medicine, New York; from Cooper LA et al. Am J Dis Child 1965; 110:416.)

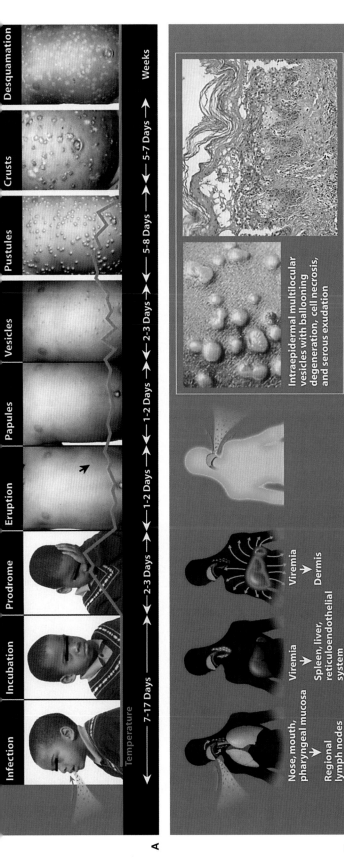

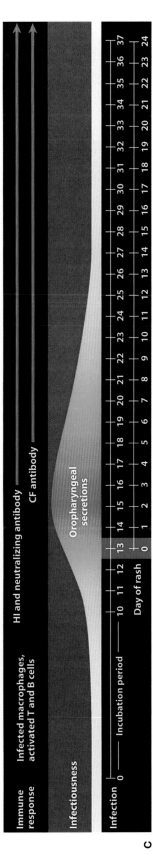

Plate 49 Clinical manifestations and pathogenesis of smallpox and the immune response. **A,** The initial phases of infection and the clinical manifestations, which include temperature spikes and progressive skin legions **B,** The pathogenesis of the infection. The photographs at the right-hand side of the panel show the characteristic features of the vesicles caused by smallpox (hematoxylin and eosin, ×90). **C,** The immune response to smallpox and the period of infectiousness. (*HI,* Hemagglutination inhibition; *CF,* complement fixation.) (*A,* Photograph of lesions courtesy of D. David Heymann, World Health Organization. From Bremen JG, Henderson DA: Diagnosis and management of smallpox. N Engl J Med 2002;346:1303. Copyright 2002 Massachusetts Medical Society. All rights reserved.)

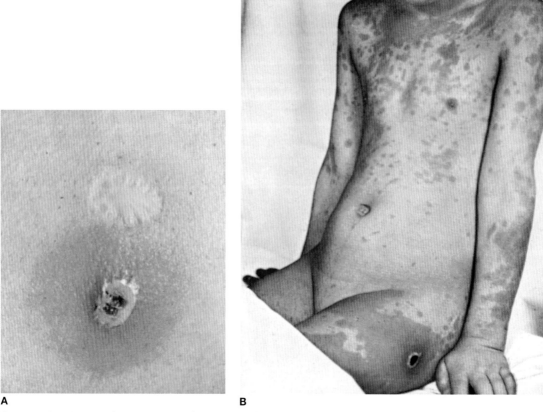

A   B

Plate 50 **A,** Primary take in a previously vaccinated person. **B,** Toxic eruption complicating vaccinia. (From Top FH, Wehrle PF, eds. Communicable and infectious diseases, ed 8. St. Louis: Mosby, 1976.)

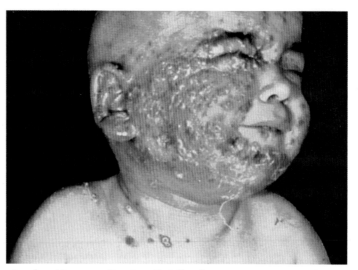

Plate 51 Excema vaccinatum. (Courtesy Dr. Otto E. Billo; from Stimson PM, Hodes HLA. Manual of the common contagious diseases. Philadelphia: Lea & Febiger, 1956.)

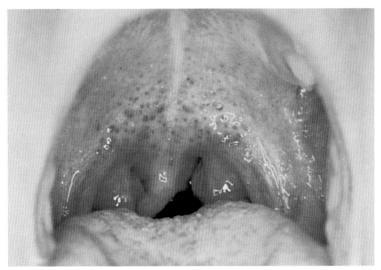

Plate 52 Marked petechial stippling of the soft palate in scarlet fever. (From Stillerman M, Bernstein SH. Am J Dis Child 1961; 101-476.)

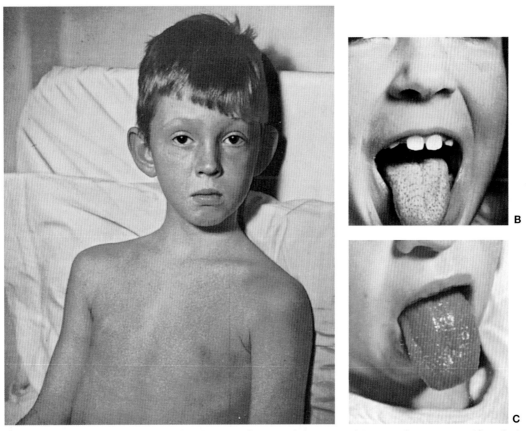

Plate 53 Scarlet fever. **A,** Punctate, erythematous rash (second day). **B,** White strawberry tongue (first day). **C,** Red strawberry tongue (third day). (Courtesy Dr. Franklin H. Top, Professor and Head of the Department of Hygiene and Preventive Medicine, State University of Iowa, College of Medicine, Iowa City, Iowa; and Parke, Davis & Company's *Therapeutic Notes*.)

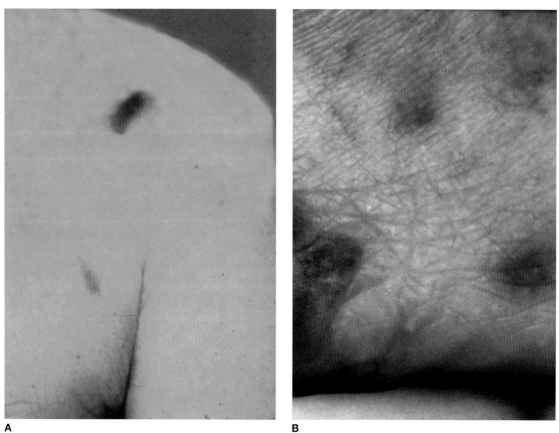

A
B
Plate 54 Lesions of Kaposi sarcoma on the shoulder (**A**) and lateral aspect of the foot (**B**) in two HIV-infected patients. (Courtesy Susan E. Cohen, MD, MPH, University of Rochester School of Medicine and Dentistry.)

the host cell via sialic acid–containing molecules on the host cell surface, whereas the neuraminidase activity is important for removing sialic acid residues from the viral and cellular surfaces (Huberman et al., 1995). The fusion protein, F, is synthesized as the inactive precursor F0, and F0 is cleaved by a host cell protease during its transit to the cell surface to produce the active protein. After this cleavage, a new hydrophobic N-terminus is exposed; this is the region directly involved in mediating fusion of the lipid bilayers. Cleavage of the F protein is required for infectivity of the virus, a fact that points to the importance of the hydrophobic fusion domain of F in the fusion process. Although the F protein is the molecule directly responsible for fusion of the lipid bilayers, the receptor-binding protein HN is also essential for cell fusion mediated by HPIV-3. Interaction of HN with its receptor is required in order for F to promote membrane fusion during viral infection (Moscona and Peluso, 1991). It has been proposed that upon binding to a sialic acid receptor, HN undergoes a receptor-induced conformational change, which in turn triggers a conformational change in F that allows fusion to occur (Lamb, 1993; Sergel et al., 1993).

Epidemiology. HPIV-1 causes large seasonal outbreaks of illness, with rises in the number of croup cases every other year (in odd-numbered years). HPIV-2 outbreaks generally follow those caused by HPIV-1. In contrast, HPIV-3 causes outbreaks each year, generally in the spring or summer (Hall, 2001).

Pathogenesis. HPIVs replicate in the epithelium of the upper respiratory tract and spread to the lower respiratory tract within 3 days. The pathogenesis in the lung has not been as well studied as it has for RSV (see the section on bronchiolitis). Epithelial cells of the small airways become infected with resultant necrosis and inflammatory infiltrates. The interplay among virus-induced cell damage, beneficial immune responses, and inflammatory responses that contribute to disease for HPIV-3 is still being resolved.

Clinical Manifestations

Croup is the most common clinical manifestation of HPIV infection. Inflammatory obstruction of the airway produces the clinical picture in all forms of infectious croup, which include acute laryngitis, laryngotracheitis, and laryngotracheobronchitis. A mild upper respiratory syndrome usually precedes the classic clinical manifestations of croup, which are produced by inflammatory obstruction of the airway in all forms of the illness. The severity and extent of the infectious process determine the sites of obstruction in the laryngotracheobronchial tree. Milder cases are characterized by hoarseness and a barking (or "croupy") cough, which is likely to be worse at night. Low-grade fever, loss of appetite, and malaise may be the only constitutional signs and symptoms. Respiratory distress is absent or minimal, and the condition responds promptly to appropriate treatment and subsides in a few days. In patients with severe acute laryngitis the infection may descend rapidly to the trachea and sometimes the bronchi, causing increased respiratory distress characterized by nasal flaring and inspiratory retractions. The site of obstruction is usually the subglottic area. Hoarseness is more marked, and breathing becomes rapid and labored, with inspiratory stridor and inspiratory retraction of the suprasternal notch, the supraclavicular spaces, the substernal region, and the intercostal spaces. The clinical condition can increase in severity to include respiratory failure with hypoxia, weakness, decreased air exchange, and ultimately death. Agitation, crying, and manipulation of the airway can aggravate the respiratory distress. Expiratory wheezes and various types of bronchitic rales are heard on auscultation of the chest. The white blood cell count is frequently normal or mildly elevated, and radiographs classically show a "steeple sign" indicative of subglottic edema.

Diagnosis

Diagnosis of HPIV infection can be made by viral isolation or by detection of antigen or nucleic acid. All three types of methods are currently available, and the detection of nucleic acid by reverse transcriptase polymerase chain reaction (RT-PCR) allows diagnosis of several respiratory viruses simultaneously. Kits for antigen detection allow for screening of children and are likely to be commonly used in the future as more therapies for pediatric respiratory viruses become available. Possibly the most important alternative diagnosis to be considered in the evaluation of suspected croup is *H. influenzae* epiglottitis, because this is a medical emergency requiring immediate therapy. Epiglottitis is marked by more rapid development, higher temperature, and greater toxicity than generally seen in viral croup (see detailed section on epiglottitis). Spasmodic croup may simulate infectious croup in many respects, but its etiology is not clearly defined. It has traditionally been distinguished from infectious croup by (1) the absence or mildness of signs of inflammation; (2) the typical remissions during the daytime; and (3) the history of previous, recurrent attacks lasting for 2 or 3 days followed by uneventful recovery.

Treatment

Novel antiviral agents for HPIV are under investigation, including molecules designed to inhibit fusion and entry of the virus, but no specific therapy was available as of June 2003. Most children with croup do not require hospitalization. Treatment is mainly supportive and aimed at maintaining the airway and hydration. Humidification of the air is often used with the aim of soothing the respiratory mucosa and loosening secretions. Avoiding agitation of the child is important, in order not to compromise the airway. If necessary, humidified supplemental oxygen (30% to 40%) may be administered by hood, mask, or nasal cannula. If respiratory distress progresses, ventilatory support may be required. Because most cases of infectious croup are viral in origin, antimicrobial agents are not indicated unless bacterial complications develop. Steroids have been shown to have a beneficial effect in the treatment of croup (Kairys et al., 1989; Orlicek, 1998; Wright et al., 2002). Nebulized steroids can be effective as well (Husby et al., 1993; Johnson et al., 1998; Klassen et al., 1994; Klassen et al., 1998). Racemic epinephrine or L-epinephrine has been successfully used for the treatment of more severe cases of croup (Kuusela and Vesikari, 1988; Waisman et al., 1992). Treatment is given at 2- to 4-hour intervals, and patients must be observed for a "rebound phenomenon," with relapse within several hours of the initial improvement.

Prevention

The development of a vaccine for the HPIVs has been hampered by the need to induce an immune response in young infants whose immature immune systems and whose maternal antibody both interfere with the development of an adequate immune response. Experimental vaccines are under evaluation, with reasonable expectation that a vaccine for HPIV-3, and perhaps also HPIV-1, will soon be feasible. Several strategies have been recently evaluated for HPIV-3 vaccines. Bovine parainfluenza type 3, attenuated in humans by nature of host range, has been shown to be infectious in seronegative recipients, with most vaccinees shedding virus or developing an immune response (Clements et al., 1996; Karron et al., 1996). Cold-adapted mutants of parainfluenza have been evaluated in both chimpanzees and in healthy infants. A cold-passaged mutant (cp45) was evaluated in seronegative chimpanzees and found to be attenuated in the upper and lower respiratory tracts. Immunized animals were resistant to wild-type HPIV-3 challenge. The vaccine was also well tolerated when given intranasally to HPIV-3–seropositive and HPIV-3–seronegative children. One dose of vaccine induced a serum hemagglutination-inhibiting antibody response in 81% of vaccinees (Hall et al., 1993; Karron et al., 1995a; Karron et al., 1995b; Karron et al., 1995c). As for RSV, it is likely that with the recent increase in our understanding of the molecular contributions to attenuation, engineered live HPIV-3 vaccines can be designed to be ideally attenuated and immunogenic (Skiadopoulos et al., 1999a; Skiadopoulos et al., 1999b; Skiadopoulos et al., 1999c; Tao et al., 1999), and that this technology will enhance our ability to rapidly develop effective HPIV candidate vaccines suitable for children in the future.

Other Etiologies of Croup

Respiratory syncytial virus. RSV is the leading cause of acute lower respiratory tract infection in young children and causes a significant percentage of croup, although it is even more commonly seen as a cause of bronchiolitis; RSV infection is discussed in detail later in the chapter. In the United States, most RSV infections occur from November to May.

Influenza virus. Influenza A and B viruses are an important cause of serious lower respiratory tract disease in children. Influenza A is an important cause of croup, as well as pneumonia and pharyngitis-bronchitis, and croup caused by influenza can be very severe. Influenza is discussed in detail later in this chapter.

Corynebacterium diphtheriae. Diphtheria caused by *C. diphtheriae* is a rare cause of croup in the United States. However, this organism may infect the larynx, trachea, and bronchi by extension from a pharyngeal infection or by primary infection and can result in a croupy cough, stridor, and hoarseness. As such, the obstruction due to diphtheria is subglottic. The leathery pseudomembrane present in the oropharynx and the bull neck of diphtheria distinguish diphtheria from other causes of croup. Nonetheless, progression of inspiratory stridor and toxicity over the course of several days should prompt the clinician to consider diphtheria in the differential diagnosis of croup. The diagnosis can be confirmed by culture of throat and tracheal aspirates.

ACUTE BRONCHIOLITIS
Etiology

RSV is the leading cause of bronchiolitis and lower respiratory tract infection in young children, accounting for 50% to 90% of all bronchiolitis hospitalizations. After RSV, HPIV type 3 and, to a lesser extent, types 1 and 2 are the most common causative agents of bronchiolitis. The rest of this section deals specifically with RSV as the major cause of bronchiolitis. Adenoviruses, rhinoviruses, influenza virus, and measles virus have been less frequently implicated as causes of bronchiolitis. These etiologic agents are described in detail in other sections of this chapter.

Respiratory syncytial virus

Classification and Structure. RSV is as a member of the genus Pneumovirus within the family Paramyxoviridae. The molecular organization of the RSV genome and the general structural features of the virus follow the paramyxovirus pattern. The virion possesses a lipid envelope with two viral glycoproteins: an attachment glycoprotein (G) and a fusion glycoprotein (F), which mediate viral attachment and cell fusion processes, respectively. Unlike other paramyxoviruses, the RSV fusion protein lacks either hemagglutinating or neuraminidase properties. RSV causes syncytia formation in infected cells, and the viral glycoproteins mediate entry and fusion at neutral pH.

Epidemiology. RSV outbreaks occur with a distinctive seasonal pattern. In temperate climates, the RSV season begins in late fall and continues until mid-spring, with a winter peak between January and March. Each community is affected every year and the attack rate in young children is high: 50% of children in their

first year of life will be infected with RSV in their first winter season, and by the age of 3, almost 100% of children will have been infected at least once. Management of the more severe respiratory manifestations often requires hospitalization.

RSV isolates are divided into two subgroups, A and B, according to variations in the antigenicity of their G proteins. A and B subgroups have been shown to cocirculate within the same community during the same season. Disease severity appears to be independent of the infecting strain.

Pathogenesis. Bronchiolitis is the result of a balance between cellular damage mediated by the viral pathogen and injury caused by the immune response of the host (Welliver, 2000). RSV (like the HPIVs) replicates initially in the nasopharyngeal epithelium and later spreads to the lower respiratory tract. Viral replication in the small airways causes inflammation, sloughing, and necrosis of bronchiolar epithelium. Edema and increased mucous secretion typically cause plugging of the small airways, atelectasis, airway narrowing, and obstruction. Primary infection with RSV tends to be the most severe. It is unclear whether this is because of immunopathologic mechanisms, immunologic immaturity, or the simple fact that the airways of the infected infants are small and vulnerable.

The immunology and immunopathogenesis of RSV infection are complex and not fully understood, although it is clear that both humoral and cellular components of the immune system contribute to both pathogenesis and protection. RSV primary infection does not confer permanent immunity. Repeated reinfection with RSV within a year of the previous infection is common in young children. Subsequent infections are usually milder, indicating protection against severe disease after primary infection. The nature of this partial protection is still not clearly defined. Secretory antibody mediates protection against upper respiratory tract infection, whereas circulating serum antibodies, particularly against F and G glycoproteins, have been shown to protect from infection and decrease progression to the lower airways (Anderson and Heilman, 1995; Falsey and Walsh, 1998). The limited degree of protection offered by maternal antibody is underscored by the fact that the peak incidence of serious RSV disease is seen in infants aged 2 to

5 months, a time of life when maternal antibody is still circulating within the infant. Nonetheless, some degree of protection may derive from maternal antibody, because infection in the first month is uncommon and higher levels of maternally derived antibody do seem to correlate with less severe illness (Glezen et al., 1981).

Attention was focused on immunopathology in RSV after children who had received formalin-inactivated RSV vaccine developed enhanced RSV disease after exposure to virus (Kim et al., 1969), and the intense inflammatory infiltrate in the lungs of vaccinated children suggested an immunopathologic cause of enhanced disease. In addition, although RSV bronchiolitis is a common disease of infants and young children and all humans are exposed to RSV early in their lives, only a few infants develop severe lung disease. Animal models have been used successfully to study the immune correlates of pathology and the basis for enhanced disease of RSV (Openshaw et al., 2001).

Several animal studies have demonstrated the role of immune responses in the pathology of RSV infection. The cotton rat model has been used for study of the vaccine-induced enhancement of RSV disease, recently to show that animals primed with formalin-inactivated virus and challenged had pulmonary viral titers $^1/_{10}$ to $^1/_{100}$ of that seen in naive animals but developed markedly accentuated lesions that included alveolitis and interstitial pneumonitis (in addition to the lesions seen in animals undergoing primary or secondary infection), which seem to be specific markers for the vaccine enhancement (Prince et al., 1999). A recent study vaccinating cotton rats with the original formalin-inactivated RSV vaccine preparation used to vaccinate children found that the histologic manifestations of enhanced disease in the cotton rat—alveolitis consisting primarily of neutrophils, and peribronchiolitis consisting primarily of lymphocytes—matched those of the two fatalities that occurred in children vaccinated with the same lot of formalin-inactivated vaccine, underscoring the importance of alveolitis as a histologic marker of immunopathologically enhanced disease (Prince et al., 2001).

The mouse model of RSV has shown the importance of T cells in enhanced lung pathology. CD4+ T cells play a major role in the immunopathogenesis of vaccine-enhanced RSV disease (Connors et al., 1992); there is a marked increase in the expression of Th2-type cytokines (interleukin [IL]-5, IL-13, IL-10) and a reduction in the expression of IL-12 in mice that were immunized with the formalin-inactivated vaccine, indicating a swing toward Th2 in the genesis of enhanced inflammation (Waris et al., 1996). Presence of IL-5 correlated with an eosinophilic infiltration in the mouse lung. In contrast, priming with live RSV resulted in a Th1 pattern of cytokine production and prevented subsequent enhanced disease (Waris et al., 1997). The mouse model has been used to dissect the contribution of different T-cell subsets and RSV proteins to the pathology of RSV infection and has shown drastically different disease outcomes, depending on the RSV protein used to prime and the cellular response (Srikiatkhachorn and Braciale, 1997). For example, in BALB/c mice the RSV surface protein G primes for an eosinophilic inflammatory response, mediated by Th2 type CD4+ T cells (Alwan et al., 1994), reminiscent of the responses seen in the formalin-inactivated RSV vaccine model (Openshaw et al., 1992). The same group showed that while transfer of cytotoxic CD8+ T lymphocytes (CTLs) to naive mice results in accelerated viral clearance, immunopathology is also greatly enhanced in mice with very active CTLs (Cannon et al., 1988), showing that in addition to Th2 cells, CTLs that are associated with Th1-type responses also contribute to the immunopathology observed in RSV-infected mice. The contribution of Th1 cells in RSV disease in humans is suggested by results that show interferon (IFN)-γ to be the most prevalent cytokine produced by RSV specific T cells, and its presence in nasopharyngeal washes of children with severe lower respiratory tract infection correlates with the severity of the disease (Bont et al., 2001).

As in the animal models, it is likely that in children cell-mediated immunity contributes to host defense against RSV but at the same time causes much of the pathologic process, and inappropriate immune responses may drive pulmonary inflammation during naturally acquired infection (Scott et al., 1978). Regulation of the response of T lymphocytes to RSV may be critical in determining the clinical outcome of RSV infection. Abnormal T-cell regulatory mechanisms may be related to a hyperactive IgE response, which contributes to an enhanced lung infiltrate. Welliver et al. (1984) have shown an inverse correlation between RSV-IgE in nasopharyngeal secretions and CD8+ cells in peripheral blood, and these cells may include those responsible for suppression of IgE production. CD8 T cells and natural killer (NK) cells are an abundant source of IFN, which inhibits the development of CD4 T cells making IL-4 and IL-5, and these cytokines are responsible for IgE production and eosinophilia (Openshaw et al., 2001).

Transmission and Infection Control. RSV is transmitted by direct inoculation of respiratory droplets and thus requires close contact with large-droplet aerosols or fomites for effective spread. RSV does not appear to be contracted by distant contact with small-particle aerosols. Because RSV is shed profusely by infected infants and may survive for hours on the skin of individuals and on environmental surfaces, it has great potential for nosocomial spread. Nosocomial RSV infection is a serious problem, because the virus can spread rapidly in the hospital environment despite routine infection-control procedures. The virus can survive on fomites such as countertops or diaper-changing stations for 4 to 7 hours, and the survival time in humid environments can exceed 24 hours. As many as 40% of hospitalized children may become infected during an RSV outbreak. In the hospital setting, these features of RSV mandate that strict isolation (gown, glove, mask) and rigorous hand-washing precautions be enforced until the child has stopped shedding RSV from the respiratory tract as documented by culture or by rapid antigen study. Additional important measures include education of caregivers and cohorting of infected patients when practical to prevent nosocomial transmission.

Clinical Manifestations of Acute Bronchiolitis

Bronchiolitis usually begins as an ordinary upper respiratory tract infection with nasal discharge, cough, slight fever, fretfulness, and loss of appetite. In a day or so the infant rapidly worsens and presents an alarming picture involving rapid labored breathing with retraction of the intercostal spaces, use of accessory respiratory muscles, cyanosis, and prostration. Increasing obstruction leads to progressive hypoxemia, which, if unrelieved, may be followed by exhaustion and death. Respirations are rapid, shallow, difficult, and often wheezy, with a rate of 60 to 80 or more per minute. Inspiratory retraction is seen in the suprasternal

notch and the intercostal and subcostal spaces. Cyanosis appears or is intensified during coughing or crying and can be continuous if the obstruction is severe.

Physical findings, often changeable, are those of overinflated lungs with hyperresonance to percussion; the diaphragm is depressed, expiration is prolonged, and wheezing is prominent. Initial hypoxemia may be followed by respiratory acidosis and hypercapnia as deterioration occurs. Hyperinflation and diffuse interstitial pneumonitis are typical chest radiography findings in severe disease.

RSV also may cause tracheobronchitis and croup (see previous discussion). Otitis media is a common manifestation of RSV infection (Okamoto et al., 1992). RSV bronchiolitis and bronchopneumonia may be found as nosocomial infections among infants and children in nurseries and pediatric wards and may also occur among day-care–center residents.

Risk factors predisposing to serious disease include underlying medical conditions such as prematurity, cardiopulmonary disease, immunodeficiency, metabolic disease, and some neuromuscular disorders. Assessment of the risk for progression to severe disease includes evaluation of underlying medical conditions and the overall clinical status of the child. An oxygen saturation less than 95% by pulse oximetry is a reliable objective predictor of progression to severe disease.

Diagnosis

Detection of viral antigen can be accomplished in several hours using commercial kits. Kits that allow screening for a panel of pediatric respiratory viruses simultaneously are likely to become very useful as additional therapies become available. Isolating or identifying the virus in respiratory tract secretions confirms the diagnosis of RSV infection. Nasopharyngeal secretions are a good source of diagnostic material, even if the disease appears to be limited to the lower respiratory tract. RSV can be detected by observation of cytopathic effect in human cell lines followed by specific immunofluorescence. Shell vial cultures allow rapid detection by immunofluorescence. Rapid identification of RSV antigen can be achieved directly in secretions using fluorescent-conjugated antibody or by enzyme-linked immunosorbent assay with a monoclonal antibody. A multiplex quantitative RT-PCR–enzyme hybridization assay that can differentiate between RSV viral subtypes A and B became available in 1998, and recently a colorimetric PCR system for specific detection of the RSV nucleocapsid gene and differentiation of viral subtypes A and B has been developed. PCR may provide a useful contribution to diagnosis and subtyping of RSV in the future.

Treatment

The treatment of acute bronchiolitis should aim to (1) relieve bronchiolar obstruction, (2) correct hypoxemia and acidosis, (3) control potential cardiac complications, (4) provide supportive measures, and (5) prevent or treat secondary bacterial infection.

Supportive therapy. Management of RSV infection is mainly supportive and symptomatic, aimed at providing adequate oxygenation and hydration. Close monitoring of the respiratory status through frequent physical examinations, pulse oximetry, and blood gas determinations is essential for evaluating the progression of the illness and further need for ventilatory support. Cardiovascular support may be required in the presence of manifestations of developing heart failure such as enlargement of the liver, gallop rhythm, change in quality of heart sounds, tachycardia, and pulmonary edema. If the patient has very severe bronchiolitis that progresses in spite of these measures, it may be necessary to provide assisted ventilation and all the support available in an intensive care unit.

Bronchodilators. The use of α- and β-adrenergic agonists remains controversial. The individual response to these therapies is variable and their use must be assessed in each individual case. A trial of inhaled bronchodilators and evaluation of the response is recommended in most cases, particularly in patients with a history of reactive airway disease or asthma. If there is no significant improvement the therapy may be discontinued.

Antinflammatory drugs. Cellular damage caused by the immune system of the host is an important component in viral bronchiolitis. Because of this element of inflammation, corticosteroids have been considered and studied for the treatment of RSV acute respiratory infection, but to date these studies have failed to demonstrate significant efficacy. Other antiinflammatory agents such as cromolyn sodium, budesonide, antileukotrienes and antikinins are currently being evaluated.

Antiviral agents. Ribavirin is a nucleoside analogue that acts to inhibit viral replication during the active replication phase of the viral life cycle. The clinical benefits of ribavirin remain controversial, and several recent trials have not reproduced the initially reported beneficial effects. More promising have been studies using ribavirin as preemptive therapy in immunocompromised patients (Adams et al., 1999). The Committee on Infectious Diseases of the American Academy of Pediatrics recently reassessed the indications for ribavirin therapy and suggests that it "may be considered" for children at high risk for serious RSV disease who are members of the following groups: (1) patients with complicated congenital heart disease (including pulmonary hypertension); (2) patients with chronic lung disease (cystic fibrosis, bronchopulmonary dysplasia); (3) premature infants (<37 weeks gestational age) and infants less than 6 weeks of age; (4) patients with underlying immunosuppressive disease or therapy (AIDS, severe combined immunodeficiency syndrome, transplant recipients); (5) severely ill infants with or without mechanical ventilation; (6) hospitalized patients at high risk for progression to severe disease because of age (<6 weeks) or underlying condition such as multiple congenital anomalies; and (7) patients with some neurologic or metabolic diseases (cerebral palsy, myasthenia gravis).

Prevention

Active immunization. Multiple obstacles have hampered the development of successful RSV vaccines. Peak incidence of severe disease occurs in young infants, whose responses to vaccines are diminished by passively acquired maternal antibody and relative immunologic immaturity. Another main obstacle is the fact that natural infection does not protect against reinfection with RSV. Additionally, the early experiences with a formalin-inactivated RSV vaccine that resulted in enhanced disease contributed to the delay in development (see the discussion of pathogenesis). In the late 1960s infants were vaccinated intramuscularly with a formalin-inactivated RSV preparation and were shown to produce both complement-fixing and neutralizing antibodies to the virus. However, when exposed to epidemic wild-type RSV, these infants experienced not protection but, rather, exaggerated disease (Kapikian et al., 1969). An explanation for this phenomenon has been considered of primary importance for future vaccine development, but none has been entirely satisfactory. Given the observation that the severity of lower respiratory tract infection decreases with repeated infections, the impetus for developing an RSV vaccine is strong. At present, several approaches to RSV vaccination are under evaluation (Dudas and Karron, 1998). Of the various approaches evaluated in animal models, two have demonstrated recent promise in clinical trials: purified F protein (PFP) subunit vaccines, and live attenuated vaccines (Dudas and Karron, 1998). Live cold-passaged, temperature-sensitive RSV vaccines (CPTS vaccines) containing many attenuating mutations are presently attractive candidates for live attenuated RSV vaccines. One such CPTS vaccine candidate has been shown to be safe and immunogenic in RSV-seronegative infants as young as 6 months of age. Subunit vaccines, while not viable for infants and therefore of limited use in the normal population, may provide a more suitable approach to vaccination in immunosuppressed populations at high risk of severe RSV infection, although these vaccines have been evaluated only in seropositive children (Dudas and Karron, 1998). One of the viral surface glycoproteins, the fusion protein (F), has been used as the antigen for development of subunit vaccines (PFP-1 and PFP-2). These vaccines have been shown to be moderately immunogenic and well tolerated in healthy seropositive children over 12 months of age, children over 12 months of age with cystic fibrosis, and children over 12 months of age with chronic lung disease of prematurity.

Immunoprophylaxis. Given the difficulty in the development of effective vaccines, the use of passive immunoprophylaxis with RSV antibody preparations is currently used to protect children at high risk for severe RSV disease. The goal of this approach is to increase the levels of neutralizing antibody in order to prevent the development of severe RSV infection. Palivizumab (Synagis, Medimmune, Inc, Gaithersburg, Maryland), a humanized monoclonal antibody directed against the RSV fusion protein, affords moderate protection to premature infants who are at high risk for severe RSV disease (American academy of Pediatrics, 1998). RSV-IG, an intravenous product prepared from pooled sera with high titers of anti-RSV antibody, has also been helpful in providing passive protection against RSV. This product also contains high antibody titers of antibody against influenza and HPIVs, and may afford broader protection than palivizumab against respiratory viral disease. RSV-IG may therefore be preferable to palivizumab for severely immunocompromised children who already receive monthly gamma-globulin infusions, since RSV-IG may be substituted for their routine infusions during RSV season. These antibody preparations have both been extensively studied and shown to be moderately effective in premature infants and in infants and children with underlying lung disease.

COMMON COLD AND COLDLIKE ILLNESS

The common cold syndrome is composed of several illnesses with overlapping clinical manifestations caused by a variety of different pathogens. Most common colds are of viral etiology, with rhinoviruses (more than 100 serotypes) accounting for over 40% of all cases. Numerous other viruses have been implicated including coronaviruses, RSV, PIVs, adenoviruses, nonpolio enterovirus, and coxsackieviruses A and B. *Mycoplasma* pneumonia, group A streptococcus, and pertussis in the catarrhal stage may manifest as an upper respiratory tract infection. This section focuses on rhinoviruses and coronaviruses as the most frequent agents of the cold.

Etiology

Rhinoviruses. Rhinovirus is the most common cause of the common cold, and as such it is perhaps the most ubiquitous agent of acute human infectious disease. Rhinoviruses are members of the Picornaviridae family of small (*pico-*) RNA viruses 20 to 30 nm in diameter. Rhinoviruses can be distinguished from the enteroviruses by their inactivation at low pH, which prevents rhinovirus survival in the stomach or intestine. The outer proteinaceous shell, or capsid, of the virus is formed by three proteins designated VP1 through VP3, and these assemble to form an icosahedral capsid protecting the single-stranded positive sense RNA genome. The virion lacks a lipid envelope, rendering it more stable to environmental forces and disinfectant processes.

The nasal epithelium is the primary site of both rhinovirus infection and symptoms. Viral entry into nasal epithelial cells is mediated by host cell receptor binding; all 102 serotypes of rhinovirus can be grouped based on their receptor use (Abraham and Colonno, 1984). The intercellular adhesion molecule-1, a transmembrane protein involved in cell adhesion and signaling, is the receptor used by 91 of these serotypes (Greve et al., 1989).

Rhinovirus infection and illness peaks in the early fall and late spring, but virus can be isolated throughout the year. Rhinovirus infection is cleared primarily by humoral immunity, and the majority of infected individuals produce neutralizing antibody to the infecting serotype. The large number of distinct serotypes results in periodic reinfection, although antibody persists in the serum for 2 to 4 years. The reduction in these reinfections as individuals grow older is most likely due to an expansion of the neutralizing antibody repertoire as the individual is exposed to an increasing number of serotypes.

Coronaviruses. Coronaviruses, members of the family Coronaviridae, are one of the etiologic agents of the common cold. Of the three serologically distinct groups, two include viruses that specifically infect humans. The virions are 100 to 200 nm in diameter and carry a single-stranded positive sense RNA genome (the largest of all RNA viruses, at 27 to 32 kb) surrounded by a lipid envelope derived from intracellular membranes. This lipid bilayer is studded with two viral glycoproteins: the spike (S) and hemagglutinin-esterase (HE) proteins. Under the electron microscope, these surface proteins give the virion the appearance of a crown (*corona* in Latin).

Spread of coronaviruses typically occurs following exposure to respiratory secretions from an infected individual. The virus binds to host cell receptors on the apical surface of epithelial cells using the S glycoprotein. After binding, S also mediates fusion of the viral envelope with the host cell plasma membrane, resulting in the release of the virion into the cytoplasm. The HE glycoprotein binds sialic acid residues that are ubiquitous on cell surfaces, and its esterase activity cleaves these residues from the surface of infected cells, thereby promoting release of newly formed virions.

Antibodies to S can neutralize viral infectivity, but clinical studies have shown that reinfection with the same serotype can occur within a year of the initial exposure. Outbreaks typically occur in the winter, and many infections pass unnoticed because of the mild symptoms and the self-limited course of natural infection.

Clinical Manifestations

The common cold is characterized by varying degrees of nasal congestion and discharge, conjunctivitis, sore throat, cough, and redness of the pharynx and tonsils without exudate. The incubation period is short; the average length is approximately 2 days, with a range of 1 to 6 days. Early symptoms include a scratchy feeling or soreness of the throat, coryza, and sneezing. Rhinorrhea and swelling of the nasal mucosa may result in obstruction of the nasal passages. The nasal discharge is initially watery, thin, and clear but often becomes mucopurulent and viscous and may persist for 10 to 14 days. Cough is usually nonproductive and appears later once the nasal symptoms subside. Headache or an uncomfortable feeling of fullness in the head is common. There may be slight fever, but the temperature rarely exceeds 38.3° C (101° F). The cervical lymph nodes may be slightly enlarged or tender. Chills, malaise, and muscular aches are not uncommon at the beginning, but they are seldom prominent nor do they persist in uncomplicated colds. The illness commonly lasts a week to 10 days, with viral shedding persisting for up to 2 to 3 weeks after the resolution of the symptoms (Winther et al., 1986).

Pathogenesis

Minor epithelial damage and structural changes have been documented in the nasal mucosa of patients with common colds, including loss of ciliated epithelial cells and increased numbers of polymorphonuclear leukocytes in the mucosa (Arruda et al., 1995; Turner et al., 1982; Winther et al., 1984). The relative absence of mucosal damage suggests that inflammatory cytokines and mediators play a significant role in the development of cold symptoms (Turner et al., 1998). Special attention has been given to IL-8 levels, which are elevated in patients infected with rhinovirus and have been shown to correlate with the severity of the symptoms (Turner et al., 1998).

Complications

The common cold may be complicated by an extension of the viral infection or by bacterial infections including otitis media, sinusitis, tonsillitis, cervical adenitis, laryngitis, bronchitis, bronchiolitis, and pneumonia. Infants and children are particularly likely to develop otitis media, making an examination of the tympanic membranes an important component of the physical exam. Secondary bacterial infections of the upper respiratory tract may occur, necessitating appropriate antimicrobial therapy to avoid complications.

Diagnosis

The typical clinical pattern of the common cold makes the diagnosis easy in most cases. Rhinitis, coryza, sneezing, scratchiness of the throat, and cough—all in the absence of pronounced constitutional symptoms—point to the common cold. There is no practical laboratory test by which the diagnosis can be confirmed, and similar clinical pictures may be presented by various other conditions. For example, allergic rhinitis may be clinically indistinguishable from the common cold. The presence of eosinophils in the nasal smear and the response to antihistamine drugs support the former diagnosis. Influenza can be distinguished by the prominence of associated constitutional symptoms and by specific diagnostic tests. Pertussis in the catarrhal stage may be confused with the common cold, as may preeruptive measles. Nasal diphtheria and foreign bodies in the nose may sometimes be mistaken for the common cold. Streptococcosis in infants under 6 months of age is characterized by nasopharyngitis associated with a thin mucopurulent discharge and irregular fever. This infection is difficult to distinguish from the common cold except by culture and by its longer duration. A diagnosis of sinusitis should also be considered in the patient with a cold that is more severe or more protracted than is usual.

Treatment

Treatment of colds remains entirely symptomatic. Antimicrobial agents do not influence the cold itself and should be reserved for treating secondary bacterial complications such as otitis media, sinusitis, and pneumonia. The occasional case of streptococcal nasopharyngitis should be treated with penicillin. Antimicrobial prophylaxis is unwarranted, and local or systemic use of decongestants such as ephedrine or phenylephrine to shrink the nasal mucosa and to prevent middle ear infection is of questionable value. It may be helpful for infants before feeding or at bedtime, but the effect is transitory and a rebound effect may occur. Antihistaminic medications are commonly used as nasal decongestants, but the effect on the rhinorrhea is modest and likely related to the anticholinergic effect rather than to the antihistaminic component of these drugs (Turner, 2001). The effectiveness of zinc dietary supplements, vitamin C, and echinacea medicinal preparations—popular remedies for treatment of colds—remains unproved despite multiple studies. Specific antiviral agents are being developed and evaluated, but to date none has been shown to have a significant effect on symptoms.

Infection Control Measures and Prevention

Rhinoviruses are transmitted by direct contact and large particle aerosols. Although isolation of the individual patient lowers the risk of spreading the disease, this procedure is not practical on a large scale. Frequent hand washing and hygiene may help in reducing the spread.

EPIGLOTTITIS

Acute epiglottitis is a life-threatening medical emergency characterized by rapid progression of stridor, drooling, fever, and toxic appearance.

Etiology

H. influenzae. Epiglottitis is nearly exclusively bacterial in origin; the etiologic agent is usually *H. influenzae*. The incidence of epiglottitis has decreased as the incidence of HIB infections has been controlled with vaccination. *H. influenzae* is a small, gram-negative pleomorphic coccobacillus and is classified based on capsular type (a-f) and nonencapsulated, nontypeable organisms. Prior to the development of conjugated *H. influenzae* type b (HIB) vaccines, HIB was the type responsible for the majority of invasive bacterial infections in children, including meningitis, pneumonia, epiglottitis, septic arthritis, occult bacteremia, cellulitis, and empyema. Since the introduction of the conjugated vaccines, the incidence of HIB disease is approximately the same as that of other capsular types. Upper respiratory tract colonization with typeable or nontypeable *H. influenzae* can be documented in 40% to 80% of children and a similar proportion of adults and serves as a reservoir for infection in the community. Antecedent upper respiratory tract infections increase the risk of colonization and subsequent infection. The major protective antigen for HIB is the capsular antigen, polyribosylribotol phosphate. The risk of invasive disease inversely correlates with the level of bactericidal antibody. Although polysaccharide antigens are not immunogenic in young children, the conjugation of oligomeric polyribosylribotol phosphate to immunogenic proteins allowed for immunogenicity of these vaccines in very young children and has resulted in a dramatic decrease in the incidence of invasive disease due to this pathogen.

Epidemiology

Epiglottitis generally occurs in the absence of meningitis or other manifestations of infection with HIB. In addition, epiglottitis occurs at a somewhat later age; the mean age for epiglottitis patients is 40 months, compared with approximately 9 months for patients with meningitis, septic arthritis, and cellulitis caused by the same organism.

Pathogenesis and Clinical Manifestations

Supraglottic obstruction develops quickly and leads to the inability to handle secretions, with resultant drooling. Epiglottitis is a medical emergency; the differentiation of this syndrome from croup is imperative. Prompt evaluation by experienced specialists such as otolaryngologists is warranted for children who exhibit symptoms suggestive of epiglottitis. Because HIB vaccine is now used widely, epiglottitis has become an uncommon illness, and clinical recognition has become more difficult yet equally important. Clinicians evaluating such patients in a primary care setting should be aware of the risks of airway obstruction and should minimize procedures that might agitate the child until trained specialists can examine the airway in a controlled environment. Children should be comforted to the extent possible, and medical intervention should be minimized until an artificial airway is established.

Children with epiglottitis usually have a rapid progression of stridor, drooling, fever, and toxic appearance. In comparison to children with epiglottitis, children with croup may have a more insidious onset of symptoms, are generally not toxic appearing, and do not have drooling and dysphagia as prominent presenting signs. The height of fever is variable in croup and may be quite high; upper respiratory symptoms are commonly associated with croup and less so with epiglottitis. The barking cough of croup occurs on expiration and is not characteristic of epiglottitis. Inspiratory stridor is characteristic of both croup and epiglottitis, although it tends to be more severe in epiglottitis. On examination, the child with epiglottitis appears anxious and may thrust the chin forward; the child is more comfortable sitting than supine. The child with croup is comfortable supine and is less anxious. Radiography is not recommended to distinguish croup from epiglottitis as the latter presents a risk for airway compromise during such evaluations. When croup is thought to be the most likely diagnosis, however, radiography can be considered. The findings characteristic of croup include the "steeple sign" indicating subglottic narrowing, while radiographic findings characteristic of epiglottitis include the "thumb sign" produced by the edematous epiglottis.

Treatment and Prevention

The acute management of epiglottitis includes maintenance of the airway, which requires placement of an artificial airway to prevent acute obstruction. Rarely, tracheostomy placement is required. Actions that minimize anxiety are appropriate until the airway is placed; the child should be held and comforted by a parent, and supplemental oxygen can be provided. Antimicrobial treatment of epiglottitis should include agents with activity against HIB. Because of the increasing frequency of β-lactamase—producing organisms, it is recommended that empiric treatment should include a third-generation cephalosporin. Alternative regimens for the penicillin-allergic child include trimethoprim-sulfamethoxazole or carbapenems. Vaccination against HIB has greatly reduced the incidence of epiglottitis. Most episodes occur in unvaccinated or partially vaccinated children (Garpenholt et al., 1999).

INFLUENZA AND INFLUENZA SYNDROMES
Epidemiology

Every year, approximately 20% of the world population is infected by influenza, resulting in significant morbidity and mortality worldwide. In the United States, influenza infections occur in epidemics each winter, generally between late December and early March. These outbreaks commonly peak for 4 to 8 weeks within a given community. Influenza is highly contagious, and school-age children have the highest attack rates of influenza (estimated to be nearly 50%). This population is believed to serve as a reservoir of virus for the community and to introduce influenza into households. Although the highest mortality rates occur among older adults, infants and younger children bear a significant burden of disease morbidity due to influenza, which occasionally surpasses RSV as a cause of pediatric admissions to the hospital (Box 29-1).

Etiology

Influenza viruses are members of the Orthomyxoviridae family, which is composed of enveloped viruses with a segmented, single-stranded RNA genome. The genome is negative-stranded; the viral messenger RNAs must be transcribed from the viral RNA segments by a viral RNA-directed RNA polymerase. The lipid envelope of influenza virus is derived from the plasma membrane of the host cell, and into this envelope are inserted the two surface glycoproteins of the virus, the receptor-binding and fusion protein hemagglutinin (HA) and the receptor-cleaving protein neuraminidase (NA). The third integral membrane protein of influenza virus is the M2 protein, which is an ion channel important for pH-mediated activation of the HA during viral entry.

The three influenza virus types—A, B, and C—infect humans, although influenza C infection rarely results in disease. Classification of influenza subtypes is based on sequence differences in the two viral surface glycoproteins: the hemagglutinin (HA) protein and the neuraminidase (NA) protein. Antigenic variation in influenza viruses occurs through two processes: antigenic drift and antigenic shift. Both influenza virus A and B undergo antigenic drift as result of point mutations in the HA and NA proteins. This antigenic variation of influenza virus requires annual vaccine reformulation. Only type A influenza virus undergoes antigenic shift. This occurs when a novel and significantly different subtype of HA or NA that circulates in an animal reservoir enters a human population without preexisting immunity. This major mechanism of antigenic variation is responsible for worldwide influenza pandemics. Global surveillance by the World Health Organization is conducted on an ongoing basis for detection of new viral strains that arise through either of these mechanisms (Centers for Disease Control and Prevention, 2000) and is the basis for the yearly selection of the strains to be included in the influenza vaccine.

Pathogenesis

Influenza viruses spread from person to person via aerosol transmission. Particles are deposited in the lower airways of the lung. The virus replicates throughout the respiratory tract, with a peak virus titer being reached on the first day of illness. Influenza viruses are sensitive to the antiviral effects of IFN, and they induce IFN during the course of infection. The virus induces an important antibody response against the surface glycoproteins HA and NA, which is important for resistance to infection with the same strain of influenza.

A day after the onset of infection, diffuse inflammation of the larynx, trachea, and bronchi occur, and desquamation of the ciliated and mucus-producing epithelial cells occurs. There is edema in the airways, along with infiltration by neutrophils and mononuclear cells. Epithelial necrosis occurs, and regeneration of the epithelium begins at the third to fifth day after infection. Resolution of the epithelial necrosis takes up to a month, and abnormalities in pulmonary function last beyond the recovery from the acute phase of illness.

Clinical Manifestations

The incubation period of influenza ranges from 24 to 72 hours. The illness is characterized by

---

BOX 29-1

GROUPS AT INCREASED RISK FOR COMPLICATIONS DUE TO INFLUENZA

- Persons >50 years old
- Residents of nursing homes and other chronic-care facilities
- Patients with chronic pulmonary and cardiac conditions
- Patients with chronic metabolic and renal diseases, hemoglobinopathies, and immunosuppression (including HIV)
- Children and teenagers on long-term aspirin therapy (increased risk for Reye's syndrome).
- Pregnant women who will be in the second or third trimester during influenza season

From Horga M-A, Caserta M, Karron R, Moscona A: Influenza virus. In Burg F, Ingelfinger J, Polin R, Gershon A: Gellis and Kagan's Current Pediatric Therapy, ed 17, Philadelphia: Saunders, 2002.

the rapid onset of symptoms in contrast with typical upper respiratory infections, which often have a more insidious presentation. Fever, chills, and rigor appear suddenly, associated with headache, prostration, and malaise. As the disease progresses, respiratory symptoms such as cough, sore throat, nasal congestion, and retrosternal pain become more prominent. Conjunctivitis, vomiting, and abdominal pain may be present. Significant myalgias are often part of the clinical syndrome, particularly localized over the cervicotrapezius region. Myositis and central nervous system (CNS) manifestations can occur. Pulmonary complications such as bronchitis or pneumonia have been estimated to occur in up to 25% of cases, particularly in immunocompromised children and other high-risk populations, such as patients with cystic fibrosis, sickle-cell anemia, diabetes, and chronic renal failure. Influenza infection is associated with otitis media in 20% to 50% of previously healthy preschool children (Belshe et al., 1998). Influenza infection is a significant cause of severe croup as well as pneumonia and pharyngitis-bronchitis in children.

Diagnosis

Most often the diagnosis of influenza is made on the basis of the clinical presentation together with evidence for presence of influenza in a given area. More recently, rapid diagnostic testing has become readily available. Rapid laboratory assays usually employ antigen, enzyme, or nucleic acid detection methods. These assays are inexpensive, with sensitivities ranging between 60% and 70% and specificities of 93% to 100% depending on the test. The results are often available in less than an hour. An early accurate diagnosis of influenza is desirable for the optimal application of antiviral agents, which should be started within 48 hours of the onset of the symptoms in order to have a significant beneficial effect. Other methods for isolation of the virus include classic tissue culture and centrifugation cultures (shell vials). Serologic testing can be used to confirm the diagnosis retrospectively, when a significant change between acute and convalescent titers is found.

Treatment

Supportive therapy. Supportive therapy aims to maintain adequate hydration and temperature control. The use of acetaminophen and other antipyretic therapy is particularly important in younger patients because of the increased risk of febrile seizures. Avoidance of salicylates is recommended because of the possible association with the development of Reye's syndrome.

Antiviral agents. Four drugs are currently available for the treatment and/or prophylaxis of influenza infections: amantadine, rimantadine, zanamivir and oseltamivir. Amantadine and rimantadine interfere with viral uncoating inside the cell, whereas zanamivir and oseltamivir are viral neuraminidase inhibitors (see below). Although the information presented below was current as of June 2003, the indications for use of the neuraminidase inhibitors are likely to expand. It is also likely that new neuraminidase inhibitors, as well as alternative formulations of existing drugs, may be available in the future. The CDC influenza Web site (http://www.cdc.gov/ncidod/diseases/flu/fluvirus.htm) is a good source for current information.

Amantadine inhibits the uncoating of viral RNA inside infected cells by blocking the ion channel formed by the influenza M2 protein, thereby preventing viral replication. It is active only against influenza A viruses. In healthy adolescents and adults, the drug is 91% efficacious in preventing influenza illness and 74% efficacious in preventing laboratory confirmed influenza infections. Studies conducted in children have extended the prophylactic benefit of amantadine in preventing influenza illness and infection to the pediatric population. Amantadine has also been shown to reduce the signs and symptoms of influenza illness in patients treated within 48 hours of the onset of disease. Amantadine-treated patients improve both subjectively and in length of fever, which resolves approximately 1 day sooner than placebo treated controls (Couch, 2000). Over 90% of amantadine is excreted unchanged by the kidneys, necessitating close monitoring and dosage adjustment based on creatinine clearance in patients with renal disease. Most commonly reported side effects involve the CNS and include nervousness, anxiety, difficulty concentrating, and lightheadedness, which usually are mild and self-limited despite continued dosing. However, more serious CNS side effects can occur, including delirium, agitation, and seizures, particularly in patients with underlying seizure disorders or psychiatric illness, those with impaired renal function, and the elderly. Administration of amantadine with antihistamines or anticholinergic medications also has been noted to increase the risk of CNS toxicity and should be avoided.

As many as 30% of patients develop viral resistance as soon as 3 days after starting a course of amantadine. Amantadine-resistant isolates of influenza A are genetically stable, can be transmitted to susceptible contacts, are equivalent in pathogenicity to wild type isolates, and can be shed for prolonged periods in immunocompromised patients taking drug. Because of this potential for resistance, the use of amantadine for treatment of influenza has been limited and is recommended for consideration by the American Academy of Pediatrics Committee on Infectious Diseases for three groups of pediatric patients (Box 29-2).

When used for treatment, amantadine should be given within 48 hours of the onset of illness. It is usually administered for 3 to 5 days or for 24 to 48 hours after symptomatic improvement; whichever is shorter. Prolonged therapy with amantadine should be avoided wherever possible to minimize the potential for development of resistant virus. Short-term prophylaxis against influenza A infections with amantadine is recommended for 2 weeks in high-risk children immunized after the start of influenza season in order to protect them from infection until vaccine immunity develops. Amantadine prophylaxis is also indicated for the entire influenza season for individuals with immunodeficiency who may not respond to vaccination, for high-risk patients who cannot receive vaccine because of allergy, for unimmunized caretakers of high-risk patients, and for any child in addition to vaccine for whom the prevention of influenza is highly desirable.

Rimantadine hydrochloride (Flumadine) is a structural analogue of amantadine and shares with amantadine a common mechanism of action. Rimantadine, like amantadine, is active only against influenza A. The drug has been demonstrated to be superior to placebo in the prophylaxis of both influenza illness and infection in healthy adolescents and young adults, with an efficacy rate of 85% and 66%, respectively. These benefits have also been documented in children and adolescents. It is essentially equivalent to amantadine in efficacy, providing a 1-day benefit in the relief of the signs and symptoms of influenza illness.

The two drugs have important differences in pharmacokinetics, adverse effects, and cost. Rimantadine is well absorbed following oral dosing and is highly metabolized by the liver before renal excretion. Thus, dosage adjustments of rimantadine are required only with severe renal disease or severe liver dysfunction. Rimantadine is associated with significantly lower rates of CNS toxicity, but it must be used with caution in patients with a history of seizure disorders (Couch, 2000). The cost of rimantadine is higher than that of amantadine. The recommended uses and dose of rimantadine in children are as for amantadine. The emergence and transmission of rimantadine-resistant isolates of influenza A virus occur at a frequency approximately equal to that seen with amantadine, and the two drugs share cross-resistance, which may further limit their use.

Zanamivir is a sialic acid transition-state analogue that acts as a specific inhibitor of the viral neuraminidase enzyme. Neuraminidase (NA), a surface glycoprotein on all influenza viruses, cleaves the cellular sialic acid residues bound to the hemagglutinin of newly formed particles and prevents viral clumping at the surface of infected cells. The function of the influenza neuraminidase is therefore necessary for multiple rounds of viral infectivity. In addition, the active site of this protein is highly conserved among all strains of influenza A and B, making it an ideal target for antiviral drugs (Couch, 2000).

The efficacy of zanamivir in the treatment of influenza has been studied in several large

---

BOX 29-2

CHILDREN IN WHOM AMANTADINE THERAPY IS RECOMMENDED

- Children with underlying chronic medical conditions (cardiac, respiratory, immunodeficiency)
- Children with severe influenza illness
- Children in special family or social situations whereby rapid improvement in symptoms or decrease in viral shedding would be highly beneficial (children with examinations, athletic competitions, household contacts that include elderly, debilitated, or immunodeficient patients)

From Horga M-A, Caserta M, Karron R, Moscona A: Influenza virus. In Burg F, Ingelfinger J, Polin R, Gershon A: Gellis and Kagan's Current Pediatric Therapy, ed 17, Philadelphia: Saunders, 2002.

controlled trials with consistent evidence of a beneficial antiviral effect (Couch, 2000). In patients with fever treated within 30 hours of onset of illness, the maximal benefit—the shortening of duration of symptoms by up to 3 days—has been observed. A similar beneficial effect of zanamivir has been demonstrated in children. In preliminary studies, zanamivir was 84% to 95% effective in preventing febrile illness due to laboratory documented influenza, with 31% to 80% efficacy against infection; however, as of June 2003 the drug has not been approved for the prophylaxis of influenza virus infections in adults or children.

Zanamivir is not orally bioavailable and is marketed as a dry powder for inhalation. It is packaged with a diskhaler and given as two oral inhalations (10 mg) twice a day for 5 days. Approximately 10% to 20% of the active compound reaches the lungs while the rest is deposited in the oropharynx. Of the total dose, 5% to 15% is absorbed and excreted in the urine. No dosage adjustment is recommended in patients with renal failure. In general, zanamivir is well tolerated, with equal numbers of patients in drug and placebo groups reporting adverse effects, of which upper respiratory and gastrointestinal complaints are most commonly noted. However, zanamivir is not generally recommended for patients with underlying respiratory disease because of postlicensure reports of wheezing and decreases on pulmonary function testing of peak expiratory flow rates of >20% in subjects receiving treatment. If such individuals use zanamivir, it is recommended that they have a fast-acting bronchodilator available and discontinue use of zanamivir if respiratory difficulty develops.

Zanamivir is licensed for the treatment of influenza A and B infections in adults and adolescents >7 years of age who have had symptoms of influenza for less than 48 hours. The major advantages to the use of zanamivir are its activity against both influenza A and B, a favorable pharmacokinetic and side effect profile, no known interaction with other medications, and antiviral activity against amantadine- and rimantadine-resistant strains. In vitro, influenza isolates have been generated that are resistant to zanamivir. Additionally, neuraminidase inhibitor–resistant influenza isolates have been occasionally recovered from immunocompromised hosts. Mutations in the conserved active site of the neuraminidase enzyme appear to mediate this resistance. Because neuraminidase function is critical to influenza virus, the changes in this enzyme associated with viral resistance have also been associated with decreased viral infectivity and virulence in animal models, suggesting that resistant strains may be less pathogenic and transmissible than wild type influenza (Couch, 2000). Based on these data, it is predicted that resistance of influenza to neuraminidase inhibitors will be infrequent and unlikely to interfere significantly with the clinical utility of this class of compounds. The drawbacks to zanamivir include cost, difficulty with administration of the drug, and the restricted use of zanamivir in children less than 7 years of age.

Oseltamivir, similar to zanamivir, exerts its antiviral effect by inhibiting influenza virus neuraminidase. In randomized controlled trials, oseltamivir has been shown to be effective both in the treatment and prophylaxis of influenza. Patients had significant reduction in the duration of viral shedding, time to resolution of symptoms, frequency of upper respiratory tract illness, and fever. The reduction in fever was apparent after the first day of therapy. Secondary complications of influenza, such as pneumonia, bronchitis, sinusitis, and otitis media, were also reduced by 50%, as was the use of physician-prescribed antibiotics in the patients given oseltamivir. Data on the treatment of influenza with oseltamivir in children 1 to 12 years of age have also been encouraging, showing a decrease in the duration of the illness by 1.5 days and a reduction in the incidence of otitis media by 43% (Couch, 2000).

Oseltamivir phosphate is the ethyl ester prodrug of the active compound, oseltamivir carboxylate, and is converted to its active form in the liver following oral dosing. Approximately 80% of the prodrug is bioavailable as the active compound, with peak plasma concentrations of oseltamivir carboxylate achieved 3 to 4 hours following a single dose. The half-life is 6 to 10 hours, with predominantly renal excretion. Dosing, therefore, needs to be modified in patients with a creatinine clearance of less than 30 mL/minute. Food does not interfere with the absorption of oseltamivir phosphate and in limited studies has been shown to reduce the nausea and vomiting associated with the use of this medication.

Like zanamivir, the benefits of the use of oseltamivir over older antiinfluenza drugs include an expanded spectrum of activity that includes influenza A and B viruses, minimal drug toxicity, and the expectation of limited viral resistance. In addition, oseltamivir is available in tablet form with good oral bioavailability and favorable pharmacokinetics, allowing for twice daily administration. Oseltamivir has been approved for prophylaxis and therapy for influenza infection. A liquid preparation has been developed for use in children. As of June 2003, oseltamivir is approved for therapy in children over 1 year of age and for prophylaxis in children over 12 years of age.

Prevention

Active immunization: inactivated influenza vaccines. Inactivated influenza vaccines are multivalent preparations containing three viral strains (two type A and one type B) likely to circulate in the forthcoming winter. The currently available preparations include a "whole virus" vaccine made from inactivated highly purified intact viral particles grown in embryonated chicken eggs. The "subvirion" vaccine adds a further step, in which the lipid-containing viral envelope has been disrupted. In addition, a purified surface antigen vaccine is also available. These last two preparations, known as *split vaccines,* should be given to children <13 years old, since the other vaccines are associated with a higher incidence of adverse effects in the younger age group.

Most vaccinated children develop high post-vaccination antibody titers. The overall effectiveness of influenza vaccine depends on the age, immunocompetence of the child, and the similarity between the viruses contained in the vaccine and those in circulation that season. The protection when challenged with a homologous virus is approximately 70% to 80% and is estimated to last only briefly—usually around 1 year.

Recommendations for the use of influenza vaccine. The Advisory Committee on Immunization Practices recommends influenza vaccine administration for any person aged >6 months at increased risk for complications due to the illness (Centers for Disease Control and Prevention, 2000). Health-care workers and persons in close contact with high-risk groups (including household contacts) should be vaccinated to decrease the risk of transmission. Women who will be beyond the first trimester of pregnancy during the influenza season should be vaccinated as well. Travelers to areas where influenza outbreaks will

be occurring should be recommended for vaccination. The vaccine can also be administered to any person aged >6 months to reduce the chance of becoming infected with influenza. The optimal time for vaccination in the United States is in early fall, from the beginning of October through mid November. However, when vaccine shortages occur (as in the 2000-2001 influenza season), immunization should be continued further into the influenza season as vaccine becomes available.

Among previously unvaccinated children aged <9 years, two intramuscular doses administered at least 1 month apart are recommended for achieving satisfactory antibody responses. If possible, the second dose should be administered before December. Children > 4 years of age can receive any of the available influenza vaccines, whereas those 6 months to 4 years of age should receive those preparations only for which safety and efficacy in this age group have been established. Adverse side effects are minimal and infrequent, limited usually to a mild illness that may include fever, malaise, myalgias, and other systemic manifestations. However, inactivated influenza vaccine contains noninfectious killed viruses, so it cannot cause influenza. Guillain-Barré syndrome has not been associated with influenza immunization in children. Inactivated influenza vaccine should not be given to individuals with a history of anaphylactic hypersensitivity to eggs or to other components of the influenza vaccine. During an acute febrile illness, administration of influenza vaccine is not recommended, although minor illnesses with or without fever particularly among children are not a contraindication.

Although infants younger than 6 months of age have been shown to be at high risk for morbidity and mortality due to influenza, the efficacy and safety of the current inactivated vaccines has not been established for this age group. The addition of young children to groups recommended for vaccination is being evaluated.

New influenza vaccines. Intranasally administered, cold-adapted, live attenuated influenza virus vaccines have recently elicited great interest in the United States. These vaccines contain live viruses that replicate in the upper respiratory tract but are unable to replicate efficiently at temperatures found in the lower respiratory tract. Therefore, although these attenuated strains are able to replicate and induce immunity, they do not produce lower respiratory tract disease. Cold-adapted influenza vaccines potentially offer advantages over inactivated vaccines such as induction of a broad mucosal and systemic immune response, ease of administration, acceptability of an intranasal route of administration (nose drops), and induction of minimal symptoms. In pediatric trials the efficacy in preventing influenza infection has been approximately 90% (Belshe et al., 1998). These vaccines have also shown efficacy in preventing febrile otitis media (Belshe et al., 1998). It is anticipated that the live attenuated influenza virus vaccines may be licensed for use in the United States in the near future.

PNEUMONIA
Etiology

A variety of pathogens are etiologic agents of pneumonia in children, including the respiratory viruses discussed above (PIVs, RSV, and influenza virus), bacterial agents including *S. pneumoniae, H. influenzae, S. aureus,* and *Streptococcus pyogenes,* atypical organisms such as *M. pneumoniae* and *Chlamydia pneumoniae,* mycobacteria, fungi, and occasionally *Legionella pneumophila, Neisseria meningitidis,* and *Bordetella pertussis.* The incidence of viral pneumonia outstrips that of bacterial and fungal pneumonia. The clinical manifestation of these various agents is dependent on the pathogen, the child's age, and the immune status. Pulmonary pathology or structural anomalies may complicate the presentation, clinical course, and management. Whereas pneumonia due to fungi is more common in immunosuppressed children, bacterial and viral pneumonia may affect both immunocompetent and immunosuppressed children. The decision to pursue radiographic and laboratory evaluation to determine the etiologic agent in otherwise healthy children depends on the degree of respiratory compromise. The evaluation of immunosuppressed patients with progressive pneumonia or pneumonitis should take place early in the course of disease and typically requires more aggressive pursuit of diagnostic procedures, including bronchoalveolar lavage or lung biopsy. This section deals specifically with several of the major agents of pneumonia; for discussion of other agents the reader is referred to other chapters of this text.

Bacterial Pneumonia

S. pneumoniae and *M. pneumoniae* are the most common pathogens causing bacterial pneumonia in immunocompetent children. *S. aureus* and *S. pyogenes* are also important pathogens, the former primarily for children less than 2 years of age. Both *S. aureus* and *S. pyogenes* pneumonia are most often complications of viral illnesses. The incidence of pneumonia due to HIB has decreased substantially with the widespread use of conjugated HIB vaccines. The etiologic agents responsible for pneumonia in children are detailed in Tables 29-2 and 29-3. The organisms responsible for pneumonia differ with the age of the patient; the causes according to age are detailed in Table 29-4.

S. pneumoniae. S. pneumoniae is the most common cause of bacterial pneumonia in children. Pneumococci are common inhabitants of the normal upper respiratory tract. Factors that predispose to invasive pneumococcal infection include preceding viral infections, bronchial obstruction, atelectasis, alteration of mucociliary function by allergy, irritants, and other agents, pulmonary congestion with cardiovascular problems, splenectomy, agammaglobulinemia, lymphocytic leukemia, sickle-cell disease, antibody deficiency states, human immunodeficiency virus (HIV) infection, and the absence of acquired immunity.

The pneumococcus is a gram-positive, lancet-shaped facultatively anaerobic organism that appears on gram stain as single cocci, pairs of lancet-shaped organisms, or chains. The polysaccharide capsule is the basis for the ability of this organism to evade phagocytosis, for stimulation of protective antibody, and for typing of pneumococci. Although 90 distinct capsular types of pneumococci have been identified, a limited number are responsible for disease in children. Among children the serotypes most commonly identified with pneumonia are 19, 23, 14, 3, 6, and 1. Antibody specific for the capsular type is protective against invasive disease. However, the protective antibodies produced are not cross-reactive; antibody to one type of pneumococcus does not protect against infection with a second pneumococcal type.

H. influenzae. H. influenzae type B (HIB) is discussed in the section on epiglottis. This organism was a major agent of pneumonia; however, introduction of the conjugated vaccines has resulted in a great decrease in the incidence of pneumonia due to this pathogen.

S. pyogenes. Group A streptococci commonly cause upper respiratory tract infections and pharyngitis but are less common causes of

TABLE 29-2	Common Causes of Community-Acquired Pneumonia in Otherwise Healthy Children
Viruses	Respiratory syncytial virus
	Influenza A or B
	Parainfluenza viruses 1, 2, and 3
	Adenovirus
	Rhinovirus[*]
	Measles virus[†]
Mycoplasma	*Mycoplasma pneumoniae*
Chlamydia	*Chlamydia trachomatis*
	Chlamydia pneumoniae[‡]
Bacteria	*Streptococcus pneumoniae*
	Mycobacterium tuberculosis
	Staphylococcus aureus[§]
	Haemophilus influenzae type b [ǁ]
	Nontypeable *H. influenzae*[†]

From McIntosh K. Community-acquired pneumonia in children. N Engl J Med 2002:346(6):429-437.
[*]Recent data from surveys that used polymerase chain reaction assays implicated rhinovirus as a cause of pneumonia. Some would question its etiologic role.
[†]Measles virus and nontypeable strains of *H. influenzae* are common causes of pneumonia in the developing world but uncommon causes in the developed world.
[‡]Among older schoolchildren and adolescents, *C. pneumoniae* may be a common cause of pneumonia. There is disagreement among studies and some concern about its role, however, in view of its frequent recovery in asymptomatic patients.
[§]Pneumonia due to *S. aureus* is now uncommon in the United States and Europe, but it is still relatively common in other areas, particularly in the developing world.
[ǁ] Pneumonia caused by *H. influenzae* type b is restricted to parts of the world where the conjugate vaccine is not widely used.

pneumonia in children. A history of antecedent viral infection is common; measles, varicella, and rubella may precede this syndrome in as many as half of affected children (Kevy and Lowe, 1961). Of 52 cases of invasive group A streptococcal infections associated with varicella, approximately 10% of affected patients developed pneumonia (Lesko et al., 2001). Pneumonia caused by this organism is frequently associated with empyema. The microbiologic, epidemiologic, and clinical characteristics of this organism are further characterized in Chapter 35.

S. aureus pneumonia is characterized by fulminant disease, frequently in a child less than 2 years of age. Staphylococcal pneumonia may present as a nosocomial problem, particularly in neonates, or as a complication of other respiratory infections such as influenza. The properties of staphylococci and the pathogenesis, pathologic and immunologic aspects, and clinical manifestations of staphylococcal infections are presented in detail in Chapter 34.

Mycobacterium tuberculosis must be considered as an etiologic agent especially in children who are foreign born or whose parents were foreign born. Clinically, tuberculosis may manifest as pneumonia unresponsive to standard antimicrobial treatment. The biology and clinical presentation of tuberculosis in children are described in detail in Chapter 39.

Atypical Bacterial Pneumonia

M. pneumoniae is the most common cause of bacterial pneumonia in school-aged children. Community spread of *M. pneumoniae* occurs in protracted outbreaks that may extend through the entire respiratory disease season. Because the organism multiplies slowly, the incubation period is long, averaging 14 days but highly variable. Carriage of viable *Mycoplasma* organisms by individual patients may last up to 3 months. As a result of this extended carriage and the relatively low rate of contagion, the period of spread in households may also last for months. *M. pneumoniae* is the most prominent single cause of pneumonia and of prolonged episodes of tracheobronchitis in school-age children and adolescents. This is particularly true in otherwise well children who do not have underlying chronic disorders. *M. pneumoniae* should also be considered in wheezing-associated illness. The infection is

TABLE 29-3	Uncommon Causes of Community-Acquired Pneumonia in Otherwise Healthy Children
Viruses	Varicella zoster virus
	Coronaviruses
	Enteroviruses (coxsackievirus and echovirus)
	Epstein-Barr virus
	Mumps virus
	Herpes simplex virus (in newborns)
	Hantavirus[*][†]
Chlamydia	*Chlamydia psittaci*[†]
Coxiella	*Coxiella burnettii*[†]
Bacteria	*Streptococcus pyogenes*
	Anaerobic mouth flora (Streptococcus milleri, Peptostreptococcus)
	Non–type b (but typeable) *Haemophilus influenzae*
	Bordetella pertussis[‡]
	Klebsiella pneumoniae
	Escherichia coli
	Listeria monocytogenes
	Neisseria meningitidis (often group Y)
	Legionella
	Pseudomonas pseudomallei[*]
	Francisella tularensis[†§]
	Brucella abortus[†]
	Leptospira[†]
Fungi	*Coccidoides immitis*[*]
	Histoplasma capsulatum[*]
	Blastomyces dermatitidis[*]

Modified from McIntosh K. Community-acquired pneumonia in children. N Engl J Med 2002:346(6):429-437.
[*]This organism should be included in the differential diagnosis as a cause of pneumonia only if there is a history of residence in or travel to an area of endemic infection.
[†]This organism should be included in the differential diagnosis only if there is a history of possible or definite exposure to a particular animal reservoir or, in the case of *Brucella* species or *F. tularensis*, a concern regarding exposure to an agent of bioterrorism.
[‡]Most infants and children with clinically significant pertussis do not have pneumonia.
[§]This organism should be included in the differential diagnosis only if there is a history of possible or definite contact with insect vectors or a concern regarding exposure to an agent of bioterrorism.

rarely severe enough to require hospitalization. However, children with sickle-cell disease and other conditions may have severe and life-threatening pneumonias in which no other causative agents may be identified.

C. pneumoniae is a frequent cause of community-acquired pneumonia in children. Sero-prevalence data and PCR suggest that the illness is most common in school-age children. *Chlamydia trachomatis* and *Ureaplasma urealyticum* may both be associated with neonatal pneumonia, usually not accompanied by fever.

L. pneumophila. Legionnaire's disease is rare in children. The Centers for Disease Control and Prevention reports usually list fewer than 2% of cases in children less than 19 years of age. Because the illness occurs

with enhanced morbidity and mortality in the aged and in the immunocompromised, more cases may be recognized in pediatric populations with underlying disorders such as cancer, immunodeficiency, and hematologic malignancies. Although *L. pneumophila* pneumonia is primarily a disease of immunosuppressed children, both nosocomial and community-acquired cases have been described in children (Brady, 1989; Green and Wald, 1996). Nosocomial neonatal legionellosis has been described, as has legionellosis acquired during a water birth.

Coxiella burnettii (formerly *Rickettsia burnettii*) is the cause of Q fever, an acute illness frequently associated with a pneumonitis acquired through contact with parturient animals including cats, cattle, and sheep.

| TABLE 29-4 | Microbial Causes of Community-Acquired Pneumonia in Childhood, According to Age |

Age grouping and cause	Salient clinical features
Birth to 20 Days[*]	
Group B streptococci	Pneumonia part of early-onset sepsis; disease usually very severe, bilateral, diffuse
Gram-negative enteric bacteria	Infection often nosocomial, therefore often not seen until after 1 week of age
Cytomegalovirus	Pneumonia part of systemic cytomegalovirus infection; other signs of congenital infection usually present
Listeria monocytogenes	Pneumonia part of early-onset sepsis; identify the virus by PCR of nasopharyngeal secretions
3 Weeks to 3 Months	
Chlamydia trachomatis	Caused by maternal genital infection; causes afebrile, progressive, subacute interstitial pneumonia
Respiratory syncytial virus	Peak incidence at 2 to 7 months of age; usually characterized by wheezing (hard to differentiate bronchiolitis from pneumonia); rhinorrhea usually profuse; midwinter or early spring
Parainfluenza virus type 3	Very similar to disease caused by respiratory syncytial virus infection, but affects slightly older infants and is not epidemic in the winter
Streptococcus pneumoniae	Probably the most common cause of bacterial pneumonia, even in this young age group
Bordetella pertussis	Primarily causes bronchitis, but also causes pneumonia in severe cases
Staphylococcus aureus	A much less common cause of pneumonia now than in former years; causes severe disease, often with complicated effusion
4 Months to 4 Years	
Respiratory syncytial virus, parainfluenza viruses, influenza virus, adenovirus, rhinovirus	Most common cause of pneumonia in the younger children in this age group
S. pneumoniae	Most likely cause of lobar or segmental pneumonia, but may cause other forms as well
Haemophilus influenzae	Type b infection almost eliminated in areas with wide vaccine use; type b, other types, and nontypeable forms common in the developing world
Mycoplasma pneumoniae	Causes pneumonia primarily in the older children in this age group
Mycobacterium tuberculosis	Important cause of pneumonia in areas with a high prevalence of infections with this organism
5 to 15 Years	
M. pneumoniae	Chief cause of pneumonia in this age group; radiographic appearance variable
Chlamydia pneumoniae	Still controversial, but probably an important cause in older children in this age group
S. pneumoniae	Most likely cause of bacterial pneumonia, but probably causes other forms as well
M. tuberculosis	Pneumonia particularly common in areas with a high prevalence of infections with this organism; may be exacerbated at the onset of puberty and by pregnancy

From McIntosh K. Community-acquired pneumonia in children. N Engl J Med 2002;346(6):429-437.
PCR, Polymerase chain reaction.
[*]Causes are listed roughly in the descending order of frequency.

Viral Pneumonia

Several of the most important agents of viral pneumonia in children have been discussed above in the sections on croup, bronchiolitis, and influenza syndromes: RSV, HPIV types 1 to 3, and influenza virus. Additional important agents that will be discussed in this section are adenovirus and hantavirus.

Adenovirus. The family Adenoviridae consists of two genera, of which one, Mastadenovirus, includes viruses infecting humans and other mammals. These viruses were first identified in primary cultures of adenoid tissue and therefore were later named *adenoviruses.* The human adenoviruses are classified into six subgroups (designated A through F) based on their capacity for hemagglutination, and within these subgroups 51 serotypes have been identified in neutralization studies. Of these 51 serotypes, less than half produce disease in humans; in the pediatric population, respiratory manifestations of adenovirus infection include acute febrile pharyngitis (serotypes 1 through 3 and 5 through 7), pharyngoconjunctival fever (serotypes 3, 7, and 14), pneumonia (serotypes 1 through 3 and 7), and a syndrome similar to pertussis (serotype 5). These manifestations account for approximately 5% to 10% of all respiratory illness in children. A typical adenoviral infection produces cough, nasal congestion, and coryza and is often accompanied by systemic symptoms such as headache, fever, chills, malaise, and myalgia. In addition to respiratory symptoms, epidemic conjunctivitis and pharyngoconjunctival fever can result. Adenoviruses are the causal agents in approximately 10% of pediatric pneumonia cases.

Adenoviruses package a linear double-stranded DNA genome within an icosahedral capsid approximately 70 to 100 nm in diameter. The capsid structure is formed from 252 subunits, or capsomeres, of two distinct types: *hexons* (240) and *pentons* (12), so termed because each is surrounded by seven or five identical subunits, respectively. Fiber proteins extend from the penton capsomeres and interact with host cell receptors. Adenoviruses initially infect and replicate within nonciliated respiratory epithelium (ciliated respiratory epithelium does not contain the receptor proteins necessary for virus entry). The infection process is initiated upon virus binding to two host cell receptor proteins. One interaction occurs between the capsid fiber proteins and the coxsackievirus and adenovirus receptor (CAR) proteins on the host cell surface (Bergelson et al., 1997). All human adenoviral subgroups except subgroup B utilize these CAR proteins as attachment receptors (Roelvink et al., 1998). In addition to this primary binding interaction, the penton bases from which the fiber proteins project bind to cellular integrin molecules to provide another attachment interaction (Wickham et al., 1993).

Adenoviral infections typically elicit the production of both subgroup- and serotype-specific antibodies, but only the latter serve to neutralize viral infection. These neutralizing antibodies are raised against antigenic sites on the hexon and fiber proteins of the viral capsid.

Although neutralizing antibodies are produced in response to infection, several products of adenoviral replication serve to modulate the host's antiviral immunity. The virus is able to override the host cell defense and continue to appropriate cellular translation machinery for the production of viral proteins. There are no antiviral compounds yet available, the adenoviral vaccine used in the past by the U.S. military is no longer routinely administered to military personnel, and there is no licensed adenovirus vaccine for use in the pediatric population.

Hantavirus. Hantavirus pulmonary syndrome (HPS) was first recognized in the United States in May 1993, when public health officials in New Mexico were alerted to an outbreak of serious respiratory infection in the Four Corners region of the state. The illness, which mainly affected healthy young adults and some teenagers, was characterized by a prodrome of fever, myalgia, and some gastrointestinal symptoms. This was followed by respiratory failure and substantial mortality. Postmortem examinations revealed lymphocytic interstitial pulmonary infiltrates and intraalveolar edema. Using PCR, Nichol and colleagues (1993) were able to implicate an agent now termed *Sin Nombre Virus* (SNV). By early 1996, 131 cases of HPS had been confirmed in the United States (Centers for Disease Control and Prevention, 1996). Case fatalities rates approximate 50%, which, coupled with an apparently low rate of seroprevalence, implicate SNV as one of the most pathogenic and virulent of human viruses.

SNV is a member of the hantavirus genus of the bunyavirus family, a group known to cause hemorrhagic pulmonary syndrome or hemorrhagic fever with renal syndrome (HFRS).

Members of this family are generally spherical, enveloped particles measuring 80 to 120 nm in diameter containing three strands of negative-sense RNA. At least 5 genera and 700 species infecting animals and plants are recognized. Other human pathogens belonging to the family include California encephalitis virus, sandfly fever viruses, and Korean hemorrhagic fever virus. The Bayou virus, Black Creek Canal virus, and the New York virus have also been associated with sporadic cases of HFRS. Although the natural host of SNV, the deer mouse, is found throughout the United States, the great majority of the cases have been clustered in the Southwest. In other areas of the country, the closely related hantavirus species have various rodents as their natural hosts. Rodents are chronically infected and asymptomatic. Direct contact with infected rodents, droppings, nests, saliva, or urine results in human infection, with an incubation period ranging from 1 to 6 weeks after exposure. The syndrome is characterized by a febrile prodrome of 3 to 7 days, accompanied by gastrointestinal symptoms and early throm- bocytopenia and leukocytosis with a left shift. The most characteristic manifestation is abrupt onset of major pulmonary edema accompanied by cardiac depression and hypotension. Diagnosis is made primarily by enzyme-linked immunosorbent assay (ELISA) detection of IgM antibodies that are present at the onset of the cardiopulmonary manifestations. Treatment is supportive. In a controlled clinical trial, ribavirin was shown to decrease mortality (Chapman et al., 2002).

Miscellaneous Agents and Specific Pneumonia Syndromes

Hospital-acquired pneumonia. Admission to an intensive care unit, chronic illness, mechanical ventilation, surgery, and burns are risk factors for hospital-acquired pneumonia in children. Most episodes are viral in etiology; RSV is the most common pathogen. Gram-negative pathogens, including *Escherichia coli, Klebsiella pneumoniae,* and *Pseudomonas aeruginosa,* are the most common bacterial pathogens; mortality in patients with disease due to gram-negative organisms is high. Pneumonia due to gram-positive organisms such as *S. aureus* and *Staphylococcus epidermidis* is less frequently associated with mortality (Zar and Cotton, 2002).

Aspiration pneumonia. Aspiration pneumonia occurs in children with CNS or neuromuscular disease or in those incapable of handling respiratory secretions. Such children are often brought to the emergency rooms of general or children's hospitals from chronic-care facilities because of fever, toxicity, or respiratory distress. Aspiration of food or secretions is almost always the source of the problem.

Pneumonia due to agents of bioterrorism. The specter of massive aerosol release is the most frightening and potentially most effective implementation of agents of bioterrorism. Such release would likely result in multitudes of people developing pulmonary manifestations of infection with agents such as *Bacillus anthracis, F. tularensis,* or *Yersinia pestis.* The release of an agent of bioterrorism is suspected when the route of exposure to the pathogen is unusual, when disease occurs that is unusual for a geographic area or transmission season, when disease is due to an agent that is transmitted by a vector not present in the local area, and when there is intelligence of a potential attack. Additionally, development of simultaneous outbreaks in noncontiguous geographic areas and diseases with zoonotic impact, such as the pathogens above, all suggest attack. Several factors place children at unique risk during bioterrorist attack, such as their rapid respiratory rate, their relatively large surface-area–to-mass ratio, their thin skin, and their closeness to the ground, should the agent be denser than air (American Academy of Pediatrics 2000).

The pulmonary manifestations of each agent are characteristic, if not pathognomonic. Large numbers of previously healthy people presenting with fulminant pneumonia is suggestive of exposure to bioterrorist agents.

Y. pestis remains endemic in the southwestern United States. The most common vector for human infection is the rodent flea. Pneumonic plague can be primary or it can be due to exposure to other patients with pneumonic plague, to aerosolization of the organism, or to exposure to the agent developed as a bioweapon. Secondary pneumonic plague develops after systemic spread of bubonic or septicemic plague. Cough, fever, bloody sputum, and prominent gastrointestinal symptoms are characteristic of pneumonia due to *Y. pestis.* Cervical buboes may be present but are uncommon in primary pneumonic plague. Sepsis, shock, and organ failure may ensue; the purpura and acral cyanosis of plague are late findings. The finding of gram-negative organisms in the sputum of previously healthy children with these characteristic findings is highly suggestive of pneumonic plague. Characteristic chest radiographs reveal pneumonic consolidation. Blood cultures are positive in as many as 96% of patients with plague. Blood should be sent for PCR and detection of F-1 antigen. *Y. pestis* can be spread by the aerosolized secretions of a patient with pneumonic plague; these patients should be on droplet precautions for the first 3 days of antimicrobial treatment. The treatment of choice for pneumonic plague includes streptomycin or gentamicin; ciprofloxacin, doxycycline, or chloramphenicol are alternative therapies in the setting of massive exposures and casualties.

Tularemia is a disease of wild animals and may be transmitted by the bite of a blood-sucking insect or by exposure to contaminated carcasses or water sources. This hardy organism may persist in mud, water, or carcasses. The bulk of naturally acquired human cases are due to exposure to rabbits or ticks.

Once inhaled, *F. tularensis* parasitizes phagocytic and nonphagocytic cells. The organism survives and multiplies intracellularly, and cell-mediated immune responses play a primary role in control of the infection. Characteristic humoral immune responses are more important for diagnostic purposes. Histologic examination of infected tissues is characterized by mononuclear cell infiltration with pyogranulomatous pathology. Initial examination may reveal focal necrosis with a surrounding inflammatory infiltration. Subsequent granulomatous formation, characterized by recruitment of epithelioid cells, lymphocytes and multinucleated giant cells surrounded by areas of necrosis, may resemble caseating necrosis typical of tuberculosis and other mycobacteria.

Tularemic pneumonia may develop after laboratory exposure, exposure to a contaminated carcass, or exposure to weaponized pathogen. Pneumonia due to tularemia typically presents as an atypical pneumonia that may be accompanied by pleural effusion and hilar adenopathy. The laboratory findings of thrombocytopenia, elevated transaminases and elevated phosphatase levels and sterile pyuria support the clinical diagnosis of tularemia.

B. anthracis, the causative agent of anthrax, is a gram-positive, spore-forming, nonmotile zoonotic bacillus. *B. anthracis* spores can survive for years in the environment; consequently, infection most often manifests as cutaneous disease contracted from handling contaminated hides. Inhalational anthrax, a hemorrhagic thoracic lymphadenitis and mediastinitis, occurs after exposure to aerosolized organisms, typically from contaminated soil or carcasses. Dissemination to the meninges is common. Known to be weaponized as part of the Soviet Union's bioweapon program, massive aerosolization at a public event or large gathering of people was the delivery method thought to be most likely prior to the attacks of 2001. The anthrax attacks beginning in October 2001 demonstrated that aerosolization of anthrax spores could occur after manipulation of envelopes containing fine spores. Although inhalational anthrax had previously been thought to be uniformly fatal, the rapid recognition of disease allowed for 54% survival of 11 patients with inhalational anthrax. Of concern, though, was the fact that the severity of disease, including microangiopathic hemolytic anemia with renal involvement, coagulopathy, and hyponatremia, encountered in a 7-month-old infant with cutaneous anthrax raises the possibility that children may suffer severe systemic involvement despite limited disease.

Immunocompromised hosts and special settings. In recent years there has been a tremendous increase of the immunosuppressed population resulting from the increasing numbers of patients undergoing solid organ and bone marrow transplantation and to HIV infection. Immunocompromised patients or normal hosts exposed to special geographic or ecologic settings may develop respiratory infections caused by viruses, bacteria, or fungi that are not commonly considered in the differential diagnosis. Fungal agents to be considered include *Blastomyces, Cryptococcus, Histoplasma, Mucor, Coccidioides, Candida*, and *Aspergillus* species. Parasites—including *Ascaris, Pneumocystis, Toxoplasma*, and *Strongyloides* species—have all been reported to cause pneumonias in these patients. Viruses including RSV, parainfluenza, and influenza can cause significant morbidity and mortality, particularly in patients undergoing bone marrow transplantation or receiving intense immunosuppression because of solid organ transplantation. CMV can cause severe interstitial pneumonitis. *Pneumocystis carinii* may cause an invasive pneumonia with bilateral alveolar disease. *P. carinii* pneumonia is extremely prevalent among patients with immunosuppressive conditions, including HIV infection. Enterobacteriaceae have assumed an increasingly important role in pneumonias of children with immune suppression and in patients on broad-spectrum antibiotics for other reasons.

In certain parts of the world, several mycotic infections—coccidioidomycosis, blastomycosis, and histoplasmosis—are relatively common and may be manifested by an influenza-like illness or by atypical pneumonia. The acquired forms of toxoplasmosis, caused by the protozoan parasite *Toxoplasma gondii*, include a syndrome characterized by fever, maculopapular rash, and pneumonia. These infections have been noted more frequently as opportunistic respiratory pathogens among immunosuppressed hosts. Atypical pneumonia may accompany Q fever caused by *C. burnettii*. Other bacteria such as *Y. pestis* and *F. tularensis* may cause plague and tularemia, respectively, in patients who have been exposed to infected animal hosts (*F. tularensis*) or fleas from infected animals (*Y. pestis*) while camping or hunting. Infections with *M. tuberculosis* are discussed in detail in Chapter 39.

Epidemiology and Pathogenesis

The incidence of pneumonia varies with age; it is more common in children less than 5 years of age than in older children.

Host defense of the respiratory tract includes physical barriers, local host immune response, and systemic immune response. Viral respiratory tract infection, drugs, uremia, or other conditions that impair these defenses may precede bacterial pneumonia. Filtration and humidification are important physical barriers in the upper respiratory tract; the epiglottis and cough reflex protect the lower respiratory tract from contamination with viral and bacterial agents. Mucociliary transport further protects the respiratory tract. The respiratory secretions play an important role in the local immune responses as they include secretory IgA, lysozyme, interferons, and alveolar macrophages. The latter can ingest and kill invading bacteria. Pneumonia can occur by hematogenous spread of organisms, as in secondary pneumonic plague after septicemic plague, or when local defenses are impaired or overcome by the virulence of the organism or the size of the inoculum.

Clinical Manifestations and Diagnosis

The clinical diagnosis of pneumonia is supported by the findings of fever, tachypnea, and crackles on lung examination. For many patients evaluated in the outpatient setting, this evaluation is sufficient. The decision to pursue further diagnostic workup, including complete blood count, chest radiograph, and blood culture, is based on the degree of toxicity and illness of the child at presentation. The most reliable indicator that the chest radiograph will be positive for pneumonia is the clinical finding of tachypnea; approximately two thirds of patients with pneumonia have tachypnea. Tachypnea is not a specific finding, though, and can be present because of a variety of illnesses.

Although the diagnosis and management of bacterial pneumonia in immunocompetent children rarely includes identification of the specific pathogen, aggressive pursuit of a microbiologic diagnosis is warranted for children with severe or complicated pneumonia. Attempts to determine the etiology in most patients will be limited because of a number of factors. For example, assays developed to identify the pathogen by latex agglutination of urine specimens suffer from a lack of sensitivity, and blood cultures are positive in less than a third of children with bacterial pneumonia. The risks of the invasive procedures required to identify the bacterial pathogen limit the use of such procedures to specific populations, such as children with parapneumonic collections or those with underlying immune defects. Isolation of a potential bacterial pathogen in the upper respiratory tract generally does not prove its etiologic involvement, as potential bacterial pathogens such as *S. pneumoniae*, *H. influenzae*, and staphylococci frequently colonize the upper respiratory tract of both ill and healthy children. Identification of the most probable pathogen often rests on clinical recognition of presenting signs, symptoms, and clinical course.

As with other bacterial infections, a toxic appearance is suggestive of bacterial etiology. Evidence of severe respiratory distress such as grunting may be seen in both bacterial and viral pneumonia but is suggestive of bacterial etiologies. Splinting may be present, particularly in patients with pleural effusions or empyema. Chest radiographs with dense consolidation and evidence of necrosis are suggestive of bacterial pneumonia, as are those that show parapneumonic effusions. An elevated absolute neutrophil count and C-reactive protein are also characteristic of bacterial pneumonia.

Clinical evidence may not be sufficient to differentiate between viral and bacterial etiologies. Conjunctivitis and otitis media are more often associated with bacterial than viral pneumonia (Ramsey et al., 1986), and wheezing is more commonly associated with viral etiologies (Forgie et al., 1991; Turner et al., 1987). The chest radiograph does not allow differentiation of bacterial from viral pneumonia when radiographs are compared in a blinded fashion (Courtoy et al., 1989; McCarthy et al., 1981). Elevated C-reactive protein (CRP) and absolute neutrophil count are more reliable indicators of bacterial pneumonia than clinical and radiologic evidence, nonetheless (Korppi et al., 1997; McIntosh, 2002). Pneumonia due to *S. aureus* tends to be rapidly progressive. Both *S. aureus* and *S. pyogenes* pneumonia are often complicated by empyema or effusion that may appear very early in the course of infection. The presence of pneumatoceles on chest radiograph, especially in a child less than 2 years of age, suggests *S. aureus* pneumonia.

Pursuit of a microbiologic diagnosis is indicated for complicated or severe pneumonia. Unusual pathogens or those presenting in an epidemiologic pattern suggestive of bioterrorism should also be aggressively investigated. Table 29-5 details a guide to preferred diagnostic techniques for the diagnosis of specific pathogens. In general, blood cultures should be obtained for all patients hospitalized for pneumonia and for patients thought to be toxic appearing who are treated on an outpatient basis. Latex agglutination suffers from a lack of sensitivity and should be reserved for patients who are pretreated, especially if their disease is complicated.

A range of disease severity, from mild cough and low-grade fever to severe disease with multiorgan failure, is characteristic of *L. pneumophila* infections. The syndrome usually starts with nonspecific symptoms and high fever. Cough may be only mildly productive and associated with chest pain and hemoptysis. Associated gastrointestinal symptoms are common; typically watery diarrhea is described. *L. pneumophila* is fastidious and difficult to grow in vitro. As a result, most diagnostic studies rely on serologic techniques for antibody increases, on demonstration of the organism in infected tissues using special strains, or on detection of antigenuria.

Mycoplasmal infection differs clinically from "typical" pneumococcal pneumonia in that it has a gradual onset with fever, sore throat, and cough as major complaints. Physical findings of pulmonary infection, rales, and rhonchi may be more severe than would be expected from the general examination. Radiologic findings are generally those of bronchopneumonia involving the lower lobes unilaterally or bilaterally. Hospitalization generally is not required. Children with *M. pneumoniae* infection also may be seen initially with localized tracheobronchitis and with cough and rhonchi in the absence of pulmonary infiltrates. Numerous extrarespiratory signs and symptoms associated with *M. pneumoniae* have been reported. Stevens-Johnson syndrome (erythema multiforme bullosa) is the most frequently observed complication and is the most firmly linked to *M. pneumoniae*. Neurologic syndromes such as meningoencephalitis, transverse myelitis, and Guillain-Barré syndrome have been temporally associated with clinically diagnosed atypical pneumonia.

Neonatal pneumonia, typically without fever, is suggestive of *Chlamydia trachomatis* or *U. urealyticum*. Staccato cough is characteristic of both, but the presence of conjunctivitis in this setting suggests the former organism. Onset of disease occurs between 3 weeks and 3 months of age.

Q fever is characterized by sudden onset of fever, chills, headache, malaise, and weakness; the condition progresses to include cough and chest pain, with a clinical picture resembling atypical pneumonia. Pneumonia due to Q fever may behave as an atypical pneumonia, a rapidly progressive pneumonia, or an incidental finding in a patient presenting with prolonged fever characteristic of the infection. On laboratory examination, most patients will have mild transaminase elevation, and a minority will be jaundiced. The diagnosis of Q fever is usually confirmed by serologic assay, as most laboratories do not have the capability to isolate the pathogen. PCR-based assays are investigational. Several serologic assays have been based on several techniques including microimmunofluorescence, microagglutination, complement fixation, and ELISA.

Although inhalational anthrax is not well described in children, the clinical description of

TABLE 29-5	Microbiologic Diagnosis of Pneumonia in Children	
Microorganism	Preferred diagnostic methods	Comments
Viruses		
Respiratory syncytial virus	Identify the virus in nasopharyngeal secretions; the best test is the immuno fluorescence assay, solid-phase immunoassay, or PCR assay	Viral culture is also helpful, but results may not be available for several days. Comparison of antibody levels during the acute phase and convalescence adds little useful information. In cases of adenoviral infection, serotyping may be useful
Influenza virus A or B Parainfluenza viruses 1, 2, and 3 Adenovirus		
Rhinovirus	Identify the virus by PCR of nasopharyngeal secretions	The etiologic connection is not well established
Measles virus	Identify the virus by immunofluorescence assay of nasopharyngeal secretions, or measure at least a quadrupling of serum antibody levels between the acute phase and convalescence.	The clinical diagnosis may be quite specific
Varicella-zoster virus	Identify the virus by immunofluorescence assay of skin lesions, or measure at least a quadrupling of serum antibody levels between the acute phase and convalescence.	The clinical diagnosis is usually quite specific
Hantavirus	Identify the virus in nasopharyngeal secretions or antibody in serum. IgM or IgG antibodies may be found at presentation.	Hantavirus infection is sufficiently uncommon that the finding of antibody in one serum sample is essentially diagnostic of the infection
Cytomegalovirus Epstein-Barr virus	Identify IgM antibodies in the serum during the acute phase or at least a quadrupling of serum antibody levels between the acute phase and convalescence.	Finding virus in upper airway secretions is not valuable with respect to the diagnosis, since both cytomegalovirus and Epstein-Barr virus may be found in normal subjects
Chlamydia		
Chlamydia trachomatis	Identify the organism in nasopharyngeal secretions by culture or PCR assay	An IgM antibody test may be helpful
Chlamydia pneumoniae	Identify the organism in nasopharyngeal secretions by culture or PCR assay, or measure at least a quadrupling of serum antibody levels between the acute phase and convalescence	Etiologic connection in young children is not well established; the evidence is more convincing with respect to adolescents
Chlamydia psittaci	The finding of at least a quadrupling of serum antibody levels between the acute phase and convalescence is diagnostic	
Coxiella		
Coxiella burnettii	The finding of at least a quadrupling of serum antibody levels between the acute phase and convalescence is diagnostic	

Continued

TABLE 29-5	Microbiologic Diagnosis of Pneumonia in Children—Cont'd

Microorganism	Preferred diagnostic methods	Comments
Mycoplasma		
Mycoplasma pneumoniae	The finding of cold agglutinins (titer > 1:128) or IgM antibody in serum late in the acute phase or early in convalescence is helpful, as is a positive PCR assay of secretions from a throat or a nasopharyngeal swab	The finding of at least a quadrupling of serum antibody levels between the acute phase and convalescence is diagnostic
Bacteria		
Streptococcus pneumoniae	Identify bacteria in culture of blood or pleural fluid	Culture of blood or pleural fluid is clearly an insensitive method, but there are not as yet any established alternatives in children
Haemophilus influenzae Streptococcus pyogenes Staphylococcus aureus Gram-negative enteric bacteria Mouth anaerobes Group B streptococci Neisseria meningitidis		
Bordetella pertussis	Identify bacteria in culture, immunofluorescence assay, or PCR assay of nasopharyngeal secretions	
Francisella tularensis	The finding of at least a quadrupling of serum antibody levels between the acute phase and convalescence is diagnostic	Culture of blood or sputum for this organism requires special medium and may pose a danger of infection to laboratory workers
Legionella pneumophila and other Legionella species	Identify bacteria in culture of sputum or tracheal aspirate or antigen in urine; or measure at least a quadrupling of serum antibody levels between the acute phase and convalescence	Culture of the organism requires special medium; urinary antigen tests can detect only L. pneumophila antigen
Brucella abortus	Identify bacteria in culture of blood or measure at least a quadrupling of serum antibody levels between the acute phase and convalescence	
Mycobacterium tuberculosis	Identify bacteria in culture of sputum or gastric aspirates, with or without a positive test for tuberculosis with purified protein derivative	Culture of bronchoalveolar lavage fluid is also specific but somewhat less sensitive; PCR assay is more useful for the identification of the bacterium than for the detection of it
Fungi		
Histoplasma capsulatum	Identify organism by staining or culture of respiratory tract secretions; or measure serum IgM antibody, or at least a quadrupling of serum antibody levels between the acute phase and convalescence	Histoplasma antigen is sometimes detectable in urine
Blastomyces dermatitidis Coccidoides immitis		

From McIntosh K. Community-acquired pneumonia in children. N Engl J Med 2002:346(6):429-437.
PCR, Polymerase chain reaction.

the first 10 intentional inhalational anthrax cases of 2001 added to our understanding of common clinical findings in this disease. Systemic symptoms, including profound, drenching sweating, was common in this cohort. In contrast to earlier descriptions of inhalational anthrax, the period of improvement between the initial phase, which includes myalgia, malaise, fatigue, and fever, and the septicemic phase was either very brief or not noted. Although this early phase has been described as flulike, patients with inhalation anthrax rarely complain of the rhinorrhea and nasal congestion characteristic of influenza and influenza-like illnesses. Additionally, all patients with inhalational anthrax had abnormal radiographs, including mediastinal widening, paratracheal fullness, hilar fullness, pleural effusions, and parenchymal infiltrates; influenza is associated with pneumonia in only 1% to 5% of adults and with pneumonia or bronchiolitis in 2% to 25% of children. The peripheral white blood cell count was not remarkable in early disease; most were normal or only slightly elevated. All patients who had not received antibiotics had positive blood culture in early disease, but antibiotic treatment rapidly sterilized blood cultures. All patients developed pleural effusions; large and progressive pleural effusions were common, and seven patients required drainage.

Aspiration pneumonia is typically described in neurologically impaired children or those that require emergency intubation. Progression of infiltrates, sometimes associated with fever, in an intubated or compromised child should suggest aspiration pneumonia. The presence of pathogens in tracheal fluid in the absence of increases in infiltrates, polymorphonuclear cells in the tracheal fluid, or requirements for ventilation may represent colonization rather than infection. The secretions of ventilated patients may harbor pathogens as soon as 24 hours after intubation (Sole et al., 2002). *Streptococcus* species and other oral anaerobes are associated with community-acquired aspiration pneumonia, whereas gram-negative bacilli such as *Klebsiella, Pseudomonas*, and *Proteus* as well as *S. aureus* are commonly associated with hospital-acquired aspiration pneumonia.

Treatment

The decision to treat pneumonia with antimicrobial agents and the choice of agent are determined in large part by the age of the child, as the most likely responsible organism differs by age group.

Pneumonia in the very young infant is unusual, but when is does occur, is likely to be due to perinatally acquired pathogens. Older infants (3 weeks to 3 months of age), particularly those with conjunctivitis and a staccato cough, are more likely to have *C. trachomatis*, and treatment with a macrolide is indicated. *B. pertussis* rarely causes pneumonia; treatment of this organism with a macrolide is appropriate.

A macrolide antibiotic is also a "first-line" agent for the child between the ages of 5 and 15 who presents with illness suggestive of *M. pneumoniae* or *C. pneumoniae*. Clinically, these children present with cough and low-grade fever. Both agents are associated with wheezing, but this is not a constant finding. The radiographic findings for both of these atypical bacteria may be indistinguishable from bacterial pneumonia.

When bacterial pneumonia is suspected in the acutely ill child, or in patients with sepsis in conjunction with pneumonia, empiric treatment with antimicrobial agents that are effective against bacterial pathogens is indicated. The choice of agent is age dependent; Table 29-6 details appropriate regimens based on the age of the patient and the decisions made regarding hospitalization. Young infants who present with pneumonia associated with sepsis should be treated with ampicillin and gentamicin. The addition of a third-generation cephalosporin can be considered for severely ill infants. The agents recommended for the treatment of bacterial pneumonia have not changed substantially, in spite of increasing resistance of respiratory pathogens, especially *S. pneumoniae*. The third-generation cephalosporins, with their excellent tissue penetration, remain effective choices for the treatment of bacterial pneumonia. This recommendation is based on a series of studies documenting that the outcome was not changed when ß-lactam antibiotics were used to treat pneumonia due to penicillin nonsusceptible *S. pneumoniae* (minimum inhibitory concentration [MIC] = 0.1) (Freij et al., 1984). It is important to note that most patients in these studies were infected with organisms whose penicillin susceptibility was in the intermediate range (MIC = 0.1 to 1.0 g/ml). The results when a resistant organism is present are conflicting (Choi and Lee, 1998; Laupland

TABLE 29-6 Suggested Drug Treatments for Community-Acquired Pneumonia in Children, According to Whether They Are Hospitalized

Age-group	Outpatient	Inpatient, without lobar or lobular infiltrate, pleural effusion, or both	Inpatient, with signs of sepsis, alveolar infiltrate, large pleural effusion, or all three
Birth to 20 Days	Admit patient	Administer ampicillin and gentamicin, with or without cefotaxime	Administer IV ampicillin and gentamicin, with or without IV cefotaxime*
3 Weeks to 3 Months	If patient is afebrile, give oral erythromycin (30-40 mg/kg of body weight/day in 4 divided doses) or oral azithromycin (1 dose of 10 mg/kg, then 5 mg/kg/day for 4 days) Admit patient if fever or hypoxia is present	If patient is afebrile, administer IV erythromycin (40 mg/kg of body weight/day in 4 divided doses given 6 hours apart).† If patient is febrile, add cefotaxime (200 mg/kg/day in 3 divided doses given 8 hours apart)	Administer IV cefotaxime (200 mg/kg/day in 3 divided doses given 8 hours apart)*‡
4 Months to 4 Years	Administer oral amoxicillin (80-100 mg/kg/day in 3 or 4 divided doses)	In cases of apparent viral pneumonia, no antibiotics should be given; otherwise, consider treatment with IV ampicillin (200 mg/kg/day in 4 divided doses given 6 hours apart)	Administer IV cefotaxime (200 mg/kg/day) or IV cefuroxime (150 mg/kg/day in 3 divided doses given 8 hours apart)*‡
5 to 15 years	Administer oral erythromycin (30-40 mg/kg/day in 4 divided doses) or oral azithromycin (1 dose of 10 mg/kg, then 5 mg/kg/day for 4 days). In children older than 8 years of age, consider oral doxycycline (4 mg/kg/day in 2 divided doses)	Administer IV erythromycin (40 mg/kg/day in 4 divided doses given 6 hours apart) or IV azithromycin (5 mg/kg/day in 2 divided doses given 12 hours apart) In children older than 8 years of age, consider IV doxycycline (4 mg/kg/day in 2 divided doses given 12 hours apart) If there is strong evidence of a bacterial cause (e.g., high white-cell count, chills, or no response to outpatient therapy with a macrolide) add ampicillin	Administer IV cefotaxime (200 mg/kg/day) or IV cefuroxime (150 mg/kg/day in 3 divided doses given 8 hours apart.‡ Consider adding IV azithromycin if patient is not doing well.

From McIntosh K. Community-acquired pneumonia in children. N Engl J Med 2002:346(6):429-437.

IV, Intravenous.

*Staphylococcal pneumonia is unusual; however, if cultures of blood or pleural fluid grow *Staphylococcus aureus*, or in other exceptional circumstances, oxacillin or, in areas where methicillin-resistant *S. aureus* is a reasonable possibility, vancomycin should be added.

†In infants younger than 6 weeks of age, treatment with azithromycin (5 mg/kg/day in two divided doses given 12 hours apart) should be considered in view of reports of hypertrophic pyloric stenosis in infants who received erythromycin.

‡Some experts suggest treatment with ampicillin (200 to 300 mg per kilogram per day intravenously in four divided doses given 6 hours apart) in patient who have lobar and therefore most likely pneumococcal pneumonia.

et al., 1998). β-Lactamase inhibitors do not increase the efficacy of these agents for pneumococcal disease, as the mechanism of resistance is through alteration of penicillin-binding proteins (PBPs). The decreased affinity for penicillin by these PBPs can be overcome by increasing the concentration of the penicillin; so high-dose amoxicillin (80 mg/kg) remains the treatment of choice for the treatment of outpatients with suspected pneumonia due to pyogenic bacteria. Once a specific organism is identified as the etiologic agent, specific therapy can be administered.

Because approximately 30% of HIB isolates are resistant to ampicillin as a result of the production of a-lactamases, initial therapy for invasive *H. influenzae* disease should include a third-generation cephalosporin, such as cefotaxime or ceftriaxone or ampicillin and chloramphenicol. Although ampicillin resistance due to altered PBPs has been described, this continues to constitute a minority of clinical isolates (Jones et al., 2002). Erythromycin is effective in shortening the symptomatic duration of mycoplasmal pneumonia. Although treatment may not eradicate the organism, and shedding may continue for weeks, clinically significant relapses are unusual. Tetracycline and doxycycline are available for older children and adolescents. Azithromycin and clarithromycin are likely at least as effective as erythromycin and have fewer side effects but are considerably more expensive. Although quinolones are also effective and can be considered for older adolescents, these drugs are relatively costly. Macrolides are also the treatment of choice for pneumonia due to *C. trachomatis* and *B. pertussis*. Both in vitro and in vivo *L. pneumophila* may be sensitive to erythromycin, which has been used with some success among patients. Q fever is usually treated with erythromycin or doxycycline if the child is older than 8 years of age.

Therapy of aspiration pneumonia should be directed against the gingival and oropharyngeal aerobic and anaerobic flora in community-acquired cases. Many physicians choose a broad-spectrum agent such as ampicillin-sulbactam, but high doses of penicillin G (300,000 U/kg /day) are an alternative. Because of the increasing frequency of penicillin-resistant anaerobes, clindamycin should be considered in patients whose pneumonia does not respond to penicillin derivatives. Clindamycin or metronidazole, supplemented with high-dose penicillin, may be appropriate for patients with aggressive presentation of aspiration pneumonia. In patients who have been on prolonged antibiotic therapy or those with nosocomially acquired aspiration pneumonia, the addition of coverage for such agents as gram-negative aerobic bacilli and staphylococci may be warranted. Therapy may be prolonged, particularly if abscess formation occurs, but surgical drainage is seldom mandatory.

The treatment of choice for pneumonic plague includes streptomycin or gentamicin. For mass exposures or for very mild, early disease, doxycycline, ciprofloxacin or chloramphenicol can be considered. The choice to use the latter agents in young children should be assessed based on the risks and benefits. Because of the severity of the disease and the late recognition of the etiologic agent, morbidity and mortality due to pneumonic plague approach 30% in treated patients and 100% in untreated patients.

The treatment of choice for tularemia includes streptomycin, amikacin, or gentamicin. Initial treatment may be associated with a Jarisch-Herxheimer reaction. Imipenem with cilastatin and fluoroquinolones are considered second-line therapy. Treatment with tetracycline or chloramphenicol is associated with an increased risk of relapse. The initial treatment of inhalational anthrax includes either doxycycline or ciprofloxacin. Once the susceptibility of the organism has been determined, amoxicillin can be considered.

Empyema and pleural effusions

Empyema and pleural effusions may complicate pneumonia; in one study as many as 80% of children with pneumonia due to *S. aureus* developed empyema. The incidence of effusion due to other pathogens ranges from 40% for *S. pneumoniae* to 11% for viral pathogens. The interpretation of such statistics is confounded by the fact that most series include children who have required hospitalization; most patients do not require hospitalization. Nonetheless, the appropriate management of pleural effusions and empyema is a recurring issue in pediatric pneumonia.

Pathogenesis. Pleural effusions develop because of the inflammatory response to replication of microorganisms in the alveoli resulting in endothelial injury and capillary permeability, and allowing for escape of interstitial pulmonary fluid into the pleural space. The excess production of fluid overwhelms the absorptive capacity of the lymphatics in the parietal pleura, resulting in fluid accumulation.

Bacterial invasion of the pleural fluid promotes a neutrophilic influx and subsequent fibropurulent reaction characterized by a decrease in pleural fluid pH and glucose with an increase in the pleural fluid lactate dehydrogenase (LDH). Fibrin deposition occurs because of this inflammatory response. Whereas in early phases this deposition may serve to restrict lung expansion, in later phases, as fibroblasts invade the pleura, organization into a fibrinous peel may ensue.

Clinical manifestations. Physical examination findings suggestive of pleural effusion include decreased breath sounds, dullness to percussion, the presence of a pleural rub, and mediastinal shift. Splinting may also be present.

Diagnosis. Differentiation of transudative from exudative effusions requires biochemical characterization of the fluid. Pleural protein to serum protein ratio is less than 0.5 in transudates and greater than 0.5 in exudates; the ratio of serum to pleural lactate dehydrogenase is 0.6 or less in transudates and over 0.6 in exudates. Empyema, the collection of pus in the pleural space, is characterized by a pH less than 7.1, a glucose level less than 40 and an LDH of more than 1,000 IU/ml in the pleural space.

Treatment. Pleural effusions are usually managed by drainage with or without insertion of a chest tube. When empyema develops, chest tube insertion or other drainage procedure is warranted. Certain findings such as loculation and pleural effusion leukocyte count predict treatment failure and argue for early surgical intervention. Video-assisted thoracic surgery (VATS) allows for less invasive approaches to the management of empyema and appears to be particularly effective in the fibrinopurulent stage, when it can be used to break up loculations and allow for continuous drainage. When compared with thoracotomy, VATS offers similar success rates with substantially improved resolution of disease, length of hospitalization, and, less importantly, long-term cosmesis. VATS should be considered when a large-bore chest tube does not result in complete resolution of pleural effusion after 2 days. Ultrasound- or computed tomography (CT)–guided drainage can be considered in this group of patients when the risk of anesthesia is thought to be prohibitive (Chen et al., 2002; Yim, 1999).

Prevention. Parapneumonic collections are a complication of bacterial pneumonia; prevention of the primary pathology through immunization including both the conjugated *H. influenzae* and *S. pneumoniae* vaccines is appropriate. Early intervention, as described under treatment, may decrease the length of hospitalization when these collections do occur.

SINUSITIS

Sinusitis refers to inflammation of the mucosa of the paranasal sinuses and the nasal epithelium. Sinusitis is classified as acute when symptoms are present for less than 4 weeks, subacute if symptoms are present for 1 to 3 months, and chronic when symptoms are present for over a month (Conrad and Jenson, 2002). The etiology includes viral and bacterial infectious agents, allergic rhinosinusitis, and chemical or irritating agents. However, the term has become synonymous with bacterial sinusitis and is currently a major cause of outpatient antibiotic overprescription. More recently, the increased threat of emerging antibiotic-resistant bacteria has forced a change in approach to this syndrome, with increasing emphasis on accurate diagnosis and conservative use of antimicrobial agents. Nevertheless, invasive bacterial sinusitis remains a common respiratory infection in children and if untreated may progress into invasive intracranial disease.

Etiology and Pathogenesis

Bacterial sinusitis and otitis media share similar etiologic agents and pathogenic mechanisms. These pathogens are part of normal colonizing respiratory flora such as *S. pneumoniae*, *H. influenzae*, and *Moraxella catarrhalis*. In the pediatric age group, inflammation caused by viral or allergic rhinosinusitis often precedes bacterial superinfection. In the paranasal sinuses, a ciliated epithelium lined with mucus clears invading bacteria though an opening into the nasopharynx. Obstruction and failure of the sweeping mechanism leads to bacterial overgrowth, infection, and potential tissue invasion. Further progression of bacterial tissue invasion may lead to mastoiditis and brain abscess.

S. pneumoniae is the most common etiology of bacterial sinusitis, accounting for up to 66%

of cases (Brooks et al., 2000). The bacteriology of this pathogen is described earlier in this chapter and in detail in Chapter 35. *H. influenzae* is the second most prevalent pathogen and accounts for 20% to 30% of cases. The biology of this pathogen is described earlier in this chapter and in detail in Chapter 14.

M. (Branhamella) catarrhalis appears on gram-stain as plump gram-negative cocci or paired short rods and is a frequent causative agent of acute otitis media and sinusitis. The organism has also been associated with bronchopneumonia in infants with underlying lung damage (Berg et al., 1987). *M. catarrhalis* colonizes the respiratory tract and has no other known animal reservoir. Carriage of the organism is most common in very young children and is highly seasonal, with prevalence greatest in the fall and winter. Colonization is most frequent in the presence of respiratory tract symptoms, although *M. catarrhalis* is not thought to cause such symptoms. At present, approximately 85% of *M. catarrhalis* isolates produce β-lactamase and thus are resistant to penicillin and ampicillin. No other resistance factors are found with any frequency. Clinical isolates of *M. catarrhalis* are highly susceptible to erythromycin and to cefixime (Verduin et al., 2002). In addition, the β-lactamase produced by this agent may be inhibited by the β-lactamase inhibitors clavulanate and sulbactam; combinations containing these drugs would also be effective in treating infections caused by *M. catarrhalis*. Clinical features of sinusitis caused by *M. catarrhalis* do not differ from those associated with other agents. Disseminated infection and pyogenic complications have not been described, even when drugs (such as ampicillin) with limited in vitro activity against the resistant strains were widely used. Rarely, *M. catarrhalis* is an agent of other infections such as bacteremia, meningitis, endocarditis, and ophthalmia neonatorum.

Diagnosis

Currently, there is no reliable noninvasive diagnostic method to differentiate bacterial sinusitis from that caused by other agents. Needle puncture with aspiration and culture of the sinus contents is the most reliable method to establish the diagnosis; however, this invasive procedure is impractical and unnecessary for the diagnosis and management of uncomplicated sinusitis (Conrad, 2002). Clinical criteria are frequently used, but several studies have shown little predictive value for the presence of underlying bacterial infection. Duration of rhinorrhea has been found to be one of the most consistent parameters (Conrad, 2002). In children, persistence of rhinorrhea and cough for more than 10 to 14 days may point to the presence of acute bacterial sinusitis (Dowell et al., 1998). The presence of high fever, purulent nasal discharge, localized pain around the sinuses, and facial swelling may further point to the presence of bacterial infection. X-ray images and CT scans may aid in the diagnosis of sinusitis, but they must be interpreted carefully because mucosal changes may be found in 30% of asymptomatic persons.

Treatment

Because bacterial sinusitis may be self-limited, it is reasonable to limit antibiotic treatment for children whose symptoms persist for 10 to 14 days in the absence of complications. Given that 50% to 60% of bacterial sinusitis episodes will improve without treatment, initial choices of antibiotics should be limited to the narrowest spectrum agent effective against the anticipated pathogens (Brooks et al., 2000). Amoxicillin remains an effective choice for bacterial sinusitis, despite the presence of β-lactamase in many isolates of *H. influenzae* and nearly all isolates of *M. catarrhalis* (Giebink, 1994). Trimethoprim-sulfamethoxazole is a reasonable choice for the β-lactam allergic child, as are azithromycin and clarithromycin (American Academy of Pediatrics, 2001). If clinical improvement does not occur within 48 to 72 hours, or if symptoms recur after treatment, a β-lactamase stable agent such as amoxicillin-clavulanate or a β-lactamase stable cephalosporin with activity against *S. pneumoniae* can be considered. No clinical trials have documented the superiority of extended spectrum cephalosporins over amoxicillin. High-dose amoxicillin or clindamycin can be considered because of their activity against penicillin-resistant pneumococcus. The latter agent will not be effective against *M. catarrhalis* or *H. influenzae*. The duration of treatment depends on clinical response. Most children can be effectively treated if antibiotics are administered for 7 to 10 days after clinical improvement or resolution of symptoms; this typically results in a 10- to 14-day course. Prolonged therapy is indicated only if the resolution of signs and symptoms is delayed.

ACUTE TONSILLOPHARYNGITIS

Acute tonsillopharyngitis is one of the most common bacterial illnesses of childhood. Many bacterial and viral agents can cause tonsillopharyngitis as a sole manifestation or as part of a syndrome (Bisno, 2001). Viral agents, such as rhinoviruses, coronaviruses, adenoviruses, influenza, and parainfluenza, frequently cause tonsillopharyngitis associated with other upper or lower respiratory manifestations. Primary infection with herpes simplex viruses can manifest as gingivitis, stomatitis, and pharyngitis. Herpangina caused by coxsackievirus A and acute retroviral syndrome due to HIV infection can result in pharyngitis. Finally, tonsillopharyngitis is part of the infectious mononucleosis syndrome caused by Epstein-Barr virus and cytomegalovirus. Bacterial causes include group A hemolytic *Streptococcus*, group C hemolytic *Streptococcus*, *Neisseria gonorrhoeae*, *C. diphtheriae*, *Chlamydia*, and *Mycoplasma*.

Acute tonsillopharyngitis with exudate or membrane is characterized by fever, sore throat, tonsillar and pharyngeal reddening and edema, and the presence of an exudate or membrane. A varying degree of cervical lymph node enlargement may be present. Group A hemolytic *Streptococcus* is by far the most common agent causing exudative tonsillopharyngitis, accounting for 15% to 30% of cases in children. Rarely, group C hemolytic *Streptococcus* and *C. diphtheriae* are the cause. The special features of disease caused by this pathogen need to be kept in mind to make possible early diagnosis (Chapter 6). Membranous tonsillitis is a frequent manifestation of infectious mononucleosis (Chapter 9) and is also seen in military recruits, infants, and children up to age 3 years with adenovirus infection. Antimicrobial therapy (discussed in detail in Chapter 35) is indicated for patients with exudative pharyngitis caused by group A hemolytic streptococcus. A 10-day course of penicillin remains the treatment of choice, since the organism remains uniformly susceptible. The aim of the therapy is to prevent suppurative and nonsuppurative complications and, if given early in the course, shorten the clinical course. If the diphtheria bacillus is suspected or is proved the responsible agent, therapy with diphtheria antitoxin in addition to penicillin or erythromycin (see Chapter 6) should be instituted. Antibiotics are of no value in the treatment of infectious mononucleosis or adenovirus infection.

Acute tonsillopharyngitis with vesicles or ulcers is characterized by fever, sore throat, and vesicles or shallow white ulcers 2 to 4 mm in diameter on the anterior fauces, palate, and buccal mucous membrane. It most commonly is caused group A coxsackieviruses. A primary infection with herpes simplex virus is usually characterized by stomatitis and gingivitis rather than tonsillopharyngitis (Chapter 15). Gingivitis is not associated with group A coxsackieviruses. Antimicrobial agents are of no value in the treatment of these infections.

SEVERE ACUTE RESPIRATORY SYNDROME (SARS)

For information on SARS, see Appendix C, p. 1001.

BIBLIOGRAPHY

Abraham G, Colonno RJ. Many rhinovirus serotypes share the same cellular receptor. J Virol 1984;51:340-345.

Adams RJ, et al. Preemptive use of aerosolized ribavirin in the treatment of asymptomatic pediatric marrow transplant patients testing positive for RSV. Bone Marrow Transplant 1999;24:661-664.

Alwan WH, Kozlowska WJ, et al. Distinct types of lung disease caused by functional subsets of antiviral T cells. J Exp Med 1994;179:81-89.

American Academy of Pediatrics. Prevention of respiratory syncytial virus infections: indications for the use of palivizumab and update on the use of RSV-IGIV. American Academy of Pediatrics Committee on Infectious Diseases and Committee of Fetus and Newborn. Pediatrics 1998;102:1211-1216.

American Academy of Pediatrics. Committee on Environmental Health and Committee on Infectious Diseases. Chemical-biological terrorism and its impact on children: a subject review. Pediatrics 2000;105:662-670.

American Academy of Pediatrics. Clinical practice guidelines: management of sinusitis. Pediatrics 2001;108:798-808.

Anderson LJ, Heilman CA. Protective and disease-enhancing immune responses to respiratory syncytial virus. J Infect Dis 1995;171:1-7.

Apalsch AM, Green M, et al. Parainfluenza and influenza virus infections in pediatric organ transplant recipients. Clin Infect Dis 1995;20:394-399.

Arruda E, Boyle TR, et al. Localization of human rhinovirus replication in the upper respiratory tract by in situ hybridization. J Infect Dis 1995;171:1329-1333.

Belshe R, Mendelman P, et al. The efficacy of live attenuated, cold-adapted, trivalent, intranasal influenza virus vaccine in children. N Engl J Med 1998;338:1405-1412.

Berg RA, Bartley DL. Pneumonia associated with *Branhamella catarrhalis* in infants. Pediatr Infect Dis J 1987;6:569-573.

Bergelson JM, Cunningham JA, et al. Isolation of a common receptor for Coxsackie B viruses and adenoviruses 2 and 5. Science 1997;275:1320-1323.

Bisno AL. Acute pharyngitis. N Engl J Med 2001;344: 20X5-211.

Bont L, Heijnen CJ, et al. Local interferon-gamma levels during respiratory syncytial virus lower respiratory tract infection are associated with disease severity. J Infect Dis 2001;184:355-358.

Brady MT. Nosocomial Legionnaire's disease in a children's hospital. J Pediatr 1989;115:46-50.

Brooks I, Gooch WM 3rd, et al. Medical management of acute bacterial sinusitis. Recommendations of a clinical advisory committee on pediatric and adult sinusitis. Ann Otol Rhinol Laryngol 2000;suppl 182:2-20.

Cannon MJ, Openshaw PJ, et al. Cytotoxic T cells clear virus but augment lung pathology in mice infected with respiratory syncytial virus. J Exp Med 1988;168:1163-1168.

Centers for Disease Control and Prevention. Prevention and control of influenza: recommendations of the Advisory Committee on Immunization Practices (ACIP). MMWR Morb Mortal Wkly Rep 2000;49.

Chanock RM. Control of pediatric viral diseases: past successes and future prospects. Pediatr Res 1990;27:S39-S43.

Chapman LE, Ellis BA, et al. Discriminators between hantavirus-infected and -uninfected persons enrolled in a trial of intravenous ribavirin for presumptive hantavirus pulmonary syndrome. Clin Infect Dis 2002;34:293-304.

Chen LE, Langer JC, et al. Management of late-stage parapneumonic empyema. J Pediatr Surg 2002;37:371-374.

Choi EH, Lee HJ. Clinical outcome of invasive infections by penicillin-resistant *Streptococcus pneumoniae* in Korean children. Clin Infect Dis 1998;26:1346-1354.

Clements ML, Makhene MK, et al. Effective immunization with live attenuated influenza A virus can be achieved in early infancy. Pediatric Care Center. J Infect Dis 1996;173:44-51.

Connors M, Kulkarni AB, et al. Pulmonary histopathology induced by respiratory syncytial virus (RSV) challenge of formalin-inactivated RSV-immunized BALB/c mice is abrogated by depletion of CD4+ T cells. J Virol 1992;66:7444-7451.

Conrad DA, Jenson HB. Management of acute bacterial rhinosinusitis. Curr Opin Pediatr 2002;14:86-90.

Couch R. Prevention and treatment of influenza. N Engl J Med 2000;343:1778-1787.

Courtoy I, Lande AE, et al. Accuracy of radiographic differentiation of bacterial from nonbacterial pneumonia. Clin Pediatr (Phila) 1989;28:261-264.

Dowell SF, Schwartz B, et al. Appropriate use of antibiotics for URIs in children: Part I. Otitis media and acute sinusitis. The Pediatric URI Consensus Team. Am Fam Physician 1998;58:1113-1118, 1123.

Dudas RA, Karron RA. Respiratory syncytial virus vaccines. Clin Microbiol Rev 1998;11:430-439.

Falsey AR, Walsh EE. Relationship of serum antibody to risk of respiratory syncytial virus infection in elderly adults. J Infect Dis 1998;177:463-466.

Forgie IM, O'Neill KP, et al. Etiology of acute lower respiratory tract infections in Gambian children: I. Acute lower respiratory tract infections in infants presenting at the hospital. Pediatr Infect Dis J 1991;10:33-41.

Freij BJ, Kusmiesz H, et al. Parapneumonic effusions and empyema in hospitalized children: a retrospective review of 227 cases. Pediatr Infect Dis 1984;3:578-591.

Garpenholt O, Hugosson S, et al. Epiglottitis in Sweden before and after introduction of vaccination against *Haemophilus influenzae* type b. Pediatr Infect Dis J 1999;18:490-493.

Giebink GS. Childhood sinusitis: pathophysiology, diagnosis and treatment. Pediatr Infect Dis J 1994;13(suppl 1):S55-S58; S63-S65.

Glezen WP, Paredes A, et al. Risk of respiratory syncytial virus infection for infants from low-income families in relationship to age, sex, ethnic group, and maternal antibody level. J Pediatr 1981;98:708-715.

Green M, Wald ER, et al. Field inversion gel electrophoretic analysis of *Legionella pneumophila* strains associated with nosocomial legionellosis in children. J Clin Microbiol 119;34:175-176.

Greve JM, Davis G, et al. The major human rhinovirus receptor is ICAM-1. Cell 1989;56:839-847.

Hall CB. Respiratory syncytial virus and parainfluenza virus. N Engl J Med 2001;344:1917-1928.

Hall SL, Sarris CM, et al. A cold-adapted mutant of parainfluenza virus type 3 is attenuated and protective in chimpanzees. J Infect Dis 1993;167:958-962.

Huberman K, Peluso R, et al. The hemagglutinin-neuraminidase of human parainfluenza virus type 3: role of the neuraminidase in the viral life cycle. Virology 1995;214:294-300.

Husby S, Agertoft L, et al. Treatment of croup with nebulised steroid (budesonide): a double blind, placebo controlled study. Arch Dis Child 1993;68:352-355.

Johnson DW, Jacobson S, et al. A comparison of nebulized budesonide, intramuscular dexamethasone, and placebo for moderately severe croup. N Engl J Med 1998;339:498-503.

Jones ME, Karlowsky JA, et al. Apparent plateau in beta-lactamase production among clinical isolates of *Haemophilus influenzae* and *Moraxella catarrhalis* in the United States: results from the LIBRA Surveillance initiative. Int J Antimicrob Agents 2002;19:119-123.

Kairys SW, Olmstead EM, et al. Steroid treatment of laryngotracheitis: a meta-analysis of the evidence from randomized trials. Pediatrics 1989;83:683-693.

Kapikian AZ, Mitchell RH, et al. An epidemiologic study of altered clinical reactivity to respiratory syncytial (RS) virus infection in children previously vaccinated with an inactivated RS virus vaccine. Am J Epidemiol 1969;89:405-421.

Karron RA, Makhene M, et al. Evaluation of a live attenuated bovine parainfluenza type 3 vaccine in two- to six-month-old infants. Pediatr Infect Dis J 1996;15:650-654.

Karron RA, Steinhoff MC, et al. Safety and immunogenicity of a cold-adapted influenza A (H1N1) reassortant virus vaccine administered to infants less than six months of age. Pediatr Infect Dis J 1995a;14:10-16.

Karron RA, Wright PF, et al. A live attenuated bovine parainfluenza virus type 3 vaccine is safe, infectious, immunogenic, and phenotypically stable in infants and children. J Infect Dis 1995b;171:1107-1114.

Karron RA, Wright PF, et al. A live human parainfluenza type 3 virus vaccine is attenuated and immunogenic in healthy infants and children. J Infect Dis 1995c;172:1445-1450.

Kevy S, Lowe B. Streptococcal pneumonia and empyema in childhood. N Engl J Med 1961;264:898-903.

Kim HW, Canchola JG, et al. Respiratory syncytial virus disease in infants despite prior administration of antigenic inactivated vaccine. Am J Epidemiol 1969;89: 422-434.

Klassen TP, Craig WR, et al. Nebulized budesonide and oral dexamethasone for treatment of croup: a randomized controlled trial. JAMA 1998;279:1629-1632.

Klassen TP, Feldman ME, et al. Nebulized budesonide for children with mild-to-moderate croup. N Engl J Med 1994;331:285-289.

Korppi M, Heiskanen-Kosma T, et al. White blood cells, C-reactive protein and erythrocyte sedimentation rate in pneumococcal pneumonia in children. Eur Respir J 1997;10:1125-1129.

Kuusela AL, Vesikari T. A randomized double-blind, placebo-controlled trial of dexamethasone and racemic epinephrine in the treatment of croup. Acta Paediatr Scand 1988;77:99-104.

Lamb R. Paramyxovirus fusion: a hypothesis for changes. Virology 1993;197:1-11.

Laupland KB, Davies HD, et al. Predictors and outcome of admission for invasive *Streptococcus pneumoniae* infections at a Canadian children's hospital. Clin Infect Dis 1998;27:597-602.

Lesko SM, O'Brien KL, et al. Invasive group A streptococcal infection and nonsteroidal antiinflammatory drug use among children with primary varicella. Pediatrics 2001;107:1108.

McCarthy PL, Spiesel SZ, et al. Radiographic findings and etiologic diagnosis in ambulatory childhood pneumonias. Clin Pediatr (Phila) 1981;20:686-691.

McIntosh K. Community-acquired pneumonia in children. N Engl J Med 2002;346:429-437.

Moscona A, Peluso RW. Fusion properties of cells persistently infected with human parainfluenza virus type 3: participation of hemagglutinin-neuraminidase in membrane fusion. J Virol 1991;65:2773-2777.

Murphy BR. Current approaches to the development of vaccines effective against parainfluenza viruses. Bull World Health Org 1988;66:391-397.

Nichol ST, Spiropoulou CF, et al. Genetic identification of a hantavirus associated with an outbreak of acute respiratory illness. Science 1993;262(5135):914-917.

Okamoto Y, Kudo K, et al. Detection of genomic sequences of respiratory syncytial virus in otitis media with effusion in children. Ann Otol Rhinol Laryngol Suppl 1992;157:7-10.

Openshaw PJ, Clarke SL, et al. Pulmonary eosinophilic response to respiratory syncytial virus infection in mice sensitized to the major surface glycoprotein G. Int Immunol 1992;4:493-500.

Openshaw PJ, Culley FJ, et al. Immunopathogenesis of vaccine-enhanced RSV disease. Vaccine 2001;20(suppl 1):S27-S31.

Orlicek SL. Management of acute laryngotracheobronchitis. Pediatr Infect Dis J 1998;17:1164-1165.

Prince G, Prieels J-P, et al. Pulmonary lesions in primary respiratory syncytial virus infection, reinfection and vaccine-enhanced disease in the cotton rat (*Sigmodon hispidus*). Lab Invest 1999;79:1385-1392.

Prince GA, Curtis SJ, et al. Vaccine-enhanced respiratory syncytial virus disease in cotton rats following immunization with Lot 100 or a newly prepared reference vaccine. J Gen Virol 2001;82(part 2):881-888.

Ramsey BW, Marcuse EK, et al. Use of bacterial antigen detection in the diagnosis of pediatric lower respiratory tract infections. Pediatrics 1986;78:1-9.

Roelvink PW, Lizonova A, et al. The coxsackievirus-adenovirus receptor protein can function as a cellular attachment protein for adenovirus serotypes from subgroups A, C, D, E, and F. J Virol 1998;72:7909-7915.

Scott R, Kaul A, et al. Development of in vitro correlates of cell-mediated immunity to respiratory syncytial virus infection in humans. J Infect Dis 1978;137:810-817.

Sergel T, McGinnes LW, et al. The attachment function of the Newcastle disease virus hemagglutinin-neuraminidase protein can be separated from fusion promotion by mutation. Virology 1993;193:717-726.

Skiadopoulos MH, Surman S, et al. Identification of mutations contributing to the temperature-sensitive, cold-adapted, and attenuation phenotypes of the live-attenuated cold-passage 45 (cp45) human parainfluenza virus 3 candidate vaccine. J Virol 1999a;73:1374-1381.

Skiadopoulos MH, Surman SR, et al. Attenuation of the recombinant human parainfluenza virus type 3 cp45 candidate vaccine virus is augmented by importation of the respiratory syncytial virus cpts530 L polymerase mutation. Virology 1999b;260:125-135.

Skiadopoulos MH, Tao T, et al. Generation of a parainfluenza virus type 1 vaccine candidate by replacing the HN and F glycoproteins of the live-attenuated PIV3 cp45 vaccine virus with their PIV1 counterparts. Vaccine 1999c;18:503-510.

Sole ML, Poalillo FE, et al. Bacterial growth in secretions and on suctioning equipment of orally intubated patients: a pilot study. Am J Crit Care 2002;11:141-149.

Srikiatkhachorn A, Braciale TJ. Virus-specific memory and effector T lymphocytes exhibit different cytokine responses to antigens during experimental murine respiratory syncytial virus infection. J Virol 1997;71: 678-685.

Tao T, Skiadopoulos MH, et al. A live attenuated chimeric recombinant parainfluenza virus (PIV) encoding the internal proteins of PIV type 3 and the surface glycoproteins of PIV type 1 induces complete resistance to PIV1 challenge and partial resistance to PIV3 challenge. Vaccine 1999;17:1100-1108.

Turner RB. The treatment of rhinovirus infections: progress and potential. Antiviral Res 2001;49:1-14.

Turner RB, Hendley JO, et al. Shedding of infected ciliated epithelial cells in rhinovirus colds. J Infect Dis 1982;145: 849-853.

Turner RB, Lande AE, et al. Pneumonia in pediatric outpatients: cause and clinical manifestations. J Pediatr 1987;111:194-200.

Turner RB, Weingand KW, et al. Association between interleukin-8 concentration in nasal secretions and severity of symptoms of experimental rhinovirus colds. Clin Infect Dis 1998;26:840-846.

Verduin CM, Hol C, et al. *Moraxella catarrhalis*: from emerging to established pathogen. Clin Microbiol Rev 2002;15:125-144.

Waisman Y, Klein BL, et al. Prospective randomized double-blind study comparing L-epinephrine and racemic epinephrine aerosols in the treatment of laryngotracheitis (croup). Pediatrics 1992;89:302-306.

Waris ME, Tsou C, et al. Respiratory syncytial virus infection in BALB/c mice previously immunized with formalin-inactivated virus induces enhanced pulmonary inflammatory response with a predominant Th2-like cytokine pattern. J Virol 1996;70:2852-2860.

Waris ME, Tsou C, et al. Priming with live respiratory syncytial virus (RSV) prevents the enhanced pulmonary inflammatory response seen after RSV challenge in BALB/c mice immunized with formalin-inactivated RSV. J Virol 1997;71:6935-6939.

Welliver RC. Immunology of respiratory syncytial virus infection: eosinophils, cytokines, chemokines and asthma. Pediatr Infect Dis J 2000;19:780-783, 784-785; 811-813.

Welliver RC, Kaul TN, et al. Defective regulation of immune responses in respiratory syncytial virus infection. J Immunol 1984;133:1925-1930.

Wickham TJ, Mathias P, et al. Integrins alpha v beta 3 and alpha v beta 5 promote adenovirus internalization but not virus attachment. Cell 1993;73:309-319.

Winther B, Farr B, et al. Histopathologic examination and enumeration of polymorphonuclear leukocytes in the nasal mucosa during experimental rhinovirus colds. Acta Otolaryngol Suppl 1984;413:19-24.

Winther B, Gwaltney JM Jr, et al. Sites of rhinovirus recovery after point inoculation of the upper airway. JAMA 1986;256:1763-1767.

Wright RB, Pomerantz WJ, et al. New approaches to respiratory infections in children. Bronchiolitis and croup. Emerg Med Clin North Am 2002;20:93-114.

Yim A. Paradigm shift in empyema management. Chest 1999;115:611-612.

Zar HJ, Cotton MF. Nosocomial pneumonia in pediatric patients: practical problems and rational solutions. Paediatr Drugs 2002;4:73-83.

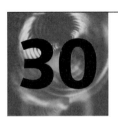

30 RUBELLA (GERMAN MEASLES)

ANNE A. GERSHON

Rubella is an acute infectious disease characterized by minimal or absent prodromal symptoms; a 3-day rash; and generalized lymph node enlargement, particularly of the postauricular, suboccipital, and cervical lymph nodes. Before 1941 rubella was important chiefly because it was responsible for epidemics in schools and military installations and because it was frequently confused with measles and scarlet fever. Since 1941 a great deal of interest has been focused on this disease because of the association of rubella during pregnancy with an increased incidence of congenital malformations. Since the widespread use of live attenuated rubella vaccine in the United States beginning in the late 1960s, rubella has become an unusual disease occurring mainly in irregular mini-epidemics, especially among the unvaccinated.

ETIOLOGY

Rubella is caused by a virus that is present in the blood and nasopharyngeal secretions of patients with the disease. Based on his transmission studies with rhesus monkeys, Hess postulated in 1914 that rubella was caused by a virus. This observation was confirmed in 1938, when Hiro and Tasaka produced the disease in children by inoculating them with filtered nasal washings obtained from patients during the acute phase of rubella. In 1942 Habel et al. also successfully transmitted rubella to the rhesus monkey, using nasal washings and blood. Reports by Anderson in 1949 and by Krugman et al. in 1953 confirmed Hiro and Tasaka's findings. Krugman et al. (1953) and Krugman and Ward (1954) also demonstrated that virus was present in the blood 2 days before and on the first day of rash and proved conclusively that rubella can occur without a rash. The cultivation of rubella virus in tissue culture was reported independently and simultaneously by

two groups. In 1962 Weller and Neva observed a cytopathic effect in human amnion cells. At the same time, Parkman et al. (1962) isolated the virus in cultures of African green monkey kidney tissue.

Rubella virus is a moderately large single-stranded RNA virus. On the basis of its biochemical, biophysical, and ultrastructural properties, rubella virus is classified in the family Togavirus, which contains the genus Alphavirus (which includes many arboviruses) and the genus Rubivirus, of which rubella virus is the only agent. The clinical and laboratory behavior of rubella virus, however, is more like that of the paramyxoviruses. It does not require a vector for transmission, and there is no RNA sequence homology between rubella virus and other togaviruses. Its nucleocapsid is 30 nm in diameter, and it is surrounded by a lipid envelope, 60 to 70 nm in diameter, that contains glycoproteins. The nucleocapsid protein consists of four polypeptides. The envelope glycoprotein consists of E1 and E2 glycopeptides. Hemagglutination inhibition and neutralizing antibodies react with the E1 peptides (Dorsett et al., 1985). Rubella virus is highly sensitive to heat, to extremes of pH, and to a variety of chemical agents. It is rapidly inactivated at $56°$ C and at $37°$ C. However, at $4°$ C the virus titer is relatively stable for 24 hours.

Rubella virus has been cultivated in a variety of tissue cultures. Cytopathic effect has been observed in a variety of cell cultures, including primary African green monkey kidney (AGMK), rabbit kidney (RK13), and Vero cells. Rubella virus strains belong to one serologic type. Rubella antigens have been prepared in several tissue culture systems and form the basis for practical serologic tests such as hemagglutinin inhibition and enzyme immunoassays. Using reverse transcription–polymerase chain reaction

(PCR), it is possible to characterize differences in the E1 nucleotide sequences that reflect rubella viruses from different geographic locations (Frey et al., 1998).

POSTNATALLY ACQUIRED RUBELLA
Clinical Manifestations

The first symptoms of rubella occur after an incubation period of approximately 16 to 18 days, with a range of 14 to 21 days. The typical clinical course is illustrated in Figure 30-1. In the child the first sign of illness is the appearance of the rash. In adolescents and adults, however, the eruption is preceded by a 1- to 5-day prodromal period characterized by low-grade fever, headache, malaise, anorexia, mild conjunctivitis, coryza, sore throat, cough, and lymphadenopathy. These symptoms rapidly subside after the first day of rash. The enanthem of rubella, described by Forschheimer in 1898, may be observed in many patients during the prodromal period or on the first day of rash. It consists of reddish spots, pinpoint or larger in size, located on the soft palate. In patients with scarlet fever the soft palate may be covered with punctate lesions, and in patients with measles it may have a red, blotchy appearance; these lesions are indistinguishable from the enanthem of rubella. The so-called Forschheimer spots are thus not pathognomonic for rubella and do not have the same diagnostic significance as Koplik's spots in measles.

Lymph node involvement. Observations of patients with experimentally induced rubella or during epidemics indicate that lymph node enlargement may begin as early as 7 days before onset of rash. There is generalized lymphadenopathy, but the suboccipital, postauricular, and cervical nodes are most commonly involved. The swelling and tenderness are most apparent and severe on the first day of rash. Subsequently, the tenderness subsides within 1 or 2 days, but the palpable enlargement of the nodes may persist for several weeks or more. The extent of the lymphadenopathy may be extremely variable; occasionally it may even be absent. At times, splenomegaly also may be noted during the acute stage of the disease. Nevertheless, involvement of the suboccipital, postauricular, and cervical lymph nodes is not pathognomonic for rubella. Lymphadenopathy is also associated with diseases such as measles, chickenpox, adenovirus infections, and infectious mononucleosis.

Exanthem. The rash, particularly in children, may be the first obvious indication of illness. It appears first on the face and then spreads downward rapidly to the neck, arms, trunk, and extremities. The eruption appears, spreads, and disappears more quickly than does the rash of measles (Figure 30-2). By the end of

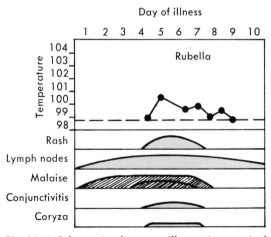

Fig. 30-1 Schematic diagram illustrating typical course of rubella in children and adults. Lymph nodes begin to enlarge 3 to 4 days before rash. Prodromal symptoms (malaise) are minimal in children *(shaded area)*. In adults there may be a 3- to 4-day prodrome *(hatched area)*. Conjunctivitis and coryza, if present, are usually minimal and accompany the rash.

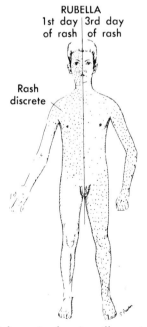

Fig. 30-2 Schematic drawing illustrating development and distribution of rubella rash.

the first day the entire body may be covered with the discrete pink-red maculapules. On the second day, the rash begins to disappear from the face, and the lesions on the trunk may coalesce to form uniform red blush that may resemble the rash of mild scarlet fever. The lesions on the extremities, however, remain discrete and generally do not coalesce. In the typical case the rash has disappeared by the end of the third day. If the eruption has been intensive, there may be some fine, branny desquamation; usually there is none.

The characteristic pink-red lesions of rubella differ from the purple-red lesions of measles and the yellow-red lesions of scarlet fever. In rubella the lesions are generally discrete and may or may not coalesce; if they do, a diffuse erythematous blush results. In contrast, the lesions of measles, particularly around the head and neck, tend to coalesce and form irregular blotches with crescentic margins. The similarities and differences between the eruptions of rubella and those of scarlet fever have been referred to previously. The circumoral area also differs in these two diseases; in rubella the rash involves this area, and in scarlet fever there is circumoral pallor.

The duration and extent of the rash may be variable. The eruption, which as a rule lasts for 3 days, may persist for 5 days or may be so evanescent that it disappears in less than a day. In an unknown number of instances, rubella may even occur without a rash. The incidence of subclinical rubella infections is approximately 25%.

Fever. In children the temperature may be either normal or slightly elevated. Fever, if present, rarely persists beyond the first day of rash and is usually low grade. A typical temperature course is illustrated in Figure 30-1. During epidemics, patients with rubella occasionally have temperatures as high as 40° C (104° F). In adolescents and adults there may be low-grade fever during both the prodromal period and the first day of rash.

Hematologic manifestations. Generally, the white blood cell count is low but it may be normal. Occasionally there may be an increased percentage of abnormal lymphocytes or a decrease in platelets.

Diagnosis

Confirmatory Clinical Factors. A diagnosis of rubella is suggested by the appearance of a maculopapular eruption beginning on the face, progressing rapidly downward to the trunk and extremities, and subsiding within 3 days. Prodromal symptoms are minimal or absent, fever is low grade or absent, and lymphadenopathy precedes the appearance of the rash. A history of exposure, if available, is helpful.

Detection of causative agent. As indicated in Figure 30-3, rubella virus may be recovered from the pharynx as early as 7 days before the onset of rash and as late as 14 days after onset of rash. As indicated in Figure 30-3, virus may be recovered from the pharynx with regularity within 5 days after the onset of rash; however, viremia that is present before the onset of rash is rarely documented after the onset of rash. Rubella virus infection may also be documented by PCR, in which rubella-specific oligonucleotide primers are used to reverse transcribe cDNA, which is then amplified by PCR and detected by Southern blotting. This type of assay has also been useful to identify the geographic origin of rubella virus, so that it is possible to identify imported rubella virus in patients with infections in the United States. PCR has been useful in the documentation of congenital rubella in infants and also in the detection of rubella in products of conception and amniotic fluid (Chernesky and Mahoney 1999).

Serologic tests. The pattern of appearance and persistence of rubella virus–neutralizing, complement-fixing (CF), and hemagglutination inhibition (HI) antibody is shown in Figure 30-3. Antibody is usually detectable by the third day of rash, and peak levels are reached approximately 1 month later. CF antibody may be short lived, declining to nondetectable levels within a year or more after infection. Neutralizing and HI antibodies usually persist for life. The HI antibody test has the advantages of high sensitivity and early availability of results. Other assays that are used include latex agglutination and indirect immunofluorescence. The most commonly used test today is an enzyme-linked immunosorbent assay (ELISA), which can be used to measure IgG and IgM antibodies to rubella. For serologic diagnosis the acute-phase serum should be obtained as early as possible after onset of rash, and convalescent-phase serum should be collected 2 to 4 weeks later. Acute rubella may be diagnosed by a fourfold or greater rise in titer of

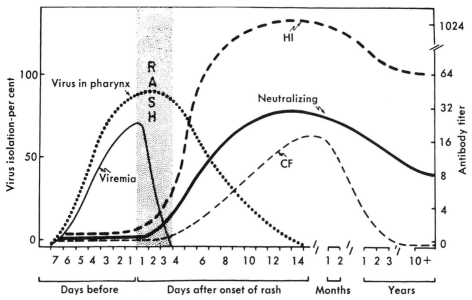

Fig. 30-3 Natural history of postnatal rubella. Pattern of virus excretion and antibody response. (Modified from Cooper LZ, Krugman S: Arch Ophthalmol 1967;77:434.)

IgG antibodies in paired acute-phase and convalescent-phase serum specimens or by the presence of rubella-specific IgM antibodies in one serum specimen. False-negative and false-positive IgM reactions may occur, however. In addition, true positive IgM reactions may be demonstrated in primary infections and reinfections (Chernesky and Mahoney, 1999).

Differential diagnosis. Other diseases that may mimic rubella include toxoplasmosis, scarlet fever, modified measles, roseola (caused by human herpesvirus–6 infection), fifth disease (erythema infectiosum, caused by parvovirus infection), and enteroviral infections. Additional information is discussed in Chapter 45.

Complications

Rubella in childhood is rarely followed by complications. Secondary bacterial infections, which are so common in measles, are not encountered in rubella. The following complications have been observed, especially during epidemics.

Arthritis. Joint involvement in adolescents and adults with rubella is much more common than is generally appreciated. It usually develops just as the rash is fading on the second to third day of illness. Either one or more of the larger and smaller joints may be involved. The arthritis may be manifested by a return of fever and either transient joint pain without swelling or massive effusion into one or more joint spaces.

These manifestations usually clear spontaneously within 5 to 10 days but may on occasion take several weeks to resolve. However, chronic arthritis that lasts for longer periods following rubella is exceedingly rare (Chantler et al., 1985).

Rubella arthritis with involvement of the knees, ankles, or elbows may simulate the polyarthritis of rheumatic fever. When there is fusiform swelling of the fingers, it may resemble rheumatoid arthritis. In a study of 10 female patients with rubella arthritis of the small- and medium-sized joints that lasted 1 week, positive latex fixation tests for rheumatoid factor were demonstrated in 9 of the 10 patients with arthritis, compared with only two of seven patients who had rubella without arthritis (Johnson and Hall, 1958). However, in another study of 14 women observed for a 2- to 5-year follow-up period after experiencing rubella arthritis, none showed any clinical manifestations suggesting rheumatoid disease (Kantor and Tanner, 1962). During an epidemic of rubella in a London suburb, Fry et al. (1962) observed arthritis in 15% of 74 adults with rubella; they detected arthritis in 33% of 40 females and in 6% of 34 males. During an epidemic of rubella in Bermuda in 1971, joint manifestations were observed in 25% of children under the age of 11 years and in 52% of patients 11 years of age or older (Judelsohn and

Wyll, 1973). Rubella virus has been isolated from joint fluid taken from patients with acute rubella arthritis and from peripheral blood of those with chronic rubella arthritis.

Encephalitis. Complications of rubella in the central nervous system (CNS) are extremely rare. Encephalitis is less commonly encountered after rubella than after measles or varicella. The incidence usually cited is 1 in 6,000 cases of rubella. The clinical manifestations are similar to those observed in other types of postinfectious encephalitis. Complete recovery is generally the rule, but fatalities have been reported. Observations by Kenny et al. in 1965 indicated that demyelinization apparently is not a feature of rubella encephalopathy. Neurologic abnormalities are minor and occur infrequently, and intellectual function is generally unaffected if the patient survives. However, electroencephalographic abnormalities are relatively common and persistent.

Purpura. Thrombocytopenic and nonthrombocytopenic purpura may, in rare instances, complicate rubella. In addition to a reduction in platelet count, there is usually prolonged bleeding time and increased capillary fragility. In some reported cases the clinical manifestations have included one or more of the following disorders: cutaneous hemorrhages; epistaxis; bleeding gums; hematuria; bleeding from the intestinal tract; and, rarely, cerebral hemorrhage. Most patients become symptom free within 2 weeks, and the platelet count returns to normal values. Thrombocytopenia may last from weeks to months; it may be associated with long-term sequelae if there is bleeding into organs such as the eye and the brain.

Prognosis

The prognosis is almost uniformly excellent. Rubella is one of the most benign of all infectious diseases in children. However, the rare complications of encephalitis and thrombocytopenic purpura may alter the prognosis. Many reported deaths attributed to rubella infection reflect errors in diagnosis. Immunosuppressed patients have not been reported to be at increased risk from rubella, as they are for measles.

Immunity

Active immunity. One attack of rubella is generally followed by permanent immunity. Although some so-called second attacks represent errors in diagnosis, it is now recognized that clinical reinfections can occur, although rarely, with this virus. Viremia is believed to be rare in reinfections. Active immunity is induced by infection after natural exposure or immunization. As indicated in Figure 30-3, rubella-neutralizing antibody may persist for many years after infection.

Passive immunity. Neutralizing antibodies for rubella are present in gamma globulin. Passive immunization of an exposed susceptible pregnant woman, however, does not prevent infection of her fetus and development of the congenital rubella syndrome. Rubella, like measles and mumps, is rarely observed in the early months of life because of transplacentally acquired immunity.

Epidemiologic Factors

Rubella is worldwide in distribution. It is endemic in most large cities where vaccination is not routine. In such areas, localized epidemics occur at irregular intervals compared with the fairly consistent periodicity of measles. During the prevaccine era, major epidemics occurred at 6- to 9-year intervals. Rubella outbreaks usually occur during the spring months in the temperate zones. The extensive and routine use of live attenuated rubella vaccine since licensure in 1969 has had a major impact on the epidemiology of the disease. The last epidemic in the United States occurred in 1964. During the subsequent 28 years there was a progressive decrease in the number of reported cases of rubella. Major epidemics of the disease have been eliminated in the United States. Today most rubella occurs in foreign-born individuals, especially Hispanics born in Central and South America, who were not immunized against the disease (Reef et al., 2002).

An enzyme immunoassay was used to measure antibodies to rubella virus in the third National Health and Nutrition Examination Survey (NHANES III), conducted from 1988 to 1994, which studied the incidence of immunity to rubella in the U.S. population. Overall, rubella seropositivity rates were 92% in persons aged 6 to 11 years, 83% in persons aged 12 to 19 years, 85% in persons aged 20 to 29 years, 89% in persons aged 30 to 39 years, and more than 92% in persons 40 years of age and older (Dykewicz et al., 2001).

The age distribution of rubella during the prevaccine era was striking. It was rare in infancy and uncommon in preschool-age children. There was an unusually high incidence of the disease in older children, adolescents, and young adults. Rubella was a constant problem in boarding schools, colleges, and military installations. A significant number of workdays were lost as a result of outbreaks among military personnel.

In the United States during the late 1990s, the highest incidence of rubella was reported in individuals aged 20 to 29 years, with an increase in cases in women. In the United States, from 1996 to 1999, rubella was reported in 281 women of childbearing years, 26% of whom were pregnant at rash onset, mostly in the first or second trimester. Most of these women were of Latin American origin (Reef et al., 2002). A large reported outbreak that occurred in Nebraska in 1999 reflects these findings: those infected were mostly young adults who were unimmunized and were born in Latin American countries (Danovaro-Holliday et al., 2000). Transmission mainly occurred in the workplace (a meat-packing plant) and was facilitated by crowded working conditions. Other reported groups with low levels of immunity to rubella include the Amish, who have also been reported to have high rates of congenital rubella in the vaccine era (Mellinger et al., 1995). In countries where rubella vaccine is not used routinely, for example, in many countries in Central and South America, the incidence of congenital rubella continues to be high, even in nonepidemic years (Irons et al., 2000). The development of congenital rubella syndrome in the United States today is not due to exposure to the virus in immunized women whose immunity is waning, but rather to the occurrence of the disease in unimmunized pregnant women.

Rubella appears to be spread via the respiratory route. The disease has been transmitted with nasopharyngeal secretions obtained from patients with rubella on the first day of the rash. The period of infectivity probably extends from the latter part of the incubation period to the end of the third day of the rash.

Isolation and Quarantine

Isolation and quarantine precautions generally are not warranted. However, outbreaks of rubella have been a problem among hospital and medical personnel in several states, including New York (McLaughlin and Gold, 1979),

California, and Colorado (Edell et al., 1979). During the New York experience a male physician with rubella exposed 170 persons, including susceptible pregnant patients. These episodes created a difficult problem for institutions and staff—a problem that is prevented today by the following measure: (1) routine screening of both male and female medical personnel caring for patients who may be pregnant, and (2) immunization of those with no detectable rubella antibody.

Treatment

Symptomatic treatment. In many instances, rubella is asymptomatic and requires no treatment at all. Even if the child has a low-grade fever, bed rest may be unnecessary. Headache, malaise, and pain in the lymph nodes can be easily controlled with acetaminophen. No specific antiviral therapy is available.

Treatment of complications. Arthritis is usually well controlled by aspirin. Bed rest is advised if there is fever or involvement of the weight-bearing joints. A patient with encephalitis should be treated in the same way as a patient with measles encephalitis (see the section on encephalitis in Chapter 20). Corticosteroid therapy and platelet transfusions may be indicated in severe cases of thrombocytopenic purpura.

CONGENITAL RUBELLA

Congenital rubella was identified as a clinical entity more than a century after the disease was first recognized. In 1941 Gregg reported the occurrence of congenital cataracts among 78 infants born after maternal rubella infection acquired during the 1940 epidemic in Australia. More than half of these infants had congenital heart disease. Since 1941 Gregg's report of the rubella syndrome has been amply confirmed. The occurrence of rubella during the first trimester of pregnancy has been associated with a significantly increased incidence of congenital malformations, stillbirths, and abortions. The epidemic of rubella in the United States in 1964 was followed by the birth of an estimated 20,000 infants with the congenital rubella syndrome. Between 1995 and 1999, despite widespread vaccination in the United States, from 38 to 220 cases of rubella were reported annually to the Centers for Disease Control and Prevention, most the result of mini-outbreaks. These cases occurred in settings such as the workplace, colleges, and cruise ships. During this 5-year period there were 110 cases of confirmed congenital rubella syndrome. Most of these infants were born to women who were young (median age 23 years), Hispanic, foreign born, and unimmunized. The recognition of this problem has led to recommendations for more intensive programs for immunization of susceptible women before they become pregnant and more intensive efforts toward immunization of high-risk groups in general (Lee et al., 1992). It is thought nevertheless that we are on the verge of elimination of rubella and the congenital rubella syndrome from the United States (Reef et al., 2002).

Pathogenesis

Studies by many investigators have provided evidence to support the following concept of the natural history of congenital rubella. As indicated in Figure 30-3, viremia is present for several days before onset of rash. Maternal viremia may be followed by a placental infection and subsequent fetal viremia, leading to a disseminated infection involving many fetal organs. Timing is the crucial element in the pathogenesis of congenital rubella. A fetal infection probably will be chronic and persistent if it is acquired during the early weeks and months of pregnancy. However, after the fourth month of gestation, the fetus apparently is no longer highly susceptible to the chronic infection that is characteristic of intrauterine rubella during the first 8 to 12 weeks.

The pathogenesis of rubella embryopathy is not entirely clear. Studies in human embryonic tissue culture cells have indicated that rubella infection was associated with inhibition of mitosis and an increased number of chromosomal breaks (Plotkin et al., 1965). Autopsies of infants with congenital rubella revealed hypoplastic organs with a subnormal number of cells (Naeye and Blanc, 1965). Consequently, it is likely that rubella embryopathy may be caused by (1) inhibition of cellular multiplication; (2) chronic, persistent infection during the crucial period of organogenesis; or (3) a combination of both factors.

Clinical Manifestations

Intrauterine growth retardation, cataracts, microcephaly, deafness, congenital heart disease, and mental retardation characterized the classic rubella syndrome described by Gregg and others in the 1940s. Extensive studies of this syndrome during the 1964 rubella epidemic in the United States shed new light on this problem. The availability of specific virus isolation and serologic techniques provided information that revealed a broader spectrum of this disease. Intrauterine rubella infection may be followed by spontaneous abortion of the infected fetus, stillbirth, live birth of an infant with single or multiple malformations, or birth of a normal infant. The various manifestations of congenital rubella are listed in Box 30-1. It is clear that the consequences of rubella infection during pregnancy are varied and unpredictable. Virtually every organ may be involved—singly, multiply, transiently, or progressively and permanently.

BOX 30-1

MANIFESTATIONS OF CONGENITAL RUBELLA

Growth retardation (low birth weight)
Eye defects
- Cataracts
- Glaucoma
- Retinopathy
- Microphthalmia
Deafness
Cardiac defects
- Patent ductus arteriosus
- Ventricular septal defect
- Pulmonary stenosis
- Myocardial necrosis
Central nervous system defects
- Psychomotor retardation
- Microcephaly
- Encephalitis
- Spastic quadriparesis
- Cerebrospinal fluid pleocytosis
- Mental retardation
- Progressive panencephalitis
Hepatomegaly
Hepatitis
Thrombocytopenic purpura
Splenomegaly
Bone lesions
Interstitial pneumonitis
Diabetes mellitus
Psychiatric disorders
Thyroid disorders
Precocious puberty

Neonatal manifestations. A variety of clinical manifestations may be present during the first weeks of life. Low birth weight in relation to period of gestation is common. Thrombocytopenic purpura characterized by a petechial and purpuric eruption may occur in association with other transient conditions, such as hepatosplenomegaly, hepatitis, hemolytic anemia, bone lesions (metaphyseal rarefaction), and bulging anterior fontanelle with or without pleocytosis in the cerebrospinal fluid (CSF). These transient manifestations may occur in association with the classic cardiac, eye, hearing, and CNS defects. An infant with neonatal thrombocytopenic purpura characterized by the typical "blueberry muffin" skin lesions is shown in Plate 48.

Cardiac defects. Patent ductus arteriosus, with or without pulmonary artery stenosis, and atrial and ventricular septal defects are the most common cardiac lesions. Clinical evidence of congenital heart disease may be present at birth or delayed for several days. Other cardiac manifestations include myocardial involvement, as indicated by electrocardiographic findings, and necropsy evidence of extensive necrosis of the myocardium. Many infants have tolerated the cardiac lesions with little difficulty; others have developed congestive heart failure in the first months of life.

Eye defects. Cataracts, unilateral or bilateral, are common consequences of congenital rubella. They appear as pearly white nuclear lesions, frequently associated with microphthalmia. The cataracts may be too small at birth to be visible on casual examination. A careful ophthalmoscopic examination with a +8 lens held 15 to 20 cm from the eye may reveal an early cataract. Rubella glaucoma is a less common eye lesion, and it may be clinically indistinguishable from hereditary infantile glaucoma. It may be present at birth, or it may appear after the neonatal period. The cornea is enlarged and hazy, the anterior chamber is deep, and ocular tension is increased. Glaucoma that requires prompt surgical therapy must be differentiated from transient corneal clouding. Retinopathy is the most common eye manifestation of congenital rubella. It is characterized by discrete, patchy, black pigmentation that is variable in size and location. Retinopathy does not affect visual acuity if the lesions do not involve the macular area. The presence of this lesion is a valuable aid in the clinical diagnosis of congenital rubella.

Hearing loss. Deafness may be the only manifestation of congenital rubella. It may be unilateral but is usually bilateral. It is probably caused by maldevelopment and possibly by degenerative changes in the cochlea and organ of Corti. Hearing loss may be severe or so mild that it is overlooked unless detected by an audiometric examination. Severe bilateral hearing loss is responsible for speech defects.

CNS involvement. Psychomotor retardation is a common manifestation of congenital rubella. In severe cases the brain is the site of a chronic, persistent infection, as indicated by the presence of pleocytosis, increased concentration of protein, and rubella virus in the CSF for as long as 1 year after birth. Microcephaly is a well-known manifestation (Desmond et al., 1967). The most common consequence of CNS involvement is mental retardation (mild or profound). Behavioral disturbances and manifestations of minimal cerebral dysfunction also are common. Less common are severe spastic diplegia and autism.

Progressive rubella panencephalitis was described in four patients with congenital rubella (Townsend et al., 1975; Weil et al., 1975). Severe, progressive, neurologic deterioration was noted during the second decade of life. In two patients there was progression of spasticity, ataxia, intellectual deterioration, seizures, and subsequent fatality. Other findings included (1) high levels of rubella antibody in serum and CSF, (2) increased levels of CSF protein and gamma globulin, (3) histopathologic changes in the brain, and (4) isolation of rubella virus from a brain biopsy of one of the patients. In some ways this syndrome resembled subacute sclerosing panencephalitis, a rare complication of measles.

Diagnosis

The presence of congenital rubella should be suspected under the following circumstances: (1) a history of possible rubella or exposure to rubella during the first trimester of pregnancy, and (2) the presence of one or more of the various manifestations of congenital rubella listed in Box 30-1. However, final confirmation of the diagnosis is dependent on virus isolation or immunologic procedures.

Demonstration of the virus. Rubella virus has been cultured from pharyngeal secretions, urine, CSF, and virtually every tissue and organ in the body. Infants with congenital rubella may remain chronically infected for many weeks or months. As indicated in Figure 30-4, the incidence of virus shedding decreases with advancing age. Most infants with congenital rubella are no longer shedding virus and have a normal pattern of serum immunoglobulins by 1 year of age. However, infants with severe dysgammaglobulinemia may shed virus for a more prolonged period. Isolation of virus from the blood is very rare. Viremia has been observed chiefly in infants with immunologic disorders. Biopsied tissues or blood and cerebrospinal fluid have also been used to demonstrate rubella antigens with monoclonal antibodies and for detection of rubella RNA by in situ hybridization and PCR (Bosma et al., 1995).

Immunologic response. The immunologic response to an intrauterine infection is shown in Figure 30-5. It differs significantly from the response to rubella acquired postnatally. The chief difference lies in the pattern of virus excretion and antibody response. In rubella acquired after birth, virus excretion is transient, rarely persisting for more than 2 or 3 weeks (Figure 30-3); in contrast, virus shedding may persist for many months after birth in congenital rubella. As indicated in Figure 30-5, the serum of an infant with congenital rubella contains actively acquired IgM-specific antibody and passively acquired maternal IgG antibody. Several months later, transplacentally acquired IgG is no longer detectable, and high levels of IgM may be present. By the end of 1 year, actively acquired IgG apparently is the dominant rubella antibody. Consequently, the presence and persistence of rubella antibody in the serum of an infant 5 to 6 months of age or older and the identification of the antibody in early infancy as IgM are indicative of congenital rubella infection.

The pattern of persistence of HI antibody following congenital rubella is different from that following naturally acquired infection. Detectable levels of antibody persist for many years in most children after a natural rubella infection. However, approximately 20% of children with congenital rubella by age 5 years may no longer have detectable rubella HI antibody (Cooper et al., 1971).

Differential Diagnosis

Cytomegalovirus infection, congenital toxoplasmosis, and congenital syphilis also may be characterized by the following manifestations of

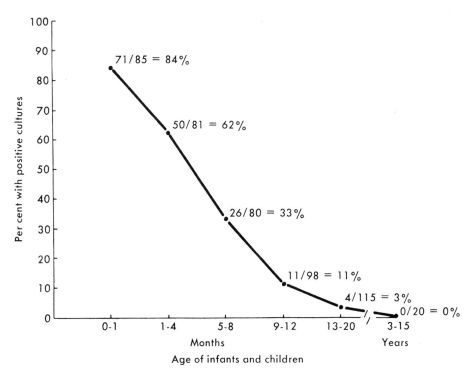

Fig. 30-4 Incidence of rubella virus excretion by age in infants with congenital rubella. (From Cooper LZ, Krugman S: Arch Ophthalmol 1967;77:434.)

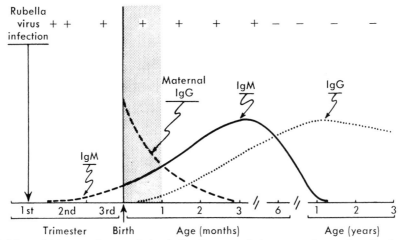

Fig. 30-5 Natural history of congenital rubella. Pattern of virus excretion and antibody response.

congenital rubella: thrombocytopenic purpura, jaundice, hepatosplenomegaly, and bone lesions. Herpes simplex virus infection may show the same manifestations, with the exception of bone lesions and a vesicular skin rash. The diagnosis may be clarified by the presence of other findings more compatible with congenital rubella, such as congenital cataract, glaucoma, patent ductus arteriosus, or maternal history of rubella. The precise diagnosis should be confirmed by specific laboratory tests.

Prognosis

Neonatal thrombocytopenic purpura carries a poor prognosis. The mortality rate exceeded 35% after the first-year follow-up of a large group of infants (Cooper and Krugman, 1967). The usual causes of death were sepsis, congestive heart failure, and general debility. In the absence of purpura the mortality rate was approximately 10%. Deaths usually occurred during the first 6 months of life. The prognosis is excellent for children with minor defects.

There has been a long-term follow-up of approximately 500 children born with the congenital rubella syndrome in New York City during the epidemic from 1964 to 1965. In their twenties, these patients could be divided into three groups: approximately one third were relatively normal; one third were mildly to moderately incapacitated; and the remainder were profoundly handicapped, requiring institutional care. Patients with congenital rubella syndrome have had difficulty in developing social skills, especially after leaving special educational units as young adults. Suicide attempts

have not been uncommon. Approximately 15% of patients with congenital rubella syndrome have developed insulin-dependent diabetes, presumably as a result of an autoimmune mechanism. Long-term follow-up studies from Australia have yielded similar findings (McIntosh et al., 1992).

Epidemiologic Factors

The incidence of congenital rubella is dependent on the immune status of women of childbearing age and the occurrence of significant epidemics. The risk associated with maternal rubella infection has been variously estimated. An evaluation of several prospective studies indicates that the risk of congenital malformations after maternal rubella is as follows: (1) 30% to 50% during the first 4 weeks of gestation, (2) 25% during the fifth to eighth weeks of gestation, and (3) 8% during the ninth to twelfth weeks of gestation. The overall risk of malformations from rubella during the first trimester is approximately 20%. There is a slight risk of deafness when rubella occurs during the thirteenth to sixteenth weeks.

Isolation and Quarantine

Isolation of infants with congenital rubella. The primary aim of isolation procedures is to prevent rubella infection in susceptible pregnant women. Infants with congenital rubella may shed virus for many weeks or months after birth. Intimate contact is generally required for the transmission of rubella. Accordingly, potentially susceptible pregnant women should avoid close exposure to these infants.

Isolation in the hospital. Infants suspected of having congenital rubella should be admitted to a separate room designated as the isolation unit. Personnel assigned to this area should be selected on the basis of their childbearing potential and immune status. Isolation should be continued until the infant is ready to go home.

Isolation in the home. No special precautions are necessary for the parents and young sibling contacts. Potentially susceptible female visitors to the home should avoid physical contact with the infant during the contagious period. If laboratory facilities are available for identification of rubella virus, infants should be considered contagious until negative cultures have been obtained. As indicated in Figure 30-4, evidence of virus shedding may disappear by 1 month of age in some infants; on the other hand, it may persist for a year or more in a small number of infants. If laboratory facilities are not available, the data shown in Figure 30-4 may be used as a guide for the estimation of period of contagion. In general, there is some correlation between the severity of the infection and the duration of virus shedding. Infants with severe involvement usually shed virus much longer than infants with minimal involvement.

PREVENTIVE MEASURES

Live attenuated rubella vaccine was licensed in the United States in 1969 (Enders, 1970); the vaccine currently available is RA 27/3, licensed in 1979, which is propagated in human diploid cells and is more immunogenic (particularly with regard to stimulation of secretory immunity) than previously licensed vaccines. The current vaccine strategy is to immunize all infants at 12 to 15 months of age with measles-mumps-rubella (MMR) vaccine and to administer a second dose of MMR during childhood between 4 and 6 years of age (Watson et al., 1998; Zimmerman et al., 2001). Two doses of monovalent rubella vaccine may also be administered to anyone who is thought to be susceptible to the infection and is not pregnant (Zimmerman, 2001). It is especially important that hospital workers of either sex be immune to rubella to avoid possible nosocomial transmission. It is likely that, years following immunization, antibody titers may be undetectable but that protection against infection is the rule. At present there is little if any evidence of significant waning immunity to rubella years after

immunization. Although rubella vaccine has not been associated with the congenital syndrome, vaccination is contraindicated in pregnant women and pregnancy should be avoided for at least 1 month following rubella vaccination. Rubella-susceptible children whose mothers are also rubella-susceptible should be immunized, because individuals who are vaccinated do not shed rubella virus or transmit the virus to susceptible individuals (Fleet et al., 1972; Fleet et al., 1974; Halstead and Diwan, 1971; Klock et al., 1972). Although it is not recommended that rubella vaccine be given to immunosuppressed persons, no adverse effects of rubella vaccine have been reported in such individuals who have been vaccinated. Rubella vaccine has been safely given to children with HIV infection. Occasionally, rubella vaccine may be associated with arthralgia or arthritis, especially in young women. Rubella vaccination can result in a chronic arthritis on very rare occasion; episodes of arthritis in vaccinees are usually self-limited, lasting only about 1 week (Cooper et al., 1969; Smith et al., 1987; Tingle et al., 1986; Weibel, 1996).

Although vaccine-induced titers are generally lower than those following natural rubella, vaccine-induced immunity usually protects against both clinical illness and viremia after natural exposure (Krugman, 1977). Rare reports have indicated that viremic reinfection following exposure may occur in vaccinated individuals with low levels of detectable antibody, but there are also rare reports of clinical reinfection and fetal infection following natural immunity (Boué et al., 1971; Cusi et al., 1991; Davis et al., 1971; Horstmann et al., 1979; O'Shea et al., 1994).

Persons can be considered immune to rubella only if they have documentation of (1) laboratory evidence of rubella immunity or (2) adequate immunization with at least 1 dose of rubella vaccine on or after the first birthday. Clinical diagnosis of rubella is not reliable and should not be considered in assessing immunity to rubella.

BIBLIOGRAPHY

Anderson SG. Experimental rubella in human volunteers. J Immunol 1949;62:29.

Bosma TJ, Corbett KM, Eckstein MB, et al. Use of PCR for prenatal and postnatal diagnosis of congenital rubella. J Clin Microbiol 1995;33:2881.

Boué A, Nicolas A, Montagnon B. Reinfection with rubella in pregnant women. Lancet 1971;1:1251.

Centers for Disease Control and Prevention. Notice to readers: revised ACIP recommendation for avoiding pregnancy after receiving a rubella-containing vaccine. MMWR 2001;50:1117.

Chantler JK, et al. Persistent rubella virus infection associated with chronic arthritis in children. N Engl J Med 1985;313:1117.

Chernesky MA, Mahoney JB. Rubella virus. In PR Murray (ed) Manual of Clinical Microbiology. Washington, D.C.: ASM Press, 1999.

Cooper LZ, et al. Neonatal thrombocytopenic purpura and other manifestations of rubella contracted in utero. Am J Dis Child 1965;110:416.

Cooper LZ, et al. Transient arthritis after rubella vaccination. Am J Dis Child 1969;118:218.

Cooper LZ, Florman AL, Ziring PR, Krugman S. Loss of rubella hemagglutination inhibition antibody in congenital rubella. Am J Dis Child 1971;122:397.

Cooper LZ, Krugman S. Clinical manifestations of postnatal and congenital rubella. Arch Ophthalmol 1967;77:434.

Cusi MG, et al. Serological evidence of reinfection among vaccinees during rubella outbreak. Lancet 1991;336:1071.

Danovaro-Holliday MC, LeBaron CW, Allensworth C, et al. A large rubella outbreak with spread from the workplace to the community. JAMA 2000;284:2733.

Davis WJ, et al. A study of rubella immunity and resistance to reinfection. JAMA 1971;215:600.

Desmond MM, et al. Congenital rubella encephalitis. J Pediatr 1967;71:311.

Dorsett PH, Miller DC, Green KY, et al. Structure and function of rubella virus proteins. Rev Infect Dis 1985;7:S150.

Dykewicz CA, Kruszon-Moran D, McQuillan GM, et al. Rubella seropositivity in the United States, 1988-1994. Clin Infect Dis 2001;33:1279.

Edell TA, et al. Rubella in hospital personnel and patients, Colorado. MMWR Morb Mortal Wkly Rep 1979;28:325.

Enders JF. Rubella vaccination. N Engl J Med 1970;283:161.

Fleet WF Jr, et al. Exposure of susceptible teachers to rubella vaccines. Am J Dis Child 1972;123:28.

Fleet WF Jr, et al. Fetal consequences of maternal rubella immunization. JAMA 1974;227:621.

Frey TK, Abernathy ES, Bosma TJ, et al. Molecular analysis of rubella virus epidemiology across three continents, North America, Europe, and Asia, 1961-1997. J Infect Dis 1998;178:642.

Fry J, Dillane JB, Fry L. Rubella, 1962. Br Med J 1962;2:833.

Gregg NM. Congenital cataract following German measles in the mother. Trans Ophthalmol Soc Aust 1941;3:35.

Gregg NM, et al. Occurrence of congenital defects in children following maternal rubella during pregnancy. Med J Aust 1945;2:122.

Habel K, et al. Transmission of rubella to *Macacus mulatta* monkeys. Public Health Rep 1942;57:1126.

Halstead S, Diwan AR. Failure to transmit rubella virus vaccine: a close contact study in adults. JAMA 1971;215:634.

Hess AF. German measles (rubella): an experimental study. Arch Intern Med 1914;13:913.

Hiro Y, Tasaka S. Die Röteln sind eine Virus-krankheit. Monatsschr Kinderheilkd 1938;76:328.

Horstmann DM, et al. Rubella: reinfection of vaccinated and naturally immune persons exposed in an epidemic. N Engl J Med 1970;283:771.

Irons B, Lewis MJ, Dahl-Regis M, et al. Strategies to eradicate rubella in the English speaking Caribbean. Am J Pub Health 2000;90:1545-1549.

Johnson RE, Hall AP. Rubella arthritis: report of cases studied by latex tests. N Engl J Med 1958;258:743.

Judelsohn RG, Wyll SA. Rubella in Bermuda: termination of an epidemic by mass vaccination. JAMA 1973;223:401.

Kantor TG, Tanner M. Rubella arthritis and rheumatoid arthritis. Arthritis Rheum 1962;5:378.

Kenny FM, Michaels RH, Davis KS. Rubella encephalopathy: later psychometric, neurologic, and encephalographic evaluation of seven survivors. Am J Dis Child 1965;110:374.

Klock LE, et al. A clinical and serological study of women exposed to rubella vaccinees. Am J Dis Child 1972;123:465.

Krugman S. Present status of measles and rubella immunization in the United States: a medical progress report. J Pediatr 1977;90:1.

Krugman S, Ward R. The rubella problem. J Pediatr 1954;44:489.

Krugman S, Ward R, Jacobs KG, Lazar M. Studies on rubella immunization. I. Demonstration of rubella without rash. JAMA 1953;151:285.

Lee SH, et al. Resurgence of congenital rubella syndrome in the 1990s. JAMA 1992;267:2616.

McIntosh ED, et al. A fifty-year follow up of congenital rubella. Lancet 1992;340:414.

McLaughlin MD, Gold LH. The New York rubella incident: a case for changing hospital policy regarding rubella testing and immunization. Am J Public Health 1979;69:287.

Mellinger AK, et al. High incidence of congenital rubella syndrome after a rubella outbreak. Pediatr Infect Dis J 1995;14:573.

Naeye RL, Blanc W. Pathogenesis of congenital rubella. JAMA 1965;194:1277.

O'Shea S, et al. Rubella reinfection; role of neutralizing antibodies and cell-mediated immunity. Clin Diagn Virol 1994;2:349.

Parkman PD, Buescher EL, Artenstein MS. Recovery of rubella virus from army recruits. Proc Soc Exp Biol Med 1962;111:225.

Plotkin SA, Boué A, Boué JG. The in vitro growth of rubella virus in human embryonic cells. Am J Epidemiol 1965;81:71.

Reef SE, Frey TK, Theall K, et al. The changing epidemiology of rubella in the 1990s: on the verge of elimination and new challenges for control and prevention. JAMA 2002;287:464.

Smith CA, et al. Rubella virus and arthritis. Rheum Dis Clin North Am 1987;13:810.

Tingle AJ, Allen M, Petty RE. Rubella-associated arthritis. I. Comparative study of joint manifestations associated with natural rubella and RA 27/3 rubella immunization. Ann Rheum Dis 1986;45:110-114.

Townsend JJ, et al. Progressive rubella panencephalitis: late onset after congenital rubella. N Engl J Med 1975;292:990.

Watson JC, Hadler SC, Dykewicz CA, et al. Measles, mumps, and rubella–vaccine use and strategies for elimination of measles, rubella, and congenital rubella syndrome and control of mumps: Recommendations of the Advisory Committee on Immunization Practices (ACIP). MMWR Recomm Rep 1998;47:1-67.

Weibel 1 RE, Benor DE. Chronic arthropathy and musculoskeletal symptoms associated with rubella vaccines: a review of 124 claims submitted to the National Injury Compensation Program. Authritis Rheum 1996; 39:1529–1534 .

Weil ML, et al. Chronic progressive panencephalitis due to rubella virus stimulating SSPE. N Engl J Med 1975;292:994.

Weller TH, Neva FA. Propagation in tissue culture of cytopathic agents from patients with rubella-like illness. Proc Soc Exp Biol Med 1962;111:215.

Zimmerman LA, Reef SE, McCauley MM. Control and prevention of rubella: evaluation and management of suspected outbreaks, rubella in pregnant women, and surveillance for congenital rubella syndrome. MMWR Recomm Rep 2001;50:1-23.

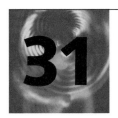

31 SEPSIS IN THE NEWBORN

MORVEN S. EDWARDS AND CAROL J. BAKER

Classically defined, neonatal sepsis or septicemia is a clinical syndrome in the first month of life manifested by systemic signs of infection and isolation of a pathogen from the bloodstream (Baker, 1986). Both clinical and laboratory definitions have been proposed (Gaynes et al., 1996). Primary bloodstream infection is documented in some healthy-appearing newborns (Wiswell et al., 1995), and in other neonates clinical sepsis without bacteremia occurs, especially if the mother has received antimicrobial agents before delivery. The improved survival of very low–birth-weight infants has rendered the postnatal age limit of 1 month impractical. It is recognized that "neonatal" sepsis occurs at least until the postconceptual age of 1 month post term and occasionally longer in the extremely low–birth-weight infant. For the purpose of this review, the neonatal period will include both the first month of life for the term infant and 1 month after hospital discharge for those infants born prematurely. The clinical presentation and management of sepsis will consider both types of infants.

Reported incidence rates for proved neonatal sepsis range from 1 to 8 cases per 1,000 live births (Stoll et al., 1996b). The incidence and the case-fatality rates both are inversely related to birth weight and to gestational age. Case-fatality rates have fallen dramatically in the past quarter century in association with improved early recognition and technologic and therapeutic advances in the care of newborn infants, especially those born before 37 weeks of gestation.

Two patterns based on age at onset of signs of sepsis have been recognized historically. The designations early-onset and late-onset neonatal sepsis, originally applied to neonatal group B streptococcal infections (Baker et al., 1973) were later used for neonatal listeriosis and subsequently for sepsis caused by other pathogens. These remain useful designations, because there are distinguishing characteristics such as risk factors, source of acquisition of infecting organisms, and clinical presentation that vary with the postnatal age at onset (Table 31-1). The term *very late–onset* has come into increasingly common use to designate a third category of neonatal sepsis. These infants usually are extremely low–birth-weight survivors who remain hospitalized for several weeks after birth. The major factor enhancing sepsis risk in these infants is the ongoing violation of anatomic and mucosal barriers to infection by the intravascular access catheters required for their care, prolonged exposure to antimicrobial agents, and ongoing immature host defense mechanisms. Despite the frequency with which very late–onset infection occurs, the associated fatality rate is low, estimated at less than 5%.

ETIOLOGY

Ongoing surveillance for the past three quarters of a century has documented shifts in the etiologic agents causing neonatal sepsis. Group A *Streptococcus* was the predominant pathogen in the 1930s and 1940s; this was replaced in the 1950s by *Escherichia coli*. The late 1950s and early 1960s witnessed outbreaks of *Staphylococcus aureus* sepsis (Freedman et al., 1981). *E. coli* experienced a resurgence in the late 1960s, and group B *Streptococcus*, then newly recognized as a human pathogen, appeared. In the 1970s several centers noted that the overall incidence of neonatal sepsis had increased, as group B *Streptococcus* added to rather than supplanted infections caused by *E. coli*.

For the past 30 years group B *Streptococcus* has remained the most frequent pathogen causing early-onset neonatal sepsis (Table 31-2). The

TABLE 31-1 Patterns of Neonatal Sepsis

Characteristic	Early onset	Late onset	Very late onset
Onset	Less than 7 days of age (usually first 48 h)	7 to 30 days	30 days to discharge
Gestation	25% <37 weeks	Often full term	Usually <30 weeks
Risk factors	Maternal intrapartum complications common	Often none	Prematurity
Source of organism	Maternal genital tract	Maternal genital tract, nosocomial, or community	Nosocomial, community
Usual clinical presentation	Nonspecific signs or respiratory distress	Focal or nonspecific signs	Focal or nonspecific signs
Case-fatality ratio	10%-20%	5%-10%	<5%

overall prevalence of *E. coli* sepsis has declined, but it remains the second most common causative agent and the most frequent gram-negative organism. Recognition that shifts do occur has prompted ongoing surveillance of bloodstream isolates in the newborn (Gladstone et al., 1990). Among gram-positive organisms, group B streptococci dominated in the early 1980s and are still the dominant cause of early-

onset cases. Other streptococci, including occasional group A, C, or G streptococci, viridans streptococci, *Enterococcus*, and *Streptococcus pneumoniae*, are less frequent causal agents.

Among gram-negative organisms, a multi-center report of very low–birth-weight neonates (401 to 1500 g) admitted to the 12 National Institute of Child Health and Human Development (NICHD) Neonatal Research

TABLE 31-2 Etiologic Agents in Early-Onset Neonatal Sepsis

Organism	PERCENT OF PATIENTS BY YEAR STUDIED			
	1966 to 1978[*]	1979 to 1988[†]	1991 to 1993[‡]	1996 to 1999[§]
Gram-Positive Organisms				
Group B *Streptococcus*	46	55	31	45
Enterococcus	3	4	0	3
Viridans streptococci	1	2	9	6
Other streptococci	3	3	7	5
Staphylococcus aureus	2	1	3	5
Coagulase-negative staphylococci	0	1	7	0
Gram-Negative Organisms				
Escherichia coli	23	14	16	23
Klebsiella or *Klebsiella-Enterobacter*	5	1	5	5
Haemophilus influenzae	6	8	11	3
Other gram-negatives	4	4	10	3
Other, Mixed, or Nonspecified	7	7	1	2
TOTAL (number of infants)	100 (137)	100 (93)	100 (147)	100 (170)

[*]Data from Freedman et al.: Am J Dis Child 1981;135:140. Refers to infants born at Yale–New Haven Hospital who were less than 48 hours of age at time of culture.
[†]Data from Gladstone et al.: Pediatr Infect Dis J 1990;9:820. Refers to infants born at Yale–New Haven Hospital who were 4 days of age or less at time of culture.
[‡]Data from Stoll et al.: J Pediatr 1996a;129:72. Refers to very low–birth-weight infants (≤1500 g) from whom cultures were obtained within 72 hours of life.
[§]Data from Baltimore RS et al. Pediatrics 2001; 108:1094, Refers to infants in the Connecticutt statewide surveillance program who were 6 days of age or less at the time of culture.

Network centers during a 32-month period from 1991 to 1993 noted *E. coli* to be the dominant early-onset pathogen (Stoll et al., 1996a). Nontypeable *Haemophilus influenzae* was recognized as an early-onset pathogen in the 1970s, and it accounts for approximately 1% to 3% of cases.

In the 1990s, a shift in serotype prevalence among group B streptococci occurred. A newly recognized serotype, type V, was observed and now causes approximately 15% of cases of infection overall (Harrison et al., 1998). Taken together, group B *Streptococcus* serotypes Ia, III, and V account for nearly 85% of disease-causing strains in infancy (Zaleznik et al., 1999). *Listeria monocytogenes* is conspicuously absent from listings of agents causing early-onset neonatal sepsis. Although it is a "classic" pathogen, it remains an uncommon one. In our inborn delivery service of approximately 9,000 infants yearly, one or two cases of listeriosis are documented. Some of these are linked epidemiologically to contaminated dairy products. Although it is eclipsed in frequency by the more common pathogens, *Listeria* is an etiologic agent to consider because its clinical and epidemiologic features are distinctive.

In contrast to the relatively modest shifts in early-onset etiologic agents, the pathogens causing late-onset sepsis in the newborn infant have shifted dramatically over the decades (Table 31-3). Coagulase-negative staphylococci have become the single most frequent cause of late-onset sepsis in low–birth-weight neonates (Gaynes et al., 1996). In the series reported by Gladstone et al. (1990), coagulase-negative staphylococci accounted for 19% of all late-onset and 43% of very late–onset infection. Coagulase-negative staphylococci comprised a majority of cases in collaborative studies conducted during the 1990s (Makhoul et al., 2002; Stoll et al., 1996b). It is likely that this shift has been caused by a change in the population at risk, with its lower birth weight and gestational age, and not by a change in virulence of these commensals. The need for prolonged use of central venous catheters in the very low–birth-weight infant enhances the risk for catheter-associated bacteremia that often is caused by coagulase-negative staphylococci.

S. aureus continues to be an important cause of late-onset neonatal sepsis. Focal signs of infection usually are evident, and the likelihood that infecting isolates will be methicillin

TABLE 31-3 Etiologic Agents in Late-Onset Neonatal Sepsis				
	PERCENT OF PATIENTS BY YEAR STUDIED			
Organism	*1966 to 1978*[*]	*1979 to 1988*[†]	*1991 to 1993*[‡]	*1995 to 1998*[§]
Gram-Positive Organisms				
Coagulase-negative staphylococci	0	21	55	47
Staphylococcus aureus	9	7	9	4
Enterococcus	3	9	5	3
Group B *Streptococcus*	10	6	2	0
Other	0	5	2	1
Gram-Negative Organisms				
Enterobacter or *Klebsiella*	23	16	8	19
Escherichia coli	37	21	4	3
Pseudomonas	4	6	2	4
Other	2	2	4	6
Candida spp.	0	6	7	11
Other, mixed, or nonspecified	12	1	2	2
TOTAL (number of infants)	100 (197)	100 (110)	100 (2355)	100 (1453)

[*]Data from Freedman et al.: Am J Dis Child 1981;135:140. Refers to infants born at or transported to Yale–New Haven Hospital who were more than 48 hours and less than 30 days old at time of culture.
[†]Data from Gladstone et al.: Pediatr Infect Dis J 1990;9:820. Refers to infants who were 5 or more days of age when cultures were obtained.
[‡]Data from Stoll et al.: J Pediatr 1996a;129:63. Refers to very low–birth-weight (VLBW) infants (≤1500 g) who were more than 72 hours of age when cultures were obtained.
[§]Data from Makhoul IR et al. Pediatrics 2003; 109:34. Refers to VLBW infants who were more than 72 hours of age when cultures were obtained.

resistant has increased. This concern requires knowledge of susceptibility patterns of *S. aureus* isolates in a particular intensive care unit. Enterococci emerged as prominent late-onset pathogens in the 1990s. These intrinsically low-virulence organisms are increasingly encountered in infants with late-onset sepsis (Dobson and Baker, 1990; McNeeley et al., 1996; Stoll et al., 1996b). Their plasmid-mediated and intrinsic capacities to acquire resistance to commonly employed antimicrobial agents, including vancomycin, pose a substantial threat to the newborn (Murray, 1990). Debilitated hosts, such as those with necrotizing enterocolitis and those requiring prolonged central vascular access, are at substantial risk for enterococcal infection. Group B streptococci causing late-onset sepsis may have been acquired vertically at time of delivery or nosocomially through hand contact in the nursery (Noya et al., 1987).

Taken as a group, gram-negative organisms are less likely to cause late-onset sepsis than in the past. Those commonly encountered, including *Enterobacter*, *Klebsiella*, *Pseudomonas*, and *Serratia* species, may exhibit multiple antibiotic resistance patterns. Nosocomial acquisition is the rule, and each of these organisms has been documented as a cause of nursery outbreaks (Campbell et al., 1992; Cook et al., 1980).

Fungal infections, especially those caused by *Candida* and *Aspergillus*, are encountered with increasing frequency in the nursery as late-onset pathogens. *Candida albicans* and *Candida parapsilosis* are the most common species, but others, such as *Candida tropicalis* and *Candida glabrata*, also are reported (Kossoff et al., 1998). *Aspergillus* species may cause a sepsislike presentation or a focal infection, such as a distinctive invasive dermatitis (Rowen et al., 1992). Because the presenting features often are indistinguishable from those of bacterial disease, these fungi should be considered as potential pathogens and appropriate diagnostic procedures should be initiated.

PATHOLOGY

Newborn infants with overwhelming early-onset sepsis often have such a rapidly fatal course that there has been insufficient time elapsed for evidence of an inflammatory response histologically. The cause of death in these patients usually is irreversible shock.

Accompanying findings may include periventricular leukomalacia and intraventricular hemorrhage, scattered areas of hepatic necrosis, and renal or adrenal hemorrhage or necrosis (Klein, 2001). The histopathologic findings in the lungs of newborns with fatal early-onset sepsis have been defined for infection caused by group B streptococci. These organisms may colonize hyaline membranes without accompanying pneumonitis. Alternatively there may be histologic evidence of extensive acute pneumonia or of mild diffuse or focal pneumonia with or without evidence of surfactant deficiency.

With late-onset infection, focal inflammation in affected organ systems often is evident. The most important of these is meningitis, in which exudate may be found around the base of the brain and involving the ependymal and subependymal tissues. Often, widespread vasculitis, hemorrhage, and venous thromboses are found. Gram-negative enteric pathogens, and less often group B streptococci, may cause central nervous system devastation, with hemorrhagic meningoencephalitis often followed by widespread necrosis and liquefaction of the brain.

PATHOGENESIS

The pathogenesis of neonatal sepsis is modulated by factors that are extrinsic to the infant and by those that are intrinsic. For early-onset infection, maternal obstetric events are the key extrinsic factors that affect infection risk, whereas for late-onset infection, the iatrogenic factors required to sustain life in low–birth-weight infants dominate.

Extrinsic Factors

Heading the list of extrinsic factors that predispose to early-onset infection is preterm delivery. The risk of early-onset sepsis is increased 10 to 15 times if gestation is less than 37 weeks. This relates in part to the role of transplacentally acquired maternal IgG, because active IgG transport does not begin until 32 weeks of gestation. Risk to the infant also is inversely related to duration of membrane rupture. Rupture of membranes more than 18 hours predisposes to acquisition of infection by the ascending route. An infant born to a woman with intraamniotic infection or chorioamnionitis has a 1% to 5% chance of developing early-onset sepsis. This risk increases to 5% to 15% if prematurity or prolonged rupture of membranes coexist. Premature rupture of membranes before onset of labor at any gestation also increases the risk for early-onset sepsis. Intrapartum maternal fever, within 24 hours before or after delivery, often heralds maternal infection including chorioamnionitis, bacteremia, or endometritis caused by organisms that also may cause early-onset sepsis (e.g., group B *Streptococcus* or *E. coli*).

Women with group B streptococci isolated from the urine during pregnancy usually are heavily colonized with these organisms and are at increased risk for delivering an infant with early-onset infection. Sepsis risk for group B *Streptococcus* also is enhanced when infants are born to women less than 20 years of age or to those who have received no prenatal care (Schuchat et al., 1994). Other significant correlates with neonatal disease are black or Hispanic ethnicity and a birth weight less than 2,500 g (Zaleznik et al., 1999).

Intrauterine monitoring devices or abrasions resulting from obstetric forceps may provide a portal of entry for maternal genital organisms to invade. The actual risk probably is quite small. Because internal monitors nearly always are used in the setting of other potential maternal risk factors, such as prolonged labor or membrane rupture, separating the risk attributable to this variable is difficult.

A consideration of extrinsic factors for late-onset sepsis differs when the neonate is admitted to the hospital from home. These infants typically were born at term, without known maternal risk factors for infection, and then develop signs of sepsis at 7 to 30 days of age. In contrast, the long-term intensive care nursery resident usually has undergone numerous invasive procedures including endotracheal intubation, umbilical vessel catheterization, placement of a central or percutaneous vascular device, transcutaneous oxygen monitoring, feeding tube placement, and frequent blood sampling. Each of these may promote bloodstream invasion by organisms colonizing skin or mucous membranes. In addition, the frequent use of antimicrobial agents, often for prolonged courses based on suspected or proved infection, enhances the risk for overgrowth of commensals (including *Candida*) and colonization with microorganisms resistant to frequently administered agents (e.g., ampicillin, gentamicin, cephalosporins).

Intrinsic Factors

Humoral immunity in the full-term newborn consists almost entirely of maternal IgG, providing an array of antibodies qualitatively similar to and quantitatively slightly higher than maternal. Maternal IgG is proportionately decreased in the preterm infant. Although passive transport occurs as early as 8 weeks of gestation, active transport does not begin until about 32 weeks. Very low–birth-weight (<1500 g) infants have relatively low IgG concentrations that decline to less than 100 mg/dl by age 3 to 4 months and gradually increase beginning at 24 weeks of age when endogenous production begins. IgA and IgM are not transported transplacentally, but the fetus has the capacity to synthesize these immunoglobulins in response to intrauterine infection; without this stimulus, however, endogenous production mirrors the delayed postnatal synthesis noted for IgG.

Complement proteins are important in humoral immune defense, particularly against bacterial pathogens. These proteins are not transplacentally transferred but are synthesized in the fetal liver as early as the first trimester. At term, classical complement pathway component concentrations in serum are similar to or slightly lower than those in older infants or adults. Levels of alternative pathway components, including factor B and properdin, range from 30% to 60% of adult normal values in full-term infants and are proportionately lower in preterm infants. Because the classical pathway usually is initiated by antigen-antibody complexes, deficient function may be caused by the lack of an appropriate initiating factor. Although the integrity of the complement pathways may be intact in the neonate, varying degrees of functional impairment have been described. For example, aberrant function of the thioester bond has been proposed as an explanation for low quantities of functional C3 in term and preterm newborns (Zach and Hostetter, 1989).

The monocyte-macrophage system consists of circulating monocytes and tissue macrophages of the reticuloendothelial system. The function of macrophages in the reticuloendothelial system of the neonate has not been extensively studied. However, damaged erythrocytes are not removed efficiently from the circulation. Because the terminal saccharides of some neonatal pathogens (*E. coli* and group B streptococci) and senescent red blood cells are quite similar, a deficiency in reticuloendothelial system–mediated bacterial clearance is presumed. The number of circulating monocytes is normal, but their chemotaxis is impaired. Mixed mononuclear cells from newborn infants are deficient in their ability to produce interferon-γ or interleukin-8 in response to group B streptococci when their function is compared with that of cells from adults (Joyner et al., 2000; Rowen et al., 1995). In contrast, comparable amounts of tumor necrosis factor-α (TNF-α) are produced by monocytes from neonates and adults (Williams et al., 1993). Gram-positive and gram-negative bacteria induce TNF-α biosynthesis through a pathway that involves p38 mitogen-activated protein kinase and increased activation of nuclear factor-κβ (Vallejo et al., 2000).

The number of circulating neutrophils is elevated in both premature and full-term infants at birth, peaking at 12 hours and returning to baseline by 72 hours of age. Increased numbers of immature neutrophils are found in neonatal sepsis. These reflect release from the neutrophil storage pool, which is more rapidly depleted in the newborn than in the older infant and in the premature than the full-term infant (Christensen et al., 1982). A number of functional defects have been described for neonatal neutrophils, including adherence, aggregation, movement, phagocytosis, and intracellular killing (Hill, 1987). The current consensus is that "stress-ing" of neutrophils by insults such as sepsis or hypoxemia decreases phagocytic activity for gram-negative and bactericidal activity for both gram-positive and gram-negative organisms. A myriad of developmental defects in signal transduction, cytoskeletal rigidity, oxidative metabolism, and cell surface receptor upregulation, to name several, contribute to the observed abnormalities in functional capacity of the neonatal neutrophil.

CLINICAL MANIFESTATIONS

The clinical manifestations of neonatal sepsis characteristically are subtle and generalized (Table 31-4). A minimal deviation from the baseline state should be viewed as a possible sign of infection. Even when focal infection exists, this often is not evident early in the course, and repeated physical examinations with special attention to the skin, soft tissues, joints, and abdomen are necessary.

Alterations in Temperature

Fever is not reliably present in neonates with septicemia. Among the 455 infants comprising the four case series summarized in Table 31-4, fever was a presenting feature in only one half. The generally accepted definition of fever is a rectal temperature exceeding 38.0° C (100.4° F). Bonadio (1987) found that none of 54 infants less than 4 weeks of age with a history of fever, but who were afebrile at evaluation in the emergency department, had sepsis. In contrast,

TABLE 31-4	Clinical Signs of Neonatal Sepsis in 455 Newborn Infants
Clinical sign	*Percentage of infants with sign*
Hyperthermia	51
Hypothermia	15
Lethargy	25
Irritability	16
Respiratory distress	33
Apnea	22
Cyanosis	24
Jaundice	35
Hepatomegaly	33
Anorexia	28
Vomiting	25
Abdominal distention	17
Diarrhea	

From Klein JO. Bacterial sepsis and meningitis. In Remington JS, Klein JO (eds). Infectious diseases of the fetus and newborn infant, ed 5. Philadelphia: Saunders, 2001.

15% of infants with documented fever at presentation had serious bacterial infection. As with older children, the magnitude of fever is predictive of seriousness of bacterial infection (Bonadio et al., 1990). A substantial subset of newborns, particularly premature infants, is more likely to develop hypothermia as a manifestation of sepsis. Often hypothermia persists despite all attempts to correct potential external contributing factors. Taken together, two thirds of neonates with sepsis can be expected to manifest alterations in the core body temperature.

Nonspecific Signs of Sepsis

Often it is a mother or a member of the nursing staff who first observes that an infant is "off his feeds," "sleeping more than usual," "fussy," or "just not right." The very nonspecificity of these signs is a hallmark of neonatal sepsis. Tachycardia or bradycardia, hypotension, or poor peripheral perfusion are later and more ominous, sometimes irreversible, signs suggesting neonatal sepsis. Although these on occasion may suggest focal infection involving the myocardium or pericardium, more often they indicate generalized sepsis with secondary cardiac dysfunction rather than cardiac disease.

Respiratory Signs

Respiratory abnormalities, including signs such as tachypnea, grunting, retractions, cyanosis, and nasal flaring, are suggestive of sepsis, either in the presence or absence of coexisting pulmonary immaturity. Apnea in an otherwise asymptomatic full-term infant is a sensitive, although late, sign of early-onset sepsis caused by group B streptococci.

Hepatic Signs

Jaundice, usually manifested as unconjugated hyperbilirubinemia, is a frequent finding, occurring in one third of neonates with proven gram-positive or gram-negative sepsis. Hepatomegaly, often striking, is observed with the same frequency. One must remember that a liver edge palpable up to 2 cm below the right costal margin is normal for full-term newborns.

Gastrointestinal Signs

Gastrointestinal signs are common in neonates with sepsis. Decreased feeding, weak suck, vomiting, or gastric residuals after nasogastric tube feeding often are observed (Table 31-4).

Abdominal distention is possibly related to intestinal ileus. Early in the course, it may be difficult to distinguish between infants who have sepsis without an intestinal focus and those with an intraabdominal process, such as necrotizing enterocolitis. Diarrhea is relatively uncommon, but guaiac-positive stools may be observed either with necrotizing enterocolitis or with sepsis.

Central Nervous System Signs

Meningitis less frequently accompanies neonatal sepsis than was the case in the 1980s. This most likely is a result of earlier initiation of empiric therapy (Shattuck and Chonmaitree, 1992). In describing the changing spectrum of group B streptococcal infection, Yagupsky et al. (1991) documented meningitis in only 15% of infants. More recent data suggest that this has been reduced to 3% of infants with early-onset infection (Schrag et al., 2000). Most infants with early-onset meningitis have nonspecific findings, including episodes of tachycardia or bradycardia, acidosis, irritability, or lethargy. Specific central nervous system signs, such as seizures, hypertonia or hypotonia, or bulging of the anterior fontanelle, are found in a minority. These are observed proportionately more often in late-onset meningitis. Overall, seizures occur in 40% of neonates with meningitis, full or bulging fontanelle in 28%, and nuchal rigidity in 15% (Klein, 2001). Seizures typically are subtle and focal.

Cutaneous and Mucous Membrane Signs

The skin and mucous membranes should be examined carefully for the clues that accompany infection in a minority of infants. These are distinctive enough that their presence often establishes a provisional diagnosis. Careful examination may reveal a pustular lesion, suggesting staphylococcal infection, or a focus of infection such as a soft-tissue abscess at a former intravenous or surgical site, omphalitis, or arthritis, focal sites from which a specimen for culture should be obtained as a part of the diagnostic evaluation. The nodular or necrotic-centered lesions typical of ecthyma gangrenosum suggest gram-negative sepsis caused by *Pseudomonas aeruginosa* or *Serratia marcescens*. However, similar lesions also have been observed in disseminated fungal infection. On occasion, these nodular lesions may have the appearance of a "cold abscess." A distinctive cutaneous presentation consisting of erythematous plaquelike or scaly lesions is characteristic of invasive fungal dermatitis caused by *C. albicans, Aspergillus*, and occasionally other fungal saphrophytes in premature infants (Rowen et al., 1992). Listeriosis may be accompanied by small, noninflammatory pustular or papular, well-circumscribed cutaneous lesions. The finding of vesicular lesions on the skin or mucous membranes is virtually pathognomonic of herpes simplex, although similar lesions may be observed with neonatal varicella, coxsackievirus infections or some noninfectious dermatologic disorders. Petechial and purpuric lesions are more often manifestations of generalized sepsis with thrombocytopenia or disseminated intravascular coagulopathy than of embolic phenomena, especially in premature infants with fragile blood vessels and thin integument.

DIAGNOSIS
Microbiologic Techniques

The gold standard establishing the diagnosis of neonatal sepsis is the isolation of a pathogen from one or more blood cultures. The minimum blood volume required depends on the intensity of bacteremia (inoculum size). In newborn infants the optimal blood volume for culture is at least 0.75 to 1.0 ml (Neal et al., 1986). Documentation of sepsis will be "missed" in 10% to 15% of infected infants when only one blood culture is obtained, but most experts feel that it is not practical or feasible to defer therapy while a second blood specimen is obtained. In those infants with a clinical course consistent with sepsis and a single sterile blood culture, sepsis is presumed and a course of therapy is completed.

Improvements in laboratory devices to monitor incubating blood cultures from newborn infants and in culture media have reduced the time required for detection of positive blood culture results. One computer-assisted, automated blood culture system identified 77%, 89%, and 94% of all 455 microorganisms at 24, 36, and 48 hours of incubation, respectively, in aerobic cultures obtained from full-term and preterm infants (Garcia-Prats et al., 2000). In another study, virtually all organisms (28 of 29) categorized as definite pathogens were identified within 48 hours (Kurlat et al., 1989). If the laboratory reports a negative culture, consideration can be given to reducing the duration of empiric therapy to 24 to 36 hours in term, asymptomatic infants undergoing evaluation for suspected early-onset sepsis because of the presence of maternal risk factors. With suspected late-onset infection, some *S. epidermidis* and yeast are not identified from blood cultures until after 48 hours of incubation.

Because the most frequent signs in neonates with proven meningitis are not specific for the central nervous system, a lumbar puncture is recommended in the evaluation of all neonates with possible sepsis. If the infant's condition is unstable, the procedure can be deferred and the infant should be treated as if there were coexistent meningitis until the clinical condition permits exclusion of this diagnosis. In one review, 6 of 39 infants (38%) with culture-proved meningitis caused by group B streptococci, *S. aureus*, or gram-negative rods had negative blood cultures (Visser and Hall, 1980).

It has been noted that meningitis is infrequently documented in healthy-appearing full-term infants evaluated at birth because maternal risk factors are reported (Fielkow et al., 1991) or in preterm infants with symptoms of respiratory distress (Weiss et al., 1991). Some experts propose omission of the lumbar puncture in evaluating such infants. However, Wiswell et al. (1995) observed that up to one-third of cases of meningitis in neonates less than 7 days of age would have been "missed" or delayed if examination of the cerebrospinal fluid had been omitted. The decision to perform a lumbar puncture is one that requires consideration of the limited risk of the procedure against the benefit of documenting the diagnosis of meningitis, a diagnosis that dictates a different approach to management and prognosis. Based on currently available data, we believe that a lumbar puncture should always be performed to exclude meningitis, ideally when the infant undergoes initial evaluation for sepsis before illness progression will not permit this procedure or soon after appropriate specific and supportive therapy is initiated for the presumptive diagnosis of meningitis.

Culture of urine is not recommended in evaluation of early-onset sepsis, because positive cultures reflect bacteremia rather than true infection. By contrast, urine obtained by catheterization or suprapubic bladder aspiration should always be a part of the evaluation of infants for late-onset infection because this may be the primary source of sepsis (Visser and Hall, 1979). Cultures from body surfaces, such as the ear canal, nasopharynx, umbilicus, or rectum, have no role in the evaluation of possible neonatal sepsis. They are poorly predictive of blood culture results and add unnecessary expense (Evans et al., 1988).

Laboratory Aids

Because clinical signs of sepsis are subtle and culture results may not be available for up to 48 hours, a number of sepsis screening tests, employed singly or together, have been proposed to aid in the diagnosis of and duration of therapy for suspected neonatal sepsis. Although these may provide useful information, none has proved sufficiently sensitive to reliably predict infection. Clinical judgment ultimately dictates which infants require evaluation and empiric treatment for neonatal sepsis. However, the screening tests summarized in Table 31-5 may provide information to assist in decision making.

The complete blood count (CBC) is the most thoroughly evaluated and easily performed sepsis screening test. White blood cell (WBC) count reference values are defined and provide range of normal values within the first hours and days of age (Klein, 2001). When consid-

ered independently of age, a WBC more than $20,000/mm^3$ or less than $5,000/mm^3$ identifies infants at risk for sepsis. A low total neutrophil (PMN) count of less than $4,000/mm^3$ suggests depletion of bone marrow reserves and may be an early indicator of overwhelming sepsis. The sensitivity of the ratio of the absolute number of immature to total PMNs (I:T ratio) is modest, but its negative predictive value is high. Nonetheless, initiation of empiric antimicrobial therapy in a healthy, full-term neonate for one of the above abnormalities is infrequent. Thus, these WBC indices should be used in the context of maternal risk factors, infant gestational age, and clinical status.

Hepatocytes stimulated by interleukin-1 rapidly synthesize large amounts of proteins collectively known as acute phase reactants (Klein, 1994). Some have been studied extensively in the evaluation of neonatal sepsis and are included in Table 31-5. None is a sufficiently sensitive indicator of neonatal sepsis to advocate its routine use.

The proinflammatory cytokines, including interleukin-1β, interleukin-6, TNF-α, and leukotriene B4, are elicited early in the course of bacterial infection being produced by peripheral blood monocytes, macrophages, and neutrophils.

TABLE 31-5	Screening Tests for Sepsis: Uses and Limitations	
Test	*Findings supporting possible infection*	*Comment(s)*
Total white blood cell (WBC) count	$<5,000/mm^3$ or $>20,000/mm^3$	Less than half of those with finding have proved infection
Total neutrophil (PMN) count	$<4,000/mm^3$	Particularly useful in first hours of life
Total immature PMN count	$>1,100/mm^3$ (cord blood); $>1,500/mm^3$ (12 h); $>600/mm^3$ (>60 h)	Relatively insensitive; finding unusual in uninfected infants
Immature to total PMN ratio (I:T ratio)	>0.2	Sensitivity 30%-90%; good negative predictive value
Platelet count	$<100,000/mm^3$	Insensitive, nonspecific, and late finding
C-reactive protein (CRP)	>1.0 mg/dl	Sensitivity 50%-90%
Erythrocyte sedimentation rate (ESR)	>5 mm/h (first 24 h); age in days plus 3 mm/h (through age 14 days); 10-20 mm/h (>2 wk of age)	Individual laboratories must establish normal values; normal value varies inversely with hematocrit
Fibronectin	<120-145 µg/ml	Sensitivity 30%-70%
Haptoglobin	>10 mg/dl (cord blood); >50 mg/dl (after delivery)	Unreliable because of poor sensitivity

From Edwards MS, Baker CJ. Bacterial infections in the neonate. In Long SS, Pickering LK, Prober CG (eds). Principles and practice of pediatric infectious diseases, ed 2. New York: Churchill Livingstone, 2002.

Several investigators have documented elevations of one or more of these cytokines or their receptors in neonatal sepsis (Spear et al., 1995; Vallejo et al., 1996; Williams et al., 1993). Whether these responses occur early and reliably enough in the course of neonatal sepsis to warrant their use as diagnostic tests awaits additional study.

The acute-phase C-reactive protein (CRP) is synthesized in the liver in response to inflammatory cytokines. The elevation of CRP provides a relatively sensitive indicator of infection. Because of its short half-life, the return of elevated serum concentrations of CRP to the normal range (<1.0 mg/dl) may be a useful parameter to minimize the duration of antibiotic therapy in newborns with suspected bacterial infection (Philip and Mills, 2000).

TREATMENT

Treatment for suspected neonatal sepsis should be initiated promptly once diagnostic studies have been obtained. Initial therapy is dictated by the infant's age, physical location at onset of signs (community or nursery), and focus of infection, if present (Table 31-6). Antimicrobial agents are selected based on the most likely pathogens and their expected antimicrobial susceptibility patterns. The dosages suggested and their intervals of administration take into account the expected renal immaturity of neonates, especially very low–birth-weight infants.

Nonbacterial agents that may cause a sepsis syndrome also should be considered. If disseminated herpes simplex infection is a consideration in the neonate, acyclovir (20 mg/kg/8 h) should be initiated while viral culture results are pending (Kimberlin et al., 2001). Cultures (skin lesions, conjunctiva, mouth, buffy coat) usually yield the virus within 48 to 72 hours, and if the diagnosis is excluded, acyclovir therapy can be discontinued. Disseminated enteroviral infection may mimic disseminated herpes simplex infection in the neonate. Both

---

TABLE 31-6 **Empiric Antimicrobial Therapy for Suspected Neonatal Sepsis**

Clinical presentation	Intravenous antibiotic(s) (dose/kg)	Interval (h)	Expected duration
Sepsis, early-onset	Ampicillin (50 mg) plus	q8	7-10 days
	gentamicin (2.5 mg)*	q12	
Sepsis, late onset (full-term infant, community acquired)	Ampicillin (50 mg) plus	q6-8	7-10 days
	gentamicin (2.5 mg)*	q8-12	
Sepsis, late onset (inpatient)	Vancomycin (15 mg) plus	q8	10-14 days
	gentamicin (2.5 mg)* or	q8	
	amikacin (15 mg)†	q8	
Meningitis, early onset	Ampicillin (100 mg) plus	q8	14-21 days
	gentamicin (2.5 mg)* plus	q8	
	cefotaxime (50 mg)	q12	
Meningitis, late onset	Ampicillin (75 mg) plus	q6	14-21 days
	gentamicin (2.5 mg)* or	q8	
	amikacin (15 mg)† plus	q8	
	cefotaxime (50 mg)‡	q6-8	
Bone or joint infection	Vancomycin (15 mg)	q6-8	3-6 weeks
	plus gentamicin (2.5 mg)*	q8	
Suspected gastrointestinal infection	Include clindamycin (10 mg) with an aminoglycoside	q6-8	10-14 days

From Edwards MS, Baker CJ. Bacterial infections in the neonate. In Long SS, Pickering LK, Prober CG (eds). Principles and practice of pediatric infectious diseases, ed 2. New York: Churchill Livingstone, 2002.
*For birth weight <1,500 g, interval may be longer. For birth weight <1,500 g, unit dosage usually is 2.5 mg/kg and interval is determined by serum levels. If given more than 72 hours, monitor serum levels to achieve a peak of 5-10 µg/ml and a trough of <2.0 µg/ml.
†For birth weight <1,500 g, interval may be longer. Monitor serum levels to achieve a peak of 25-40 µg/ml and a trough of 5-15 µg/ml. Monitor serum levels to achieve a peak of 20-35 µg/ml and a trough of <10 µg/ml.
‡Interval is q12h (first week of life), q8h (7-28 days of age), q6h (>28 days of age).

typically appear late in the first week of life, have clinical signs similar to bacterial sepsis, and should be considered especially in full-term infants. A clue to these viral infections is the rapid onset of hepatomegaly and coagulopathy. Unfortunately, therapy for enteroviral infection is supportive as no antiviral agent is available for treatment. If disseminated candidiasis is a diagnostic consideration in the neonate with late-onset infection, amphotericin B therapy usually can be deferred until blood cultures confirm this diagnosis. Exceptions to this include neonates with invasive fungal dermatitis and necrotizing enterocolitis with fungal hyphae present by stains. When used, the initial dose of amphotericin B is 0.5 mg/kg given over a 1- to 2-hour interval, and subsequent daily doses are 1 mg/kg (higher doses are necessary when aspergillosis is proved).

The initial empiric treatment of early-onset sepsis should include ampicillin and gentamicin. This same regimen is appropriate for infants admitted from the community with presumed late-onset sepsis without an evident focus. Gentamicin serum levels need not be obtained unless therapy is continued for more than 72 hours, renal function is abnormal or unstable, or the infant has a birth weight of <1,500 g. Serum gentamicin level determination should be deferred until the fifth dose, allowing for steady state distribution equilibrium. This combination therapy provides empiric coverage for the expected pathogens causing early-onset and community-acquired late-onset infection, including group B streptococcus, *E. coli*, *Enterococcus*, and *L. monocytogenes*.

The empiric treatment of late-onset sepsis in neonates who remain hospitalized depends in part on the nosocomial pathogens prevalent in a specific nursery. Because coagulase-negative staphylococci are the most frequent gram-positive organisms causing sepsis in these infants, vancomycin should be initiated pending results of cultures. This choice also is appropriate empiric therapy for those nurseries in which methicillin-resistant *S. aureus* is endemic, as well as for group B streptococci, *Enterococcus*, and viridans streptococci. The choice of aminoglycoside depends on the gram-negative pathogens common in the nursery and their susceptibility to aminoglycosides. If blood culture surveillance for the nursery indicates uniform susceptibility to gentamicin, this considerably less expensive and well tolerated agent should be employed. If

amikacin is initiated empirically and a gentamicin-susceptible gram-negative pathogen is isolated, gentamicin should be substituted when continued aminoglycoside therapy is indicated.

Routine use of third-generation cephalosporins for empiric therapy of neonatal sepsis is not recommended. Routine use of these agents as empiric therapy for early-onset neonatal sepsis has been associated with outbreaks of infection caused by multiply antibiotic-resistant enteric pathogens (de Man et al., 2000; McCracken, 1985). When employed selectively, some third-generation cephalosporins have an important role in treatment of neonatal infection. When lumbar puncture suggests meningitis, cefotaxime should be added to the regimen to provide an extended spectrum for gram-negative enterics and to provide therapeutic cerebrospinal fluid concentrations during the interval when aminoglycosides may not have attained therapeutic serum levels. Because ceftriaxone may cause biliary sludging and contribute to hyperbilirubinemia, use of this agent usually is not appropriate in the newborn.

Several caveats apply to choice of empiric therapy when a presumed or potential focus of infection accompanies sepsis. First, ampicillin in doses appropriate for meningitis should be employed until lumbar puncture results exclude meningeal infection in infants with suspected early-onset sepsis. Second, ampicillin should be added to a vancomycin-aminoglycoside regimen if listeriosis or group B streptococcal meningitis is suspected at any age, because vancomycin concentrations in the cerebrospinal fluid may not be bactericidal for these organisms (Albanyan et al., 1998). Third, an antistaphylococcal agent, vancomycin initially, should be provided as part of the regimen whenever a soft tissue, bone, or joint focus of infection is suspected. If *S. aureus* is isolated and susceptible to oxacillin, treatment is completed using nafcillin. If necrotizing enterocolitis or another abdominal focus of infection is suspected, the empiric regimen should include an antimicrobial agent with activity against anaerobes, usually clindamycin. Fourth, for certain etiologic agents, removal of an indwelling intravascular catheter will be mandatory. These agents include *Candida*, most gram-negative enteric organisms, and any microorganism when blood cultures remain positive after 48 hours of appropriate antimicrobial therapy (Benjamin, 2001). Finally, purulent collections require drainage or sepsis may persist despite medical therapy.

Once a pathogen has been identified and its antibiotic susceptibility determined, therapy can be modified and simplified (Table 31-7). Penicillin G remains the drug of choice for proved group B streptococcal infection. The suggested dose is 200,000 units/kg/day for non-meningeal and 450,000 to 500,000 units/kg/day for meningeal infections. Because the median minimal inhibitory concentration of group B streptococci to penicillin is some ten-fold higher than that of group A streptococci, these doses are chosen to optimize adequate penetration into all tissues including cerebrospinal fluid. Because *Enterococcus* is only moderately susceptible to ampicillin and because *in vitro* and *in vivo* synergy with gentamicin has been demonstrated for many strains, the combination should be continued to complete the course of therapy. Ampicillin alone is sufficient to complete therapy for *L. monocytogenes* infections. An antistaphylococcal penicillin should always be used rather than vancomycin for treatment of susceptible *S. aureus* strains because it has superior *in vitro* activity when compared to vancomycin and because unnecessary use of vancomycin will promote emergence of vancomycin-resistant *Enterococcus* and staphylococci.

Monotherapy can be used to complete treatment for many enteric gram-negative infections. For example, ampicillin may be employed for susceptible *E. coli* strains. Often an aminoglycoside is appropriate for the treatment of *Klebsiella* infections. Because strains of *Enterobacter cloacae* or *S. marcescens* rapidly may develop resistance to β-lactam antibiotics,

treatment regimens should include an aminoglycoside alone or in combination with a β-lactam, such as cefotaxime. However, the β-lactam chosen should not be employed as monotherapy. Similarly, combination therapy including an aminoglycoside and cephalosporin (e.g., ceftazidime) or an antipseudomonal penicillin is indicated for the treatment of infections caused by *P. aeruginosa*. Extended-spectrum β-lactamase-producing *E. coli* and *Klebsiella pneumoniae* are becoming increasingly prevalent in intensive care unit patients. Close monitoring of susceptibility profiles of invasive gram-negative isolates, judicious use of antimicrobial agents, and attention to barrier precautions and hand hygiene are important precautions to prevent outbreaks in neonatal units (Lautenbach et al., 2001).

Therapy should be continued for a total of 10 days for clinically suspected and proved neonatal sepsis. A minimum of 14 days of therapy is appropriate if gram-positive meningitis is documented, and a minimum of 21 days is required if the etiology is a gram-negative organism. A blood culture should be performed to document resolution of bacteremia 24 to 48 hours into antimicrobial therapy. Persistent bacteremia suggests an ongoing focus of infection (e.g., an intravascular catheter or infected thrombus) or inadequate therapy.

The duration of amphotericin B treatment for invasive fungal infection usually is a total dose of 25 to 30 mg/kg. Newborn infants usually tolerate amphotericin B without complications, but renal function and serum potassium should be monitored daily during the first several days of therapy. Renal tubular wasting of potassium may occur, but this adverse effect

TABLE 31-7   Antimicrobial Therapy of Proved Newborn Sepsis

Organism	Antibiotics of choice
Group B streptococci	Penicillin
Enterococcus	Ampicillin (if susceptible) plus gentamicin, or vancomycin plus gentamicin
Listeria monocytogenes	Ampicillin ± gentamicin
Staphylococci, coagulase positive	Vancomycin
Staphylococcus epidermidis	Vancomycin
Escherichia coli, Klebsiella, Citrobacter	Ampicillin and/or aminoglycoside or cefotaxime
Enterobacter, Serratia	Aminoglycoside in combination with a β-lactam antibiotic
Pseudomonas aeruginosa	Aminoglycoside plus ceftazidime or aminopenicillin
Anaerobic enteric organisms	Clindamycin or piperacillin

will occur in the first week of therapy. If potassium levels and renal function remain normal, monitoring can be liberalized to twice weekly. If the diagnosis of disseminated fungal infection can be excluded by renal ultrasound, ophthalmologic examination, and echocardiogram to exclude a large vessel thrombus at the tip of an indwelling catheter site, and if all blood cultures are sterile after catheter removal, a shorter course of amphotericin B therapy (approximately 10 mg/kg) is sufficient for catheter-related fungemia (Butler et al., 1990). Other antifungal agents, including lipid formulations of amphotericin B, have not been studied sufficiently to provide guidance regarding optimal dose and interval, safety, and efficacy. Their use in neonates is not recommended (American Academy of Pediatrics, 2003).

Supportive Therapy

Supportive therapy is important in the management of neonatal sepsis. Fluids and electrolytes should be carefully monitored, and hypovolemia and electrolyte abnormalities should be corrected. Shock, hypoxia, and metabolic acidosis should be identified and managed appropriately. Anticipatory ventilatory support should be employed so that adequate oxygenation of tissues is ensured. Hypoglycemia should be treated promptly. Monitoring for hyperbilirubinemia should be carried out so that phototherapy can be initiated early enough to obviate the need for exchange transfusion. Adequate caloric intake, sometimes as parenteral nutrition, is required to provide positive nitrogen balance so that tissue healing can be optimized.

Neonatal sepsis may be complicated by the development of disseminated intravascular coagulopathy. Monitoring of prothrombin and partial thromboplastin times, platelet count, hemoglobin, and fibrin-split products is important so that fresh frozen plasma, platelet, red blood cell, or whole blood transfusion can be judiciously employed.

Neutropenia caused by neutrophil storage pool depletion is associated with a poor prognosis in neonatal sepsis (Strauss, 2000). Clinical trials employing neutrophil transfusions met with variable results (Baley, 1988; Cairo, 1989), and, because of logistic considerations and concerns regarding transmission of blood-borne pathogens, leukocytes infrequently are administered. Recent technologic

advances suggest that stimulation of neonatal hematopoiesis through the administration of granulocyte colony-stimulating factor may promote improvement of neonatal neutrophil number and function, but use of these growth factors is still considered experimental.

The adjunctive treatment of neonatal sepsis with intravenous immunoglobulin (IGIV) containing specific antibodies holds therapeutic promise. Development of "pathogen-specific" products, whether polyclonal IGIV or monoclonal, would permit administration of small volumes but at potentially effective doses. Such products are under development.

PREVENTION

Potential approaches for the prevention of neonatal sepsis include prenatal interventions that promote delivery of full-term rather than premature infants, intrapartum or postpartum chemoprophylaxis, and immunoprophylaxis to confer IgG-mediated passive immunity for infants during the interval of maximum risk from maternal or nosocomial pathogens.

Although provision of prenatal care as a measure to reduce prematurity is conceptually simple, its implementation is socially complex. Furthermore, modern reproductive methods have led to an increase in the number of multiple births known to enhance the likelihood of preterm birth. A decline in the rate of preterm deliveries would reliably reduce the incidence of early-onset neonatal sepsis and would substantially drop that for late-onset nosocomial sepsis. Regarding the latter, infection control measures to minimize risk from disruption of skin and mucous membrane defense barriers and transmission of nosocomial pathogens should be encouraged. Among these, hand hygiene remains crucial.

Maternal intrapartum antibiotic prophylaxis (IAP) has been the focus of preventive measures for group B streptococcal infection (American Academy of Pediatrics, 1992). This approach was based on the randomized, controlled trial reported by Boyer and Gotoff (1986) in which intrapartum ampicillin given to high-risk women who were carriers of group B streptococci significantly reduced both early-onset disease and vertical transmission of group B streptococci. These and other controlled clinical trial data provided the basis for formulating initial guidelines for use of IAP to prevent early-onset group B streptococcal disease (American

Academy of Pediatrics, 1992). These were modified and expanded to identify candidates for IAP based either on culture screening for group B streptococci (vaginal and rectal sites) at 35 to 37 weeks gestation or on the presence of one or more risk factors (without culture screening) enhancing risk for early-onset group B streptococcal disease in the neonate (American College of Obstetricians and Gynecologists, 1996; American Academy of Pediatrics, 1997; Centers for Disease Control and Prevention, 1996). The maternal risk factors included labor onset or membrane rupture before 37 weeks of gestation, intrapartum fever ($\geq$38.0° C), and rupture of membranes 18 hours or longer before delivery. Women either with previous delivery of an infant with group B streptococcal disease or with group B streptococcal bacteriuria during pregnancy would always receive prophylaxis.

An active population-based surveillance has documented a 65% decrease in the incidence of early-onset group B streptococcal infection, from 1.7 per 1,000 live births in 1993 to 0.6 per 1,000 in 1998 (Schrag et al., 2000), an interval coinciding with the implementation consensus recommendations for maternal IAP. Despite this steep decline, in 1998 some 2,000 infants were projected to acquire early-onset group B streptococcal infection yearly in the United States. The estimated proportion of preventable early-onset group B streptococcal disease approximates 80% for the culture screening–based and 40% for the risk-based approaches (Rosenstein and Schuchat, 1997). These estimates have been verified by clinical studies conducted since the publication of the 1996 Centers for Disease Control and Prevention guidelines (Davis et al., 2001; Gilson et al., 2000; Hafner et al., 1998; Main and Slagle, 2000; Schrag et al., 2002). Updated guidelines now recommend universal culture screening for the prevention of early-onset group B streptococcal disease in neonates (CDC, 2002). The risk-based approach should be employed only in circumstances where culture screening results are not available before delivery.

The preferred regimen for maternal IAP is penicillin G, 5 million units administered intravenously initially, followed by 2.5 million units every 4 hours until delivery. Penicillin is preferable to ampicillin to discourage emergence of ampicillin-resistant *E. coli* infections in infancy (Schuchat et al., 2000). Penicillin-allergic women who are not at high risk for anaphylaxis should receive cefazolin 2 g intravenously initially and 1 g every 8 hours. For those penicillin-allergic women at high risk for anaphylaxis, clindamycin susceptibility testing, if feasible, should be performed, and if susceptibility is documented clindamycin can be used for IAP (900 mg intravenously initially and 600 mg every 8 hours). If this information is not available, vancomycin should be employed. Whatever the agent selected, the most important predictor of the efficacy of IAP is that it be administered 4 or more hours before delivery (applies only to penicillin, ampicillin, or cefazolin).

The updated 2002 guidelines clarify some aspects of the management of infants born to women who receive IAP (CDC, 2002). First, there is no evidence suggesting that IAP delays the clinical expression of early-onset group B streptococcal infection. Thus, a healthy infant with at least 38 weeks gestation and whose mother received at least 4 hours of IAP prior to delivery may be discharged home as early as 24 hours if all other discharge criteria have been met and a parent has ready access to medical care for the neonate. Next, the revised 2002 guidelines suggest that if a woman has received antimicrobial therapy for suspected chorioamnionitis, her newborn should have a full diagnostic evaluation and initiation of empiric therapy for all potential early-onset sepsis pathogens pending culture results, because in this circumstance the administration of antibiotics to the mother constitutes early treatment for infection rather than prophylaxis. A detailed algorithm for infant management is summarized in the 2003 Red Book of the American Academy of Pediatrics.

Information is limited concerning chemoprophylaxis for prevention of early-onset gram-negative sepsis. One trial conducted in Central America evaluated the effect of a single 1-g dose of intrapartum ceftriaxone compared with no treatment (Sáez-Llorens et al., 1995). Infants born to women given ceftriaxone were colonized with gram-negative bacilli (as well as group B streptococci) at a lower rate than untreated women, and there was a trend toward a lower incidence of culture-proved early-onset sepsis. Additional data are required before this approach can be recommended.

The frequent occurrence of catheter-related late-onset infection caused by coagulase-negative staphylococci has prompted the evaluation of low-dose vancomycin added to parenteral alimentation solution to prevent nosocomial gram-positive infection (Kacica et al., 1994; Spafford et al., 1994). Although a dramatic and significant reduction in the rate of catheter-related sepsis was observed, this form of chemoprophylaxis is not recommended. Concerns for development of vancomycin resistance outweigh any potential advantage.

The use of immunoprophylaxis to prevent neonatal sepsis is attractive. This approach is preferable to chemoprophylaxis because it obviates concerns regarding complications of antimicrobial use and development of resistance. A number of promising studies preceded the assessment in two prospective large clinical trials designed to determine the role of standard preparations of IGIV prophylaxis in reducing nosocomial infections in very low–birth-weight infants. One found that prophylactic use of IGIV failed to reduce the incidence of hospital-acquired infections in infants weighing <1,500 g at birth (Fanaroff et al., 1994), whereas the other showed that IGIV effected a significant reduction in the risk of nosocomial infection (Baker et al., 1992). Differences in the distribution of infectious agents, as well as the pathogen-specific content of the IGIV preparations employed, may account for the conflicting conclusions of these two trials. Currently, IGIV is not recommended for the routine prophylaxis of very low–birth-weight infants.

Even if 100% efficacious, any postpartum immunoprophylactic approach to prevention of neonatal sepsis will have nominal impact on early-onset disease. The use of maternal immunization to impart passive protection for the neonate is a realistic goal. Clinical trials of protein-polysaccharide vaccines for group B streptococci have been initiated (Baker et al., 1999; Baker et al., 2000; Baker and Rench, 2001; Paoletti et al., 2001). The model of maternal immunization for prevention of neonatal sepsis has seen success in the prevention of neonatal tetanus, and it holds promise for application not only to group B streptococcal disease but also for other bacterial pathogens causing sepsis in the newborn infant.

BIBLIOGRAPHY

Albanyan EA, Baker CJ. Is lumbar puncture necessary to exclude meningitis in neonates and young infants?: Lessons from the cellulitis-adenitis syndrome group B *Streptococcus*. Pediatrics 1998;102:985-986.

American Academy of Pediatrics Committee on Infectious Diseases. 2003 Red Book: Report of the Committee on Infectious Diseases, ed 26. Elk Grove Village, Ill: American Academy of Pediatrics, 2003.

American Academy of Pediatrics Committee on Infectious Diseases and Committee on Fetus and Newborn. Guidelines for prevention of group B streptococcal (GBS) infection by chemoprophylaxis. Pediatrics 1992;90:775-778.

American Academy of Pediatrics Committee on Infectious Diseases and Committee on Fetus and Newborn. Revised guidelines for prevention of early-onset group B streptococcal (GBS) infection. Pediatrics 1997;99:489-496.

American College of Obstetricians and Gynecologists Committe on Obstetric Practice. Prevention of early-onset group B streptococcal disease in newborns. [Opinion 173] Washington DC, 1996, ACOG. Int J Gynaecol Obstet 1996;173:1-12.

Baker CJ. Neonatal sepsis: an overview. Clinical use of intravenous immunoglobulins. London: Academic Press, 1986.

Baker CJ. Neonatal sepsis: an overview. In Imbach P (ed). Immunotherapy with Intravenous Immunoglobulins. London: Academic Press, 1991.

Baker CJ, Rench MA. Safety and immunogenicity of group B streptococcal (GBS) type III capsular polysaccharide (CPS)-tetanus toxoid (III-TT) conjugate vaccine in pregnant women. Clin Infect Dis 2001;33:1151(A370).

Baker CJ, Barrett FF, Gordon RL, Yow MD. Suppurative meningitis due to streptococci of Lancefield group B: a study of 33 infants. J Pediatr 1973;82:724-729.

Baker CJ, Melish ME, Hall RT, et al. Intravenous immune globulin for the prevention of nosocomial infection in low–birth-weight neonates. N Engl J Med 1992;327:213-219.

Baker CJ, Paoletti LC, Rench MA, et al. Use of capsular polysaccharide-tetanus toxoid conjugate vaccine for type II group B *Streptococcus* in healthy women. J Infect Dis 2000;182:1129-1138.

Baker CJ, Paoletti LC, Wessels MR, et al. Safety and immunogenicity of capsular polysaccharide-tetanus toxoid conjugate vaccines for group B streptococcal types Ia and Ib. J Infect Dis 1999;179:142-150.

Baley JE. Neonatal sepsis: the potential for immunotherapy. Clin Perinatol 1988;15:755-771.

Baltimore RS, Huie SM, Meek JI, et al. Early-onset neonatal sepsis in the era of group B streptococcal prevention. Pediatrics 2001;108:1094-1098.

Benjamin DK Jr, Miller W, Garges H, et al. Bacteremia, central catheters, and neonates: when to pull the line. Pediatrics 2001;107:1272-1276.

Blumberg HM, Stephens DS, Modansky M, et al. Invasive group B streptococcal disease: the emergence of serotype V. J Infect Dis 1996;173:365-373.

Bonadio WA. Incidence of serious infections in afebrile neonates with a history of fever. Pediatr Infect Dis J 1987;6:911-914.

Bonadio WA, Romine K, Gyuro J. Relationship of fever magnitude to rate of serious bacterial infections in neonates. J Pediatr 1990;116:733-735.

Boyer KM, Gotoff SP. Prevention of early-onset neonatal group B streptococcal disease with selective intrapartum chemoprophylaxis. N Engl J Med 1986;314:1665-1669.

Butler KM, Rench MA, Baker CJ. Amphotericin B as a single agent in the treatment of systemic candidiasis in neonates. Pediatr Infect Dis J 1990;9:51-59.

Cairo MS. Neutrophil transfusions in the treatment of neonatal sepsis. Am J Pediatr Hematol Oncol 1989; 11:231-232.

Campbell JR, Diacovo T, Baker CJ. *Serratia marcescens* meningitis in neonates. Pediatr Infect Dis J 1992;11: 881-886.

Centers for Disease Control and Prevention. Prevention of perinatal group B streptococcal disease: a public health perspective. MMWR Morb Mortal Wkly Rep 1996;45:1-24.

Centers for Disease Control and Prevention, Prevention of perinatal group B streptococcal disease: revised guidelines from CDC. MMWR 2002;51(RR-11):1-22.

Cook LN, Davis RS, Stover BH. Outbreak of amikacin-resistant Enterobacteriaceae in an intensive care nursery. Pediatrics 1980;65:264-268.

Davis RL, Hasselquist MB, Cardenas V, et al. Introduction of the new Centers for Disease Control and Prevention group B streptococcal prevention guideline at a large West Coast healthy maintenance organization. Am J Obstet Gynecol 2001;184:603-610.

de Man P, Verhoeven BAN, Verbrugh HA, et al. An antibiotic policy to prevent emergence of resistant bacilli. Lancet 2000;355:973-978.

Dobson SRM, Baker CJ. Enterococcal sepsis in neonates: features by age at onset and occurrence of focal infection. Pediatrics 1990;85:165-171.

Edwards MS, Baker CJ. Bacterial infections in the neonate. In Long SS, Pickering LK, Prober CG (eds). Principles and Practice of Pediatric Infectious Diseases. New York: Churchill Livingstone, 1997.

Evans ME, Schaffner W, Federspiel CF, et al. Sensitivity, specificity, and predictive value of body surface cultures in a neonatal intensive care unit. JAMA 1988;259: 248-252.

Fanaroff AA, Korones SB, Wright LL, et al. A controlled trial of intravenous immune globulin to reduce nosocomial infections in very-low–birth-weight infants. N Engl J Med 1994;330:1107-1113.

Fielkow S, Reuter S, Gotoff SP. Cerebrospinal fluid examination in symptom-free infants with risk factors for infection. J Pediatr 1991;119:971-973.

Freedman RM, Ingram DL, Gross I, et al. A half century of neonatal sepsis at Yale, 1928 to 1978. Am J Dis Child 1981;135:140-144.

Garcia-Prats JA, Cooper TR, Schneider VF, et al. Rapid detection of microorganisms in blood cultures of newborn infants utilizing an automated blood culture system. Pediatrics 2000;105:523-527.

Gaynes RP, Edwards JR, Jarvis WR, et al. Nosocomial infections among neonates in high-risk nurseries in the United States. Pediatrics 1996;98:357-361.

Gilson GJ, Christensen K, Romero H, et al. Prevention of group B *Streptococcus* early-onset neonatal sepsis: comparison of the Centers for Disease Control and Prevention screening-based protocol to a risk-based protocol in infants at greater than 37 weeks' gestation. J Perinatol 2000;20:491-495.

Gladstone IM, Ehrenkranz RA, Edberg SC, et al. A ten-year review of neonatal sepsis and comparison with the previous fifty-year experience. Pediatr Infect Dis J 1990;9: 819-825.

Hafner E, Sterniste W, Rosen A, et al. Group B streptococci during pregnancy: a comparison of two screening and treatment protocols. Am J Obstet Gynecol 1998;179: 677-681.

Harrison LH, Elliott JA, Dwyer DM, et al. Serotype distribution of invasive group B streptococcal isolates in

Maryland: implications for vaccine formulation. Maryland Emerging Infections Program. J Infect Dis 1998;177:998-1002.

Hill HR. Biochemical, structural, and functional abnormalities of polymorphonuclear leukocytes in the neonate. Pediatr Res 1987;22:375-382.

Joyner JL, Augustine NH, Taylor KA, et al. Effects of group B streptococci on cord and adult mononuclear cell interleukin-12 and interferon-γ mRNA accumulation and protein screen. J Infect Dis 2000;182: 974-977.

Kacica MA, Horgan MJ, Ochoa L, et al. Prevention of gram-positive sepsis in neonates weighing less than 1500 grams. J Pediatr 1994;125:253-258.

Kimberlin DW, Lin C-Y, Jacobs RF, et al. Safety and efficacy of high-dose intravenous acyclovir in the management of neonatal herpes simplex virus infections. Pediatrics 2001;108:230-238.

Klein JO. Neonatal sepsis. Semin Pediatr Infect Dis 1994;5:3-8.

Klein JO. Bacterial sepsis and meningitis. In Remington JS, Klein JO (eds). Infectious Diseases of the Fetus and Newborn Infant, ed 5. Philadelphia: Saunders, 2001.

Kossoff EH, Buescher ES, Karlowicz MG. Candidemia in a neonatal intensive care unit: trends during fifteen years and clinical features of 111 cases. Pediatr Infect Dis J 1998;17:504-508.

Kurlat I, Stoll BJ, McGowan JE Jr. Time to positivity for detection of bacteremia in neonates. J Clin Microbiol 1989;27:1068-1071.

Lautenbach E, Patel JB, Bilker WB, et al. Extended-spectrum β-lactamase-producing *Escherichia coli* and *Klebsiella pneumoniae*: risk factors for infection and impact of resistance on outcomes. Clin Infect Dis 2001;32:1162-1171.

Main EK, Slagle T. Prevention of early-onset invasive neonatal group B streptococcal disease in a private hospital setting: the superiority of the culture-based protocol. Am J Obstet Gynecol 2000;182:1344-1354.

Makhoul IR, Sujov P, Smolkin T, et al. Epidemiological, clinical, and microbiological characteristics of late-onset sepsis among very low birth weight infants in Israel: a national survey. Pediatrics 2002;109:34-39.

McCracken GH Jr. Use of third-generation cephalosporins for treatment of neonatal infections. Am J Dis Child 1985;139:1079-1080.

McNeeley DF, Saint-Louis F, Noel GJ. Neonatal enterococcal bacteremia: an increasingly frequent event with potentially untreatable pathogens. Pediatr Infect Dis J 1996;15:800-805.

Murray BE. The life and times of the enterococcus. Clin Microbiol Rev 1990;3:46-65.

Neal PR, Kleiman MB, Reynolds JK, et al. Volume of blood submitted for culture from neonates. J Clin Microbiol 1986;24:353-356.

Noya FJD, Rench MA, Metzger TG, et al. Unusual occurrence of an epidemic of type Ib/c group B streptococcal sepsis in a neonatal intensive care unit. J Infect Dis 1987;155:1135-1144.

Paoletti LC, Rench MA, Kasper DL, et al. Effects of alum adjuvant or a booster dose on immunogenicity during clinical trials of group B streptococcal type III conjugate vaccines. Infect Immun 2001;69:6696-6701.

Philip AG, Mills PC. Use of C-reactive protein in minimizing antibiotic exposure: Experience with infants initially admitted to a well-baby nursery. Pediatrics 2000;106:E4.

Rosenstein NE, Schuchat A. Opportunities for prevention of perinatal group B streptococcal disease: a multistate surveillance analysis. Obstet Gynecol 1997;90:901-906.

Rowen JL, Correa AG, Sokol DM, et al. Invasive aspergillosis in neonates: report of five cases and literature review. Pediatr Infect Dis J 1992;11:576-582.

Rowen JL, Smith CW, Edwards MS. Group B streptococci elicit leukotriene B4 and interleukin-8 from human monocytes: neonates exhibit a diminished response. J Infect Dis 1995;172:420-426.

Sáez-Llorens X, Ah-Chu MS, Castaño E, et al. Intrapartum prophylaxis with ceftriaxone decreases rates of bacterial colonization and early-onset infection in newborns. Clin Infect Dis 1995;21:876-880.

Schrag SJ, Zell ER, Lynfield R, et al. A population-based comparison of strategies to prevent early-onset group B streptococcal disease in neorates. N Engl J Med 2002, 347:233-234.

Schrag SJ, Zywicki S, Farley MM, et al. Group B streptococcal disease in the era of intrapartum antibiotic prophylaxis. N Engl J Med 2000;342:15-20.

Schuchat A, Deaver-Robinson K, Plikaytis BD, et al. Multistate case-control study of maternal risk factors for neonatal group B streptococcal disease. Pediatr Infect Dis J 1994;13:623-629.

Schuchat A, Zywicki SS, Dinsmoor MJ, et al. Risk factors and opportunities for prevention of early-onset neonatal sepsis: a multicenter case-control study. Pediatrics 2000;105:21-26.

Shattuck KE, Chonmaitree T. The changing spectrum of neonatal meningitis over a fifteen-year period. Clin Pediatr 1992;31:130-136.

Spafford PS, Sinkin RA, Cox C, et al. Prevention of central venous catheter–related coagulase-negative staphylococcal sepsis in neonates. J Pediatr 1994;125:259-263.

Spear ML, Stefano JL, Fawcett P, et al. Soluble interleukin-2 receptor as a predictor of neonatal sepsis. J Pediatr 1995;126:982-985.

Stoll BJ, Gordon T, Korones SB, et al. Early-onset sepsis in very low birth weight neonates: a report from the National Institute of Child Health and Human Development Neonatal Research Network. J Pediatr 1996a;129:72-80.

Stoll BJ, Gordon T, Korones SB, et al. Late-onset sepsis in very low birth weight neonates: a report from the National Institute of Child Health and Human Development Neonatal Research Network. J Pediatr 1996b;129:63-71.

Strauss RG. Blood banking and transfusion issues in perinatal medicine. In Christensen RD (ed). Hematologic problems of the neonate. Philadelphia; Saunders, 2000, pp. 405-425.

Vallejo JG, Baker CJ, Edwards MS. Interleukin-6 production by human neonatal monocytes stimulated by type III group B streptococci. J Infect Dis 1996;174:332-337.

Vallejo JG, Kneufermann P, Mann DL, et al. Group B *Streptococcus* induces TNF-α gene expression and activation of the transcription factors NF-κβ and activator protein-1 in human cord blood monocytes. J Immunol 2000;165:419-425.

Visser VE, Hall RT. Urine culture in the evaluation of suspected neonatal sepsis. J Pediatr 1979;94:635-638.

Visser VE, Hall RT. Lumbar puncture in the evaluation of suspected neonatal sepsis. J Pediatr 1980;96:1063-1066.

Weiss MG, Ionides SP, Anderson CL. Meningitis in premature infants with respiratory distress: role of admission lumbar puncture. J Pediatr 1991;119:973-975.

Williams PA, Bohnsack JF, Augustine NH, et al. Production of tumor necrosis factor by human cells in vitro and in vivo, induced by group B streptococci. J Pediatr 1993;123:292-300.

Wiswell TE, Baumgart S, Gannon CM, et al. No lumbar puncture in the evaluation for early-onset neonatal sepsis: will meningitis be missed? Pediatrics 1995;95:803-806.

Yagupsky P, Menegus MA, Powell KR. The changing spectrum of group B streptococcal disease in infants: an eleven-year experience in a tertiary care hospital. Pediatr Infect Dis J 1991;10:801-808.

Zach TL, Hostetter MK. Biochemical abnormalities of the third component of complement in neonates. Pediatr Res 1989;26:116-120.

Zaleznik DF, Rench MA, Hillier S, et al. Invasive disease due to group B *Streptococcus* in pregnant women and neonates from diverse population groups. Clin Infect Dis 1999;30:276-281.

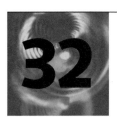

32 SEXUALLY TRANSMITTED DISEASES

Margaret R. Hammerschlag, Sarah A. Rawstron, and Kenneth Bromberg

Sexually transmitted diseases (STDs) include a wide range of infections and conditions that are transmitted mainly by sexual activity. The "classic" STDs, gonorrhea and syphilis, currently are being overshadowed by a new set of STDs that are not only more common, but more difficult to diagnose and treat. These "new" STDs include infections caused by *Chlamydia trachomatis*, human papillomavirus (HPV), and human immunodeficiency virus (HIV). Physicians are confronted by particularly complex social and clinical problems caused by STDs in neonates and infants, in abused older children, and in adolescents. Rapid application of new technology to the diagnosis of STDs has led to a growing array of diagnostic laboratory tests that require critical evaluation. This chapter presents a comprehensive overview of STDs in neonates, infants, older children, and adolescents.

STDs AND SEXUAL ABUSE OF CHILDREN

Sexual assault is a violent crime that affects men, women, and children of all ages. STDs can be transmitted during sexual assault. In children the isolation of a sexually transmitted organism may be the first indication that abuse has occurred. However, most sexually abused children are not initially seen with genital complaints. Unfortunately, the presence of an STD is frequently viewed as a shortcut to prove abuse. Although the presence of a sexually transmissible agent in a child beyond the neonatal period is suggestive of sexual abuse, exceptions do occur. For example, rectal and genital infection with *C. trachomatis* in young children may be due to persistent perinatally acquired infection, which may persist for up to 3 years. The use of STDs as indicators of sexual abuse is further complicated by inappropriate use of certain diagnostic tests such as tests for *C. trachomatis* antigen or misidentification of other bacteria as *Neisseria gonorrhoeae*. A much higher standard of accuracy must be used for children than for adults because identification of an STD in a child will have legal and social, as well as medical, implications.

Epidemiology of Sexual Abuse in Children

The incidence and prevalence of sexual abuse of children are difficult to estimate, in major part because much sexual abuse in childhood escapes detection. Several relatively extensive studies of sexual abuse of children in the United States have examined sex, race, and age-dependent variables. Patterns of childhood sexual abuse appear to depend on the sex and age of the victim (Glaser et al., 1989). Approximately 80% to 90% of abused children are female, with mean ages of 7 to 8 years. Most (75% to 85%) have been abused by a male assailant—adult or minor—known to the child. This individual is most likely a family member, especially the father or father substitute (stepfather, mother's boyfriend), uncle, or other male relative (Rimsza and Niggemann, 1982). Victims of unknown assailants usually are older than the children abused by a known person, and the abuse usually involves only a single episode. In contrast, abuse by family members or acquaintances usually involves multiple episodes over periods of time ranging from 1 week to years. Most victims describe a single type of sexual activity, but more than 20% have experienced multiple types of forced sexual acts. Vaginal penetration occurs in approximately 50% and anal penetration in one third of female victims. More than 50% of male victims have experienced anal penetration. Other types of sexual activity include orogenital contact (in 20% to 50% of victims) and fondling. Children who are abused by a known assailant usually experience less trauma than victims of assault by a stranger.

Risk of Infection

An accurate determination of the risk of sexually transmitted conditions in victims of sexual abuse has been hindered by a variety of factors. First, the prevalence of sexually transmitted infections may vary regionally and among different populations within the same region. Second, few studies have attempted to differentiate between infections resulting from abuse and those that existed before the abuse occurred. The presence of preexisting infection in adults is usually related to prior sexual activity (Jenny et al., 1990). In children, preexisting infection may be related to prolonged colonization after perinatal acquisition, inadvertent nonsexual spread, prior peer sexual activity, or prior sexual abuse (Glaser et al., 1989). Finally, incubation periods for STDs range from a few days for N. gonorrhoeae to several months for HPV. The incubation periods and timing of an examination after an episode of abuse are critically important in detecting infections. Multiple episodes of abuse increase the risk of infection, probably by increasing the number of contacts with an infected individual. In most cases the site of infection is consistent with the child's history of assault (Rimsza and Niggemann, 1982). Rates of infection also vary with the type of assault initially described. Vaginal or rectal penetration is more likely to lead to detectable infection than is fondling (Tilelli et al., 1980; White et al., 1983). However, the majority of children who are abused have no physical complaints related to either trauma or infection.

GONORRHEA

Since 1995, gonorrhea has become the second most frequently reported infectious disease after chlamydial infection in the United States. The World Health Organization estimates that there are approximately 100 million gonorrheal infections each year throughout the world. The reported number of cases of gonorrhea in the United States in 1998 was 355,131. This number has been decreasing yearly since a peak of 1 million cases in 1978, until 1997 through 1998, when the rates increased over 10% in women and 7.4% in men (Centers for Disease Control and Prevention, 2000). This increase may be due in part to changes in screening and reporting practices and what appears to be an increase in unsafe sexual behavior, especially among men who have sex with men. Many cases escape detection and contribute to the silent reservoir of infection in males and females. In 1998, gonococcal infections were most common in the 15- to 19-year age group (Centers for Disease Control and Prevention, 2000), making this a significant pediatric infection, and not solely an adult infection.

Gonorrhea is an inflammatory disease of the mucous membranes of the genitourinary tract that occurs only in humans. It is caused by N. gonorrhoeae, which first was described by Neisser in 1879. The most common portal of entry is the genitourinary tract, and the organism may then cause various inflammatory diseases of adjacent tissues such as cervicitis, salpingitis, and vulvovaginitis in children. The newborn may acquire the organism during delivery when direct contact with contaminated vaginal secretions leads to conjunctivitis. Bacteremia may occur, leading most commonly to the arthritis-dermatitis syndrome and, rarely, endocarditis and meningitis. Other manifestations of infection in children include gonococcal proctitis and pharyngitis. However, many gonococcal infections (15% to 44%) in children are asymptomatic (De Jong, 1986; Ingram et al., 1992).

Bacteriology

N. gonorrhoeae is a nonmotile non–spore forming, gram-negative coccus that characteristically grows in pairs (diplococci), with flattened adjacent sides in the configuration of "coffee beans." All Neisseria species, including Neisseria meningitidis, rapidly oxidize dimethyl- or tetramethyl-paraphenylene diamine, the basis of the diagnostic oxidase test. The cell envelope of N. gonorrhoeae is similar to that of other gram-negative bacteria. Specific surface components of the envelope have been related to adherence, tissue and cellular penetration, cytotoxicity, and evasion of host defenses, both systemically and at the mucosal level.

Pili. Pili are filamentous projections that traverse the outer membrane of the organism and are composed of repeating protein subunits (pilin). When N. gonorrhoeae is grown on translucent agar, various colonial morphologies can be seen. Fresh clinical isolates initially form colony types P+ and P++ (formerly called T1 and T2). These organisms have numerous pili extending from the cell surface. After 20 to 24 hours, P– (formerly T3 and T4) colonies—in which the cells are nonpiliated—predominate. These nonpiliated organisms are not virulent. The shift between P+ or P++ and P– colony types is termed *phase variation* and is mediated by chromosomal rearrangement (Segal et al., 1985). The protein that constitutes pili (pilin) has regions of considerable antigenic variability between strains of *N. gonorrhoeae*. Single strains of *N. gonorrhoeae* also can produce pili of different antigenic composition (antigenic variation), which has made the possibility of a pilus-based vaccine against *N. gonorrhoeae* less feasible. Piliated gonococci are better able to attach to human mucosal surfaces than nonpiliated organisms. Pili also contribute to killing by neutrophils (Britigan et al., 1985).

Outer membrane. The gonococcus has a cell envelope like other gram-negative bacteria; it consists of three layers: an inner cytoplasmic membrane, a middle peptidoglycan cell wall, and an outer membrane. The outer membrane contains lipooligosaccharide (LOS), phospholipid, and a variety of proteins. One of them is protein I, which functions as a porin and is believed to play an important role in pathogenesis. Preliminary data suggest that it may facilitate endocytosis of the organism or otherwise trigger invasion. Protein I is also the basis of the most commonly used gonococcal serotyping system because there is consistent antigenic variation between different strains (Knapp et al., 1984). Certain *N. gonorrhoeae* protein I serovars are associated with resistance of the organism to the bactericidal effect of normal nonimmune serum and an increased propensity to cause bacteremia. Gonococcal LOS is an endotoxin that differs from the polysaccharide of most gram-negative bacteria in that it lacks O-antigenic side chains. Some components of LOS are also related to resistance of *N. gonorrhoeae* to serum bactericidal activity. LOS also demonstrates interstrain antigenic variations, which are the basis of another serotyping system (Apicella, 1976).

Strain Typing

Characterization of gonococcal strains recently has been based on two primary methods—auxotyping and serology. Auxotyping is based on the differing requirements for specific nutrient or cofactors, which are genetically stable characteristics. It is done by examining the ability of strains of the organism to grow on chemically defined media that lack these factors (Catlin, 1973). More than thirty auxotypes have been identified. Common types include prototrophic (Proto) strain, also known as *zero* or *wild-type* strain; proline-requirement (Pro) strain; and strains that require arginine, hypoxanthine, and uracil (AHU strain). The most widely based serotyping system is based on protein I, as described previously. There are two major subgroups—IA and IB—which can be classified further into serovars based on coagglutination with a panel of monoclonal antibodies (Knapp et al., 1984). Combining typing strains with auxotyping and serology has been helpful in studying the epidemiology of gonococcal infection both geographically and temporally (Ahmed et al., 1992). It has been especially helpful in analyzing patterns of antibiotic resistance (Hook et al., 1987).

Genetics

Many strains of *N. gonorrhoeae* possess a 24.5-mD conjugative plasmid and can therefore conjugally transfer other non–self-transferable plasmids. Many strains also carry a plasmid that specifies production of a TEM-1 type β-lactamase; the two most common plasmids of this type have molecular weights of 3.2 and 4.4 mD. Gonococci that carry the 24.5-mD conjugative plasmid with the tetM transposon inserted have high-level resistance to tetracycline, with minimum inhibitory concentration (MIC) greater than 16 mg/L, and this can be readily transferred to other gonococci. This tetM determinant functions by encoding for a protein that protects ribosomes from the effect of tetracycline. All gonococci also contain a small cryptic plasmid (2.6 mD) whose function is unknown.

Antibiotic resistance in *N. gonorrhoeae* may also be mediated by chromosomal mutations, which are not transferable by plasmids. Chromosomal resistance to β-lactam antibiotics and the tetracyclines appears to result from a series of minor mutations that reduce the permeability of the outer membrane or alter penicillin-binding protein 2, reducing its affinity for penicillin (Johnson and Morse, 1988). Chromosomal resistance to quinolones has been localized to multiple mutations in genes coding for the bacterial DNA gyrase and typoisomerase enzymes (Zenilman, 2002).

Pathology and Pathogenesis

Stratified squamous epithelium can resist invasion by the gonococcus, whereas columnar epithelium is susceptible to it. This difference accounts for the absence of lesions in the adult vagina and on the external genitalia of both sexes. The susceptibility of columnar epithelium leads to infection of the urethra, prostate gland, seminal vesicles, and epididymis in males. In females, infection occurs primarily in the urethra, Skene's and Bartholin's glands, cervix, and fallopian tubes. Gonorrhea can occur in males or females without signs or symptoms (Amstey and Steadman, 1976). The primary infection can also occur in the rectal or pharyngeal mucosa of either sex. The alkaline pH of secreted mucus and the lack of estrogen permit vaginal infections with overt vulvovaginitis to occur in the prepubertal girl (Hook and Holmes, 1985). Gonococci attach to the mucosal epithelium and then penetrate between and through the epithelial cells to reach the subepithelial connective tissue by the third or fourth day of infection. An inflammatory exudate quickly forms beneath the epithelium. In the acute phase of infection, numerous leukocytes (many with phagocytosed gonococci) are present in the lumen of the urethra, causing a characteristic profuse yellow-white discharge in males. In the absence of specific treatment the inflammatory exudate in the subepithelial connective tissue is replaced by macrophages and lymphocytes. Direct extension of the infection occurs through the lymphatic vessels and less often through the blood vessels. Acute urethritis is the most common manifestation in males, and the infection can then spread to the posterior urethra, Cowper's glands, seminal vesicles, prostate, and epididymis, which leads to perineal, perianal, ischiorectal, or periprostatic abscesses. Rarely, in young boys (Fleisher et al., 1980) and in adults, penile edema may be seen. In teenage and adult males, acute prostatitis can result in prostatic abscess or chronic prostatitis. Acute epididymitis is the most frequent complication of gonococcal infection.

In females, primary infection most frequently affects the columnar epithelium of the postpubertal cervix, and the histopathologic appearance resembles that of the male urethra. Spread of infection to the fallopian tubes may be acute or subacute, without signs and symptoms, and sometimes it is extremely difficult to diagnose. Acute stages can result in peritonitis.

As a rule, the infection is confined to the pelvis. The end result of untreated or inadequately treated salpingitis is complete or partial obstruction of the tubes, which often leads to tubal pregnancy or sterility. Pelvic inflammatory disease (PID) is an especially common complication of gonorrhea in female adolescents, and when it occurs in this age range, it is especially likely to result in infertility (see the discussion of pelvic inflammatory disease and salpingitis later in this chapter) (Hook and Holmes, 1985).

Clinical Manifestations

In pregnancy. The effects of gonococcal disease on the infant may begin before delivery, because there is evidence that gonococcal disease in pregnant women may have an adverse effect on both the mother and the infant. Edwards et al. (1978) observed 19 women with intrapartum gonorrhea. They had a significantly greater occurrence of premature rupture of membranes, prolonged rupture of membranes, chorioamnionitis, and premature delivery. Other studies have shown an alarming incidence of perinatal deaths and abortions. In addition to the effect on the fetus, postpartum complications in the mother are common. Therefore the diagnosis of gonococcal disease should be sought and controlled during pregnancy. To obtain control, the following issues should be considered:

- Recurrent infection after an initial episode during pregnancy is very common. Therefore specimens for culture should be obtained in later pregnancy from the woman who is infected in early pregnancy.
- Many mothers conceive their first child while they are teenagers, an age range in which gonococcal disease has a particularly high prevalence and in which the young women may look to their pediatrician for medical care.
- Gonococcal disease is especially dangerous to women because PID is a relatively frequent complication (see the discussion of pelvic inflammatory disease and salpingitis).

In Infancy. Gonococcal ophthalmia is the most common form of gonorrhea in infants and results from perinatal contamination of infants by their infected mothers during parturition. Transmission rates of 42% have been observed (Laga et al., 1986b). An initially nonspecific conjunctivitis with serosanguineous discharge is rapidly replaced by a thick, purulent exudate. Corneal ulceration and iridocyclitis appear unilaterally or bilaterally. Unless therapy is initiated promptly, perforation of the cornea may occur, leading to blindness. Ophthalmia neonatorum, formerly a leading cause of blindness, has been controlled by prophylaxis with silver nitrate or with antimicrobial agents such as erythromycin and tetracycline. Crede's original study in 1881 reported that 2% silver nitrate prophylaxis reduced the incidence of gonococcal ophthalmia from 10% to 0.5%. Neonatal ocular prophylaxis is not 100% effective; failures occur with every regimen (Bernstein et al., 1983; Laga et al., 1988; Rothenberg, 1979). The infant possibly is more likely to acquire the infection despite prophylaxis if there has been premature rupture of membranes (Handsfield et al., 1973). A more recent study of neonatal ocular prophylaxis in the United States suggests that prenatal screening and treatment of pregnant women has had a significant impact on the prevention of gonococcal ophthalmia (Hammerschlag et al., 1989). Bacitracin and sulfonamides are ineffective for prophylaxis (Rothenberg, 1979).

Other manifestations seen in newborns are other local infections such as scalp abscesses (associated with scalp electrodes) or systemic infections caused by gonococcemia and subsequent seeding of the organism to other areas—for example, sepsis, arthritis, meningitis and pneumonia. Gonococcal infections may also be asymptomatic, with positive cultures from oropharynx, vagina, and rectum.

In young children. Gonococcal vulvovaginitis is the most common gonococcal disease in children. It must be distinguished bacteriologically from vulvovaginitis caused by other agents by isolating *N. gonorrhoeae* from a vaginal swab; an endocervical culture is not necessary. In preadolescent girls the vaginal exudate may be minimal and may be confused with a benign discharge (Michalowski, 1961). Symptoms referable to the urinary tract (dysuria) may predominate. *N. gonorrhoeae* rarely may be spread by sexual play among children, but the index case has usually been a victim of abuse (Potterat et al., 1986). It may cause purulent vulvovaginitis in girls or urethritis in boys. Gonococcal ophthalmia may also occur as a result of autoinoculation from a genital site.

It is generally recommended that all children suspected of being sexually abused have cultures obtained from genitals, rectum, and phar-

ynx (Centers for Disease Control and Prevention, 2002). This recommendation originated in part because of the high predictive value of the presence of gonococcal infection with the occurrence of sexual abuse and because several studies suggested that many of these infections were asymptomatic, even vaginal infections (De Jong, 1986). Shapiro et al. (1999) identified *N. gonorrhoeae* in 4 (9%) of 43 girls less than 12 years of age who had vaginitis but in whom sexual abuse was not suspected. However, most children being evaluated for sexual abuse are not symptomatic, and because recent studies have found the rates of gonococcal infection in abused children to be <3% (Beck-Sagué and Solomon, 1999; Ingram et al., 1992; Ingram et al., 1997; Ingram et al., 2001; Siegel et al., 1995), it has been suggested that selective criteria could be used to determine which children suspected of being sexually abused should be screened rather than screening every child to avoid the trauma and expense of obtaining unnecessary cultures. In 1991 the American Academy of Pediatrics (AAP) Committee on Child Abuse and Neglect suggested that routine cultures and screening of all children for gonorrhea were not necessary or recommended because the yield of positive cultures was very low in asymptomatic prepubertal children, especially those with histories of fondling only. The AAP suggested that testing be done when "epidemiologically indicated or when the history and/or physical findings suggest the possibility of oral, genital, or rectal contact." In 1995, Siegel et al. applied a modification of these criteria to children being evaluated for suspected sexual abuse at Children's Hospital Medical Center in Cincinnati. The modified criteria were as follows:

- The victim had a history of genital discharge or contact with the perpetrator's genitalia.
- The victim had a genital discharge or trauma on examination.
- The victim had a history of consensual sexual activity.
- The victim was postpubertal (Tanner III).
- The victim had sexual contact with a perpetrator known to have an STD.
- There was a family member with an STD.

They evaluated 855 children (704 girls and 151 boys) over a 1-year period. Of 379 girls tested for gonorrhea, 12 (3.2%) had positive results; all had either vaginal discharge or a history of vaginal penetration. All the prepubertal girls had symptomatic vaginal discharges. Subsequently, Ingram et al. (1997) evaluated these criteria to determine if they would have accurately detected all cases of vaginal gonococcal infection in their population. Of 2,898 girls seen over a 10-year period, 2,731 (94%) had vaginal cultures obtained for *N. gonorrhoeae*; 84 (2.9%) had positive cultures, 80 of whom had a vaginal discharge. The four remaining girls who were asymptomatic included two with a history of vaginal intercourse with an alleged perpetrator with gonorrhea—one had *N. gonorrhoeae* isolated from her urine culture, and the other had a preteenaged sister with gonorrhea. Thus all of the 84 girls with vaginal gonorrhea would have been identified using the selective screening criteria recommended by the AAP. The validity of this risk assessment algorithm was confirmed in a subsequent study from the same group, where all children with gonorrhea and/or chlamydial infection were identified, whereas they avoided testing of the 56% of children who did not have infection (Ingram et al., 2001). Although it appears that one can use these selective criteria for vaginal specimens in girls, there are insufficient data to support their use for rectal and pharyngeal infection or genital infections in boys. Rectal and pharyngeal infections with *N. gonorrhoeae* are more likely to be asymptomatic in children (De Jong, 1986; Groothius et al., 1983).

Ascending pelvic infection may occur in prepubertal females (Burry, 1971), and it may occur in the absence of significant vaginal discharge. The main signs of early disease are dysuria and vaginal discharge. When gonococcal infection spreads from the cervix into the fallopian tubes, it is characterized by lower abdominal pain. The onset of acute salpingitis or PID may be abrupt and must be distinguished from acute appendicitis, cystitis, pyelonephritis, cholecystitis, and ectopic pregnancy (see the discussion of pelvic inflammatory disease and salpingitis).

In adolescents. Gonococcal infections are now most common in the 15- to 19-year age-group (Centers for Disease Control and Prevention, 2000). Among adolescent girls, the most frequent presenting symptoms are those of cervicitis (vaginal discharge and intermenstrual bleeding) and urethritis (dysuria). However, many girls have only mild symptoms, and many infections are asymptomatic (32% in one study of adolescent girls [Biro et al.,

1995]). Coinfection with *C. trachomatis* is common (about one third of patients with gonococcal infections are coinfected with *C. trachomatis* [Biro et al., 1995]). Abdominal pain is usually a manifestation of PID and is not associated with uncomplicated gonococcal infection.

In teenage males the onset of gonococcal urethritis is marked by sudden burning on urination occurring 2 days to 2 weeks after sexual exposure, similar to the presentation in adult males. This is followed by a mucopurulent discharge from the urethra. Involvement of the prostate gland is manifested by retention of urine, pain, and fever. Epididymitis may also occur, characterized by severe pain, tenderness, and swelling. Asymptomatic infection can also occur and is seen in approximately 2% of asymptomatic adolescent boys screened for gonorrhea (Hein et al., 1977; Smith et al., 1986).

Extragenital Manifestations

Disseminated gonococcal infection. Disseminated gonococcal infection (DGI) results from gonococcal bacteremia and occurs in 0.5% to 3% of patients with gonorrhea (Holmes et al., 1971). The strains of *N. gonorrhoeae* associated with DGI are usually very susceptible to penicillin, are resistant to the bactericidal action of nonimmune serum, have the AHU–auxotype, and belong to several specific protein 1A serovars (Knapp and Holmes, 1975). Individuals with deficient terminal components of complement (C5, C6, C7, or C8) are more susceptible to DGI and meningococcal bacteremia (Petersen et al., 1979). Approximately 5% of patients with DGI have this deficiency. Other host risk factors apparently associated with an increased risk of dissemination include female sex, menstruation, pharyngeal gonorrhea, and pregnancy (Holmes et al., 1971). DGI can result from a primary infection at any site including cervix, urethra, anal canal, pharynx, and conjunctiva. The most common clinical manifestation of DGI is the arthritis-dermatitis syndrome. Joint symptoms are seen at initial presentation of DGI in more than 90% of patients (Handsfield, 1975). The arthralgias may be migratory and may involve more than one joint. The most commonly involved joints are the knees, ankles, wrists, elbows, and the small joints of the hands and feet. The symptoms range from mild to severe and include arthralgias with no inflammation to arthritis with synovial effusion and even joint destruction. Tenosynovitis is frequent (O'Brien et al., 1983). A characteristic rash consisting of discrete papules and pustules, often with a hemorrhagic or necrotic component, is also present in 50% to 75% of patients. Usually 5 to 40 lesions are present, occurring primarily on the extremities, and ranging from 1 to 20 mm (Barr and Danielsson, 1971). The polyarthropathy and dermatitis frequently resolve spontaneously if not treated. However, arthritis may persist and progress, usually in one or two joints, most commonly the knee, ankle, elbow, or wrist. At this stage the clinical picture is that of septic arthritis. DGI is the leading cause of infective arthritis in young adults. Studies of septic arthritis in children have found that *N. gonorrhoeae* is the third most frequent organism in children over 3 years of age and the most frequent in children over 11 years of age (Nelson, 1972). Some patients can develop gonococcal septic arthritis without prior polyarthritis or dermatitis. Most clinical manifestations of DGI are secondary to the bacteremia, although immune complexes and other immunologic mechanisms may be contributory to some cases. Patients usually have fever and some systemic toxicity, although it is frequently mild and often absent. It has been hypothesized that DGI consists of an early bacteremic stage that leads to a septic joint stage if left untreated (Handsfield, 1975; O'Brien et al., 1983), although not all patients fit this picture. Some bacteriologic findings are consistent with this hypothesis; for example, blood cultures are often positive in the early phase, and joint fluid may be culture positive in the later stage. Positive blood and synovial fluid cultures are almost always mutually exclusive (O'Brien et al., 1983). The organism may also be detected by immunochemical methods in biopsy specimens from about 60% of the skin lesions (Tronca et al., 1974), but cultures and Gram stains are positive in only 10% of cases. Overall, approximately 50% of patients with DGI will have positive cultures of the blood or synovial fluid, but *N. gonorrhoeae* can be recovered from a mucosal site (e.g., pharynx, rectum) in at least 80% of patients, an important consideration when evaluating a child with suspected septic arthritis. The differential diagnosis of DGI includes meningococcemia; other infectious arthritis; and an entire range of inflammatory arthritides, including Reiter's

syndrome. Infrequent but serious complications of DGI include infective endocarditis, meningitis, osteomyelitis, and pneumonia.

Perihepatitis. Gonococcal perihepatitis (Fitz-Hugh-Curtis syndrome) results from extension of infection from salpingitis to the capsule and outer surface of the liver. It should be considered in female patients with right upper quadrant pain, palpable liver, abnormal liver function tests, and adnexal and uterine cervical tenderness. A positive endocervical culture for *N. gonorrhoeae* supports the diagnosis.

Conjunctivitis. Conjunctivitis beyond the newborn period follows direct spread of the gonococcus, usually via fingers contaminated with genital secretions. It rarely results from gonococcemia. Conjunctivitis is often severe with profuse purulent discharge, chemosis, eyelid edema, and ulcerative keratitis, and presentations may mimic orbital cellulitis (Lewis et al., 1990).

Oropharyngitis. Gonococcal oropharyngitis is common among homosexuals (Weisner et al., 1973) and among children who are victims of sexual abuse. Infection follows orogenital contact. Pharyngitis is usually asymptomatic and is detected on routine screening (Groothius et al., 1983). Pharyngeal cultures are positive in 15% (Nelson et al., 1976) to 54% (Groothius et al., 1983) of children with genital gonococcal infections. Rarely, pharyngeal infections are symptomatic (Abbott, 1973).

Anorectal gonorrhea. Rectal infections are common in girls, probably because of the proximity of the vagina and the possibility of contamination of the anus with vaginal discharge. Rectal cultures may be positive in up to 50% of girls with positive vaginal cultures (Nelson et al., 1976). Most rectal infections are asymptomatic and are detected by routine screening, but occasionally there are symptoms (Speck, 1971). The symptoms are a purulent rectal discharge with rectal pain, blood, or mucus in the stool and perianal itching or burning.

Diagnosis

The Gram stain for diagnosis of gonorrhea is considered to be positive if typical gram-negative diplococci are seen in association with polymorphonuclear leucocytes. A positive Gram stain from a male urethral specimen is highly sensitive and specific for gonococcal infection. However, in females, the adult cervix and the vagina of prepubertal children may be colonized with other *Neisseria* species, rendering the Gram stain less reliable. Similarly, Gram-stained smears of rectum and pharynx are not useful to determine infection at these sites.

In younger children, because of medical and legal implications, the importance of an accurate microbiologic diagnosis cannot be overemphasized. Gram stain of the vaginal discharge in a child with suspected gonorrhea is not accurate and has a poor predictive value for the diagnosis of gonorrhea. Diagnostic specimens of the pharynx, rectum, and vagina or urethra should be taken and immediately plated onto selective media appropriate for isolation of *N. gonorrhoeae* (e.g., Thayer-Martin media) and then placed in an atmosphere enriched with carbon dioxide, which is done most easily using an extinction candle jar. Isolation of gonococci from sites containing many saprophytic organisms (vagina, cervix, pharynx, and rectum) is enhanced if selective media containing antibiotics (e.g., Thayer-Martin media) are used; these media inhibit most of the normal flora and permit only the growth of gonococci and meningococci. Specimens from other usually sterile sites (blood, synovial fluid, or cerebrospinal fluid [CSF]) should be inoculated only onto nonselective (antibiotic free) media such as enriched chocolate agar. *N. gonorrhoeae* organisms are gram-negative, oxidase-positive diplococci, and their presence should be confirmed with additional tests, including rapid carbohydrate tests, enzyme-substrate tests, and rapid serologic tests. Failure to perform appropriate confirmatory tests may lead to misidentification of other organisms as *N. gonorrhoeae*. Whittington et al. (1988) found that 14 of 40 presumptive gonococcal isolates sent to the Centers for Disease Control (CDC) for confirmation had been misidentified as *N. gonorrhoeae*. Misidentified organisms included other *Neisseria* species, *Moraxella catarrhalis*, and *Kingella denitrificans*. The CDC (2002) recommends that confirmation of an organism as *N. gonorrhoeae* should include at least two procedures that use different principles (e.g., biochemical, enzyme-substrate, serologic, or DNA probe). In addition, it is recommended that isolates be preserved to allow additional or repeated analyses.

Although culture of *N. gonorrhoeae* is well standardized and widely available, there have always been concerns about the loss of viability during transport to the laboratory. Enzyme immunoassays (EIAs) for detection of *N. gonorrhoeae* were introduced in the 1980s but were not satisfactory in terms of sensitivity or specificity. In the late 1980s, a nonamplified DNA probe was introduced (PACE 2, Gen-Probe, San Diego, California). The overall sensitivity of the DNA probe compared with that of culture of endocervical specimens from women has been on the order of 95%. Data are similar for male urethra, with sensitivities of 98.8% to 100% and specificities >99% compared with culture. There are now four nucleic acid amplification tests (NAATs) approved by the U.S. Food and Drug Administration (FDA) for the detection of *N. gonorrhoeae* in clinical specimens: polymerase chain reaction (PCR) (Amplicor, Roche Molecular Diagnostics, Pleasanton, California); transcription mediated amplification (TMA) (GenProbe, San Diego, CA); and strand displacement amplification (SDA) (ProbeTec, Becton Dickson, Franklin Lakes, New Jersey). PCR and SDA are DNA amplification tests; TMA is an RNA amplification assay. A fourth NAAT, ligase chain reaction (LCR) (LCX assay, Abbott Diagnostics, Abbott Park, IC) was withdrawn from the market by the manufacturer in 2002 because of poor quality control. Currently NAATs are approved for cervical swabs from women, urethral swabs from men and urine from men and women. None of these tests are approved or recommended by the manufacturers for rectal specimens from adults and they are not approved for rectogenital specimens or urine from children. Several of these assays are also available in a multiplexed format for detection of *N. gonorrhoeae* and *C. trachomatis* in the same specimen (Morse, 2001). Unlike the experience with NAATs for detection of *C. trachomatis*, the performance of these assays have not been dramatically better than standard culture methods for detection of *N. gonorrhoeae*, especially in low prevalence populations (CDC, 2002a, 2002b). In one study of the use of the coamplification PCR with genital and urine specimens from men and women attending STD clinics in the United States, the sensitivities and specificities for detection of *N. gonorrhoeae* in urine from males and females compared with those of culture were 94.4% and 98.5%, and 90% and 95.9%, respectively. The prevalences of gonorrhea among men and women were 17.4% and 7.8%, respectively. Discrepant specimens were all resolved by repeat PCR testing with a confirmatory 16SrRNA assay. However, another multicenter evaluation from Europe of more than 3,000 women attending non-STD clinics where the prevalence of *N. gonorrhoeae* was only 0.3% found only 9 positive samples by coamplification PCR. None of the positive PCR results could be confirmed by the 16SrRNA PCR. The CDC recommends that only culture be used for detection of *N. gonorrhoeae* in children being evaluated for suspected sexual abuse (Centers for Disease Control and Prevention, 2002a).

Treatment

During the 20 years before 1976, all *N. gonorrhoeae* strains were sensitive to penicillin, but a gradual increase had been noted in the mean MIC. The first reports of penicillinase-producing *N. gonorrhoeae* (PPNG) arising in the Far East occurred in the 1970s. PPNG strains have accounted for more than 30% of isolates of *N. gonorrhoeae* in the United States (Schwarcz et al., 1990). Because children acquire their infections from adults, parallel increases in PPNG infections in children were also found (Rawstron et al., 1989). There has also been a similar increase in tetracycline-resistant *N. gonorrhoeae* (TRNG). The CDC (1987) defines any area that has a rate of PPNG higher than 3% over a 3-month period as a hyperendemic area for PPNG and recommends that all infections be treated with penicillinase-resistant antibiotics. These resistant strains cause the same disease spectrum as penicillin-sensitive organisms. In 1983 an outbreak of chromosomally mediated penicillin-resistant gonococci was reported from North Carolina; subsequently, it has occurred in other areas of the country (Hook et al., 1987). These organisms, which do not produce penicillinase, are rare in children. Quinolone-resistant *N. gonorrhoeae* has emerged as a major problem in Southeast Asia and the Pacific Rim (Knapp et al., 1997). Quinolone-resistant strains account for approximately 10% of isolates in Hong Kong and the Philippines. As many as 50% of isolates from some Far Eastern countries now exhibit decreased susceptibility to quinolones. Quinolone-resistant strains of *N. gonorrhoeae* have been detected sporadically in the United States, often associated epidemiologically with the Far East (Centers for Disease Control and Prevention, 2002a). Although strains of *N. gonorrhoeae* with decreased susceptibility to ceftriaxone do occur (Schwebke et al., 1995), no documented clinical treatment failures have been observed related to decreased gonococcal susceptibility to ceftriaxone in the United States (Gorwitz et al., 1993).

Prevention of neonatal infection. Endocervical cultures for gonococci should be obtained from all pregnant women as an integral part of prenatal care at the first prenatal visit. A second culture late in pregnancy should be obtained from women who are at high risk of gonococcal infection.

Prevention of gonococcal ophthalmia. Routine preventive prophylaxis of gonococcal ophthalmia includes (1) 1% silver nitrate (with no irrigation with saline solution, which might reduce efficacy); or (2) ophthalmic ointments containing tetracycline (1%) or erythromycin (0.5%) (Centers for Disease Control and Prevention, 2002). Use of bacitracin ointment (not effective) and penicillin drops (sensitizing) is not recommended. Data on use of povidone-iodine are limited; initial studies suggested less efficacy. Silver nitrate is no longer manufactured in the United States.

Management of infants born to mothers with untreated gonococcal infection. The infant born to a mother with untreated gonorrhea should have orogastric and rectal cultures taken routinely and blood cultures taken if the infant is symptomatic. A full-term infant should receive a single injection of ceftriaxone (50 mg/kg intravenously [IV] or intramuscularly [IM], not to exceed 125 mg). Although ceftriaxone is not usually given to newborn infants, it is indicated in this specific setting.

Neonatal Disease

Gonococcal ophthalmia. Infants with gonococcal ophthalmia should be hospitalized. They should receive a single dose of ceftriaxone (25 to 50 mg/kg/day, maximum dose 125 mg IV or IM) (Centers for Disease Control and Prevention, 2002; Laga et al., 1986a). Cefotaxime (25 mg/kg IV or IM every 12 hours for 7 days) is an alternative treatment. Infants with gonococcal ophthalmia should receive eye irrigations with buffered saline solution until the discharge is cleared. Additional topical therapy is not indicated. Simultaneous infection with *C. trachomatis* has been reported and should be considered in infants who do not respond satisfactorily. Both mother and infant should be tested for chlamydial infection.

Complicated infection. Infants with arthritis, abscess, and septicemia should be treated by hospitalization and administration of ceftriaxone at 25 to 50 mg/kg IV or IM once daily for 7 days. Meningitis should be similarly treated with ceftriaxone, with treatment extending for 10 to 14 days.

Childhood Disease Beyond Infancy

Children with uncomplicated gonococcal vulvovaginitis, cervicitis, urethritis, pharyngitis, or proctitis should be treated with ceftriaxone (125 mg IM once) (Centers for Disease Control and Prevention, 2002) whether lighter or heavier than 45 kg. Using lidocaine as a diluent for the ceftriaxone injection reduces the pain of the injection (Schichor et al., 1994). Children who cannot tolerate ceftriaxone may be treated with spectinomycin (40 mg/kg, maximum 2 g) IM in a single dose (Rettig et al., 1980). Spectinomycin is not as effective in treating pharyngeal gonorrhea (Judson et al., 1985). The source of the infection must be identified, which may be facilitated by hospitalization (Ingram et al., 1982). Children with DGI (bacteremia or arthritis) should be treated with ceftriaxone (50 mg/kg, maximum 1 g, once daily for 7 days). Meningitis requires the same therapy, except the maximum dose is 2 g and duration of therapy is 10 to 14 days. All children with rectogenital gonorrhea should also be evaluated for coinfection with *Chlamydia*. The newer expanded-spectrum oral cephalosporins such as cefixime are effective as a single dose (oral) in adults but have not yet been evaluated in children.

Gonococcal Infections in Adolescents

Single-dose efficacy is a major consideration in treatment of gonococcal infections, especially in adolescents. Another important factor is coinfection with *C. trachomatis*, which can be documented in up to 45% of adolescents with gonorrhea in some populations. For teenagers over 12 years of age, treatment should follow the recommended regimens for adults with one exception: Quinolones are not approved for use in children up to 18 years of age. The first-line regimen for treatment of uncomplicated gonococcal infection adults recommended by the CDC (2002a) is cefixime (400 mg orally, single dose); ciprofloxacin (500 mg orally, single dose); single-dose ceftriaxone (125 mg IM); or a single-dose oral quinolone (ciprofloxacin, 500 mg, ofloxacin, 400 mg, levofloxacin, 250 mg, or

gatifloxacin, 400 mg). However, cefixime is no longer available, as the manufacturer ceased production in 2002. Each regimen should also include a regimen effective against possible coinfection with *C. trachomatis* (Stamm et al., 1984) such as azithromycin (1 g orally in a single dose) or doxycycline (100 mg orally, 2 times a day for 7 days). Quinolone regimens may be used only if the adolescent is more than 18 years old. Because of the possibility of quinolone-resistant *N. gonorrhoeae*, these regimens are no longer recommended for the treatment of gonorrhea in Hawaii and should not be used to treat infections that may have been acquired in Asia or the Pacific (including Hawaii) (Centers for Disease Control and Prevention, 2002). Recent data from the CDC's Gonococcal Isolate Surveillance Project from several sites in California are also demonstrating an increased prevalence of quinolone resistance in the state and further suggest that use of quinolones in California is also probably not advisable.

Alternative injectable regimens for individuals who cannot tolerate ceftriaxone are spectinomycin (2 g IM in a single dose); cefotaxime (500 mg IM once); ceftizoxime (500 mg IM once); and cefoxitin (2 g IM once with probenecid, 1 g orally). All these regimens should also be followed by single-dose azithromycin or a 7-day course of doxycycline.

PID AND SALPINGITIS

Vaginal infection of females who are adolescent or younger may progress to involve the fallopian tubes or may disseminate to the pelvis. PID is composed of a spectrum of inflammatory disorders of the upper genital tract in women and may include endometritis, salpingitis, tuboovarian abscess, and pelvic peritonitis. *N. gonorrhoeae* and *C. trachomatis* are implicated in most cases; however, microorganisms that can be part of the vaginal flora, such as anaerobes, *Gardnerella vaginalis*, *Haemophilus influenzae*, enteric gram-negative rods, and *Streptococcus agalactiae*, are also involved (Eschenbach et al., 1975; Mardh, 1980). Some experts believe that genital mycoplasmas such as *Mycoplasma hominis* and *Ureaplasma urealyticum* also play a role in the etiology of PID.

PID in adolescents is particularly likely to result in infertility and is the single most common cause of infertility in young women (Gates, 1984; Shafer et al., 1982; Westrom, 1980). A confirmed diagnosis of salpingitis and a more accurate bacteriologic diagnosis are made by laparoscopy. Because laparoscopy is not always available, the diagnosis of PID is often based on imprecise clinical findings and culture of specimens from the lower genital tract. Cultures of women with acute PID have recovered *N. gonorrhoeae* from the endocervix from approximately 35% to 80% of cases and from a smaller proportion of samples of fallopian tube aspirates (Eschenbach et al., 1975).

Risk factors for PID and acute salpingitis include young age at acquisition of gonococcal disease, a history of previous PID, multiple sexual partners, and use of an intrauterine device (IUD) for contraception. Approximately 15% of teenagers who develop gonorrhea progress to PID (Westrom, 1980). Diagnosing PID may be difficult, and the differential diagnosis includes numerous other conditions of the lower abdomen, including appendicitis, ectopic pregnancy, cholecystitis, mesenteric adenitis, pyelonephritis, and septic abortion. Misdiagnosis of PID is common, and it is one of the more common causes of medically nonindicated laparotomy. As mentioned previously, laparoscopy assists in establishing a diagnosis. The clinical diagnosis of PID is imprecise. Data indicate that a clinical diagnosis of symptomatic PID has a positive predictive value for salpingitis of 65% to 90% when compared with laparoscopy as the standard. Recommendations by Shafer et al. (1982) suggest that a clinical diagnosis of PID be supported by presence of lower abdominal pain and tenderness, cervical motion tenderness, and adnexal tenderness. Fever, leukocytosis, elevated sedimentation rate, and adnexal mass observed through abdominal ultrasound support the diagnosis. Culdocentesis, if performed, may reveal evidence of purulent reaction in the peritoneal cavity. The outcome for fertility probably is improved with prompt and vigorous therapy.

The CDC (2002a) recommends that empiric treatment of PID should be instituted on the basis of the presence of all of the following three minimum clinical criteria for pelvic inflammation and in the absence of a cause other than PID:
- Lower abdominal tenderness
- Adnexal tenderness
- Cervical motion tenderness

When severe clinical signs are present a more elaborate diagnostic evaluation is warranted.

These additional criteria may be used to increase the specificity of the diagnosis:

Routine criteria
- Oral temperature > 101° F (38.3° C)
- Abnormal cervical or vaginal discharge
- Presence of white blood cells on saline microscopy of vaginal secretions
- Elevated erythrocyte sedimentation rate
- Elevated C-reactive protein
- Laboratory documentation of infection with *N. gonorrhoeae* or *C. trachomatis*

Most specific criteria
- Histopathologic evidence of endometritis on endometrial biopsy
- Tuboovarian abscess on transvaginal sonography or magnetic resonance imaging (MRI)
- Laparoscopic abnormalities consistent with PID

Treatment and prevention of salpingitis and PID. Detailed recommendations are contained in the "Sexually Transmitted Diseases Treatment Guidelines," published by the CDC as a supplement to the Morbidity and Mortality Weekly Report. The last edition was published in 2002, and the following recommendations are based on this edition. Treatment regimens must provide empiric, broad-spectrum coverage of likely pathogens. Antimicrobial coverage should include *N. gonorrhoeae*, *C. trachomatis*, gram-negative facultative bacteria, anaerobes, and streptococci. In female adolescents treatment of gonorrhea with drug regimens that are effective against gonococci but not chlamydiae has led to a high incidence of residual salpingitis and, in males, of urethritis, both associated with continued disease caused by chlamydia (Stamm et al., 1984). No single therapeutic regimen has been established for women with PID. Selection of a regimen depends on availability of a drug, cost, patient acceptance, and regional differences in antimicrobial susceptibility of the likely pathogens.

Many experts recommend that all patients with PID be hospitalized so that therapy with parenteral antibiotics can be given under supervision. Indications for hospitalization for therapy of PID include the following:
- Surgical emergencies such as appendicitis or ectopic pregnancy cannot be excluded.
- The patient is pregnant.
- The patient does not respond clinically to oral antimicrobial therapy.

- The patient is unable to follow or tolerate an outpatient regimen.
- The patient has severe illness, nausea and vomiting, or high fever.
- The patient has a tuboovarian abscess.

The first-line inpatient regimen recommended by the CDC is cefoxitin, 2 g IV every 6 hours; or cefotetan, 2 g IV every 12 hours, plus doxycycline, 100 mg orally or IV every 12 hours for at least 48 hours after the patient demonstrates substantial clinical improvement, after which doxycycline, 100 mg orally, bid, should be continued for a total of 14 days. The alternate regimen is clindamycin, 900 mg IV every 8 hours, plus gentamicin, loading dose IV or IM (2 mg/kg) followed by a maintenance dose (1.5 mg/kg) every 8 hours. This regimen should also be continued for 48 hours after the patient demonstrates substantial clinical improvement, followed by doxycycline, 100 mg orally, bid, or clindamycin, 450 mg, orally qid, for a total of 14 days. Other alternative regimens include ofloxacin 400 mg IV every 12 hours or levofloxacin 500 mg IV once daily, with or without metronidazole 500 mg IV every 8 hours or ampicillin/sulbactam 3 g IV every 6 hours plus doxycycline 100 mg orally or IV every 12 hours. Outpatient regimens include ofloxacin 400 mg orally every 12 hours or levofloxacin 500 mg orally once daily, with or without metronidazole 500 mg orally every 12 hours for 14 days or ceftriaxone 250 mg IM once or cefoxitin 2 g IM plus probenecid 1 g orally as a single dose, or other parenteral third-generation cephalosporin (cefotaxime or ceftizoxime) plus doxycycline 100 mg orally twice daily for 14 days with or without metronidazole 500 mg orally twice daily for 14 days.

Follow-up. Patients should demonstrate significant clinical improvement, including defervescence and reduction in direct or rebound tenderness and adnexal tenderness within 72 hours of the start of treatment. Patients who do not improve may require hospitalization, additional diagnostic tests, and/or surgical intervention. Because of the risk of persistent *C. trachomatis* infection, patients should be retested 7 to 10 days after completing treatment. Some experts also recommend screening for *C. trachomatis* and *N. gonorrhoeae* 4 to 6 weeks after completion of treatment. Evaluation and treatment of the sex partners of women with PID is very important because of the risk of reinfection.

There is a high likelihood of urethral gonococcal or chlamydial infection in the partner. The CDC (2002) recommends that sex partners should be treated empirically with regimens effective against *C. trachomatis* and *N. gonorrhoeae* regardless of the apparent etiology of PID in their partner.

SYPHILIS

The incidences of primary and secondary syphilis continue to decline after having reached epidemic proportions in the United States in the early 1990s. Rates of primary and secondary syphilis have reached the lowest levels since reporting began in 1941 (2.5/100,000 population in 1999, compared with 20.3/100,000 in 1990) (Centers for Disease Control and Prevention, 2001a). Although syphilis rates typically fluctuate over time, these low rates are encouraging. However, focal outbreaks continue, including recent outbreaks among men who have sex with men (Centers for Disease Control and Prevention, 2001b). In addition, worldwide, syphilis remains a problem, and rates have risen sharply in Eastern Europe in Russia and former states of the Soviet Union (Renton, 1998).

The number of babies with congenital syphilis is known to parallel closely the rates of primary and secondary syphilis among women of childbearing age. The number of babies with congenital syphilis reported to the CDC reached a peak of 4,410 in 1991, a 1-year lag from the peaks of primary and secondary syphilis. The number of babies with congenital syphilis has gradually fallen to 529 cases in 2000 (Centers for Disease Control and Prevention, 2001c). A change in congenital syphilis definition in 1988 (see surveillance definition in Centers for Disease Control, 1990) increased the totals by including "at risk" babies as well as those with fully documented infections (Cohen et al., 1990). This definition change makes direct comparison of numbers more difficult; however, there has been a clear decrease over time with the new definition. The epidemiology of syphilis has also changed over time. The epidemic in the early 1990s was associated with increases of crack and cocaine use among the urban poor, with exchange of sex for drugs (Centers for Disease Control, 1988). Unfortunately, because much of this sexual activity was anonymous, contact tracing and treatment of sexual partners—the usual methods of containing syphilis—became increasingly difficult, undoubtedly impeding elimination of this disease. Rates of early syphilis have remained disproportionately high in the South and among non-Hispanic blacks (St. Louis et al., 1996).

Children of any age can have syphilis, which may be congenital or acquired. Physicians taking care of children should be aware of the signs and symptoms of acquired and congenital syphilis.

Bacteriology

Treponema pallidum is the causative agent of syphilis. It is a thin, delicate organism, varying in length from 5 to 15 μm, with a width of 0.15 μm, which means it is not visible by light microscopy. *T. pallidum* has tight spirals every 1.1 μm along its length, appearing like a helical coil (Hovind-Hougen, 1983). When seen through darkfield microscopy, it exhibits a spiral movement, with flexion around its midportion. The organism divides slowly, only every 30 hours, and cannot be cultured on artificial media. Tissue culture does not sustain the growth of *T. pallidum* for long periods (Jenkin and Sander, 1983), and inoculation into rabbits is the only reliable means for cultivating this organism. Humans are the only natural host, although several mammals (including rabbits and monkeys) can be infected.

Pathogenesis

The central problem in understanding the pathogenesis of syphilis is that, although there is a vigorous host response to infection, treated disease has a minimal effect on resistance to reinfection, and the infection may persist for life. The treponemes initially invade the body through microscopic abrasions produced by sexual intercourse or other physical activity or via the placenta to the newborn. Approximately one third of people who have sex with infected partners will become infected. The treponemes attach to cells by one end, although no specialized receptor site has been seen on electron microscopy (Hovind-Hougen, 1983). Once inside the epithelial layer, the organisms replicate locally. The host responds first with an influx of polymorphonuclear neutrophil leukocytes (PMNs). The *T. pallidum* undergoes rapid phagocytosis (Musher et al., 1983), probably because host IgG is present on the surface of the organism (Alderete and Baseman, 1979). Lymphocytes soon replace the PMNs (Baker-

Zander and Sell, 1980). By the time the patient comes to clinical attention, a variety of antibodies usually are detected. However, the occurrence of secondary syphilis at the same time that the antibody titers are their highest indicates that the host antibody response to infection is not effective, since the localized disease comes under control at the same time that the manifestations of generalized infection appear. However, at this time the host is immune to intradermal challenge with *T. pallidum* (Musher, 1984). The host eventually suppresses the infection, and there are no clinically apparent lesions, although the organism is not necessarily eradicated from the body; *T. pallidum* can be isolated from patients years after infection.

Acquired Syphilis

Acquired syphilis in childhood appears to follow a course similar to that in adults. Although most recognized syphilitic disease of children is congenital, syphilis can be acquired at any age. Acquired syphilis in preadolescent children represents the result of sexual abuse or assault until proven otherwise, although sexually active adolescents may acquire the disease through consensual sexual activity.

Primary syphilis. Primary syphilis is characterized by a painless chancre that appears at the site of contact 10 to 90 days after exposure (average, 21 days). A chancre looks like a rounded, firm ulcer with a rubbery base and well-defined margins. The lesion is usually single and most commonly is found on the glans penis of the male and on the cervix or external genitalia of the female. It can also be found on the scrotum, anus, rectum, lips, tongue, tonsil, nipple, and fingers. Primary lesions in women often go unnoticed, since they may not be visible. Chancres persist for 3 to 6 weeks, then heal spontaneously. They usually are accompanied by regional lymphadenopathy. The lymph nodes are painless, not tender, not fluctuant, rubbery in consistency, and often bilaterally enlarged with genital lesions.

The diagnosis of primary syphilis can be made definitively by a positive darkfield examination or a reactive direct fluorescent antibody test for *T. pallidum* (DFA-TP). In addition, serologic tests for syphilis should be performed. However, nontreponemal serologic tests are reactive in less than 80% of patients presenting with primary syphilis. The treponemal tests (e.g., fluorescent treponemal antibody absorption [FTA-ABS]) become reactive earlier, with approximately 90% of patients initially seen with primary syphilis having reactive tests (Duncan et al., 1974). Therefore, if primary syphilis is suspected, the laboratory should be instructed to perform the treponemal test even if the nontreponemal or reagin test (rapid plasma reagin [RPR] or VDRL) is nonreactive. However, patients with a previously reactive treponemal test may be reactive for life, so the results may not be specific for a particular episode of genital ulcer disease (Romanowski et al., 1991).

Secondary syphilis. The secondary manifestations usually appear 3 to 6 weeks after the appearance of the chancre and 6 weeks to several months after the initial contact. The primary lesion may still be evident or may have healed when the secondary lesions appear. Signs and symptoms commonly include local or generalized rash, generalized adenopathy, malaise, fever, headache, and pharyngitis. Less common manifestations are condylomata lata (not to be confused with condyloma acuminata or genital warts, caused by HPV), mucous patches of the mouth, and alopecia. This is a systemic infection, and it is not unusual to find pleocytosis or increased protein in the CSF of patients with secondary syphilis. Lukehart et al. (1988) isolated *T. pallidum* from 10 (30%) of 33 patients with secondary syphilis, with four of these patients having normal CSF values. Therefore patients with central nervous system (CNS) involvement with *T. pallidum* can have normal CSF values. Nevertheless, it is neither routine nor recommended to perform lumbar punctures on patients with secondary syphilis, because CNS involvement is so common it is considered a part of the disease.

The skin rash is usually macular or maculopapular and rarely pustular. The rose-pink rash spreads to involve the whole body, including palms and soles, and darkens to a dull red color; it is usually not pruritic. *T. pallidum* can be demonstrated in any mucous or cutaneous lesion but is found most easily in moist lesions. The diagnosis is usually confirmed by serology during this stage, and serologic tests are virtually always reactive with high titers (>1:16). Secondary syphilitic manifestations usually resolve in 3 to 12 weeks.

Other conditions that may resemble primary and secondary syphilis include carcinoma, scabies, lichen planus, psoriasis, drug reactions, Behçet's syndrome, Reiter's syndrome, pityriasis rosea, and tinea versicolor. Because the rash is so similar, when a diagnosis of pityriasis rosea is made, a test should be performed to exclude syphilis.

Latent syphilis. After the secondary lesions resolve, the stage of latent syphilis begins. The latent stage is arbitrarily divided into early latency (syphilis of less than 1 year's duration) and late latency (syphilis of more than 1 year's duration). During early latency approximately 25% of patients with untreated syphilis will have relapses of secondary syphilis. Late latency is the stage during which tertiary manifestations can occur. By definition, latent syphilis is clinically inapparent, and the diagnosis is usually made by a reactive serologic finding in the absence of any primary or secondary symptoms. All untreated cases of syphilis are latent at some time during the course of the disease; indeed, the disease may be latent for the duration of the infection or the life of the patient. Approximately one third of infected untreated individuals develop late syphilitic manifestations, with characteristic CNS, cardiovascular, or gummatous lesions. Approximately two thirds of untreated infected individuals do not have any problems later, although more than half remain serologically reactive. However, historically these patients have had a shorter life expectancy than normal. Patients who have latent syphilis for more than 4 years are rarely contagious to their sexual partners, but pregnant women can transmit the disease to the fetus even after having latent syphilis for many years. The likelihood of transmission is directly related to the duration of infection, with secondary syphilis being the most infectious.

Late syphilis. Late syphilis is an uncommon entity in the postantibiotic era among adults and is extremely uncommon in children. Late syphilis is asymptomatic in the majority of people but may manifest as neurosyphilis, cardiovascular syphilis, or gummas. Gummas probably represent a hypersensitivity phenomenon. The other lesions of late syphilis are those of a vascular disease, with obliterative endarteritis of terminal arterioles and small arteries, which results in inflammatory and necrotic changes. Patients can have more than one late manifestation of syphilis.

Neurosyphilis. The essential pathologic process of all types of neurosyphilis is obliterative endarteritis, usually of terminal vessels, with associated parenchymatous degeneration. Neurosyphilis may be divided into the following groups, depending on the type and degree of CNS pathologic condition: asymptomatic; meningeal; meningovascular; and parenchymatous, consisting of paresis or tabes dorsalis. Optic atrophy is a serious complication of neurosyphilis and is detected by examination of the peripheral visual fields. Pupillary changes may be seen in late neurosyphilis; the classic change is the Argyll Robertson pupil, which is small and irregular and fails to react to light but responds normally to accommodation effort.

Asymptomatic Neurosyphilis. The patient with asymptomatic neurosyphilis is usually seen because of a reactive serologic finding without signs or symptoms of CNS involvement. However, the CSF shows an increase in number of cells and total amount of protein and a reactive CSF VDRL test.

Meningeal Neurosyphilis. Acute syphilitic meningitis usually appears within a year of infection as acute hydrocephalus, cranial nerve palsies, or focal cerebral involvement. The CSF shows pleocytosis, increased protein, and a reactive CSF VDRL.

Meningovascular Neurosyphilis. In patients with meningovascular neurosyphilis, definite signs and symptoms of CNS damage are present, indicating cerebrovascular occlusion; infarction; and encephalomalacia with focal neurologic signs, depending on the size and location of the lesion. The CSF is always abnormal, with pleocytosis, increase in amount of protein, and a reactive CSF VDRL.

Parenchymatous Neurosyphilis. This form of neurosyphilis appears as paresis or tabes dorsalis. The manifestations of paresis can be myriad and are always indicative of widespread damage to the parenchyma. Personality changes range from minor ones to obvious psychosis. Focal neurologic signs are uncommon. Results of the CSF studies are invariably abnormal, the number of cells and the concentration of protein are increased, and the CSF VDRL is reactive.

Cardiovascular syphilis. The damage in patients with cardiovascular syphilis is caused by medial necrosis of the aorta, with aortic dilation often extending into the valve commissures. The essential signs are those of aortic insufficiency or saccular aneurysm of the thoracic aorta.

Syphilitic gummas. Gummas are nonspecific granulomatous-like lesions. They most commonly are found in skin or bone and less commonly in mucosae, viscera, and muscle. They are usually benign, although they may cause serious problems if located in vital areas.

Congenital Syphilis

Congenital syphilis is a disease caused by maternal syphilis. Infection results from transplacental infection of the developing fetus from a mother with spirochetemia. An untreated syphilitic pregnant woman can transmit infection to the fetus at any clinical stage of her disease, although transmission is more likely with early infection. Fiumara et al. (1952) found that 50% of mothers with untreated primary or secondary syphilis had babies with congenital syphilis. The transmission to the fetus declined to 40% in early latent syphilis and 10% in late latent syphilis. Stillbirth is a frequent outcome of untreated syphilitic pregnancies. Wendel (1988) found that one half of babies with congenital syphilis were stillborn. Rawstron et al. (1997) found that most stillbirths associated with reactive maternal syphilitic serologic conditions during an outbreak had detectable *T. pallidum,* thus proving infection. However, evidence of fetal damage such as abortion is rare before the eighteenth week of gestation. Pathologic examination of tissues obtained from therapeutic abortions before 12 weeks of gestation have shown that treponemal organisms are present in fetuses from mothers who have untreated syphilis (Harter and Benirschke, 1976). No inflammatory response has been seen unless gestation is 15 weeks or more. Fetal immunoimmaturity and the inability to recognize *T. pallidum* antigens are probably responsible for the lack of damage caused by syphilis in fetuses at less than 18 weeks gestation.

The major factor associated with congenital syphilis is lack of or inadequate treatment for maternal syphilis, with no prenatal care an important risk factor (Mascola et al., 1984b, Rawstron et al., 1993). Congenital syphilis is a preventable disease if the mother receives appropriate therapy early in pregnancy. However, treatment does not guarantee that the baby will not be infected (Conover et al., 1998), particularly if therapy is given late in pregnancy (Mascola et al., 1984a; Rawstron and Bromberg, 1991a) or if the mother has early stage syphilis and a high nontreponemal titer (Sheffield et al., 2002). A woman who has been adequately treated with penicillin and followed with quantitative serologic testing and who has no evidence of reinfection does not need retreatment with each subsequent pregnancy. However, a study by Warner et al. (2001) found that more than one third of prenatal syphilis infections were repeat infections. Thus any pregnant woman with syphilis, past or present, should be reevaluated carefully, and if any doubt exists about the adequacy of previous treatment or the presence of active infection, a course of treatment should be given to prevent congenital syphilis.

The signs and symptoms of congenital syphilis are divided arbitrarily into early manifestations, which appear in the first 2 years of life, and late manifestations, which emerge any time thereafter. The outcome of untreated fetal infection is variable. Intrauterine death (stillbirth) occurs in an estimated 25% to 50% of infections. Historically, perinatal death has occurred in another 25% to 30% of untreated infected babies, although perinatal death is less common now, since many deaths in the past were due to prematurity (Wendel, 1988), but recent data suggest mortality associated with congenital syphilis remains significant (Gust, 2001). Those infants who survive have a broad spectrum of manifestations.

Early congenital syphilis. The abnormal physical and laboratory findings in patients with early congenital syphilis are varied. The onset may be before birth to approximately 3 months of age, with most cases occurring within the first 5 weeks of age. Some babies are so severely infected that they are stillborn, and some die in the early neonatal period despite the use of antibiotics. However, not all newborns are symptomatic. A baby with congenital syphilis may appear normal at birth only to appear later (delayed onset) with multiorgan system involvement (Taber and Huber, 1975). Some neonates have only hepatosplenomegaly, with or without jaundice, and some are totally asymptomatic but have evidence of bone involvement on roentgenograms or abnormal lumbar puncture results. Because most congenital syphilis is now discovered during the newborn hospital stay after suspicion is raised by a reactive serologic finding in the mother or baby, the current presentation of congenital syphilis is different from that described formerly in the literature (Fiumara, 1975). More babies who are asymptomatic but have abnormal tests indicative of infection are found. In the past these infants probably would have presented later with symptoms. Recent publications have downplayed the value of bone roentgenograms and CSF examinations in the diagnosis of congenital syphilis (Beeram et al., 1996; Risser and Hwang, 1996), but it is likely that the incidence of congenital syphilis in these populations was low. During epidemics of syphilis, women of childbearing age can remain seroreactive for long periods of time if not treated early in their infections. In addition, information about this treatment may not be easily available, giving the false impression that these women have untreated syphilis. Because these studies did not employ either *T. pallidum* detection or specific IgM determination, their conclusions should be suspect. It is reasonable to accept the utility of roentgenograms (Ingraham, 1935) and CSF VDRL determinations based on their sensitivity and specificity from both the preantibiotic era and other epidemics. Only studies that create an independent standard for congenital syphilis diagnosis can be used to refute the historically determined utility of these recommended tests.

Skeletal System. The roentgenographic changes in the bones are of diagnostic value because of their frequency and early appearance. They are present in approximately 50% to 95% of babies with congenital syphilis (Hira et al., 1985). The changes often are present at birth but may not appear until the first few weeks of life. Some have suggested that roentgenograms would be of most value at 1 month of age but this suggestion is not usually practical. The bony changes include osteochondritis and periostitis; metaphyseal changes are most common. The findings are symmetric and self-limited and heal in approximately 6 months, with or without therapy. The skeletal lesions are usually asymptomatic but are occasionally painful, so much so that the child will refuse to move the affected limb (pseudoparalysis of Parrot). The femur and tibia are most often involved, and a radiologic study of the knee is recommended when screening for syphilis. On x-ray films the earliest changes are revealed in the metaphysis and are seen as transverse, sawtooth, radiodense bands of provisional calcification, with an underlying zone of osteoporosis, which is seen as radiolucent bands. Irregular areas of increased density and rarefaction produce the moth-eaten appearance on the x-ray film. The classic Wimberger's ("cat-bite") sign consists of a focal defect in the medial proximal tibial epiphysis and is caused by destructive osteitis. Periostitis appears later than osteochon- dritis and is seen on x-ray films as multiple layers of periosteal new bone formation. Radiologic findings in patients with congenital syphilis are shown in Figures 32-1, 32-2, and 32-3.

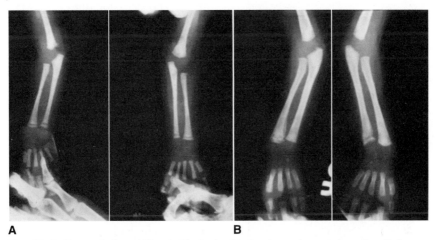

A   **B**

Fig. 32-1 Congenital syphilis. **A,** Typical wide horizontal metaphyseal radiolucent bands. **B,** Destructive syphilitic metaphysitis of the radius and ulna in a 6-week-old infant. Note subperiosteal reaction.

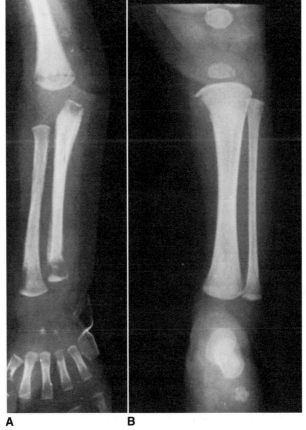

A   **B**

Fig. 32-2 Congenital syphilis. **A,** Panosteitis in an infant 9 weeks old. Metaphysitis is present and subperiosteal bone is appearing. **B,** Radiolucent area of the medial aspect of the proximal tibial metaphyses. This is called *Wimberger's sign.*

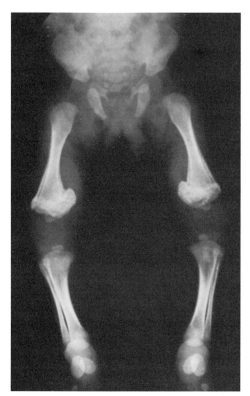

Fig. 32-3 Congenital syphilis. Diaphysitis with abundant callus formation secondary to pathologic fractures through the metaphyseal lesions. The lesions healed, and there were no sequelae.

Rhinitis. Rhinitis was a common manifestation historically but is uncommon now. It is not usually present at birth but appears after the first week of life. It initially is seen as severe and intractable rhinorrhea, which is often bloody and may be associated with a hoarse cry caused by laryngitis. Treponemes can be easily identified by darkfield microscopy or immunofluorescent antibody testing of the nasal material.

Rash. Historically, the syphilitic rash typically appeared 1 or 2 weeks after the rhinitis, but it is more common now to see the rash without preceding rhinitis. The typical eruption is maculopapular and consists of small, dark-red spots, but bullous eruptions can also occur. The rash commonly is present on the back, perineum, extremities, palms, and soles. The rash lasts 1 to 3 months without treatment, and the lesions may be covered by a fine, silvery scale and be followed by desquamation. The rash usually fades to leave coppery residual pigmentation.

Constitutional Symptoms. The most common finding with early congenital syphilis is hepatosplenomegaly. Jaundice may be associated

with it because of hepatic dysfunction, which is manifest by an increase in conjugated bilirubin (Srinivasan et al., 1983). Generalized lymphadenopathy may occur, although it is more common in historical cases. Infants may have fevers and occasionally nephrosis or nephritis. Choroiditis and iritis are uncommon.

The laboratory findings include a Coombs-negative hemolytic anemia with leukopenia or leukocytosis and thrombocytopenia. Congenital syphilis is one of the causes of a leukemoid reaction. Lumbar puncture may reveal a reactive CSF VDRL, with increased protein and pleocytosis, although most babies clinically have no findings of CNS involvement. Michelow et al, (2002) used rabbit infectivity testing (RIT) to detect *T. pallidum* in CSF of infants with congenital syphilis. They found that a combination of CSF VDRL, white blood cell count (WBC), and protein had a low sensitivity (85%) and specificity (65%) compared with RIT. Three of 17 infants with spirochetes detected in the CSF by RIT were not identified by conventional CSF tests (but other findings of congenital syphilis), and one infant with normal results on conventional diagnostic evaluation also had treponemes identified in the CSF by RIT. This highlights the limitations of conventional diagnostic tests for congenital syphilis. No single test identified infants who had congenital syphilis or those with treponemes identified in the CSF. We have detected *T. pallidum* in the unremarkable CSF of infants with congenital syphilis by immunofluorescent antigen detection.

The congenital syphilis of neonates and infants may resemble other intrauterine infections, including toxoplasmosis, rubella, cytomegalovirus, and herpes simplex virus. Other conditions that may resemble congenital syphilis in newborns include bacterial sepsis, blood group incompatibility, battered child syndrome, "periostitis" of prematurity, neonatal hepatitis, and osteomyelitis.

The placenta is a useful organ to examine when looking for congenital syphilis. The presence of necrotizing funisitis suggests congenital syphilis (Fojaco et al., 1989). The placenta may also be large and bulky and have the characteristic findings of focal villitis, endovascular and perivascular proliferation of vessels, and relative immaturity of villi (Russell and Altshuler, 1974). Increased placental thickness diagnosed by ultrasound was seen in 17 of 24 fetuses diagnosed with congenital syphilis by Hollier et al.

(2001). Identification of *T. pallidum* (either whole organisms or genetic material) in tissue specimens or by RIT is the only accepted method for making a confirmed diagnosis of congenital syphilis.

Late congenital syphilis. Late manifestations of congenital syphilis are the result of scarring from the early systemic disease and include involvement of the teeth, bones, eyes, and eighth nerve (Fiumara and Lessell, 1983); gummas in the viscera, skin, or mucous membranes; and neurosyphilis (Digre et al., 1991; Wolf and Kalangu, 1993). Late syphilis is very rare in the antibiotic era.

Teeth. Characteristic changes are found in the permanent upper-central incisors, which present a notched appearance of the biting edges; these are called *Hutchinson's teeth*. First molars with maldevelopment of the cusps are known as *mulberry* or *Moon's molars* (Figures 32-4 and 32-5).

Interstitial Keratitis. Interstitial keratitis is the most common late lesion. It may appear at any age between 4 and 30 years or later, but characteristically it appears when the patient is close to puberty. It first manifests with unilateral photophobia, pain, and blurred vision. A ground-glass appearance may develop in the cornea, accompanied by vascularization of the adjacent sclera. These changes become bilateral and lead to blindness. Penicillin treatment is ineffective, but steroid treatment can help prevent loss of vision.

Eighth Nerve Deafness. Hearing loss is usually sudden and appears in children around 8 to 10 years of age. Hutchinson's triad consists of interstitial keratitis accompanied by neural deafness and typical Hutchinson's teeth (Karmody and Schuknecht, 1966).

Neurosyphilis. The same manifestations of neurosyphilis seen in patients with acquired syphilis can occur in those with congenital syphilis,

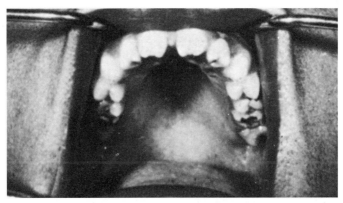

Fig. 32-4 Hutchinson's teeth. Note the notched edges and screwdriver shape of the central incisors.

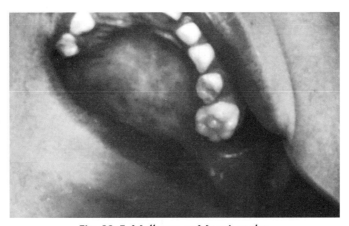

Fig. 32-5 Mulberry or Moon's molar.

although symptomatic neurosyphilis is very rare. Paresis is seen more frequently and tabes dorsalis less frequently in the congenital form than in the acquired form of the disease.

Bone Changes. Bone changes include sclerosing lesions, saber shins, frontal bossing, and the gummatous or destructive lesion of saddle nose. Perforation of the hard palate is almost pathognomonic of congenital syphilis.

Clutton's Joint. Clutton's joint is painless arthritis of the knees and, rarely, other joints. It usually is first seen around puberty.

Cutaneous Lesions. Rhagades represent scarring from persistent rhinitis during infancy and are rarely seen today.

Laboratory Procedures in the Diagnosis of Syphilis

There are two main ways of diagnosing syphilis. The first is to detect treponemes using darkfield or immunofluorescent methods (or RIT in research laboratories). The second is to detect antibodies formed in response to a treponemal infection, using nontreponemal and treponemal antibody tests.

Dark-field examination. The diagnosis of syphilis can be made by a reactive darkfield examination of appropriate specimens. This test requires a compound microscope equipped with a darkfield condenser with which the specimen is illuminated by reflected light against a dark background. A reactive diagnosis can be made by an experienced worker on the basis of characteristic morphologic aspects and motility. Darkfield examination is most productive during primary, secondary, and early congenital syphilis when lesions are present. Gloves should be worn when examining suspected syphilitic lesions and when performing darkfield examinations. Lesions should be cleaned thoroughly with physiologic saline solution with no additives. The lesion should then be squeezed and scraped firmly to collect serum rather than blood. Aspirated material from involved regional lymph nodes also can be examined for *T. pallidum*. The specimen must be viewed within 5 to 10 minutes to detect motile treponemes. If the result of the initial darkfield examination is negative, it should be repeated on at least 2 successive days to confirm a negative result.

Immunofluorescent antigen detection. Alternative methods to detect *T. pallidum* in lesions are direct and indirect fluorescent antibody (FA) tests for *T. pallidum*. These tests use either monoclonal or polyclonal antibodies against *T. pallidum* that are directly fluorescein tagged or use a second fluorescein-tagged antibody to detect the primary antibody-antigen complex (Yobs et al., 1964). The advantage of immunofluorescent methods over darkfield microscopy is that slides are more permanent and can be mailed to reference laboratories for review by experts if the volume of patients seen is too small to warrant having a darkfield microscope (Bromberg et al., 1993).

Nontreponemal tests. The serologic diagnosis of syphilis uses two general types of tests: nontreponemal (reaginic) and treponemal. The nontreponemal tests use cardiolipin and lecithin as antigen. The antibody measured has been termed *reagin,* which has no relationship to the reaginic IgE in allergic patients. Antibody appears in the blood 1 to 3 weeks after the chancre appears or approximately 4 to 6 weeks after the infection. The nontreponemal tests commonly used today are the VDRL test and the RPR test. The RPR test uses a modified VDRL antigen. The RPR test is inexpensive and quantitated and can be well controlled. The height of the titer tends to correlate with disease activity, rising with new infection and falling after treatment. A change of one doubling dilution is within laboratory error and therefore not significant. Changes of two dilutions (fourfold changes, e.g., 1:2 increasing to 1:8) are considered significant when assessing disease activity. However, these tests are not specific for syphilis and may also be reactive in patients with collagen-vascular disease, liver disease, and other conditions.

Reactive nontreponemal serologic results are found in approximately 80% of patients with primary syphilis, 100% of patients with secondary syphilis, and 95% of patients with early latent syphilis, but only 70% of patients with late latent or late (tertiary) syphilis (Sparling, 1971). Thus, false-negative serologic findings using nontreponemal tests is a problem in very early and again in later stages of untreated syphilis. With adequate treatment the nontreponemal tests should become nonreactive 6 to 12 months after primary syphilis and 12 to 24 months after secondary syphilis (Fiumara, 1980). Romanowski et al. (1991) found that it took much longer for titers to become nonreactive. Patients with later stages of syphilis who are treated take longer for their titers to fall and may never revert to having nonreactive results on nontreponemal tests; thus they may continue to have low titers for life, or be "serofast."

Treponemal tests. The FTA-ABS test is an indirect antibody test that uses *T. pallidum* as the antigen. The FTA-ABS test is quite sensitive and specific when used as a confirmatory test (Deacon et al., 1966). It is technically more difficult than the nontreponemal tests and is used for confirmation of reactive nontreponemal tests. The results of this test are reported as reactive, minimally reactive, or nonreactive, and they are not quantitated. The treponemal tests become reactive earlier in primary syphilis than do nontreponemal tests and, once reactive, can remain so for life, even after appropriate therapy.

The microhemagglutination assay for antibodies to *T. pallidum* (MHA-TP or TPHA) is a qualitative hemagglutination test that uses sheep erythrocytes as carriers for the *T. pallidum* antigen. False-reactive tests are very uncommon with both FTA-ABS and MHA-TP when they are used to confirm a reactive nontreponemal test. When treponemal tests are used as screening tests, they have lower specificity. Patients with lupus may have false-reactive FTA-ABS, MHA-TP, and nontreponemal tests. A newer test using gelatin particles instead of erythrocytes as a carrier for the *T. pallidum* (*T. pallidum* particle agglutination [TPPA] assay) appears to be at least as sensitive (Pope et al., 2000) and is being used as a replacement for the MHA-TP in some laboratories (Young, 2000). New tests on the horizon using recombinant technology are being evaluated for use as both screening (Young et al., 1998) and confirmatory tests (Fears et al., 2001).

Some laboratories are no longer using the two-step approach described above but are using newer treponemal antigen-based EIAs such as the CAPTIA Syphilis-G test (Trinity Biotech, Jamestown, New York) (Halling et al., 1999; Young et al., 1989) and others (Schmidt et al., 2000; Young et al., 2000) as initial screening tests. Reactive screening tests need to be confirmed with another treponemal test different from the one used for screening, for example, TPHA if an EIA is used for screening (Egglestone and Turner, 2000; Young, 2000), as well as a quantitative test to assess disease activity (RPR or VDRL). These treponemal EIAs have advantages such as automation, lack

of prozone phenomena, and increased sensitivity in late stages of disease.

T. pallidum IgM tests have been used in the diagnosis of congenital syphilis because, unlike IgG, IgM does not cross the placenta. Therefore, detection of specific IgM in a baby is a strong indication of infection. There are various kinds of *T. pallidum* IgM tests, but none is widely available, and none is currently recommended by the CDC (Centers for Disease Control and Prevention, 2002) or other experts (Sanchez, 1998). The original *T. pallidum* IgM, an immunofluorescent test described by Scotti and Logan (1968), had too many false-reactive (10%) and false-negative (up to 35%) results for widespread clinical use (Kaufman et al., 1974). Newer IgM tests have been evaluated in congenital syphilis (Stoll et al., 1993), with sensitivities of 73% to 88% in symptomatic babies. Western blot tests have been used for research purposes and apparently are sensitive and specific for evaluating babies with congenital syphilis, although only small numbers of babies have been evaluated using this technique (Grimprel et al., 1991; Sanchez et al., 1989; Sanchez et al., 1992; Sanchez et al., 1993). None of these IgM tests can detect all babies with syphilis, because some babies are so recently infected that they have no IgM present at delivery. Thus a combination of antigen or DNA detection along with IgM might present the best strategy for diagnosing or identifying them (Bromberg et al., 1993).

Diagnosis of congenital syphilis. The diagnosis of congenital syphilis in the newborn period can be difficult. Both the nontreponemal and treponemal tests measure IgG antibody and therefore do not distinguish disease in the infant from maternally derived antibody. The minority of babies with congenital syphilis are symptomatic at birth. Although some infants will develop symptoms later if left untreated, some may never become symptomatic. Unfortunately, there is no "gold standard" test for congenital syphilis. A combination of physical findings, radiologic results, laboratory tests, and ancillary tests is used to screen for and diagnose congenital syphilis. In the past clinicians waited for the development of symptoms, but in present-day practice this is unwise because of the high probability of losing the patient to follow-up. In the diagnosis of congenital syphilis, therefore, it is best to err on the side of overdiagnosis and overtreatment

(Box 32-1). The 2002 CDC guidelines recommend that infants should be evaluated for congenital syphilis if they are born to mothers with reactive nontreponemal and treponemal tests. Evaluation and treatment of the baby depend on physical examination findings and nontreponemal titer in the baby and the history of maternal syphilis therapy and follow-up.

The CDC (Centers for Disease Control and Prevention, 2002a) recommends that every baby

---

BOX 32-1

CONGENITAL SYPHILIS

Clinical Description

A condition caused by infection in utero with *Treponema pallidum*. A wide spectrum of severity exists, and only severe cases are clinically apparent at birth.

An infant (<2 years) may have signs such as hepatosplenomegaly, characteristic skin rash, condyloma lata, snuffles, jaundice (nonviral hepatitis), pseudoparalysis, anemia, or edema (nephrotic syndrome and/or malnutrition). An older child may have stigmata such as interstitial keratitis, nerve deafness, anterior bowing of shins, frontal bossing, mulberry molars, Hutchinson's teeth, saddle nose, rhagades, or Clutton's joints.

Laboratory Criteria for Diagnosis

Demonstration of *T. pallidum* by darkfield microscopy, fluorescent antibody, or other specific stains in specimens from lesions, placenta, umbilical cord, or autopsy material.

Case Classification

Presumptive

The infection of an infant whose mother had untreated or inadequately treated* syphilis at delivery regardless of signs in the infant; or the infection of an infant or child who has a reactive treponemal test for syphilis and any one of the following:

- Any evidence of congenital syphilis on physical examination.
- Any evidence of congenital syphilis on long bone roentgenogram.
- A reactive cerebrospinal fluid (CSF) VDRL.
- An elevated CSF cell count or protein (without other cause).
- A reactive test for fluorescent treponemal antibody absorbed-19S-IgM antibody.

Confirmed

A case (among infants) that is laboratory confirmed.

Comment

Congenital and acquired syphilis may be difficult to distinguish when a child is seropositive after infancy. Signs of congenital syphilis may not be obvious, and stigmata may not yet have developed.

Abnormal values for CSF VDRL, cell count, and protein, as well as IgM antibodies, may be found in either congenital or acquired syphilis. Findings on long bone roentgenograms may help, since roentgenographic changes in the metaphysis and epiphysis are considered classic for congenitally acquired disease. The decision may ultimately be based on maternal history and clinical judgment. The possibility of sexual abuse should be considered.

For reporting purposes, congenital syphilis includes cases of congenitally acquired syphilis among infants and children, as well as syphilitic stillbirths.

Syphilitic Stillbirth

Clinical case definition

A fetal death that occurs after a 20-week gestation or in which the fetus weighs >500 g, and the mother had untreated or inadequately treated* syphilis at delivery.

Comment

For reporting purposes, syphilitic stillbirths should be reported as cases of congenital syphilis.

From Centers for Disease Control, October 19, 1990.

*Inadequate treatment consists of any nonpenicillin therapy or penicillin given <30 days before delivery.

born to a mother with a reactive nontreponemal and treponemal test be evaluated as follows:

1. Quantitative nontreponemal (RPR/VDRL) test should be performed on the baby's serum (not cord blood). A treponemal test in the baby is not necessary, because the mother's reactive treponemal test confirms the nontreponemal test is due to syphilis.
2. Infants should be thoroughly examined for evidence of congenital syphilis (e.g., nonimmune hydrops, jaundice, hepatosplenomegaly, rhinitis, skin rash, and/or pseudoparalysis of an extremity).
3. Pathologic examination of the placenta or umbilical cord using specific fluorescent antitreponemal antibody staining is suggested.
4. Darkfield microscopy or DFA staining of suspicious lesions or body fluids should also be performed.

Further evaluation of the baby and treatment depend on the results of the above examination and the history of maternal therapy and follow-up.

Scenario 1. A baby with an abnormal physical examination consistent with congenital syphilis or a nontreponemal titer fourfold higher than the mother's (in our experience an uncommon event) or detection of treponemes in the baby by darkfield or immunofluorescent antibody tests should be further evaluated with CSF analysis of VDRL, cell count, protein, complete blood count with differential and platelet count and other tests as indicated (long bone x-ray examination, chest x-ray examination, liver function tests, cranial ultrasound, ophthalmologic examination, and auditory brainstem response). These infants require 10 days of parenteral penicillin (see regimens below).

Scenario 2. If the infant has a normal physical examination and nontreponemal titer that is the same as or less than fourfold the maternal titer, then further evaluation depends on the history of maternal therapy. The infant requires evaluation (CSF VDRL, glucose, protein, complete blood count plus differential and platelet count, and long bone x-ray examination) under any of the following conditions:

- The mother was not treated, was inadequately treated, or has no documentation of treatment.
- The mother was treated with erythromycin or another nonpenicillin regimen.
- The mother was treated less than 4 weeks before delivery.

- The mother has early syphilis and has a nontreponemal titer that has either not decreased fourfold or has increased fourfold.

Scenario 3. Infant has a normal examination and has a titer the same as or less than fourfold maternal titer. Maternal treatment was adequate, with appropriate penicillin regimen administered more than 4 weeks before delivery with appropriate fall in titer. In this case, the baby does not need to be evaluated according to the CDC.

Scenario 4. Infants with normal physical examination and nontreponemal titer the same as or less than fourfold maternal titer do not need to be evaluated if the mother was treated before pregnancy and her titer remained low and stable before and during pregnancy and at delivery (VDRL ≤ 1:2; RPR ≤ 1:4).

Note that the maternal history and treatment must be well documented for any of the scenarios in which the infant is not evaluated or treated.

It is also recommended that an infant not be released from the hospital until the serologic status of the mother is known because one third of babies born to mothers with reactive serologic findings have nonreactive cord blood serologic findings (Miller et al., 1960; Rawstron and Bromberg, 1991b). Therefore maternal serologic testing is preferred over cord blood testing in screening for congenital syphilis at delivery.

Treatment

T. pallidum is exquisitely sensitive to penicillin, with an MIC of 0.005 to 0.01 μg/ml as defined by rabbit experimentation (Eagle et al., 1950). Effective therapy for syphilis has been aimed at maintaining an MIC of 0.03 units/ml (0.018 μg/ml) for 7 to 10 days (Idsoe et al., 1972) because of the slow dividing time of *T. pallidum* (every 30 hours). Thus therapy is designed to achieve and maintain several times the necessary inhibitory levels. Penicillin remains the drug of choice because there is no evidence of resistance of *T. pallidum* to penicillin, and it has minimal toxicity and established efficacy in treating syphilis.

Congenital syphilis. Who should be treated? The decision to treat rests on the results of the evaluation of the baby described previously and the history of syphilis and treatment in the mother. Infants with abnormalities on evaluation (scenario 1) or those born to mothers with inadequately treated syphilis (scenario 2) should be treated, even when the evaluation is "normal."

How they should be treated? In scenario 1 treatment of congenital syphilis is the same regardless of whether or not there are CSF abnormalities, because patients can have neurosyphilis and normal CSF values. Treatment should be with aqueous crystalline penicillin G (50,000 units/kg/dose) administered every 12 hours during the first 7 days of life and then every 8 hours (100,000 to 150,000 units/kg/day) thereafter. An alternative, which perhaps is preferable because of its ease of administration, is procaine penicillin (50,000 units/kg/day), given as 1 IM dose daily (McCracken and Kaplan, 1974). The length of therapy for both regimens is 10 days. If more than 1 day of therapy is missed, the entire therapy should be restarted. The CDC prefers a full 10-day course of penicillin, even if ampicillin was initially given for suspected sepsis, and close serologic follow-up is recommended if agents other than penicillin are used. However, we have included the ampicillin doses used as part of the initial "sepsis workup" as part of a total 10-day treatment course in a number of babies without any problems or known failures.

All infants in scenario 2 are also treated, although another treatment option is offered here. In addition to the treatment for scenario 1, the option of a single dose of benzathine penicillin G (50,000 units/kg/dose IM) is given for infants who are fully evaluated (including lumbar puncture, x-ray examination, and complete blood count with platelets) and have negative results. However, some specialists and we prefer 10 days of therapy for all babies in this group, regardless of evaluation results. If an infant in scenario 2 does not undergo a full evaluation, or the lumbar puncture is uninterpretable because of contamination of CSF with blood, then treatment with 10 days of parenteral penicillin is recommended. Some experts do not like to use benzathine penicillin G in babies with congenital syphilis because CSF levels are subtherapeutic (Speer et al., 1977) and treatment failures, although not common, have been documented (Beck-Sagué and Alexander, 1987). If follow-up of these patients is a problem, they should be treated with procaine penicillin for 10 days. Some programs have treated these infants with procaine penicillin at home administered by visiting nurses. These programs have the secondary benefit of providing needed parenting education.

Infants in scenario 3 can be treated with one intramuscular dose of benzathine penicillin G (50,000 units/kg); alternatively, some specialists would not treat these infants, but would follow them closely, performing repeat serologic tests. Similarly in scenario 4, there are 2 options: no treatment but close follow-up, or a single dose of benzathine penicillin G, particularly if follow-up is uncertain.

Treatment beyond the newborn period. After the newborn period, all children with syphilis should have a lumbar puncture performed, and birth and maternal records should be reviewed to assess whether the infection is congenital or acquired. Any child who is thought to have congenital syphilis or who has neurologic involvement should be treated with aqueous crystalline penicillin G (50,000 units/kg/dose) every 4 to 6 hours for 10 days. Older children with acquired syphilis and normal neurologic results may be treated with benzathine penicillin G (50,000 units/kg IM) up to the adult dose of 2.4 million units for primary or secondary syphilis. If the child has latent syphilis of unknown duration, 3 doses of benzathine penicillin (50,000 units/kg/dose [maximum 2.4 million units per dose]) at weekly intervals should be given. Penicillin is the only recommended treatment for children with syphilis; therefore, if there is a history of penicillin allergy, children and all pregnant women should be skin tested and desensitized if necessary (Zenker and Rolfs, 1990; Wendel et al., 1985).

Adolescents with syphilis. Treatment of adolescents with syphilis should be similar to that of adults at the same stage of disease. Primary, secondary, and early latent syphilis of less than 1 year's duration should be treated with benzathine penicillin G (50,000 units/kg), with a maximum of 2.4 million units IM in 1 dose. An alternative regimen for penicillin-allergic patients is doxycycline (100 mg orally twice a day for 2 weeks).

Adolescents with late latent syphilis of more than 1 year's duration should be treated with benzathine penicillin G (150,000 units/kg total, with a maximum of 7.2 million units total) administered as 3 doses of 50,000 units/kg IM (maximum of 2.4 million units) given 1 week apart for 3 consecutive weeks. Alternative therapy for penicillin-allergic patients is doxycycline in the same doses used for patients with early syphilis but given for 4 weeks instead of 2 weeks.

Neurosyphilis. Recommended treatment for neurosyphilis in adults is aqueous penicillin G,

3 to 4 million units every 4 hours IV (18 to 24 million units per day) for 10 to 14 days. Alternative therapy is procaine penicillin (2.4 million units IM daily) with probenecid (500 mg orally 4 times a day) for 10 to 14 days. Many experts also recommend benzathine penicillin G (2.4 million units IM weekly for 3 doses) after finishing either of the foregoing treatment regimens.

Jarisch-Herxheimer reaction. Jarisch-Herxheimer reaction is an acute febrile reaction that may occur after any therapy for syphilis. The reaction consists of a fever, which is usually accompanied by headache and myalgia, that commonly lasts less than 24 hours. Pregnant women may have associated contractions and should be warned about this possibility. There is no treatment recommended except for antipyretic agents if necessary.

Follow-up. Infants with congenital syphilis should be followed with serologic tests every 2 to 3 months. If the baby did not receive therapy, follow-up should also include serologic testing at 1 and 2 months to ensure that titers are falling. Nontreponemal titers should decline by 3 months and usually disappear by 6 months of age in the absence of infection. If titers are stable or increasing, the child should be reevaluated and retreated. Treponemal titers will eventually become negative in the absence of infection. A child that retains a reactive treponemal titer after the expected time of maternal antibody disappearance has had congenital syphilis. The timing of disappearance of maternal antibodies in these babies is not clear. The 2002 CDC guidelines state that maternal antibodies can be present for up to 15 months, and that a reactive treponemal titer after 18 months is diagnostic of congenital syphilis. Published data on follow-up of babies born to mothers with reactive syphilis serology are limited (Chang et al., 1995; Rawstron et al., 2001). Chang found that 84% of uninfected children born to mothers with syphilis had VDRL seroreversion by 6 months, and 100% by 12 months, with TPHA seroreversion by 12 months in 95% and FTA-ABS seroreversion by 12 months in 100%. Rawstron et al. found that a reactive FTA-ABS was retained after 12 and 15 months in many (but not all) babies with congenital syphilis, although FTA-ABS reactivity declined with time, and almost half of the children with reactive FTA-ABS at 12 months had not been identified as having congenital

syphilis in the newborn period (although they were treated). The CDC recommends no retreatment of a child with a reactive FTA-ABS at 18 months (and nonreactive nontreponemal titer) and adequate therapy as a newborn. However, if the nontreponemal test is reactive at this time, the CDC recommends reevaluation and treatment. Close follow-up of children born to mothers with syphilis is very important, and documentation of a reactive treponemal test after adequate treatment of congenital syphilis may be very important if syphilis screening is performed at a later date for potential sexual abuse or as part of adolescent sexual health screening.

Infants who had reactive findings on the initial lumbar puncture should have repeat lumbar punctures every 6 months until the CSF examination is normal.

Syphilis and HIV Disease

The epidemic of early syphilis in the United States in the late 1980s overlapped with the HIV epidemic. Early observations (Musher et al., 1990) found that HIV coinfection with syphilis caused the following: failure to respond to treatment within the expected time; relapse after treatment; and the frequent appearance of early neurosyphilis, especially after conventional doses of benzathine penicillin. However, systematic study of patients coinfected with syphilis and HIV in a prospective multicenter randomized controlled trial (Rolfs et al., 1997; Rompalo et al., 2001) of enhanced versus standard therapy for syphilis revealed few significant differences associated with HIV coinfection. The clinical manifestations of primary and secondary syphilis differed only in the more frequent development of multiple ulcers in patients with primary syphilis who were HIV reactive, and the more frequent occurrence of manifestations of secondary syphilis concomitantly with genital ulcers in those who were HIV reactive. Serologic response to treatment among HIV-infected patients with primary and secondary syphilis was slower, but clinically defined treatment failures were uncommon and enhanced therapy did not improve outcome regardless of HIV status.

There have been no documented treatment failures among either pregnant women who are HIV reactive with syphilis or their offspring, although the congenital syphilis rate was almost 50 times higher in a group of mothers in Texas with syphilis and HIV (Schulte et al.,

2001). At this time the CDC recommends no change in therapy for patients with early syphilis in HIV-infected patients, although some experts recommend additional benzathine penicillin treatments (three doses as recommended for late syphilis), and some experts recommend CSF examination before treatment of HIV-infected persons with early syphilis and intensified therapy if CNS syphilis is diagnosed. These patients should be followed very closely for signs of treatment failure. Any patient with syphilis should have HIV testing, because both of these diseases may be present in the same patient. In regard to the management of infants born to HIV reactive and RPR reactive mothers, although there are no data, it is our recommendation that these infants be treated as if they had CNS involvement.

Syphilis and Sexual Abuse

Syphilis is not commonly found among sexually abused children (Table 32-1). However, it has been reported in a few instances. White et al. (1983) detected six cases among 108 of 409 prepubertal children on whom serologic tests were performed. Five children were asymptomatic and had additional STDs, and only one was symptomatic with chancres. De Jong (1986) found only 1 out of 532 abused children had a reactive serologic test for syphilis. Children are seen with the same signs and symptoms as adults with syphilis. Ginsberg (1983) described three patients with acquired syphilis, one of whom was initially seen with a primary chancre and two with rashes of secondary syphilis. Ackerman (1972) similarly observed three abused children with rashes of condylomata lata of secondary syphilis. More recent case reports of four young children with acquired syphilis (Christian 1999; Connors 1998), also presented with condyloma lata, rashes of secondary syphilis, and latent syphilis. Evaluation of some of the cases was confounded by a history of possible congenital syphilis, highlighting the importance of follow-up of children born to mothers with syphilis to determine their serologic outcomes. It is recommended that a serologic test for syphilis be performed on every child suspected of being sexually abused and that the test also be repeated after 12 weeks.

CHLAMYDIA TRACHOMATIS
Biology of Chlamydiae

The order Chlamydiales is composed of a group of obligate intracellular parasites with a unique developmental cycle with morphologically distinct infectious and reproductive forms. All members of the order have a gram-negative envelope without peptidoglycan, share a genus-specific lipopolysaccharide antigen, and use host adenosine triphosphate (ATP) for the synthesis of chlamydial protein. Originally the order contained one genus, *Chlamydia*, with four recognized species: *C. trachomatis*, *Chlamydia psittaci*, *Chlamydia pneumoniae*, and *Chlamydia pecorum*, with *C. trachomatis* and *C. pneumoniae* being the most important as human pathogens. Recent taxonomic analysis using the 16S and 23S rRNA genes have found

| TABLE 32-1 | Prevalence of Syphilitic, Gonorrheal, and Chlamydial Infections in Sexually Abused Children: Selected Studies |

Study (year)	Number tested	NUMBER (%) POSITIVE		
		Syphilis	Gonorrhea	Chlamydia
Rimsza and Niggemann (1982)	285	0	21 (7)	NS
White et al. (1983)	409	6 (1)	46 (11)	NS
De Jong (1986)	532	1 (0.2)	25 (5)	NS
Hammerschlag et al. (1984)	51	0	5 (10)	2 (4)
Ingram et al. (1984)	50	NS	10 (20)	3 (6)
Ingram et al. (1992)	1538	1 (0.1)	41 (3)	18 (1)
Siegel et al. (1995)	423	0	12 (2.8)	11 (2.6)
Sicoli (1995)	316	NS	7 (2.1)	NS
Embree et al. (1996)	138	NS	2 (1.5)	2 (1.5)
Ingram et al. (2001)	3040	NS	37 (1.2)	25 (0.8)

NS, Not stated.

TABLE 32-2	Serovars of *Chlamydia trachomatis*
Serovar	Disease
A, B, Ba, C	Hyperendemic blinding trachoma
D, E, F, G, H, I, J, K	Neonatal inclusion conjunctivitis
	Infantile pneumonitis
	Nongonococcal urethritis
	Mucopurulent cervicitis and salpingitis
	Proctitis
	Epididymitis
L1, L2, L3	Lymphogranuloma venereum

that the order Chlamydiales contains at least four distinct groups at the family level and that within the order Chlamydiaceae are two distinct lineages (Everett et al., 1999). This analysis has suggested splitting the genus *Chlamydia* into two genera, *Chlamydia* and *Chlamydophila*. Two new species, *Chlamydia muridarum* (formerly the agent of mouse pneumonitis—MoPn) and *Chlamydia suis* would join *C. trachomatis*. *Chlamydophila* would contain *C. pecorum*, *C. pneumoniae*, and *C. psittaci* and three new species split off from *C. psittaci*: *Chlamydia abortus*, *Chlamydia caviae* (formerly *C. psittaci* Guinea pig conjunctivitis strain) and *Chlamydia felis*. There are fifteen known serotypes of *C. trachomatis* (Table 32-2).

Chlamydiae have a gram-negative envelope without detectable peptidoglycan, although recent genomic analysis has revealed that both *C. trachomatis* and *C. pneumoniae* encode for proteins forming a nearly complete pathway for synthesis of peptidoglycan, including penicillin-binding proteins (Rockey et al., 2000). This may be the basis for the so-called "chlamydial peptidoglycan paradox," as it has been known for decades that chlamydia development is sensitive to ß-lactam antibiotics. Chlamydiae also share a group-specific lipopolysaccharide antigen and utilize host adenosine triphosphate for the synthesis of chlamydial protein. Although chlamydiae are auxotrophic for three of four nucleoside triphosphates, they do encode functional glucose-catabolizing enzymes, which can be used for generation of ATP. As with peptidoglycan synthesis, for some reason these genes are turned off. This may be related to their adaptation to the intracellular environment. All chlamydiae also encode an abundant protein called the *major outer membrane protein* (MOMP or OmpA) that is surface exposed in *C. trachomatis* and *C. psittaci*, but apparently not in

C. pneumoniae. The MOMP is the major determinant of the serologic classification of *C. trachomatis* and *C. psittaci* isolates. Chlamydiae are susceptible to antibiotics that interfere with DNA and protein synthesis, including tetracyclines, macrolides, and quinolones.

Chlamydiae have a unique developmental cycle with morphologically distinct infectious and reproductive forms: elementary body (EB) and reticulate body (RB) (Figure 32-6). EBs, 200 to 400 nm in diameter, attach to the host cell by a process of electrostatic binding and are taken into the cell by endocytosis that is not dependent on the microtubule system. Within the host cell the EB remains within a membrane-lined phagosome. Fusion of the phagosome with the host cell lysosome does not occur. The EBs then differentiate into reticulate bodies that undergo binary fission. After approximately 36 hours, the reticulate bodies differentiate into

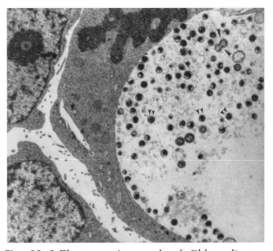

Fig. 32-6 Electron micrograph of *Chlamydia trachomatis* inclusions at 48 hours, demonstrating reticulate body undergoing binary fission *(arrows)* and elementary bodies *(double arrows)*.

EBs. At approximately 48 hours, release may occur by cytolysis or by a process of exocytosis or extrusion of the whole inclusion, leaving the host cell intact. Infection can proceed without causing significant cellular damage. Thus there is a biologic basis for the prolonged subclinical infection, which is a hallmark of human chlamydial disease. Because the organisms are obligate intracellular parasites, they are actively infecting cells rather than simple colonizers, which have no interaction with the host cells.

Epidemiology

C. trachomatis is the most prevalent infectious disease and sexually transmitted infection in the United States today. There were 656,721 cases of *C. trachomatis* infection reported in 1999 (Centers for Disease Control and Prevention, 2001a). The prevalence of chlamydial infection is more weakly associated with socioeconomic status, urban or rural residence, and race or ethnicity than gonorrhea and syphilis. Prevalences of *C. trachomatis* infection are consistently greater than 5% among sexually active, adolescent, young adult women attending outpatient clinics, regardless of the region of the country, location of the clinic (urban or rural), or the race or ethnicity of the population (Table 32-3). The highest prevalences are seen in females 15 to 19 years of age and commonly exceed 10%. In contrast, infection rates in males in the same age range are frequently much less—often only one third to one half the rates in females in the same population. The reasons for this disparity are not clear. One possible explanation is that the sexual partners of these girls are often adult men. Infection with *C. trachomatis* is usually asymptomatic and of long duration. If a pregnant woman has active infection during delivery, the infant can acquire the infection and is at risk to develop either conjunctivitis or pneumonia (Alexander and Harrison, 1983). Rarely, children acquire chlamydial infection as a result of sexual abuse.

Infections in Adolescent and Adult Males

C. trachomatis is the single most frequently identifiable cause of nongonococcal urethritis in men, accounting for 30% to 40% of all episodes, or 1.5 million episodes annually. The usual incubation period is 5 to 10 days. Nongonococcal urethritis generally causes less dysuria and less profuse, less purulent urethral exudate than gonorrhea. However, in the individual patient it may be difficult to differentiate between chlamydial and gonococcal infection (Chacko and Lovchik, 1984). Most men develop symptoms after *C. trachomatis* infection, but a large proportion may have prolonged, clinically inapparent infection. The presence of four or more PMNs per high-power field (hpf) on a Gram stain of an intraurethral smear or more than 15 PMNs per hpf in the sediment of a first-voided urine specimen is evidence of urethritis even in the absence of frank discharge (Chambers et al., 1987).

C. trachomatis can also cause proctitis among homosexual men. If the infection is due to a lymphogranuloma venereum (LGV) strain, the individual may develop proctocolitis that is difficult to differentiate from Crohn's disease both clinically and histopathologically. *C. trachomatis* can also cause epididymitis in young men. It has been estimated that one diagnosed case of epididymitis caused by *C. trachomatis* occurs for every eighteen diagnosed episodes of uncomplicated chlamydia-related urethritis in men aged 15 to 34 years. Overall, *C. trachomatis* causes 50% of epididymitis among men 15 to 34 years of age (Hammerschlag, 1989).

Infections in Adolescent and Adult Females

Nonpregnant women. Most cervical infections with *C. trachomatis* in women are asymptomatic and of long duration (Eagar et al., 1985). Sexually active adolescent women have one of the highest reported rates of chlamydial infection, often exceeding 10% to 15%. A recent study from Canada found that after implementation of a chlamydia control program in 1987, the annual incidence of chlamydial infection was highest among females from 15 to 24 years of age (3,418 cases per 100,000 residents) (Orr et al., 1994). Recurrent infection occurred in 13.4% of patients and was also more common in women and patients from 15 to 24 years of age. In the United States, Blythe et al. (1992) found that 38.4% of adolescent women had recurrent infection within 9 months of their initial chlamydial infection. Similar results were recently reported by Orr et al. (2001) who found that 60% of adolescent men and 73% of adolescent women infected with *C. trachomatis* and/or *N. gonorrhoeae* at enrollment were reinfected within 7 months. Although *C. trachomatis* has been associated with mucopurulent cervicitis, the majority of women have no specific physical clinical findings.

TABLE 32-3	Selected Studies on Prevalence of STDs in Adolescents			
Study (date)	Location	Infection	Sex	Percent
Chacko and Lovchik (1984)	Baltimore	Chlamydia trachomatis	M	35
			F	23
Golden et al. (1984)	Brooklyn	C. trachomatis	F	10.2
		Gonorrhea	F	9.7
		Syphilis	F	3
Saltz et al. (1981)	Cincinnati	C. trachomatis	F	22
		Gonorrhea	F	3
Fraser et al. (1982)	Oklahoma City	C. trachomatis	F	8
		Gonorrhea	F	12
Fisher et al. (1987)	Suburban New York City	C. trachomatis	F	14.5
Chambers et al. (1987)	San Francisco	C. trachomatis	M	30
		Gonorrhea	M	4
Blythe et al. (1988)	Indianapolis	C. trachomatis	F	25
		Gonorrhea	F	5.5
Moscicki et al. (1990)	San Francisco	C. trachomatis	F	8
		HPV	F	18
Fisher et al. (1991)	Suburban New York City	HPV	F	32
Hammerschlag et al. (1993)	Brooklyn	C. trachomatis	F	21.8
	Birmingham, Alabama		F	18.5
			M	9.4
Gaydos et al. (1998)	Baltimore	C. trachomatis	F	15.4
Oh et al. (1998)	Birmingham, Alabama (Detention Center)	C. trachomatis	F	28.3
			M	8.8
			F	13.1
			M	2.8
Cohen et al. (1999)	New Orleans	C. trachomatis	F	11.5
			M	6.2
		Gonorrhea	F	2.5
			M	1.2
Burstein et al. (2001)	Mid-Atlantic States (Washington, D.C., Maryland, Virginia)	C. trachomatis	F	14.2
			M	19.1

HPV, Human papillomavirus.

Among the many possible complications of chlamydial infection, the most important in female patients is acute salpingitis. Several studies and histopathologic reports from Scandinavia indicate a very strong causal association between *C. trachomatis* and salpingitis (Mardh, 1980). Later clinical and animal studies from the United States using aggressive culture methods, including cultures from the fallopian tubes, have confirmed the European experience (Bowie and Jones, 1981; Patton, 1985; Wasserheit et al., 1986). The organism is probably responsible for at least 20% of salp-

ingitis cases in the United States. Studies from Sweden and the United States indicate that approximately one in four patients admitted to the hospital with acute salpingitis has upper genital tract infection with *C. trachomatis,* confirmed by isolation of the organism from the fallopian tubes. The presence of *C. trachomatis* in the cervix of a woman with PID does not necessarily imply that the organism will be present in the tubes, but it is very suggestive. Investigators from Sweden found that 19 of 53 women with salpingitis had cervical chlamydial infection and that of those who had cervical infection and laparoscopy, six of seven grew *C. trachomatis* from the cultures from the fallopian tubes (Mardh, 1980). Why ascending infection develops in some women with cervical infection is not known. Salpingitis is 10 times more likely to occur in a sexually active 15-year-old girl than in a sexually active 25-year-old woman (Westrom, 1980). In addition to being more prevalent than gonococcal infections, chlamydial salpingitis apparently has a more severe clinical outcome. Compared with patients with gonococcal salpingitis or nonchlamydial, nongonococcal salpingitis, patients with chlamydial salpingitis have a less acute presentation, are less often febrile, have a longer history of symptoms, have a higher erythrocyte sedimentation rate, and have more tubal inflammation (Cromer and Heald, 1987). In addition, chlamydial salpingitis is more likely to lead to infertility. Infertility rates of 13% after one episode of salpingitis, 36% after two episodes, and 75% after three or more episodes have been reported (Westrom, 1980). Case-control studies have documented a consistent association between high titers of antibody to *C. trachomatis* and tubal obstruction (Brunham et al., 1986; Westrom, 1980). Studies in animals have shown that *C. trachomatis* infects and subsequently destroys the tubal mucosa (Patton, 1985). A similar microscopic and pathologic appearance of the tubes has been found in several patients from whom *C. trachomatis* was isolated. This pattern of repeated infections leading to fibrosis and eventual scarring is also seen in another human chlamydial infection—trachoma. Studies have demonstrated that screening women 18 to 34 years of age for cervical chlamydial infection and treating them will prevent subsequent PID (Scholes et al., 1996). This study showed a nearly 60% reduction in disease in the women who were screened and treated compared with a group of women that was not offered routine screening.

Another serious complication of chlamydial salpingitis is an increased risk of ectopic pregnancy, which is related directly to the oviduct damage. Many women who have had an ectopic pregnancy give no history of PID, but over 20% have histopathologic and serologic evidence of chlamydial infection (Brunham et al., 1986).

Pregnant women. In the United States the prevalence of *C. trachomatis* infection in pregnant women ranges from a low of 2% to more than 30%, depending on the population studied (Hammerschlag, 1989). Chlamydial infection during pregnancy has been inconstantly linked to prematurity. The overall relationship, when found, has been weak, and the mechanism is not understood (Harrison et al., 1983). Late (>72 hours) endometritis occurs consistently in 10% to 30% of women with chlamydial infections after induced abortion. *C. trachomatis* apparently is an important cause of postabortion complications.

Infections in Infants

Pregnant women who have cervical infection with *C. trachomatis* can transmit the infection to their infants, who may subsequently develop neonatal conjunctivitis or pneumonia. Epidemiologic evidence strongly suggests that the infant acquires chlamydial infection from the mother during vaginal delivery (Alexander and Harrison, 1983). Infection after cesarean section is rare and usually occurs after early rupture of the amniotic membrane. No evidence supports the idea of postnatal acquisition from the mother or other family members. Approximately 50% to 75% of infants born to infected women will become infected at one or more anatomic sites, including the conjunctiva, nasopharynx, rectum, and vagina.

Conjunctivitis. Inclusion conjunctivitis, or inclusion blennorrhea, is probably the major clinical manifestation of perinatally acquired chlamydial infection. The risk of developing chlamydial conjunctivitis after vaginal delivery in an infant born to a mother with active cervical chlamydial infection ranges from 20% to 50% (Alexander and Harrison, 1983). *C. trachomatis* was the most common identifiably infectious cause of neonatal conjunctivitis in the United States, accounting for 17% to more than 40% of cases. However, the incidence of perinatal chlamydial infection, including conjunctivitis, has dramatically declined following the introduction of widespread screening and treatment of maternal chlamydia infection.

The incubation period is usually 5 to 14 days but may be shorter if the membranes rupture prematurely. The clinical presentation is variable, ranging from minimal conjunctival injection with scant mucopurulent discharge to a more severe presentation with chemosis, pseudomembrane formation, and marked palpebral swelling. The conjunctivae are frequently very friable and may bleed when stroked with a swab. Although conjunctivitis may initially be unilateral, it frequently becomes bilateral. If not treated, the infection may persist for weeks. Chlamydial conjunctivitis in infants is not a follicular conjunctivitis as seen in classic endemic trachoma. Approximately 50% of infants with chlamydial conjunctivitis are also infected in the nasopharynx.

Pneumonia. The nasopharynx is the most frequent site of perinatally acquired chlamydial infection. Approximately 70% of infected infants have positive cultures at that site. Most of these nasopharyngeal infections are asymptomatic and may persist for 3 years or more. *C. trachomatis* pneumonia develops in approximately 30% of infants with nasopharyngeal infection. In those who develop pneumonia the presentation and clinical findings are very characteristic. The children usually are initially seen at 4 to 12 weeks of age. A few cases have been seen initially as early as 2 weeks of age, but no infant cases have been seen beyond 4 months. The infants frequently have a history of cough and congestion, with an absence of fever. On physical examination the infant is tachypneic, and rales are heard on auscultation of the chest; wheezing is distinctly uncommon. There are no specific radiographic findings except hyperinflation (Figure 32-7) (Beem and Saxon, 1977; Harrison et al., 1978). A review of chest roentgenograms of 125 infants with *C. trachomatis* pneumonia found bilateral hyperinflation and diffuse infiltrates (with a variety of radiographic patterns, including interstitial,

reticular, and nodular ones); atelectasis; and bronchopneumonia. Lobar consolidation and pleural effusions were not seen (Radkowski et al., 1981). Significant laboratory findings include peripheral eosinophilia ($\geq$300 cells/cm^3) and elevated serum immunoglobulin levels.

C. trachomatis is rarely isolated from the lungs of infants with chlamydia pneumonia, leading some to believe that an immune mechanism is involved in pathogenesis (Alexander and Harrison, 1983). Histopathologic studies have not revealed any characteristic features. Biopsy material has shown pleural congestion and near-total alveolar and partial bronchiolar mononuclear consolidation with occasional eosinophils, granular pneumocytes, and focal aggregations of neutrophils. Marked necrotic changes are evident in the bronchioles. Follow-up studies have suggested that infantile chlamydial pneumonia may be associated with pulmonary function test abnormalities and respiratory symptoms 7 to 8 years after recovery from the acute illness (Weiss et al., 1986).

Infections in Older Children

C. trachomatis has not been associated with any specific clinical syndrome in older infants and children. It has been suggested that the isolation of *C. trachomatis* from a rectal or genital site in children without prior sexual activity may be a marker of sexual abuse. Although evidence for other modes of spread such as through fomites is lacking for this organism, perinatal maternal-infant transmission resulting in vaginal or rectal infection has been

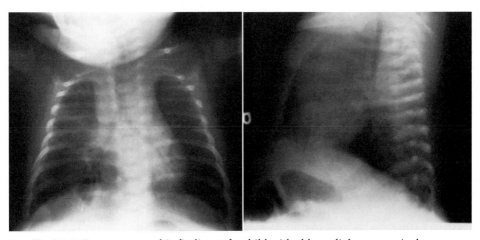

Fig. 32-7 Roentgenographic findings of a child with chlamydial pneumonia demonstrating hyperinflation and atelectasis.

documented, with prolonged infection lasting for periods up to 2 years. Pharyngeal infection for up to 3 years has also been observed. Schachter et al. (1986a) have detected subclinical rectal and vaginal infection in 14% of infants born to chlamydia-positive women; some infants were still culture positive at 18 months of age.

Reporting of vaginal infection with *C. trachomatis* in prepubertal children was uncommon before 1980. The possibility of sexual contact frequently was not discussed. In 1981 Rettig and Nelson reported concurrent or subsequent chlamydial infection in 9 of 33 (27%) prepubertal children with gonorrhea. This rate compares with those of 11% to 62%, depending on the study, of concurrent infection in men and women. *C. trachomatis* was not found in any of 31 children presenting with urethritis or vaginitis that was not gonococcal. No information was given about possible sexual activity.

Data from surveys published from 1988 to 1996 have identified rectogenital chlamydial infection in 0.4% to 11.1% of sexually abused children when the children were routinely cultured for the organism (Beck-Sagué and Solomon, 1999) (Table 32-1). Most of those with chlamydial infection were asymptomatic. In two earlier studies that had control groups, similar percentages of control patients were infected (Hammerschlag et al., 1984; Ingram et al., 1984). The control group in one study was composed of children who were referred also for evaluation of possible sexual abuse but were found to have no history of sexual contact and siblings of abused children. The mean age of this group was 4.5 years, compared with 7.5 years for the group with a history of sexual contact, which suggests a bias related to the inability to elicit a history of sexual contact from young children. In the second study the control group was selected from a well-child clinic. Three girls in this group had positive chlamydial cultures; two who had positive vaginal cultures were sisters who had been sexually abused 3 years previously and had not received interim treatment with antibiotics. The implication of this observation was that these children were infected for at least 3 years and were totally asymptomatic. The remaining control child had *C. trachomatis* isolated from her throat and rectum; no history of sexual contact could be elicited. Ingram et al. (1992) reviewed the results of *C. trachomatis* cultures among 1,538 children, 1 to 12 years of

age, being evaluated for possible sexual abuse who were seen between May 1981 and November 1991. The overall rate of chlamydial infection during this period was 1.2%. Most were asymptomatic and almost all had a definite history of sexual contact. One 31-month-old girl had no history of sexual contact; *C. trachomatis* was isolated from her rectal and vaginal specimens. Her mother was known to have chlamydial infection when she was pregnant, and her daughter had culture-positive chlamydial conjunctivitis at 8 weeks of age. This probably represents persistent perinatally acquired infection.

The possibility of prolonged vaginal or rectal carriage in the sexually abused group was minimized in the study by Hammerschlag et al. (1984) because the chlamydial cultures obtained at the initial examination were negative and the infection was detected only at follow-up examination 2 to 4 weeks later. However, the two abused girls who developed chlamydial infection were victims of a single assault by a stranger. In the setting of repeated abuse by a family member over long periods of time, development of infection would be difficult to demonstrate.

Lymphogranuloma Venereum

LGV is a systemic STD caused by the LGV biovars of *C. trachomatis* (L1, L2, L3). Approximately 20 cases of LGV have been reported in children. Fewer than 1,000 cases are reported in adults in the United States each year. Unlike the trachoma biovar, LGV strains have a predilection for lymph node involvement. The clinical course of LGV can be divided into three stages: (1) the primary lesion, a painless papule on the genitals, which usually is very transient; (2) lymphadenitis or lymphadenopathy; and (3) the tertiary stage. The time of presentation for most patients is during the second stage, with enlarging, painful buboes, usually in the groin, as the presenting sign. The nodes may break down and drain. This is more likely to occur in male patients. In female patients the lymphatic drainage of the vulva is to the retroperitoneal nodes. Fever, myalgia, and headache are also common. The tertiary stage includes the genitoanorectal syndrome, with rectovaginal fistulas, rectal strictures, and urethral destruction. Diagnosis can be made by culture of *C. trachomatis* from a bubo aspirate or serologically. Most patients with LGV have complement fixation (CF) titers greater than 1:16. The recommended therapy is 2 to 3 weeks of either tetracycline or sulfisoxazole.

Diagnosis

The definitive diagnosis of genital chlamydial infection had been isolation of the organism in tissue culture—from the urethra in men and the endocervix in women. Care should be taken to obtain cells, not discharge. The most commonly used tissue culture system is McCoy cells treated with cycloheximide. After a 48- to 72-hour incubation period the cultures are confirmed by staining the inclusions, preferably with a fluorescein-conjugated monoclonal antibody. Characteristic intracytoplasmic inclusions should be visible. Although many centers now perform *C. trachomatis* cultures, there is no standardization of methods or designated reference laboratories. Alternately, a nonculture method can be used. The introduction of NAATs has been the most important advance in the field of chlamydia diagnostics since tissue culture replaced inoculation of eggs for culture and isolation of *C. trachomatis* from clinical specimens. Because nucleic acid amplification is exquisitely sensitive, theoretically capable of detecting as little as a single gene copy, and highly specific, it offers the opportunity to use noninvasive sampling, e.g., of urine. There are now three NAATs approved by the FDA for the detection of *C. trachomatis* in clinical specimens: PCR, TMA, and SDA. A fourth NAAT, LCR, was withdrawn from the market by the manufacturer in 2002. Currently NAATs are approved for cervical swabs from women, urethral swabs form men, and urine from men and women. None of these tests are approved or recommended by the manufacturers for rectal specimens from adults and they are not approved for rectogenital specimens from children.

NAATs are more sensitive than culture for detection of *C. trachomatis* in genital specimens in adults, detecting an additional 25% to 30% over culture (Black, 1997, Morse, 2001). Multiple studies in adults have demonstrated sensitivities of >80% to 100% compared with 65% to 88% for culture, while maintaining high specificities (95% to 100%) (Black, 1997, Morse, 2001). Although all these assays are approved for use with urine from women, the sensitivities are lower than those of endocervical swabs. Practically all of these studies have been done in high prevalence populations (3% to 15%). However, despite high sensitivities and specificities, false-positive and false-negative results can occur. False-negative results due to inhibitors of DNA polymerase is more of a problem than false-positive results due to amplicon carryover. Inhibitors appears to be more frequent in cervical specimens. There are no inhibition controls included with any of the currently available kits.

Other types of nonculture tests currently available include DFA tests, in which chlamydial EBs are identified directly on a specimen smear stained with a conjugated antichlamydial monoclonal antibody, EIAs, and DNA probe. Sensitivities for these assays compared with those of culture range from 60% to 80% (Black, 1997). Use of these tests has been decreasing as NAATs have become more available and price competitive.

Serologic testing is not helpful for the diagnosis of chlamydial infections in adults. Because most infections in adolescents and adults are asymptomatic, it would be difficult to demonstrate either seroconversion or rises in titers. Serosurveys of populations of sexually active adults have found prevalences of antichlamydial antibody in more than 20% of individuals. The most widely available serologic test is the CF test. This genus-specific test is most useful for the diagnosis of LGV. Unfortunately, it is not sensitive enough for use in oculogenital infections caused by the trachoma biovar in adults or children. The microimmunofluorescence (MIF) test is species specific and sensitive but is available only at a limited number of research laboratories.

Chlamydial conjunctivitis and pneumonia in infants. Culture of chlamydia from the conjunctivae or nasopharynx is diagnostic. The nasopharyngeal specimens can be obtained with a posterior swab or by aspirate. The use of Dacron-tipped swabs with either wire or plastic shafts is preferred. The DFA and EIA tests can also be used for conjunctival and nasopharyngeal specimens. These tests are very successful with conjunctival specimens, with sensitivities and specificities exceeding 90% (Hammerschlag, 1994). Performance with nasopharyngeal specimens has not been as good; sensitivity compared with culture can be as low as 30%. Preliminary evaluation of PCR suggests that this assay is as sensitive as culture for detection of *C. trachomatis* in conjunctival specimens (Hammerschlag et al., 1997).

Chlamydial infections in older children. Because of the medical and legal implications, culture is the only approved method for the diagnosis of rectal and genital chlamydial infections in prepubertal children (Centers for Disease Control and Prevention, 2002). Culture means isolation of the organism in tissue culture with confirmation by visual identification of the characteristic inclusions, preferably with FA staining. Nonculture methods, especially DFAs and EIAs, cannot be used in this setting. Few data are available about the use of these tests in rectal and genital specimens from prepubertal children, and the information that is available suggests that they are neither sensitive nor specific (Hammerschlag et al., 1988; Hauger et al., 1988; Porder et al., 1989). The CDC suggests that a NAAT can be used, but only if culture is not available and any positive NAAT result can be confirmed with another NAAT that uses another genetic target (Centers for Disease Control and Prevention, 2002a).

Treatment

Uncomplicated genital infection in adolescent and adult males and nonpregnant women. The treatment of choice is azithromycin (1 g as a single oral dose) or doxycycline (100 mg orally, twice a day for 7 days) (Centers for Disease Control and Prevention, 2002a). The results of numerous clinical trials indicate that azithromycin and doxycycline are equally efficacious (Ridgway, 1997). Alternative regimens include erythromycin base 500 mg orally 4 times a day for 7 days; erythromycin ethylsuccinate 800 mg orally 4 times a day for 7 days; and ofloxacin 300 mg orally twice a day or levofloxacin 500 mg orally once daily, both for 7 days. Other quinolones either are not reliable effective against chlamydial infection or have not been adequately evaluated.

Follow-up testing is not recommended routinely. *C. trachomatis* DNA can be detected in endocervical specimens for ≥9 days after treatment (Gaydos et al., 1998). Studies among female adolescents have demonstrated high rates of subsequent chlamydial infection among women tested several months after treatment, presumably because of reinfection resulting from contact with an untreated or new sexual partner (Orr et al., 2001). Adolescents should be retested in 3 to 6 months, especially those whose behavior places them at greater risk of reinfection.

C. trachomatis in pregnancy. The CDC currently recommends either erythromycin base, at the dosage given above, or amoxicillin 500 mg orally 3 times daily for 7 days (Centers for

Disease Control and Prevention, 2002). Alternative regimens include erythromycin base 250 mg orally 4 times daily for 14 days or erythromycin ethylsuccinate, at the dose given in the preceding section, or half dose for 14 days. None of these erythromycin regimens have been extensively evaluated, and poor tolerance may reduce the compliance to 50% or less in some populations (Schachter et al., 1986b). Azithromycin, 1 g orally as a single dose, is also recommended as an alternative regimen. Limited preliminary data suggest that azithromycin is well tolerated, safe, and effective (Jacobson, et al., 2001; Kacmar, et al., 2001).

Chlamydial conjunctivitis and pneumonia in infants. Oral erythromycin suspension (ethylsuccinate or stearate; 50 mg/kg/day for 14 days) is the therapy of choice for chlamydial conjunctivitis and pneumonia in infants. It provides better and faster resolution of the conjunctivitis and treats any concurrent nasopharyngeal infection, which will prevent the potential development of pneumonia. Additional topical therapy is not needed (Heggie et al., 1985). Erythromycin administered at the same dose for 2 to 3 weeks is the treatment of choice for pneumonia and results in clinical improvement and elimination of the organism from the respiratory tract. Use of erythromycin suspensions in the early neonatal period (≤14 days of age) has been associated with the subsequent development of hypertrophic pyloric stenosis (Honein et al., 1999; Mahon et al., 2001). Erythromycin therapy instituted after 2 weeks of age appears to associated with a lower risk. Data on use of other macrolides for this indication, including clarithromycin and azithromycin, are limited. A preliminary study found that azithromycin suspension, 20 mg/kg, orally once daily for 3 days was as effective as 14 days of erythromycin ethylsuccinate for treatment of chlamydial conjunctivitis (Hammerschlag et al., 1998).

Although an initial study suggested that neonatal ocular prophylaxis with erythromycin ointment would prevent the development of chlamydial ophthalmia, subsequent studies have not confirmed this (Bell et al., 1987; Hammerschlag et al., 1989). It appears that neither ocular prophylaxis with silver nitrate nor erythromycin and tetracycline ointments or drops are effective for the prevention of neonatal chlamydial conjunctivitis or pneumonia. The identification and treatment of pregnant women before delivery is the optimal method of prevention of chlamydial infection in infants (Centers for Disease Control and Prevention, 2002a).

Older children. Chlamydial infections in older children can be treated with oral erythromycin (50 mg/kg/day, 4 times a day orally to a maximum of 2 g/day for 7 to 14 days) or azithromycin 1 g orally as a single dose, if the children weigh ≥45 kg and are less than 8 years of age. Children older than 8 years of age may be treated with 1 g azithromycin or doxycycline (2 to 4 mg/kg/day divided into 2 doses orally for 7 days).

BACTERIAL VAGINOSIS

Bacterial vaginosis (nonspecific vaginitis) is a polymicrobial infection characterized by the overgrowth of *G. vaginalis* and several anaerobic bacteria and by depletion of *Lactobacillus* species. The diagnosis of bacterial vaginosis is made by examination of the vaginal secretions for clue cells (vaginal epithelial cells heavily covered with bacteria) (Figure 32-8), the development of a fishy odor after the addition of 10% potassium hydroxide to vaginal secretions ("whiff test"), and a vaginal pH greater than 4.5 (Amsel et al., 1983; Thomason et al., 1990). Examination of a Gram stain of vaginal fluid for bacterial morphotypes associated with bacterial vaginosis, a predominance of small Gram-negative or Gram-variable rods (*G. vaginalis*) and curved Gram-negative to Gram-variable rods (*Mobilluncus* species), along with a decrease in large Gram-positive rods (*Lactobacillus* species) can be diagnostic (Joesoef et al., 1999).

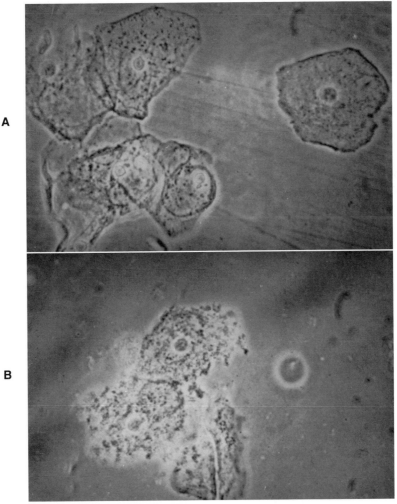

Fig. 32-8 A, Photomicrograph of a wet mount, demonstrating normal vaginal epithelial cells. **B,** Photomicrograph of wet mount containing clue cells, which are epithelial cells studded with bacteria.

Although bacterial vaginosis is very common in adult women, it has been diagnosed infrequently in children (Table 32-4). One possible reason is that prior studies of pediatric populations have concentrated on the isolation of G. vaginalis and have not routinely examined vaginal secretions for clue cells or odor. The CDC has stated that cultures for G. vaginalis are not useful and are not recommended for the diagnosis of this syndrome because it is nonspecific. Studies in children have suggested that G. vaginalis may be part of the normal vaginal flora (Hammerschlag et al., 1985). Bartley et al. (1987) examined a group of sexually abused children and a group of control children. Although G. vaginalis was isolated from the vaginal cultures of 14.6% of the abused girls, it was also found in 4.2% of the controls. Presence of G. vaginalis was not associated with vaginal discharge in these children. Another study reported finding G. vaginalis in vaginal specimens from 37% of non–sexually active postmenarcheal girls (median age, 15.9 years; range, 13 to 21 years) (Shafer et al., 1985). Ingram et al. (1992) isolated G. vaginalis from 5.3% of a group of children with confirmed sexual contact and/or gonorrhea or chlamydial infection; 4.9% of a group of children evaluated for possible abuse, but not confirmed; and 6.4% of a group of normal children seen as controls. Although some practitioners have suggested that the presence of G. vaginalis is an indicator of sexual abuse, the preceding data suggest otherwise.

Data from adults suggest that acquisition of bacterial vaginosis is related to sexual activity. In a major study, Amsel et al. (1983) diagnosed bacterial vaginitis in 69 of 397 females consecu-tively coming to a student health center gynecology clinic. They failed to demonstrate the disease among 18 patients who had no history of previous sexual intercourse. Four of these sexually inexperienced patients had positive vaginal cultures for G. vaginalis, which suggests that other organisms or factors are involved in the sexual transmission of bacterial vaginitis. Other investigators have found that male partners of women with bacterial vaginosis have a high prevalence of urethral colonization with G. vaginalis.

Minimal data exist on the prevalence of bacterial vaginosis in sexually abused female children. Hammerschlag et al. (1985) obtained paired vaginal wash specimens from 31 girls within 1 week and 2 or more weeks after sexual assault. None had bacterial vaginosis as defined by the presence of both clue cells and a positive whiff test at the initial examination. Vaginal pH was not used as a diagnostic criterion because the normal pH range in prepubertal girls is not well defined. At follow-up examination, 4 (13%) of the 31 girls had bacterial vaginosis. Two girls were asymptomatic. Treatment with metronidazole was followed by clinical improvement. None of the 23 controls (nonabused children) had bacterial vaginosis. Beck-Sagué and Solomon (1999) reviewing the literature from 1988-1996 found reported prevalence of bacterial vaginosis in girls being evaluated for sexual abuse to range from 5.2% to 13.3%, using the presence of clue cells and whiff test as diagnostic criteria.

Bacterial vaginosis apparently is also a common cause of vaginal discharge in children without sexual contact. Samuels et al. (1985) examined vaginal washes from 29 girls 3 months to 1 year of age with symptomatic vul-

TABLE 32-4	Prevalence of Trichomoniasis and Bacterial Vaginosis in Sexually Abused Children		
Study (year)	Number tested	Infection	Number (%) positive
White et al. (1983)	409	Trichomoniasis	4 (1)
De Jong (1983)	25*	Trichomoniasis	0
		Bacterial vaginosis	3 (12)
Hammerschlag et al. (1985)	31	Trichomoniasis	2 (6)
		Bacterial vaginosis	6 (19)
Ingram et al. (1992)	141*	Trichomoniasis	3 (2)
	99*	Bacterial vaginosis	7 (7)
Siegel et al. (1995)	423	Trichomoniasis	4 (0.9)
Embree et al. (1996)	138	Trichomoniasis	1 (0.7)

*Only patients with signs suggestive of vaginitis were evaluated.

vovaginitis. Bacterial vaginosis was diagnosed in nine (31%) of these children. All had a discharge, which was uniformly thin and ranged from gray-white to yellow in color, and only three (33%) of these girls had a history of sexual abuse; *N. gonorrhoeae* also was isolated from a pharyngeal culture from one child. Treatment with metronidazole resulted in reversion of the vaginal secretions to normal on follow-up examination. The relatively common occurrence of bacterial vaginosis in children may be due in part to the frequent colonization of the prepubertal vagina with anaerobes, especially *Bacteroides* species.

Treatment

Oral metronidazole (15 mg/kg/day, 3 times a day for 7 days) apparently is effective for the treatment of bacterial vaginosis in children. In addition to oral metronidazole, the CDC also recommends two topical treatments, metronidazole gel, 0.75%, one full applicator intravaginally, once a day for 5 days, or clindamycin cream, 2%, one full applicator intravaginally, once a day for 7 days (Centers for Disease Control and Prevention, 2002). There are no data on use of these topical preparations in children. Oral clindamycin is recommended as an alternative regimen in adults but there are also no data in its use in children.

TRICHOMONIASIS

Trichomonas vaginalis is a flagellated protozoan that inhabits the urogenital systems of both males and females and is considered a pathogen (Figure 32-9). The trophozoites (the only stage) are found in the urine of both sexes, in vaginal secretions, and in prostatic secretions. Approximately 5 million women in the United States have trichomoniasis, and roughly 1 million men may harbor the parasite. The infection in males is generally asymptomatic, but 25% to 50% of infected women exhibit symptoms, which include dysuria; vaginal itching and burning; and, in severe infections, a foamy, yellowish-green discharge with a foul odor.

Although nonsexual transmission of *T. vaginalis* has been reported between infected mothers and their infants at delivery, the exact risk of the infant's acquiring the infection is unknown (Al-Salihi et al., 1974). The presence of this organism in vaginal specimens from prepubertal girls strongly suggests sexual abuse; but, as with other STDs, perinatally acquired infection can be an important confounding variable. The duration of perinatally acquired trichomoniasis has been assumed to be very short—2 to 3 months after birth. We have seen two female infants with well-documented neonatal trichomonal infection that persisted for 6 and 9 months before the infants were finally treated. In most reports of infection with *T. vaginalis* in prepubertal children published before 1978, the possibility of sexual activity or abuse is not discussed (Neinstein et al., 1984). In one study of unselected girls who went to a well-child clinic, *T. vaginalis* was identified in

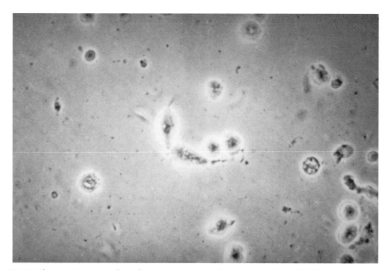

Fig. 32-9 Photomicrograph of wet mount, demonstrating *Trichomonas vaginalis* trophozoites.

two girls; both were postmenarcheal and one was sexually active. They both were symptomatic (Hammerschlag et al., 1978).

In most reported studies, wet mount examinations have been performed infrequently in asymptomatic sexually abused children and often are not performed in abused girls who have not had a vaginal discharge. Patients with trichomoniasis may be asymptomatic and have negative results from wet mount preparations (Wolner-Hanssen et al., 1989). In one study in which both wet mount examinations and cultures were used, trichomoniasis was found in 2 of 31 abused children at follow-up but not at an initial examination (Table 32-4). *T. vaginalis* was not identified in the children who served as controls. Trichomonads are not infrequently seen in urine collected for other purposes. If the specimen is obtained with a urinary collection bag—as is done frequently in young children, especially girls—the trichomonads may have originated in the vagina or may represent fecal contamination.

Trichomonas hominis, a commensal species that can inhabit the colon, is considered nonpathogenic. The only way the two *Trichomonas* species can be differentiated is by the presence of an undulating membrane that extends most of the length of the organism in *T. hominis* but only half the length of the organism in *T. vaginalis*. Old urine specimens may also be contaminated with *Bodo* species or other free-living flagellates, especially if the urinary collection vessel is open to the air and is not sterile. The presence of a trichomonad in a vaginal specimen has greater significance.

Diagnosis

Although some workers believe wet mount examinations are as efficient as culture for the diagnosis of *T. vaginalis* infection, current evidence suggests that cultivation methods are superior (Fouts and Kraus, 1980). Direct examination has a sensitivity ranging from only 38% to as high as 82%, when compared with culture (Petrin et al., 1997). The broth culture method is felt by many to be the "gold standard" for the diagnosis of trichomoniasis because it is simple to interpret and requires as few as 300 to 500 trichomonads/ml of inoculum to initiate growth (Petrin et al., 1997). However, culture requires 2 to 7 days of incubation. Although several culture media are commercially available, culture is not widely available or used.

A conjugated monoclonal antibody stain has been developed that apparently is both sensitive and specific, but available clinical data are limited. It has not yet been evaluated as an assay for the diagnosis of trichomoniasis in children (Kruger et al., 1988). Several PCR methods have also been developed for detection of *T. vaginalis,* but there are no FDA-approved, standardized assays available at this time.

Treatment

Trichomoniasis in adult women can be successfully treated with a single oral dose (2 g) of metronidazole or with 250 mg taken orally 3 times daily for 7 days, but there are no published studies of its use in children (Centers for Disease Control and Prevention, 2002). The few cases of trichomoniasis in prepubertal girls reported in the literature were treated with 7-day courses of oral metronidazole (15 to 35 mg/kg/day) (Jones et al., 1985).

HPV INFECTION

HPV, a double-stranded DNA virus, is the organism responsible for common warts and venereal warts, or condylomata acuminata. Genital papillomas in adults are transmitted by sexual intercourse. The majority is caused by HPV type 6 (HPV-6) or type 11 (HPV-11); smaller numbers are caused by types 16 (HPV-16) and 18 (HPV-18). Common skin warts and genital warts do not share HPV types.

HPV is becoming recognized as one of the most frequently occurring STDs. Studies of adolescents and young women from the San Francisco Bay area and suburban New York City done in the late 1980s found 18% to 33% of sexually active females tested positive for HPV DNA (Fisher et al., 1991; Moscicki et al., 1990). HPV represented the most common STD in that age group, followed by *C. trachomatis,* with a prevalence rate of 8%. A subsequent study by Moscicki et al. (1998) found a prevalence of HPV DNA of 20.7%. More than 80% of male partners of females with HPV are infected with HPV; most of these infections are subclinical. The cause of genital papillomas in children is less well studied, but sexual abuse by an infected adult or, less likely, contact with warts at other body sites has been suggested. HPV can also be transmitted to infants at birth, causing laryngeal papilloma (Boyd, 1990). The condylomata may affect the vulva, perineum, vaginal introitus, and periurethral areas. Girls apparently are affected twice as frequently as boys, although this may reflect a difference in patterns of reporting rather than a true epidemiologic observation (Boyd, 1990; Davis and Emans, 1989).

Clinical Manifestations

The lesions of condylomata acuminata are usually flesh-colored to purple papillomatous growths. These warts are often multiple and commonly coalesce into larger masses. In females, condylomata acuminata lesions usually occur at the posterior part of the introitus, the adjacent labia minora, and the rest of the vestibule. Less commonly, they can be found on the clitoris, perineum, vagina, cervix, anus, and rectum. In males, venereal warts are usually localized to the penis, including the shaft, prepuce, frenulum, corona, and glans. The meatus, anus, and scrotum may also be involved. Anal warts are seen most commonly in patients who have engaged in anal intercourse. In contrast, many females with anal warts report no history of anal sex, suggesting autoinoculation as a mode of transmission. The anatomic distribution may be different in prepubertal children, especially boys. Boys are less likely to have involvement of the penile shaft, prepuce, or glans—3% versus 18% to 52%—and are more likely to have perianal disease—77% versus 8% (Boyd, 1990). Female disease patterns show fewer age-related differences. Recently a new clinical and histologic type of HPV infection—subclinical HPV infection—has been described. The lesions with this type cannot be seen with the naked eye and require colposcopy, aceto-whitening, or cytologic studies for diagnosis. They can occur anywhere in the anogenital tract. In women they occur predominantly on the cervix; in men they can occur anywhere on the penis and on the perianal area, scrotum, and urethra. Recently, increasing attention has been focused on the association between HPV infection and the various genital carcinomas, particularly cervical carcinoma in women. HPV structural antigens and DNA have been found in the lesions of cervical intraepithelial neoplasia, which precedes the development of frank cervical carcinoma. HPV antigens and DNA have also been found in invasive carcinoma specimens and in specimens of anal, vulvar, vaginal, and penile carcinomas. Studies of adolescents in San Francisco have found infection with oncogenic-related HPV

types is very common (Moscicki et al., 1990). Follow-up studies of adolescent and young women with positive HPV tests have also found that approximately 70% become negative within a 24-month period (Moscicki et al., 1998).

The risk of developing genital warts in sexually abused children has not been adequately assessed because no studies have included data on long-term follow-up. However, one half of the cases of genital warts in children reported since 1976 were related to sexual abuse (De Jong et al., 1982; Neinstein et al., 1984; Seidel et al., 1979). Rock et al. (1986) examined the genital tract papillomas by molecular hybridization in five children for the presence of HPV DNA. HPV DNA was detected in each sample and consisted of HPV-6, HPV-11, or HPV-16. These types are the same as those responsible for genital warts in adults. Sexual abuse was thought likely to have occurred in three of these children. Although there was no history of maternal condylomata at the time of birth in the remaining two children, many congenital infections in women are subclinical, and flat warts of the vulva and vagina may go unnoticed by the affected individual and the physician (Bender, 1986). DNA typing in four subsequent studies reported that 5% to 20% of anogenital warts in children have skin HPV types (HPV-2, HPV-3), suggesting possible nonsexual acquisition (Cohen et al., 1990; Gibson et al., 1990; Obaleck et al., 1990; Padel et al., 1990). Gutman et al. (1992), examining vaginal washes, found HPV DNA in 5 of 15 sexually abused girls 2 to 11 years of age, compared with none of 17 controls (3 months to 5.5 years of age). The HPV types were 6, 11, and 15. The results of the wash did not correlate with the presence or absence of external anogenital warts. This was also a very small, selected population. The children in the control group were significantly younger than the cases. A larger recent study examined 70 surface swabs (introitus, throat, rectum) from 40 children, male and female, aged 1 to 16 years, who were being evaluated for suspected sexual abuse for the presence of HPV DNA (Siegfried et al., 1998). None of these children had condyloma on physical exam. HPV DNA was detected in the introital specimens from only 2 (0.5%) children, both girls, 8 and 10 years of age; both were typed as having HPV-16. *C. trachomatis* was isolated from 5 (12.5%) other children.

None of the children had positive cultures for *N. gonorrhoeae*. Additional studies should be done to evaluate the predictive value of the method for the diagnosis of HPV infection in the setting of suspected sexual abuse.

A major confounding variable in linking the presence of genital warts with sexual abuse is ruling out perinatal acquisition. Maternal HPV infection may be more common than previously thought; however, data on the prevalence of genital HPV among pregnant women are limited. Fife and colleagues (1987) detected HPV DNA in cervical scrape specimens from 11% of unselected pregnant women who went to an inner city obstetric service during the first trimester. Only 2 of the 26 women with positive specimens had genital warts. Rando and colleagues (1989) found HPV DNA in 20.9% of exfoliated cervical cells from pregnant women during the first trimester. The prevalence dramatically increased to 46% during the third trimester, but decreased to 17.5% of women postpartum. Watts et al. (1998) found that 74% of pregnant women had historical, clinical or DNA evidence of genital HPV infection during pregnancy. Studies of transmission and infection with genital HPV types during the neonatal period have given highly variable results. In 1989, Sedlacek and colleagues detected HPV DNA by Southern blot in neonatal nasopharyngeal aspirates from 11 (47.8%) of 23 infants born by spontaneous vaginal delivery to women who had HPV DNA present in their cervical scrapings. HPV DNA was also detected in the nasopharyngeal washes of 4 (22%) of 18 infants born to HPV-negative women. HPV was not detected in 2 infants of positive women who were delivered by Cesarean section. Using similar methods, Fife et al. (1990) demonstrated HPV DNA in oral cavity scrapings and foreskins from 5 (45.5%) of 11 newborn infants whose mothers were known to have HPV DNA present in the cervix during pregnancy. A subsequent study by Pakarian et al. (1994) found HPV DNA in 10 (50%) of 20 oral specimens from infants born to HPV-positive mothers and 1 (9%) of 11 infants born to HPV-negative mothers evaluated at one day of age. In contrast, HPV DNA was detected in genital specimens obtained at 6 weeks of age from 6 (30%) of 20 infants born to HPV-positive mothers compared with 2 (18%) of 11 infants born to HPV-negative mothers. The frequent detection of HPV DNA

from infants within a few days of birth may represent transient mucosal colonization. This is suggested by the findings of Pakarian et al. (1994), where the prevalence of HPV DNA among infants born to HPV-positive mothers decreased at 6 weeks of age. Conversely, the high presence of HPV DNA in infants born to HPV-negative women suggests contamination.

Data on the presence of HPV DNA in children beyond the neonatal period are also inconsistent. The results of three such studies found that the presence of HPV DNA in children born to infected mothers ranged from 1.2% to 77% (Cason et al., 1995; Puranen et al., 1996; Watts et al., 1998). The rate of HPV infection in children born to uninfected women ranged from 1% to 50%. The anatomic sites tested varied from study to study, and the study included oral, genital, and rectal specimens. Similarly, the duration of follow-up also differed from study to study. Puranen et al. (1996) examined children, 4 months to 11.3 years of age, but each child was sampled only once. Cason et al. (1995) evaluated infants born to HPV-positive and HPV-negative women at 1 day, 6 weeks, and 6 months of age. Watts et al. (1998) evaluated the children in their study at birth, 6 weeks, and 6, 12, 18, 24, and 36 months of age. The high rate of HPV DNA detected in infants born to HPV-negative mothers in the 1995 study by Cason et al.—50%—suggests the possibility of horizontal transmission between infants and care-givers.

However, the relationship between the presence of HPV DNA and the ultimate development of disease in these children is not clear. None of the infants followed by Watts et al. (1998) developed any clinical manifestations of HPV infection, specifically genital warts or laryngeal papillomatosis. Puranen et al. (1996) found minor hyperplastic growths in the oral mucosa of 21 (21%) of 98 children, but HPV DNA was detected in only one papilloma (site not specified) in one child. It is possible that the duration of follow-up in the study of Watts et al. (1998) was not long enough. However, in juvenile-onset laryngeal papillomatosis (clinical onset before puberty), 75% of cases are diagnosed before 5 years of age. The types of HPV involved are the same types responsible for the majority of genital warts: HPV-6 and HPV-11. Juvenile-onset laryngeal papillomatosis is very rare. Shah and colleagues (1986) calculated that, on the basis of crude estimates of the number of children born to infected mothers and of new cases of juvenile-onset disease, the risk of developing disease for a child born to an infected mother was one in several hundred exposures. It is felt that most genital warts in children less than 3 years of age are most likely due to perinatal acquisition. The results of these studies of perinatal transmission cast some doubt on this.

Diagnosis

Until the recent recognition that HPV infection can be inapparent, the diagnosis of condylomata acuminata was usually based on the history and appearance of the lesions. Anogenital warts must be differentiated from other papillomatous lesions, including benign and malignant neoplasms, anatomic variants, and other infectious conditions. Of the latter, the most important lesions to differentiate are condylomata lata of secondary syphilis. Because these may coexist with condylomata acuminata, obtaining serologic tests for syphilis and dark-field microscopy of suspicious or ulcerating lesions is strongly recommended. Genital lesions of molluscum contagiosum also can be confused with genital warts.

In adolescent and adult women the Papanicolaou (Pap) test commonly is used to diagnose HPV infection. The koilocyte ("balloon cell") can be seen on a Pap smear and is pathognomonic for HPV. However, there is a subjective component to reading smears, and the sampling error presents a problem. A negative Pap smear result does not rule out HPV infection. Performance of a biopsy should be considered for any puzzling lesion.

Electron microscopy can be used to identify HPV particles in biopsy specimens and may be especially useful in identifying lesions from children. However, the same problems encountered with Pap smears occur with these newer methods. Their diagnostic use may be compromised because of sampling error, insufficient material, or interference by large numbers of red or white blood cells that obscure visualization of the cervical epithelial cells. There are no data that support the use of any type-specific HPV DNA tests in the routine diagnosis or management of visible genital warts (Centers for Disease Control and Prevention, 2002). The routine use of these tests for screening to detect subclinical infection is also not recommended. Pap-test diagnosis of HPV does not always cor-

relate with the detection of HPV DNA in cervical cells. None of these methods have been evaluated in prepubertal children.

Treatment

The primary goal of treatment of HPV infection is the removal of symptomatic warts. Treatment can induce wart-free periods in most patients. However, visible genital warts often resolve on their own, remain unchanged, or increase in number. Most importantly, no evidence indicates that either the presence of genital warts or their treatment is associated with the development of cervical cancer. None of the currently available therapies is completely satisfactory for the treatment of genital warts in adults, and less information is available about treatment for children. Current recommended therapies for adults include the local application, by the patient, of podofilox 0.5% gel or imiquimod 5% cream. Provider-administered treatments include cryotherapy, podophyllin resin 10% to 25%, intralesional interferon, ablation with carbon dioxide laser, and 75% trichloroacetic acid (Centers for Disease Control and Prevention, 2002). Treatment of genital warts in children can be complicated and should be carried out in consultation with an expert.

OTHER INFECTIONS

Several other STDs deserve mention. Chancroid is caused by *Haemophilus ducreyi*, a small, nonmotile, gram-negative, non–spore forming rod. Clinically, chancroid usually is seen initially as a small, inflammatory papule on the preputial orifice or frenulum in men and on the labia, fourchette, or perianal region in women. The lesion becomes pustular and ulcerative within 2 to 3 days. An associated painful, tender inguinal adenopathy occurs in over 50% of cases. Unlike that of LGV, the characteristic ulcer of chancroid is concurrent with lymphadenopathy. Reported cases of chancroid in the United States peaked at 5,001 in 1988, but decreased to only 143 cases in 1999 (Centers for Disease Control and Prevention, 2001). No reports of chancroid in children have been found in the literature. A definitive diagnosis of chancroid requires identification of *H. ducreyi* on special culture media that is not widely available (Centers for Disease Control and Prevention, 2002). There are no FDA-approved nonculture tests, including PCR. Current recommendations for treatment are either azithromycin 1 g orally as a single dose, ceftriaxone 250 mg IM in a single dose, ciprofloxacin 500 mg orally twice daily for 3 days or erythromycin base 50 mg/kg/day in divided doses for 7 days (maximum 500 mg four times per day).

Infection with hepatitis B virus (HBV) is also an STD and may be a complication of sexual abuse (Szmuness et al., 1975) (see Chapter 11). It has been recommended that male victims of homosexual rape be screened for HBV infection. Although homosexual behavior is a well-recognized risk factor for acquiring HBV infection, a similar increased risk exists among heterosexuals with multiple sex partners. Screening for HBV probably should also be included in the medical evaluation of the child victim of sexual assault.

Consideration should also be given to screening for HIV infection in victims of sexual assault, including children (Gellert et al., 1990). Since HIV, like HBV, can be transmitted through homosexual or heterosexual activity, screening for infection may be indicated in both instances. Several individual reports have noted acquisition of HIV infection through sexual assault (Leiderman and Grimm, 1986; Gutman et al., 1991). The risk factors for HIV infection are similar to those for sexual abuse: drug abuse in parent, alcoholism, and poverty. Gellert et al. (1993) reviewed the results of HIV testing of 5,622 children suspected of being sexually abused; 28 (0.5%) were infected with HIV and lacked any alternative transmission route to that of sexual abuse. The CDC conducted a retrospective review of all reports by state and local health departments to the national HIV/AIDS surveillance system of children with either HIV or AIDS through December 1996 for a history of sexual abuse (Lindegren et al., 1998). Of 9,136 children reported with HIV or AIDS, 26 (0.3%) had a history of sexual abuse with confirmed or suspected exposure to HIV. The mean age at diagnosis of HIV infection was 8.8 years. For 17 of these children with confirmed sexual exposure to HIV, they identified 19 male perpetrators, who were either known to be HIV positive or had risk factors for HIV infection including intravenous drug use and homosexual contact. Most of these perpetrators were either a parent or relative. Sexual abuse must be considered as a potential, although infrequent, mode of transmission of HIV infection in children. If exposure to HIV is suspected, postexposure prophylaxis should be considered (Centers for Disease Control and Prevention, 2002; Merchant and Kehavarz, 2001). (Herpes simplex virus infections are discussed in Chapter 15.)

Laboratory studies that are indicated as part of the evaluation of sexually assaulted children at initial and follow-up examinations are presented in Box 32-2.

BOX 32-2

LABORATORY STUDIES INDICATED AS PART OF EVALUATION OF SEXUALLY ASSAULTED CHILDREN AT INITIAL AND FOLLOW-UP EXAMINATIONS

- Cultures for *Neisseria gonorrhoeae* (rectogenital and throat) and *Chlamydia trachomatis*—vaginal and rectal from girls, rectal from boys. A meatal specimen for *C. trachomatis* should be obtained if a urethral discharge is present)
- Wet mount preparation of vaginal swab specimen for trichomonads and bacterial vaginosis (whiff test, clue cells)
- Vaginal culture for *Trichomonas vaginalis*, if available
- Cultures of lesions for herpes simplex virus
- Serologic tests for syphilis
- Hepatitis B surface antigen[*] (if not vaccinated)
- Human immunodeficiency virus antibody[*]
- Serum sample (save frozen)

Studies should be repeated 7 days later, except for syphilis and hepatitis B serologic tests, which should be obtained 12 weeks later.

---

[*]Obtain if there is supportive epidemiologic evidence.

BIBLIOGRAPHY
STDs and sexual abuse of children (general)

Beck-Sagué CM, Solomon F. Sexually transmitted diseases in abused children and adolescent and adult victims of rape: review of selected literature. Clin Infect Dis 1999;28(suppl 1):S74-83.

Centers for Disease Control and Prevention. Sexually transmitted diseases treatment guidelines 2002. MMWR Recomm Rep 2002;51:1-84.

De Jong AR. Sexually transmitted diseases in sexually abused children. Sex Transm Dis 1986;13:123-126.

Glaser JB, Hammerschlag MR, McCormack WM. Epidemiology of sexually transmitted diseases in rape victims. Rev Infect Dis 1989;11:246-254.

Hammerschlag MR. Sexually transmitted diseases in sexually abused children: medical and legal implications. Sex Transm Infect 1998;74:167-174.

Hammerschlag MR, Alpert S, Rosner I, et al. Microbiology of the vagina in children: normal and potentially pathogenic organisms. Pediatrics 1978;62:57-62.

Ingram DL, Everett D, Lyna PR, et al. Epidemiology of adult sexually transmitted disease agents in children being evaluated for sexual abuse. Pediatr Infect Dis J 1992;11:945-950.

Jenny C, Hooton TM, Bowers A, et al. Sexually transmitted diseases in victims of rape. N Engl J Med 1990;322:713-716.

Neinstein LS, Goldenring J, Carpenter S. Nonsexual transmission of sexually transmitted diseases: an infrequent occurrence. Pediatrics 1984;74:67-75.

Rimsza ME, Niggemann EH. Medical evaluation of sexually abused children: a review of 311 cases. Pediatrics 1982;69:8-14.

Seigel RM, Schubert CJ, Myers PA, et al. The prevalence of sexually transmitted diseases in children and adolescents evaluated for sexual abuse in Cincinnati: rational for limited STD testing in prepubertal girls. Pediatrics 1995;96:1090-1094.

Sicoli RA. Indications for *Neisseria gonorrhoeae* cultures in children with suspected sexual abuse. Arch Pediatr Adolesc Med 1995;149:86-89.

Tilelli JA, Turek D, Jaffe AC. Sexual abuse of children: clinical findings and implications for management. N Engl J Med 1980;302:319-323.

White ST, Coda FA, Ingram DA, et al. Sexually transmitted diseases in sexually abused children. Pediatrics 1983;72:16-21.

Gonorrhea

Abbott SL. Gonococcal tonsillitis-pharyngitis in a 5-year-old girl. Pediatrics 1973;52:287-289.

Ahmed HJ, Ilardi I, Antognoli A, et al. An epidemic of *Neisseria gonorrhoeae* in a Somali orphanage. Int J STD AIDS 1992;3:52-53.

American Academy of Pediatrics Committee on Child Abuse and Neglect. Guidelines for the evaluation of sexual abuse of children. Pediatrics 1991;87:254-260.

Amstey MS, Steadman KT. Asymptomatic gonorrhea and pregnancy. J Am Vener Dis Assoc 1976;3:14.

Apicella MA. Serogrouping the *Neisseria gonorrhoeae*: identification of four immunologically distinct acidic polysaccharides. J Infect Dis 1976;134:377.

Barr J, Danielsson D. Septic gonococcal dermatitis. Br Med J 1971;1:482-485.

Bernstein GA, Davis JP, Katcher ML. Prophylaxis of neonatal conjunctivitis: an analytic review. Clin Pediatr 1983;21:545-550.

Biro FM, Rosenthal SL, Kiniyalocts M. Gonococcal and chlamydial genitourinary infections in symptomatic and asymptomatic adolescent women. Clin Pediatr 1995;34:419-423.

Branch G, Paxton R. A study of gonococcal infection among infants and children. Public Health Rep 1965;80:347-352.

Britigan BE, Cohen MS, Sparling PF. Gonococcal infections: a model of molecular pathogenesis. N Engl J Med 1985;312:1683-1694.

Burry VF. Gonococcal vulvovaginitis and possible peritonitis in prepubertal girls. Am J Dis Child 1971;21:536-537.

Catlin BW. Nutritional profiles of *Neisseria gonorrhoeae*, *Neisseria meningitidis*, and *Neisseria lactamica* in chemically defined media and the use of growth requirements for gonococcal typing. J Infect Dis 1973;128:178-194.

Centers for Disease Control. Antibiotic-resistant strains of *Neisseria gonorrhoeae*. MMWR Morb Mortal Wkly Rep 1987;36(suppl 5):1S-18S.

Centers for Disease Control and Prevention. Summary of notifiable diseases, United States, 1999. MMWR Morb Mortal Wkly Rep 2001;48:1–104.

Centers for Disease Control and Prevention. Gonorrhea—United States, 1998. MMWR Morb Mortal Wkly Rep 2000;49:538-542.

DeJong AR. Sexually transmitted diseases in sexually abused children. Sex Transm Dis 1986;13:123-126.

Edwards LE, et al. Gonorrhea in pregnancy. Am J Obstet Gynecol 1978;132:637.

Embree JE, Lindsay D, Williams T, et al. Acceptability and usefullness of vaginal washes in premenarcheal girls as a diagnostic procedure for sexually transmitted diseases. Pediatr Infect Dis J 1996; 15:662-667.

Fleisher G, Hodge D, Cromie W. Penile edema in childhood gonorrhea. Ann Emerg Med 1980;9:314-315.

Gorwitz RJ, Nakashima AK, Knapp JS. Sentinel surveillance for antimicrobial resistance in Neisseria gonorrhoeae—United States, 1988-1991. MMWR Surveill Summ 1993;42:29-39.

Groothuis J, Bischoff MC, Javrequi LE. Pharyngeal gonorrhea in young children. Pediatr Infect Dis 1983;2:99-101.

Hammerschlag MR, Cummings C, Roblin PM, et al. Efficacy of neonatal ocular prophylaxis for the prevention of chlamydial and gonococcal conjunctivitis. N Engl J Med 1989;320:769-772.

Hammerschlag MR, Doraiswamy B, Alexander ER, et al. Are rectogenital chlamydial infections a marker of sexual abuse in children? Pediatr Infect Dis J 1984;3:100-104.

Handsfield HH. Disseminated gonococcal infection. Clin Obstet Gynecol 1975;18:131-142.

Handsfield HH, Hodson EA, Holmes KK. Neonatal gonococcal infection. JAMA 1973;225:697.

Hein K, Marks A, Cohen MI. Asymptomatic gonorrhea: prevalence in a population of urban adolescents. J Pediatr 1977;90:634-635.

Holmes KK, Counts GW, Beaty HN. Disseminated gonococcal infection. Ann Intern Med 1971;74:979.

Hook EW III, Holmes KK. Gonococcal infections. Ann Intern Med 1985;102:229-243.

Hook EW III, Judson FN, Handsfield HH. Auxotype/serovar diversity and antimicrobial resistance of *Neisseria gonorrhoeae* in two mid-sized American cities. Sex Transm Dis 1987;14:141-146.

Ingram DL, Evenett VD, Flick LA, et al. Vaginal gonococcal cultures in sexual abuse evaluations: evaluation of selective criteria for preteenaged girls. Pediatrics 1997; 99:E8.

Ingram DL, White ST, Durfee MR, et al. Sexual contact in children with gonorrhea. Am J Dis Child 1982;136:994-996.

Ingram DM, Miller WC, Schoenbach VJ, et al. Risk assessment for gonococcal and chlamydial infections in young children undergoing evaluation for sexual abuse. Pediatr 2001;107:e73-e80.

Johnson SR, Morse SA. Antibiotic resistance in *Neisseria gonorrhoeae*: genetics and mechanisms of resistance. Sex Transm Dis 1988;15:217-224.

Judson FN, Ehret JM, Handsfield HH. Comparative study of ceftriaxone and spectinomycin for treatment of pharyngeal and anorectal gonorrhea. JAMA 1985;253:1417-1419.

Kam KM, Wong PW, Cheung MM, et al. Quinolone-resistant *Neisseria gonorrhoeae* in Hong Kong. Sex Transm Dis 1996;23:103-108.

Knapp JS, Fox KK, Trees DL, et al. Fluoroquinolone resistance in *Neisseria gonorrhoeae*. Emerg Infect Dis 1997;3:33-39.

Knapp JS, Holmes KK. Disseminated gonococcal infections caused by *Neisseria gonorrhoeae* with unique nutritional requirements. J Infect Dis 1975;132:204.

Knapp JS, Tam MR, Nowinski RC, et al. Serological classification of *Neisseria gonorrhoeae* with use of monoclonal antibodies to gonococcal outer membrane protein I. J Infect Dis 1984;150:44-48.

Laga M, Naamara W, Brunham RC, et al. Single-dose therapy of gonococcal ophthalmia neonatorum. N Engl J Med 1986a;315:1382-1385.

Laga M, Nzanze H, Brunham RC, et al. Epidemiology of ophthalmia neonatorum in Kenya. Lancet 1986b; 2:1145-1149.

Laga M, Plummer FA, Piot P, et al. Prophylaxis of gonococcal and chlamydial ophthalmia neonatorum. N Engl J Med 1988;318:653-657.

Lewis LS, Glauser TA, Joffe MD. Gonococcal conjunctivitis in prepubertal children. Am J Dis Child 1990; 144:546-548.

McClure EM, Stack MR, Tanner T, et al. Pharyngeal culturing and reporting of pediatric gonorrhea in Connecticut. Pediatrics 1986;78:509-510.

Michalowski B. Difficulties of diagnosis and treatment of gonorrhea in young girls. Br J Vener Dis 1961;37:142-144.

Morse SA. New tests for sexually transmitted diseases. Curr Opin Infect Dis 2001;14:45-51.

Nelson JD. The bacterial etiology and antibiotic management of septic arthritis in infants and children. Pediatrics 1972;50:437-440.

Nelson JD, Mohs E, Dajani AS, Plotkin SA. Gonorrhea in preschool and school-aged children: a report of the prepubertal gonorrhea cooperative study group. JAMA 1976;236:1359.

O'Brien JP, Goldenberg DL, Rice P. Disseminated gonococcal infection: a prospective analysis of 49 patients and a review of the pathophysiology and immune mechanisms. Medicine 1983;62:395-406.

Oh MK, Smith KR, O'Cain M, et al. Urine-based screening of adolescents in detention to guide treatment for gonococcal and chlamydial infections. Arch Pediatr Adolesc Med 1998;152:52-56.

Petersen BH, Lee TJ, Synderman R, et al. *Neisseria meningitidis* and *Neisseria gonorrhoeae* bacteremia associated with C6, C7, or C8 deficiency. Ann Intern Med 1979;90:917-920.

Potterat JJ, Markewich GS, King RD, et al. Child-to-child transmission of gonorrhea: report of asymptomatic genital infection in a boy. Pediatrics 1986;78:711-712.

Rawstron SA, Hammerschlag MR, Gullans C, et al. Ceftriaxone treatment of penicillinase-producing *Neisseria gonorrhoeae* infections in children. Pediatr Infect Dis 1989;8:445-448.

Rettig PJ, Nelson JD, Kusmiess H. Spectinomycin therapy for gonorrhea in prepubertal children. Am J Dis Child 1980;134:559-563.

Rothenberg R. Ophthalmia neonatorum due to *Neisseria gonorrhoeae*: prevention and treatment. Sex Transm Dis 1979;6:187-191.

Schichor A, Bernstein B, Weinerman H, et al. Lidocaine as a diluent for cetriaxone in the treatment of gonorrhea. Arch Pediatr Adolesc Med 1994;148:72-75.

Schwarcz SK, Whittington WL. Sexual assault and sexually transmitted diseases: detection and management in adults and children. Rev Infect Dis 1990;12:S682-S690.

Schwebke JR, Whittington W, Rice RJ, et al. Trends in susceptibility of *Neisseria gonorrhoeae* to ceftriaxone from 1985 through 1991. Antimicrob Agents Chemother 1995;39:917-920.

Segal E, Billyard E, So M, et al. Role of chromosomal rearrangement in *Neisseria gonorrhoeae* pilus phase variation. Cell 1985;40:293-300.

Shapiro RA, Schubert CJ, Siegel RM. *Neisseria gonorrhoeae* in girls younger than 12 years of age evaluated for vaginitis. Pediatr 1999;104:e72-e77.

Sicoli RA, Losek JD, Hudlett JM, Smith D. Indications for *Neisseria gonorrheae* cultures in children with suspected sexual abuse. Arch Pediatr Adolesc Med 1995; 49:86-89.

Smith JA, Linder CW, Jay S. Isolation of *Neisseria gonorrhoeae* from the urethra of asymptomatic adolescent males. Clin Pediatr (Phila) 1986;25:566-568.

Speck WT, Lawsky AR. Symptomatic anorectal gonorrhea in an adolescent female. Am J Dis Child 1971;122:438-439.

Stamm WE, Guinan ME, Johnson C, et al. Effect of treatment regimens for *Neisseria gonorrhoeae* on simultaneous infection with *Chlamydia trachomatis*. N Engl J Med 1984;310:545-549.

Tronca E, Handsfield HH, Weisner PJ, Holmes KK. Demonstration of *Neisseria gonorrhoeae* with fluorescent antibody in patients with disseminated gonococcal infection. J Infect Dis 1974;129:583-586.

Weisner PJ, Tronca E, Bonin P, et al. Clinical spectrum of pharyngeal gonococcal infection. N Engl J Med 1973;288:181-185.

Whittington WL, Rice RJ, Biddle JW, Knapp JS. Incorrect identification of *Neisseria gonorrhoeae* from infants and children. Pediatr Infect Dis 1988;7:3-10.

Zenilman JM. Update on quinolone resistance in *Neisseria gonorrhoeae*. Curr Infect Dis Rep 2002;4:144-147.

PID and salpingitis

Bowie WR, Jones H. Acute pelvic inflammatory disease in outpatients: association with *Chlamydia trachomatis* and *Neisseria gonorrhoeae*. Ann Intern Med 1981;95:685-688.

Cromer BA, Heald FP. Pelvic inflammatory disease associated with *Neisseria gonorrhoeae* and *Chlamydia trachomatis*: clinical correlates. Sex Transm Dis 1987;14:125-129.

Eschenbach DA, Buchanan TM, Pollock HM, et al. Polymicrobial etiology of acute pelvic inflammatory disease. N Engl J Med 1975;293:166-171.

Gates W. Sexually transmitted organisms and infertility: the proof of the pudding. Sex Transm Dis 1984;11:113-116.

Mardh PA. An overview of infectious agents of salpingitis, their biology, and recent methods of detection. Am J Obstet Gynecol 1980;138:933-951.

Patton DL. Immunopathology and histopathology of experimental chlamydial salpingitis. Rev Infect Dis 1985;7:746-753.

Scholes D, Stergachis A, Heidrich FE. Prevention of pelvic inflammatory disease by screening for cervical chlamydial infection. N Engl J Med 1996;334:1362-1366.

Shafer M-A, Irwin CE, Sweet RL. Acute salpingitis in the adolescent female. J Pediatr 1982;100:339-350.

Walters MD, Gibbs RS. A randomized comparison of gentamicin-clindamycin and cefoxitin-doxycycline in the treatment of acute pelvic inflammatory disease. Obstet Gynecol 1990;75:867-872.

Wasserheit JN, Bell TA, Kiviat NB, et al. Microbial causes of proven pelvic inflammatory disease and efficacy of clindamycin and tobramycin. Ann Intern Med 1986;104:187-193.

Westrom L. Incidence, prevalence, and trends of acute pelvic inflammatory disease and its consequences in industrialized countries. Am J Obstet Gynecol 1980;138:880-892.

Wolner-Hanssen P, Eschenbach D, Paavonen J, et al. Treatment of pelvic inflammatory disease: use of doxycycline with an appropriate β-lactam while we wait for better data. JAMA 1986;256:3262-3263.

Syphilis

Ackerman AB, Goldfaden G, Cosmides JC. Acquired syphilis in early childhood. Arch Dermatol 1972;106:92-93.

Alderete JF, Baseman JB. Surface-associated host proteins on virulent *Treponema pallidum*. Infect Immun 1979;26:1048.

Baker-Zander S, Sell S. A histopathologic and immunologic study of the course of syphilis in the experimentally infected rabbit: demonstration of long-lasting cellular immunity. Am J Pathol 1980;101:387.

Beck-Sagué C, Alexander ER. Failures of benzathine penicillin G therapy in early congenital syphilis. Pediatr Infect Dis 1987;6:1061-1064.

Beeram MR, Chopde N, Dawood Y, et al. Lumbar puncture in the evaluation of possible asymptomatic congenital syphilis in neonates. J Pediatr 1996;128:125-129.

Bromberg K, Rawstron S, Tannis G. Diagnosis of congenital syphilis by combining *Treponema pallidum*–specific IgM detection with immunofluorescent antigen detection for *T. pallidum*. J Infect Dis 1993;168:238-242.

Centers for Disease Control. Continuing increase in infectious syphilis, United States. MMWR Morb Mortal Wkly Rep 1988;37:35-37.

Centers for Disease Control. Case definitions for public health surveillance. MMWR Recomm Rep 1990;39:36.

Centers for Disease Control and Prevention. Outbreak of syphilis among men who have sex with men—Southern California, 2000. MMWR Morb Mortal Wkly Rep 2001b;50:117-120.

Centers for Disease Control and Prevention. Summary of notifiable diseases, United States 1999. MMWR Morb Mortal Wkly Rep 2001a;48;1-104.

Centers for Disease Control and Prevention. Congenital syphilis—United States, 2000. MMWR Morb Mortal Wkly Rep 2001c;50:573-577.

Centers for Disease Control. Sexually transmitted diseases treatment guidelines 2002. MMWR Recomm Rep 2002a;51:1-84.

Chang SN, Chung K-Y, Lee M-G, Lee JB. Seroreversion of the serological tests for syphilis in the newborns born to treated syphilitic mothers. Genitourin Med 1995;71:68-70.

Christian CW, Lavelle J, Bwll LM. Preschoolers with syphilis. Pediatrics 1999;103;e4

Cohen DA, Boyd D, Pabhudas I, Mascola L. The effects of case definition, maternal screening, and reporting criteria on rates of congenital syphilis. Am J Public Health 1990;80:316-317.

Connors JM, Schubert C, Shapiro R. Syphilis or abuse: making the diagnosis and understanding the implications. Pediatr Emerg Care 1998;14:139-142

Conover CS, Rend CA, Miller GB, Schmid GP. Congenital syphilis after treatment of maternal syphilis with a penicillin regimen exceeding CDC guidelines. Infect Dis Obstet Gynecol 1998;6:134-137.

Deacon WE, Lucas JB, Price EV. Fluorescent treponemal antibody–absorption (FTA-ABS) test for syphilis. JAMA 1966;198:624.

Digre KA, White GL, Cremer SA, Massanari RM. Late-onset congenital syphilis: a retrospective look at University of Iowa hospital admissions. J Clin Neuroophthalmol 1991;11:1-6.

Duncan WC, Knox JM, Wende RD. The FTA-ABS test in dark field–reactive primary syphilis. JAMA 1974;228:859-860.

Eagle H, Fleischman R, Muselman AD. The effective concentration of penicillin in vitro and in vivo for streptococci, pneumococci, and *Treponema pallidum*. J Bacteriol 1950;59:625-643.

Egglestone SI, Turner AJL for the PHLS Syphilis Serology Working Group. Serological diagnosis of syphilis. Communicable Disease and Public Health. 2000;3:158-162.

Fears MB, Pope V. Syphilis fast latex agglutination test, a rapid confirmatory test. Clin Diagn Lab Immunol 2001;8:841-842

Fiumara NJ. Syphilis in newborn children. Clin Obstet Gynecol 1975;18:183-189.

Fiumara NJ. Treatment of primary and secondary syphilis. Serological response. JAMA 1980;243:2500-2502.

Fiumara NJ, Fleming WL, Downing JG, Good FL. The incidence of prenatal syphilis at the Boston City Hospital. N Engl J Med 1952;247:48-52.

Fiumara NJ, Lessell S. The stigmata of late congenital syphilis: an analysis of 100 patients. Sex Transm Dis 1983;10:126-129.

Fojaco RM, Hensley GT, Moskowitz L. Congenital syphilis and necrotizing funisitis. JAMA 1989;261:1788-1790.

Ginsberg CM. Acquired syphilis in prepubertal children. Pediatr Infect Dis 1983;2:232-234.

Grimprel E, Sanchez PJ, Wendel GD, et al. Use of polymerase chain reaction and rabbit infectivity testing to detect *Treponema pallidum* in amniotic fluid, fetal and neonatal sera, and cerebrospinal fluid. J Clin Microbiol 1991;29:1711-1718.

Gust DA, Levine WC, St. Louis ME, et al. Mortality associated with congenital syphilis in the United States, 1992-1998. Pediatrics 2002;109:e79.

Halling VW, Jones MF, Bestrom JE, et al. Clinical comparison of the *Treponema pallidum* CAPTIA Syphilis-G enzyme immunoassay with the Fluorescent Treponemal Antibody Absorption Immunoglobulin G assay for syphilis testing. J Clin Microbiol 1999;37:3233-3234.

Harter CA, Benirschke K. Fetal syphilis in the first trimester. Am J Obstet Gynecol 1976;124:705.

Hira SK, Bhat GJ, Patel JB, et al. Early congenital syphilis: clinicoradiologic features in 202 patients. Sex Transm Dis 1985;12:177-183.

Hollier LM, Harstad TW, Sanchez PJ, et al. Fetal syphilis: clinic and laboratory characteristics. Obstet Gynecol 2001;97:947-953.

Hovind-Hougen K. Morphology. In Shell RF, Musher DM (eds). Pathogenesis and Immunology of Treponemal Infection. New York: Marcel Dekker, 1983.

Idsoe O, Guthie T, Willcox RR. Penicillin in the treatment of syphilis. Bull World Health Org 1972;47(suppl):1-68.

Ingraham NR. The diagnosis of infantile congenital syphilis during the period of doubt. Am J Syph Neurol 1935;19:547-580.

Jenkin HW, Sander PL. In vitro cultivation of *Treponema pallidum*. In Shell RF, Musher DM (eds). Pathogenesis and Immunology of Treponemal Infection. New York: Marcel Dekker, 1983.

Karmody CS, Schuknecht HP. Deafness in congenital syphilis. Arch Otolaryngol 1966;83:44-53.

Kaufman RE, Olansky DC, Wiesner PJ. The FTA-ABS (IgM) test for neonatal congenital syphilis: a critical review. J Am Venereol Dis Assoc 1974;1:79-84.

Lukehart SA, Hook EW III, Baker-Zander SA, et al. Invasion of the central nervous system by *Treponema pallidum*: implications for diagnosis and treatment. Ann Intern Med 1988;109:855-862.

Mascola L, Pelosi R, Alexander CE. Inadequate treatment of syphilis in pregnancy. Am J Obstet Gynecol 1984a;150:945-947.

Mascola L, Pelosi R, Blount JH, et al. Congenital syphilis: why is it still occurring? JAMA 1984b;252:1719-1722.

McCracken GH Jr, Kaplan JM. Penicillin treatment for congenital syphilis. JAMA 1974;228:855.

Michelow IC, Wendel GD, Norgard MV, et al. Central nervous system infection in congenital syphilis. New Engl J Med 2002;346:1792-1798.

Miller JL, Meyer PG, Parrott NA, Hill JH. A study of the biologic falsely reactive reactions for syphilis in children. J Pediatr 1960;57:548-552.

Musher DM. Biology of *Treponema pallidum*. In Holmes KK, Mardh PA, Sparling PF, Wiesner PJ (eds). Sexually Transmitted Diseases. New York: McGraw-Hill, 1984.

Musher DM, et al. The interaction between *Treponema pallidum* and human polymorphonuclear leucocytes. J Infect Dis 1983;147:77.

Musher DM, Hamill RJ, Baughn RE. Effect of human immunodeficiency virus (HIV) infection on the course of syphilis and on the response to treatment. Ann Intern Med 1990;113:872-881.

Pope V, Fears MB, Morrill WE, Castro A, Kikkert SE. Comparison of the Serodia *Treponema pallidum* Particle Agglutination, Captia Syphilis-G, and SpiroTek Reagin II tests with standard test techniques for diagnosis of syphilis. J Clin Microbiol 2000;38:2543-2545

Rawstron SA, Bromberg K. Failure of recommended maternal therapy to prevent congenital syphilis. Sex Transm Dis 1991a;18:102-106.

Rawstron SA, Bromberg K. Comparison of maternal and newborn serologic tests for syphilis. Am J Dis Child 1991b;145:1383-1388.

Rawstron SA, Jenkins S, Blanchard S, et al. Maternal and congenital syphilis in Brooklyn, NY. Epidemiology, transmission, and diagnosis. Am J Dis Child 1993;147:727-731.

Rawstron SA, Mehta S, Marcellino L, et al. Congenital syphilis and Fluorescent Treponemal Antibody Test reactivity after the age of 1 year. Sex Transm Dis 2001;28:412-416.

Rawstron SA, Vetrano J, Tannis G, Bromberg K. Congenital syphilis: detection of *Treponema pallidum* in stillborns. Clin Infect Dis 1997;24:24-7.

Renton AM, Borisenko KK, Meheus A, Gromyko A. Epidemics of syphilis in the newly independent states of the former Soviet Union. Sex Transm Infect 1998;74:165-166.

Risser WL, Hwang LY. Problems in the current case definition of congenital syphilis. J Pediatr 1996;129:499-505.

Rolfs RT, Joesoef MR, Henershot EF, et al. A randomized trial of enhanced therapy for early syphilis in patients with and without human immunodeficiency virus infection. New Engl J Med 1997;337:307-314.

Romanowski B, Sutherland R, Fick GH, et al. Serologic response to treatment of infectious syphilis. Ann Intern Med 1991;114:1005-1009.

Rompalo AM, Joesoef MR, O'Donnell JA, et al. Clinical manifestations of early syphilis by HIV status and gender. Results of the Syphilis and HIV study. Sex Transm Dis 2001;28:158-165.

Russell P, Altshuler G. Placental abnormalities of congenital syphilis. Am J Dis Child 1974;128:160-163.

Sanchez PJ. Laboratory tests for congenital syphilis. Pediatr Infect Dis J1998;17:70-71.

Sanchez PJ, McCracken GH Jr, Wendel GD, et al. Molecular analysis of the fetal IgM response to *Treponema pallidum* antigens: implications for improved serodiagnosis of congenital syphilis. J Infect Dis 1989;159:508-517.

Sanchez PJ, Wendel GD, Norgard MV. IgM antibody to *Treponema pallidum* in cerebrospinal fluid of infants with congenital syphilis. Am J Dis Child 1992;146:1171-1175.

Sanchez PJ, Wendel GD Jr, Grimprel E, et al. Evaluation of molecular methodologies and rabbit infectivity testing for the diagnosis of congenital syphilis and neonatal central nervous system invasion by *Treponema pallidum*. J Infect Dis 1993;167:148-157.

Schmidt BL, Edjlalipour M, Luger A. Comparative evaluation of nine different enzyme-linked immunosorbent assays for the determination of antibodies against

Treponema pallidum in patients with primary syphilis. J Clin Microbiol 2000;38:1279-1282.

Schulte JM, Burkham S, Hamaker D, et al. Syphilis among HIV-infected mothers and their infants in Texas from 1988-1994. Sex Transm Dis 2001;28:315-320.

Scotti AT, Logan LL. A specific IgM antibody test in neonatal congenital syphilis. J Pediatr 1968;73:242-243.

Shah AM, Boby KFJ, Karande SC, et al. Late onset congenital syphilis. Indian Pediatr 1995;32:795-798.

Sheffield JS, Sanchez PJ, Morris G, et al. Congenital syphilis after maternal treatment for syphilis during pregnancy. Am J Obstet Gynecol 2002;186:569-573.

Sparling PF. Diagnosis and treatment of syphilis. N Engl J Med 1971;284:642.

Speer ME, Taber LH, Clark DB, Rudolph AJ. Cerebrospinal fluid levels of benzathine penicillin G in the neonate. J Pediatr 1977;9:996.

Srinivasan G, Ramamurthy RS, Bharathi A, et al. Congenital syphilis: a diagnostic and therapeutic dilemma. Pediatr Infect Dis 1983;2:436-441.

St. Louis ME, Farley TA, Aral SO. Untangling the persistence of syphilis in the South. Sex Transm Dis 1996;23:11-14.

Stoll BJ, Lee FK, Larsen S, et al. Clinical and serologic evaluation of neonates for congenital syphilis: continuing diagnostic dilemma. J Infect Dis 1993;167:1093-1099

Taber LH, Huber TW. Congenital syphilis. Prog Clin Biol Res 1975;3:183.

Warner L, Rochat RW, Fichtner RR, et al. Missed opportunities for congenital syphilis prevention in an urban Southeastern hospital. Sex Transm Dis 2001;28:92-98.

Wendel GD. Gestational and congenital syphilis. Clin Perinatol 1988;15:287-303.

Wendel GD Jr, Sanchez PJ, Peters MT, et al. Identification of *Treponema pallidum* in amniotic fluid and fetal blood from pregnancies complicated by congenital syphilis. Obstet Gynecol 1991;78(5 pt 2):890-895.

Wendel GD, Stark BJ, Jamison RB, et al. Penicillin allergy and desensitization in serious infections during pregnancy. N Engl J Med 1985;312:1229-1232.

Wolf B, Kalangu K. Congenital neurosyphilis revisited. Eur J Pediatr 1993;152:493-495.

Yobs AR, Brown L, Hunter EF. Fluorescent antibody technique in early syphilis. Arch Pathol 1964;77:220-225.

Young H. Guidelines for serological testing for syphilis. Sex Transm Infect 2000;76:403-405.

Young H, Aktas G, Moyes A. Enzywell recombinant enzyme immunoassay for the serological diagnosis of syphilis. Int J STD AIDS 2000;11:288-291.

Young H, Moyes A, de Ste Croix I, McCillan A. A new recombinant antigen latex agglutination test (Syphilis Fast) for the rapid serological diagnosis of syphilis. Int J STD AIDS 1998;9:196-200.

Young H, Moyes A, McMillan A, Robertson DHH. Screening for treponemal infection by a new enzyme immunoassay. Genitourin Med 1989;65:72-78.

Zenker PN, Rolfs RT. Treatment of syphilis, 1989. Rev Infect Dis 1990;12(suppl 6):S590.

Chlamydia trachomatis infections

Alexander ER, Harrison HR. Role of *Chlamydia trachomatis* in perinatal infection. Rev Infect Dis 1983;5:713-719.

Beem MO, Saxon EM. Respiratory tract colonization and a distinctive pneumonia syndrome in infants infected with *Chlamydia trachomatis*. N Engl J Med 1977;296:306-310.

Bell TA, Sandstrom KI, Gravett MG, et al. Comparison of ophthalmic silver nitrate solution and erythromycin ointment for prevention of natally acquired *Chlamydia trachomatis*. Sex Transm Dis 1987;14:195-200.

Black CM. Current methods of laboratory diagnosis of *Chlamydia trachomatis* infections. Clin Microbiol Rev 1997;10:160-184.

Blythe MJ, Katz BP, Batteiger BE, et al. Recurrent genitourinary chlamydia infection in sexually active adolescents. J Pediatr 1992;121:487-493.

Blythe MJ, Katz BP, Caine VA. Historical and clinical factors associated with *Chlamydia trachomatis* genitourinary tract infection in female adolescents. J Pediatr 1988;112:1000-1004.

Brunham RC, Binns B, McDowell J, Paraskevas M. *Chlamydia trachomatis* infection in women with ectopic pregnancy. Obstet Gynecol 1986;67:722-726.

Burstein GR, Snyder MH, Conley D, et al. Adolescent chlamydia testing practices and diagnosed infections in a large managed care organization. Sex Transm Dis 2001;28:477-483.

Centers for Disease Control and Prevention. Screening tests to detect *Chlamydia trachomatis* and *Neisseria gonorrheae* infection—2002. MMWR 2002b;51(No. RR-15):1-39.

Centers for Disease Control and Prevention. Summary of notifiable diseases, United States, 1999. MMWR Morb Mortal Wkly Rep 2001;48:1-104.

Chacko MR, Lovchik JC. *Chlamydia trachomatis* infection in sexually active adolescents: prevalence and risk factors. Pediatrics 1984;73:836-840.

Chambers CV, Shafer MA, Adger H, et al. Microflora of the urethra in adolescent boys: relationship to sexual activity and nongonococcal urethritis. J Pediatr 1987;110:314-321.

Cohen DA, Nsuami M, Martin DH, et al. Repeated school-based screening for sexually transmitted diseases: a feasible strategy for reaching adolescents. Pediatrics 1999;104:1281-1285.

Eagar RM, Beach RK, Davidson AJ. Epidemiologic and clinical factors of *Chlamydia trachomatis* in black, Hispanic and white female adolescents. West J Med 1985;143:3-41.

Everett KDE, Bush RM, Anderson AA. Emended description of the order Chlamydiales, proposal of Parachlamydiaceae fam. nov. and Simkaniaceae fam. nov., each containing one monotypic genus, revised taxonomy of the family Chlamydiaceae, including a new genus and five new species, and standards for identification of organisms. Int J Syst Bacteriol 1999;49:425-440.

Fisher M, Swenson PD, Risucci D, Kaplan MH. *Chlamydia trachomatis* in suburban adolescents. J Pediatr 1987;111:617-620.

Fraser JJ, Rettig PJ, Kaplan DW. Prevalence of cervical *Chlamydia trachomatis* and *Neisseria gonorrhoeae* in female adolescents. Pediatrics 1982;71:333-336.

Gaydos CA, Crotchfelt KA, Howell MR, et al. Molecular amplification assays to detect chlamydial infections in urine specimens from high school female students and to monitor the persistence of chlamydial DNA after therapy. J Infect Dis 1998;177:417-424.

Golden N, Hammerschlag M, Neuhoff S, Gleyzer A. Prevalence of *Chlamydia trachomatis* cervical infection in female adolescents. Am J Dis Child 1984;138:562-564.

Hammerschlag MR. Chlamydial infections. J Pediatr 1989;114:727-734.

Hammerschlag MR. *Chlamydia trachomatis* in children. Pediatr Ann 1994;32:349-353.

Hammerschlag MR, Ajl S, Laraque D. Inappropriate use of nonculture tests for the detection of *Chlamydia trachomatis* in suspected victims of child sexual abuse: a continuing problem. Pediatrics 1999;104:1137-1139.

Hammerschlag MR, Cummings C, Roblin P, et al. Efficacy of neonatal ocular prophylaxis for the prevention of chlamydial and gonococcal conjunctivitis. N Engl J Med 1989;320:769-772.

Hammerschlag MR, Doraiswamy B, Alexander ER, et al. Are rectogenital chlamydial infections a marker of sexual abuse in children? Pediatr Infect Dis J 1984;3:100-104.

Hammerschlag MR, Gelling M, Roblin PM, et al. Treatment of neonatal chlamydial conjunctivitis with azithromycin. Pediatr Infect Dis J 1998;17:1049-1050.

Hammerschlag MR, Golden NH, Oh MK, et al. Single dose of azithromycin for the treatment of genital chlamydia infections in adolescents. J Pediatr 1993;122:961-965.

Hammerschlag MR, Rettig PJ, Shields ME. False-positive results with the use of chlamydial antigen detection tests in the evaluation of suspected sexual abuse in children. Pediatr Infect Dis 1988;7:11-14.

Hammerschlag MR, Roblin PM, Gelling M, et al. Use of polymerase chain reaction for the detection of *Chlamydia trachomatis* in ocular and nasopharyngeal specimens from infants with conjunctivitis. Pediatr Infect Dis J 1997;16:293-297.

Harrison HR, Alexander ER, Weinstein L, et al. Cervical *Chlamydia trachomatis* and mycoplasmal infections in pregnancy: epidemiology and outcomes. JAMA 1983;250:1721-1727.

Harrison HR, English MG, Lee CK, Alexander ER. *Chlamydia trachomatis* infant pneumonia. N Engl J Med 1978;298:702-708.

Hauger SB, Brown J, Agre F, et al. Failure of MicroTrak to detect *Chlamydia trachomatis* from genital tract sites of prepubertal children at risk for sexual abuse. Pediatr Infect Dis 1988;7:660-661.

Heggie AD, Jaffe AC, Stuart LA, et al. Topical sulfacetamide vs oral erythromycin for neonatal chlamydial conjunctivitis. Am J Dis Child 1985;139:564-566.

Heggie AD, Lumicao GG, Stuart LA, et al. *Chlamydia trachomatis* infection in mothers and infants. Am J Dis Child 1981;135:507-511.

Honein MA, Palozzi LJ, Himelright IM, et al. Infantile hypertrophic pyloric stenosis after pertussis prophylaxis with erythromycin: a case review and cohort study. Lancet 1999;354:2101-2105.

Ingram DL, Runyan DK, Collins AD, et al. Vaginal *Chlamydia trachomatis* infection in children with sexual contact. Pediatr Infect Dis J 1984;3:97-99.

Jacobson GF, Autry AM, Kirby RS et al. A randomized controlled trial comparing amoxicillin and azithromycin for the treatment of *Chlamydia trachomatis* in pregnancy. Am J Obstet Gynecol 2001;184:1352-1356.

Kacmar J, Cheh E, Montagno A, et al. A randomized trial of azithromycin versus amoxicillin for the treatment of *Chlamydia trachomatis* in pregnancy. Infect Dis Obstet Gynecol 2001;9:197-202.

Mahon BE, Rosenman MB, Kleiman MB. Maternal and infant use of erythromycin and other macrolides antibiotics as risk factors for infantile hypertrophic pyloric stenosis. J Pediatr 2001;136:380-384.

Orr DP, Johnston K, Brizendine E, et al. Subsequent sexually transmitted infection in urban adolescents and young adults. Arch Pediatr Adolesc Med 2001;155:947-953.

Orr P, Sherman E, Blanchard J, et al. Epidemiology of infection due to *Chlamydia trachomatis* in Manitoba, Canada. Clin Infect Dis 1994;19:876-883.

Porder K, Sanchez N, Roblin PM, et al. Lack of specificity of Chlamydiazyme for detection of vaginal chlamydial infection in prepubertal girls. Pediatr Infect Dis 1989;8:358-360.

Radkowski MA, Kranzler JK, Beem MO, Tippk MA. Chlamydia pneumonia in infants: radiography in 125 cases. Am J Roentgenol 1981;137:703-706.

Rettig PJ, Nelson JD. Genital tract infection with *Chlamydia trachomatis* in prepubertal children. J Pediatr 1981;99:206-210.

Ridgway GL. Treatment of chlamydial genital infection. J Antimicrob Chemother 1997;40:311-314.

Rockey DD, Lenart J, Stephens RS. Genome sequencing and our understanding of chlamydiae. Infect Immun 2000;68:5473-5479.

Saltz GR, Linnemann CC, Brookman RR, et al. *Chlamydia trachomatis* cervical infections in female adolescents. J Pediatr 1981;98:981-985.

Schachter J, Grossman M, Sweet RL, et al. Prospective study of perinatal transmission of *Chlamydia trachomatis*. JAMA 1986a;255:3374-3377.

Schachter J, Sweet RL, Grossman M, et al. Experience with the routine use of erythromycin in pregnancy. N Engl J Med 1986b;314:276-279.

Stamm WE, Guinan ME, Johnston C, et al. Effect of treatment regimens for *Neisseria gonorrheae* on simultaneous infection with *Chlamydia trachomatis*. N Engl J Med 1984;310: 545-549.

Turrentine MA, Newton ER. Amoxicillin or erythromycin for the treatment of antenatal chlamydial infection: a metaanalysis. Obstet Gynecol 1995;86:1021-1025.

Weiss SG, Newcomb RW, Beem MO. Pulmonary assessment of children after chlamydial pneumonia of infancy. J Pediatr 1986;108:661-664.

Bacterial vaginosis

Amsel R, Tolter PA, Spiegel CA, et al. Nonspecific vaginitis: diagnostic criteria and microbial and epidemiologic associations. Am J Med 1983;74:14-22.

Bartley DL, Morgan L, Rimsza MA. *Gardnerella vaginalis* in prepubertal girls. Am J Dis Child 1987;141:1014-1017.

Hammerschlag MR, Cummings M, Doraiswamy B, et al. Nonspecific vaginitis following sexual abuse in children. Pediatrics 1985;75:1032-1031.

Ingram DL, White ST, Lyna PR, et al. *Gardnerella vaginalis* infection and sexual contact in female children. Child Abuse Neglect 1992;16:847-853.

Joesoef MR, Schmid GP, Hillier SL. Bacterial vaginosis: review of treatment options and potential clinical indications for therapy. Clin Infect Dis 1999;28(suppl 1): S57-S65.

Samuels P, Hammerschlag MR, Cummings M, et al. Nonspecific vaginitis is an important cause of vaginitis in children (abstract 391). Presented at the 25th Interscience Conference on Antimicrobial Agents and Chemotherapy, Minneapolis, 1985.

Shafer M-A, Sweet RL, Ohm-Smith MJ, et al. Microbiology of the lower genital tract in postmenarcheal adolescent girls, differences by sexual activity, contraception, and presence of nonspecific vaginitis. J Pediatr 1985;107:974-981.

Spiegel CA, Amsel R, Holmes KK. Diagnosis of bacterial vaginosis by direct Gram stain of vaginal fluid. J Clin Microbiol 1983;18:170-177.

Thomason JL, Velbart SM, Anderson RJ, et al. Statistical evaluation of diagnostic criteria for bacterial vaginosis. Am J Obstet Gynecol 1990;162:155-160.

Trichomoniasis

Al-Salihi FL, Curram JP, Wang JS. Neonatal *Trichomonas vaginalis*: report of three cases and review of the literature. Pediatrics 1974;53:196-200.

Fouts AC, Kraus SJ. *Trichomonas vaginalis*: reevaluation of its clinical presentation and laboratory diagnosis. J Infect Dis 1980;141:137-143.

Jones JG, Yamauchi T, Lambert B. *Trichomonas vaginalis* infestation in sexually abused girls. Am J Dis Child 1985;139:846-847.

Kruger JN, Tam MR, Stevens CE, et al. Diagnosis of trichomoniasis: comparison of conventional wet-mount examination with cytologic studies, cultures, and monoclonal antibody staining of direct specimens. JAMA 1988;259:1223-1227.

Petrin D, Delgaty K, Bhatt R, et al. Clinical and microbiological aspects of *Trichomonas vaginalis*. Clin Microbiol Rev 1998;11:300-312.

Wolner-Hanssen P, Krieger JN, Stevens CE, et al. Clinical manifestations of vaginal trichomoniasis. JAMA 1989;261:571-576.

HPV infection

Bauer HM, Greer CE, Chambers JC, et al. Genital human papillomavirus infection in female university students as determined by a PCR-based method. JAMA 1991;265:472-477.

Bender ME. New concepts of condyloma acuminata in children. Arch Dermatol 1986;122:1121-1124.

Boyd AS. Condylomata acuminata in the pediatric population. Am J Dis Child 1990;144:817-824.

Cohen BA, Honig P, Androphy E. Anogenital warts in children. Arch Dermatol 1990;126:1575-1580.

Cason J, Kaye JN, Jewers RJ, et al. Perinatal infection and persistence of human papillomavirus types 16 and 18 in infants. J Med Virol 1995;47:209-218.

Davis AJ, Emans SJ. Human papillomavirus infection in the pediatric and adolescent patient. J Pediatr 1989;115:1-9.

DeJong AR, Weiss JC, Brent RL. Condyloma acuminata in children. Am J Dis Child 1982;136:704-706.

Fife KH, Bubalo F, Boggs DL, et al. Perinatal exposure of newborns to HPV: detection by DNA amplification. UCLA Symposia on Molecular and Cellular Biology 1990;124:73-76.

Fife KH, Rogers RE, Zwickl BW. Symptomatic and asymptomatic cervical infections with human papilloma-virus during pregnancy. J Infect Dis 1987;156:904-911.

Fisher M, Rosenfeld WD, Burk RD. Cervicovaginal human papillomavirus infection in suburban adolescents and young adults. J Pediatr 1991;119:821-825.

Gibson PE, Gardner SD, Best SJ. Human papillomavirus types in anogenital warts of children. J Med Virol 1990;30:142-145.

Gutman LT, St Claire KK, Everett VD, et al. Cervical-vaginal and intra-anal human papillomavirus infection of young girls with external genital warts. J Infect Dis 1994;170:339-344.

Gutman LT, St Claire KK, Hermann-Giddens ME, et al. Evaluation of sexually abused and nonabused young girls for intravaginal human papillomavirus infection. Am J Dis Child 1992;146:694-699.

Jenison SA, Yu X, Valentine JM, et al. Evidence of prevalent genital-type human papillomavirus infections in adults and children. J Infect Dis 1990;162:60-69.

Moscicki A-B, Palefsky J, Gonzales J, et al. Human papillomavirus infection in sexually active adolescent females: prevalence and risk factors. Pediatr Res 1990;28:507-513.

Moscicki A-B, Shiboski S, Broering J, et al. The natural history of human papillomavirus infection as measured by repeat DNA testing in adolescent and young women. J Pediatr 1998;132:211-284.

Obaleck S, Jablonska S, Favre M, et al. Condylomata acuminata in children: frequent association with human papillomaviruses responsible for cutaneous warts. J Am Acad Dermatol 1990;23:205-213.

Padel AF, Venning VA, Evans MF, et al. Human papillomaviruses in anogenital warts in children; typing by in situ DNA hybridization. Br Med J 1990;300:1491-1494.

Pakarian F, Kaye J, Cason J, et al. Cancer associated human papillomaviruses: perinatal transmission and persistence. Br J Obstet Gynaecol 1994;101:514-517.

Puranen M, Yliskoski M, Saarikoski S. Vertical transmission of human papillomavirus from infected mothers to their newborn babies and persistence of the virus in childhood. Am J Obstet Gynecol 1996;174:694-699.

Rando RF, Lindheim S, Hasty L, et al. Increased frequency of detection of human papillomavirus deoxyribonucleic acid in exfoliated cervical cells during pregnancy. Am J Obstet Gynecol 1989;161:50-55.

Rock B, Noghashfar Z, Barnett N, et al. Genital tract papillomavirus infection in children. Arch Dermatol 1986;122:1129-1132.

Sedlacek TV, Lindheim S, Eder C, et al. Mechanism for human papillomavirus transmission at birth. Am J Obstet Gynecol 1989;161:55-59.

Seidel J, Zonana J, Tolten E. Condylomata acuminata as a sign of sexual abuse in children. J Pediatr 1979;95:553-554.

Shah K, Kashima H, Polk BF, et al. Rarity of cesarean delivery in cases of juvenile-onset respiratory papillomatosis. Obstet Gynecol 1986;68:795-799.

Siegfried E, Rasnick-Conley J, Cook S, et al. Human papillomavirus screening in pediatric victims of sexual abuse. Pediatrics 1998;101:43-47.

Watts DH, Koutsky LA, Holmes KK, et al. Low risk of perinatal transmission of human papillomavirus: results from a prospective cohort study. Am J Obstet Gynecol 1998;178:365-373.

Other infections

Gellert GA, Durfee MJ, Berkowitz CD. Developing guidelines for HIV antibody testing among victims of pediatric sexual abuse. Child Abuse Neglect 1990;14:9-17.

Gellert GA, Durfee MJ, Berkowitz CD, et al. Situational and sociodemographic characteristics of children infected with human immunodeficiency virus from pediatric sexual abuse. Pediatrics 1993;91:39-44.

Gutman LT, St Claire KK, Weedy C, et al. Human immunodeficiency virus transmission by child sexual abuse. Am J Dis Child 1991;145:137-141.

Leiderman BA, Grimm KT. A child with HIV infection. JAMA 1986;256:3094.

Lindegren ML, Hanson IC, Hammett TA, et al. Sexual abuse of children: intersection with the HIV epidemic. Pediatrics 1998;102:e46-e56.

Merchant RC, Kehavarz R. Human immunodeficiency virus post-exposure prophylaxis for children and adolescents. Pediatrics 2001;108:e38-e51.

Szmuness W, Much MI, Prince AM, et al. On the role of sexual behavior in the spread of hepatitis B infection. Ann Intern Med 1975;83:489-495.

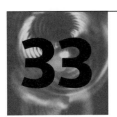

33 SMALLPOX AND VACCINIA

SAMUEL L. KATZ

In a prefatory paragraph to this chapter in the previous edition of this text, the editors offered an apologetic explanation for continuing to include a chapter on a disease that had been declared eradicated 20 years previously. However, both the historic significance of the disease as well as the beginning use of vaccinia virus as a vector for genes of other agents justified its continued inclusion. Anxiety regarding bioterrorism in the late 1990s (Henderson et al., 1999), followed by the events of September and October 2001 in the United States surrounding the destruction of the World Trade Center in New York City and later the deliberate circulation of anthrax spores, have precipitated a heightened national and global concern regarding bioterrorism; variola is identified as one of the prime possible agents. Although the only acknowledged variola virus is stored at the Centers for Disease Control and Prevention (CDC) in Atlanta, Georgia and at the State Scientific Center of Virology and Biotechnology (VEKTOR) in Novosibirsk, in the Russian Federation, concerns and reports that smallpox virus has found its way to a number of other nations enhances anxiety regarding its accidental escape or deliberate use (Alibek, 1999). Destruction of the virus remaining in the U.S. and Russian repositories has been postponed repeatedly and currently is on hold (Stone, 2002). Abundant new information has been disseminated among public health installations, health-care workers, and others regarding smallpox (Centers for Disease Control and Prevention, 2002; Meltzer et al., 2001), and the U.S. Government has issued contracts for several hundred million doses of smallpox vaccine (vaccinia) to augment its current (early 2003) stockpile of approximately 100 million doses. Recent investigations have demonstrated that the original vaccine (pre-

pared in 1981 and 1982) can be diluted 1:5 or 1:10 while retaining its ability to confer a primary vaccinial response (Frey et al., 2002). Universal smallpox vaccination in the United States was halted in 1971 and 1972 and in the ensuing decade in all other countries throughout the world. Except for selected laboratory workers and some military groups, individuals born after 1972 have never received smallpox vaccination. With resumption of vaccination, most individuals under age 31 years are receiving their primary exposure to the agent. Residual immunity among those older persons who were vaccinated early in life remains uncertain and is the subject of current discussion and investigation (Cohen, 2001). This strikingly altered setting warrants a more complete consideration of the epidemiologic, clinical, and other aspects of variola and vaccinia.

For at least 3,000 years smallpox was a widespread illness with serious morbidity and mortality. Nations in Africa and the Asian subcontinent reported millions of eases annually as recently as 1967. In that year the World Health Organization (WHO) began its 10-year program of smallpox eradication. On October 26, 1977, Ali Maow Maalin, a cook in the district hospital at Merka, Somalia, had the onset of his smallpox rash. He will go down in history as the last known patient with endemic smallpox. In the year after Maalin's recovery, the only known smallpox victims acquired their infections as the result of a laboratory contamination in Birmingham, England. The WHO Assembly in 1980 received the documentation of the final global eradication of smallpox, an achievement unique in the history of the interaction between human beings and the microorganisms of their environment.

Several hundred episodes of suspected endemic smallpox have been reported to WHO since the case of Ali Maow Maalin, but none has been verified. Instead, they proved to be chickenpox, herpes simplex, monkeypox, drug eruptions, or other skin disorders. Of special note is monkeypox, which has been reported from West and Central Africa (Hutin et al., 2001). Originally recovered from monkeys who became ill in captivity, the virus has been responsible for human illness closely resembling smallpox, usually in children with no history of previous smallpox vaccination. Secondary spread among humans is unusual, but several generations of cases have been documented (Breman, 2000). Sporadic cases of human monkeypox are reported and may result from direct transmission via the handling of carcasses of monkeys who have died from the infection or from eating infected squirrels (Ivker, 1997).

SMALLPOX (VARIOLA MAJOR; VARIOLA MINOR OR ALASTRIM; VARIOLOID)

Smallpox is an acute, highly contagious, usually preventable rash disease caused by poxvirus variola, a specific agent immunologically related to vaccinia virus.

Variola major, variola minor or alastrim, and varioloid are the three chief forms of the disease. Variola major is classic smallpox. It has a high mortality that varies as follows according to the type of lesions: discrete, 5% to 10%; confluent, 50% to 75%; hemorrhagic, 80% to 100%. Variola minor, or alastrim, is a mild type of smallpox occurring in nonvaccinated persons. It is caused by a less virulent strain of the virus that breeds true. The mortality is usually under 1% except in rare instances in which the rash may become confluent or hemorrhagic. Varioloid is a mild form of smallpox occurring in previously vaccinated persons who have partial immunity. This mild disease may be caused by a virulent strain of the virus that is capable of causing variola major in a nonimmunized contact.

ETIOLOGY

The Poxviridae family is a group of large, complex DNA viruses with a multitude of individual agents. A number of the viruses can initiate human infection, but only variola (smallpox) has been of worldwide significance. The other agents are of importance in various species, including monkeys, camels, sheep, rabbits, swine, buffalo, goats, cows, mice, and turkeys, canaries, pigeons, and other birds. Variola and vaccinia are members of the genus Orthopoxvirus; others in the genus are cowpox and monkeypox. Humans are the only host for variola and there is no vector-borne transmission, so there is no sylvan or other occult reservoir.

Smallpox and vaccinia viruses are morphologically indistinguishable and closely related immunologically. The elementary bodies can be identified in smears of vesicular fluid stained by the Paschen, Giemsa, or Gutstein method. Under the electron microscope virions are seen to be brick shaped or ovoid and approximately 200×300 nm. Aggregates of these bodies in the cytoplasm of infected host cells form the so-called Guarnieri bodies, measuring approximately 10 μm in diameter. The viral genome is a single linear double-stranded DNA contained within a core that, in turn, is enclosed by an external coat of lipid and protein surrounding one to two lateral bodies as well. The complete genome of smallpox has been cloned and sequenced (LeDuc and Jahrling, 2001; Shchelkunov, 1995). Ropp et al. (1995) reported rapid identification of smallpox and its differentiation from vaccinia by polymerase chain reaction.

Smallpox and vaccinia viruses can be grown on the chorioallantoic membranes of embryonated eggs. Each produces characteristic plaques that can be inhibited by the addition of specific antiserum to the virus. Inoculation of a scarified rabbit's cornea with the virus is followed by keratoconjunctivitis with histologic evidence of typical Guarnieri's bodies. The viruses grow in tissue cultures derived from various mammalian cells. Cytopathic changes generally appear later with smallpox virus (5 to 6 days) than with vaccinia virus (1 to 2 days).

The viruses are very stable, and their viability is retained in the dry state. Smallpox and vaccinia crusts have been shown to contain active virus after more than 1 year at room temperature (Downie and Dumbell, 1947).

Infection with smallpox and vaccinia viruses stimulates the production of four types of antibody: antihemagglutinin, complement fixing antibodies, neutralizing antibodies, and antibodies that inhibit agar gel precipitation. Levels of antihemagglutinin and complement-fixing antibodies rise significantly by the end of the second week of illness or vaccination; they persist for several months. Neutralizing antibodies develop later but persist for years.

PATHOGENESIS

The virus first invades the upper respiratory tract, where it multiplies locally in the oropharyngeal and respiratory mucosa. It then spreads to the regional lymphatics and nodes, from which it enters the bloodstream. Following a brief asymptomatic viremia, virus replicates in the reticuloendothelial system, leading to a secondary viremia with widespread dissemination of virus to the capillary endothelium of the skin, the mucous membranes of the oropharynx, and multiple organs (spleen, liver, kidneys, lungs, and bone marrow) (Fenner et al., 1988).

Virus has been isolated from the blood of patients as early as 1 day before onset of rash and as late as the eighth day of illness. All stages of the skin lesions from maculopapules to crusts are productive of active virus. Pharyngeal secretions also are positive by the first day of rash. Transmission generally occurs through close direct contact, with inhalation of infected droplet nuclei, although rare instances of apparent airborne transmission have been reported within hospital settings (Wehrle et al., 1970). Oral lesions ulcerate, releasing large titers of virus, during the first week after onset of rash. Secondary attack rates among susceptible individuals in close contact to such a patient range from 25% to 75%.

PATHOLOGY

The lesions most commonly observed are those of the skin and mucous membranes of the oropharyngeal area and upper respiratory tract. At autopsy, however, there may be evidence of widespread dissemination of virus, with areas of focal necrosis in the liver, spleen, testes, lungs, and other organs.

Histopathologically, the skin lesions begin in the epithelial cells, which first show evidence of edema followed by degeneration of the cytoplasm. These foci develop into vacuoles that are separated by a lacework of reticular fibers. The fluid in the vacuoles becomes infiltrated by polymorphonuclear leukocytes and bacteria, and these, combined with necrotic tissue, are responsible for pustule formation. The reticular fibers rupture, the lesion becomes umbilicated, and as the fluid is absorbed, a crust forms. The scab, which is made up of cellular exudate and destroyed tissue, separates and falls off. After approximately 2 weeks, there is complete epithelial regeneration. The inflammatory reaction extends down into the corium. It is the damage to this layer of skin that influences scar formation although some lesions may heal without scarring. The typical acidophilic intracytoplasmic inclusion bodies (Guarnieri's bodies) are present in the epithelial cells.

CLINICAL MANIFESTATIONS
Variola Major

The incubation period of classic smallpox (variola major) is 12 days, with a range of 8 to 16 days. The typical clinical course (Plate 49) is characteristically biphasic, with a prodromal or toxemic period and an eruptive period (Henderson, 1999).

Prodromal period. The disease usually begins abruptly with chills, fever, headache, backache, and severe malaise. Vomiting occurs, particularly in children, who are also more prone to develop seizures than chills. The temperature rises to levels above 40° C (104° F), and the symptoms become more intense by the end of the second day. The patient exhibits an extreme toxicity, marked prostration, and occasionally delirium, stupor, or coma. Within the next 24 hours a striking improvement begins. The temperature falls to lower levels—37.8° to 38.3° C (100° to 101° F)—and by the end of the third day the patient begins to feel and look better. At this time, however, sore throat, cough, and rash appear.

In some cases a transient eruption may develop during the prodromal period. It may be petechial, morbilliform, or scarlatiniform, with characteristic bathing-trunks distribution. In most instances it disappears within 1 to 2 days.

The duration of the prodromal period is 2 to 4 days. In most instances it is terminated by the end of the third day, as the patient seems to improve concomitantly with the development of the rash.

Period of eruption. The first lesions appear on the mucous membranes of the mouth, throat, and respiratory tract usually 1 day before rash is noted. The enanthem begins as painful ulcers on the buccal, pharyngeal, and bronchial mucosa, causing the symptoms of sore throat, hoarseness, and cough.

The exanthem appears first on the face and forearms, then spreads to the upper arms and trunk, particularly the back, and finally reaches the lower extremities. The initial skin lesions are macules and are first detected on the third or fourth day of illness. They rapidly become papular within a matter of hours. The papules, 4 mm

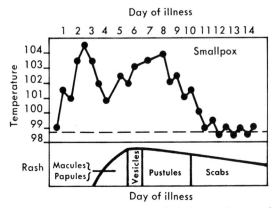

Fig. 33-1 Schematic diagram depicting evolution of smallpox rash.

in diameter, have a shotty feel on palpation and erupt over a 2- to 3-day period. By the end of the sixth day, the papules develop into vesicles that measure up to 6 mm in diameter and are usually surrounded by red areolae. Between the seventh and ninth days, the vesicles become pustules, measuring up to 8 mm in diameter.

During the pustular stage, the temperature begins to rise again and the constitutional symptoms return, now aggravated by the intensely painful lesions. At this time the patient presents a dramatic picture of a miserable person whose face is intensely inflamed, edematous, and distorted by a mass of pustules. On the tenth day,

the pustules begin to rupture, then to dry, and finally to form crusts (Figure 33-1).

The temperature and constitutional symptoms finally subside by the end of the second week. The desiccation of the lesions is accompanied by intense pruritus and is followed by a 1- to 2-week period of desquamation of the scabs.

A patient with full-blown smallpox presents the following characteristics:

- The lesions in any one regional area are in the same stage of development.
- The lesions have a typical order of appearance: (1) the face; (2) the upper extremities, beginning distally; (3) the trunk, particularly the back; and (4) the lower extremities, beginning distally.
- The lesions have a peripheral distribution. There is a greater concentration of lesions over the more distal areas such as the face, forearms and hands, and legs and feet. The lesions are more sparse and discrete on the trunk, arms, and thighs (Figure 33-2).

An attack of classic smallpox in an unvaccinated person may vary considerably in severity. A convenient classification is one based on the character of the lesions and correlated with case fatality rates: (1) ordinary-discrete, less than 10%; (2) ordinary-semiconfluent, 25% to 50%; (3) ordinary-confluent, 50% to 75%; (4)

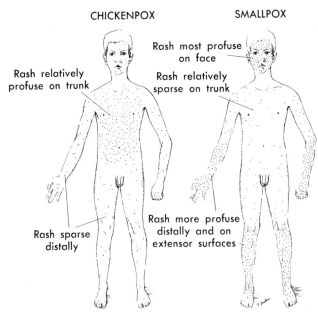

Fig. 33-2 Schematic drawing illustrating differences in distribution of chickenpox and smallpox rashes.

flat, greater than 90%; (5) hemorrhagic, nearly 100%; and (6) modified (altered by previous vaccination), less than 20% (Koplan and Foster, 1979). Discrete lesions are usually associated with milder constitutional symptoms, lower temperatures, and a more benign course. Hemorrhagic lesions, however, usually herald a severe and potentially fatal disease complicated by disseminated intravascular coagulation.

Hemorrhagic lesions in smallpox may develop early or late in the disease. In purpura variolosa the hemorrhages occur during the prodromal period. This type of so-called black smallpox is characterized by a fulminating course, associated with hemorrhages into the skin and from the mucous membranes, and usually by fatal termination before the period of eruption (variola sine eruptione). In variola hemorrhagica pustulosa the hemorrhages occur later, during the vesicular or pustular stages.

Variola Minor or Alastrim

This benign type of smallpox is caused by a less virulent strain of the virus. The incubation period is prolonged to approximately 15 days, with a range of 12 to 20 days. Generally, the prodromal period is relatively mild. The rash is typically discrete and tends to progress through the various stages more rapidly than in variola major. However, the rash has the characteristic peripheral distribution. The constitutional symptoms are not severe.

Varioloid

Varioloid has a clinical picture that may be indistinguishable from variola minor. It is a modified form of smallpox occurring in partially immune persons. The severity of the symptoms and extent of the rash vary with the patient's residual immunity.

Blood Picture

During the early prodromal period, there is granulocytopenia with a relative increase in lymphocytes. Later, during the eruptive phase, there may be significant leukocytosis with a predominance of polymorphonuclear leukocytes.

DIAGNOSIS

Historically, smallpox was recognized with ease during an epidemic or after a known contact. The diagnosis was generally made on the basis of suggestive clinical features and specific laboratory tests when available.

Suggestive Clinical Features

Some suggestive clinical features are as follows: (1) history of exposure, (2) acute illness and toxic condition with hyperpyrexia, prostration, severe backache, and possibly a prodromal rash with bathing-trunks distribution, (3) biphasic temperature curve, and (4) centrifugally distributed focal eruption progressing from macule to papule to vesicle to pustule and to crusting, with lesions in the same stage in any one general area.

Specific Laboratory Tests

Specific tests were helpful, particularly in doubtful or atypical cases. The most commonly employed techniques when available were electron microscopy (EM), gel diffusion, and the inoculation of the chorioallantoic membrane of embryonated hens' eggs. EM was the most rapid and reliable diagnostic method in experienced hands. The diagnostic procedures were employed to detect virus, to demonstrate specific antigen in focal lesions, and to demonstrate a rise in antibody level during the course of the illness.

Microscopic examination for elementary bodies. Material obtained from maculopapular or vesicular skin lesions can be stained by the Gispen or Gutstein method. Elementary bodies may be identified within an hour by an experienced person. EM, if available, can be used to identify the typical brick-shaped virus; this does not differentiate variola from vaccinia.

Serologic tests. Antibody is detectable 4 or 5 days after onset of disease. Complement fixation, hemagglutination inhibition, and gel precipitation assays were most often employed in the past. Paired serum specimens collected at 5- to 10-day intervals should be tested for a rise in antibody titer. Enzyme-linked immunosorbent assays are under development (LeDuc and Jahrling, 2001).

Electron microscopic examination. Scrapings, crusts, or fluid contents of skin lesions should be examined for presence of poxvirus.

Virus isolation. Material obtained from lesions at any stage is inoculated onto the chorioallantoic membrane of an embryonated egg. Smallpox virus produces plaques that are grossly and histologically different from vaccinia virus. Various human and other primate cell culture systems are also susceptible to variola virus.

Differential Diagnosis

The prodromal stage of smallpox may simulate a variety of infectious diseases, including influenza, pneumonia, meningitis, malaria, and typhoid fever. If a prodromal eruption is present, measles, scarlet fever, and meningococcemia have to be considered.

During the eruptive period the differential diagnosis will vary with the stage and character of the lesions. The following diseases may be confused with smallpox.

Chickenpox. The prodromal period is minimal or absent in chickenpox. Lesions appear in crops, rapidly progressing from macule to papule to vesicle to crust. Distribution is centripetal, with lesions in all stages in any one regional area.

Monkeypox. Since 1970 sporadic cases of human monkeypox infections have been reported in Central Africa (Hutin et al., 2001), especially among children who have never received smallpox vaccination that will protect against the virus. Because the clinical manifestations are so similar to those of smallpox, laboratory confirmation is required to distinguish them (Breman and Henderson, 1998). Case fatality rates among unprotected children have been as high as 15%. Human-to-human transmission is unusual and unsustained, but secondary attack rates of 9% have been claimed, although on careful investigation some alleged cases have turned out to be chickenpox.

Measles. During the early eruptive phase, the maculopapular eruption on the face of a patient with smallpox may simulate the rash of measles. The typical Koplik's spots and subsequent course of the rash are diagnostic of measles.

Rickettsialpox. Rickettsialpox is a mild illness with the following triad of manifestations: (1) a primary eschar, (2) a grippelike syndrome, and (3) a discrete papulovesicular eruption.

Eczema herpeticum or vaccinatum. In eczema herpeticum or vaccinatum there may be a history of vaccination or of contact with either a vaccinated person or one with a herpetic lesion. The eruption is chiefly confined to the areas of exfoliation. Stained scrapings of herpetic skin lesions reveal giant cells with intranuclear inclusions.

Disseminated herpes simplex infection. In this infection there is no prodrome as a rule, the lesions have no typical distribution but are vesicular, not pustular, and the diagnosis is usually made by laboratory tests that identify herpes simplex virus. Patients are often immunocompromised.

Pustular rashes of syphilis. The constitutional symptoms with pustular rashes of secondary syphilis are not striking. Spirochetes can be demonstrated in the lesions, and serologic tests will have positive results. Lesions are not vesicular but progress from macules to papules to pustules slowly over several weeks.

Erythema multiform eruptions (including Stevens-Johnson syndrome and drug rashes). In erythema multiforme eruptions there is usually no prodromal illness; lesions may be present in various stages, with maculopapules, vesicles, and bullae symmetrically distributed with a predilection for extensor surfaces of the extremities. Mucous membrane involvement is marked and may include oral and genital areas.

COMPLICATIONS
Bacterial

Bacterial complications may involve the skin and respiratory tract, with the development of impetigo, furuncles, cellulitis, and pneumonia. These infections may serve as a focus for subsequent septicemia, osteomyelitis, or septic arthritis. Secondary infected focal lesions on the bulbar conjunctiva may be followed by keratitis and corneal ulceration.

Nonbacterial Complications

Nonbacterial complications may occur in the respiratory tract and the central nervous system. Focal lesions may cause laryngeal edema, with obstruction of the airway. A demyelinating encephalitis or a peripheral neuritis may occasionally be observed. Psychoses also have been described after smallpox.

Smallpox in pregnancy is frequently followed by abortion and occasionally by congenital infection.

PROGNOSIS

The prognosis of smallpox depends on factors that are related to the causative agent, the host, and the disease.

Causative Agent

Infections caused by strains of variola major virus are generally more severe than those caused by alastrim or variola minor viruses. During the importation outbreaks of smallpox in Europe in the 1960s the case fatality rate was 50% among unvaccinated persons. On the other hand, disease acquired during an outbreak of alastrim carried a good prognosis, with a mortality of less than 1%.

Host

The prognosis is less favorable for patients at the extremes of life. Infants, the elderly, and pregnant women have the highest fatality rates. The more recently the patient has been vaccinated, the milder the disease is likely to be. Unvaccinated persons have a poorer prognosis.

Disease

A mild prodrome usually heralds a benign disease with a good prognosis. Overwhelming toxemia and prostration during the first few days are usually associated with a high mortality. The gravity of the prognosis increases with the development of encephalitis or septicemia.

IMMUNITY

There is no natural immunity to smallpox or vaccinia. Newborn infants may have transplacentally acquired antibodies.

Active immunity is acquired by either an attack of the disease or vaccination. Permanent protection is the rule after either smallpox or alastrim; very rarely, second attacks may occur. Smallpox vaccination is followed by variable immunity ranging from 1 to 20 years (Mack, 1972). The efficacy and duration of the immune response depend on a number of factors, including (1) the technique of vaccination, (2) the potency of the vaccine, (3) the number of previous vaccinations, and (4) the immunocompetence of the person.

After vaccination, antihemagglutinin, complement-fixing, and virus-neutralizing antibodies appear and can be detected between the tenth and thirteenth days. Protection may be achieved by vaccination within 3 to 4 days of exposure.

EPIDEMIOLOGIC FACTORS

In 1967, WHO began a program of global smallpox eradication. Before that time, smallpox was worldwide in distribution. In 1945 the majority of the world's population lived in areas where smallpox was endemic. By 1966, 43 countries reported smallpox to WHO, but in only 28 of them was the disease endemic. In 1976 only two countries, Ethiopia and Somalia, reported smallpox. By autumn of 1977 there were no known endemic areas in the world (Fenner et al., 1988).

Season and climate appeared to affect the incidence of smallpox in certain areas where the disease was endemic. In the temperate zone the number of cases increased in the winter months. In the tropics the disease was most prevalent during the hot, dry months.

Age had no effect on the susceptibility to smallpox in a community of unvaccinated people. The disease attacked persons in all age groups, from newborn infants to the elderly. Infants in utero were also susceptible. The age incidence of smallpox in an area was governed chiefly by the vaccination status of the population.

Sex distribution was also dependent on the vaccinal state. Males and females were equally susceptible.

The transmission occurred through direct and indirect contact. A typical case of variola major was infective from the onset of illness until the last scab was shed, possibly a month or more later. Epidemiologic and virus isolation studies, however, have indicated that smallpox is most infective in the first few days after the onset of the rash.

The disease was spread by respiratory droplets, and infected dry crusts were also a dangerous source (Wolff and Croon, 1968). An important source of infection was a case of unrecognized attenuated smallpox that was erroneously diagnosed as chickenpox. Some cases of varioloid that were clinically indistinguishable from varicella were nonetheless potential sources of infection.

TREATMENT

Patients with smallpox or suspected of having smallpox should be admitted to a hospital or institution if rigid isolation procedures can be enforced. In the past there was no specific therapy for smallpox, but recent advances in antiviral chemotherapy offer some optimism. Cidofovir, a cyclic derivative of ribavirin, has been studied for the treatment of cytomegalovirus and other serious herpes virus infections, especially in immunocompromised patients, but it carries the liabilities of bioavailability only via intravenous infusion and the risk of nephrotoxicity. Bray et al. (2000) have demonstrated its protective efficacy against cowpox virus in a murine model. More recently a related compound, hexadecyloxypropyl-cidofovir (HDP-CDV), has been shown to block variola virus replication in cell cultures and to protect mice in vivo from the lethality of cowpox (Hostetler et al., 2002). HDP-CDV can be administered orally and has an alleged potency far greater than that of cidofovir.

Supportive therapy is extremely important. Difficulty in swallowing caused by pharyngeal lesions causes many patients to refuse fluids and food. Parenteral therapy may be difficult because of the extensive eruption on the extremities. An indwelling polyethylene catheter for gavage is extremely useful. In this way, fluid, electrolyte, nutritional, and caloric requirements can be maintained.

Headache, hyperpyrexia, backache, and other symptoms require appropriate analgesic therapy. The eyes should be carefully cleansed with physiologic saline solution.

Severe hemorrhagic smallpox is frequently complicated by shock. In such instances the use of volume expanders, pressor agents, and other similar measures are required.

PREVENTIVE MEASURES

The most efficient way to prevent smallpox was to vaccinate everyone living in an area where the disease was endemic. To be most effective, vaccination should be done *before* exposure. Contacts should be vaccinated as soon as possible. In India the attack rate of persons vaccinated *after* exposure was reported to range between 10% and 40%.

Vaccinia immune globulin has been used in conjunction with smallpox vaccine for susceptible intimate contacts. Reports from India indicated that the combination reduced both the attack rate of the contacts and the mortality of the cases. The recommended dosage of the vaccinia immune globulin was 0.12 to 0.24 ml/kg of body weight; administered intramuscularly 12 to 24 hours after vaccination or revaccination (Kempe, 1960). Smallpox vaccination is discussed in more detail later in this chapter.

Bauer and colleagues reported an advance in the control of smallpox in 1963 (Bauer et al., 1963). They investigated the effect of N-methylisatin-β-thiosemicarbazone in the prophylaxis of smallpox in house contacts of patients in Madras hospitalized with the disease. Among 1,101 contacts who were given the drug, only three mild cases occurred; in contrast, among 1,126 comparable controls, 78 cases occurred and 12 patients died (Bauer et al., 1970). This compound was given orally, and it appeared to protect unvaccinated persons even

though it sometimes was given late in the incubation period. Side effects were limited to nausea and vomiting. Currently it is unavailable.

Isolation, Quarantine, and Control

The control of smallpox is not an individual problem; it is a community-wide, national, and international problem. Isolation, quarantine, and control procedures are currently being reviewed in the context of a potential bioterrorism event.

In the event of recognition of a case of smallpox, all contacts should be vaccinated as soon as possible, not more than 2 or 3 days after exposure. Subsequent decisions regarding more extensive programs of "ring" vaccination or mass administration will be the responsibility of public health authorities (Centers for Disease Control and Prevention, 2002; Henderson et al., 1999).

VACCINIA

Vaccinia is an acute infectious disease caused by smallpox vaccination or by the accidental contact of abraded skin with infective material. It is characterized by the development of a localized lesion that progresses in sequence from papule to vesicle to pustule to crust. Fever and regional lymphadenitis may develop during the vesicular or pustular stage. The infection stimulates the production of antibodies that are protective against smallpox (Coneybeare, 1951).

HISTORY

In 1798 Edward Jenner published his classic report that proved that cowpox was protective against smallpox. The relationship between cowpox and smallpox had been apparent to farmers and other country folk of England for many years. They had observed that persons developing cowpox lesions were subsequently protected against smallpox. On May 14, 1796, Jenner performed his crucial and historic experiment. He inoculated the arm of an 8-year-old boy (James Phipps) with material obtained from the cowpox lesion of a milkmaid's hand (Sarah Nelmes). A typical pox lesion developed on the boy's arm. Subsequently, on July 1, 1796, the boy was inoculated with pustular material from an active case of smallpox. Again, there was a local lesion but no disease. These studies were extended by Jenner, who inoculated active smallpox material into 10 persons with a history of cowpox: again, no disease resulted. He thus established that cowpox, an extremely mild and benign disease, protected against smallpox. It was not until 1798 that he published his work (Jenner, 1896).

Jenner's observations were subsequently confirmed in the United States by Benjamin Waterhouse, who, on July 8, 1800 vaccinated his 5-year-old son, Daniel, who earned the distinction of being the first person to be inoculated with cowpox virus in this country. Daniel's father subsequently inoculated him with smallpox virus, which failed to cause disease, thus indicating immunity.

Variolation has a history that dates back centuries before vaccination. The inoculum in variolation was smallpox virus itself. The result was usually an attenuated case of smallpox. Lady Mary Wortley Montague introduced this type of protection into England in 1717. Through her influence this procedure became popular in England and later was introduced into America and used by Cotton Mather and Zabdiel Boylston during a 1721 epidemic in Boston. Because its results were quite variable, it never was universally accepted. Finally, it was replaced by vaccination with cowpox virus and then by vaccination with vaccinia.

ETIOLOGY

The original material used by Jenner probably was cowpox virus. Cowpox virus has been postulated to be a variant of smallpox virus produced by passage through cattle. Similarly, the repeated passage of the agent through man and laboratory animals has produced a strain, vaccinia virus, that is distinct from the other poxviruses—variola major, variola minor, and cowpox (Baxby, 1977).

Vaccinia virus is morphologically indistinguishable from cowpox and smallpox viruses. Except for tissue culture preparations used by the Japanese and the Dutch, nearly all the vaccinia used in the global smallpox eradication program was grown in the traditional calfskin method. Various strains of virus were used including the Lister in Europe, Temple of Heaven in China, Patwadanger in India, and New York City Board of Health in the United States. They were all of equal efficacy, with perhaps some minor variation in frequency and severity of reactions. The new vaccines currently under production are all of cell culture derivation.

CLINICAL MANIFESTATIONS

The clinical manifestations of vaccinia are dependent for the most part on the immune status of the individual. Two types of reactions may result from a successful vaccination: a "major" response (pustular lesion or an area of definite induration or congestion surrounding a central lesion, scab, or ulcer 6 to 8 days after vaccination), or an "equivocal" response.

Major Response

The inoculated site becomes reddened and pruritic 3 days after vaccination. It becomes papular on the fourth day and vesicular by the fifth or sixth day. A red areola surrounds the vesicle, which becomes umbilicated and then pustular by the eighth to the eleventh day. By this time the red areola has enlarged tremendously. The pustule begins to dry, the redness subsides, and the lesion becomes crusted between the second and third week. By the end of the third week, the scab falls off; leaving a permanent scar that at first is pink in color but eventually becomes white.

At the end of the first week, between the vesicular and pustular phases, there may be a variable amount of fever, malaise, and regional lymphadenitis. These symptoms usually subside within 1 to 2 days and are more likely to occur in older children and adults than in infants.

Accelerated, Modified, or Vaccinoid Reaction

Revaccination of a partially immune person is followed by an attenuated form of vaccinia with the following characteristics: (1) usually there is no fever or constitutional symptoms; (2) a papule appears by the third day, becomes vesicular by the fifth to seventh day, and dries shortly thereafter; (3) the vesicle and its red areola are relatively small; and (4) the scar, if present, is usually insignificant and disappears within a year or two.

The absence of a reaction does not mean that the person is immune. In most instances, either the vaccine is not potent or the technique is at fault. Occasionally a papule may result from needle trauma. Consequently, when there is doubt, it is wise to repeat the vaccination.

In order to evaluate a vaccination, it would be ideal to inspect the lesion daily. When this is not practical, the optimum times of inspection are the third, seventh, and fourteenth days.

VACCINATION PROCEDURES
Methods

The recommended method of vaccination is multiple puncture (15 strokes) with a bifurcated needle, on the outer aspect of the arm over the insertion of the deltoid muscle.

Precautions

Because vaccination is generally an elective procedure, it should be postponed in instances of intercurrent infection. Primary vaccination of infants, children, or adults with eczema or other types of exfoliative dermatitis may be complicated by eczema vaccinatum, a severe and potentially fatal disease. Vaccination should be deferred until the skin lesions clear. Infants with eczema may acquire vaccinia by contact with recently vaccinated siblings or parents. Consequently, either the infant or the vaccinated members of the family should avoid contact until the danger of infection has passed. A nonocclusive dressing may be applied to prevent accidental inoculation or autoinoculation.

In summary, it is recommended that vaccination, when indicated, be given over the insertion of the deltoid muscle with the bifurcated needle multiple puncture technique and a fully potent vaccine.

Immunity

Immunity develops between the eighth and eleventh days after vaccination. Antihemagglutinin, complement-fixing, and virus-neutralizing antibodies are demonstrable between the tenth and thirteenth days. Vaccination within 48 to 72 hours after exposure to smallpox has been shown to be protective in most cases (Henderson and Fenner, 2001).

Duration of immunity is extremely variable; it may range between 3 and 10 years, but some retrospective studies suggest more prolonged protection (Cohen, 2001; Mack, 1972). During the mass vaccination program in New York City in 1947, a random sampling of 25,000 of the 5 million vaccinated persons indicated that 74% had successful takes, suggesting susceptibility to smallpox. Revaccination at 3-year intervals was generally recommended to maintain optimum immunity.

Complications

Secondary bacterial infection. The local lesion may be secondarily infected with staphylococci or streptococci, causing cellulitis. Formerly a common complication, tetanus is practically unheard of today. Not a single case occurred among the 5 million people who were vaccinated in New York City in 1947.

Accidental infection. Autoinoculation by means of scratching an active lesion may produce secondary pocks over various parts of the body. The site of inoculation governs the severity of this complication. For example, a lesion of the eye with corneal involvement may result in ulceration, scarring, and blindness.

Toxic eruptions. An erythema multiform type of eruption occasionally occurs between the seventh and tenth days at the height of the vaccinia reaction. The rash may be generalized or localized to a particular area. It usually clears within 3 to 5 days. It is thought to be due to a sensitivity reaction. This rash is most often seen in infants vaccinated before their first birthdays.

Generalized vaccinia. This potentially serious complication develops between the seventh and fourteenth days after vaccination and may initially be indistinguishable from the so-called toxic eruptions. However it progresses to a more generalized rash, with crops of lesions simulating a primary vaccination. Healing without scars takes place rapidly, being completed at the same time as the healing of the primary vaccinia lesion.

Eczema vaccinatum. This potentially fatal complication of vaccinia developed in infants with eczema who have been either vaccinated or exposed to an active case of vaccinia (Kempe, 1960). The disease is characterized by high fever, severe toxicity, and an extensive vesicular and pustular eruption chiefly confined to the area of dermatitis. Healthy areas of skin also may become involved. The mortality may be significant.

Progressive vaccinia (vaccinia necrosum; prolonged vaccinia; vaccinia gangrenosa). This highly fatal complication is fortunately rare. The initial vaccinal lesion fails to heal and progresses to involve more and more areas of adjacent skin. The necrosis of the tissues continues to extend, often over a period of months. Metastatic lesions may develop in other parts of the skin, bones, and other viscera. This complication has been observed in patients with profound immunologic disorders, particularly those with markedly compromised cellular immune function (e.g., severe combined immunodeficiency). Among current populations it might be anticipated in individuals with acquired immunodeficiency syndrome (Barlett, 2003) and others undergoing therapy or prophylaxis that results in marked immune suppression (e.g., transplantation; malignancies, especially lymphomas and leukemia; therapies with high-dose antimetabolites, corticosteroids, alkylating agents, radiation). Treatment has been attempted with VIG and with N-methylisatin-β-thiosemicarbazone (Barbero et al., 1955). Cases have been too infrequent to evaluate therapy in an acceptable fashion.

Postvaccinal encephalitis. Postvaccinal encephalitis is a serious but fortunately rare complication. The incidence of encephalitis after the vaccination of 5 million people in New York City in 1947 was 0.9 per 100,000. Four of the reported patients died, and at necropsy there was no evidence of encephalitis; other causes of death were found. Consequently, the true incidence was less than 0.9 per 100,000. The incidence of postvaccinal encephalitis in Sweden from 1947 to 1954 was 1.9 per 100,000. Surveillance of complications of smallpox vaccination in the United States in 1968 revealed 2.9 cases of encephalitis per 1 million primary vaccinations; the highest incidence, 6.5 per 1 million, was observed in infants less than 12 months old.

The clinical picture is the same as that in other postinfectious encephalitides. The usual manifestations are fever, headache, vomiting,

meningeal signs, paralyses, drowsiness, coma, or convulsions. The spinal fluid contains an increased number of mononuclear cells and an increased amount of protein. Pathologically, the brain shows the same type of perivascular infiltration and demyelination as occurs in encephalitis complicating measles and chickenpox. The mortality may be as high 30% to 40%.

MYOCARDITIS, PERICARDITIS

With the primary vaccination in 2003 of 240,000 Department of Defense personnel (mainly healthy, young troops) and the revaccination of approximately 40,000 adult civilians (mainly healthcare workers and other possible first responders to a suspected case of smallpox) there have been a small number of cardiac events noted within 5 to 10 days of vaccination (CDC, 2003). These have been acute pericarditis, myocarditis, or both. Duration has been brief and patients have recovered fully. These complications had not been noted in the United States when vaccinia (prior to discontinuation in the 1970s) was routinely administered to infants and adult recipients received revaccination. However, cardiac complications had been reported in Europe (MacAdam, 1962).

These complications (Lane et al., 1969) are far more common following a primary vaccination rather than revaccination (Table 33-1).

TABLE 33-1 **Rates of Reported Complications Associated With Vaccinia Vaccination (Cases/Million Vaccinations)**[*]

Age (yr) and status	Autoinoculation or contact inoculation	Generalized vaccinia	Eczema vaccinatum	Progressive vaccinia	Postvaccinal encephalitis
Primary					
<1	507.0	394.4	14.1	–	42.3
1-4	577.3	233.4	44.2	3.2	9.5
5-19	371.2	139.7	34.9	–	8.7
≥20	606.1	212.1	30.3	–	–
Overall rates	529.2	241.5	38.5	1.5	12.3
Revaccination					
<1	–	–	–	–	–
1-4	109.1	–	–	–	–
5-19	47.7	9.9	2.0	–	–
≥20	25.0	9.1	4.5	6.8	4.5
Overall rates	42.1	9.0	3.0	3.0	2.0

[*]Modified from Lane JM, et al: N Engl J Med 1969;281:307.

TREATMENT

Primary vaccinia requires no treatment. Dressings are unnecessary but may be employed to reduce the likelihood of accidental contact. Fever and pain in the arm may be treated with appropriate doses of antipyretics. Superimposed pyogenic infections may require antimicrobial therapy. Patients with eczema vaccinatum or progressive vaccinia need intensive supportive therapy; patients should receive VIG, 0.6 ml per kilogram of body weight intramuscularly. In general, the treatment of encephalitis is the same as that of other encephalitides.

PREVENTIVE MEASURES

Most complications of vaccinia are preventable. Vaccination is contraindicated under the following circumstances: evidence of eczema or other chronic forms of exfoliative dermatitis in the vaccinated person or a close contact or altered immune states from disease or immunosuppressive therapy.

An experimental attenuated vaccinia virus vaccine was used by Kempe (Kempe, 1967) for the primary vaccination of more than 1,000 patients suffering from eczema. The vaccination was well tolerated; local and systemic reactions were not significant, and there was no evidence of virus dissemination. The success of the WHO smallpox eradication program obviated the need for this product, and no data could be obtained regarding its efficacy.

In 1971 the U.S. Public Health Service accepted the recommendation of its Advisory Committee on Immunization Practices that routine smallpox vaccination in the United States be discontinued. Since that time, smallpox vaccination has been limited to several selected groups. Until 1976, it was still recommended for health-care workers in case of an unexpected hospital exposure to an importation. Since 1980 it has been recommended for laboratory personnel working with nonvariola orthopoxviruses (Advisory Committee on Immunization Practices, 2001). Military personnel in some settings also were vaccinated (Haim et al., 2000). Wyeth Laboratories, the sole U.S. source of vaccinia, ceased production in 1981, and the remaining stockpile of vaccine (15.4 million doses) was transferred to the jurisdiction of CDC. On March 28, 2002, Aventis Pasteur, a French vaccine firm, announced that it had donated to the U.S. government an additional 85 million doses of vaccinia previously stored at its Connaught Laboratories subsidiary in Swiftwater, Pennsylvania (Connally, 2002). Current contracts for a new smallpox vaccine rely on a cell culture–grown virus, which may become available in 2003-2004 (Rosenthal et al., 2001). Rather than the previous calf-lymph preparation, these new vaccines will be propagated in MRC-5 or Vero cell cultures. Additional investigations are under way to apply modern serologic and genomic methods in smallpox diagnosis, to further investigate the pathogenesis of smallpox, and to develop new antiviral drugs (LeDuc and Jahrling, 2001).

BIBLIOGRAPHY

Advisory Committee on Immunization Practices (ACIP). Vaccinia (smallpox) vaccine. MMWR Recomm Rep 2001;50:1-25.

Alibek K. Biohazard. New York: Random House, 1999.

Barbero GJ, Gray A, Scott TF McN, Kempe CH. Vaccinia gangrenosa treated with hyperimmune vaccinal gamma-globulin. Pediatrics 1955;16:609.

Bartlett JG. Smallpox vaccination and patients with human immunodeficiency virus infection or acquired immunodeficiency syndrome. Clin Infect Dis 2003;36:468-471.

Bauer DJ, St. Vincent L, Kempe CH, Downie AW. Prophylactic treatment of smallpox contacts with N-methylisatin-β-thiosemicarbazone (compound33T57). Lancet 1963;2:494.

Bauer DJ, et al. Prophylaxis of smallpox with methisazone. Am J Epidemiol 1970; 90:130.

Baxby D. The origins of vaccinia virus. J Infect Dis 1977;136:453.

Bray M, Martinez M, Smee DF, et al. Cidofovir protects mice against lethal aerosol or intranasal cowpox virus challenge. J Infect Dis 2000;181:10-19.

Breman JG. Monkeypox: an emerging infection for humans? In Scheld WM, Craig WA, Hughes JM (eds). Emerging Infections. Washington, D.C.: ASM Press, 2000.

Breman JG, Henderson DA. Poxvirus dilemmas—monkeypox, smallpox, and biologic terrorism. N Engl J Med 1998;339:556-559.

Centers for Disease Control and Prevention. Adverse events following civilian smallpox vaccination—United States, 2003. MMWR 2003;52:278-284.

Centers for Disease Control and Prevention. Interim Smallpox Response Plan and Guidelines [on CD-ROM]. Atlanta, Georgia: Centers for Disease Control and Prevention, 2002.

Cohen J. Smallpox vaccinations: how much protection remains? Science 2001;294:985.

Coneybeare ET. Smallpox immunization. Practitioner 1951;167:215.

Connally C. Aventis to donate smallpox vaccine. Washington Post. March 30, 2002: AO2.

Downie AW, Dumbell KR. Survival of variola virus in dried exudate and crusts from smallpox patients. Lancet 1947;1:550.

Fenner F, Henderson DA, Arita I, et al. (eds). Smallpox and Its Eradication. Geneva, Switzerland: World Health Organization, 1988.

Frey SE, Couch RB, Tacket CO, et al. Clinical responses to undiluted and diluted smallpox vaccine in vaccinia naïve individuals. N Engl J Med 2002;346 (in press).

Haim M, Gdalevich M, Mimouni D, et al. Adverse reactions to smallpox vaccine: the Israeli defense force experience, 1991 to 1996. Mil Med 2000;165:287-289.

Henderson DA. Smallpox: clinical and epidemiologic features. Emerg Infect Dis 1999;5:537-539.

Henderson DA, Fenner F. Recent events and observations pertaining to smallpox virus destruction in 2002. Clin Infect Dis 2001;33:1057-1059.

Henderson DA, Inglesby TV, Bartlett JG, et al. Smallpox as a biological weapon. JAMA 1999;281:2127-2137.

Hostetler KY, Beadle J, Huggins J, Kern E. Presentation at 15th International Conference on Antiviral Research, Prague, March 2002.

Hutin YJF, Williams RJ, Malfait P, et al. Outbreak of human monkeypox, Democratic Republic of Congo, 1996-1997. Emerg Infect Dis 2001;7:434-438.

Ivker R. Human monkeypox hits beleaguered Zaire. Lancet 1997;349:709.

Jenner E. An inquiry into the causes and effects of the variolae vacciniae, a disease discovered in some of the western counties of England, particularly Gloucestershire, and known by the name of cowpox. Reprinted by Cassell and Co, Ltd, 1896. (Available in pamphlet vol 4232, Army Medical Library, Washington, D.C..)

Kempe CH. Studies on smallpox and complications of smallpox vaccination. Pediatrics 1960;26:176.

Kempe CH. Attenuated vaccinia in the elective primary vaccination of eczema patients (abstract). 77th Annual Meeting of the American Pediatric Society, Atlantic City, NJ, April 26-29, 1967.

Koplan JP, Foster SO. Smallpox: clinical types, causes of death, and treatment. J Infect Dis 1979;140:440

Lane JM, Ruben FL, Neff JM, Millar JD. Complications of smallpox vaccination, 1968. N Engl J Med 1969;281:1201.

Lane JM, Ruben FL, Neff JM, Millar JD. Complications of smallpox vaccination, 1968: results of ten statewide surveys. J Infect Dis 1970;122:303-309.

LeDuc JW, Jahrling PB. Strengthening national preparedness for smallpox: an update. Emerg Infect Dis 2001;7:155-157.

MacAdam DB, Whitaker W. Cardiac complications after vaccination for smallpox. Brit Med J 1962;1099-1100.

Mack TM. Smallpox in Europe, 1950-1971. J Infect Dis 1972;125:161-169.

Meltzer MI, Damon I, LeDuc JW, Millar JD. Modeling potential response to smallpox as a bioterrorism weapon. Emerging Infect Dis 2001;7:959-969.

Ropp SL, Jin Q, Knight JC, et al. PCR strategy for identification and differentiation of smallpox and other orthopoxvirus. J Clin Microbiol 1995;33:2069-2076.

Rosenthal SR, Merchlinsky, Kleppinger C, Goldenthal KL. Developing new smallpox vaccines. Emerg Infect Dis 2001;7:920-926.

Shchelkunov SN. Functional organization of variola major and vaccinia virus genomes. Virus Genes 1995;10:55-71.

Stone R. Smallpox. WHO puts off destruction of U.S., Russian Caches. Science 2002;295:598-599.

Wehrle PF, Posch J, Richter KH, et al. An airborne outbreak of smallpox in a German hospital and its significance with respect to other recent outbreaks in Europe. Bull World Health Org 1970;43:669-679.

Wolff HL, Croon JJAB. The survival of smallpox virus in natural circumstances. Bull World Health Org 1968;38:492-493.

World Health Organization. Declaration of global eradication of smallpox. Wkly Epidemiol Rev 1980;55:145-152.

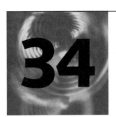

34
STAPHYLOCOCCAL INFECTIONS

ALICE S. PRINCE

*S*taphylococcus aureus is a major cause of infection in infants, children, and adults. It is particularly common in the pediatric population as a cause of skin and soft tissue infection, ranging from impetigo, furuncles, and wound infections to septic arthritis and osteomyelitis. Staphylococci are also frequently associated with major systemic infections such as septicemia, endocarditis, and toxic shock syndrome (TSS) and cause disease in both normal hosts and immunocompromised hosts. Coagulase-negative staphylococci are a common clinical problem and are currently the most frequent cause of bacteremia in hospitalized patients, particularly in the neonate or child with an indwelling intravascular device.

ETIOLOGY
Microbiology

Staphylococci are catalase-producing gram-positive organisms that often grow in clusters, as suggested by the term *staphylococci,* which is derived from the Greek, meaning "bunch of grapes." These are hardy organisms that can persist on surfaces for long periods of time and grow well on artificial media under both aerobic and anaerobic conditions. Colonies often produce a yellow pigment. *S. aureus* ferments a variety of sugars, including mannitol, under anaerobic conditions and tolerates high concentrations of NaCl. The ability to produce coagulase differentiates *S. aureus* from the less virulent coagulase-negative staphylococci such as *Staphylococcus saprophyticus, Staphylococcus haemolyticus,* and *Staphylococcus epidermidis.* The cell wall of *S. aureus* is composed primarily of peptidoglycan, repeating subunits of N-acetyl muramic acid and N-acetyl glucosamine, and teichoic acid, a polymer of repeating units of glycerol-phosphate and protein A.

The cell wall components of *S. aureus* are important in pathogenesis because they can elicit specific responses by the host immune system.

PATHOGENESIS

Staphylococci are ubiquitous organisms that may be considered as part of the commensal flora in some settings or may act as virulent pathogens. The expression of specific bacterial virulence factors and the nature of the host immune response contribute to the nature of the pathogen-host interaction. Many staphylococcal components interact directly with specific host targets. Peptidoglycan components bind to toll-like receptors, especially TLR2, on host cells and activate proinflammatory cytokine and chemokine responses through the stimulation of NF-κB dependent genes (Takeuchi et al., 2000; Yoshimura et al., 1999). This serves to recruit and activate neutrophils at the site of the infection. Upon exposure to *S. aureus,* endothelial cells and mononuclear leukocytes are stimulated to initiate a cascade of cytokine production in a manner analogous to that following lipopolysaccharide stimulation by gram-negative organisms, with the elaboration of interleukin (IL)-1β and IL-6 (Soell et al., 1995; Yao et al., 1995). Many strains also express a capsular polysaccharide that may contribute to virulence; organisms that express certain capsular polysaccharides (types 5 and 8) are more frequently associated with bacteremia and sepsis, and these capsular polysaccharides activate endothelial IL-8 expression, a major neutrophil chemokine.

Staphylococci express several classes of adhesins that mediate binding to host extracellular matrix materials, such as fibronectin, fibrinogen vitronectin, laminin, and collagen. The expression of such adhesins helps to explain the

627

association of *S. aureus* and soft-tissue infections. Specific staphylococcal surface proteins bind to the RGD (arginine-glycine-aspartate) sequence of fibronectin. Staphylococcal clumping factor mediates attachment of the organisms to platelets (Siboo et al., 2001). In response to the environmental milieu, the organisms coordinately express a number of specific virulence factors that enable them to establish a nidus of infection. Staphylococcal fibronectin binding proteins mediate invasion of host tissues, and *S. aureus* can persist and replicate within host cells, a privileged site which escapes many antibiotics and antibodies. These organisms can grow in biofilms, in which the expression of extracellular polysaccharides is upregulated in response to diffusible molecular signals (Arciola et al., 2001). Staphylococci in biofilms have a peculiar colonial morphology and slow growth and are therefore relatively resistant to antibiotics and phagocytosis. Alternatively, under different conditions, *S. aureus* can cause local tissue damage because of the expression of exoproducts and disseminate via the bloodstream once infection is established.

Staphylococci are capable of causing disease by three major mechanisms: direct destruction of tissue associated with the activity of numerous secreted exoenzymes, production of intoxication syndromes in which staphylococcal exotoxins enter the circulation and act at sites in the host distant from the source of the infection, and induction of multisystem disease by widespread T-cell activation and cytokine release resulting from the expression of staphylococcal superantigens (Lowy, 1998). Local staphylococcal infections are characterized by suppuration, eliciting a neutrophil response. These bacteria produce numerous factors that impede phagocytosis. Much of the local pathology associated with staphylococcal infection is due to expression of secreted exoproducts, including lipase; phospholipase; the hemolysins α, β, γ, and Δ; and hyaluronidase, enzymes that enable the organism to break down host tissues, including the extracellular matrix components. Coagulase, an enzyme that triggers the final steps in the coagulation cascade to produce fibrin, is produced by *S. aureus*, enabling the organism to wall itself off from the blood supply of the host. Protein A, a major component of staphylococcal cell walls, binds the Fc portion of immunoglobulin chains, thereby blocking the ligand for internalization of organisms by phagocytic cells and effectively thwarting efficient phagocytosis. Staphylococci also produce catalase, which converts H_2O_2 to water and oxygen, destroying one of the important antibacterial products generated by neutrophils. In patients with chronic granulomatous disease of childhood, who are unable to generate superoxide, catalase production allows *S. aureus* to persist in the absence of effective phagocytic killing. Other defects in phagocytic function—such as Job's syndrome, Chédiak-Higashi syndrome, and Wiskott-Aldrich syndrome—similarly predispose to staphylococcal infections.

Staphylococcal toxins that cause exfoliation have been well characterized (Ladhani et al., 1999). The exfoliatins (ETA and ETB) are responsible for dermatologic lesions characterized by erythema and desquamation caused by the splitting of the desmosomes that link epidermal cells. Exfoliatin (ETB) production is historically associated with organisms of phage group II and is plasmid encoded. ETB is associated with staphylococcal scalded skin syndrome, a disease of infants and young children. ETA is a chromosomal enzyme found in several different phage groups.

Staphylococci also produce several toxins that act as superantigens. These are antigens that bind to MHC class II molecules and interact with specific Vβ chains of the T-cell receptor causing excessive T-cell activation and multiorgan pathology (Davis et al., 1980). These antigens do not require processing and are able to interact superficially with components of the Vβ chain alone, not in the context of the usual antigen-binding groove of the T-cell receptor. Thus, these antigens can activate entire classes of T cells bearing specific Vβ domains. This T-cell activation results in the amplification of these clones; the activation of monocytes; and the release of numerous cytokines, including IL-2; IL-4; IL-6; interferon (IFN)-γ; tumor necrosis factor (TNF)-α; and IL-1β, with consequent effects on multiple organ systems. The staphylococcal toxins TSST-1 and TSST-2 associated with TSS (Kappler et al., 1989) (described later in this chapter) and the staphylococcal enterotoxin B, a cause of staphylococcal food poisoning, are superantigens. The expression of these toxins is highly regulated. TSST-1, for example, is expressed under conditions of low Mg^{++}; thus staphylococci in a milieu in which the divalent cations are depleted, as might occur in proximity to a hyperabsorbent synthetic tampon, upregulate the expression of these genes.

EPIDEMIOLOGY

The usual source of staphylococcal infection is colonization of the nares (Peacock et al., 2001). Persistent nasal carriage, strain-specific factors, and host susceptibility all contribute to the pathogenesis of infection. Clinical studies in surgical patients have demonstrated that preoperative nasal colonization with this organism is associated with a significantly higher rate of surgical wound infection (Kluytmans et al., 1995). The organisms can be aerosolized from the anterior nares or, more commonly, spread by interpersonal contact. Small breaks in the skin can become infected, or the organisms can disseminate via a nosocomial route from hospital personnel to patients. Careful hand washing is of utmost importance in preventing spread of infection.

Numerous molecular techniques have been developed to track the epidemiology of hospital outbreaks of staphylococcal infection. Comparison of restriction endonuclease fragment polymorphisms using pulsed field gel electrophoresis facilitates strain identification and has been extremely useful in identifying outbreaks of infection from a common source (Villari et al., 2000). Molecular typing has been of great importance in nursery epidemics of staphylococcal disease, such as scalded skin syndrome, pustulosis, and bullous impetigo. Historically, phage typing was used to trace the source of these organisms. However, because staphylococci often contain numerous transferable genetic elements, such as plasmids, transposons, and phages, molecular typing has become the standard for epidemiologic studies.

CLINICAL SYNDROMES CAUSED BY S. AUREUS

Skin and Soft Tissue Infections

One of the most common manifestations of *S. aureus* infection is localized infection of the skin, including small, localized infections such as impetigo, paronychia, and furuncles. Organisms gain access to the skin structures following nasal colonization or from small breaks in the skin. Local replication of organisms producing the exoproducts and toxins described earlier causes a localized infection of the contiguous connective tissue. The peptidoglycan of *S. aureus* heralds a brisk immunologic response with the local accumulation of macrophages and polymorphonuclear leukocytes. Thrombosis of the small surrounding blood vessels occurs with the deposition of fibrin, a consequence of staphylococcal coagulase. As this process continues, a central area of necrotic tissue with dead and dying phagocytes and bacteria is surrounded by a fibrinous capsule, that is, a small abscess. Thus a small, localized infection such as impetigo may progress to cellulitis and development of an abscess.

Impetigo. Impetigo, particularly bullous impetigo, is most often caused by *S. aureus*. The infection usually begins with a small area of erythema that progresses into bullae filled with cloudy fluid. These rupture and heal with crust formation. Impetigo is most common in the summer months in temperate climates and is a common complication of insect bites and varicella. Topical treatment with mupirocin is usually adequate; however, children with extensive impetiginized varicella are at significant risk for superinfection with *S. aureus* or group A streptococci, which requires systemic therapy.

Folliculitis. This is common superficial staphylococcal infection involving the hair follicle. Clinically, folliculitis presents as a tender pustule surrounding a hair follicle and can usually be managed with local treatment.

Staphylococcal furuncles and carbuncles. Staphylococcal furuncles and carbuncles represent more extensive local staphylococcal infections of the skin and traditionally involve areas of the skin with hair follicles, such as the neck, axillae, and buttocks. These localized infections extend into the subcutaneous tissues and are actually small abscesses containing abundant amounts of purulent material. They respond promptly to drainage.

Hydradenitis suppurativa. An infection of the sweat glands of the skin, hydradenitis suppurativa usually is caused by *S. aureus*. This is most often seen in moist areas such as the axillae or in the folds in the perineal and genital region. These lesions may spontaneously rupture and heal with scarring.

Mastitis. *S. aureus* is a well-recognized cause of mastitis, which occurs both in nursing mothers (animals and human) and newborn infants. The ability of most strains of *S. aureus* to produce lipase is thought to contribute to the pathogenesis of this infection. Patients present with erythema, swelling, and tender induration of the breast, and some may progress to have systemic symptoms of fever and malaise. These infections occasionally evolve to frank abscess formation and require prompt systemic antistaphylococcal therapy.

Staphylococcal lymphadenitis. A common infection in children, staphylococcal lymphadenitis presents as a tender, erythematous mass in the cervical chain of lymph nodes with accompanying fever. Cervical adenitis was traditionally considered a complication of streptococcal pharyngitis; however, staphylococci are often the cause of these infections, although the possibility of mycobacterial infection should also be considered. Surgical drainage of staphylococcal lymphadenitis is preferable if lesions are fluctuant. More often the involved area is indurated and not amenable to drainage. In these cases, treatment with antistaphylococcal antibiotics is usually successful, although complete resolution of all swelling may take weeks.

Skin Diseases Caused by Staphylococcal Toxins

Staphylococcal scalded skin syndrome was originally described as an exfoliative dermatitis of infants by Ritter von Rittershain. The disease is caused by staphylococci that produce an exfoliative toxin (Ladhani et al., 1999; Melish and Glasgow, 1970). In infants the disease causes generalized erythema, which progresses to bullae formation, followed by generalized desquamation (Gooch and Britt, 1978) (Figures 34-1 and 34-2). The skin becomes extremely friable, and even gentle stroking leads to desquamation (Nikolsky's sign). Histopathologically, the skin separates intradermally at the stratum granulosum layer. Clinically, staphylococcal scalded skin syndrome is similar to a disease in adults characterized by Lyell and termed *toxic epidermal necrolysis* (TEN), and analogous pathology can be seen in some drug hypersensitivity reactions as well. However, TEN can be differentiated from staphylococcal scalded skin syndrome by intraepithelial splitting at the dermoepidermal junction. In staphylococcal scalded skin disease, cultures of the skin are usually negative for staphylococci, although a distant site of infection, such as the umbilical stump or the nasopharynx, may yield the organism. The infants have systemic signs of infection with fever and irritability and

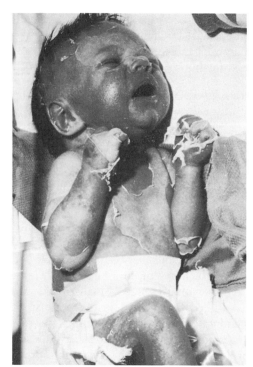

Fig. 34-1 Newborn infant with scalded skin syndrome in exfoliative stage. (From Melish ME, Glasgow LA: N Engl J Med 1970;282:1114. Reprinted by permission.)

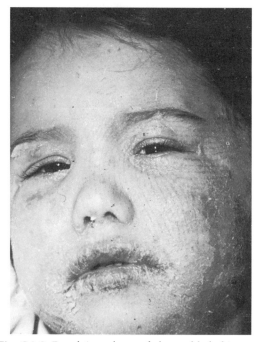

Fig. 34-2 Resolving phase of the scalded skin syndrome in a 2-year-old girl undergoing secondary desquamation. Large, thick flakes of dried skin are concentrated particularly about the mouth. (From Melish ME and Glasgow LA: N Engl J Med 1970; 282:1114. Reprinted by permission.)

occasionally may be septic. Treatment involves the administration of antistaphylococcal antibiotics and supportive care with attention to the fluid deficits caused by loss of the epidermal barrier.

Diseases Caused by Staphylococcal Superantigens

Staphylococcal TSS was first characterized by Todd, who observed seven children with a severe multisystem illness characterized by high fever, scarlatiniform rash, vomiting, diarrhea, renal and hepatic dysfunction, disseminated intravascular coagulation, and shock (Wiesenthal and Todd, 1984). This syndrome is similar to the previously described staphylococcal scarlet fever syndrome. A large increase in cases has been noted in young, previously healthy women who use hyperabsorbent tampons. During their menses while using tampons, these women develop fever, vomiting, diarrhea, myalgias, and a characteristic "sunburn" type of rash. This rash progresses to a generalized desquamation, usually involving the palms and soles (Davis et al., 1980). S. aureus is isolated from the tampon or vagina, or from another site in the cases of non–menstrual-associated TSS, as originally described by Todd. These staphylococci produce a toxin (Schlievert et al., 1981), TSST-1 or TSST-2, which acts as a superantigen, activating whole classes of T cells bearing specific Vβ chains, without specificity for the α chain or the antigen binding groove of the T-cell receptor. TSST-1 can also induce the expression of IL-1β and TNF-α by mononuclear cells. Thus the manifestations of the disease are those of excessive T-cell activation and cytokine release. The diagnosis can be made clinically in a patient with fever, rash, hypotension, and signs of multisystem involvement. Treatment of TSS should focus on reversing shock and hypotension, removing the focus of the staphylococcal infection, and treatment with antistaphylococcal antibiotics to prevent further expression of the toxin. Association with toxin-producing staphylococci should be made by screening for the TSST-1 gene. Most susceptible hosts lack antibody to TSST-1.

Staphylococcal Enterotoxins

Staphylococcal enterotoxin type B is another superantigen that is associated with outbreaks of gastrointestinal disease. This is typically associated with outbreaks in which a common food source is contaminated by an individual carrying the staphylococci. The toxin-producing organisms proliferate in food that is uncooked or only partially cooked (custards, potato salad) and not properly refrigerated. Patients experience an acute onset of vomiting and watery diarrhea 2 to 6 hours after ingestion. Symptoms are generally self-limited, and supportive therapy is usually sufficient. Antimicrobial agents are not necessary. The staphylococcal enterotoxins can also be associated with a TSS-like syndrome.

Illnesses Caused by S. aureus

Septicemia. Sepsis caused by S. aureus can occur in both normal (Hieber et al., 1977; Hill et al., 2001; Shulman and Ayoub, 1976) and immunocompromised hosts (Donowitz et al., 200; Ladisch and Pizzo, 1978). As ubiquitous organisms, staphylococci gain access to the blood after colonization of indwelling plastic catheters or other foreign bodies, through breaks in the skin, or from frank infection of wounds. Once the organisms reach the vascular endothelium, they are able to induce the expression of cytokines, including IL-6 and IL-1β (Yao et al., 1995). Thus, in a manner analogous to that of the gram-negative organisms, in which LPS or endotoxin triggers the expression of inflammatory mediators, staphylococcal cell wall components can similarly initiate an immune response by activating proinflammatory chemokine and cytokine expression by both endothelial cells as well as by professional immune cells. High-grade bacteremia follows, with the usual signs of fever and tachycardia in an acutely ill patient. Although uncomplicated staphylococcal bacteremia may occur in previously well patients, including adolescents (Shulman and Ayoub, 1976) the organisms can seed other sites, causing local complications.

Endocarditis. Endocarditis is a major complication of staphylococcal septicemia. In a review of endocarditis in the pediatric age group, S. aureus was the most common pathogen isolated, accounting for 39% of 62 cases, and was associated with central nervous system complications and the need for surgical intervention more often than other pathogens (Saiman et al., 1993). S. aureus endocarditis is a well-known complication of congenital heart disease. This entity can present in a previously well child with asymptomatic cardiac pathology such as mitral valve prolapse or with an asymptomatic ventricular septal defect. These lesions (1) produce turbulent blood flow that causes a reactive focus on the cardiac endothelium, providing a nidus for fibrin and platelet deposition; and (2) expose fibronectin receptors. During transient bacteremia, staphylococci can lodge in these fibrinous lesions, bind to fibronectin, and proliferate. Patients are acutely ill at presentation, often with septic shock and petechiae, and are found to have positive blood cultures for *S. aureus*. Embolic phenomena are common with this disease and may include pulmonary emboli; renal emboli; and central nervous system involvement with significant sequelae, including stroke (Figure 34-3). Treatment of these patients includes detailed hemodynamic assessment and two-dimensional echocardiography, which may help to document the nature and size of vegetations. Because *S. aureus* endocarditis can be a fulminant disease that results in destruction of the infected valve, valvular replacement can be an important therapeutic option. For hemodynamically stable patients not actively embolizing from their infection, treatment with antimicrobial agents can be curative.

Another group of patients at risk for staphylococcal endocarditis are those with indwelling vascular access devices. This is a common problem in oncology patients receiving chemotherapy, organ transplant patients (Patterson et al., 1998), and neonates who are dependent on such catheters for parenteral nutrition. Infections can occur at the skin site of the intravascular device and then seed the catheter, or they may occur on the catheter itself, because of the organisms' ability to grow in biofilms on foreign bodies (Vuong et al., 2000). Some of these infections, particularly those due to coagulase-negative staphylococci, can be managed without removal of the catheter. However, persistent *S. aureus* bacteremia is associated with significant sequelae (Benjamin et al., 2001). Patients who are acutely ill and at risk of embolizing from this source should be treated with prompt removal of the catheter and a course of antistaphylococcal drugs.

Pulmonary infections. Pulmonary infections caused by *S. aureus* can arise as complications of septicemia or may result from aspiration of these organisms, often in a nosocomial setting. Staphylococci activate both mucin secretion and the production of cytokines by airway epithelial cells (Heyer et al., 2002). In young infants, staphylococcal pneumonia usually pre-

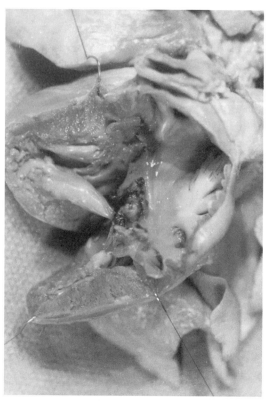

Fig. 34-3 Vegetation on the systemic (tricuspid) valve of a 15-month-old patient with hypoplastic left-heart syndrome. The cause of death was a cerebral vascular accident caused by septic emboli and a mycotic aneurysm.

sents with high fever, respiratory distress, and pulmonary infiltrates. The radiographic findings progress to dense consolidation, followed by pneumatocele formation, consisting of multiple thin-walled abscesses with air fluid levels (Chartrand and McCracken, 1982). Areas of consolidation may extend to the pleura, causing empyema (Figure 34-4). Several methods are available to evacuate purulent material from the pleural space, to reexpand the lung, and to control the infection. Percutaneous drainage, under ultrasound or computed tomographic guidance, is often effective if performed early in the course of the disease, before multiple loculated areas develop. The instillation of urokinase to act as a thrombolytic agent has been advocated. It is also possible to perform video-assisted thoracoscopy to lyse adhesions and facilitate drainage of purulent material (Bryant and Salmon, 1996). This is likely to be a safe and effective procedure preferable to a formal decortication, and there is increasing experience with children. Thoracoscopy may be performed early in the course of empyema, before extensive adhesions develop. These therapeutic alternatives provide much more flexibility in the management of empyema than the relatively rigid guidelines offered for decorti-

cation in traditional teachings. Resolution of fever and pleural reaction may take weeks. Open thoracotomy and decortication is still an alternative therapy that may be needed less often as physicians accrue experience in

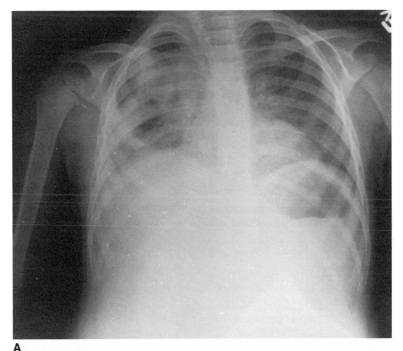

A

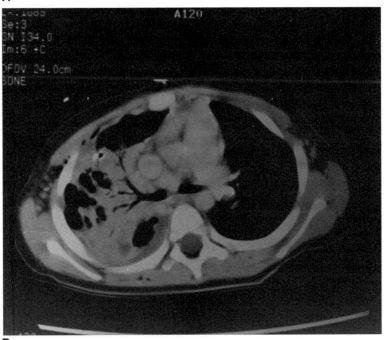

B

Fig. 34-4 A, Chest radiograph demonstrating staphylococcal empyema with areas of consolidation scattered throughout the right lung. **B,** Mediastinal window on an axial computed tomographic scan at the level of the take-off of the right middle lobe bronchus shows areas of consolidation and abscess (pneumatocele) formation. The top of the empyema can be seen adjacent to the spine.

treating children with alternative, less invasive techniques.

Bone and joint infections. A common complication of staphylococcal bacteremia in children, 90% of the cases of bone and joint infections occur in patients under 15 years of age (Faden and Grossi, 1991; Lew and Waldvogel, 1997). Staphylococcal osteomyelitis occurs most often in the metaphyseal portions of the long bones, particularly the tibia, femur, and humerus. It is proposed that organisms lodge in the long capillary loops that perfuse the metaphysis, where blood flow is relatively sluggish and there are few phagocytic cells. Organisms slowly replicate, and symptoms are often delayed until there is a significant degree of bone destruction. Presenting signs and symptoms in children include fever and bony tenderness; infants demonstrate irritability, limpness, or refusal to walk. Laboratory data are not usually diagnostic. The white blood cell count may not be elevated, although the erythrocyte sedimentation rate is usually high. The diagnosis of acute hematogenous osteomyelitis can be made by radionuclide scan using ^{99}Tc phosphonate, which demonstrates areas of bone turnover, or by magnetic resonance imaging MRI (Figure 34-5). Plain radiographs of the involved area do not show the classic changes of periosteal new bone formation until the infection has been present for 10 to 14 days. Rupture of a focus of osteomyelitis into a contiguous joint space can result in a septic arthritis, as in the hip or shoulder. Patients have local signs of soft tissue swelling and limited range of movement. Diagnosis is made by aspiration of the joint. Because of the virulence of *S. aureus*, septic arthritis of the hip usually requires open drainage to prevent destruction of the joint. Repeated needle aspirations of the knee may provide adequate drainage.

Septic arthritis. *S. aureus* infection may also cause an acutely swollen joint with signs of erythema, warmth, tenderness, and swelling without any bony involvement. The organisms seed the joint space through hematogenous dissemination. This diagnosis is confirmed by the aspiration of purulent joint fluid with polymorphonuclear leukocytes, high protein content, and the recovery of staphylococci. However, in cases of hematogenous septic arthritis, the plain radiographs and ^{99}Tc scans of the surrounding bones are negative. Treatment with prompt drainage and antibi-

otics usually results in excellent cure rates. Several studies have demonstrated excellent cure rates for staphylococcal bone and joint infections treated with oral antimicrobial agents if the organisms are susceptible to the usual antistaphylococcal agents and if patients are compliant with therapy.

Pyomyositis. Pyomyositis is another soft-tissue infection often caused by *S. aureus*. Although this entity is most often described in tropical regions, it is also seen in normal and immunocompromised patients in temperate climates (Christin and Sarosi, 1992). This is a primary infection of the skeletal muscle, most often involving the larger muscles of the extremities; it is thought to arise in areas of traumatized skeletal muscle. Presenting signs and symptoms include muscle tenderness, cramping, pain, and fever. The diagnosis can be suggested by ultrasonography, although computed tomography and especially magnetic resonance imaging will differentiate hematomas, tumors, and abscesses. Treatment consists of appropriate antibiotics and usually is expedited by drainage.

Methicillin-resistant S. aureus. Methicillin-resistant *S. aureus* (MRSA) has become an increasingly common cause of infection in the community as well as in hospitalized patients (Fergie and Pucell, 2001; Hussain et al., 2001). Although first recognized as a major cause of nosocomial infection associated with indwelling intravascular catheters, MRSA strains are associated with highly variable rates of infection in the community, ranging from 2.5% to 47% of *S. aureus* isolates. Patients with nasal carriage of MRSA are at increased risk of developing an infection caused by these organisms (Kluytmans et al., 1995). In addition, MRSA may be isolated from the sputum of cystic fibrosis patients who have been treated with multiple courses of antistaphylococcal antibiotics.

MRSA expresses *mecA*, a gene that encodes a mutant penicillin-binding protein, PBP2b, not found in methicillin-susceptible strains of staphylococci (Hartmann and Tomacz, 1984). Many clinical microbiology laboratories routinely screen for *mecA* using gene probes. This altered penicillin binding protein has diminished affinity for penicillin. Thus, the usual concentrations of the antistaphylococcal penicillins do not significantly impair the activity of PBP2b, and the organism is not killed. The gene *mecA* is part of a transposon and can be found

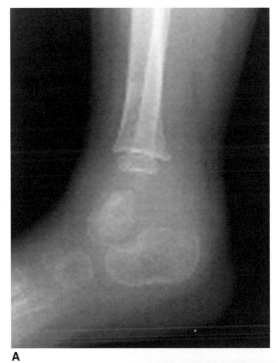

A

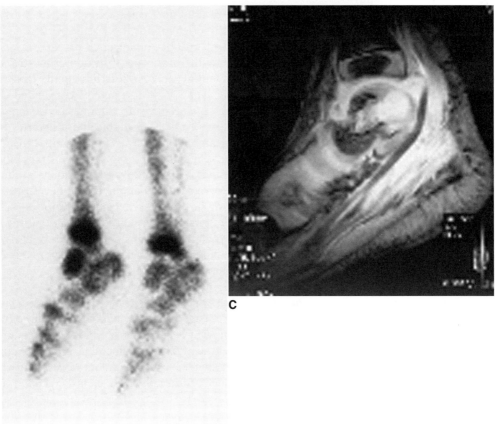

B

C

Fig. 34-5 Radiologic imaging of staphylococcal osteomyelitis of the right talus. **A,** A plain radiograph of the ankle demonstrates bony destruction and an irregular border of the talus. **B,** ^{99}Tc bone scan shows an area of increased uptake of the radionuclide in the right talus. **C,** The appearance of the bone on magnetic resonance imaging demonstrates bone destruction surrounded by a dense inflammatory response and fluid collection.

in methicillin-resistant coagulase-negative staphylococci as well (Spratt, 1994). As discussed in the following section, therapy of infections caused by MRSA requires administration of antibiotics that do not interact with these mutant target sites.

Vancomycin-resistant strains and isolates with "intermediate" susceptibility to vancomycin have also been described and associated with clinical infection (Smith et al., 1999). Although not as widespread as the vancomycin-resistant enterococci, these strains are a major concern.

THERAPY OF INFECTIONS CAUSED BY *S. AUREUS*

There are numerous antimicrobial agents with activity against the staphylococci. Because *Staphylococcus* is a major pathogen, there has been a long-standing interest in the development of effective antistaphylococcal agents. These agents include parenteral drugs, oral compounds, topical agents, fixed combinations, and antimicrobial glycopeptides with activity against MRSA and coagulase-negative staphylococci. Because virtually all strains of *S. aureus* produce β-lactamase with penicillinase activity, the antistaphylococcal agents must be stable to these enzymes. The antistaphylococcal penicillins for parenteral use (methicillin, oxacillin, and nafcillin) all contain bulky side groups to protect the integrity of the β-lactam ring. Each has slightly different pharmacologic properties and side effects, but they have comparable activity against most clinical isolates. The addition of a β-lactamase inhibitor such as clavulanate, sulbactam, or tazobactam to the penicillins amoxicillin, ticarcillin, ampicillin, or piperacillin, respectively, results in broad-spectrum penicillins that are also highly active against β-lactamase–producing staphylococci. Oral agents such as Augmentin (clavulanic acid + amoxicillin), cloxacillin, and dicloxacillin are available for therapy of infections that can be treated with oral drugs.

Most first-generation and some second-generation cephalosporins (including cephalothin, cefazolin, cefamandole, and cefuroxime) also have excellent antistaphylococcal activity by virtue of the poor activity of most staphylococcal β-lactamases against the cephalosporin nucleus. Any of these parenteral β-lactam agents should be effective against serious staphylococcal infections caused by susceptible organisms. Imipenem, a carbapenem, is also highly active against most strains of *S. aureus*. There are numerous oral cephalosporin derivatives that have excellent antistaphylococcal activity (Rodriguez and Weidermann, 1994). These include cephalexin, cefaclor, and cefuroxime. The second- and third-generation oral cephalosporins, in general, have less antistaphylococcal activity than the older drugs. Cefuroxime axetil does have good antistaphylococcal activity and is available in a liquid form.

Other classes of antimicrobial agents also possess excellent antistaphylococcal activity. The macrolides (including erythromycin, clarithromycin, azithromycin, and clindamycin) all can be used for the oral therapy of staphylococcal infection, and some MRSA strains are susceptible to macrolides. Similarly, the fluoroquinolones, particularly ciprofloxacin, have excellent antistaphylococcal activity and have been used in selected settings where a β-lactam antibiotic cannot be used. Several of these agents can be administered parenterally, as well as by the oral route. The addition of rifampin, an antibiotic that interferes with RNA polymerase activity, also may be considered for the therapy of difficult staphylococcal infections, because it is lipid soluble and penetrates widely throughout the intracellular compartments and the central nervous system (Brackbill and Brophy, 2001). However, resistance to rifampin develops rapidly and it should never be used as a single agent. The aminoglycosides, such as gentamicin, also have excellent antistaphylococcal activity but in general are only used for an additive or synergistic effect in infections that are difficult to treat, or they are occasionally used topically.

For severe life-threatening infections, particularly in areas in which MRSA is found, vancomycin is the drug of choice for presumptive treatment of staphylococcal infection until an organism is isolated and its susceptibility established. Although the β-lactam agents are considered to be the drugs of choice for serious staphylococcal infection, the increased numbers of strains with altered penicillin-binding proteins and the hyperexpression of penicillinases have resulted in the widespread use of vancomycin for staphylococcal infections. Newer glycopeptide antibiotics such as linezolid have excellent activity against MRSA and can be used instead of vancomycin (Stevens et al.,

2000). For the treatment of endocarditis or other infections with persistent bacteremia, combination therapy—such as the addition of rifampin (which can accumulate within phagocytic cells) to vancomycin or a β-lactam agent—may be useful. Aminoglycosides can be used similarly, although this class of drugs is associated with nephrotoxicity.

INFECTIONS CAUSED BY COAGULASE-NEGATIVE STAPHYLOCOCCI
Microbiology

Coagulase-negative staphylococci such as those belonging to the *S. epidermidis* group are ubiquitous bacteria, part of the commensal flora of both normal and immunocompromised hosts. They are common nosocomial pathogens causing infection in patients with indwelling intravascular devices, especially oncology and transplant patients, and in multiply instrumented patients in an intensive care setting and are a major cause of infection in neonates (Benjamin et al., 2001; Gray, 1995; Huebner and Goldmann, 1999). Although these staphylococci lack the virulence factors that enable *S. aureus* to be such an effective pathogen, they express extracellular polysaccharides, form biofilms, and efficiently colonize foreign bodies. The coagulase-negative staphylococci are differentiated from *S. aureus* on the basis of their lack of coagulase, lack of β-hemolysis of blood agar plates, and inability to ferment mannitol. They often contain extrachromosomal DNA and can exchange plasmids and transposons with *S. aureus*; the *mecA* gene, which confers methicillin resistance in *S. aureus*, is also found at a high frequency in coagulase-negative staphylococci. Because these staphylococci are isolated from normally sterile sites with increasing frequency, clinical laboratories can identify many of the strains previously grouped only as "coagulase-negative staphylococci." *S. epidermidis*, *S. saprophyticus*, and *S. haemolyticus* have been recognized as causes of human disease, along with other members of this group.

Nosocomial Infections

These ubiquitous organisms are the most frequent cause of nosocomial infection and are responsible for significant morbidity and increased cost of hospitalization (Gray, 1995; Hueber and Goldmann, 1999; Rupp and Archer, 1994). The vast majority of these infections are attributed to infections related to intravascular devices, most commonly intravenous catheters in neonates. Because of the indolence of these infections, they can go undetected for relatively long periods of time. The coagulase negative staphylococci form biofilms that are relatively resistant to eradication (Gotz et al., 2000). Organisms in biofilms grow very slowly and therefore are relatively resistant in vivo to antimicrobial agents that act only on dividing organisms (such as the β-lactams). Polymorphonuclear leukocytes are relatively ineffective in ingesting bacteria that are part of a biofilm. Virtually all indwelling catheters become colonized by these organisms, but symptomatic infections are infrequent. It is postulated that bacteremia occurs when large numbers of organisms are present and are intermittently shed into the bloodstream. This bacteremia may be accompanied by clinical signs of fever or hypothermia, cardiovascular instability, or glucose intolerance. These findings are particularly common in premature neonates, with bacteremia and sepsis caused by coagulase-negative staphylococci necessitating line removal (Benjamin, 2001). Older patients with bacteremia caused by these organisms may have transient fever but generally have few clinical signs indicative of a systemic infection. Treatment of these infections without removal of the indwelling catheter is often successful using vancomycin because these organisms invariably have altered penicillin binding proteins with low affinity for the β-lactam antibiotics.

The coagulase-negative staphylococci are a common source of bacteremia in neonates—particularly low–birth-weight, premature infants (Gray, 1995). Epidemiologic studies suggest that, like *S. aureus*, specific endemic strains of coagulase-negative staphylococci can cause clusters of nosocomial infections in neonatal intensive care units (Hueber and Goldman, 1999; Lyytikainen et al., 1995). In addition to the clinical symptoms caused by bacteremia, infections caused by the coagulase-negative staphylococci are a significant cause of neonatal morbidity, prolonging the length and cost of hospitalization of the small infants.

Endocarditis

Although increasing numbers of pediatric patients with congenital heart disease undergo operative repair, there has been a corresponding increase in the prevalence of endocarditis caused by coagulase-negative staphylococci

(Saiman et al., 1993). These organisms do not generally infect native valves but cause an indolent, subacute picture in patients with prosthetic valves and conduits. Unlike the fulminant infections associated with *S. aureus*, these bacteremias may be difficult to document because of the intermittent administration of antibiotics in these high-risk patients. In addition, single positive blood cultures for coagulase-negative staphylococci are often considered contaminants if endocarditis is not considered to be part of the differential diagnosis. Thus, if this diagnosis is to be entertained, it is important to draw several blood cultures and use echocardiography (including two-dimensional techniques) and esophageal leads to try to make a diagnosis. These patients can also present with worsening congestive heart failure and embolic phenomena, although this is less common than in the adult population. Children with central venous catheters, particularly neonates, can also develop cardiovascular infections caused by coagulase-negative staphylococci in the presence of native valves. This can be a complication of a patent ductus arteriosus, or it can be secondary to jet flow lesions and endothelial damage accompanying unrepaired ventricular septal defects.

Central Nervous System Infections

Coagulase-negative staphylococci are the most common cause of cerebrospinal fluid (CSF) shunt infection, accounting for more than 50% of incidences. It is likely that most of these infections are caused by organisms that colonize the shunt at the time of surgery, although infection tracking up from the sutures at an infected wound site can also occur. CSF shunts in young infants are most commonly infected, and most infections occur within the first few months following placement (Jordan et al., 1980). Nosocomial strains of *S. epidermidis* are most commonly isolated from the CSF and can cause a relatively indolent infection characterized by fever and shunt malfunction but only rarely with signs of meningismus or peritonitis. Examination of the CSF usually reveals pleocytosis, and cultures are positive for the staphylococci. Particularly in infants, increased protein and low glucose levels may be present but are milder than expected in infection caused by other bacterial species. Treatment invariably requires removal of the infected hardware and high doses (vancomycin at 60 to 70 mg/kg of

body weight) to achieve levels in the CSF in the absence of a brisk inflammatory response. Some clinicians advocate the use of rifampin plus vancomycin, since rifampin penetrates into the CSF.

Urinary Tract Infection

S. saprophyticus has been recognized to be a cause of urinary tract infection (UTI) in adolescent girls (Jordan et al., 1980), although its prevalence and significance have been debated. *S. saprophyticus* UTIs lead to the same signs and symptoms as the more widely recognized infections caused by *Escherichia coli*. Patients present with dysuria and are found to have pyuria and hematuria. *S. saprophyticus* can be differentiated from other staphylococcal species by resistance to novobiocin, production of urease, and specific pattern of carbohydrate utilization. Screening tests for UTI would be positive for leukocyte esterase activity but negative for nitrites. *S. saprophyticus* is rarely a cause of UTI outside of this group of young, healthy, sexually active women. However, when *S. saprophyticus* is recovered from the urine in this setting it should not be considered commensal flora, but instead treated as a pathogen. These organisms are usually susceptible to several antimicrobial agents, including trimethoprim-sulfamethoxazole.

PREVENTIVE MEASURES

Because staphylococci are ubiquitous organisms, it is difficult to prevent the infections associated with them. The use of topical antimicrobial agents such as mupirocin to eradicate nasal carriage in high-risk patients has been advocated (Lowy, 1998). Specific recommendations have been provided by the American Heart Association for the use of prophylactic antibiotics to prevent endocarditis in specific clinical settings (Dajani et al., 1997). Careful hand washing is of paramount importance in preventing person-to-person spread of the organism from contaminated secretions. It is important to consider the susceptibility of different hosts to these bacteria. The risk of nosocomial staphylococcal infection is much greater and is of greater consequence in a neonatal nursery than among older children. Patients in intensive care units with multiple venous access devices or large surgical incisions are also at greater risk for hospital-acquired staphylococcal infection. Control of nosocomial outbreaks of staphylococcal disease requires the coordinated efforts of all medical personnel involved and the input of the hospital epidemiologist.

BIBLIOGRAPHY

Arciola CF, Baldassarri L, Montanaro G. Presence of *icaA* and *icaD* genes and slime production in a collection of staphylococcal strains from catheter-associated infections. J Clin Microbiol 2001;39:2151-2156.

Benjamin DK, Miller W, Garges H, et al. Bacteremia, central catheters and neonates, when to pull the line. Pediatrics 2001;107:1272-1276.

Brackbill M, Brophy G. Adjunctive rifampin therapy for central nervous system staphylococcal infections. Ann Pharmacother 2001;35:765-769.

Bryant RE, Salmon CJ. Pleural empyema. Clin Infect Dis 1996;22:747-764.

Chartrand SA, McCracken GH. Staphylococcal pneumonia in infants and children. Pediatr Infect Dis 1982; 1:19-23.

Christin L, Sarosi GA. Pyomyositis in North America: case reports and review. Clin Infect Dis 1992;15:668-677.

Dajani AS, Taubert KA, Wilson W, et al. Prevention of bacterial endocarditis: recommendations by the American Heart Association. Clin Infect Dis 1997;25:1448-1458.

Davis JP, Chesney PJ, LaVenture M. Toxic-shock syndrome: epidemiologic features, recurrence, risk factors, and prevention. N Engl J Med 1980;303:1429-1435.

Donowitz GR, Maki DG, Crnich CJ, et al. Infections in the neutropenic patient—new views of an old problem. Hematology 2001:113-139.

Faden H, Grossi M. Acute osteomyelitis in children: reassessment of etiologic agents and their clinical characteristics. Am J Dis Child 1991;145:65-69.

Fergie JE, Purcell K. Community-acquired methicillin-resistant *Staphylococcus aureus* infections in South Texas children. Pediatr Infect Dis J 2001;20:860-863.

Gooch JJ, Britt EM. *Staphylococcus aureus* colonization and infection in newborn nursery patients. Am J Dis Child 1978;132:893-896.

Gotz F, Heilman C, Cramton SE. Molecular basis of catheter associated infections by staphylococci. Adv Exp Med Biol 2000;485:103-111.

Gray JE. Coagulase-negative staphylococci bacteremia among very low birth weight infants: relation to admission illness severity, resource use, and outcome. Pediatrics 1995;95:225-230.

Hartmann BM, Tomacz A. Low-affinity penicillin binding protein associated with β-lactam resistance in *Staphylococcus aureus*. J Bacteriol 1984;158:513-518.

Heyer G, Saba S, Adamo R, et al. *Staphylococcus aureus agr* and *sarA* functions are required for invasive infection but not inflammatory responses in the lung. Infect Immun 2002;70:127-133.

Hieber JP, Nelson JA, McCracken GH. Acute disseminated staphylococcal disease in childhood. Am J Dis Child 1977;131:181-185.

Hill PC, Wong CG, Voss LM, et al. Prospective study of 125 cases of *S. aureus* bacteremia in children in New Zealand. Pediatr Infect Dis J 2001;20:868-874.

Hueber J, Goldmann DA. Coagulase-negative staphylococci: role as pathogens. Ann Rev Med 1999;50:223-236.

Hussain FM, Boyle-Vavra S, Daum RS. Community-acquired methicillin-resistant *Staphylococcus aureus* colonization in healthy children attending an outpatient pediatric clinic. Pediatr Infect Dis J 2001;20:763-767.

Jain A, Daum RS. Staphylococcal infections in children: part 1. Pediatr Rev 1999;20:183-191.

Jordan PA, Irvani A, Richard GA, et al. Urinary tract infection caused by *Staphylococcus saprophyticus*. J Infect Dis 1980;142:510-515.

Kappler J, Kotzin B, Herron J, et al. V beta-specific stimulation of human T cells by staphylococcal toxins. Science 1989;244:811-813.

Kluytmans JA, Mouton JW, Ijzerman EP, et al. Nasal carriage of *Staphylococcus aureus* as a major risk factor for wound infections after cardiac surgery. J Infect Dis 1995;171:216-219.

Ladhani S, Joannou CL, Lochrie DP, et al. Clinical, microbial, and biochemical aspects of the exfoliative toxins causing staphylococcal scalded-skin syndrome. Clin Microbiol Rev, 1999;12:224-242.

Ladisch S, Pizzo PA. *S. aureus* sepsis in children with cancer. Pediatrics 1978;61:231-234.

Lew DP, Waldvogel FA. Osteomyelitis. N Engl J Med 1997;336:999-1007.

Lowy FD. *Staphylococcus aureus* infections. N Engl J Med 1998;339:520-523.

Lyytikainen O, Saxen H, Ryhanen R, et al. Persistence of a multiresistant clone of *Staphylococcus epidermidis* in a neonatal intensive care unit for a four-year period. Clin Infect Dis 1995;20:24-29.

Melish ME, Glasgow LA. The staphylococcal scalded skin syndrome: development of an experimental model. N Engl J Med 1970;282:1114.

Patterson DL, Dominguez EA, Chang FY, et al. Infective endocarditis in solid organ transplant recipients. Clin Infect Dis 1998;26:689-694.

Peacock SJ, de Silva I, Lowy FD. What determines nasal carriage of *S. aureus* ? Trends Microbiol 2001;9:605-610.

Pople IK, Bayston R, Haywood R. Infection of cerebrospinal fluid shunts in infants: a study of etiological factors. J Neurosurg 1992;77:29-36.

Rodriguez WJ, Wiedermann BL. The role of newer oral cephalosporins, fluoroquinolones, and macrolides in the treatment of pediatric infections. Adv Pediatr Infect Dis 1994;9:125-140.

Rupp ME, Archer GL. Coagulase-negative staphylococci: pathogens associated with medical progress. Clin Infect Dis 1994;19:231-245.

Saiman L, Prince A, Gersony W. Pediatric infective endocarditis in the modern era. J Pediatr 1993;122:847-853.

Schlievert PM, Shands KN, Dan BB, et al. Identification and characterization of an exotoxin from *S. aureus* associated with toxic-shock syndrome. J Infect Dis 1981;143:509.

Shulman ST, Ayoub EM. Severe staphylococcal sepsis in adolescents. Pediatrics 1976;58:59-66.

Siboo IR, Cheung AL, Bayer AS, Sullam PM. Clumping factor A mediates binding of *Staphylococcus aureus* to human platelets. Infect Immun 2001;69:3120-3127.

Smith TL, Pearson ML, Wilcox KR, et al. Emergence of vancomycin resistance in *Staphylococcus aureus,* The Glycopeptide-Intermediate *Staphylococcus aureus* Working Group. N Engl J Med 1999;340:493-501.

Soell M, Diab M, Haan-Archipoff G, et al. Capsular polysaccharide types 5 and 8 of *Staphylococcus aureus* bind specifically to human epithelial (KB) cells, endothelial cells, and monocytes and induce release of cytokines. Infect Immun 1995;63:1380-1386.

Spratt B. Resistance to antibiotics mediated by target alterations. Science 1994;264:388-393.

Stevens DL, Smith LG, Bruss JB, et al. Randomized comparison of linezolid (PNU-100766) versus oxacillin-dicloxacillin for treatment of complicated and soft tissue infections. Antimicrob Agents Chemother 2000;44:3408-3413.

Takeuchi O, Hoshino K, Akira S. TLR2-deficient and MyD88-deficient mice are highly susceptible to *Staphylococcus aureus* infection. J Immunol 2000;165:5392-5396.

Villari P, Sarnataro C, Iacuzio L. Molecular epidemiology of *Staphylococcus epidermidis* in a neonatal intensive care unit over a three-year period. J Clin Microbiol 2000;38:1740-1746.

Vuong C, Saenz HL, Gotz F, Otto M. Impact of the *agr* quorum-sensing system on adherence to polystyrene in *Staphylococcus aureus*. J Infect Dis 2000;182:1688-1693.

Wiesenthal AM, Todd JK. Toxic shock syndrome in children aged 10 years or less. Pediatrics 1984;74:112-117.

Yao L, Bengualid V, Lowy FD, et al. Internalization of *Staphylococcus aureus* by endothelial cells induces cytokine gene expression. Infect Immun 1995;63:1835-1839.

Yoshimura A, Lien E, Ingalls RR, et al. Recognition of gram-positive bacterial cell wall components by the innate immune system occurs via Toll-Like Receptor 2. J Immunol 1999;163:1-5.

35

STREPTOCOCCAL INFECTIONS

JAMES K. TODD

Streptococci are common causes of bacterial infection in infancy and childhood. *Streptococcus pyogenes* (group A *Streptococcus*) is the most common bacterial cause of acute pharyngitis and severe skin infection and also causes a wide variety of other suppurative infections as well as nonsuppurative sequelae such as rheumatic fever and glomerulonephritis.

MICROBIOLOGY AND PATHOGENESIS

Streptococci are aerobic gram-positive cocci that divide in pairs, forming chains of variable lengths. They are initially classified on the basis of their ability to hemolyze red blood cells: those with hemolysins producing complete hemolysis (β-hemolytic), those producing partial (green) hemolysis (α-hemolytic), and those producing no hemolysis (γ-hemolytic). Group A streptococci grow readily on sheep blood agar and, with rare exception, are β-hemolytic because of their production of two soluble hemolysins: streptolysins S and O. Group A streptococci often grow well anaerobically or in the presence of increased CO_2, and such conditions may enhance hemolysin production. Because other aerobic gram-positive organisms—notably *Staphylococcus aureus*—also are β-hemolytic, the colonies can be further characterized by a negative catalase reaction, that is, the absence of response in the presence of H_2O_2. Staphylococci are catalase positive and produce vigorous bubbling in the presence of H_2O_2 (Todd, 1982).

Hemolysis alone does not define pathogenicity among the various species of streptococci; there are many β-hemolytic streptococci found in the mouth and intestinal tract that are not common causes of human disease. Lancefield developed immunologic methods to distinguish between β-hemolytic streptococci on the basis of differences in carbohydrate components within the cell wall, identifying streptococcal groups A through H and K through V (Lancefield, 1933). Group A *Streptococcus* (*S. pyogenes*) appears to be the most virulent of these groups, although group B *Streptococcus* (*Streptococcus agalactiae*) is well known as a cause of newborn bacteremia and meningitis. Although streptococci can be readily classified in the laboratory by rapid tests (e.g., latex agglutination) that detect these group-specific immunologic differences, group A *Streptococcus* can also be presumptively identified by inhibition of its growth on primary plates by a 0.04-unit bacitracin disk and by a simple chemical reaction (PYR test) that results in the hydrolysis and color reaction of L-pyrrolidonyl arylamidase (Oberhofer, 1986; Roe et al., 1984). Other streptococci are usually bacitracin resistant, and most, except for enterococci, are PYR negative.

The group A streptococci have many associated virulence factors that play roles in causing disease (Table 35-1) (Cunningham, 2000). In addition to the group-specific carbohydrate, the group A streptococcal cell wall also contains several antigenic proteins labeled M, T, and R. Group A β-hemolytic streptococci can be categorized into more than 80 immunologically distinct types that are based on differences in the M protein. These proteins appear to be a major virulence factor, playing a role in attachment to epithelial cells and resistance to phagocytosis (Ashbaugh et al., 2000). M-typing is still the method of choice for identifying strains commonly associated with the propensity to cause certain group A streptococcal diseases (e.g., rheumatogenic strains—types 1, 3, 5, 16, 18; nephritogenic strains—types 2, 49, 55, 57, 59, 60, 61; severe invasive streptococcal syndrome strains—types 1, 3). M protein—specific (emm) gene sequences show the same strain specificity as the immunologically

TABLE 35-1	Virulence Factors Associated With Group A Streptococcal Infections		
Factor	*Location*	*Action*	*Pathophysiology*
Hyaluronic acid	Capsule	Mucoid strains	Resists phagocytosis
M-protein	Cell wall	Attachment	Colonization, resists phagocytosis
Lipoteichoic acids/proteins	Cell wall	Attachment	Colonization
DNase B	Soluble	DNA lysis	Spreading factor
Streptokinase	Soluble	Fibrinolysin	Spreading factor
Hyaluronidase	Soluble	Cleaves ground substance	Spreading factor
Proteinase	Soluble	Protein cleavage	Necrotizing factor
Pyrogenic exotoxin A-C	Soluble	TNF, IL-1 stimulator	Scarlet fever toxin
			Toxic shock syndrome

TNF, Tumor necrosis factor; *IL,* interleukin.

detected proteins and may provide a faster and more complete method for identifying strains (Facklam et al., 1999). Lipoteichoic acid, another cell wall constituent, promotes colonization by binding to fibronectin on the surface of epithelial cells. The hyaluronic acid capsule resists phagocytosis and has been associated with invasive infection.

In addition to the cell wall components that play a major role in cell attachment and resistance to host defenses, group A streptococci excrete a number of exoproteins that act as either systemic toxins or locally invasive enzymes. The extracellular products of greatest clinical significance are pyrogenic (formerly erythrogenic) exotoxins (A, B, and C), streptokinase, DNase, hyaluronidase, and proteinase. Pyrogenic exotoxins are associated with the rash of scarlet fever—the rash being enhanced by host cellular response to the toxin and mitigated by host antibody (Schlievert et al., 1979). Immunity to one pyrogenic toxin does not prevent disease resulting from another. The pyrogenic exotoxins also act as superantigens by stimulating clonal expansion of lymphocytes (McCormick et al., 2001). The resultant release of interleukin (IL)-1 and tumor necrosis factor (TNF) is thought to mediate the hypotension of streptococcal toxic shock illness. Streptococcal pyrogenic exotoxin A has partial amino acid homology with staphylococcal enterotoxin B, which is associated with staphylococcal toxic shock syndrome (TSS). Several of these streptococcal enzymes act as "spreading factors," facilitating the rapid spread of group A streptococci through tissue planes: streptokinase lyses fibrin, DNase B helps liquefy pus, and hyaluronidase breaks down ground substance. Proteinase, in

particular, is associated with tissue destruction of the necrotizing cellulitis and fasciitis of severe invasive streptococcal syndrome (Talkington et al., 1993).

Antimicrobial resistance to the β-lactam antibiotics has not been reported in group A streptococci, whereas increasing resistance to the macrolides (erythromycins) seems to be directly related to the amount of specific agent use in the community (Macris et al., 1998; Martin et al., 2002; Seppala et al., 1997). Clindamycin resistance is uncommon but does occur. The tetracyclines and sulfonamides are not useful in treatment; trimethoprim-sulfamethoxazole is actually used in blood agar plates to selectively encourage growth of group A streptococci, so it also should not be used in the treatment of clinical infections.

In a mouse model, Eagle reported the failure of penicillin to cure animals with deep tissue infection. This so-called Eagle effect was confirmed by Stevens, who also demonstrated an improved cure rate in infected mice with erythromycin and especially clindamycin (Stevens et al., 1988). Susceptibility testing is not ordinarily necessary for group A streptococcal strains isolated from noninvasive infections but should be considered for strains isolated from patients with severe invasive streptococcal syndrome, especially if non-β-lactam antibiotics (e.g., clindamycin) are used for first-line treatment (Zimbelman et al., 1999).

IMMUNITY

The immune response to group A streptococci can be both protective against invasive disease and potentiating for its nonsuppurative complications (e.g., rheumatic fever, glomerulonephritis) (Stollerman, 2001). Acquired humoral immunity to symptomatic pharyngeal infection is directed at the M protein, although patients may remain colonized in spite of otherwise protective antibody levels (Ashbaugh et al., 2000). Immunity, which is type specific, may be induced either by carriage of the organism or by overt infection. The risk of streptococcal disease appears to decrease during adult life in part as immunity develops to the more prevalent serotypes. Early antimicrobial treatment of group A streptococcal pharyngitis with the penicillins may decrease this antibody response, resulting in an increased recurrence rate with the homologous strain, which may persist despite treatment in 20% to 40% of treated patients (Pichichero et al, 1987).

Antibody to the pyrogenic exotoxins is protective against scarlet fever and TSS caused by organisms producing the homologous toxin (McCormick et al., 2000). Passive administration of IVIG has been reported to mitigate some clinical manifestations of severe invasive streptococcal syndrome (Kaul et al., 1999). Antibodies develop 4 to 8 weeks after streptococcal infection to streptolysin O (ASO), DNase B (AOB), hyaluronidase, or streptokinase and may be useful in the diagnosis of recent group A streptococcal disease, usually only necessary when rheumatic fever or poststreptococcal glomerulonephritis is considered. Low titer antibody levels may also be found in 30% of colonized children. Multiple antibody tests may be required, because the ASO titer is more often elevated in rheumatic fever and the ADB titer is more often elevated in glomerulonephritis associated with skin infection.

Rheumatic fever appears to be the result of an infection caused by certain "rheumatogenic" streptococcal strains in genetically predisposed hosts who respond with an atypical immune response (Gibofsky et al., 1998). There is an increased incidence of rheumatic fever and rheumatic heart disease among members of certain family groups (Visentainer et al., 2000). The immune response cross-reacts with some human tissues (e.g., heart, synovium, skin, central nervous system) resulting in immunologic damage that leads to clinical manifestations. The latent period, usually 1 to 3 weeks between the onset of the actual group A streptococcal infection and the onset of symptoms of acute rheumatic fever, lends support to an immunologic mechanism of tissue damage.

EPIDEMIOLOGY

Group A streptococcal disease is common world wide. The organism is often found as part of the normal flora (10% to 20%) in the mouths of asymptomatic school-age children and less frequently in the anus or vagina. Because there are many different streptococcal strains, local disease incidence and manifestations reflect the virulence factors of the strains that are present in the community (Kaplan et al., 2001). Cycles of group A streptococcal strains and consequently the diseases they cause are well known to occur both locally and globally (Denny, 1994). After a sustained global outbreak of severe invasive streptococcal syndrome in the nineteenth century there was a gradual decrease in incidence in the twentieth century, until the incidence of severe disease from group A streptococci increased again in the late 1980s and 1990s associated with M-types 1 and 3—strains not commonly isolated in prior decades (Wheeler et al., 1991). Likewise a prolonged decrease in the incidence of rheumatic fever was noted in the United States until outbreaks associated with particular rheumatogenic strains (M18) were reported beginning in the middle 1980s (Veasy et al., 1994).

In addition to strain variation, other influences on streptococcal disease include the patient's age, season of the year, and contact history. Infants have a low incidence, perhaps because of transplacental acquisition of type-specific antibodies and a low density of pharyngeal receptors for streptococcal binding. Superficial streptococcal infection of the skin is most common in children younger than 6 years, whereas streptococcal pharyngitis is most common in school-age children. The incidence of streptococcal pharyngitis is higher in temperate climates and appears to increase in cold weather—typically during the school year, when interaction with carriers is promoted by close, intense contact. Impetigo is more prevalent in tropical climates.

Group A streptococci are generally spread from person to person. Transmission of streptococci is generally enhanced by close contact in the home, school, military installation, or other institution. Acquisition from an infected individual is most common during the acute illness and decreases during the colonization stage, which may last weeks to months. Pharyngeal infection may be spread by droplets, whereas skin infection may be spread by direct contact with skin lesions or oral secretions.

CLINICAL MANIFESTATIONS

Like many organisms, group A streptococci seem to have an affinity (trophism) for certain cells and anatomic sites; in this case those include the posterior oropharynx, anal mucosa, and vaginal mucosa (Lilja et al., 1999). These are common sites where the carrier state can be established. Once attached, organisms of the particular strain of group A *Streptococcus* may have additional virulence factors that cause local inflammation in nonimmune patients. The clinical manifestations of subsequent infection are determined by these virulence factors (Figure 35-1), the portal of entry, and the age and immune response of the patient, resulting in three different categories of group A streptococcal infection: localized suppurative, invasive, and nonsuppurative infections.

Localized Suppurative Infections

Streptococcal tonsillopharyngitis. Streptococcal pharyngitis and tonsillitis are most common in children 5 to 13 years of age, during the school year, and in temperate climates. The high incidence in school-age children is due in part to the opportunity for exposure that schools provide, but more importantly may be due to the development of increasing concentrations of streptococcal receptors in the posterior pharynx that are not as prevalent in infants and younger children.

Physical findings consistent with but not diagnostic of group A streptococcal pharyngitis (Plate 52) include tonsillar exudates, palatal petechiae, bilateral cervical lymphadenitis, and/or a scarlet fever rash. Of those patients who are symptomatic, approximately one third will have severe symptoms with fever, severe sore throat, and bilateral cervical lymphadenitis; these are the patients who are likely to clinically improve with early antimicrobial treatment. The remainder may have various combinations of low-grade fever, sore throat, and dysphagia; response to antimicrobial treatment is much less predictable in these patients (Nelson, 1984). Many carriers of group A streptococci have no history of recent pharyngeal symptoms, emphasizing the wide spectrum of infection.

Although group A streptococci are the most common bacterial cause of pharyngitis, approximately two thirds of all cases are caused by viruses (e.g., adenovirus, Epstein-Barr virus, influenza virus). Given that 20% of these patients may be carriers of group A streptococci, the diagnosis of group A streptococcal pharyngitis must rely on a combination of clinical and laboratory findings. In many countries, patients are treated based solely on clinical findings; however, depending on the criteria used, rates of false-positive and false-negative diagnosis based solely on clinical judgment may be as high as 30%. In the United States it has been a long-time practice to use office-based laboratory tests to identify group A

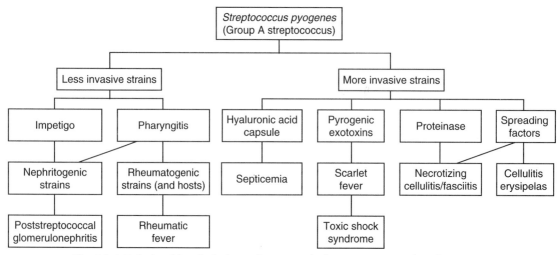

Fig. 35-1 Relationship of virulence factors with diseases associated with group A streptococcal strains.

streptococci in children with sore throat (Breese, 1969). Based on the recommendations of the Committee on Infectious Diseases of the American Academy of Pediatrics, patients with acute onset of sore throat and any combination of fever, headache, pain on swallowing, enlarged tender anterior cervical lymph nodes, or exposure to group A streptococci should be tested (American Academy of Pediatrics, 2000). The Committee also concludes that patients with symptoms of cough, runny nose, hoarseness, conjunctivitis, or diarrhea are more likely to have a viral illness and should not routinely be tested.

The accuracy of throat cultures and rapid antigen tests is highly dependent on the quality of the throat specimen, which must contain pharyngeal and tonsillar secretions, and on the experience of the person performing the test (Brien and Bass, 1985). Vigorous swabbing of the tonsils and the posterior pharyngeal wall will yield the best specimen, presumably by increasing the inoculum size (Kurtz et al., 2000). Agar plates containing sheep blood should be used for culture. Various commercial media incorporate antibiotics into the sheep blood agar plates to selectively enhance the growth of group A streptococci; these require careful quality control but may increase the recovery rate by 30% (Tolliver et al., 1987). Anaerobic or CO_2-enhanced aerobic conditions enhance recovery of group A streptococci but are impractical in an office setting. Cultures that are negative for group A streptococci after 24 hours should be incubated for a second day to optimize recovery of group A streptococci. The number of colonies of group A streptococci on the agar culture plate does not accurately differentiate streptococcal infection from the carrier state, so patients with a positive culture who meet clinical criteria should be treated (Kaplan, 1980). False-negative culture results occur in fewer that 10% of symptomatic patients when a throat swab specimen is obtained properly and cultured.

Because the culture process may require several days of incubation to rule-out group A streptococci, rapid antigen detection tests for the detection of group A streptococci have been developed and are commonly used. Few head-to-head comparative studies of these products have been done, and studies evaluating individual products report sensitivities that range from 70% to 99% (Radetsky et al., 1987; Roe et al.,

1995). This variation in sensitivity may be due to differences in study design and the "gold standard" used. When rigorous culture gold standards are applied, using multiple swab sampling and multiple culture plates with selective media, sensitivities of single rapid antigen tests tend to be lower than if a single culture plate is used. This has led the Red Book Committee to recommend that when a patient suspected on clinical grounds of having group A streptococcal pharyngitis has a negative result of a rapid streptococcal test, a throat culture should be obtained to ensure that the patient does not have group A *Streptococcus* infection (American Academy of Pediatrics, 2000). Although this is the correct stratagem for maximizing the detection of group A streptococci, it is not practical in the current highly regulated office laboratory setting. Better sampling strategies and rapid antigen products need to be developed and validated against rigorous standards that will meet or exceed the Academy's benchmark.

Suppurative complications of streptococcal pharyngitis. Group A streptococcal pharyngitis may occasionally be associated with otitis, sinusitis, and/or peritonsillar cellulitis or abscess caused by the same organism (see below). Early treatment of pharyngitis may decrease the incidence of these complications (Del Mar, 2000).

Sinusitis and Otitis. Unlike *Haemophilus influenzae* type B, *Streptococcus pneumoniae*, and *S. aureus*, group A streptococci are not common inhabitants of nasal normal flora. Because the pathogenesis of otitis and sinusitis is secondary to obstruction of the internal auditory tube and sinus ostia with subsequent trapping of normal flora, group A streptococci are only an occasional cause of sinusitis and otitis. Early treatment of streptococcal pharyngitis may reduce the incidence of these complications.

Streptococcal Febrile Nasopharyngitis. *Streptococcosis* is an old term that nonetheless includes some important, and yet diverse, disease manifestations caused by group A streptococci, including streptococcal febrile nasopharyngitis and reactive arthritis. Streptococcal febrile nasopharyngitis is a syndrome that can affect infants and young children. The syndrome lasts a week or longer and is characterized by acute fever with serosanguineous or mucopurulent drainage from the nose, often with impetiginous crusting around the nares. These clinical findings are not organism specific, as they also can be seen associated with *H. influenzae* type B and pneumococcus (Todd et al., 1984). More diagnostic is a gram stain that demonstrates polymorphonuclear leukocytes (PMNs) associated with gram-positive cocci in chains. Treatment with an oral penicillin or cephalosporin is appropriate. Similar findings may be seen in older children with group A streptococcal sinusitis.

Pneumonia. Overall, group A *Streptococcus* is an uncommon cause of pneumonia in children, but when present pneumonia may be rapidly progressive with severe consequences. It may be focal but often is bilateral and diffuse. Empyemas are common, and pleurocentesis often yields a thin, watery fluid that continues to flow when a chest tube is inserted and does not loculate as do empyemas resulting from other causes; this is probably because of the production of 'spreading factors' produced by the organisms that break down DNA and fibrin. The lung is a common focus of infection in patients with streptococcal TSS (Wheeler et al., 1991).

Perineal infection. In young children, group A *Streptococcus* is a common cause of perineal disease, including vaginitis in prepubertal girls and perianal infection (Mogielnicki et al., 2000). Specific group A *Streptococcus* strains may have a trophism for this area. Patients with vaginitis may have a serous discharge with marked erythema and irritation of the vulvar area, often accompanied by discomfort in walking and in urination. Perianal streptococcal infection is underrecognized (Combs, 2000). This is a common site of group A streptococcal colonization and may produce local itching, pain, blood-streaked stools, erythema, and proctitis.

Superficial skin infection. The most common form of skin infection (pyoderma) due to group A streptococci is impetigo characterized by superficial, honey-colored, crusting lesions around the nose and mouth (Dajani et al., 1972; Ferrieri et al., 1972). Colonization of the skin may precede impetigo by about 10 days and may lead to subsequent pharyngeal colonization with the same strain. Streptococcal strains causing impetigo have been associated with an increased incidence of subsequent poststreptococcal glomerulonephritis.

Severe invasive streptococcal syndrome. Certain strains of group A *Streptococcus* produce enzymes and/or toxins that cause more severe streptococcal infection (Figure 35-1).

Box 35-1 shows the definition for severe invasive streptococcal syndrome (SISS). The major clinical findings in SISS include puerperal sepsis, severe scarlet fever, necrotizing fasciitis, TSS, and septicemia (Working Group on Severe Streptococcal Infections, 1993). The streptococcal pyrogenic exotoxins have been associated with scarlet fever and streptococcal TSS, and the streptococcal proteinase has been associated with necrotizing cellulitis, fasciitis, and myositis (Talkington et al., 1993). Since 1990, strains producing these exoproteins (especially M-type 1) have been associated with an increase in SISS in many parts of the world. Successful treatment of these severe forms of group A streptococcal disease requires early recognition and aggressive therapy.

Deep soft-tissue infection. Group A *Streptococcus* is particularly adapted to causing soft-tissue infection, requiring a much smaller initial inoculum than most organisms. A minor break in the skin caused by an insect bite, varicella lesion, or scratch is sufficient to provide a portal of entry for the organism. Once under the skin the streptococcal spreading factors facilitate further invasion and spread.

Erysipelas is an acute, well-demarcated infection of the skin that spreads rapidly through the superficial lymphatics. The lesion is usually solitary, erythematous, and indurated with advancing margins and raised, firm borders. Streptococcal cellulitis is a deeper lesion than erysipelas, involving the skin and subcutaneous tissue. It is an often painful, erythematous, indurated infection of the skin and subcutaneous tissues. Some streptococcal strains produce a proteinase that is associated with a more severe, necrotizing cellulitis, fasciitis, or myositis that rapidly spreads, with a tissue-destructive process that causes necrosis of involved soft tissues including skin, fat, fascia, and muscle

---

BOX 35-1

CLINICAL MANIFESTATIONS OF SEVERE, INVASIVE STREPTOCOCCAL INFECTION

- Toxic shock syndrome
- Septicemia (with or without focal infection)
- Scarlet fever
- Necrotizing cellulitis or fasciitis
- Puerperal sepsis

(Talkington et al., 1993). This may be associated with varicella which, besides providing a portal of entry, seems to alter the immune response to the streptococcus (Lesko et al., 2001). Surgical exploration is often necessary if the lesion is poorly perfused or progressing, frequently demonstrating necrotic tissue with vascular thrombosis. Sequential débridement may be necessary to identify viable, bleeding margins (Zimbelman et al., 1999). Concomitant streptococcal TSS (see below) may occur.

Bacteremia or sepsis. Group A streptococcal bacteremia may follow either localized soft-tissue infection or respiratory infection (e.g., pharyngitis, otitis media, sinusitis, pneumonia) in previously healthy or immunocompromised (e.g., because of malnutrition or malignancy) patients (Wheeler et al., 1991). Sepsis may be rapidly progressive, leading to a toxic shock with hypotension, fever, leukocytosis, disseminated intravascular coagulation (DIC), and peripheral gangrene. Metastatic foci may result in meningitis, brain abscess, osteomyelitis, septic arthritis, and peritonitis.

Scarlet fever. Scarlet fever is the result of infection by group A streptococci that elaborate any of three pyrogenic (erythrogenic) exotoxins. The primary focus of infection is most commonly pharyngitis, but infection may be secondary to a wound or skin infection (surgical scarlet fever) or have some other focus. The onset is acute and is characterized by fever, chills, vomiting, headache, and toxicity (Figure 35-2). A generalized sunburnlike, "scarlatiniform" exanthem soon becomes apparent accentuated in the axillae, groin, and neck and is characterized by punctate red macules or fine papules that blanch on pressure (Figure 35-3; Plate 53). Petechiae may be present, especially on the distal extremities. In some individuals, it may feel like coarse sandpaper. Areas of hyperpigmentation that do not blanch with pressure may appear in the deep creases, particularly in the antecubital fossae (i.e., Pastia lines). The cheeks appear flushed, with sparing of the area around the mouth (i.e., circumoral pallor). The pharynx is inflamed, and the tonsils are hyperemic and edematous and may be covered with a gray-white exudate. The tongue may be edematous and reddened initially, with a white coating through which protrude red papillae (i.e., white strawberry tongue). After several days the white coat desquamates, leaving a red tongue studded with prominent papillae (i.e.,

red strawberry tongue, raspberry tongue). The palate and uvula may be reddened and covered with petechiae.

As shown in Figure 35-2, the exanthem and enanthem of scarlet fever tend to parallel the fever course, lasting 5 to 7 days in the untreated patient; early antibiotic treatment may mitigate the physical findings. Desquamation begins on the face in fine flakes toward the end of the first week and continues over the trunk, ultimately involving the hands and feet.

The exanthem of streptococcal scarlet fever is not diagnostic of a streptococcal infection; other organisms can cause a similar rash,

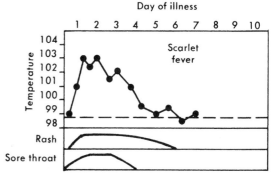

Fig. 35-2 Schematic diagram of a typical case of untreated uncomplicated scarlet fever. The rash usually appears within 24 hours of onset of fever and sore throat.

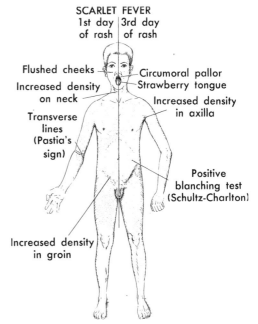

Fig. 35-3 Schematic drawing illustrating development and distribution of scarlet fever rash.

including several toxigenic stains of *S. aureus* and *Arcanobacterium haemolyticum* (Karpathios et al., 1992; Lina et al., 1997). The severity of illness and presence or absence of a strawberry tongue can help narrow the differential diagnosis; in general, the streptococcal pyrogenic exotoxins and TSST-1 produced by *S. aureus* cause a strawberry tongue as well as a scarlatiniform rash, whereas *A. haemolyticum* and exfoliatin-producing strains of *S. aureus* do not. Because of this difficulty in distinguishing the causative agent, when the cause of illness is uncertain it may be prudent to treat patients with scarlet fever with a cephalosporin or β-lactamase–resistant penicillin. Scarlet fever must also be differentiated from other exanthematous diseases, including measles, rubella, human parvovirus disease, and other viral exanthems. Kawasaki syndrome should also be considered, especially in younger children.

Streptococcal toxic shock syndrome. Box 35-2 shows the definition of streptococcal TSS (Working Group on Severe Streptococcal Infections, 1993). It is associated with streptococcal strains that produce the pyrogenic exotoxins and is characterized by hypotension accompanied by multi–organ-system dysfunction (kidney, lung, DIC, necrotizing soft-tissue infection, scarlet fever). It is often clinically indistinguishable from staphylococcal TSS until results of cultures are obtained. A focus of group A streptococcal infection can usually be identified (e.g., bacteremia, pneumonia, cellulitis) (Wheeler et al., 1991). Symptomatic pharyngitis is commonly absent, and throat cultures may be negative for streptococci in spite of isolation of the organism from other sites.

Treatment of suppurative group A streptococcal infections. The goals of therapy are to decrease symptoms and prevent septic, suppurative, and nonsuppurative complications. Penicillin is the drug of choice for the treatment of most streptococcal infections (American Academy of Pediatrics, 2000). All strains of group A β-hemolytic streptococci isolated to date have been sensitive to concentrations of penicillin (and many cephalosporins) achievable in vivo. Variable levels of resistance to erythromycin have been reported, depending on the frequency of the use of that antibiotic, and rarely resistance to clindamycin (Martin et al., 2002). The "eagle effect" has been described, in which failure to respond to penicillin treatment occurs because of slowly growing organisms at

---

BOX 35-2

DEFINITION OF STREPTOCOCCAL TOXIC SHOCK SYNDROME

Hypotension or shock plus two or more of the following:
- Renal impairment
- DIC
- Liver impairment
- ARDS
- Scarlet fever rash
- Soft-tissue necrosis

Definite Case

Clinical criteria plus group A streptococci from normally sterile site

Probable Case

Clinical criteria plus group A streptococci from nonsterile site

---

ARDS, acute respiratory distress syndrome; *DIC*, disseminated intravascular coagulation.

---

the site of deep group A streptococcal infections (e.g., necrotizing fasciitis) (Stevens et al., 1988).

The rationale for treatment of group A streptococcal pharyngitis falls into three separate categories: the mitigation of acute symptoms, prevention of suppurative sequelae, and prevention of nonsuppurative sequelae. A metaanalysis of the effect of antimicrobial treatment on 11,452 cases of sore throat reached the following conclusions (Del Mar et al., 2000):

1. *Acute symptoms*: Antibiotics shorten the duration of symptoms of pharyngitis, but by a mean of only about half of 1 day at day 3 (the time of maximal effect), and by about 8 hours overall. One study suggests that children with more severe symptoms (e.g., high fever, tender lymphadenitis) are more likely to show the clinical benefits of treatment. Another study reported the superiority of antibiotic treatment over nonsteroidal antiinflammatory therapy.

2. *Suppurative complications*: Treatment of group A streptococcal pharyngitis results in a 75% reduction in the incidence of resultant acute otitis media, a 50% reduction in the incidence of acute sinusitis, and

an 80% reduction in peritonsillar cellulitis and abscess.

3. *Nonsuppurative complications*: The incidence of rheumatic fever is reduced by 70%, and there is a trend indicating protection against acute glomerulonephritis, although the latter is debated.

Blood and tissue levels of penicillin sufficient to kill streptococci should be maintained for at least 10 days (American Academy of Pediatrics, 2000). Children with streptococcal pharyngitis can be treated with penicillin (250 to 500 mg/dose two to three times a day) for 10 days. Amoxicillin once per day for 10 days may be equally effective. A single intramuscular injection of a long-acting benzathine penicillin G (600,000 U for children <60 lb and 1,200,000 U for children ≥60 lb) may be more effective for treatment or prevention of relapse and is indicated for all noncompliant patients or those with nausea, vomiting, or diarrhea.

Erythromycin (40 mg/kg/24 h), clindamycin (30 mg/kg/24 h), or the first-generation cephalosporins may be used for treating streptococcal pharyngitis in patients who are allergic to penicillin. Increases in erythromycin resistance have been reported to be associated with increased use of the drug in the community. Generally, relapse rates are lower with regimens other than penicillin. Tetracyclines and sulfonamides should not be used for treatment, although sulfonamides may be used for prophylaxis of rheumatic fever. Recently, successful treatment with shorter courses (5 days) of azithromycin or cefpodoxime has been reported.

Bacteriologic treatment failure, defined as persistence of streptococci after a complete course of penicillin, occurs in up to 40% of children and is more common with oral penicillin therapy (Kaplan and Johnson, 2001). It may be due to poor compliance, reinfection, presence of β-lactamase–producing oral flora, tolerant streptococci, or presence of a carrier state. Persistent carriage of streptococci predisposes some patients to symptomatic relapse, especially if treated with penicillin early in the clinical course (Pichichero et al., 1997). Repeating the throat culture after a course of penicillin therapy is generally not recommended in asymptomatic children. The carrier state is common (5% to 20%) and is thought not to be highly contagious (Kaplan, 1980). Throat cultures in children who have symptoms incompatible with streptococcal infection (acute rhinorrhea, cough, hoarseness) may be misleading. It may be difficult to distinguish recurrent streptococcal infection from viral infections in a streptococcal carrier. In such cases clindamycin is probably the best drug for eradication of the carrier state (Kaplan and Johnson, 2001).

Patients with severe scarlet fever, streptococcal bacteremia, pneumonia, meningitis, deep soft-tissue infections, erysipelas, streptococcal TSS, or complications of streptococcal pharyngitis should be treated parenterally with penicillin. The dose and duration of therapy must be tailored to the nature of the disease process, with daily doses as high as 400,000 U/kg/24 h required in the most severe infections. A recent study suggests that deep or necrotizing infections may require the addition of a second antibiotic (e.g., clindamycin) to ensure complete killing of bacteria and a decrease in toxin production (Zimbelman et al., 1999). TSS may require additional therapies that may include aggressive fluid management, IVIG, and/or steroids (American Academy of Pediatrics, 1998). Exploratory surgery and débridement is indicated early in children with progressive or necrotizing soft-tissue disease, and often a second look is required to assure viable margins.

Nonsuppurative Sequelae of Group A Streptococcal Infection

Several diseases have been associated with the immune response to prior group A streptococcal infection, including reactive arthritis, rheumatic fever, and acute poststreptococcal glomerulonephritis. An important element of the diagnosis of these diseases is the ability to document the occurrence of a recent group A streptococcal infection. The organism may grow on throat or skin culture, but, if not, it may be necessary to measure antibody levels to one or more streptococcal products. The immunologic response of the host after streptococcal infection is usually assessed by measuring ASO and ADB titers. Demonstrating a rise in titer between acute and convalescent sera is the best evidence of prior infection. Such a rise may be modified or abolished by early, effective antibiotic therapy. A single ASO titer greater than 166 Todd units occurs in more than 80% of untreated children with streptococcal pharyngitis within the first 3 to 6 weeks after infection but may also be seen in 30% of long-term carriers. ASO titers may be very high in patients with rheumatic fever but are not usually increased in patients with glomerulonephritis.

Individuals with impetigo may elicit a strong anti-DNase (deoxyribonuclease) B reaction, which begins to rise 6 to 8 weeks after infection. When it is essential to document a recent streptococcal infection, antibody titers to several streptococcal products should be considered (e.g., ASO, ADB, and antihyaluronidase [AH]).

Reactive arthritis. In older children reactive arthritis (in the past included in the designation *streptococcosis*) may be secondary to a focus of group A *Streptococcus* infection elsewhere (usually the throat) resulting in nonmigratory arthritis, with a lack of response to aspirin or nonsteroidal antiinflammatory agents, and sometimes the presence of extraarticular manifestations, like vasculitis or glomerulonephritis (Jansen et al., 1999; Moon et al., 1995). This may be mediated by an autoimmune response causing synovitis similar to rheumatic fever. The patient should be evaluated carefully for signs of major manifestations of rheumatic fever, because evidence suggests that the risk of cardiac damage is quite low in reactive arthritis, and long-term penicillin prophylaxis may not be necessary.

Rheumatic fever. Rheumatic fever is the major cause of valvular heart disease in the world. It is no longer common in the United States and Western Europe, although there have been periodic, localized resurgences associated with the isolation of more rheumatogenic streptococcal strains (Veasy et al., 1994). It remains common in developing countries and socially and economically disadvantaged groups. Rheumatic fever is most frequently observed in school-age children and closed populations such as military recruits—those most susceptible to group A streptococcal throat infections. There appear to be genetic differences in rheumatic susceptibility among humans, presumably because of related differences in their immune response to streptococcal antigens (Gibofsky et al., 1998).

The symptoms of rheumatic fever generally follow 2 to 3 weeks after a streptococcal throat infection that often may be subclinical. There is no single specific clinical manifestation or laboratory test that establishes the diagnosis of

rheumatic fever, and severity of symptoms may range from severe to very mild. The current recommendations of the American Heart Association detail the Jones criteria for the diagnosis of the initial attack of rheumatic fever (Table 35-2) (American Heart Association, 1992). They require two major criteria (carditis, migratory polyarthritis, subcutaneous nodules, erythema marginatum, chorea), or one major and two minor criteria (Table 35-2). These criteria must be coupled with evidence of a recent streptococcal infection (culture, antibody titer rise). It is important to be accurate in the definition of major criteria. The arthritis is migratory and affects multiple (usually larger) joints. It usually responds quickly to low-dose salicylate therapy. Signs of carditis include pericarditis, myocarditis, or valvular insufficiency. It is still debated if the latter must be documented clinically or the criterion can be met with subclinical evidence of valvular regurgitation as detected by two-dimensional Doppler echocardiography. Chorea occurs much later than other manifestations; emotional lability or a change in school performance is a frequent finding. The rash of erythema marginatum can be mistaken for the rash seen with Lyme disease. It occurs very infrequently and usually is characterized by serpiginous, erythematous lesions over the trunk. Subcutaneous nodules are also uncommon, with pea-sized lesions that are firm and nontender, characteristically seen on the extensor surfaces of the knees and elbows and over the spine.

The minor manifestations are much less specific (Table 35-2). Most children with an infection of any kind will have some of these findings, so the documentation of one or more specific major criteria is essential if a diagnosis of rheumatic fever is being considered.

It is important to note that there must be evidence of a preceding group A streptococcal infection documented by a positive throat culture, a history of scarlet fever, or elevated streptococcal antibodies such as ASO, ADB, or AH; elevation of at least one of these three antibodies is found in more than 95% of patients with rheumatic fever.

There are three categories of patients who may be diagnosed as having acute rheumatic fever even in the absence of two major criteria or one major and two minor criteria, as required by the revised Jones criteria. These include strongly considering rheumatic fever

TABLE 35-2	The Jones Criteria for Diagnosis of the Initial Attack of Rheumatic Fever

Major criteria[*]	Minor criteria
Carditis	Fever
Polyarthritis, migratory	Arthralgia
Erythema marginatum	Elevated acute-phase reactants (ESR, CRP)
Chorea	Prolonged P-R interval on an electrocardiogram
Subcutaneous nodules	

Plus

Evidence of a preceding group A streptococcal infection (culture, rapid antigen, antibody rise or elevation)

From Special Writing Group of the Committee on Rheumatic Fever, Endocarditis, and Kawasaki Disease of the Council on Cardiovascular Disease in the Young of the American Heart Association: Guidelines for the diagnosis of rheumatic fever. JAMA 1992;268:2069.
CRP, C-reactive protein; *ESR,* erythrocyte sedimentation rate.
[*]Two major criteria or one major and two minor criteria plus evidence of a preceding streptococcal infection indicate a high probability of rheumatic fever. In the three special categories listed below, the diagnosis of rheumatic fever is acceptable without two major or one major and two minor criteria. However, only for a and b can the requirement for evidence of a preceding streptococcal infection be ignored.
   a. Chorea, *if other causes have been excluded.*
   b. Insidious or late-onset carditis *with no other explanation.*
   c. Rheumatic recurrence: In patients with documented rheumatic heart disease or prior rheumatic fever the presence of one major criterion, or of fever, arthralgia, or elevated acute-phase reactants suggests a presumptive diagnosis of recurrence. Evidence of previous streptococcal infection is needed here.

if chorea or indolent carditis is present with no other likely cause. In addition, a recurrence of rheumatic fever should be considered in patients with prior rheumatic fever or rheumatic heart disease who have evidence of a recent streptococcal infection with one major or two minor criteria. Patients with a previous history of rheumatic fever or rheumatic valvular heart disease should be carefully evaluated for infective endocarditis before the diagnosis of recurrent rheumatic fever is made. The major complication of acute rheumatic fever is the development of stenotic valvular heart disease, usually of the mitral or aortic valves.

All patients presenting with acute rheumatic fever should be treated for a group A streptococcal infection at the time the diagnosis is made, whether or not the organism is initially isolated from the patient. There are three systemic manifestations of acute rheumatic fever for which therapy is given acutely. These are arthritis, carditis, and Sydenham's chorea. Salicylates provide prompt and dramatic relief for the patient with the arthritis of acute rheumatic fever. In patients with congestive heart failure or other significant manifestations of carditis, corticosteroids may be effective. A variety of therapies (valproic acid, diazepam, carbamazepine, halperidol) may prove effective

in mitigating the symptoms of Sydenham's chorea (Genel et al., 2002). There is no definitive evidence that the use of any of these drugs is beneficial in preventing the subsequent development of rheumatic heart disease.

There are two modes of prevention for acute rheumatic fever: primary prophylaxis and secondary prophylaxis. Primary prophylaxis refers to antibiotic treatment of acute streptococcal infection to prevent an initial attack of rheumatic fever (see discussion of treatment, above).

Secondary prophylaxis refers to the prevention of infection of the upper respiratory tract with group A streptococci in people who have already had a previous attack of acute rheumatic fever (American Academy of Pediatrics, 2000). The recommended methods of secondary prophylaxis include regular (every 3 to 4 weeks) injections of intramuscular benzathine penicillin G, daily administration of oral penicillin, daily administration of oral sulfadiazine, or daily oral administration of erythromycin. Regular injections of intramuscular benzathine penicillin G are preferable to oral secondary prophylaxis because of better compliance. The duration of secondary prophylaxis is not clearly defined. Recommendations range from 5 years after the most recent attack or when the patient reaches the twenty-first birthday, whichever is longer, to at least 10 years in patients with residual rheumatic valvular heart disease and at least until the age of 40.

Pediatric autoimmune neuropsychiatric disorders associated with streptococcal infections. Recently a link between group A streptococcal infection and childhood-onset obsessive-compulsive disorder and Tourette's syndrome has been proposed. It has been named *pediatric autoimmune neuropsychiatric disorders associated with streptococcal infections* (PANDAS) (Bottas and Richter, 2002). The analogy with Sydenham's chorea, as well as positive results of culture and serologic data, have been cited as support for a causative role of group A streptococci. The impact of both primary penicillin treatment and secondary prophylaxis on this disorder has not been clearly established, although clinical benefits of early treatment have been claimed (Garvey et al., 1999; Murphy and Pichichero, 2002)

Poststreptococcal glomerulonephritis. Acute poststreptococcal glomerulonephritis (APSGN) is characterized by edema, hypertension, hematuria, and hypocomplementemia in association with evidence of a recent group A streptococcal infection (McPhaul and Mullins, 1976). It is most common in the summer or fall in preschool and school-age children, occurring days to weeks after streptococcal pyoderma or pharyngitis. Only certain "nephritogenic" strains of group A *Streptococcus* are associated with APSGN, presumably causing a host humoral response that results in antigen-antibody complex deposition in the kidney. Therapy is supportive and also includes antibiotic treatment of the streptococcal infection. Most patients recover completely.

ULTIMATE PREVENTION OF GROUP A STREPTOCOCCAL INFECTION

Current strategies for the prevention of group A streptococcal infection and its attendant complications (e.g., rheumatic fever, TSS) are hampered by the diversity of its strains, virulence factors (Figure 35-1), and clinical presentations; by the diagnostic confusion caused by the carrier state; by the difficulty of early diagnosis and treatment; and by the logistics of long-term prophylaxis. These are problems that only a vaccine can solve, but further work must be done to identify the appropriate antigens that will result in protective immu-

nity without increasing the risk of adverse autoimmune effects (Brandt and Good, 1999; Dale, 1999).

BIBLIOGRAPHY

Ashbaugh CD, Moser TJ, Shearer MH, et al. Bacterial determinants of persistent throat colonization and the associated immune response in a primate model of human group A streptococcal pharyngeal infection. Cell Microbiol 2000;2:283-292.

American Academy of Pediatrics. Committee on Infectious Diseases. Severe invasive group A streptococcal infections: a subject review. Pediatrics 1998;101:136-140.

American Academy of Pediatrics. Group A streptococcal infections. In Pickering LK (ed). 2000 Red Book: Report on the Committee on Infectious Diseases. Elk Grove Village, Ill: American Academy of Pediatrics, 2000:526-536.

American Heart Association. Guidelines for the diagnosis of rheumatic fever. Jones Criteria, 1992 update. Special Writing Group of the Committee on Rheumatic Fever, Endocarditis, and Kawasaki Disease of the Council on Cardiovascular Disease in the Young of the American Heart Association. JAMA 1992;268:2069-2073.

Bottas A, Richter MA. Pediatric autoimmune neuropsychiatric disorders associated with streptococcal infections (PANDAS). Pediatr Infect Dis J 2002;21:67-71.

Brandt ER, Good MF. Vaccine strategies to prevent rheumatic fever. Immunol Res 1999;19:89-103.

Breese BB. Culturing beta hemolytic streptococci in pediatric practice observation after twenty years. J Pediatr 1969;75:164-166.

Brien JH, Bass JW. Streptococcal pharyngitis: optimal site for throat culture. J Pediatr 1985;106:781-783.

Combs JT. Perianal streptococcal disease. Clin Pediatr (Phila) 2000;39:500.

Cunningham MW. Pathogenesis of group A streptococcal infections. Clin Microbiol Rev 2000;13:470-511.

Dajani AS, Ferrieri P, Wannamaker LW. Natural history of impetigo. II. Etiologic agents and bacterial interactions. J Clin Invest 1972;51:2863-2871.

Dale JB. Group A streptococcal vaccines. Infect Dis Clin North Am 1999;13:227-243.

Del Mar CB, Glasziou PP, Spinks AB. Antibiotics for sore throat. Cochrane Database Syst Rev 2000:D000023.

Denny FW Jr. A 45-year perspective on the streptococcus and rheumatic fever: the Edward H. Kass Lecture in infectious disease history. Clin Infect Dis 1994;19:1110-1122.

Facklam R, Beall B, Efstratiou A, et al. emm typing and validation of provisional M types for group A streptococci. Emerg Infect Dis 1999;5:247-253.

Ferrieri P, Dajani AS, Wannamaker LW, Chapman SS. Natural history of impetigo. I. Site sequence of acquisition and familial patterns of spread of cutaneous streptococci. J Clin Invest 1972;51:2851-2862.

Garvey MA, Perlmutter SJ, Allen AJ, et al. A pilot study of penicillin prophylaxis for neuropsychiatric exacerbations triggered by streptococcal infections. Biol Psychiatry 1999;45:1564-1571.

Genel F, Arslanoglu S, Uran N, Saylan B. Sydenham's chorea: clinical findings and comparison of the efficacies of sodium valproate and carbamazepine regimens. Brain Dev 2002;24:73-76.

Gibofsky A, Kerwar S, Zabriskie JB. Rheumatic fever. The relationships between host, microbe, and genetics. Rheum Dis Clin North Am 1998;24:237-259.

Jansen TL, Janssen M, Traksel R, de Jong AJ. A clinical and serological comparison of group A versus non-group A streptococcal reactive arthritis and throat culture negative cases of post-streptococcal reactive arthritis. Ann Rheum Dis 1999;58:410-414.

Kaplan EL. The group A streptococcal upper respiratory tract carrier state: an enigma. J Pediatr 1980;97:337-345.

Kaplan EL, Johnson DR. Unexplained reduced microbiological efficacy of intramuscular benzathine penicillin G and of oral penicillin V in eradication of group a streptococci from children with acute pharyngitis. Pediatrics 2001;108:1180-1186.

Kaplan EL, Wotton JT, Johnson DR. Dynamic epidemiology of group A streptococcal serotypes associated with pharyngitis. Lancet 2001;358:1334-1337.

Karpathios T, Drakonaki S, Zervoudaki A, et al. *Arcanobacterium haemolyticum* in children with presumed streptococcal pharyngotonsillitis or scarlet fever. J Pediatr 1992;121:735-737.

Kaul R, McGeer A, Norrby-Teglund A, et al. Intravenous immunoglobulin therapy for streptococcal toxic shock syndrome—a comparative observational study. The Canadian Streptococcal Study Group. Clin Infect Dis 1999;28:800-807.

Kurtz B, Kurtz M, Roe M, Todd J. Importance of inoculum size and sampling effect in rapid antigen detection for diagnosis of *Streptococcus pyogenes* pharyngitis. J Clin Microbiol 2000;38:279-281.

Lancefield RC. A serological differentiation of human and other groups of hemolytic streptococci. J Exp Med 1933;57:571.

Lesko SM, O'Brien KL, Schwartz B, et al. Invasive group A streptococcal infection and nonsteroidal antiinflammatory drug use among children with primary varicella. Pediatrics 2001;107:1108-1115.

Lilja M, Silvola J, Raisanen S, Stenfors LE. Where are the receptors for *Streptococcus pyogenes* located on the tonsillar surface epithelium? Int J Pediatr Otorhinolaryngol 1999;50:37-43.

Lina G, Gillet Y, Vandenesch F, et al. Toxin involvement in staphylococcal scalded skin syndrome. Clin Infect Dis 1997;25:1369-1373.

Macris MH, Hartman N, Murray B, et al. Studies of the continuing susceptibility of group A streptococcal strains to penicillin during eight decades. Pediatr Infect Dis J 1998;17:377-381.

Martin JM, Green M, Barbadora KA, Wald ER. Erythromycin-resistant group A streptococci in schoolchildren in Pittsburgh. N Engl J Med 2002;346:1200-1206.

McCormick JK, Tripp TJ, Olmsted SB, et al. Development of streptococcal pyrogenic exotoxin C vaccine toxoids that are protective in the rabbit model of toxic shock syndrome. J Immunol 2000;165:2306-2312.

McCormick JK, Yarwood JM, Schlievert PM. Toxic shock syndrome and bacterial superantigens: an update. Annu Rev Microbiol 2001;55:77-104.

McPhaul JJ Jr, Mullins JD. Glomerulonephritis mediated by antibody to glomerular basement membrane. Immunological, clinical, and histopathological characteristics. J Clin Invest 1976;57:351-361.

Mogielnicki NP, Schwartzman JD, Elliott JA. Perineal group A streptococcal disease in a pediatric practice. Pediatrics 2000;106:276-281.

Moon RY, Greene MG, Rehe GT, Katona IM. Poststreptococcal reactive arthritis in children: a potential predecessor of rheumatic heart disease. J Rheumatol 1995;22:529-532.

Murphy ML, Pichichero ME. Prospective identification and treatment of children with pediatric autoimmune neuropsychiatric disorder associated with group A streptococcal infection (PANDAS). Arch Pediatr Adolesc Med 2002;156:356-361.

Nelson JD. The effect of penicillin therapy on the symptoms and signs of streptococcal pharyngitis. Pediatr Infect Dis J 1984;3:10-13.

Oberhofer TR. Value of the L-pyrrolidonyl-beta-naphthylamide hydrolysis test for identification of select grampositive cocci. Diagn Microbiol Infect Dis 1986;4: 43-47.

Pichichero ME. Sore throat after sore throat after sore throat. Are you asking the critical questions? Postgrad Med 1997;101:205-206.

Pichichero ME, Casey JR, Mayes T, et al. Penicillin failure in streptococcal tonsillopharyngitis: causes and remedies. Pediatr Infect Dis J 2000;19:917-923.

Pichichero ME, Disney FA, Talpey WB, et al. Adverse and beneficial effects of immediate treatment of Group A beta-hemolytic streptococcal pharyngitis with penicillin. Pediatr Infect Dis J 1987;6:635-643.

Radetsky M, Solomon JA, Todd JK. Identification of streptococcal pharyngitis in the office laboratory: reassessment of new technology. Pediatr Infect Dis J 1987;6: 556-563.

Roe M, Kishiyama C, Davidson K, et al. Comparison of BioStar Strep A OIA optical immune assay, Abbott TestPack Plus Strep A, and culture with selective media for diagnosis of group A streptococcal pharyngitis. J Clin Microbiol 1995;33:1551-1553.

Roe MH, Tolliver PR, Lewis PL, Todd JK. Primary plate identification of group A *Streptococcus* on a selective medium. Efficiency in an office practice. Am J Dis Child 1984;138:589-591.

Schlievert PM, Bettin KM, Watson DW. Reinterpretation of the Dick test: role of group A streptococcal pyrogenic exotoxin. Infect Immun 1979;26:467-472.

Seppala H, Klaukka T, Vuopio-Varkila J, et al. The effect of changes in the consumption of macrolide antibiotics on erythromycin resistance in group A streptococci in Finland. Finnish Study Group for Antimicrobial Resistance. N Engl J Med 1997;337:441-446.

Stevens DL, Gibbons AE, Bergstrom R, Winn V. The Eagle effect revisited: efficacy of clindamycin, erythromycin, and penicillin in the treatment of streptococcal myositis. J Infect Dis 1988;158:23-28.

Stollerman GH. Rheumatic fever in the 21st century. Clin Infect Dis 2001;33:806-814.

Talkington DF, Schwartz B, Black CM, et al. Association of phenotypic and genotypic characteristics of invasive *Streptococcus pyogenes* isolates with clinical components of streptococcal toxic shock syndrome. Infect Immun 1993;61:3369-3374.

Todd JK. Throat cultures in the office laboratory. Pediatr Infect Dis J 1982;1:265-270.

Todd JK, Todd N, Damato J, Todd WA. Bacteriology and treatment of purulent nasopharyngitis: a double blind, placebo-controlled evaluation. Pediatr Infect Dis 1984;3:226-232.

Tolliver PR, Roe MH, Todd JK. Detection of group A Streptococcus: comparison of solid and liquid culture media with and without selective antibiotics. Pediatr Infect Dis J 1987;6:515-519.

Veasy LG, Tani LY, Hill HR. Persistence of acute rheumatic fever in the intermountain area of the United States. J Pediatr 1994;124:9-16.

Visentainer JE, Pereira FC, Dalalio MM, et al. Association of HLA-DR7 with rheumatic fever in the Brazilian population. J Rheumatol 2000;27:1518-1520.

Wheeler MC, Roe MH, Kaplan EL, et al. Outbreak of group A streptococcus septicemia in children. Clinical, epidemiologic, and microbiological correlates. JAMA 1991;266:533-537.

Working Group on Severe Streptococcal Infections. Defining the group A streptococcal toxic shock syndrome. Rationale and consensus definition. JAMA 1993;269:390-391.

Zimbelman J, Palmer A, Todd J. Improved outcome of clindamycin compared with beta-lactam antibiotic treatment for invasive *Streptococcus pyogenes* infection. Pediatr Infect Dis J 1999;18:1096-1100.

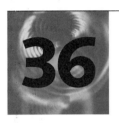

36 TETANUS (LOCKJAW) AND NEONATAL TETANUS

CATHERINE WILFERT AND PETER HOTEZ

Clostridium tetani produces a potent, soluble exotoxin that is responsible for the clinical manifestations of tetanus. Tetanus, or "lockjaw," is an acute toxemia characterized by tonic spasms of voluntary muscles and a high fatality rate. *C. tetani* infection usually occurs at a break in the skin, which may be trivial or unrecognized, but the infection also can complicate burns, puerperal infections, and infections of the umbilical stump (tetanus neonatorum) and can occur after certain surgical operations, in which the source of infection may be contaminated sutures, dressings, or plaster. The illness begins with tonic spasms of the skeletal muscles and is followed by paroxysmal contractions. The muscle stiffness involves the jaw (lockjaw) and neck first and later becomes generalized. In the United States, fewer than 60 cases have been reported annually for the past 5 years. However, in developing countries tetanus is a leading cause of death in childhood. The World Health Organization estimates that in 1999 there were 377,000 deaths from tetanus, most of which occurred during the neonatal period (neonatal tetanus [NT]). NT is one of the world's leading killers of infants. More than one-half of the deaths resulting from NT occur in South Asia.

ETIOLOGY

The tetanus bacillus is a long, thin (2 to 5 μm × 3 to 8 μm), motile, gram-positive anaerobic rod. Older cultures of these organisms and smears from wounds frequently stain as gram-negative microbes, and this result may be confusing to the uninitiated. These organisms may develop a terminal spore that does not take the Gram stain and gives the bacterium a drumstick appearance. The spores are very resistant to heat and the usual antiseptics, and they may persist in tissues for many months in a viable,

although dormant, state. Under anaerobic conditions the organisms are easily isolated on blood agar or in cooked meat broth. The organism does not ferment carbohydrates, does not usually liquefy gelatin, and produces little change in litmus milk.

The bacilli are widely distributed in soil; street dust; and the feces of some horses, sheep, cattle, dogs, cats, rats, guinea pigs, and chickens. Consequently, manure-containing soil may be highly infectious. In agricultural areas a significant number of normal human adults may harbor the organisms, and agricultural workers have a higher incidence of infection. The spores have also been found in contaminated heroin.

Tetanus bacilli produce a potent neurotoxin that is one of the most toxic substances known; the mouse LD_{50} of highly purified preparations is between 0.1 and 1 ng/kg (Schiavo et al., 1995). Tetanus neurotoxin derives its potency by virtue of its absolute specificity for neuronal cells and its target intracellular catalytic activity. It resembles other clostridial neurotoxins in that the molecule is synthesized as a single inactive polypeptide chain of 150 kDa without a leader sequence: Release of the neurotoxin occurs as a consequence of bacterial lysis in the host. Exposure and cleavage of a protease-sensitive loop within the molecule generates an active heterodimer composed of a 100-kDa heavy chain and a 50-kDa light chain joined by a disulfide bond. New evidence suggests that the light chain is catalytically active as a zinc metalloprotease. Once inside the host target cell the metalloprotease degrades specific protein components of the host neuroexocytosis apparatus. The major protease substrates are membrane proteins of synaptic vesicles, including synaptobrevin (also called VAMP), SNAP-25, and syntaxin.

PATHOGENESIS

The portal of entry is usually the site of a minor puncture wound or scratch, and the organism can proliferate only if the oxidation-reduction (Eh) potential is lower than that of normal living tissues. Deep puncture wounds, burns, and crush or other injuries that promote favorable conditions for the growth of anaerobic organisms may be followed by tetanus. Occasionally, no apparent portal of entry can be found. Under these circumstances the site of infection may have been the alimentary tract.

When conditions are favorable, the bacilli multiply at the site of primary inoculation and produce toxin. Toxin then travels centripetally in the axoplasm of the alpha motor fibers and accumulates in the motor neurons in the membrane-bound endoplasmic reticulum. In 1902, Marie and Morax proposed this route of access of toxin to the central nervous system, as did Meyer and Ransome in 1903. It was shown experimentally that toxin was not lethal if the local motor nerves were severed. Toxin is neutralizable when it is free and is only partially neutralizable when it is on the cell surface. Pinocytosis, internalizing the toxin, renders it nonneutralizable. Thus, fixation of toxin to nerves and its internalization result in irreversible effects. Cleavage of host neuronal cell membrane proteins by the catalytically active neurotoxin results in a persistent and sustained blockade of neuroexocytosis. The neuronal blockade then results in the uncontrolled spread of impulses, hyperreflexia, and constant muscle contraction. The strongest muscles, usually extensors, exert the greatest effects. The toxin also affects the sympathetic nervous system.

PATHOLOGY

There are no specific pathologic lesions caused by the infectious agent or toxin. Secondary effects of the muscular contractions may include vertebral fractures, pneumonia, and hemorrhages into the muscles.

CLINICAL MANIFESTATIONS

The incubation period is variable, with a usual range of 5 to 14 days; however, it may be as short as 1 day or as long as 3 or more weeks. The appearance of the site of infection, if obvious, provides no clue to the impending toxemia. The disease begins insidiously, with progressively increasing stiffness of the voluntary muscles; generally, the muscles of the jaw and neck are involved first. Within 24 to 48 hours after the onset of the disease, rigidity may be fully developed and may spread rapidly to involve the trunk and extremities. With spasm of the jaw muscles, trismus (lockjaw) develops. The wrinkling of the forehead and distortion of the eyebrows, and the angles of the mouth produce a peculiar facial appearance called *risus sardonicus* (sardonic grin). The neck and back become stiff and arched (opisthotonos). The abdominal wall is boardlike, and the extremities are usually stiff and extended.

Painful paroxysmal spasms that persist for a few seconds or several minutes may be provoked by the most trivial kind of visual, auditory, or cutaneous stimuli, such as bright lights, sudden noises, and movement of the patient. Risus sardonicus and opisthotonos are most marked during these spasms. Initially the spasms occur at infrequent intervals, with complete relaxation between attacks. Later the spasms occur more often and are more prolonged and more painful. Involvement of the muscles of respiration, laryngeal obstruction caused by laryngospasm, or accumulation of secretions in the tracheobronchial tree may be followed by respiratory distress, asphyxia, coma, and death. Involvement of the bladder sphincter leads to urinary retention.

The manifestations of sympathetic nervous system involvement may include labile hypertension, tachycardia, peripheral vasoconstriction, cardiac arrhythmias, profuse sweating, hypercapnia, increased urinary excretion of catecholamines, and late-appearing hypotension.

During the illness the patient's sensorium is usually clear. The fever is generally low grade or absent. Patients who recover are usually afebrile. After a period of weeks the paroxysms decrease in frequency and severity and gradually disappear. Generally, the trismus is the last symptom to subside. Patients with fatal disease are usually febrile, with death occurring in most instances before the tenth day of illness.

The spinal fluid in patients with tetanus is normal. The peripheral white blood cell count may be normal or slightly elevated. Most patients with tetanus show the generalized manifestations described previously. Occasionally, however, generalized tetanus may be preceded by cephalic tetanus. In this case the incubation period is only 1 to 2 days; it follows a head injury or otitis media, and the patient has a poor prognosis (Bagratuni, 1952). This form of tetanus is characterized by involvement of various cranial nerves, especially the seventh, but the third, fourth, ninth, tenth, and twelfth may be affected also. Cephalic tetanus can occur without subsequent generalized disease.

Neonatal Tetanus

The onset of NT usually begins when the newborn infant is 3 to 10 days old (5.6 ± 2.8 days in a recent review of 73 cases of NT in Turkey [Yaramis and Tas, 2000]) and is manifested by difficulty in sucking and by excessive crying. Soon the jaw becomes too stiff for the infant to suck, and swallowing becomes difficult. Shortly thereafter, stiffness of the body appears, and intermittent jerking spasms may begin. Variable degrees of trismus; sustained, tonic, or rigid states of muscle contraction; and spasms or convulsions occur. The spasms occur spontaneously or in response to stimuli with variable frequency. Deep-tendon reflex activity may be increased, or the deep tendons may show no response during testing because of constant generalized stiffness. Opisthotonos may be absent or so extreme that the head almost touches the heels. The cry varies from a repeated, short, mildly hoarse cry to a strangled-sounding voiceless noise. The patient's color may be normal, cyanotic, or pale from hypoxia and impending shock. Severe spasms may be followed by flaccidity, anoxia, and exhaustion.

■ **Case 1** A 13-day-old male infant was brought to Children's Hospital of Los Angeles with respiratory arrest. The infant was born at another hospital to a gravida 5, para 5 mother. On the second day of life, the patient left the other hospital. On the tenth day the umbilical stump fell off and purulent drainage was observed at the site. On the thirteenth day the infant had trismus, was irritable, and refused feedings. On the morning of the fourteenth day, the day of admission to Children's Hospital, the infant was febrile, his body was rigid, his respirations were noisy, and he was drooling. He had frequent spasms of the extremities and the body triggered by external stimuli. The mouth was locked in an open position. Respirations were shallow, and an inspiratory rattle was heard that was suggestive of laryngospasm.

Gram-positive rods and spores were present in pus from the umbilicus. Treatment included human tetanus antitoxin (TAT); surgical débridement of the umbilical stump; tracheostomy; reduction of environmental stimuli; and the use of diazepam (Valium), meprobamate, phenobarbital, thorazines, and antibiotics (see below). The infant received feedings by gavage, and the bladder was emptied by Credé's method.

The patient's condition improved steadily. Spasms decreased in frequency and stopped altogether after 4 weeks. The use of medications was also discontinued and the patient was discharged after 48 days in the hospital.

■ **Case 2** A 16-year-old white female was admitted to Duke University Medical Center (DUMC) in March 1991 because of jaw tightness, tongue rolling, and neck stiffness of 1 day's duration. Approximately 3 weeks before admission a rusty fishhook had been caught in her scalp. She had received no immunizations for the past 10 years. The referring physician had recognized trismus, opisthotonos, and risus sardonicus. He had administered tetanus immune globulin, intubated her, and had her transported to DUMC. Her temperature was 36.1° C (97° F); pulse, 35; respirations, 16; and blood pressure, 125/60.

She was sedated and paralyzed with pancuronium (Pavulon). She required respirator-assisted ventilation for 10 days, and she received parenteral antibiotics, tetanus immune globulin, and tetanus toxoid. No bacterial pathogens were identified, and there was no wound to culture. She recovered completely and was discharged 17 days after admission.

DIAGNOSIS

The development of trismus, risus sardonicus, generalized tonic rigidity, and spasms in a patient with a clear sensorium and a recent history of trauma is highly suggestive of a diagnosis of tetanus. The recovery of C. *tetani* from the wound confirms the diagnosis; however, in most instances the organism is not detected.

DIFFERENTIAL DIAGNOSIS
Side Reaction to Phenothiazines

Among the extrapyramidal neurologic syndromes that may accompany the use of some phenothiazine drugs are acute dystonic reactions, with facial grimacing, torticollis, and muscle rigidity. They disappear with discontinuation of the drug.

Tetany

In patients with tetany, trismus is usually absent, but carpopedal spasms and laryngospasm may be present. Low blood calcium content confirms the diagnosis.

Peritonsillar Abscess

Peritonsillar abscess, a febrile painful condition, usually is accompanied by trismus. However, there are no generalized muscular spasms.

Encephalitis

Patients with viral and postinfectious encephalitides rarely have trismus, do not have clear minds as a rule, and usually have abnormal spinal fluid findings.

Rabies

Continuous tonic seizures are not present in patients with rabies; the seizures are usually intermittent and clonic. Trismus is rarely observed.

Strychnine Poisoning

Relaxation between convulsions is usually complete in patients with strychnine poisoning. When trismus occurs, it occurs late.

COMPLICATIONS

The interference with pulmonary ventilation by laryngospasm, respiratory muscle spasm, or accumulation of secretions may be followed by pneumonia and atelectasis. Vertebral compression fractures and lacerations of the tongue may follow a seizure.

PROGNOSIS

Tetanus remains a very serious disease. The declines in incidence (Figure 36-1) and mortality rate of tetanus over the past two decades have been parallel, resulting in minor changes in the case fatality rate. In patients who survive, recovery is complete—without sequelae if supportive measures have provided adequate ventilation. The prognosis is significantly affected by the following factors.

Age

The highest mortality rate is found among patients in the extremes of life. For neonates the case fatality rate is 66%, and for persons 50 years of age or older it is 70%. In contrast, for patients 10 to 19 years old, the case fatality rate is 10% to 20%.

Incubation Period

The median incubation period of fatal and non-fatal tetanus cases with known wounds was 6.2 and 7.6 days, respectively, in 1968 and 1969. Christie (1969) believes that a more reliable guide to the prognosis is the length of the period of onset, defined as the interval between the first evidence of trismus and the first generalized convulsion. If this period is shorter than 48 hours, the attack probably will be severe; if the interval is longer, the illness will be milder. Nevertheless, the course of tetanus cannot be predicted until the severity and frequency of the convulsions have been made clear. It is easy to be misled in the first day or two. Mortality in NT is also higher if the incubation period is less than 4 days.

Fever

In mild or moderately severe cases of tetanus, fever is not a common finding. In patients with involvement of the brain stem, fever or hyperpyrexia is often present. Afebrile patients have a better chance of recovery. This is also true in NT.

Extent of Involvement

In patients with local tetanus the symptoms are confined to the wound area, and the prognosis

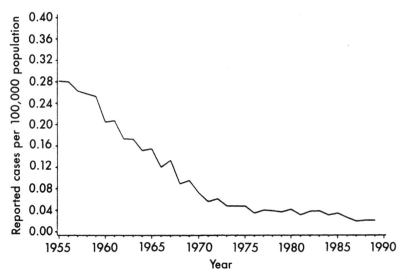

Fig. 36-1 Tetanus by year in the United States, 1955 to 1989. (From MMWR Morb Mortal Wkly Rep 1990;38:41.)

is usually good. Generalized involvement, however, is followed by a more serious outcome. Tetanus following penetrating injury has a higher mortality than infection following abrasions. Mortality is lower in otogenic tetanus. The manifestations of tetanus that correlate significantly with a poorer prognosis are convulsion and spasms (Patel and Mehta, 1999).

Antitoxin Therapy

In general, antitoxin therapy does not significantly affect the prognosis. Toxin usually has been fixed and is not available for neutralization. However, antitoxin may modify the disease if it is given during the incubation period or very early in the course of the illness.

EPIDEMIOLOGIC FACTORS

Tetanus is worldwide in distribution. Reported cases of tetanus in the United States from 1955 to 1989 are shown in Figure 36-1. The spores are widely disseminated in soil and in animal feces. Tetanus spores or toxin can contaminate a variety of biologic and surgical products, such as vaccines, sera, and catgut. Unimmunized persons of all ages and both sexes are equally susceptible. In spite of the ubiquity of C. tetani, tetanus is a relatively rare occurrence, but NT is still a serious problem in developing countries, where it is the cause of between 8% and 69% of neonatal mortality. Southern Asia and sub-Saharan Africa are especially affected. In India, NT is, after septicemia, the leading cause of neonatal mortality. More than 300,000 infants die annually from NT. Community-based surveys have identified risk factors for NT, including the omission of maternal tetanus toxoid immunization during pregnancy, home delivery, unhygienic cutting of the umbilical cord, the application of an unhygienic dressing to the umbilical stump (including ghee, a type of clarified butter, particularly when it is heated with cow dung fuel [Bennet et al., 1999]), and a history of NT after an earlier delivery (Galazka and Gasse, 1995). Thus the disease can be prevented in newborns by immunizing women either during or before pregnancy and increasing the proportion of deliveries that are attended by trained individuals. In fact, with available tools of modern aseptic technique and active immunization, tetanus is a disease that could be eliminated. The WHO estimates that in 1992 immunization and clean delivery prac-

tices prevented 686,000 neonatal deaths from tetanus (Galazka and Gasse, 1995). Many of these efforts were achieved through the Expanded Programme on Immunization.

IMMUNITY

It is estimated that 0.01 U of antibody to C. tetani toxin in serum is protective in humans. Maternal IgG antibodies, if present, are transmitted through the placenta. This passively acquired immunity is, however, of short duration, because maternal globulins are metabolized by the infant. The administration of tetanus toxoid to infants, children, and adults stimulates the production of antibodies that provide protection against the effects of toxin. This protective level can be maintained by periodic booster injections. Elderly patient who have not received a recent booster may be at particularly high risk for tetanus. Patients recovering from tetanus should be actively immunized because the extremely potent toxin may not stimulate an antibody response in the patient.

TREATMENT
Control of Muscular Spasms

The patient should be admitted to a quiet, darkened room where all possible auditory, visual, tactile, or other stimuli are reduced to a minimum. The first priority in the management of muscular spasms should be the administration of appropriate drugs to reduce the number and severity of spasms.

Diazepam is a valuable drug because it effectively controls spasms and hypertonicity without depressing the cortical centers. The recommended dosage for infants under 2 years of age is 8 mg/kg of body weight per day given in doses of 2 to 3 mg every 3 hours. Alternatively, for infants an initial dose of 0.1 to 0.2 mg/kg, intravenously (IV), is used to relieve an acute spasm, followed by a continuous IV infusion of 15 to 40 mg/kg/day (Gerdes, 1995). After 5 to 7 days the dose can be tapered by 5 to 10 mg/day and then given by the orogastric route. Vecuronium with mechanical ventilation may be required to control spasms (Singhi et al., 2001). Phenobarbital and morphine may also be used as an adjunctive therapy, with the understanding that it be administered only in a controlled, intensive setting because of the risk of apnea.

Antitoxin Therapy

After adequate sedation has been achieved, human tetanus immune globulin (TIG) should be given in a single dose (3,000 to 6,000 U, intramuscularly). Lower doses of 500 U may be appropriate for NT. Although not approved by the Food and Drug Administration, intravenous immune globulin (IVIG) contains antibodies to tetanus and can be considered if TIG is not available. The standard dose of IVIG for other indications is 400 to 500 mg/kg (Gerdes, 1995). In some countries where human immune globulin is unavailable, equine TAT should be given if the sensitivity reactions to horse serum are negative. The antitoxin is given intravenously and intramuscularly, half the dose via each route. For neonates it may be necessary to delay active immunization with tetanus toxoid for 4 to 6 weeks following the administration of TIG.

Antimicrobial Therapy

Oral or intravenous metronidazole (30 mg/kg per day, given at 6-hour intervals) is effective in reducing the number of vegetative forms of *C. tetani*. Parenteral penicillin G is an alternative drug.

Surgical Treatment

After the patient has been sedated and has received antitoxin, any wound should be thoroughly cleansed and débrided. Extensive surgical excision is usually not indicated.

Supportive Treatment

Good medical and nursing care must minimize stimuli that may precipitate a convulsion. Procedures such as catheterization or placement of indwelling lines should be carried out at a time when any sedative is exerting its maximal effect. Such procedures preferably are performed early in the course of clinical illness. In addition, care should be taken to anticipate and prevent complications such as aspiration pneumonia, lower-bowel obstruction resulting from fecal impaction, urinary retention, and decubitus ulcers. Adequate sedation may prevent a compression fracture of the vertebra. Respiratory support is essential, and intubation or tracheostomy with respirator ventilation may be required. High-quality intensive care during the first week (i.e., early intubation, mechanical ventilation, and neuromuscular blockade [pancuronium or its equivalent]) is an essential component of the management of a neonate with tetanus.

Tracheostomy

The combination of heavy sedation, difficulty in swallowing, laryngospasm, and accumulation of secretions leads to obstruction of the airway. A relatively low mortality rate of 10% was reported by Edmondson and Flowers (1979), who treated 100 patients with tetanus in an intensive care unit. Intubation can be lifesaving.

PREVENTIVE MEASURES
Active Immunization

Because many cases of tetanus follow minor abrasions and lacerations that are ignored, control of the disease can best be achieved by active immunization with toxoid before exposure. All infants should be immunized routinely with tetanus toxoid that is incorporated with diphtheria toxoid and pertussis vaccine. The usual basic series of the triple antigen should consist of five doses of tetanus and diphtheria toxoid–containing vaccine. The initial three doses are given as DTaP administered at 2-month intervals beginning at approximately 2 months of age. A fourth dose is recommended 6 to 12 months after the third dose, usually at 15 to 18 months of age. An additional dose of DTaP is necessary before school entry, usually at 4 to 6 years of age, unless the fourth dose was given after the fourth birthday. DTaP can be given concurrently with other vaccines. For specific recommendations regarding children who have missed one or more vaccinations or who have started their vaccinations at a time later than the typical schedule, the reader is advised to consult the Report of the Committee on Infectious Diseases of the American Academy of Pediatrics (Red Book, 2003). Infant survivors of NT still require active immunization against tetanus.

After the initial immunization series is completed, a booster dose of tetanus toxoid (given as dT) should be given at 11 to 12 years of age and no later than by 16 years of age, and every 10 years thereafter. If more than 5 years have elapsed since the last dose, a booster of dT should be considered for persons who are going to high risk areas or on wilderness expeditions where tetanus boosters may not be available.

The WHO has recently adopted the goal of eliminating NT worldwide in developing countries through a strategy of administering at least two properly spaced doses of toxoid (given as dT if available) to women of childbearing age in high-risk areas. Typically, the two doses of dT should be administered at least 4 weeks apart, and the second dose should be given at least 2 weeks before delivery. The strategy relies on the stimulation of maternal antibodies that will passively protect newborns at birth. Unfortunately, many lots of toxoid produced in developing countries are of inadequate potency; fewer than half of the nations that produce toxoid have a functional national control authority to monitor vaccine production and quality (Dietz et al., 1996). Immunization with tetanus toxoid or dT is not contraindicated during pregnancy. In the event of an injury, administration of an additional booster dose of tetanus toxoid may be indicated; a protective antitoxin level is usually achieved within 1 week. It is common practice to use dT instead of tetanus toxoid alone in a child 7 years or older, so that adequate levels of diphtheria immunity are also maintained. Children younger than 7 years should receive DTaP (unless pertussis vaccine is contraindicated). A booster dose can provoke an adequate response after a 10-year lapse since the last injection. In severe, crush, and heavily contaminated wounds (particularly, compound skull fractures), human TIG (250 U) should be given intramuscularly in conjunction with the toxoid. This procedure should prevent a potential short-incubation period disease. Patients recovering from tetanus may not be immune; therefore they should be actively immunized with tetanus toxoid. Recent studies suggest that there is minimal, if any, risk of inducing Guillain-Barré syndrome following administration of tetanus toxoid (Tuttle et al., 1997).

Passive Immunization

Persons who have not been actively immunized should be protected with human TIG in the event of an injury. When TIG is required for wound prophylaxis, it is given intramuscularly (250 U). The dose used for prophylaxis is different from the treatment dose.

Care of a Wound

A wound should be cleansed thoroughly, foreign bodies and necrotic tissues should be removed, and the area should be débrided when indicated. Wounds containing devitalized tissue and those resulting from crush and avulsion injuries, as well as burns, are particularly prone to contamination with *C. tetani*.

BIBLIOGRAPHY

Adams JM, Kenny JD, Rudolph AJ. Modern management of tetanus neonatorum. Pediatrics 1979;64:472.

Armitage P, Clifford R. Prognosis in tetanus: use of data from therapeutic trials. J Infect Dis 1978;138:1-8.

Bagratuni L. Cephalic tetanus: with report of a case. BMJ 1952;1:461.

Bennett J, Ma C, Traverso H, et al. Neonatal tetanus associated with topical umbilical ghee. Int J Epidemiol 1999;28:1172.

Bizzini B. Tetanus toxin. Microbiol Rev 1979;43:224-240.

Bjerregaard P, Steinglass R, Mutie DM, et al. Neonatal tetanus mortality in coastal Kenya: a community survey. Int J Epidemiol 1993;22:163-169.

Brand DA, Acampora D, Gottlieb ZD, et al. Adequacy of antitetanus prophylaxis in six hospital emergency rooms. N Engl J Med 1983;309:636-640.

Brooks VB, Asanuma H. Action of tetanus toxin in the cerebral cortex. Science 1962;137:674.

Brooks VB, Curtis DR, Eccles JC. Mode of action of tetanus toxin. Nature 1955;175:120.

Christie AB. Infectious diseases: epidemiology and clinical practice. Baltimore: Williams & Wilkins, 1969.

Corradin G, Watts C. Cellular immunology of tetanus toxoid. Curr Top Microbiol Immunol 1995;195:77-87.

Dietz V, Milstien JB, van Loon F, et al. Performance and potency of tetanus toxoid: implications for eliminating neonatal tetanus. Bull World Health Org 1996;74:619-628.

Edmondson RS, Flowers MW. Intensive care in tetanus: management, complications, and mortality in 100 cases. BMJ 1979;1:1401.

Edsall G. Specific prophylaxis of tetanus. JAMA 1959;171:417.

Edsall G. Passive immunization. Pediatrics 1963;32:599.

Eidels L, Proia RL, Hart DA. Membrane receptors for bacterial toxins. Microbiol Rev 1983;47:596-620.

Einterz EM, Bates ME. Caring for neonatal tetanus patients in a rural primary care setting in Nigeria: a review of 237 cases. J Trop Pediatr 1991;37:179-181.

Galazka A, Gasse F. The present status of tetanus and tetanus vaccination. Curr Top Microbiol Immunol 1995;195:31-53.

Gerdes JS. Tetanus neonatorum. In Burg FD, Ingelfinger JR, Wald ER, Polin RA (eds). Gellis & Kagan's Current Pediatric Therapy, ed 15. Philadelphia: Saunders, 1995.

Goyal RK, Neogy CN, Mathur GP. A controlled trial of antiserum in the treatment of tetanus. Lancet 1966;2:1371.

Hlady WG, Bennett JV, Samadi AR, et al. Neonatal tetanus in rural Bangladesh: risk factors and toxoid efficacy. Am J Public Health 1992;82:1365-1369.

Kaeser HE, Sauer A. Tetanus toxin: a neuromuscular blocking agent. Nature 1969;223:842.

Kerr JH, et al. Involvement of the sympathetic nervous system in tetanus: studies on 82 cases. Lancet 1968;2:236.

Kessimer JG, Habig WH, Hardegree MC. Monoclonal antibodies as probes of tetanus toxin structure and function. Infect Immun 1983;42:942-948.

Laird WJ, Aronson W, Silver RP, et al. Plasmid-associated toxigenicity in *Clostridium tetani*. J Infect Dis 1980;142:623.

Levine L, Edsall G. Tetanus toxoid: what determines reaction proneness? J Infect Dis 1981;144:376.

Lichtenhan JB, Kellerman RD, Richards JF. Tetanus. A threat to elderly patients. Postgrad Med 1992;15:59.

Looney JM, Edsall G, Ispen J Jr, Chasen WH. Persistence of antitoxin levels after tetanus toxoid inoculation in adults and effects of a booster dose after intervals. N Engl J Med 1956;254:6.

Marie A, Morax V. Recherches sur l'absorption de la toxine tetanique. Ann Inst Pasteur 1902;16:818.

McCracken GH Jr, Dowell DL, Marshall FN. Double-blind trial of equine antitoxin and human immune globulin in tetanus neonatorum. Lancet 1971;1:1146.

Meyer H, Ransome F. Untersuchungen uber den Tetanus. Arch Exp Pathol Pharmakol 1903;49:369.

Patel JC, Mehta BC. Tetanus: study of 8,697 cases. Indian J Med Sci 1999;53:393.

Pratt EL. Clinical tetanus: a study of 56 cases, with special reference to methods of prevention and a plan for evaluating treatment. JAMA 1945;129:1243.

Rubbo SD, Suri JC. Passive immunization against tetanus with human immune globulin. BMJ 1962;2:79.

Rubinstein HM. Studies on human tetanus antitoxin. Am J Hyg 1962;76:276.

Schiavo G, Rossetto O, Tonello F, Montecucco C. Intracellular targets and metalloprotease activity of tetanus and botulism neurotoxins. Curr Top Microbiol Immunol 1995;195:257-274.

Singhi S, Jain V, Subramanian C. Post-neonatal tetanus: issues in intensive care management. Indian J Pediatr 2001;68:267.

Smolens J, Vogt A, Crawford MN, Stokes J Jr. The persistence in the human circulation of horse and human tetanus antitoxins. J Pediatr 1961;59:899.

Stanfield JP, Gall D, Braden PM. Single dose-antenatal tetanus immunization. Lancet 1973;1:215.

Tuttle J, Chen RT, Rantala H, Cherry JD, et al. The risk of Guillain-Barré syndrome after tetanus-toxoid–containing vaccines in adults and children in the United States. Am J Public Health 1997;87:1919.

Veronesi R. Clinical observations on 712 cases of tetanus subject to four different methods of treatment: 18.2 percent mortality rate under a new method of treatment. Am J Med Sci 1956;232:629.

World Health Organization. World Development Report 2000, Geneva, 2000, WHO.

Yaramis A, Tas MA. Neonatal tetanus in the southeast of Turkey: risk factors, and clinical and prognostic aspects. Review of 73 cases, 1990-1999. Turk J Pediatr 2000;42:272.

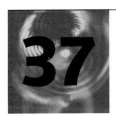

37 TICK-BORNE DISEASES

EUGENE D. SHAPIRO

Infections that are recognized as being transmitted by ticks in the United States have been increasing in both number and importance (Centers for Disease Control and Prevention, 2002; Fishbein and Dennis, 1995; Parola and Raoult, 2001; Spach et al., 1993). They include infections that have long been recognized, such as Rocky Mountain spotted fever and tick-borne relapsing fever, as well as "emerging" infections such as Lyme disease, ehrlichiosis, and babesiosis. A number of viruses, notably Powassan virus and the virus that causes Colorado tick fever in the United States, the virus that causes Congo-Crimean hemorrhagic fever in Africa, and the virus that causes tick-borne encephalitis in central Europe, also are transmitted by ticks. These viral illnesses are not covered in this chapter.

LYME DISEASE

Lyme disease is the most common vector-borne disease in the United States. Extensive publicity about the illness in the lay press, which at times has been accompanied by near hysteria about its risks and its complications, has resulted in anxiety about the illness (among physicians as well as among both patients and parents) that is out of proportion to the morbidity that it causes (Aronowitz, 1991; Shapiro and Gerber, 2000; Steere, 1989; Steere, 2001; Sigal, 1994). The clinical manifestations of Lyme disease are protean. This fact, coupled with the practical difficulties of confirming the diagnosis in many patients, has led to many misconceptions about both the symptoms and the prognosis of patients with Lyme disease—misconceptions that are reinforced by a high frequency of misdiagnosis of Lyme disease in persons with symptoms due to other conditions (Feder and Hunt, 1995; Reid et al., 1998; Sigal and Patella, 1992; Steere et al., 1993).

Etiology and Epidemiology

Lyme disease is caused by the spirochete *Borrelia burgdorferi*, a fastidious, microaerophilic bacterium that replicates very slowly and requires special, complex media for in vitro growth (Benach et al., 1983; Burgdorfer et al., 1982; Steere et al., 1983). Its cell membrane is covered by flagella and a loosely associated outer membrane. The major outer-surface proteins include OspA, OspB, and OspC (which are highly charged basic proteins of molecular weights of about 31, 34, and 23 kd, respectively), as well as the 41-kd flagellar protein, and are important targets for the immune response of humans. Based on studies of its DNA, the organism has been subclassified into several genospecies: *B. burgdorferi* sensu stricto, *B. garinii*, and *B. afzelii* (Shapiro and Gerber, 2000). In the United States, only *B. burgdorferi* sensu stricto has been isolated from humans. In contrast, there is substantial variability among isolates of *B. burgdorferi* from humans in Europe, most of which are either *B. garinii* or *B. afzelii*.

B. burgdorferi is transmitted by ticks of the *Ixodes* species. In the United States the common vectors are *Ixodes scapularis* (the black-legged tick), commonly called the deer tick, in both the Northeast and the upper Midwest, and *Ixodes pacificus* (the Western black-legged tick) on the Pacific Coast (Lane et al., 1991).

The life cycle of *I. scapularis* consists of three stages—larva, nymph, and adult—that develop during a 2-year period (Lane et al., 1991). The adult female lays eggs in the spring. The larvae emerge in the early summer. Most larvae (98%) are born uninfected with *B. burgdorferi*, because transovarial transmission rarely occurs. The larvae feed on a wide variety of small mammals, such as *Peromyscus leucopus* (the white-footed mouse), which are natural reservoirs for *B. burgdorferi*. A deer tick may become infected with *B. burgdorferi* by feeding on a mouse or another small mammal that is infected with the spirochete. The tick emerges the following spring as a nymph. In this stage the tick (if it is infected with *B. burgdorferi*) may transmit the infection to humans. Indeed, it is at this stage of development that the tick is most likely to transmit infections to humans (Nadelman et al., 2001), presumably because the nymphs are active at times that humans are most likely to be in tick-infested areas and because they are very small and difficult to recognize. Alternatively, if the nymph is uninfected with *B. burgdorferi*, it may subsequently become infected if it feeds on an infected host. The nymphs molt in the late summer or fall and then reemerge as adults. If the adult is infected, it also may transmit *B. burgdorferi* to humans. The female spends the winter on an animal host, a favorite being white-tailed deer (hence the name *deer tick*). In the spring the females lay their eggs and die, thereby completing the 2-year life cycle.

There are a number of factors associated with the risk of transmission of *B. burgdorferi* from ticks to humans. First, a tick has to be infected to be able to transmit the organism. The proportion of infected ticks varies greatly both by geographic area and by the stage of the tick in its life cycle. *I. pacificus* often feeds on lizards, which are not a competent reservoir for *B. burgdorferi*. Consequently, only 1% to 3% of these ticks, even in the nymphal and adult stages, are infected with *B. burgdorferi*. As a result, Lyme disease is rare in the Pacific states. By contrast, *I. scapularis* feeds on small mammals that are competent reservoirs for *B. burgdorferi*. As a result, in highly endemic areas the rates of infection of deer ticks are, approximately, 2% for larvae, 15% to 30% for nymphs, and 37% to 50% for adults.

B. burgdorferi is transmitted when an infected tick inoculates saliva into the blood vessels of the skin of its host. The risk of transmission of *B. burgdorferi* from infected deer ticks has been shown to be related to the duration of feeding. It takes hours for the mouth parts of ticks to implant fully in the host, and much longer (days) for the tick to become fully engorged. In infected ticks, *B. burgdorferi* is found primarily in the midgut of the tick, but as the tick feeds and becomes engorged, the bacteria migrate to the salivary glands, from which they can be transmitted to the host.

Experiments with animals have shown that infected nymphal-stage ticks must feed for 48 hours or longer, and infected adult ticks must feed for 72 hours or longer before the risk of transmission of *B. burgdorferi* becomes substantial (Piesman et al., 1987; Piesman et al., 1991; Piesman, 1993). These experimental results have been corroborated in a study of humans, in which the duration of feeding by nymphal-stage ticks was estimated for a proportion of the subjects (Nadelman et al., 2001). The risk of Lyme disease was 0% among persons bitten by nymphs that had fed for <72 hours but was 25% among persons bitten by nymphs that had fed for ≥72 hours. Approximately 75% of persons who recognize that they have been bitten by a deer tick remove the tick <48 hours after it has begun to feed (Falco et al., 1996). This explains why only a small proportion of persons who recognize that they've been bitten by deer ticks subsequently develop Lyme disease. Indeed, the risk of Lyme disease is greater from unrecognized bites, because in such instances the tick is able to feed for a longer time.

There is substantial evidence that the risk of Lyme disease after a recognized deer tick bite, even in hyperendemic areas, is only from 1% to 3% (Nadelman et al., 2001; Shapiro et al., 1992). A double-blind randomized trial of antimicrobial prophylaxis for ticks bites conducted in Westchester County, New York, found that a single, 200-mg dose of doxycycline was 87% effective in preventing Lyme disease in adults and adolescents, although the 95% confidence interval around this estimate of efficacy was wide (the lower bound was 25% or less, depending on the method used) (Nadelman et al., 2001). In that study, the only persons who developed Lyme disease had been bitten by nymphal-stage ticks that were at least partially engorged; among recipients of placebo, the risk of Lyme disease among persons bitten by an engorged nymphal-stage tick was 9.9%, whereas it was 0% for bites by all larval and adult deer ticks. Unfortunately, the expertise to identify the species, stage, and degree of engorgement of a tick, and thereby to assess the degree of risk, is rarely available to persons who are bitten. Many "ticks" are actually spiders, lice, scabs, or dirt, and thus cannot transmit Lyme disease. Consequently, routine use of antimicrobial agents to prevent Lyme disease in persons who are bitten by a deer tick, even in highly endemic areas, is still not generally recommended because the overall risk of Lyme disease is low (1% to 3%), treatment for Lyme disease, if it does develop, is very effective, and a substantial proportion of patients who take doxycycline develop nausea and/or vomiting (Shapiro, 2001). Although some argue in favor of antimicrobial prophylaxis for persons with bites associated with high risk (e.g., a nymphal-stage tick that has fed for >48 hours), estimates of the duration of feeding by patients are unreliable (Schwartz et al., 1993). Moreover, selective treatment of persons with "high-risk" tick bites assumes that the species, stage, and degree of engorgement of the ticks can be readily ascertained, which usually is not the case; special training and equipment are necessary. In the unusual instance in which doxycycline prophylaxis is used (e.g., in a patient who removes a fully engorged nymphal-stage deer tick in an endemic area), only a single dose of doxycycline (200 mg) should be prescribed, and it should taken with food to minimize nausea.

Ascertainment of whether the tick is infected, using tests such as the polymerase chain reaction (PCR) assay, is not recommended. Although testing ticks with PCR may provide important epidemiologic information, the predictive value for infection of humans of either a positive or a negative PCR test result is unknown. The result may be positive even if only very few organisms are present, and it provides no information about the duration of feeding, a key determinant of the risk of transmission. In addition, the problems of both false-positive results due to contamination with amplification products and false-negative results due to inhibition of the PCR by substances (such as blood) in the sample limit the test's validity.

Although Lyme disease occurs throughout the world, most cases occur in a few highly endemic areas. In the United States, most cases occur in southern New England, New York, New Jersey, Pennsylvania, Minnesota, and Wisconsin (Figure 37-1) (Centers for Disease Control and Prevention, 2002). In Europe, most cases occur in the Scandinavian countries and in central Europe (especially in Germany, Austria, and Switzerland), although cases have been reported from throughout the region.

Although there has been an increase in frequency and an expansion of the geographic distribution of Lyme disease in the United States in recent years, the incidence of Lyme disease even in endemic areas varies substantially both from region to region and within local areas (Centers for Disease Control and Prevention, 2002). Information about the incidence of the disease is complicated by reliance, in most instances, on passive reporting of cases as well as by the

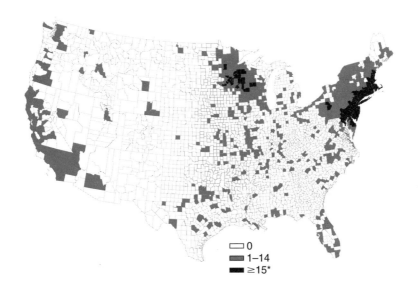

0
1–14
≥15*

*Total number of cases from these counties represented 90% of all cases in 2000.

Fig. 37-1 Number of cases of Lyme disease—United States, 2000. Total number of cases from counties with ≥15 cases represented 90% of all cases. (From MMWR Morb Mortal Wkly Rep 2002;51:29-31.)

high frequency of misdiagnosis of the disease. Furthermore, studies have indicated that some patients who develop serologic evidence of recent infection with *B. burgdorferi* are asymptomatic (Hanrahan et al., 1984; Steere et al., 1986).

A total of 17,730 cases of Lyme disease were reported to the Centers for Disease Control and Prevention (CDC) by 44 states and the District of Columbia in 2000 (a 9% increase from 1999) (Centers for Disease Control and Prevention, 2002) (Figure 37-2). Approximately 90% of the reported cases occurred in just 124 counties (Figure 37-1).

Clinical Manifestations

Lyme disease generally is divided into three clinical stages: early localized disease, early disseminated disease, and late disease (Shapiro and Gerber, 2000; Steere, 1989). The first clinical manifestation of Lyme disease is the typical annular rash, erythema migrans (Figure 37-3) at the site of the bite. The onset of the rash usually occurs 7 to 14 days after the bite, with a reported range of from 3 to 32 days. The initial lesion occurs at the site of the bite. The rash most often is uniformly erythematous, although it may appear as a target lesion with variable degrees of central clearing. Occasionally there may be a vesicular or necrotic center. The rash may be itchy, painful, or asymptomatic. There may or may not be associated systemic symptoms such as fever, myalgia, headache or malaise. Untreated, the rash gradually expands

(hence the name "migrans") to an average diameter of 15 cm, although lesions larger than 30 cm can occur. Without treatment it will remain present for 2 weeks or longer.

A substantial proportion of children with Lyme disease (about one third) develop early-disseminated disease, the most common manifestation of which is multiple erythema migrans, which is a consequence of bacteremia with dissemination of organisms to multiple sites in the skin. Secondary lesions usually are smaller than the primary lesion and are often accompanied by fever, myalgia, headache, and fatigue; conjunctivitis and lymphadenopathy also may develop. Occasionally, when the erythema migrans rash resolves, new evanescent lesions, which usually are small (1- to 3-cm) erythematous annular lesions, appear transiently over a period of several weeks at differ-

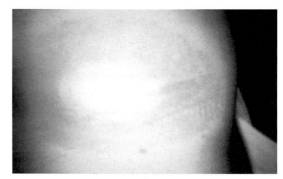

Fig. 37-3 Erythema migrans.

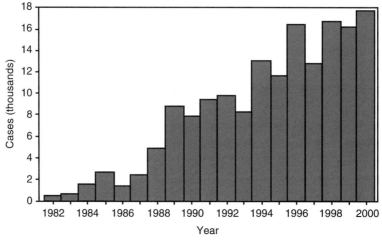

Fig. 37-2 Number of cases of Lyme disease—United States, 1982-2000. (From MMWR Morb Mortal Wkly Rep 2002;51;29-31.)

ent sites. Aseptic meningitis may occur (about 1% of patients). Carditis, usually marked by varying degrees of heart block, also may occur at this stage of Lyme disease, although it is rare (<1% of patients).

Focal neurologic involvement, in particular cranioneuropathy, also is a manifestation of this stage of the illness. Paralysis of the seventh cranial nerve is relatively common in children (3% to 5% of patients) and may be the only manifestation of Lyme disease. Paralysis usually lasts from 2 to 8 weeks before it resolves completely. Rarely, palsy resolves only partially or not at all. There is no evidence that the clinical course of the facial palsy is affected by antimicrobial treatment (the goal of treatment of affected children is to treat or to prevent other manifestations of Lyme disease). Radiculoneuritis, manifesting as radicular pain with motor and sensory abnormalities of peripheral nerves, has been reported, although it is more common among adults and in Europe.

The usual manifestation of late Lyme disease (which occurs in about 7% of patients) is oligoar-ticular arthritis; it usually occurs months after the initial infection. The large joints, especially the knee (which is affected in more than 90% of cases), are usually involved (Eichenfield et al., 1986; Gerber et al., 1996). Although the affected joint is swollen and tender, the patient usually does not experience the exquisite pain that is typical of acute bacterial arthritis. Joint swelling usually resolves within 1 to 2 weeks (although it may last for several weeks) before recurring (in virtually all untreated patients), often in other joints. After treatment is begun, the arthritis usually abates over 4 to 7 days, although in some patients it may take 2 to 6 weeks before the symptoms completely resolve. Rarely, arthritis recurs in treated patients, but it usually resolves with retreatment. Chronic arthritis can occur, primarily among patients with DR-2, DR-3 or DR-4 HLA-types (Steere et al., 1990). The pathogenesis of this chronic, recurrent arthritis is most likely autoimmune (Gross et al., 1998). Late manifestations of Lyme disease of the central nervous system (CNS) rarely have been reported in children.

In the largest prospective study of children with Lyme disease that has been reported (a community-based study of 201 children with Lyme disease in Connecticut who were enrolled from April 1992 through November 1993), the median age of the children was 7 years (Gerber et al., 1996). The initial (presenting) manifestations of Lyme disease in these children were single erythema migrans (66%), multiple erythema migrans (23%), arthritis (7%), facial palsy (3%), aseptic meningitis (1%) and carditis (0.5%). Erythema migrans was more likely to occur on either the head or neck in younger children and on the extremities in older children, a finding similar to those reported from Europe. As in studies of primarily adults, only about one third of the children with a single erythema migrans rash had positive serology for *B. burgdorferi* at the time of presentation, whereas almost 90% of the children with multiple erythema migrans were seropositive. Of the patients with a single erythema migrans rash, 45% had had a recognized tick bite in the preceding month, but in only about half of these children was the recognized bite at the site of the rash (which indicates that the infection was transmitted by a different, unrecognized tick).

Congenital Lyme Disease

Because clinical syndromes caused by congenital infection have been recognized with other spirochetal infections such as syphilis, there has been concern about the possible transmission of *B. burgdorferi* from an infected pregnant woman to her fetus. Although case reports have been published in which *B. burgdorferi* has been identified from abortuses and from a few live-born children with congenital anomalies, the placentas, the abortuses, and the tissues from affected children in which the spirochete was identified did not show histologic evidence of inflammation. In addition, no consistent pattern of congenital malformations (as would be expected in a "syndrome" due to congenital infection) has been identified. In two small longitudinal studies of pregnant women who developed Lyme disease that were conducted by the CDC and in another study conducted in the Czech Republic, the occasional adverse outcomes that occurred (such as spontaneous abortion) could not be attributed to infection with *B. burgdorferi*. In addition, two serosurveys conducted in endemic areas found no difference in the prevalence of congenital malformations among the offspring of women with serum antibodies against *B. burgdorferi* and the offspring of those without such antibodies (Nadal et al., 1989; Williams et al., 1988). In the most comprehensive study of Lyme disease in pregnancy, investigators prospectively studied

2,000 pregnant women in Westchester County, New York (Strobino et al., 1993). Although the number of exposed women was relatively small, no association was found between a mother's exposure to *B. burgdorferi* either before conception or during pregnancy and fetal death, prematurity, or congenital malformations.

To assess the frequency of clinically significant neurologic disorders attributable to congenital infection with *B. burgdorferi*, Gerber conducted a survey of all pediatric neurologists in areas of the country in which Lyme disease is endemic (Connecticut, Rhode Island, Massachusetts, New York, New Jersey, Wisconsin, and Minnesota) (Gerber and Zalneraitis, 1994). Of the 162 pediatric neurologists who responded to the survey (92%), none had seen a child with a clinically significant neurologic disorder that was attributed to congenital Lyme disease or whose mother had Lyme disease during her pregnancy. Thus, there is no definitive evidence that *B. burgdorferi* causes congenital disease. If it does occur, congenital Lyme disease is extremely rare. Transmission of Lyme disease through breast-feeding has not been documented.

Diagnosis

The diagnosis of Lyme disease, especially in the absence of the characteristic rash, may be difficult, because the other clinical manifestations of Lyme disease are not specific. Clinically, seventh nerve palsy due to Lyme disease is indistinguishable from idiopathic Bell's palsy, and Lyme meningitis may mimic viral meningitis. The manifestations of Lyme arthritis may be indistinguishable from arthritis due to other causes in children, such as juvenile rheumatoid arthritis or HLA-B27 arthritis. Even the diagnosis of erythema migrans sometimes may be difficult, because the rash initially may be confused with nummular eczema, cellulitis, granuloma annulare, an insect bite, or tinea (ringworm). However, the relatively rapid expansion of erythema migrans helps to distinguish it from these other conditions.

Because the sensitivity of culture for *B. burgdorferi* is poor and it is necessary for patients to undergo an invasive procedure such as a biopsy or a lumbar puncture to obtain appropriate tissue or fluid for culture, such tests are indicated only in rare circumstances. Likewise, although preliminary studies in research laboratories suggest that PCR assay is a promising diagnostic test (Rosa and Schwan, 1989), its accuracy

when used under nonexperimental conditions (especially in commercial laboratories rather than in research laboratories) has not been established. Consequently, the confirmation of either early disseminated or late Lyme disease by the laboratory usually rests on the demonstration of antibodies to *B. burgdorferi* in the patient's serum. It is well documented that the sensitivity and specificity of antibody tests for Lyme disease vary substantially. The accuracy of prepackaged commercial kits is much poorer than that of tests performed by reference laboratories that maintain tight quality control and regularly prepare the materials that are used in the test (Bacterial Zoonoses Branch, 1991; Bakken et al., 1992; Bakken et al., 1997).

The use of Western immunoblots improves the specificity of serologic testing for Lyme disease (Dressler et al., 1993). Official recommendations from the Second National Conference on Serologic Diagnosis of Lyme Disease suggest that clinicians use a two-step procedure when ordering antibody tests for Lyme disease: first, a sensitive screening test, either an enzyme-linked immunosorbent assay (ELISA) or an immunofluorescent assay (IFA), and, if that result is positive or equivocal, a Western immunoblot to confirm the result (Centers for Disease Control and Prevention, 1995). If the ELISA or the IFA is negative, an immunoblot is not necessary. Of course, antibody tests are not useful for the diagnosis of early-localized Lyme disease, because only a minority of patients with single erythema migrans will have a positive test.

As with any diagnostic test, the predictive value of antibody tests for Lyme disease (even of very accurate tests) is highly dependent on the prevalence of the infection among patients who are tested. Unfortunately, because many patients as well as many physicians have the erroneous impression that nonspecific symptoms alone (e.g., headache, fatigue, or arthralgia) may be manifestations of Lyme disease, parents of children with only nonspecific symptoms frequently demand that a child be tested for Lyme disease (and some physicians routinely order tests for Lyme disease on such patients). Lyme disease will be the cause of the nonspecific symptoms in very few such children, if any. However, because the specificity of even excellent antibody tests for Lyme disease rarely exceeds 90% to 95%, some of the test results in children without specific signs or symptoms of Lyme disease will be positive; the vast majority of these (>90%) will be false-positive results (Seltzer and Shapiro, 1996; Tugwell et al., 1997). Nevertheless, an erroneous diagnosis of Lyme disease based on the results of these tests frequently is made, and such children often are treated unnecessarily with antimicrobial agents. In addition, even if a symptomatic patient has a serologic test that is positive for antibodies to *B. burgdorferi*, it is possible that Lyme disease may not be the cause of that patient's symptoms. In addition to the possibility that the positive test result is false (by far the most common occurrence), the patient may have been infected with *B. burgdorferi* previously, and the patient's symptoms may be unrelated to that previous infection. In the latter instance, the positive test is accurate, but the test is "falsely positive" in terms of the cause of the patient's symptoms. Once serum antibodies to *B. burgdorferi* develop, they may persist for many years (both IgG and IgM antibodies) despite adequate treatment and clinical cure of the disease (Feder et al., 1992; Hilton et al., 1997; Kalish et al., 2001). In addition, because a substantial proportion of people who become infected with *B. burgdorferi* never develop symptoms, in endemic areas there will be a background rate of seropositivity among patients who have never had clinically apparent Lyme disease. When patients with previous Lyme disease (whether asymptomatic and untreated or clinically apparent and adequately treated) develop any kind of symptoms and are tested for antibodies against *B. burgdorferi*, their symptoms may erroneously be attributed to active Lyme disease. For all of these reasons, misdiagnosis is a common clinical problem (Feder and Hunt, 1995; Reid et al., 1998; Seltzer and Shapiro, 1996; Sigal 1994; Sigal 1996; Sigal and Patella, 1992; Steere et al., 1993).

Treatment

Recommendations for the treatment of children with Lyme disease have been extrapolated from studies of adults, because no clinical trials of treatment have been conducted among children (Shapiro and Gerber, 2000; Wormser et al., 2000). Either doxycycline or amoxicillin are used to treat most manifestations of Lyme disease, except that meningitis and severe carditis are treated with parenterally administered penicillin or ceftriaxone. Children <9 years of age should not be treated with doxycycline because it may cause permanent discoloration of their teeth. Cefuroxime is an effective alternative agent. The macrolides (including erythromycin and azithromycin) are somewhat less effective clinically than these agents, though they are alternatives for persons who cannot take any of the above-cited drugs. Jarisch-Herxheimer reactions, manifest as increased temperature with myalgia and arthralgia as a result of release of toxins as organisms are killed shortly after antimicrobial treatment is begun, occur infrequently.

Symptoms such as fatigue, arthralgia, and myalgia sometimes persist for some time after completion of a course of treatment for Lyme disease. These nonspecific symptoms (which may accompany or follow more specific symptoms and signs of Lyme disease but almost never are the sole presenting manifestations of Lyme disease) generally resolve over a period of weeks to months. There is no evidence that such symptoms are related to persistence of the organism. Likewise, there is no evidence that repeated courses of antimicrobial agents speed the resolution of such symptoms. Indeed, the results of two double-blind, randomized clinical trials of treatment of persons who believed that they had "chronic Lyme disease" after being treated for an episode of Lyme disease indicated that the outcomes of such persons who underwent long-term treatment with antibiotics (3 months, 1 month of which was with ceftriaxone) was no better than the outcomes of controls treated with placebo (Klempner et al., 2001). Finally, antibodies against *B. burgdorferi* will persist for many years after successful treatment of symptoms (Kalish et al., 2001). There is no reason routinely to obtain follow-up tests of antibody concentrations against *B. burgdorferi*.

Prognosis

Despite the widespread misconception that Lyme disease is difficult to treat successfully and that chronic symptoms and clinical recurrences are common, in fact, the most common reason for failure of treatment is misdiagnosis (i.e., the patient actually does not have Lyme disease). Likewise, Lyme disease does not require either multiple courses or prolonged treatment (although retreatment is recommended for the occasional patient with late disease who develops objective signs of relapse, such as frank arthritis). Nonspecific symptoms such as arthralgia or fatigue that occur long after treatment should not be attributed to failure of treatment.

The prognosis for children treated for Lyme disease is excellent (Shapiro, 2002). In a review of 65 children who were treated for erythema migrans, at follow-up a mean of more than 3 years later all of the children were well and none had developed symptoms of late Lyme disease (Salazaar et al., 1993). In a larger, prospective follow-up study of 201 children with newly diagnosed Lyme disease of all stages (though most had early-localized or early-disseminated disease), at follow-up a mean of 2.5 years later all of the children were clinically cured (Gerber et al., 1996). The long-term prognosis for patients who are treated for late Lyme disease also is excellent. Although recurrences of arthritis do occur rarely, especially among patients with the DR-2, DR-3, or DR-4 HLA-type, most children who are treated for Lyme arthritis are permanently cured (Adams et al., 1994; Salazaar et al. 1993). One group of investigators performed neuropsychologic tests on children with Lyme disease up to 4 years after they were treated and found no evidence of any long-term sequelae of the infection (Gerber et al., 1998). Other investigators who conducted a community-based study of the long-term outcomes of persons with Lyme disease also found no evidence of impairment of normal functioning in children 4 to 11 years after they were diagnosed with Lyme disease (Seltzer et al., 2000).

Prevention

In endemic areas it is very common for children to be bitten by deer ticks. Such bites often engender tremendous anxiety. However, the overall risk of acquiring Lyme disease is low (approximately 1% to 3%) even in areas in which Lyme disease is endemic. Furthermore, treatment of the infection, if it develops, is highly effective. Consequently, the routine administration of antimicrobial prophylaxis for persons who have been bitten by a deer tick is not recommended (as discussed above). The routine testing of ticks that have been removed from humans for infection with *B. burgdorferi* also is not recommended, because the predictive value of a positive test for infection in the human host is unknown.

A more reasonable approach to preventing Lyme disease is to wear appropriate protective clothing (such as lightweight long pants) when entering tick-infested areas and to check for and to remove ticks after spending time in such areas. Insect repellants may provide temporary protection, but they may be absorbed from the skin and, if used frequently or in large doses, they may produce significant toxicity, especially in children.

A vaccine for Lyme disease that uses recombinant outer surface protein A (rOspA) as the antigen is approved for persons 15 to 70 years of age (Advisory Committee on Immunization Practices, 1999; Steere et al., 1998). LYMErix (GlaxoSmithKline, Research Triangle Park, North Carolina) contains 30 µg of purified rOspA lipidated protein combined with 0.5 mg of aluminum adjuvant. The efficacy of Lyme vaccine in preventing clinically apparent Lyme disease was 49% (95% confidence interval: 15% to 69%) in the first year, after two doses (Steere et al., 1998). After the third dose, the vaccine's efficacy in preventing symptomatic Lyme disease was 76% (95% confidence interval: 58% to 86%). Three doses of the vaccine are required for optimal protection in adults (the vaccine is more immunogenic in children [Feder et al., 1999; Sikand et al., 2001]); the second dose is given one month after the first dose and the third dose is given 12 months after the first dose. Preliminary data suggest that other immunization schedules (e.g., 0, 1, 6 months or 0, 1, 2 months) are safe and induce antibody responses similar to the 0, 1, 12–month schedule.

This rOspA vaccine has a unique mode of action. OspA is expressed by *B. burgdorferi* that reside in the midguts of ticks; expression of OspA is later downregulated in response to a blood meal. Because ticks must become engorged with blood before they transmit the organism, the human host who becomes infected with *B. burgdorferi* has little exposure to the OspA protein (at least in the early stages of infection). When an immunized host is bitten by a tick infected with *B. burgdorferi*, the host's vaccine-induced antibodies against OspA are ingested by the tick. Antibody-dependent killing of *B. burgdorferi* occurs within the tick, thereby preventing transmission to the host. However, because the host is not directly exposed to the OspA antigen, boosting of the immune response to OspA through natural exposure does not occur. Consequently, it is likely that additional booster doses of the vaccine would be needed to maintain immunity. Studies suggest that Lyme disease is cost effective only if the patient's risk of Lyme disease is extremely high (>1%/year) (Shadick et al., 2001). Official recommendations were that the vaccine should be *considered* for persons in endemic areas who are at increased risk of Lyme disease because of either occupational or recreational exposure. For most people the potential benefits of the vaccine (compared with other protective measures, including early diagnosis and treatment of Lyme disease) were outweighed by its cost and adverse side effects; the risk of Lyme disease is relatively low for most people in endemic areas, the vaccine was expensive, the vaccine was associated with a high rate of minor adverse effects such as pain and swelling at the site of the injection (it has not been shown to cause serious adverse effects [Lathrop et al., 2002]), and multiple doses of the vaccine are likely to be required. In early 2002, the manufacturer announced that it no longer would make Lyme vaccine because it was not profitable.

Coinfections

Both babesiosis and human granulocytic ehrlichiosis are also transmitted by the deer tick. Consequently, coinfection with either or both of these infections can occur (Nadelman et al., 1997; Thompson et al., 2001; Wang et al., 2000). Detailed discussion of each of these infections can be found later in this chapter. Although coinfection in children clearly does occur, in most cases it is subclinical (it is not apparent that child has more than just Lyme disease), and the outcomes of persons with coinfection appear not to be different from the outcomes of persons with Lyme disease alone (unless the patient is immunocompromised).

RELAPSING FEVER

There are two different vectors, ticks and lice, that transmit the bacteria that cause relapsing fever in humans. Louse-borne relapsing fever, caused by *Borrelia recurrentis*, is transmitted by the body louse, *Pediculus humanus*. This section focuses on tick-borne recurrent fever.

Etiology and Epidemiology

The *Borrelia* organisms that cause recurrent fever are fastidious, microaerophilic spirochetal bacteria that are characterized morphologically by coarse and irregularly shaped coils and were first identified in 1873 in the blood of a patient with recurrent fever. Tick-borne relapsing fever is caused by many different species of *Borrelia*, including *Borrelia duttonii*, *Borrelia hermsii*, *Borrelia parkeri*, and *Borrelia mazzottii*. These bacteria are able to change the antigenic structure of their surface proteins by transposition of structural genes on a linear plasmid, which allows them temporarily to elude host defenses and results in "relapsing fever" in infected humans (Barbour et al., 1983; Barbour et al., 2000; Plasterk et al., 1985; Stoenner et al., 1982). The bacteria reversibly change their major outer surface protein when transmitted from ticks to mammals (Schwan and Hinnebusch, 1998). The resolution of symptomatic stages of the illness correlates with peaks in the concentrations of antibodies against the specific antigens of the circulating strain. The bacteria cause a vasculitis, with a predilection for capillaries and small arterioles of any organs, especially the reticuloendothelial system, the bone marrow, and the CNS.

Tick-borne relapsing fever is transmitted by various species of soft ticks of the genus *Ornithodoros*. Many small animals (chipmunks, rats, mice, squirrels, and others) serve both as reservoirs for these species of *Borrelia* and as hosts for *Ornithodoros* ticks (Felsenfeld, 1965). There is variable transovarial transmission of the bacteria to larval stages of the ticks and there is a well-established enzootic cycle in certain areas of the United States. The ticks thrive in warm, humid environments and at altitudes of 1,500 to 6,500 feet. Unlike the hard *Ixodes* ticks that transmit *B. burgdorferi* and *Babesia microti*, which feed for days, soft ticks feed for a much shorter time (5 to 30 minutes), yet are able to transmit the bacteria during this relatively brief period. Although there is some uncertainty as to the exact mode of transmission, it is generally believed that transmission occurs when either excrement or saliva from an infected tick comes into contact with the wound produced by the tick's bite. The ticks often feed at night. Although humans are the only hosts for *B. recurrentis* (the cause of louse-borne recurrent fever), humans are incidental hosts for the bacteria that cause tick-borne relapsing fever. Humans become infected when they enter or live in environments in which the ticks thrive, such as old cabins and caves.

Tick-borne recurrent fever has a worldwide distribution. The disease is endemic in parts of East Africa, Asia, and South America. In the United States most cases occur in rural areas in the Western states. Outbreaks have occurred among spelunkers and in tourists who stayed in log cabins at Grand Canyon National Park and elsewhere (Boyer et al., 1977; Dworkin et al., 1998; Edall et al., 1979; Trevejo et al., 1998).

Clinical Manifestations

Tick-borne and louse-borne relapsing fevers are indistinguishable from each other clinically, although tick-borne disease tends to have more (although less severe) recurrences (Dworkin et al., 1998; Horton and Blaser, 1985; Le, 1980; Southern and Sanford, 1969). It is thought that the symptoms of relapsing fever begin from 5 to 10 days after exposure, with the sudden onset of fever and chills, usually accompanied by headache, myalgia, arthralgia, photophobia, and cough. Petechiae, purpura, conjunctivitis, nuchal rigidity, hepatosplenomegaly, and jaundice are common. This phase of the illness is associated with bacteremia, which usually lasts for from 3 to 7 days, after which the fever rapidly resolves.

In the subsequent phase of the illness patients are afebrile or have only low-grade fever and often have a diffuse maculopapular rash accompanied by diaphoresis, extreme fatigue, and, occasionally, hypotension. During this phase of the illness cultures of the blood are sterile. It is presumed that organisms multiply and develop antigenically different strains in the spleen or the liver. The relapse phase of the illness (which usually occurs 5 to 7 days after the primary bacteremia resolves) is again marked by the rapid onset of high fever and chills. In untreated patients, three to five relapses may occur.

Laboratory Findings and Diagnosis

Laboratory findings are nonspecific and usually include leukocytosis (with a shift to the left) and a markedly elevated erythrocyte sedimentation rate, as well as a mononuclear pleocytosis in the CSF. To make the diagnosis, awareness of the epidemiologic history is important. A history of recent visits to caves, old cabins, or other environments where rodents are common should make one consider relapsing fever in the differential diagnosis of patients with unexplained, persistent, or relapsing fever.

Routine cultures of the blood are not useful in making the diagnosis of relapsing fever because special media are required for the bacteria to grow. However, during the febrile phases of relapsing fever the concentrations of the organism in the blood are very high, and the diagnosis often can be made by examining smears of the peripheral blood by darkfield microscopy or by examining smears stained with Wright's stain, Giemsa stain, or acridine orange.

Treatment and Prognosis

Tetracycline is the drug of choice for treating relapsing fever. In children younger than 8 years of age erythromycin and penicillin are other options. Treatment is administered four times a day for 7 to 10 days. If vomiting is severe, the initial dose of the antimicrobial agent may be administered intravenously, although this may induce a severe Jarisch-Herxheimer reaction (the result of the release of toxins in association with lysis of the spirochetes). These reactions may be prevented by treatment with antibodies against tumor necrosis factor–α (Fekade et al., 1996).

Relapsing fever usually resolves even in untreated patients. Death is rare, although it does occasionally occur as a result of a ruptured spleen, severe hepatitis, myocarditis, or cerebral hemorrhage. Long-term sequelae are uncommon among those who survive. Iridocyclitis may result in scars and impaired vision. Pregnant women who become infected often abort, in most instances because of thrombocytopenia and retroplacental hemorrhage.

Prevention

The primary means of preventing tick-borne relapsing fever is the avoidance of the ticks that transmit this disease. The use of insecticides around the inner walls of old wooden buildings and huts (where ticks often are found) may help to prevent the disease (Talbert et al., 1998).

TULAREMIA

Tularemia is caused by *Francisella tularensis*, a small, fastidious, pleomorphic gram-negative coccobacillus. The bacterium was named after Edward Francis, who conducted early studies of tularemia, and can be acquired either from ticks or by direct contact with the organism (Francis, 1925). Because of the potential for transmission of infection by aerosol, there has been increased interest in the potential use of this bacterium as an agent for bioterrorism (Dennis et al., 2001).

Etiology and Epidemiology

There are two biovars of *F. tularensis*: type A and the less virulent type B. These strains were characterized on the basis of biologic rather than antigenic differences, although PCR-based diagnostic methods are being developed (Johansson et al., 2000). Both biovars are prevalent in the United States. Biovar A, found only in North America, is found in rabbits and in ticks (primarily *Amblyomma americanum*—the Lone Star tick—in the southern and southeastern states; *Dermacentor variabilis*—the dog tick—in eastern states; and *Dermacentor andersoni*—the wood tick—in western states) (Hopla, 1974). The reservoir for biovar B is primarily water-dwelling rodents, such as beavers and muskrats. It is found throughout the world in temperate areas of the northern hemisphere and often causes subclinical infections.

F. tularensis is highly infectious; exposure to as few as 10 organisms can cause infection in humans. *F. tularensis* infects humans through either the skin (typically from the bite of an infected tick or through a wound) or the mucosa (e.g., via the conjunctivae or the upper respiratory tract). Transmission may occur via tick bites (about 50% of cases), via either bites from or direct contact with tissues of infected animals, via inhalation of organisms, or via the ingestion of infected meat or contaminated water. From 100 to 300 cases of tularemia are reported to the CDC each year, most of which occur in the southern states (Guerrant et al., 1976; Taylor et al., 1991).

Clinical Manifestations

The clinical manifestations of tularemia depend, in large part, on the route of inoculation (Feldman et al., 200; Jacobs and Narain, 1983; Jacobs et al., 1985; Perez-Castrillon et al., 2001). Ulceroglandular tularemia (the most common form of the illness) is a result of inoculation of the organism from an infected tick. The incubation period of tularemia transmitted by ticks is 3 to 7 days (Evans et al., 1985). This form of the illness is characterized by an ulcer at the site of the bite, as well as local and regional lymph nodes that are tender and enlarged. Fever and other systemic symptoms may accompany the illness. Without treatment, the ulcer at the site of the bite may persist for weeks. Rarely, tick-borne disease may cause a flulike illness without involvement of either the skin or the lymph nodes. Oculoglandular tularemia devel-ops from primary infection of the conjunctivae (often from fingers that were contaminated through contact with infected animals, usually rabbits). Ingestion of contaminated foods may cause oropharyngeal tularemia (which may simulate diphtheria), gastrointestinal tularemia (marked by diarrhea and abdominal pain) or a typhoidal form of tularemia that is associated with fever and a sepsislike picture. Pneumonia, which may rapidly be fatal, is due to inhalation of aerosolized organisms. Any form of the illness may be characterized by the sudden onset of fever, headache, chills, myalgia, and fatigue. However, the severity of tick-borne illness is highly variable and sometimes may be mild and self-limited (Markowitz et al., 1985).

Diagnosis

Because of the substantial risk to laboratory personnel, most laboratories will not culture the organism, although it may grow on media used for other bacteria. Consequently, the diagnosis of tularemia is usually based on the presence of agglutinating antibodies to *F. tularensis*. A four-fold increase in concentration of agglutinins between acute and convalescent sera is considered to be diagnostic of infection. A single titer of ≥1:160 in a patient with a history and clinical symptoms compatible with tularemia strongly suggests the diagnosis. Tests that use PCR to detect the organisms in the blood have been developed (Dolan et al., 1998; Fulop et al., 1996; Johansson et al., 2000a; Junhui et al., 1996; Long et al., 1993; Sjostedt et al., 1997).

Treatment and Prognosis

Because agglutinins may not appear until near the end of the second week after infection begins, if tularemia is suspected the patient should be treated empirically. Streptomycin was once the treatment of choice, although gentamicin or amikacin may be equally effective (Enderlin et al., 1994). Newer studies indicate that fluoroquinolones such as ciprofloxacin may be as effective as parenteral agents, with fewer side effects (Johansson et al., 2000b; Limaye and Hooper, 1999). Patients usually have a clinical response to treatment within 48 hours, and should be treated for 7 to 10 days. Most patients who receive antimicrobial treatment have a complete recovery. The mortality rate of patients with tularemia is about 3%; fatalities occur primarily in patients with either pneumonia or the typhoidal form of the disease.

Prevention

Minimizing exposure to ticks, wearing gloves when handling game, and fully cooking meat all should reduce the risk of developing tularemia. A live attenuated vaccine has proved useful for lowering the risk of infection of the respiratory tract in workers who are exposed in the laboratory, but it is not effective for tick-borne disease (Burke, 1977). Efforts to develop new vaccines are ongoing (Khlebnikov et al., 1996; Waag et al., 1996).

BABESIOSIS

Babesiosis, a zoonosis first described in humans in 1957, is caused by intraerythrocytic protozoa and has many clinical features in common with malaria (Homer et al., 2000).

Etiology and Epidemiology

Many different species of *Babesia* infect a variety of domestic and wild animals throughout the world. In the United States *B. microti*, a piroplasm of rodents, is the principal cause of human infection, which occurs primarily in the northeastern and midwestern states (Eskow et al., 1999). The organism is transmitted by *I. scapularis* (the deer tick), which also transmits *B. burgdorferi*, the cause of Lyme disease. As with *B. burgdorferi*, rodents such as the white-footed mouse serve as reservoirs for *B. microti*. Consequently, coinfection with *B. microti* and *B. burgdorferi* (and sometimes with *Ehrlichia* as well) occurs with some frequency in the northeastern and midwestern states (Krause et al., 1996c; Magnarelli et al., 1995; Thompson et al., 2001). Babesiosis has been transmitted via blood transfusion (McQuiston et al., 2000; Mintz et al., 1991). Babesial infection usually is asymptomatic or it causes a mild, flulike illness that is not recognized as babesiosis. Serosurveys suggest that children may be infected more often than adults (Krause et al., 1992). In the western United States there have been rare reports of human babesiosis caused by *Babesia gibsoni* (WA-1) or by similar Babesia (Persing et al., 1995). In Europe *Babesia divergens*, a parasite of cattle, also infects humans.

Babesia have solid pyriform shapes and frequently are arranged in pairs. It is possible to infect a variety of animals experimentally; removal of the spleen often increases both the duration and the severity of infection. Microscopic study of an extensively parasitized patient during illness has shown that usually one to four of the basophilic parasites are seen in infected red blood cells, but as many as 5 to 12 parasites per cell are present. Different developmental stages of the parasite, including ring, ameboid, and other forms, can be seen even within a single cell. Extracellular merozoites are present singly or in a syncytial structure. Free ribosomes, endoplasmic reticulum, and small dense bodies may be seen in the cytoplasm of merozoites, with a single large membrane-limited dense body (rhoptry). Trophozoites are surrounded by a single plasma membrane. Early in the course of illness red blood cells show changes in their cell membranes, with protrusions and perforations.

Clinical Manifestations

Symptoms of babesiosis begin 1 to 9 weeks after the tick bite. Typical signs and symptoms include intermittent fever as high as 40° C and chills, sweats, myalgia, arthralgia, nausea, or vomiting (Hatcher et al., 200; Reubush et al., 1977; Sun et al., 1983; White et al., 1998). The physical examination often is normal (except for fever) or reveals only mild splenomegaly or hepatomegaly. About half of the patients have abnormal liver function tests. Thrombocytopenia is also common. Invasion of erythrocytes by *B. microti* and subsequent lysis may result in mild to moderately severe hemolytic anemia with an elevated reticulocyte count. Unlike malaria, the illness is not marked by periodicity of symptoms.

In most immunocompetent persons the illness is indistinguishable from an acute viral infection, so the diagnosis rarely is made. However, immunocompromised patients, particularly those without a spleen, may have severe infection, with up to 90% of the red blood cells parasitized. These patients may develop severe hemolysis, shock, thrombocytopenia, and disseminated intravascular coagulation.

Diagnosis

Babesiosis can be diagnosed by microscopic identification of the organisms on either thick or thin smears of blood that are stained with either Giemsa or Wright's stains, by detection of antibodies to *Babesia*, or by PCR assay (Weinberg, 2001). During the early stage of the illness, when most people seek medical attention, less than 1% of erythrocytes may be infected, so making the diagnosis may be difficult, and careful examination of multiple smears of blood is important. PCR is a potentially useful diagnostic technique that is both highly sensitive and highly specific in the setting of a research laboratory (Krause et al., 1996b; Persing et al., 1992); its value as a commercially available test has not been assessed. Of the commonly used serologic tests, the indirect IFA assay is the most accurate and reliable (Krause et al., 1994). Titers greater than 1:64 are suggestive of recent infection, but paired sera with a fourfold or greater rise in concentration of antibody confirms the diagnosis. An indirect IFA for IgM antibody also may be useful in making the diagnosis (Krause et al., 1996a). An immunoblot test for serologic diagnosis may also be sensitive and specific as well as easier to standardize than the indirect IFA assay (Ryan et al., 2001).

Treatment and Prognosis

Most infections with *B. microti* are self-limited, and patients recover without treatment. More severe infections that come to medical attention should be treated either with both quinine and clindamycin or with both atovaquone and azithromycin, which may be more effective and is better tolerated than the former regimen (Krause et al., 2000). Patients who are extremely ill often require exchange transfusion to diminish the load of parasites. The infection may be fatal in asplenic patients. Untreated, the clinical illness usually lasts from a few weeks to several months. Parasitemia, which may persist for many months, may continue even after the patient's symptoms have resolved (Krause et al., 1998). Relapse is unusual but has occurred.

Prevention

There is no vaccine available. Preliminary evidence indicates that, as with transmission of *B. burgdorferi,* an infected tick must feed for at least 48 hours before the risk of transmission becomes substantial. Consequently, examination for and prompt removal of embedded ticks may decrease the risk of infection.

DISEASES CAUSED BY RICKETTSIACEAE

Rickettsiae are obligate intracellular gram-negative bacteria that are transmitted primarily by arthropod vectors. Except for epidemic typhus, humans are the incidental hosts for most rickettsial infections. The geographic distribution of most rickettsial diseases reflects that of their vectors. Diseases such as typhus have been recognized for centuries, but not until the early twentieth century was the causative group of agents recognized when Dr. Howard T. Ricketts produced disease by injecting blood from a patient with Rocky Mountain spotted fever into a guinea pig.

The taxonomy of the family Rickettsiaceae is shown in Figure 37-4. All Rickettsiaceae grow only within cells. *Rickettsia* can be divided into three groups—typhus, spotted fever, and scrub typhus—with more than 10 different species in these groups that cause human illness. The closely related genus *Coxiella* is composed of the species *Coxiella burnetii,* which, although similar to the Rickettsieae in morphology and intracellular growth, differs in major ways. This organism produces a sporelike small cell, has very different DNA composition, and is transmitted to humans by aerosol means rather than by ticks. As a result of molecular analyses of the bacteria, in 1993 the four members of the genus *Rochalimaea* (which had been in the Rickettsiaceae family), *Rochalimaea henselae, Rochalimaea quintana, Rochalimaea elizabethae,* and *Rochalimaea vinsonii,* were renamed and moved to the genus *Bartonella* within the family Bartonellaceae.

Etiology

Rickettsiae are pleomorphic coccobacillary organisms that range from 0.3 to 0.6 μm in width and from 0.8 to 2.0 μm in length. They are gram negative but stain poorly. The organisms are best visualized with a Gimenez modification of the Macchiavello method, which stains organisms red. These bacteria have a three-layered cell wall, trilaminar plasma membrane, ribosome-like particles, and intracellular organelles. They possess both RNA and DNA, and they divide by binary fission. The genome is large, varying from 1.0 to 1.5 × 10^9 d. They have developed carrier-mediated exchange transport systems for phosphorylated compounds (ADP and ATP) similar to those of mitochondria. The genome size, DNA-DNA hybridization, and guanosine-cytosine content are similar within species of a group, but significant differences exist between groups (e.g., between *C. burnetii* and *Rickettsia prowazekii*).

All members of the genus *Rickettsia* can obtain access to cytoplasm by traversing the membrane of the host cell and are unstable outside of the cell, whereas *C. burnetii* (genus *Coxiella*) is very resistant to both heating and

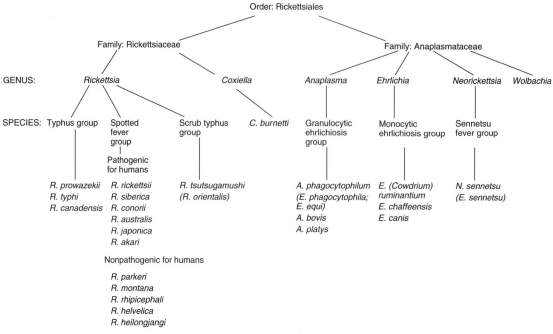

Fig. 37-4 Taxonomy of Rickettsiales.

TABLE 37-1	Rickettsiales That Cause Disease in Humans
Causative agent	*Diseases*
Rickettsia prowazekii	Epidemic typhus. Brill-Zinsser disease
Rickettsia typhi	Endemic or murine typhus
Rickettsia canadensis	?—disease similar to Rocky Mountain spotted fever
Rickettsia rickettsii	Rocky Mountain spotted fever
Rickettsia akari	Rickettsial pox
Rickettsia sibirica	North Asian tick typhus
Rickettsia australis	Queensland tick typhus
Rickettsia japonica	Japanese spotted fever
Rickettsia conorii	Boutonneuse fever
R. tsutsugamushi	Scrub typhus (chigger-borne typhus, mite-borne typhus, Japanese river fever, rural fever, tropical typhus)
Coxiella burnettii	Q fever
Neorickettsia sennetsu	Sennetsu fever
Ehrlichia chaffeensis	Human monocytic ehrlichiosis
Anaplasma phagocytophilum	Human granulocytic ehrlichiosis

drying. All members of the Rickettsiaceae family can be propagated in various tissue culture systems, embryonated eggs, laboratory animals, and certain arthropods. Generally, organisms in the typhus group grow in the cytoplasm, whereas organisms in the spotted fever group grow in both the cytoplasm and the nucleus.

The Spotted Fever Group

Rickettsiae in the spotted fever group cause a diffuse vasculitis of the small vessels that produces a rash that typically is petechial or purpuric. Any of the viscera may be involved with the clinical disease, which includes a spectrum of severity from unrecognized infection to fatal illness. Rocky Mountain spotted fever is the second most commonly reported tick-borne infection in the United States.

Rocky mountain spotted fever (tick-borne typhus)

Etiology and Epidemiology. R. rickettsii are morphologically similar to other rickettsiae. R. rickettsii and R. prowazekii have a slime layer (glycocalix), probably composed of polysaccharide and external to the cell wall, which could be antigenically important and/or related to cell attachment (Silverman et al., 1978). R. rickettsii are labile and are killed by drying at room temperature, by moist heat (≥50°C), and by formalin or phenol. R. rickettsii multiply in both the nucleus and the cytoplasm and produce demonstrable cytopathic effects. Studies with the scanning electron microscope have shown R. rickettsii exiting from cells on long cytoplasmic projections without causing lysis of the cell. Large numbers of cells become infected relatively quickly. These microorganisms live within ticks, in which they do not cause disease, and are transovarially transmitted from female ticks to their progeny. The ticks pass through three stages in their life cycle. They can acquire infection at any stage by feeding on a rickettsemic animal. The infection is maintained by the tick through its sequential stages of development: egg to larvae to nymph to adult (i.e., transtadially). The arthropods are both reservoirs and vectors of infection.

Rocky Mountain spotted fever (tick-borne typhus) occurs only in the Western Hemisphere. The disease is most prevalent in the Piedmont region of the southeastern United States and in Oklahoma. Small numbers of cases have been recognized over the years in almost every state. Approximately 2,640 cases of disease were reported to the CDC in 1998 (Figure 37-5). In the United States the reported incidence of Rocky Mountain spotted fever peaked at an annual incidence of approximately 0.5 cases per 100,000 population in the late 1970s and early 1980s and subsequently declined. Rocky Mountain spotted fever is responsible for 95% of all reported rickettsial infections in the United States (Figure 37-6). Because ticks transmit the disease, the incidence is seasonal, with most cases occurring during the peak period of exposure of humans to ticks—from April to September (D'Angelo et al., 1978;

Wilfert et al., 1984). Persons who live in rural or suburban areas are more likely to acquire disease than are persons who live in urban areas, although outbreaks have occurred in urban areas such as in New York City (Salgo et al., 1988). Very young infants (<2 years old) are rarely exposed, and illness in this age group is unusual. Persons who are outdoors in oak, hickory, and pine forests are most likely to be exposed and to acquire the disease.

Infection is transmitted to humans by ticks. Infection may be transmitted within the laboratory by aerosol (Oster et al., 1977), but aerosol transmission (which is associated with severe disease) is not known to occur in nature. Very rarely, transmission from human to human has occurred through a blood transfusion from a patient incubating disease or through an accidental stick by a needle contaminated with infected blood. The wood tick, D. andersoni, is the major vector of R. rickettsii in the western United States. D. variabilis, the dog tick, is the usual culprit in both the southeastern and the northeastern United States. Ticks obtained from vegetation (not from dogs) harbor rickettsia at varying frequencies (<1% to 10%); however, only one tick of 2,510 (0.03%) had R. rickettsii in one study conducted in North Carolina. The Lone Star tick (A. americanum) and the rabbit tick (Haemaphysalis leporispalustris) only occasionally transmit disease to humans, but they may be important in maintaining infection in animals. The infected tick must ingest a blood meal to "activate" the rickettsia, which is transmitted from the salivary glands of the tick during feeding. This phenomenon probably is related to increasing the temperature of the organism, which microscopically correlates with the presence of a microcapsular slime layer on the organism (Hayes and Burgdorfer, 1982).

Pathogenesis and Pathology. Rickettsiae initially enter the endothelial cells of small blood vessels (Silverman, 1984; Silverman and Bond, 1979). The membrane of the host cell engulfs them. Phospholipase may aid the organism in evading phagocytosis and may contribute to damage of the membrane of the host cell. In mammals organisms multiply in the vascular endothelium and smooth muscle, producing endothelial damage and occlusion of small vessels, with extravasation of blood and fluid and attendant changes in serum electrolytes (especially hyponatremia). Typhus rickettsiae increase

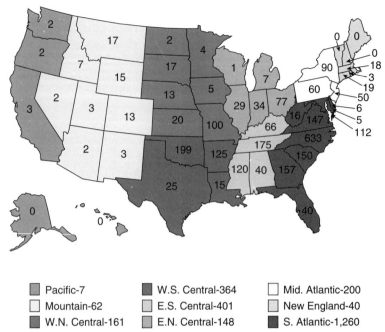

Fig. 37-5 Number of reported cases of Rocky Mountain spotted fever by state and region, 1994-1998. (From Viral and Rickettsial Zoonoses Branch. Rocky Mountain spotted fever. Centers for Disease Control and Prevention, 2000. Available at: http://www.cdc.gov/ncidod/dvrd/rmsf/Epidemiology.htm.)

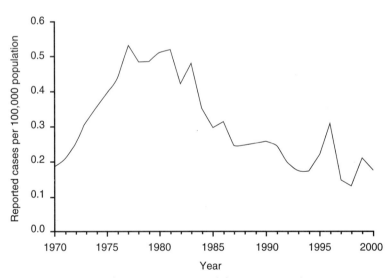

Fig. 37-6 Rocky Mountain spotted fever—reported cases per 100,000 population by year, United States, 1970–2000. (From MMWR Morb Mortal Wkly Rep 2000;49:60.)

endothelial and macrophage secretion of arachidonate-derived autocoids. Activation of the kallikrein-kinin system has been documented in humans, as has disseminated intravascular coagulation. The vasculitis is apparent in many tissues, especially the skin, CNS, heart, lungs, liver, and kidney. Severe disease can cause occlusion of larger vessels as well as gangrene. In animal models the rickettsiae themselves cause cellular damage. Cell-mediated immunity to antigens of *R. rickettsii* has been demonstrated in vitro and may contribute to eradication of organisms in tissues. The immune response of the host may also contribute to the tissue damage (Teysseire et al., 1992; Walker et al., 1993).

Clinical Manifestations. The clinical features of Rocky Mountain spotted fever have been well defined (Abramson and Givner, 1999; Thorner et al., 1998; Treadwell et al., 2000; Walker, 1995). The incubation period is usually 5 to 7 days, with a range of 3 to 12 days. The illness is characterized by a short prodromal period of headache, malaise, and myalgia. Chills may accompany the abrupt onset of fever, and the severity of myalgia and headache may increase. Usually, a rash is noted 2 to 4 days after onset of illness, although there have been reports of "spotless" and "almost spotless" fever (Sexton and Corey, 1992). It begins as a maculopapular eruption with a peripheral distribution. The skin lesions appear first on the thenar eminence and the flexor surfaces of the wrists and ankles. The rash spreads to involve the arms, legs, chest, and, finally, the abdomen. The palms and soles are nearly always affected. The lesions are at first discrete, macular, and maculopapular, and they blanch with pressure. Within 1 to 3 days the rash becomes hemorrhagic, and lesions may become confluent, with areas of necrosis at sites of maximal involvement. Gangrene of fingers, toes, genitalia, or the nose may develop (Kirkland et al., 1993). During the period of convalescence, the rash becomes pigmented, and evidence of desquamation appears over the more severely affected areas.

The illness varies in severity even without specific antimicrobial therapy. The case-fatality rate is 4%, which makes it the most common fatal tick-borne illness in the United States. Factors associated with higher mortality include increased age and an increased length of time from onset of the illness to initiation of therapy (Centers for Disease Control and Prevention, 2000; Hattwick et al., 1978; Kirkland et al., 1995). The diffuse organ involvement of this infection results in protean manifestations. Myalgia and associated elevations of muscle enzymes are common. Hepatic involvement is frequent and may produce mild to severe hepatocellular dysfunction and jaundice. The gastrointestinal manifestations include abdominal pain, vomiting, and diarrhea. Myocardial involvement, with vasculitis and inflammation, is common. The patient may have an altered sensorium or may be comatose as a result of encephalitis, and there is frequently pleocytosis in the CSF, although there usually are fewer than 100 to 200 WBC/mm^3 (Baganz et al., 1995). The peripheral WBC count is often normal, but there may be a shift to the left with prominent vacuolization of polymorphonuclear cells. Hyponatremia and mild peripheral edema are frequent consequences of the vasculitis. Increased antidiuretic hormone levels have also been observed in patients with this disease.

Illness in the most severely affected patients may last from days to weeks. Prolonged fever of 10 days to several weeks and relapse after cessation of therapy may occur. It is likely that infections that are either asymptomatic or the symptoms of which are relatively mild occur and are not recognized as Rocky Mountain spotted fever, since some persons with specific antibodies that indicate previous infection have had no known illness consistent with Rocky Mountain spotted fever.

Diagnosis. It is critical to consider the diagnosis of Rocky Mountain spotted fever in all patients in endemic areas who have symptoms that are compatible with this infection, especially during the months of peak exposure to ticks. In the absence of rash (e.g., early in the course of the illness or in the unusual patient in whom no rash develops) it is difficult to make a specific diagnosis. The differential diagnosis includes other diseases that cause similar rashes, such as meningococcemia, septic shock of any cause, erythema multiforme and other types of vasculitis, murine typhus, drug-induced rashes, and enteroviral infections. A febrile illness with the characteristic rash often constitutes enough evidence to initiate therapy because of the poor outcomes of persons with this disease in whom treatment is delayed (Archibald and Sexton, 1995; Centers for Disease Control and Prevention, 2000). Additional points in the patient's history such as a known tick bite, myalgia, headache, and hyponatremia constitute a compelling clinical constellation. Laboratory diagnosis has primarily depended on the demonstration of antibodies to *R. rickettsii*, which are rarely present during the first 3 to 5 days of illness. Accordingly, initiation of specific antimicrobial therapy should not await confirmation of diagnosis by serologic tests.

Isolation of *R. rickettsii* from the blood is expensive and time consuming because it requires cell culture or inoculation of animals. It is done in only a few research laboratories. It takes several days for a culture to become positive, so culture cannot be used for early diagnosis of infection. Early diagnosis can be made by detection of intracellular *R. rickettsii* by fluorescein-conjugated antibody in biopsies of skin lesions (Woodward et al., 1976). *R. rickettsii* are not present in areas of normal skin. Results of this test may be negative in infected patients who received antibiotics for more than 24 hours before the specimen was obtained. It is also possible to demonstrate the presence of intracellular organisms in tissues obtained at autopsy.

Diagnosis generally is made by detection of antibodies that appear during convalescence. Results of the Weil-Felix test, a test for nonspecific antibodies, often are positive in patients with Rocky Mountain spotted fever. Because of their O polysaccharide antigens, several strains of *Proteus* (OX-19, OX-2, OX-K) are agglutinated by antibodies that are induced by rickettsial infections. Antibodies may be detected after the first week of illness, and a fourfold increase is suggestive of recent infection. The test is easy to perform and is inexpensive but both its specificity and its sensitivity are poor. Specific antibody to rickettsiae can be assessed by indirect hemagglutination (IHA), microimmunofluorescence (micro-IF), latex agglutination, ELISA, and complement-fixation (CF) tests. The sensitivity of the CF test is poor, and it is no longer in general use in the United States; antibodies detected by CF may develop late, and their development may be aborted by specific antibiotic therapy. The sensitivity and specificity of IHA, micro-IF, and latex agglutination tests are comparable (Philip et al., 1977). ELISA tests that use a monoclonal antibody directed against specific antigens of *R. rickettsii* are more specific than earlier ELISA tests (Radulovic et al., 1993). An antibody rise of fourfold or greater in paired sera is diagnostic of acute infection. The presence of specific IgM antibody by immunofluorescence or ELISA suggests recent infection (Clements et al., 1983). Typical patterns of antibody titers appear over time in patients with Rocky Mountain spotted fever.

PCR also has been used successfully to diagnose Rocky Mountain fever in its early stages (Dumler and Walker, 1994; Sexton et al., 1994). However, as with its use in other infections, the use of PCR as a diagnostic test is complicated by the possibility of false-positive results due to amplicon carryover, and the sensitivity of the test is not known. Additional experience is necessary before this technique becomes a standard method for making the diagnosis.

Immunity. A single infection with *R. rickettsii* probably confers long-term immunity. Persons who have been challenged twice with *R. rickettsii* develop clinical illness only after the first exposure (DuPont et al., 1973). A spectrum of antibodies develops in response to *R. rickettsii* (Anacker et al., 1983). Crossed immunoelectrophoresis demonstrates antibody responses to multiple different antigens of the organism; it is not known which antibodies confer protection against *R. rickettsii*. Antibody coating of *R. rickettsii* is necessary for phagocytosis and killing of the organism by guinea pig peritoneal macrophages in cell culture systems. Lymphocytes from patients with prior infection have been shown in vitro to be sensitized to spotted fever group antigens. The relative importance in humans of antibody and of cell-mediated immunity in either response to infection or protection against subsequent infection are unknown.

Treatment and Prognosis. Tetracycline, doxycycline, and chloramphenicol are the drugs of choice for treating Rocky Mountain spotted fever. Fluoroquinolone antimicrobial agents, which are rickettsicidal, may also be effective, but there has not yet been enough experience with these drugs in the treatment of Rocky Mountain spotted fever to recommend them for routine use. For optimal effect, it is critical to treat patients early in the course of the illness. Although tetracycline may permanently stain teeth of children <9 years of age, reports of poorer outcomes in persons treated with chloramphenicol have led some to suggest that tetracycline or doxycycline (the effect of which on teeth is negligible after relatively short courses of treatment) should be used even in young children (Lochary et al., 1998; Purvis and Edwards, 2000). Recent studies have confirmed the superiority of tetracyclines (Cale and McCarthy, 1997; Holman et al., 2001). Patients should be treated for a minimum of 7 days.

Complications of Rocky Mountain spotted fever are more likely to occur in untreated patients and in patients in whom specific therapy is initiated after more than 4 days of clinical illness (Centers for Disease Control and Prevention, 2000; Hattwick et al., 1978; Kirkland et al., 1995). CNS sequelae do occur in a small proportion of patients (Archibald and Sexton, 1995). Occasionally, amputation of fingers and toes or of other tissues may be necessary because of gangrene (Kirkland et al., 1993). Arrhythmias have been observed as a manifestation of the myocardial involvement.

Prevention. Nonspecific measures to diminish exposure to ticks (such as use of long pants rather than shorts when walking in wooded areas) can be taken but have not been shown to be effective in preventing disease. Individuals who are exposed to ticks and tick-infested environments should inspect themselves for ticks and carefully remove any they find. A period of time is necessary for activation of *R. rickettsii* in infected ticks; therefore early removal of ticks could in theory prevent infection. Attached ticks should be removed with forceps and gentle traction. Care should be taken since tissues and feces of ticks are highly infectious if they contain *R. rickettsii*. Rocky Mountain spotted fever is not transmitted from human to human except for the unusual circumstance of blood transfusion or needle puncture. Therefore, isolation of patients is unnecessary.

There is no vaccine available for prevention of Rocky Mountain spotted fever. An early product made from egg-grown rickettsiae was used until it was shown conclusively that it failed to prevent infection. An experimental vaccine grown in cell-culture systems also was tested in experimental trials in animals and humans. Although humoral antibodies and sensitization of lymphocytes could be demonstrated, it did not protect humans from infection; therefore, studies of this vaccine have been stopped.

Rickettsialpox

Rickettsialpox is caused by *Rickettsia akari*, an organism of the spotted fever group that cross-reacts serologically with *R. rickettsii*. The disease is usually a mild febrile illness heralded by the development of a local eschar. Subsequently, a papulovesicular rash appears.

Etiology and Epidemiology. The common house mouse in the United States is infested with a mite (formerly known as *Allodermanyssus sanguineus*, and now called *Liponyssoides sanguineus*) that may be infected with *R. akari*. This organism may also be transmitted transovarially to the progeny of an infected mite. Humans enter the cycle of infection accidentally, often as the result of displacement of a rodent population by construction or during reduction of the rodent population by control programs. The mite attacks humans when its normal murine host is scare. This rickettsia has also been found in a wild Korean rodent (*Microtus fortis*).

Persons of all ages are susceptible to rickettsialpox. The majority of cases have been reported in New York City, where the disease was originally described in the Kew Gardens area of the borough of Queens in 1946 (Greenberg, 1948; Sussman, 1946). It has also been identified in West Hartford, Connecticut; Boston, Massachusetts; Philadelphia, Pennsylvania; Arkansas; Delaware; and Russia.

Clinical Manifestations. The incubation period is estimated to be 10 to 24 days. A triad of symptoms occurs in sequence: the initial eschar, a febrile illness, and a generalized papulovesicular eruption. The primary lesion at the site of the original bite of the mite is a local erythematous papule that evolves into a vesicle over a period of days and, finally, into an eschar. Most patients are not aware of either the bite or the lesion. The eschar resolves over a period of 3 to 4 weeks, and this lesion is usually associated with enlarged regional lymph nodes.

Approximately 3 to 7 days after the appearance of the eschar, fever begins abruptly. Patients often have headache, malaise, and myalgia. Within 72 hours of the onset of fever, a rash develops. There is no characteristic distribution of this rash. It may occur on any part of the body, but it only rarely involves the palms or soles. The lesions are initially maculopapular and discrete, but small vesicles form on the summit of the papules. The lesions dry and may have tiny scabs that fall off without leaving scars. The entire course of illness is approximately 2 weeks. There usually is leukopenia with relative lymphocytosis.

Because there have been no reported deaths from this disease, only skin usually is available for examination of histopathology (Dolgopol, 1948). The initial lesion is a firm nodule approximately 1 cm in diameter. It consists of a vesicle or pustule covered with dry epithelium or crust. Histologically, the vesicle is situated subepidermally and may arise from vacuolar changes of the basal layer. Mononuclear infiltration of the epidermis is seen, with a mixed polymorphonuclear mononuclear cell infiltrate in the dermis. The capillaries of the stratum cornium are dilated and surrounded by mononuclear cells, and the endothelial cells in blood vessels are swollen.

Diagnosis. Rickettsialpox may be confused with varicella (chickenpox) and is the only rickettsial disease characterized by the appearance of vesicular lesions. The presence of a primary eschar, however, differentiates it from varicella. In addition, the vesicular lesions in rickettsialpox are smaller than those in varicella and are usually situated on top of a papule. Rickettsialpox can affect persons of all ages, but varicella is more likely to occur in children. The typical crusting of varicella lesions may not be observed in many of the rickettsialpox lesions. The diffuse nature of the vesicular lesions is in contrast to the characteristic sequential eruption of varicella vesicles. This difference should also help to distinguish this illness from primary herpes simplex infection. The demonstration of multinuclear giant cells and/or isolation of either herpes simplex or varicella-zoster virus will easily distinguish these infections.

The diagnosis of rickettsialpox can be made clinically and confirmed by measurements of antibodies. Weil-Felix antibodies do not appear after infection with *R. akari*. However, more specific testing available at the CDC or at certain research laboratories can demonstrate an antibody response 1 to 2 months after the onset of illness. Because *R. rickettsii* and *R. akari* share some antigens, antibodies to *R. rickettsii* may be detected in some patients with rickettsialpox.

R. akari has been isolated from both the blood and the vesicular fluid of infected persons. Using a research laboratory or one specifically interested in the diagnosis of this infection is necessary to obtain diagnosis by culture because animals and embryonated eggs are used.

Treatment, Prognosis, and Prevention. Both tetracycline and chloramphenicol have been reported to shorten the course of the illness. Prevention is directed at control of the rodent host of the vector. Untreated rickettsialpox is a benign, self-limited, nonfatal disease. No complications have been reported.

No vaccines are available, and there is little stimulus to develop additional preventive measures because of both the mild nature and the rarity of this disease.

Other tick-borne rickettsial diseases. An illness similar to but milder than Rocky Mountain spotted fever has been ascribed to several other tick-borne rickettsiae. North Asian tick typhus, which occurs in Central Asia, Siberia, and Mongolia, is caused by *Rickettsia sibirica*. Queensland tick typhus is caused by *Rickettsia australis* and is found only in Australia. South African tick bite fever, Kenya tick typhus, Indian tick typhus, and boutonneuse fever (Mediterranean region), all of which are different names for the same illness, are caused by *Rickettsia conorii*. *Rickettsia japonica* is the causative agent of Japanese spotted fever. All four of these *Rickettsia* infect different species of Ixodes ticks and their wild animal hosts. Humans are only incidentally infected and are not important as reservoirs for these illnesses. In contrast to Rocky Mountain spotted fever, these rickettsial illnesses are characterized by a local skin lesion at the site at which the tick attaches and the formation of an eschar at the site of the bite, as with rickettsial pox. These illnesses are milder than Rocky Mountain spotted fever. Group-reactive complement-fixing antibodies have been demonstrated in response to infection with any of these four rickettsiae, but results of the Weil-Felix test are positive only occasionally. The diagnosis can be specific because the geographic distribution of the individual rickettsiae overlaps very little. These illnesses are also treated with chloramphenicol or tetracycline.

The Typhus Group

The typhus group of rickettsiae causes epidemic typhus (including recrudescent disease) and murine typhus. These organisms share a common group-specific antigen and grow within the cytoplasm of cells.

Epidemic (louse-borne) typhus

Epidemic typhus is an acute, potentially fatal infectious disease caused by *R. prowazekii* that has played an important role in history. For example, it has been estimated that in World War I more than 3 million Russians died as a result of this infection.

Etiology and Epidemiology. *R. prowazekii* is similar to the previously described rickettsial species. The organisms multiply in cytoplasm much as do classic bacteria in liquid medium. The cells in which they grow exhibit few cytopathic effects. The organism is infectious for mice, guinea pigs, and embryonated eggs. Infectivity is maintained after either lyophilization or storage at −70° C. This organism can infect both the human body louse (*P. humanus corporis*) and the head louse (*P. humanus capitis*) (Raoult and Roux, 1999). *P. humanus corporis* feeds only on humans, and lice in all stages (egg, nymph, and adult) can be present on the same host. The louse becomes infected by taking a blood meal from a person with rickettsemia. *R. prowazekii* multiplies in the epithelial cells of the intestine of the louse. After 3 to 7 days, large numbers of rickettsiae are excreted in the feces. Fortunately, lice do not transmit the rickettsiae to their progeny, and infected lice die within several weeks. An infected louse transmits disease by moving to another person and excreting feces during the blood meal. The abrasions induced by scratching provide a portal of entry for rickettsiae deposited on the skin. Rarely, infections have been acquired by inhalation of dry infective feces of the louse. Humans are the primary reservoir of infection, although flying squirrels also may harbor the organism.

Epidemic typhus occurs throughout the world. All ages and both sexes are equally susceptible. It occurs chiefly in Asia, Africa, Europe, Central America, and South America, although cases do occur rarely in the United States. During World War II the disease was epidemic in Russia, Poland, Germany, Spain, and North Africa. Conditions that promote infestation with lice, including crowding, poor hygiene, and conditions under which the same clothing is worn for prolonged periods, favor the disease. The conditions favorable for proliferation of lice are associated with war, poverty, and famine. Lice apparently seek locations where the temperature is approximately 20° C; they will abandon the host when the body temperature rises to ≥40° C.

The few sporadic cases of epidemic typhus in the United States have been associated with the flying squirrel (*Glaucomys volans*); its lice (*Neohaematopinus sciuropteri*) and fleas (*Orchopeas howardi*) are vectors that have been occasionally responsible for disease in Virginia, North Carolina, Florida, West Virginia, and other parts of the United States (Duma et al., 1981; Massung et al., 2001; Sonenshine et al., 1978).

Clinical Manifestations. After an incubation period of 7 to 14 days, epidemic typhus begins abruptly with fever, chills, headache, malaise, and generalized aches and pains. The fever and constitutional symptoms increase in severity and are followed by a rash that erupts on the fourth to sixth day of illness. The maculopapular rash appears first on the trunk near the axillae and spreads to involve the extremities. The face, palms, and soles are usually not involved. Initially, the lesions are discrete pleomorphic macules that blanch on pressure. During the second week of illness, the skin lesions become petechial and purpuric, after which brownish pigmentation develops.

In the untreated patient fever lasts for 2 weeks and then falls by lysis over a period of 2 to 3 days. Severe illness is characterized by stupor, delirium, hallucinations or excitability, marked weakness, prostration, and temporary deafness. By the second and third weeks the patient either recovers or progresses to coma and death. Early in the course of infection relative bradycardia may be present; later, tachycardia and gallop rhythm may reflect inflammation of the myocardium. Splenomegaly, albuminuria, and elevated blood urea nitrogen usually develop, and there may be leukopenia and anemia.

The primary insult is to the endothelial cells of the small blood vessels. Multiplication of the rickettsiae causes edema, deposition of both fibrin and platelets, and obstruction of the vessels, which may be followed by thrombosis, hemorrhage, and perivascular infiltration of neutrophils, macrophages, and lymphocytes. The vascular lesions are widely disseminated, but they are most numerous in the skin, myocardium, skeletal muscle, kidneys, and CNS.

Diagnosis. The diagnosis of epidemic typhus should be based on the clinical picture; appropriate therapy should not be withheld until there is laboratory confirmation of the diagnosis. Isolating *R. prowazekii* can substantiate the clinical diagnosis, but doing so is both difficult and potentially dangerous and it must be done with the use of special equipment by specially trained personnel. The organism also may be visualized in tissue and has been detected with the use of PCR (Carl et al., 1990; Massung et al., 2001). Primary isolation of *R. prowazekii* can be accomplished by inoculating blood into either guinea pigs or adult white mice or into the yolk sac of embryonated eggs. It has also been isolated from the blood by shell vial cell culture (Birg et al., 1999). Infection with *R. prowazekii* also induces the formation of antibodies that agglutinate the OX polysaccharide antigens of *Proteus vulgaris*.

These agglutinins appear in the second week after onset of illness, and agglutination is usually maximal with OX-19 strains. A fourfold rise in agglutination titers is suggestive of recent infection. CF antibodies can be detected in the third week after onset of the illness. However as with Rocky Mountain spotted fever, immunofluorescence tests and microagglutination procedures, available in specialized laboratories, are more sensitive (Ormsbee, 1977).

Treatment and Prognosis. Patients with epidemic typhus should be deloused, which can be accomplished by bathing with soap and water and with weekly dusting with 10% dichloro-diphenyltrichloroethane (DDT), 1% lindane, or another effective agent lethal to the lice. Tetracycline and chloramphenicol are the antimicrobial agents of choice for treatment. A therapeutic response usually occurs within 48 hours. Early treatment is more likely to induce a prompt clinical response.

Otitis media, parotitis, and bronchopneumonia may complicate epidemic typhus. Gangrene of portions of the extremities may also result from the vasculitis and thrombosis. Untreated epidemic typhus fever is a severe and potentially fatal infection. The mortality rate ranges from 10% to 40% and is higher in older individuals. The severe myocardial and CNS involvement is not usually followed by sequelae if the patient survives. If antimicrobial therapy is administered early in the course of the illness, death from the infection is rare.

Brill-Zinsser Disease. Recrudescent infection sometimes occurs many years after an individual has had epidemic typhus. It was first suggested in 1934 that this recurrence was a relapse of a prior infection with *R. prowazekii*. Thus the disease may occur in an individual who is living in a louse-free environment. Brill-Zinsser disease most frequently occurs in immigrants from endemic areas. As the number of survivors of World War II who are alive diminishes, the frequency of Brill-Zinsser disease in the United States has decreased, because a majority of cases occurred in this group of patients. An additional aspect of recrudescent disease is that lice that feed on affected patients can become infected and subsequently initiate another cycle of transmission. Latent human infection therefore constitutes an interepidemic reservoir. Weil-Felix antibodies usually do not develop in patients with Brill-Zinsser disease. However,

specific IgG antibodies, detected by micro-IF, aid in making the diagnosis.

Prevention. After the patient and his clothing have been cleared of lice, no isolation is necessary because the patient will not transmit disease to other persons. Contacts known to have lice also should be deloused. After that, quarantine is not necessary. Specific protein antigens of *R. prowazekii* and of *Rickettsia typhi*, antibodies against which are protective, have been characterized. These purified large polypeptides do not have significant endotoxin content. Both humoral and cellular immunity to these antigens does develop in humans after natural infection, and subunit vaccines that are composed of these antigens have been tested successfully for immunogenicity and efficacy in guinea pigs.

Murine typhus (endemic typhus, flea-borne typhus, rat typhus)

Murine typhus fever is an acute, relatively mild infection caused by *R. typhi*. It is characterized clinically by headache, fever, malaise, and a maculopapular eruption with a centripetal distribution. Essentially, it is a modified version of epidemic typhus fever.

Etiology and Epidemiology. *R. typhi* is a natural infection of rodents that is spread to humans by the rat flea (*Xenopsylla cheopis*) and the rat louse (*Polyplax spinulosus*). The vector, most frequently the rat flea, becomes infected with *R. typhi* by feeding on either a mouse or a rat that is infected. The rickettsiae multiply in cells of both the gut of the flea and in malpighian tubules. Thus infected, the flea may infect other susceptible rodents. Rickettsiae can be found in brains of infected rodents for up to several months. Fleas do not transmit *R. typhi* transovarially, so the murine hosts constitute the reservoir for the microorganisms. The infection is not transmitted by the bite of the flea. Transmission of *R. typhi* to humans occurs on occasions when the infected flea that is taking a blood meal is scratched by a human, thereby inoculating the infected feces of the flea into the excoriation. The feces of the flea are also infective if they happen to contact a mucosal surface such as the conjunctiva. *R. typhi* is very similar to *R. prowazekii* and is also infective for rats, mice, guinea pigs, and the yolk sac of embryonated eggs.

Murine typhus fever has a worldwide distribution and is endemic in many countries, including the United States. In the United

States the largest number of cases has occurred in the southern states along the Gulf of Mexico and the Atlantic seaboard and in California. In recent years the majority of reported cases in the United States have occurred in Texas. The disease occurs in areas that are infested with rats or mice; these animals tend to be present in large numbers where grains and feeds for animals are stored. The disease occurs most often during the summer months.

The incubation period of murine typhus ranges from 1 to 2 weeks. Clinically, endemic typhus is indistinguishable from a mild case of epidemic typhus. The development of fever, headache, malaise, myalgia, and a maculopapular nonpruritic skin rash that becomes apparent on the third to the fifth day of the illness are typical. The rash is usually sparse and discrete and rarely is hemorrhagic. In the untreated patient fever seldom persists for more than 2 weeks.

Diagnosis. Endemic typhus is clinically similar to but usually much milder than epidemic typhus, and the rash of endemic typhus is less likely to be hemorrhagic. If rickettsiae are isolated and injected into guinea pigs, scrotal edema develops if the organisms belong to *R. typhi* (the cause of endemic typhus), but not if they belong to *R. prowazekii*. Specific antibody measurements will establish the correct diagnosis. The distribution of the rash of endemic typhus differs from that of Rocky Mountain spotted fever; the former begins on the trunk and usually does not involve the palms and soles, whereas the latter is concentrated on the face and on the extremities (including the palms and soles). Specific antibody tests will help distinguish these two illnesses. A primary lesion usually is present with scrub typhus, which consists of a papule that progress to become a vesicle and then a scab with an ulcer. The severe febrile illness and rash could be confused with epidemic typhus. Specific antibody tests can be used to distinguish between epidemic typhus and scrub typhus. Meningococcemia usually progresses more rapidly than typhus, a fact that may be helpful in making a clinical diagnosis. The symptoms of coryza, conjunctivitis, and fever that precede the maculopapular eruption often provide a useful way to distinguish between measles and typhus. The distribution of the rash of measles, with its initial appearance on the face and neck, is different from that of typhus. Hemorrhagic lesions are uncommon in patients with measles, and the fever usually subsides after the first week of illness.

Weil-Felix agglutinins to *Proteus* OX-19 usually appear in the second week of infection. However, measurement of antibodies by micro-IF is both more sensitive and more specific. The CF assay is a standard method that is generally available but is less sensitive than micro-IF. Serologic cross-reactions among members of the typhus group occur frequently, but the concentrations to the homologous antigen usually are the greatest. Inoculation of organisms or of blood that contains organisms into the peritoneal cavity of a guinea pig produces severe vesicular lesions and scrotal swelling. *R. typhi* produces a much more severe disease in this animal than the disease caused by inoculation of *R. prowazekii*.

Treatment and Prognosis. The treatment is the same as that for epidemic typhus. This disease is transmitted only by the infected vector and does not spread directly from person to person. The reported mortality rate is <2%. Cardiac, CNS, and renal manifestations occur less frequently in patients with murine typhus than in those with epidemic typhus.

Scrub typhus

An additional group of rickettsiae, the scrub typhus group, is capable of producing a clinical illness in humans. These rickettsiae have different surface antigens classified as Karp, Gilliam, or Kato. The different antigenic types are not associated with any differences in the clinical manifestations of infection.

Etiology and Epidemiology. *Rickettsia tsutsugamushi* (or *Rickettsia orientalis*) causes scrub typhus. This rickettsia has been observed to form blebs from its outer membranes in cell culture just as do some other gram-negative organisms. The organism infects several species of *Trombicula* mites. The mites have a three-stage life cycle (i.e., larvae, nymphs, and adults). *R. tsutsugamushi* is transmitted transtadially. The larva, or chigger, is the only stage that feeds on vertebrates. After a blood meal the chigger detaches and matures into a nymph and, subsequently, into an adult. Both nymphs and adults are free-living in the soil. Therefore *Trombicula* mites are the vectors as well as the reservoirs of the rickettsial infections they transmit. Normally the chiggers feed on small mammals or ground-feeding birds. Humans accidentally enter the natural cycle of infection in areas of secondary or scrub vegetation or on beaches and deserts and in rain forests. The disease is endemic in a geographic area of approximately 5 million square miles that includes Australia, Japan, Korea, India, and Vietnam. There was significant morbidity from scrub typhus during World War II among both American and Japanese soldiers. The disease usually occurs sporadically unless a group of people is brought into an endemic mite-infested area.

Clinical Manifestations. The incubation period of scrub typhus ranges from 1 to 3 weeks. Clinical manifestations of scrub typhus are very similar to those of other rickettsial infections, with abrupt onset of fever, headache, vomiting, myalgia, and abdominal pain. A local cutaneous lesion evolves from a small indurated or vesicular lesion into an ulcerated area that is present at the time of onset of symptoms. An eschar is usually present, as is local lymphadenopathy. Approximately 1 week after the onset of fever, a macular or maculopapular rash appears and is apparent first on the trunk. Neurologic symptoms may be prominent (Kim et al., 2000; Pai et al., 1997). The disease may be fatal (Cracco et al., 2000). In epidemics, fatality rates have varied from 0% to 50%. Antimicrobial therapy is effective and prevents fatal illness. Surface antigens of the causative organism vary, so that infection with one strain of *R. tsutsugamushi* does not confer protection against other strains. Thus, clinical disease may occur more than once in a single individual.

Diagnosis. Serologic diagnosis may be difficult because different organisms express antigens that are not cross-reactive. Several antigens (usually the three strains cited above) must be used in a test such as a CF assay. A Weil-Felix reaction may be positive, with agglutinins to *Proteus* OX-K. The time course of the illness is similar to that of other rickettsial infections; antibodies become detectable in the second week of illness. Tests for agglutinins are less sensitive than is quantitation of antibodies by immunofluorescence. Newer diagnostic tests that are being developed included ELISA, PCR-based tests, and a rapid dot-blot immunoassay (Chinprasatsak et al., 2001; Land et al., 2000; Shieh et al., 1996).

Treatment and Prognosis. Tetracycline and chloramphenicol are effective therapeutic agents that inhibit the growth of rickettsiae and usually produce prompt clinical improvement. If antibiotics are discontinued too early, relapse may occur. In some areas (e.g., Northern Thailand), strains resistant to tetracycline have become prevalent (Watt et al., 1996). Rifampicin may be an effective alternative for treatment of these strains (Watt et al., 2000).

Q Fever

C. burnettii was isolated simultaneously from infected persons in Australia and from wood ticks in Montana and was identified as a member of the Rickettsiaceae in 1939 (Burnet and Freeman, 1939). The name of the disease, *Q fever*, comes from the first letter in the word *query*, which was the clinical designation for this unusual febrile illness.

Etiology and epidemiology. C. burnettii grows within cells in membrane-bound vesicles primarily in monocytes and macrophages. As an obligate intracellular organism, it parasitizes eukaryotic cells and goes through its developmental cycle in the phagolysosome. The metabolism of these organisms is active at a pH of 4.5, which is the intravacuolar pH, and is not active at a pH of 7.0. This organism therefore thrives in the usually hostile environment of the phagolysosome. Differences in surface antigens define phase I and phase II organisms, which are morphologically identical. Phase I organisms exist in nature, whereas phase II organisms develop with passage in embryonated eggs.

The ecology of *C. burnettii* is complex. One ecologic cycle involves arthropods, especially ticks, which infect a variety of vertebrates, including domestic animals but not humans. Another cycle is maintained among domestic animals (typically sheep). These animals may have inapparent infection and may shed large quantities of infectious organisms in urine, milk, and feces and from placentas. *C. burnettii* is resistant to drying, to light, and to extremes of temperature. Consequently, infectious material often becomes aerosolized. Humans and animals may become infected by inhaling the organism. Infection may also be acquired by ingestion of infected milk or by handling contaminated wool or hides. *C. burnettii* also can penetrate the skin (e.g., through a minor abrasion) and the mucous membranes. Rarely, human-to-human transmission has occurred. Q fever is an occupational risk in abattoir workers, farm workers, and persons who are employed in tanneries and in plants that produce wool or felt, as well as in persons who work in laboratories that use sheep and other livestock.

Clinical manifestations. The incubation period of Q fever is 2 to 3 weeks. Illness usually begins abruptly with fever, chills, headache, malaise, and weakness (Ruiz-Contreras et al., 1993). After 5 or 6 days of symptoms, cough and chest pain occur, and rales may be audible. Pneumonia usually is apparent on a radiograph of the chest by the third day of illness. The consolidation clears over a period of 1 to 2 weeks (Derrick, 1973). There are peribronchial and perivascular infiltrates of lymphocytes, plasma cells, and monocytes in the lungs. Fibrinous exudate fills the alveoli and bronchioles. Q fever is unique among the rickettsial diseases in that a rash is not a part of the clinical syndrome. Prolonged fever, endocarditis, and hepatitis may occur. There is a spectrum of illness; asymptomatic infection has been documented. Q fever endocarditis can occur months or years after the acute attack; persons with prosthetic valves are at increased risk of Q fever endocarditis (Fenollar et al., 2001). Organisms isolated from persons with chronic illness contain a large plasmid (QpRS), whereas a smaller plasmid (QpH1) is present in organisms isolated from persons with acute illness.

Diagnosis. The compatible clinical picture, isolation of *C. burnettii* from the blood or sputum, and serologic tests establish the diagnosis (Fournier et al., 1998). Isolation of the organism requires inoculation of blood or sputum into an animal such as a guinea pig, mouse, or hamster or into embryonated eggs or cell culture. Because of the risk of transmission in the laboratory, this procedure is available only in research laboratories accustomed to dealing with the organism. Consequently, it is more reasonable to rely on serology to confirm the diagnosis. Several state health departments perform the CF test using purified antigens. Because *C. burnettii* exists in two phases, tests have been devised that use either phase I or phase II antigens, which are useful in distinguishing acute from either chronic or past infection (antibodies to the phase II antigen are present in acute infection). Serosurveys with CF antibodies underestimate the prevalence of infection; intradermal skin tests are more sensitive. The use of ELISA for specific IgM antibody to *C. burnettii* may be helpful in diagnosing acute infection (Field et al., 1983). Likewise, plasmids of *C. burnettii* may be identified in human sera by PCR assay

(Zhang et al., 1998). Weil-Felix agglutinins do not develop in response to infection with *C. burnettii*.

Treatment and prognosis. Patients with Q fever should be treated with either tetracycline or chloramphenicol; either drug should be administered for several days after the patient has become afebrile. The clinical response to treatment often is not as dramatic as that of patients with other rickettsial infections. The mortality rate of Q fever before antimicrobial therapy was available was approximately 1%. Fatalities are extraordinarily rare if patients are treated appropriately with an antimicrobial agent; the only exception is patients with endocarditis, for whom the mortality rate is higher. Replacement of an infected heart valve with a prosthetic valve combined with long-term antimicrobial therapy may improve the prognosis for patients with endocarditis. Recombinant gamma interferon may be useful in intractable cases (Morisawa et al., 2001).

Prevention. Transmission of *C. burnettii* via milk can be prevented by pasteurizing it; otherwise, it is difficult to interrupt the transmission of infection. Laboratory personnel who work with sheep or their tissues should do their research in a separate area away from other laboratories and areas in which patients are treated. Use of seronegative flocks is another alternative; skin tests can be used to assess whether personnel have become infected previously or are at risk. Lymphocyte transformation studies and skin testing are better predictors of immunity than are measurements of antibodies because antibody-negative persons may be immune. Human beings rarely transmit disease to one another; thus isolation of the infected patient is not indicated. A vaccine composed of inactivated phase II organisms was used effectively in Public Health Service and Army laboratories, but adverse reactions precluded widespread use of the vaccine. A formalin-inactivated vaccine against phase I *C. burnettii* has been effective in workers in Australian abattoirs (Marmion et al., 1990).

EHRLICHIOSIS

Based on genetic analyses of the 16S rRNA genes, the taxonomy of the bacteria that cause ehrlichiosis recently has been revised (Figure 37-4) (Dumler and Bakken, 1995; Dumler et al., 2001; Fishbein et al., 1994; McDade,

1989). All are now considered part of the family Anaplasmataceae.

Etiology and epidemiology. Ehrlichiosis is caused by several different obligate intracellular bacteria. Based on sequencing of their 16S rRNA genes, four different genogroups exist. The organism of major importance in the first genogroup, Anaplasma, is *Anaplasma phagocytophilum* (also known as *Ehrlichia phagocytophil*), the cause of human granulocytic ehrlichiosis (HGE). *Ehrlichia equi*, which causes granulocytic ehrlichiosis in sheep, cattle, deer, and horses is also closely related. In the second genogroup, Ehrlichia, *Ehrlichia chaffeensis*, is the cause of human monocytic ehrlichiosis (HME), and *Ehrlichia canis*, is the cause of ehrlichiosis in dogs. Another genogroup, *Neorickettsia*, contains *Neorickettsia sennetsu* (*Ehrlichia sennetsu*), the cause of sennetsu fever in Japan. The final genogroup is Wolbachia.

These organisms replicate within the phagosome in the host cell and have a tropism for circulating leukocytes. Like chlamydiae, these bacteria go through developmental stages of elementary bodies, initial bodies, and morulae. The individual organisms, called *elementary bodies*, are gram-negative rods that are about 0.5 μm in diameter. They are phagocytized either by monocytes (in HME) or by granulocytes (in HGE), and phagolysosomal fusion fails to occur. The elementary bodies divide by binary fission within the phagosome and form initial bodies, which are composed of many elementary bodies and can be seen as inclusions in the cells in 3 to 5 days. These initial bodies grow further and divide during the next 7 to 12 days, so that by light microscopy the configuration resembles a mulberry, or morula. Each infected leukocyte can contain several morulae. Rupture of the infected cells releases individual elementary bodies from the broken morulae.

Ehrlichiae are transmitted by ticks. The primary vector for *E. chaffeensis* (which causes HME) is *A. americanum*, the Lone Star tick. Most cases occur in the southern and south-central United States. The vector for the agent that causes HGE is *I. scapularis*, the deer tick (Thompson et al., 2001). Most cases of HGE occur in southern New England, the upper Midwestern states (Wisconsin and Minnesota), and the mid-Atlantic states (Bakken et al., 1996; Bakken et al., 1998; Belongia et al., 2001; Centers for Disease Control and Prevention, 1998; Ijdo et al., 2000; Pancholi et al., 1995;

Schwartz et al., 1997). It also has been reported in Europe (Brouqui et al., 1995). As with most tick-borne infections in temperate climates, the highest incidence of infection occurs during the peak months of human exposure to ticks: from April to September. The agent of HGE is highly prevalent in vector ticks in endemic areas (Schwartz et al., 1997). The vector for *E. sennetsu* is unknown.

As with *B. burgdorferi* and *B. microti*, the white-footed mouse appears to be an important natural reservoir for the agent of HGE (Hodzic et al., 1998; Ravyn et al., 2001). There are conflicting data from laboratory experiments on the duration of attachment of deer ticks that is necessary before the agent of granulocytic ehrlichiosis can be transmitted, although it has been suggested that it may be transmitted more rapidly than is *B. burgdorferi* (des Vignes et al., 2001; Katavolos et al., 1998). Perinatal transmission of HGE, though extremely rare, has been documented (Horowitz et al., 1998). Congenital disease has not been described.

Clinical manifestations. In 1987 the first case of human ehrlichiosis in the United States was reported (Maeda et al., 1987). Since then, HME and HGE have been recognized with increasing frequency (Bakken et al., 1998; Barton et al., 1992; Belongia et al., 2000; Centers for Disease Control and Prevention, 1998; Harkness et al., 1991; Ijdo et al., 2000). Despite differences in the cells that they infect, the clinical manifestations of HME and HGE are similar, and they resemble the clinical manifestations of Rocky Mountain spotted fever except that few patients have a rash (Bakken and Dumler, 2001; Bakken et al., 1996; Dumler et al., 1996; Horowitz et al., 1998; Jacobs and Schutze, 1997). Fever and headache are the most common manifestations of the illness, followed by myalgia, nausea, vomiting, and arthralgia. Symptoms of involvement of the CNS may be prominent (Ratnasamy et al., 1996). Leukopenia and thrombocytopenia occur in most patients in the first week of the illness. Fishbein et al. (1987, 1989) reported leukopenia in 57% of their patients and thrombocytopenia in 85% at the time of hospitalization. More than three quarters of the patients have elevated concentrations of either alanine or aspartate aminotransferase during the course of the illness, usually during the first week. During the acute illness inclusion bodies may be seen in atypical lymphocytes, neutrophils, and monocytes. These inclusions are dark blue, round, and approximately 2 to 5 μm in diameter. Electron microscopy shows aggregates of organisms in membrane-lined vacuoles.

Sennetsu fever, described in the 1950s, is marked by the rapid onset of fever, lymphadenopathy, and atypical lymphocytosis. A rickettsia-like agent was isolated from the blood, lymph nodes, and bone marrow of an affected patient. The provisional species name associated with the organism was *R. sennetsu*; however, the organism was reclassified as *E. sennetsu* (and, more recently, *N. sennetsu*). The disease rarely has been reported outside of Japan. One serologic survey from Malaysia suggested that a substantial number of patients with febrile illnesses had antibodies to this organism. The illness occurs predominately in the summer and fall. The incubation period is approximately 14 days, with sudden onset of illness and generalized adenopathy developing within the first week of illness. The untreated illness is benign, and no fatalities or serious complications have been described.

Diagnosis. Although examination of the peripheral smear for the presence of morulae may be helpful, the sensitivity of this method of diagnosis is poor. Culture of the organisms is possible, but the procedure is difficult and not widely available (Goodman et al., 1996). Use of PCR assay to make the diagnosis is promising and is being used more widely, although, like new ELISA tests (Ijdo et al., 1999), it is not well standardized (Comer et al; 1999b; Everett at al., 1994; Felek et al., 2001; Massung et al., 1998; Walls et al., 2000). Consequently, the mainstay of diagnosis is serologic testing (Aguero-Rosenfeld et al., 2000; Comer et al., 1999a). To make a diagnosis of ehrlichiosis in a patient with a compatible clinical history, there should be a fourfold rise between acute and convalescent serum samples in the concentration of antibodies against *E. chaffeensis* (minimum titer 1:64) for HME and, for HGE (until the causative agent is identified), a similar increase in antibody concentrations (or a single titer of ≥ 1:128) against *E. equi* (Dawson et al., 1990; Dawson et al., 1991). Indirect IFA tests are the most widely used, although there may be some variation from laboratory to laboratory (Nicholson et al., 1997; Walls et al., 1999).

Treatment and prognosis. Tetracyclines are the drugs of choice to treat ehrlichiosis. Although chloramphenicol has been effective in many instances, there also are a considerable number of reports of failures of treatment with chloramphenicol. Consequently, many experts treat even young children with tetracycline or doxycycline because the risk of staining of the teeth from a short course of treatment is low and the potential benefit of the drug outweighs the small risk. Quinolones and rifamycins may also be effective (Klein et al., 1997). Rifampin has been used successfully to treat a pregnant woman with HGE (Buitrago et al., 1998).

Ehrlichiosis sometimes (but rarely) is fatal. Serosurveys indicate that unrecognized infection is far more common than severe infection (some patients have either asymptomatic or unrecognized illness) (Magnarelli et al., 1995). The illness may be prolonged in some patients, but the ultimate prognosis is excellent (Bakken and Dumler, 2000; Dumler at al., 1996).

Prevention. Measures that reduce the risk of exposure to ticks may be effective in limiting the opportunities for infection to occur. There is no effective vaccine.

BIBLIOGRAPHY
Lyme disease
Adams WV, Rose CD, Eppes SC, et al. Cognitive effects of Lyme disease in children. Pediatrics 1994;94:185-189.

Advisory Committee on Immunization Practices. Centers for Disease Control and Prevention. Recommendations for the use of Lyme disease vaccine. MMWR Recomm Rep 1999;48:1-25.

Aronowitz RA. Lyme disease: the social construction of a new disease and its social consequences. Millbank Q 1991;69:79-112.

Bacterial Zoonoses Branch. Centers for Disease Control and Prevention. Evaluation of serologic tests for Lyme disease: report of a national evaluation. Lyme disease Surveill Summ 1991;2:1-3.

Bakken LL, Callister SM, Wand PJ, et al. Interlaboratory comparison of test results for detection of Lyme disease by 516 participants in the Wisconsin State Laboratory of Hygiene/College of American Pathologists proficiency testing program. J Clin Microbiol 1997;35:537-543.

Bakken LL, Case KL, Callister SM, et al. Performance of 45 laboratories participating in a proficiency testing program for Lyme disease serology. JAMA 1992;268:891-895.

Benach JL, Bosler EM, Hanrahan JP, et al. Spirochetes isolated from the blood of two patients with Lyme disease. N Engl J Med 1983;308:740-742.

Burgdorfer W, Barbour AG, Hayes SF, et al. Lyme disease—a tick born spirochetosis? Science 1982;216:1317-1319.

Centers for Disease Control and Prevention. Recommendations for test performance and interpretation from the second national conference on serologic diagnosis of Lyme disease. MMWR Morb Mortal Wkly Rep 1995;44:590.

Centers for Disease Control and Prevention. Lyme disease—United States, 2000. MMWR Morb Mortal Wkly Rep 2002;51:29-31.

Dressler F, Whalen JA, Reinhardt BN, et al. Western blotting in the serodiagnosis of Lyme disease. J Infect Dis 1993;167:392-400.

Eichenfield AH, Goldsmith DP, Benach JL, et al. Childhood Lyme arthritis: experience in an endemic area. J Pediatr 1986;109:753-758.

Falco RC, Fish D, Piesman J. Duration of tick bites in a Lyme disease-endemic area. Am J Epidemiol 1996; 143:187-192.

Feder HM Jr, Hunt MS. Pitfalls in the diagnosis and treatment of Lyme disease in children. JAMA 1995;274: 66-68.

Feder HM Jr, Beran J, Van Hoecke C, et al. Immunogenicity of a recombinant Borrelia burgdorferi outer surface protein A vaccine against Lyme disease in children. J Pediatr 1999;135:575-579.

Feder HM Jr, Gerber MA, Luger SW, et al. Persistence of serum antibodies to Borrelia burgdorferi in patients treated for Lyme disease. Clin Infect Dis 1992;15: 788-793.

Fishbein DB, Dennis DT: Tick-borne diseases—a growing risk. N Engl J Med 1995;333:452-453.

Gerber MA, Shapiro ED, Burke GS, et al. Lyme disease in children in Southeastern Connecticut. N Engl J Med 1996;335:1270-1274.

Gerber MA, Zalneraitis EL. Childhood neurologic disorders and Lyme disease during pregnancy. Pediatr Neurol 1994;11:41-43.

Gerber MA, Zemel LS, Shapiro ED. Lyme arthritis in children: clinical epidemiology and long-term outcomes. Pediatrics 1998;102:905-908.

Gross DW, Forsthuber T, Tary-Lehmann M, et al. Identification of LFA-1 as a candidate autoantigen in treatment-resistant Lyme arthritis. Science 1998; 281:703-706.

Hanrahan JP, Benach JL, Coleman JL, et al. Incidence and cumulative frequency of endemic Lyme disease in a community. J Infect Dis 1984;150:489-496.

Hilton E, Tramontano A, DeVoti J, et al. Temporal study of immunoglobulin M seroreactivity to Borrelia burgdorferi in patients treated for Lyme borreliosis. J Clin Microbiol 1997;35:774-776.

Kalish RA, McHugh G, Granquist J, et al. Persistence of immunoglobin M or immunoglobin G antibody responses to Borrelia burgdorferi 10-20 years after active Lyme disease. Clin Infect Dis 2001;33:780-785.

Klempner MS, Hu LT, Evans J, et al. Two controlled trials of antibiotic treatment in patients with persistent symptoms and a history of Lyme disease. N Engl J Med 2001;345:85-92.

Lane RS, Piesman J, Burgdorfer W. Lyme borreliosis: relation of its causative agent to its vectors and hosts in North America and Europe. Ann Rev Entomol 1991; 36:587-609.

Lathrop SL, Ball R, Haber P, et al. Adverse event reports following vaccination for Lyme disease: December 1998-July 2000. 2002;20:1603-1608.

Nadal D, Hunziker UA, Bucher HU, et al. Infants born to mothers with antibodies against Borrelia burgdorferi at delivery. Eur J Pediatr 1989;148:426-427.

Nadelman RB, Hororwitz HW, Hsieh T-C, et al. Simultaneous human ehrlichiosis and Lyme borreliosis. N Engl J Med 1997;337:27-30.

Nadelman RB, Nowakowski J, Fish D, et al. Prophylaxis with single-dose doxycycline for the prevention of Lyme disease after an Ixodes scapularis tick bite. N Engl J Med 2001;345:79-84.

Nocton JJ, Dressler F, Rutledge BJ, et al. Detection of Borrelia burgdorferi DNA by polymerase chain reaction in synovial fluid from patients with Lyme arthritis. N Engl J Med 1994;330:229-234.

Parola P, Raoult D. Ticks and tick-borne bacterial diseases in humans: an emerging infectious threat. Clin Infect Dis 2001;32:897-928.

Piesman J. Dynamics of Borrelia burgdorferi transmission by nymphal Ixodes dammini ticks. J Infect Dis 1993;167:1082-1085.

Piesman J, Mather TN, Sinsky R. Duration of tick attachment and Borrelia burgdorferi transmission. J Clin Microbiol 1987;25:557-558.

Piesman J, Maupin GO, Campos EG, et al. Duration of adult female Ixodes dammini attachment and transmission of Borrelia burgdorferi, description of a needle aspiration isolation method. J Infect Dis 1991;163:895-897.

Reid MC, Schoen RT, Evans J, et al. The consequences of overdiagnosis and overtreatment of Lyme disease: an observational study. Ann Intern Med 1998;128:354-362.

Rosa PA, Schwan TG. A specific and sensitive assay for the Lyme disease spirochete Borrelia burgdorferi using the polymerase chain reaction. J Infect Dis 1989;160:1018-1029.

Salazaar JC, Gerber MA, Goff CW. Long-term outcome of Lyme disease in children given early treatment. J Pediatr 1993;122:591-593.

Schwartz B, Nadelman RB, Fish D, et al. Entomologic and demographic correlates of anti-tick saliva antibody in a prospective study of tick bite subjects in Westchester County, New York. Am J Trop Med Hyg 1993;48:50-57.

Seltzer EG, Gerber MA, Cartter ML, et al. Long-term outcomes of persons with Lyme disease. JAMA 2000; 283:609-616.

Seltzer EG, Shapiro ED. Misdiagnosis of Lyme disease: when not to order serologic tests. Pediatr Infect Dis J 1996;15:762-763.

Shadick NA, Liang MH, Phillips CB, et al. The cost-effectiveness of vaccination against Lyme disease. Arch Intern Med 2001;161:554-561.

Shapiro ED. Doxycycline for tick bites—not for everyone. N Engl J Med 2001;345:133-134.

Shapiro ED, Gerber MA. State-of-the-art clinical article: Lyme disease. Clin Infect Dis 2000;31:533-542.

Shapiro ED, Gerber MA, Holabird NB, et al. A controlled trial of antimicrobial prophylaxis for Lyme disease after deer-tick bites. N Engl J Med 1992;327:1769-1773.

Shapiro ED. Long-term outcomes of persons with Lyme disease. Vector Borne Zoonotic Dis 2002;2:279-281.

Sigal LH. Persisting complaints attributed to chronic Lyme disease: possible mechanisms and implications for management. Am J Med 1994;96:365-374.

Sigal LH. The Lyme disease controversy: Social and financial costs of misdiagnosis and mismanagement. Arch Intern Med 1996;156:1493-1500.

Sigal LH, Patella SJ. Lyme arthritis as the incorrect diagnosis in pediatric and adolescent fibromyalgia. Pediatrics 1992;90:523-528.

Sikand VK, Halsey N, Krause PJ, et al. Safety and immunogenicity of a recombinant Borrelia burgdorferi outer surface protein A vaccine against Lyme disease in healthy children and adolescents: a randomized controlled trial. Pediatrics 2001;108:123-128.

Spach DH, Liles WC, Campbell GL, et al. Medical progress: tick-borne diseases in the United States. N Engl J Med 1993;329:936-947.

Steere AC. Lyme disease. N Engl J Med 1989;321:586-596.

Steere AC. Lyme disease. N Engl J Med 2001;345:115-125.

Steere AC, Grodzicki RL, Kornblatt AN, et al. The spirochetal etiology of Lyme disease. N Engl J Med 1983;308:733-740.

Steere AC, Sikand VK, Meurice F, et al. Vaccination against Lyme disease with recombinant *Borrelia burgdorferi* outer-surface lipoprotein A with adjuvant. N Engl J Med. 1998;339:209-216.

Steere AC, Taylor E, McHugh GL, et al. The overdiagnosis of Lyme disease. JAMA 1993;269:1812-1826.

Steere AC, Taylor E, Wilson ML, et al. Longitudinal assessment of the clinical and epidemiological features of Lyme disease in a defined population. J Infect Dis 1986;154:294-300.

Steere C, Dwyer E, Winchester R. Association of chronic Lyme arthritis with HLA-DR4 and HLA-DR2 alleles. N Engl J Med 1990;323:219-223.

Strobino BA, Williams CL, Abid S, et al. Lyme disease and pregnancy outcome: prospective study of two thousand prenatal patients. Am J Obstet Gynecol 1993;169:367-375.

Thompson C, Spielman A, Krause PJ. Coinfecting deer-associated zoonoses: Lyme disease, babesiosis, and ehrlichiosis. Clin Infect Dis 2001;33:676-685.

Tugwell P, Dennis DT, Weinstein A, et al. Laboratory evaluation in the diagnosis of Lyme disease. Ann Intern Med 1997;127:1109-1123.

Wang TJ, Liang MH, Sangha O, et al. Coexposure to *Borrelia burgdorferi* and *Babesia microti* does not worsen the long-term outcome of Lyme disease. Clin Infect Dis 2000;31:1149-1154.

Williams CL, Benach JL, Curran AS, et al. Lyme disease during pregnancy: a cord blood serosurvey. Ann NY Acad Sci 1988;539:504-506.

Wormser GP, Nadelman RB, Dattwyler RJ, et al. Infectious Diseases Society of America practice guidelines for the treatment of Lyme disease. Clin Infect Dis 2000;31(suppl 1):S1-S14. (Also available at: www.idsociety.org)

Relapsing Fever

Barbour AG, Barrera O, Judd RC. Structural analysis of the variable major proteins of *Borrelia hermsii*. J Exp Med 1983;158:2127-2140.

Barbour AG, Carter CJ, Sohaskey CD. Surface protein variation by expression site switching in the relapsing fever agent *Borrelia hermsii*. Infect Immun 2000;68:7114-7121.

Boyer KM, Munford RS, Maupin GO, et al. Tick-borne relapsing fever: an interstate outbreak originating at Grand Canyon National Park. Am J Epidemiol 1977;105:469-479.

Dworkin MS, Anderson DE Jr, Schwan TG, et al. Tick-borne relapsing fever in the northwestern United States and southwestern Canada. Clin Infect Dis 1998;26:122-131.

Edall TA, Emerson JK, Maupin GO, et al. Tick-borne relapsing fever in Colorado. Historical review and report of cases. JAMA 1979;241:2279-2282.

Fekade D, Knox K, Hussein K, et al. Prevention of Jarisch-Herxheimer reactions by treatment with antibodies against tumor necrosis factor alpha. N Engl J Med 1996;335:311-315.

Felsenfeld O. *Borrelia*, human relapsing fever, and parasite-vector-host relationships. Bacteriol Rev 1965;29:46-74.

Horton JM, Blaser MJ. The spectrum of relapsing fever in the Rocky Mountains. Arch Intern Med 1985;145:871-875.

Le CT. Tick-borne relapsing fever in children. Pediatrics 1980;66:963-966.

Plasterk RHA, Simon MI, Barbour AG. Transposition of structural genes to an expression sequence on a linear plasmid causes antigenic variation in the bacterium *Borrelia hermsii*. Nature 1985;318:257-263.

Schwan TG, Hinnebusch BJ. Bloodstream-versus tick-associated variants of a relapsing fever bacterium. Science 1998;280:938-940.

Stoenner HG, Dodd T, Larsen C. Antigenic variation of *Borrelia hermsii*. J Exp Med 1982;156:1297-1311.

Southern PM, Sanford JP. Relapsing fever: a clinical and microbiological review. Medicine 1969;48:129-149.

Talbert A, Nyange A, Molteni F. Spraying tick-infested houses with lambda-cyhalothrin reduces the incidence of tick-borne relapsing fever in children under five years old. Trans R Soc Trop Med Hyg 1998;92:251-253.

Trevejo RT, Schriefer ME, Gage KL, et al. An interstate outbreak of tick-borne relapsing fever among vacationers at a Rocky Mountain cabin. Am J Trop Med Hyg 1998;58:743-747.

Tularemia

Burke DS. Immunization against tularemia: analysis of the effectiveness of live *Francisella tularensis* vaccine in prevention of laboratory-acquired tularemia. J Infect Dis 1977;135:55-60.

Dennis DT, Inglesby TV, Henderson DA, et al. Tularemia as a biological weapon: medical and public health management. JAMA 2001;285:2763-2773.

Dolan SA, Dommaraju CB, DeGuzman GB. Detection of *Francisella tularensis* in clinical specimens by use of polymerase chain reaction. Clin Infect Dis 1998;26:764-765.

Enderlin G, Morales L, Jacobs RF, et al. Streptomycin and alternative agents for the treatment of tularemia: review of the literature. Clin Infect Dis 1994;19:42-47.

Evans ME, Gregory DW, Schaffner W, et al. Tularemia: a 37-year experience with 88 cases. Medicine 1985;64:251-269.

Feldman KA, Enscore RE, Lathrop SL, et al. An outbreak of primary pneumonic tularemia on Martha's Vineyard. N Engl J Med 2001;345:1601-1606.

Fournier PE, Bernabeu L, Schubert B, et al. Isolation of *Francisella tularensis* by centrifugation of shell vial cell culture from an inoculation eschar. J Clin Microbiol 1998;36:2782-2783.

Fulop M, Leslie D, Titball R. A rapid, highly sensitive method for the detection of *Francisella tularensis* in clinical samples using the polymerase chain reaction. Am J Trop Med Hyg 1996;54:364-366.

Francis E. Tularemia. JAMA 1925;84:1243-1250.

Guerrant RL, Humphries MK Jr, Butler JE, et al. Tickborne oculoglandular tularemia: case report and review of seasonal and vectorial associations in 106 cases. Arch Intern Med 1976;136:811-813.

Hopla CE. The ecology of tularemia. Adv Vet Sci Compar Med 1974;18:25-53.

Jacobs RF, Condrey YM, Yamauchi T. Tularemia in adults and children: a changing presentation. Pediatrics 1985;76:818-822.

Jacobs RF, Narain JP. Tularemia in children. Pediatr Infect Dis J 1983;2:487-491.

Johansson A, Berglund L, Eriksson U, et al. Comparative analysis of PCR versus culture for diagnosis of ulceroglandular tularemia. J Clin Microbiol 2000a;38:22-26.

Johansson A, Berglund L, Gothefors L, et al. Ciprofloxacin for treatment of tularemia in children. Pediatr Infect Dis J 2000b;19:449-453.

Johansson A, Ibrahim A, Goransson I, et al. Evaluation of PCR-based methods for discrimination of Francisella species and subspecies and development of a specific PCR that distinguishes the two major subspecies of Francisella tularensis. J Clin Microbiol 2000c;38: 4180-4185.

Junhui Z, Ruifu Y, Jianchun L, et al. Detection of Francisella tularensis by the polymerase chain reaction. J Med Microbiol 1996;45:477-482.

Khlebnikov VS, Golovliov IR, Kulevatsky DP, et al. Outer membranes of a lipopolysaccharide-protein complex (LPS-17 kDa protein) as chemical tularemia vaccines. FEMS Immunol Med Microbiol 1996;13:227-233.

Limaye AP, Hooper CJ. Treatment of tularemia with fluoroquinolones: two cases and review. Clin Infect Dis 1999;29:922-924.

Long GW, Oprandy JJ, Narayanan RB, et al. Detection of Francisella tularensis in blood by polymerase chain reaction. J Clin Microbiol 1993;31:152-154.

Markowitz LE, Hynes NA, de la Cruz P, et al. Tick-borne tularemia: an outbreak of lymphadenopathy in children. JAMA 1985;254:2922-2925.

Perez-Castrillon JL, Bachiller-Luque P, Martin-Luquero M, et al. Tularemia epidemic in northwestern Spain: clinical description and therapeutic response. Clin Infect Dis 2001;33:573-576.

Sjostedt A, Eriksson U, Berglund L, et al. Detection of Francisella tularensis in ulcers of patients with tularemia by PCR. J Clin Microbiol 1997;35:1045-1048.

Taylor JP, Istre GR, McChesney TC, et al. Epidemiologic characteristics of human tularemia in the southwest-central states, 1981-1987. Am J Epidemiol 1991;133: 1032-1038.

Waag DM, Sandstrom G, England MJ, et al. Immunogenicity of a new lot of Francisella tularensis live vaccine strain in human volunteers. FEMS Immunol Med Microbiol 1996;13:205-209.

Babesiosis

Eskow ES, Krause PJ, Spielman A, et al. Southern extension of the range of human babesiosis in the eastern United States. J Clin Microbiol 1999;37:2051-2052.

Hatcher JC, Greenberg PD, Antique J, et al. Severe babesiosis in Long Island: review of 34 cases and their complications. Clin Infect Dis 2001;32:1117-1125.

Homer MJ, Aguilar-Delfin I, Telford SR 3rd, et al. Babesiosis. Clin Microbiol Rev 2000;13:451-469.

Krause PJ, Lepore T, Sikand VK, et al. Atovaquone and azithromycin for the treatment of babesiosis. N Engl J Med 2000;343:1454-1458.

Krause PJ, Ryan R, Telford S 3rd, et al. Efficacy of immunoglobulin M serodiagnostic test for rapid diagnosis of acute babesiosis. J Clin Microbiol 1996a;34:2014-2016.

Krause PJ, Spielman A, Telford SR 3rd, et al. Persistent parasitemia after acute babesiosis. N Engl J Med 1998;339:160-165.

Krause PJ, Telford SR III, Pollack RJ, et al. Babesiosis: an underdiagnosed disease of children. Pediatrics 1992;89:1045-1048.

Krause PJ, Telford SR III, Ryan R, et al. Diagnosis of babesiosis: evaluation of a serologic test for the detection of Babesia microti antibody. J Infect Dis 1994;69: 923-926.

Krause PJ, Telford S 3rd, Spielman A, et al. Comparison of PCR with blood smear and inoculation of small animals for diagnosis of Babesia microti parasitemia. J Clin Microbiol 1996b;34:2791-2794.

Krause PJ, Telford SR III, Spielman A, et al. Concurrent Lyme disease and babesiosis: evidence for increased severity and duration of illness. JAMA 1996c;275: 1657-1660.

Magnarelli LA, Dumler JS, Anderson JF, et al. Coexistence of antibodies to tick-borne pathogens of babesiosis, ehrlichiosis, and Lyme borreliosis in human sera. J Clin Microbiol 1995;33:3054-3057.

Meldrum SC, Birkhead GS, White DJ, et al. Human babesiosis in New York state: an epidemiological description of 136 cases. Clin Infect Dis 1992;15: 1019-1023.

Mintz ED, Anderson JF, Cable RG, et al. Transfusion-transmitted babesiosis: a case report from a new endemic area. Transfusion 1991;31:365-368.

Persing DH, Herwaldt BL, Glaser C, et al. Infection with a babesia-like organism in northern California. N Engl J Med 1995;332:298-303.

Persing DH, Mathiesen D, Marshall WF, et al. Detection of Babesia microti by polymerase chain reaction. J Clin Microbiol 1992;30:2097-2103.

McQuiston JH, Childs JE, Chamberland ME, et al. Transmission of tick-borne agents of disease by blood transfusion: a review of known and potential risks in the United States. Transfusion 2000;40:274-284.

Reubush TK II, Cassaday PB, Marsh HJ, et al. Human babesiosis on Nantucket Island. Ann Intern Med 1977;86:6-9.

Ryan R, Krause PJ, Radolf J, et al. Diagnosis of babesiosis using an immunoblot serologic test. Clin Diagnost Lab Immunol 2001;8:1177-1180.

Sun T, Tenenbaum MJ, Greenspan J, et al. Morphologic and clinical observations in human infection with Babesia microti. J Infect Dis 1983;148:239-244.

Thompson C, Spielman A, Krause PJ. Coinfecting deer-associated zoonoses: Lyme disease, babesiosis, and ehrlichiosis. Clin Infect Dis 2001;33:676-685.

Weinberg GA. Laboratory diagnosis of ehrlichiosis and babesiosis. Pediatr Infect Dis J 2001;20:435-437.

White DJ, Talarico J, Chang HG, et al. Human babesiosis in New York State: review of 139 hospitalized cases and analysis of prognostic factors. Arch Intern Med 1998;158:2149-2154.

Rocky Mountain spotted fever

Abramson JS, Givner LB. Should tetracycline be contraindicated for therapy of presumed Rocky Mountain spotted fever in children less than 9 years of age? Pediatrics 1990;86:123-124.

Abramson JS, Givner LB. Rocky Mountain spotted fever. Pediatr Infect Dis J 1999;18:539-540.

Anacker RL, Lissh RH, Mann RE, et al. Antigenic heterogeneity in high and low virulence strains of Rickettsia *rickettsii* revealed by monoclonal antibodies. Infect Immun 1986;51:653.

Anacker RL, Philip RN, Casper E, et al. Biological properties of rabbit antibodies to a surface antigen of *Rickettsia rickettsii*. Infect Immun 1983;40:292.

Anderson BE, Tzianabosj I. Comparative sequence analysis of a genus-common rickettsial antigen gene. J Bacteriol 1989;171:5199.

Archibald LK, Sexton DJ. Long-term sequelae of Rocky Mountain spotted fever. Clin Infect Dis 1995;20: 1122-1125.

Baganz MD, Dross PE, Reinhardt JA. Rocky Mountain spotted fever encephalitis: MR findings.
Am J Neuroradiol 1995;16(suppl):919-922.

Bradford WD, Croker BP, Tisher CC. Kidney lesions in Rocky Mountain spotted fever. Am J Pathol 1979;97:383.

Bradford WD, Hawkins HK. Rocky Mountain spotted fever in childhood. Am J Dis Child 1977;131:1228.

Cale DF, McCarthy MW. Treatment of Rocky Mountain spotted fever in children. Ann Pharmacother 1997;31: 492-494.

Centers for Disease Control and Prevention. Consequences of delayed diagnosis of Rocky Mountain spotted fever in children—West Virginia, Michigan, Tennessee, and Oklahoma, May-July 2000. MMWR Morb Mortal Wkly Rep 2000;49:885-888.

Clements ML, Dumler JS, Fiset P, et al. Serodiagnosis of Rocky Mountain spotted fever: comparison of IgM and IgG enzyme-linked immunosorbent assays and indirect fluorescent antibody test. J Infect Dis 1983;148:876.

D'Angelo LJ, Winkler WG, Bergman DJ. Rocky Mountain spotted fever in the United States, 1975-1977. J Infect Dis 1978;138:273.

Dumler JS, Walker DH. Diagnostic tests for Rocky Mountain spotted fever and other rickettsial diseases. Dermatol Clin 1994;12:25-36.

DuPont HL, Hornick RB, Dawkins AT, et al. Rocky Mountain spotted fever: a comparative study of the active immunity induced by inactivated and viable pathogenic *R. rickettsii*. J Infect Dis 1973;128:340.

Feng WC, Waner JL. Serological cross-reaction and cross-protection in Guinea pigs infected with *Rickettsia rickettsii* and *Rickettsia montana*. Infect Immun 1980;28:627.

Hattwick MAW, Retailliau H, O'Brien RJ, et al. Fatal Rocky Mountain spotted fever. JAMA 1978;240:1499.

Hayes SF, Burgdorfer W. Reactivation of *Rickettsia rickettsii* in *Dermacentor andersoni* ticks: an ultrastructural analysis. Infect Immun 1982;37:779.

Hechemy KE, Michaelson EE, Anacker RL, et al. Evaluation of latex *Rickettsia rickettsii* test for Rocky Mountain spotted fever in 11 laboratories. J Clin Microbiol 1983;18:938.

Holman RC, Paddock CD, Curns AT, et al. Analysis of risk factors for fatal Rocky Mountain spotted fever: evidence for superiority of tetracyclines for therapy. J Infect Dis 2001;184:1437-1444.

King WV. Experimental transmission of Rocky Mountain spotted fever by means of the tick. Public Health Rep 1986;21:863.

Kirkland KB, Marcom PK, Sexton DJ, et al. Rocky Mountain spotted fever complicated by gangrene: report of six cases and review. Clin Infect Dis 1993;16:629-634.

Kirkland KB, Wilkinson WE, Sexton DJ. Therapeutic delay and mortality in cases of Rocky Mountain spotted fever. Clin Infect Dis 1995;20:1118-1121.

Lochary ME, Lockhart PB, Williams WT Jr. Doxycycline and staining of permanent teeth. Pediatr Infect Dis J 1998;17:429-431.

McDade JE, Newhouse VF. Natural history of *Rickettsia rickettsii*. Ann Rev Microbiol 1986;40:287.

McDonald GA, Anacker RL, Gargjian K. Cloned gene of *Rickettsia rickettsii* surface antigen: candidate vaccine for Rocky Mountain spotted fever. Science 1987;235:83.

Oster CN, Burke DS, Kenyon RH, et al. Laboratory-acquired Rocky Mountain spotted fever: the hazard of aerosol transmission. N Engl J Med 1977;297:859.

Philip RN, Casper EA, MacCormack JN, et al. A comparison of serologic methods for diagnosis of Rocky Mountain spotted fever. Am J Epidemiol 1977;105:56.

Purvis JJ, Edwards MS. Doxycycline use for rickettsial disease in pediatric patients. Pediatr Infect Dis J 2000;19: 871-874.

Radulovic S, Speed R, Feng HM, et al. EIA with species-specific monoclonal antibodies: a novel seroepidemiologic tool for determination of the etiologic agent of spotted fever rickettsiosis. J Infect Dis 1993;168:1292-1295.

Salgo MP, Telzak EE, Currie B, et al. A focus of Rocky Mountain spotted fever within New York City. N Engl J Med 1988;318:1345-1348.

Sexton DJ, Corey GR. Rocky Mountain "spotless" and "almost spotless" fever: a wolf in sheep's clothing. Clin Infect Dis 1992;15:439-448.

Sexton DJ, Kanj SS, Wilson K, et al. The use of a polymerase chain reaction as a diagnostic test for Rocky Mountain spotted fever. Am J Trop Med Hyg 1994;50: 59-63.

Silverman DJ. *Rickettsia rickettsii*–induced cellular injury of human vascular endothelium in vitro. Infect Immun 1984;44:545.

Silverman DJ, Bond SB. Infection of human vascular endothelial cells by *Rickettsia rickettsii*. J Infect Dis 1979;26:714.

Silverman DJ, Wisseman CL. In vitro studies of rickettsia-host cell interactions: ultrastructural changes induced by *Rickettsia rickettsii* infection of chicken embryo fibroblasts. Infect Immun 1984;149:201.

Silverman DJ, Wisseman CL Jr, Waddell AD, et al. External layers of *Rickettsia prowazekii* and *Rickettsia rickettsii*: occurrence of a slime layer. Infect Immun 1978;22:233.

Teysseire N, Arnoux D, George F, et al. Von Willebrand factor release and thrombomodulin and tissue factor expression in *Rickettsia conorii*–infected endothelial cells. Infect Immun 1992;60:4388-4393.

Thorner AR, Walker DH, Petri WA Jr. Rocky Mountain spotted fever. Clin Infect Dis 1998;27:1353-1359.

Todd WJ, Burgdorfer W, Wray GP. Detection of fibrils associated with *Rickettsia rickettsii*. Infect Immun 1983;41: 1252.

Treadwell TA, Holman RC, Clarke MJ, et al. Rocky Mountain spotted fever in the United States, 1993-1996. Am J Trop Med Hyg 2000;63:21-26.

Walker DH. Rocky Mountain spotted fever: a seasonal alert. Clin Infect Dis 1995;20:1111-1117.

Walker DH, Firth WT, Edgell CJS. Human endothelial cell culture plaques induced by *Rickettsia rickettsii*. Infect Immun 1982;37:301.

Walker TS. Rickettsial interactions with human endothelial cells in vitro: adherence and entry. Infect Immun 1984; 44:205.

Walker TS, Melott GE. Rickettsial stimulation of endothelial platelet-activating factor synthesis. Infect Immun 1993;61:2024-2029.

Wells GM, Woodward TE, Fiset P, et al. Rocky Mountain spotted fever caused by blood transfusion. JAMA 1978;239:2763.

Wilfert CM, MacCormack JN, Kleeman K, et al. Epidemiology of Rocky Mountain spotted fever as determined by active surveillance. J Infect Dis 1984;150: 469-479.

Woodward TE, Pedersen SE, Oster CN, et al. Prompt confirmation of Rocky Mountain spotted fever. Identification of rickettsiae in skin tissues. J Infect Dis 1976;134:297.

Rickettsialpox

Brettman LR, Lewin S, Holzman RS, et al. Rickettsialpox: report of an outbreak and a contemporary review. Medicine 1981;60:363.

Dolgopol VB. Histologic changes in rickettsialpox. Am J Pathol 1948;24:119.

Greenberg M. Rickettsialpox in New York City. Am J Med 1948;4:866.

Huebner RJ, Jellison WL, Pomerantz C. Rickettsialpox—a newly recognized disease. IV. Isolation of a rickettsia apparently identical with the causative agent of rickettsialpox from Allodermanyssus sanguineus, a rodent mite. Public Health Rep 1946;61:1677.

Sussman LN. Kew Gardens' spotted fever. NY Med J 1946;2:27.

Wong B, Singer C, Armstrong D, Millian SJ. Rickettsialpox. Case report and epidemiologic review. JAMA 1979;242: 1998.

Typhus group

Berman SJ, Kundin WD. Scrub typhus in South Vietnam, a study of 87 cases. Ann Intern Med 1973;79:26.

Birg ML, La Scola B, Roux V, et al. Isolation of Rickettsia prowazekii from blood by shell vial cell culture. J Clin Microbiol 1999;37:3722-3724.

Brown GW, Robinson DM, Huxsall DL, et al. Scrub typhus: a common cause of illness in indigenous populations. Trans R Soc Trop Med Hyg 1976;70:444.

Carl M, Tibbs CW, Dobson ME, et al. Diagnosis of acute typhus infection using the polymerase chain reaction. J Infect Dis 1990;161:791-793.

Chinprasatsak S, Wilairatana P, Looareesuwan S, et al. Evaluation of a newly developed dipstick test for the rapid diagnosis of scrub typhus in febrile patients. Southeast Asian J Trop Med Public Health 2001;32:32-36.

Cracco C, Delafosse C, Baril L, et al. Multiple organ failure complicating probable scrub typhus. Clin Infect Dis 2000;31:191-192.

Dasch GA, Samms JR, Weiss E. Biochemical characteristics of typhus group rickettsiae with special attention to the Rickettsia prowazekii strains isolated from flying squirrels. Infect Immun 1978;19:676.

Duma RJ, Sonenshine DE, Bozeman FM, et al. Epidemic typhus in the United States associated with flying squirrels. JAMA 1981;245:2318.

Kim DE, Lee SH, Park KI, et al. Scrub typhus encephalomyelitis with prominent focal neurologic signs. Arch Neurol 2000;57:1770-1772.

Land MV, Ching WM, Dasch GA, et al. Evaluation of a commercially available recombinant-protein enzyme-linked immunosorbent assay for detection of antibodies produced in scrub typhus rickettsial infections. J Clin Microbiol 2000;38:2701-2705.

Massung RF, Davis LE, Slater K, et al. Epidemic typhus meningitis in the southwestern United States. Clin Infect Dis 2001;32:979-982.

Ormsbee RA. Serologic diagnosis of epidemic typhus fever. Am J Epidemiol 1977;105:261.

Osterman JV, Eisemann CS. Surface proteins of typhus and spotted fever group rickettsiae. Infect Immun 1978; 21:866.

Pai H, Sohn S, Seong Y, et al. Central nervous system involvement in patients with scrub typhus. Clin Infect Dis 1997;24:436-440.

Raoult D, Roux V. The body louse as a vector of reemerging human diseases. Clin Infect Dis 1999;29:888-911.

Samra Y, Shaked Y, Maier MK. Delayed neurologic display in murine typhus: report of two cases. Arch Intern Med 1989;149:949-951.

Shieh GJ, Chen HL, Chen HY, et al. ELISA-based colorimetric detection of Rickettsia tsutsugamushi DNA from patient sera by nested polymerase chain reaction. Southeast Asian J Trop Med Public Health 1996;27: 139-144.

Silpapojakul K, Chupuppakarn S, Yuthasompob S, et al. Scrub and murine typhus in children with obscure fever in the tropics. Pediatr Infect Dis 1991;10:200-203.

Sonenshine DE, Bozeman M, Williams MS, et al. Epizootiology of epidemic typhus (R. prowazekii) in flying squirrels. Am J Trop Med Hyg 1978;27:339.

Traub R, Wisseman CL. The ecology of chigger-borne rickettsiosis (scrub typhus). J Med Entomol 1974;11:237.

Watt G, Chouriyagune C, Ruangweerayud R, et al. Scrub typhus infections poorly responsive to antibiotics in northern Thailand. Lancet 1996;348:86-89.

Watt G, Kantipong P, Jongsakul K, et al. Doxycycline and rifampicin for mild scrub-typhus infections in northern Thailand: a randomised trial. Lancet 2000;356: 1057-1061.

Q fever

Amano KI, Williams JC. Sensitivity of Coxiella burnettii peptidoglycan to lysozyme hydrolysis and correlation of sacculus rigidity with peptidoglycan-associated proteins. J Bacteriol 1984;160:989.

Ascher MS, Berman MA, and Ruppanner R. Initial clinical and immunologic evaluation of a new phase I Q fever vaccine and skin test in humans. J Infect Dis 1983;148:214.

Baca OG, Paretsky D. Q fever and Coxiella burnettii: a model for host-parasite interactions. Microbiol Rev 1983;47:127.

Burnet FM, Freeman M. A comparative study of rickettsial strains from an infection of ticks in Montana (United States of America) and from Q fever. Med J Aust 1939;2:887.

Derrick EH. The course of infection with Coxiella burnettii. Med J Aust 1973;1:1051.

Fenollar F, Fournier PE, Carrieri MP, et al. Risks factors and prevention of Q fever endocarditis. Clin Infect Dis 2001;33:312-316.

Field PR, Hunt JG, Murphy AM. Detection and persistence of specific IgM antibody to Coxiella burnettii by enzyme-linked immunosorbent assay: a comparison with immunofluorescence and complement fixation tests. J Infect Dis 1983;148:477.

Fournier PE, Marrie TJ, Raoult D. Diagnosis of Q fever. J Clin Microbiol 1998;36:1823-1834.

Hart RJC. The epidemiology of Q fever. Postgrad Med J 1973;49:535.

Marmion BP, Ormsbee RA, Kyrkou M, et al. Vaccine prophylaxis of abattoir-associated Q fever: eight years' experience in Australian aborigines. Epidemiol Infect 1990;104:275-287.

Morisawa Y, Wakiguchi H, Takechi T, et al. Intractable Q fever treated with recombinant gamma interferon. Pediatr Infect Dis J 2001;20:546-547.

Ruiz-Contreras J, Montero RG, Amador JTR, et al. Q fever in children. Am J Dis Child 1993;147:300-302.

Sawyer LA, Fishbein DB, McDade JE. Q fever: current concepts. 1987;9:935-946.

Williams JC, Peacock MG, McCaul TF. Immunological and biological characterization of Coxiella burnettii, phases I and II, separated from host components. Infect Immun 1981;32:840.

Zhang GQ, Hotta A, Mizutani M, et al. Direct identification of Coxiella burnettii plasmids in human sera by nested PCR. J Clin Microbiol 1998;36:2210-2213.

Ehrlichiosis

Aguero-Rosenfeld ME, Kalantarpour F, Baluch M, et al. Serology of culture-confirmed cases of human granulocytic ehrlichiosis. J Clin Microbiol 2000;38:635-638.

Bakken JS, Dumler JS. Human granulocytic ehrlichiosis. Clin Infect Dis 2000;31:554-560.

Bakken JS, Dumler JS, Chen S-M, et al. Human granulocytic ehrlichiosis in the upper midwest United States. JAMA 1994;272:212-218.

Bakken JS, Goellner P, Van Etten M, et al. Seroprevalence of human granulocytic ehrlichiosis among permanent residents of northwestern Wisconsin. Clin Infect Dis 1998;27:1491-1496.

Bakken JS, Krueth J, Wilson-Nordskog C, et al. Clinical and laboratory characteristics of human granulocytic ehrlichiosis. JAMA 1996;275:199-205.

Barton LL, Rathore MH, Dawson JE. Infection with Ehrlichia in childhood. J Pediatr 1992;120:998-1001.

Belongia EA, Gale CM, Reed KD, et al. Population-based incidence of human granulocytic ehrlichiosis in northwestern Wisconsin, 1997-1999. J Infect Dis 2001;184:1470-1474.

Brouqui P, Dumler JS, Liehnard R, et al. Human granulocytic ehrlichiosis in Europe. Lancet 1995;346:782-783.

Buitrago MI, Ijdo JW, Rinaudo P, et al. Human granulocytic ehrlichiosis during pregnancy treated successfully with rifampin. Clin Infect Dis 1998;27:213-215.

Centers for Disease Control and Prevention. Statewide surveillance for ehrlichiosis—Connecticut and New York, 1994-1997. MMWR Morb Mortal Wkly Rep 1998;47:476-480.

Comer JA, Nicholson WL, Olson JG, et al. Serologic testing for human granulocytic ehrlichiosis at a national referral center. J Clin Microbiol 1999a;37:558-564.

Comer JA, Nicholson WL, Sumner JW, et al. Diagnosis of human ehrlichiosis by PCR assay of acute-phase serum. J Clin Microbiol 1999b;37:31-34.

Dawson JE, Fishbein DB, Eng TR, et al. Diagnosis of human ehrlichiosis with the indirect fluorescent antibody test: kinetics and specificity. J Infect Dis 1990;162:91-95.

Dawson JE, Rikihisa Y, Ewing SA, et al. Serologic diagnosis of human ehrlichiosis using two Ehrlichia canis isolates. J Infect Dis 1991;163:564-567.

des Vignes F, Piesman J, Heffernan R, et al. Effect of tick removal on transmission of Borrelia burgdorferi and Ehrlichia phagocytophila by Ixodes scapularis nymphs. J Infect Dis 2001;183:773-778.

Dumler JS, Bakken JS. Ehrlichial diseases of humans: emerging tick-borne infection. Clin Infect Dis 1995;20:1102-1110.

Dumler JS, Bakken JS. Human granulocytic ehrlichiosis in Wisconsin and Minnesota: a frequent infection with the potential for persistence. J Infect Dis 1996;173:1027-1030.

Dumler JS, Barbet AF, Bekker CP, et al. Reorganization of genera in the families Rickettsiaceae and Anaplasmataceae in the order Rickettsiales: unification of some species of Ehrlichia with Anaplasma, Cowdria with Ehrlichia and Ehrlichia with Neorickettsia, descriptions of six new species combinations and designations of Ehrlichia equi and "HGE agent" as subjective synonyms of Ehrlichia phagocytophila. Int J Syst Evol Microbiol 2001;6:2145-2165.

Everett ED, Evans KA, Henry RB, et al. Human ehrlichiosis in adults after tick exposure: diagnosis using polymerase chain reaction. Ann Intern Med 1994;120:735-737.

Felek S, Unver A, Stich RW, et al. Sensitive detection of Ehrlichia chaffeensis in cell culture, blood, and tick specimens by reverse transcription–PCR. J Clin Microbiol 2001;39:460-463.

Fishbein DB, Dawson JE, Robinson LE. Human ehrlichiosis in the United States, 1985-1990. Ann Intern Med 1994;120:736-743.

Fishbein DB, Kemp A, Dawson JE, et al. Human ehrlichiosis: prospective active surveillance in febrile hospitalized patients. J Infect Dis 1989;160:803-809.

Fishbein DB, Sawyer LA, Holland CJ, et al. Unexplained febrile illnesses after exposure to ticks. JAMA 1987;257:3100-3104.

Goodman JL, Nelson C, Vitale B, et al. Direct cultivation of the causative agent of human granulocytic ehrlichiosis. N Engl J Med 1996;334:209-215.

Gaudreault-Keener M, Manian FA, Liddell AM, et al. Ehrlichia ewingii, a newly recognized agent of human ehrlichiosis. N Engl J Med 1999;341:148-155.

Harkness JR, Ewing SA, Brumit T, et al. Ehrlichiosis in children. Pediatrics 1991;87:199-203.

Hodzic E, Fish D, Maretzki CM, et al. Acquisition and transmission of the agent of human granulocytic ehrlichiosis by Ixodes scapularis ticks. J Clin Microbiol 1998;36:3574-3578.

Horowitz HW, Aguero-Rosenfeld ME, McKenna DF, et al. Clinical and laboratory spectrum of culture-proven human granulocytic ehrlichiosis: comparison with culture-negative cases. Clin Infect Dis 1998;27:1314-1317.

Horowitz HW, Kilchevsky E, Haber S, et al. Perinatal transmission of the agent of human granulocytic ehrlichiosis. N Engl J Med 1998;339:375-378.

Ijdo JW, Meek JI, Cartter ML, et al. The emergence of another tickborne infection in the 12-town area around Lyme, Connecticut: human granulocytic ehrlichiosis. J Infect Dis 2000;181:1388-1393.

Ijdo JW, Wu C, Magnarelli LA, et al. Serodiagnosis of human granulocytic ehrlichiosis by a recombinant HGE-

44-based enzyme-linked immunosorbent assay. J Clin Microbiol 1999;37:3540-3544.

Jacobs RF, Schutze GE. Ehrlichiosis in children. J Pediatr 1997;131:184-192.

Katavolos P, Armstrong PM, Dawson JE, et al. Duration of tick attachment required for transmission of granulocytic ehrlichiosis. J Infect Dis 1998;177:1422-1425.

Klein BM, Nelson CM, Goodman JL. Antibiotic susceptibility of the newly cultivated agent of human granulocytic ehrlichiosis: promising activity of quinolones and rifamycins. Antimicrob Agents Chemother 1997;41:76-79.

Maeda K, Markowitz N, Hawley RC, et al. Human infection with *Ehrlichia canis*, a leukocytic rickettsia. N Engl J Med 1987;316:853-856.

Magnarelli LA, Dumler JS, Anderson JF, et al. Coexistence of antibodies to tick-borne pathogens of babesiosis, ehrlichiosis, and Lyme borreliosis in human sera. J Clin Microbiol 1995;33:3054-3057.

Massung RF, Slater K, Owens JH, et al. Nested PCR assay for detection of granulocytic ehrlichiae. J Clin Microbiol 1998;36:1090-1095.

McDade JE. Ehrlichiosis—a disease of animals and humans. J Infect Dis 1989;161:609-617.

Nicholson WL, Comer JA, Sumner JW, et al. An indirect immunofluorescence assay using a cell culture–derived antigen for detection of antibodies to the agent of human granulocytic ehrlichiosis. J Clin Microbiol 1997;35:1510-1516.

Pancholi P, Kolbert CP, Mitchell PD, et al. *Ixodes dammini* as a potential vector of human granulocytic ehrlichiosis. J Infect Dis 1995;172:1007-1012.

Ratnasamy N, Everett ED, Roland WE, et al. Central nervous system manifestations of human ehrlichiosis. Clin Infect Dis 1996;23:314-319.

Ravyn MD, Kodner CB, Carter SE, et al. Isolation of the etiologic agent of human granulocytic ehrlichiosis from the white-footed mouse *(Peromyscus leucopus)*. J Clin Microbiol 2001;39:335-338.

Schwartz I, Fish D, Daniels TJ. Prevalence of the rickettsial agent of human granulocytic ehrlichiosis in ticks from a hyperendemic focus of Lyme disease (letter). N Engl J Med 1997;337:49-50.

Thompson C, Spielman A, Krause PJ. Coinfecting deer-associated zoonoses: Lyme disease, babesiosis, and ehrlichiosis. Clin Infect Dis 2001;33:676-685.

Walls JJ, Aguero-Rosenfeld M, Bakken JS, et al. Inter- and intralaboratory comparison of *Ehrlichia equi* and human granulocytic ehrlichiosis (HGE) agent strains for serodiagnosis of HGE by the immunofluorescent-antibody test. J Clin Microbiol 1999;37:2968-2973.

Walls JJ, Caturegli P, Bakken JS, et al. Improved sensitivity of PCR for diagnosis of human granulocytic ehrlichiosis using epank1 genes of *Ehrlichia phagocytophila*—group Ehrlichiae. J Clin Microbiol 2000;38:354-356.

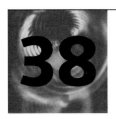

38 TOXOPLASMOSIS

Fiona Roberts, Kenneth Boyer, and Rima McLeod

Toxoplasmosis is disease caused by the ubiquitous, obligate intracellular protozoan *Toxoplasma gondii*. Infection is usually acquired orally or transplacentally, rarely by inoculation in a laboratory accident, by blood or leukocyte transfusion, or from a transplanted organ. Disease may also occur as the result of recrudescence of latent infection in immunocompromised individuals.

Clinical signs and symptoms depend in part on the host's immunologic status. In the immunologically healthy older child the acute infection may be asymptomatic, may cause self-limited lymphadenopathy with or without fatigue and malaise, or occasionally may cause significant organ damage. In the child who is immunocompromised because of acquired immunodeficiency syndrome (AIDS), organ transplantation, or cytotoxic therapy for malignancy or vasculitis, initial infection or recrudescence of latent infection may cause severe illness. The most common presentation in immunocompromised individuals is that of neurologic disease.

Congenitally acquired toxoplasmosis almost always causes morbidity and occasionally causes mortality. Most congenital infections are not recognized at birth but are manifested in later infancy, childhood, or adulthood. When infection is acquired by a mother early in gestation, transmission of the infection to her fetus occurs less frequently than when her infection is acquired later in gestation. When infection is transmitted, however, neurologic and ophthalmologic impairment is often severe. Involvement is less severe at birth in infants born to mothers who acquired the disease later in gestation. Nonetheless, although these infants usually appear normal in initial newborn examinations, 80% to 90% of them have ophthalmologic lesions by adolescence. Because *T. gondii* is a major opportunistic pathogen for patients with AIDS, congenital transmission of human immunodeficiency virus (HIV) and *T. gondii* from such mothers is an emerging problem, often causing extensive, fulminant, disseminated toxoplasmosis in the newborn infant.

Toxoplasmosis causes not only substantial morbidity and mortality for affected individuals, but also major expenditures for health care. For example, in 1975 Wilson and Remington (1980) estimated that the average lifetime cost of special care for each child with congenital toxoplasmosis was $67,000. Since the estimated incidence of congenital toxoplasmosis is 1.1 per 1,000 births, an estimated 3,300 infants are affected each year in the United States, resulting in a cost of $221,000,000 for lifetime care in 1975 dollars for infants born in just 1 year. Estimated productivity losses resulting from infection of children born in 1 year in the United States are $65 million to $1.6 billion, and estimated total preventable costs are $368 million to $8.7 billion dollars (Roberts and Frenkel, 1990; Wilson and Remington, 1980).

Congenital *Toxoplasma* infection in the fetus can be prevented by pregnant women if they avoid consumption of raw or undercooked meat and avoid accidental ingestion of material contaminated with cat feces. Serologic testing and antimicrobial therapy are important for prevention and treatment. Antimicrobial therapy given to an acutely infected mother can block transmission to her fetus (Desmonts and Couvreur, 1979). Such therapy can also cure signs of infection caused by proliferating tachyzoites in congenitally infected fetuses (Daffos et al., 1988; Hohlfeld et al., 1989); infants (McAuley et al., 1994; McGhee et al., 1992; McLeod et al., 1992; Mets et al., 1996; Patel et al., 1996; Roizen et al., 1995; Swisher et al., 1994); and immunocompromised individuals

(McLeod et al., 1979). Development of vaccines that prevent toxoplasmosis in humans and in animal reservoirs is important for prevention of this disease. A commercial vaccine is available for sheep that reduces ovine abortion resulting from toxoplasmosis (Buxton and Innes, 1995). Vaccines to prevent oocyst shedding from cats (Frenkel et al., 1991) and vaccines that potentially could protect against initial infection or disease in humans (Duquesne et al., 1990; McLeod et al., 1988; Prince et al., 1989) are still experimental.

HISTORY

In 1908 Nicolle and Manceaux described tachyzoites in spleen and liver mononuclear cells from the North African rodent *Ctenodactylus gundi*. In 1923 *T. gondii* was implicated in human disease when Janku, an ophthalmologist in Prague, found cysts containing *T. gondii* in the retina of an 11-month-old child with congenital hydrocephalus. In 1937 Wolf and Cowen described an infant with granulomatous encephalitis. The protozoan parasite causing this infection was later identified by Sabin as *T. gondii*. In 1948 Sabin and Feldman developed the Sabin-Feldman dye test, which permitted serologic testing and provided another means, in addition to histopathologic testing, for detecting disease caused by *T. gondii*. In 1970 *T. gondii* was classified among the coccidia, and it was discovered that the domestic cat and other felines were the only hosts in which the sexual form develops. In the 1960s through the 1980s the full spectrum of clinical syndromes caused by *T. gondii* was defined, as were more rational approaches to antimicrobial therapy in different clinical settings.

Recent developments in immunology and molecular and cell biology and new developments in the care of pregnant women, children, and immunocompromised individuals have led to development of improved diagnostic tests and approaches to care for patients with toxoplasmosis. Recent studies also have further elucidated the pathogenesis of the infection, facilitated diagnostic testing, contributed to the development of effective antimicrobial agents, and provided the groundwork for development of vaccines.

THE ORGANISM

T. gondii, a coccidian parasite, exists in a number of forms: tachyzoites (the rapidly proliferative form, formerly referred to as *trophozoites*);

bradyzoites (which replicate more slowly than tachyzoites and exist within tissue cysts); and oocysts (which contain highly infectious sporozoites). There are three primary clonal types of parasites (and recombinats of these) with different virulence for mice (and recent experience suggests possibly also for humans) and capacity to form cysts (Darde and Bouteille, 1988; Grigg et al 2001).

Tachyzoites

Tachyzoites (Figure 38-1, *A)* are crescent or oval in shape and are approximately 2 to 4 μm wide and 4 to 8 μm long. They stain well with either Wright's or Giemsa stain. Tachyzoites can invade and multiply in all mammalian cells. Their reproduction is by endodyogeny, a process of internal budding in which two daughter cells are formed within the parent cell. Daughter cells are released when the host cell wall is disrupted or lysed. Tachyzoites are fastidious and do not survive freezing, thawing, desiccation, or exposure to normal gastric secretions.

Bradyzoites

Bradyzoites (Figure 38-1, *B)* in tissue cysts are crescent-shaped organisms that appear similar to tachyzoites but replicate more slowly. They have unique epitopes that are not expressed by tachyzoites or sporozoites. In electron micrographs, bradyzoites differ from tachyzoites in that they have amylopectin granules, an increased number of organelles called *micronemes,* and electron-dense rhoptry organelles. Tissue cysts vary in size and contain a few to approximately 10,000 bradyzoites. Tissue cysts can be stained with periodic acid–Schiff (PAS) stain. Primary human infection can also occur by ingestion of bradyzoites within cysts in raw or undercooked meat. After ingestion the cyst wall is disrupted by pepsin or trypsin. The liberated bradyzoites can remain viable for up to 2 hours in pepsin–hydrogen chloride or as long as 6 hours in trypsin. Bradyzoites then invade the digestive tract mucosa and can disseminate throughout the body. Tissue cysts have been found in virtually every organ but appear to have greatest predilection for the retina, brain, heart, and skeletal muscle. Cysts remain viable throughout the life of the host. These tissue cysts can be a source of local or disseminated infection if the host becomes immunocompromised. Freezing to –20° C (–4° F), heating to 60° C (140° F),

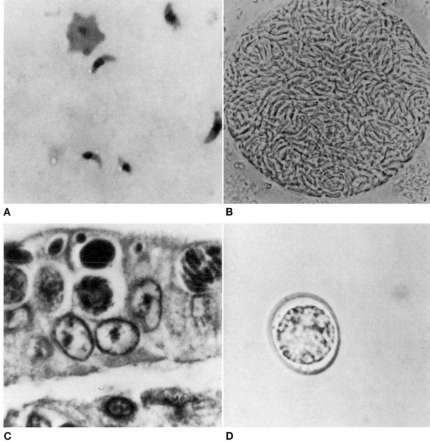

Fig. 38-1 Forms of *Toxoplasma gondii*. **A**, Tachyzoite. **B**, Bradyzoite in tissue cyst. **C**, Gametocytes in cat ileum. **D**, Unsporulated oocyst. (Modified from Dubey JP, Beattie CP. Toxoplasmosis of animals and man. Boca Raton, Fla.: CRC Press, 1988; and Gardiner CH, Fayer R, Dubey JP. An atlas of protozoan parasites in animal tissues. Washington, D.C.: U.S. Department of Agriculture, Agriculture Handbook No. 651, 1988.)

desiccation, and irradiation destroy viability of encysted bradyzoites.

Oocysts and Sporozoites

Oocysts (Figure 38-1, *C*) are oval and approximately 10 to 12 μm in diameter. They complete the life cycle of *T. gondii* within the intestine of its definitive host, cats. They are found in the cat intestine only during primary infection or, rarely, in a chronically infected cat that acquires another coccidian parasite, *Isospora* species. Oocysts can remain infectious in warm, moist soil for 1 year or more and easily resist the gastric acid barrier after ingestion. They can be killed by exposure to nearly boiling water for 5 minutes, by burning, or by contact with strong ammonia (7%) for 3 hours. Oocysts sporulate 1 to 5 days after excretion, and the sporozoites become highly infectious if they are ingested.

Life Cycle

There are two life cycles for *T. gondii*. The complete cycle—with schizogony (an asexual cycle) and gametogony (sporulating sexual cycle), which results in the formation of infectious oocysts—occurs only in members of the cat family. In all other animals only an incomplete cycle by schizogony occurs, forming tachyzoites or bradyzoites in tissue cysts. Toxoplasma organisms are acquired by susceptible cats when they eat meat (e.g., mice) that contains tissue cysts or ingest oocysts excreted by other recently infected cats (Figure 38-2). *T. gondii* then multiplies through both schizogonic and gametogonic cycles in the tips of villi in the cat's distal ileum. The time of the first appearance of oocysts in cat feces depends on the form of *T. gondii* ingested: 3 to 5 days after ingestion of *T. gondii* tissue cysts; 7 to 10 days after ingestion of *T. gondii*

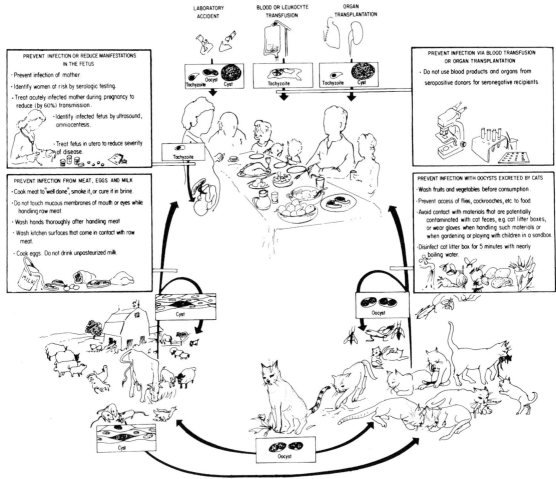

Fig. 38-2 Life cycle of *Toxoplasma gondii* and prevention of acquisition by humans. Infection of older children and adults occurs primarily after ingestion of cysts in undercooked meat or oocysts excreted by cats or by the fetus transplacentally from an acutely infected mother. After ingestion, organisms invade the intestinal epithelium, either hematogenously or through lymphatics, and are spread to other tissues; when there is a normal immune response, they form cysts. Rarely, infection is acquired by blood or leukocyte transfusion, in a transplanted organ, or via a laboratory accident. (Modified from McLeod and Remington. In Behrman RL, Vaughan VC III, Nelson WE [eds]. Nelson's textbook of pediatrics, ed 14. Philadelphia, Saunders, 1990.)

tachyzoites; and 20 to 24 days after the ingestion of *T. gondii* oocysts. For a brief 1- to 3-week period, an acutely infected cat can excrete 10^7 to 10^9 oocysts per day.

EPIDEMIOLOGY

The prevalence of *Toxoplasma* infection in cats and in tissue cysts in meat used for human consumption varies widely, depending in part on locale. In early studies in the United States, 50% of domestic cats were seropositive. In a study in Costa Rica where the overall antibody prevalence in people was 60%, over 20% of 237 cats were shedding oocysts when examined, and 60% overall were infected as shown by either oocyst shedding or *T. gondii*–specific antibody (Ruiz and Frenkel, 1980). *T. gondii* has been isolated from the skeletal muscle of 23% of market pigs and 42% of breeder pigs in the United States. The prevalence in Czechoslovakia ranged from 43% to 73%. Sheep used for human consumption had a prevalence rate of 4% to 22% in California. Cattle apparently are infected less commonly than sheep or pigs in the United States, Europe, and New Zealand. The combined prevalence rates range from 1% to 33%. The prevalence of infection in humans is also highly variable, depending in part on locale and age. Highest rates of seropositivity occur in El Salvador, Tahiti, and France, where the prevalence of seropositivity is greater than 90% by the fourth decade of life. In the United Kingdom and in the United States approximately 10% of the population has IgG antibody at 10 years of age, 20% at 20 years, and 50% at 70 years. The prevalence of infection lessens in colder regions, in hot and arid climates, and at high elevations. There is no significant difference in prevalence between men and women. One study showed that in Erecim, Brazil 18% of the 80% of seropositive individuals had toxoplasmic chorioretinitis and/or retinal scars (Glasner, 1992).

There have been clusters of cases of toxoplasmosis or *T. gondii* infection (1) caused by common exposures in a riding stable or by exposure to water, (2) associated with eating similarly prepared meat, and (3) in families. Data in experimental animals demonstrate significant immunogenetic differences in the manifestations of infection in mice (Brown and McLeod, 1990). Recent work suggests that genetics also influences human toxoplasmosis (Mack et al., 1999; McLeod et al., 1996; Suzuki et al., 1996). Congenital toxoplasmosis occurs when the mother acquires the infection for the first time during pregnancy. The risk of infection in an obstetric population depends on two factors: (1) the incidence of primary infection in the population as a whole, and (2) the proportion of women of childbearing age who have not been previously infected.

In the relatively few studies of prevalence of *Toxoplasma* antibodies in pregnant women, there is geographic variation. In the United States, 39% of 23,000 pregnant women in the Collaborative Perinatal Project had *T. gondii*–specific serum antibody. Other studies indicate a varying incidence of seropositivity in women of childbearing age in the United States: Denver, 3%; Palo Alto, California, 10%; Chicago, 12%; Boston, 14%; and Birmingham, Alabama, 30% (Remington et al., 1995). Seroprevalence studies of women of childbearing age from other nations or cities outside the United States also demonstrate variability in rates of seropositivity: Thailand, 3%; Australia, 4%; Japan, 6%; Scotland, 13%; London, 20%; Poland, 36%; Belgium, 53%; and Paris, 73%. Published estimates for the incidence of congenital toxoplasmosis range from 0.1 to 10 per 1,000 live births. Approximations per 1,000 births for individual cities are as follows: Birmingham, Alabama, 0.12; London, 0.07 to 0.25; Glasgow, Scotland, 0.46 to 0.93; Basel, Switzerland, 1; Brussels, 2; Melbourne, 2; and Vienna, 6 to 7. Sera from 330,000 newborns in Massachusetts and New Hampshire were tested using the double-sandwich (DS) IgM enzyme-linked immunosorbent assay (ELISA) of Remington and Naot, and the incidence of seropositivity using this test was 1 per 10,000 live births.

Acute maternal infection is transmitted to the fetus in approximately 40% of cases. Incidence and severity of congenital infection depend in part on the time of acquisition of infection during pregnancy (Table 38-1). By the last weeks of gestation the incidence of transmission to the fetus approaches 100%. The severity of manifestations of infection at birth decreases the later in gestation the infection is acquired. Approximately half of the infected infants detected in serologic screening programs who were initially believed normal based on routine newborn evaluations had one or more signs of infection apparent with more complete evaluations. Almost all infected infants have some evidence of infection (e.g., chorioretinitis) by adolescence if untreated or treated for only 1 month.

TABLE 38-1   Inverse Relationship Between Incidence of Fetal Infection and Severity of Fetal Damage Following Acutely Acquired Maternal Infection With *T. gondii* at Different Stages of Gestation

Trimester of pregnancy	Fetuses infected (%)	Severity of illness
1	17	Most severe
2	25	Intermediate
3	65	Least severe or subclinical

Data from Remington JS, Desmonts G. In Remington JS, Klein JO (eds). Infectious diseases of the fetus and newborn infant, ed 3. Philadelphia: Saunders, 1990.

PATHOGENESIS

After acquisition by the older child or adult (usually through the gastrointestinal tract), organisms invade cells directly or are phagocytosed by leukocytes. Within these cells, organisms multiply, cause cell lysis, and are spread throughout the body hematogenously or through the lymphatics. Organisms can infect every mammalian cell. Proliferation of tachyzoites results in rupture of infected cells and eventually in areas of localized tissue necrosis surrounded by infiltrates of inflammatory cells. The eventual outcome of acute infection depends on the host's immune response. Cysts form in immunocompetent hosts, in whom both cellular and humoral immunity is intact. Cyst formation can be demonstrated as early as the seventh day after infection. Cysts can persist in many organs and tissues after immunity is acquired; thus *T. gondii* remains in tissues for the life of the host.

In immunodeficient individuals and in some apparently immunologically normal individuals the acute infection is not contained by an effective immune response; it may cause marked destruction of the host's tissues, leading to, for example, pneumonitis, myocarditis, or necrotizing encephalitis. Encysted organisms may also cause recrudescent disease in previously immunocompetent patients. Such previously latent infection is the major source of disease caused by *T. gondii* in patients with AIDS, transplant recipients, and older children who develop new or recrudescent chorioretinitis as a sequela of congenital *T. gondii* infection.

When a pregnant woman acquires *T. gondii*, tachyzoites are hematogenously spread to the placenta. The organism then can be transmitted transplacentally directly to the fetus during gestation or at birth. Overall, in approximately 60% of cases, maternal acute infection does not result in fetal infection. However, as stated previously, almost all infected infants have manifestations of infection (e.g., chorioretinitis) by adolescence if they are untreated. It has been suggested that the differences in rates of transmission during gestation depend on placental blood flow, virulence of the *T. gondii* strain, possibly genetic susceptibility of the patient, and the number of organisms hematogenously spread to the placenta. As in other congenital infections, the greater severity of toxoplasmic infection acquired early in gestation relates to the sensitivity of early fetal organs to damage by intracellular parasites, the placental barrier separating the fetus from the mother's humoral and cell-mediated immune responses, and the fetus's intrinsic immunologic immaturity. The most profoundly affected babies frequently exhibit specific immunologic tolerance in the perinatal period (McLeod et al., 1990).

PATHOLOGY

Information about pathologic changes observed in toxoplasmosis in humans is largely derived from lymph node biopsies, from autopsy data described in fatal congenital infections, and from immunodeficient individuals. Limited information is available on the pathologic changes in immunocompetent individuals because acute infection is usually asymptomatic or self-limited in such persons. Tachyzoites and tissue cysts are only rarely observed in conventionally stained sections. Tachyzoites may be observed with Wright's or Giemsa stain but are best demonstrated with the immunoperoxidase technique. Tissue cysts stain well with PAS stain, silver impregnation stains, and immunoperoxidase techniques.

Lymph Nodes

In acute acquired lymphadenopathic toxoplasmosis (Figure 38-3) there is a characteristic triad of (1) reactive follicular hyperplasia, with (2) irregular clusters of epithelioid histiocytes, and (3) monocytoid B cells that distend the subcapsular and trabecular lymph node sinuses (Dorfman and Remington, 1973). Tachyzoites and tissue cysts are only very rarely demonstrable in affected nodes, but *T. gondii* DNA may be identified in tissue sections by the polymerase chain reaction (PCR) (reviewed by Roberts and McLeod, 1999).

Eye

Single or multiple foci of tissue necrosis in the retina and choroid are the earliest manifestations of *T. gondii* involvement of the eye. Secondary changes such as vitritis, iridocyclitis, and cataracts are complications of the chorioretinitis. Organisms first lodge in the capillaries of the inner layer of the retina, invade the endothelium, and extend to adjacent tissues. An intense local inflammatory reaction develops, with (1) edema, and (2) infiltration of lymphocytes, plasma cells, mononuclear cells, and occasionally eosinophils. Both intracellular and extracellular tachyzoites and tissue cysts may

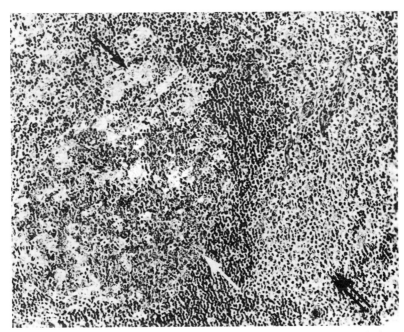

Fig. 38-3 Lymph node biopsy showing characteristic lymph node pathology in lymphadenitis caused by *Toxoplasma*. Epithelioid cells *(black arrow)* encroach upon and blur margins of germinal center *(white arrow)*. There is focal distension of subcapsular and trabecular sinuses by "monocytoid" cells *(double black arrows)*. Irregular clusters of epithelioid cells are scattered throughout paracortical lymphoid stroma. (Modified from Dorfman RF, Remington JS: N Engl J Med 1973;287(17):878-881.)

be seen. After resolution of the active infection, scarring is characterized by an area of gliosis with a hyperpigmented border resulting from disruption and proliferation of the pigmented retinal epithelium (reviewed by Roberts and McLeod, 1999).

Central Nervous System

Along with involvement of the eye, congenital toxoplasmosis most often involves the central nervous system (CNS). In the CNS there may be acute and focal or multifocal diffuse meningoencephalitis, with cellular necrosis, microglial nodules, and perivascular mononuclear inflammation. In patients with congenital infection, secondary vascular thrombosis may produce extensive areas of necrosis, often several centimeters in diameter. The basal ganglia are often severely involved, and scattered cortical lesions are often seen as well. Large areas of necrosis in congenital toxoplasmosis may lead to sloughing of periventricular tissue, which causes obstruction of the aqueduct of Sylvius or foramen of Monro and subsequent hydrocephalus. The protein count of such ventricular

fluid is high (grams per deciliter) and contains large amounts of *T. gondii* antigen. Eventually, necrotic brain tissue may calcify, giving rise to the typical findings in conventional radiographs and computed tomography (CT) scans.

In cases of acute CNS infection acquired postnatally or with immunocompromise, there is focal or diffuse meningoencephalitis with necrosis and microglial nodules. In immunocompromised patients, such as infants and children with both congenital toxoplasmosis and AIDS, the major finding is necrotizing encephalitis in both acute and recrudescent disease.

Other Sites

Rarely, *T. gondii* infection gives rise to interstitial pneumonitis. The myocardium is a frequent site for necrosis, inflammation, and encysted organisms. Acute and chronic pericarditis have also been described. Infection of kidney (and antigen-antibody complex–mediated glomerulonephritis), spleen, liver, adrenals, pancreas, stomach, intestine, thyroid, thymus, testes, ovaries, and skin also have been described (reviewed in Remington et al., 2001).

CLINICAL MANIFESTATIONS

Acute Acquired Toxoplasmosis in Apparently Immunologically Normal Older Children and Adults

Infection acquired after birth is generally asymptomatic in 80% to 90% of immunologically normal persons, including pregnant women. Those with clinically apparent disease generally have lymphadenopathy with or without a "mononucleosis-like" illness. Rarely, severe systemic disease or specific organ involvement (e.g., encephalitis or chorioretinitis) occurs.

Lymphadenopathy is the most commonly recognized clinical manifestation of acute acquired toxoplasmosis (McCabe et al., 1987). Lymphadenitis can be generalized, but in approximately two thirds of patients only one area is affected. Cervical lymph nodes are the most frequently involved. However, axillary, inguinal, retroperitoneal, and mesenteric lymph nodes may also be involved. Lymph nodes generally measure 0.5 to 3.0 cm and can be tender or nontender. They are often firm, discrete, smooth, and mobile, but they do not suppurate or ulcerate. Although self-limited, lymphadenopathy can persist or recur for up to 1 year. Retroperitoneal or mesenteric node involvement with fever may mimic appendicitis. Toxoplasmic lymphadenopathy often raises concern about lymphoma or other malignancy. Appropriate serologic testing can differentiate this condition and avert the need for lymph node biopsy.

Occasionally, lymphadenopathy is accompanied by a constellation of symptoms suggestive of infectious mononucleosis, or these symptoms may occur alone. This infection also has a self-limited course; however, fatigue and lymphadenopathy may persist for months to a year. It usually ends with complete recovery.

Significant systemic disease can occur. Onset may be insidious, with weakness and malaise that persist for 6 to 10 days, followed by fever, rash, and symptoms of pneumonia or hepatitis. Temperature may be as high as 41° C (105.8° F). Abdominal pain may be present. A maculopapular, generalized rash may occur. It appears similar to that of Rocky Mountain spotted fever except that the palms of the hands and the soles of the feet are spared. These skin lesions are bright red to pale pink and may blanch with pressure. Signs of pneumonia may appear simultaneously with the rash or later. Roentgenographic examination of the chest may show irregular areas of increased density in the lower lobes or only accentuation of the hilar or lower-lobe markings.

Systemic toxoplasmosis in immunologically normal individuals has also been manifested as hepatitis, polymyositis, pericarditis with effusion, myocarditis, or meningoencephalitis. Toxoplasmic meningoencephalitis has been characterized by headache, vomiting, seizures, focal neurologic signs, and transitory confusion (Townsend et al., 1975). Temperature is not always elevated at the onset. Lymphadenopathy and splenomegaly are present in some cases. Cerebrospinal fluid (CSF) has increased numbers of white blood cells (WBCs), particularly mononuclear cells. Protein and glucose concentrations are normal or simulate those of bacterial meningitis. The patient's condition may steadily deteriorate, ending in death or survival with residual brain damage manifested by seizures or focal neurologic deficits. Complete recovery without residua has also been described.

Infection in the Immunocompromised Individual

Immunocompromised patients, such as those with AIDS, malignancy, autoimmune disease and its therapy, and solid organ or bone marrow transplants, are at risk for severe toxoplasmosis. In most cases, toxoplasmosis is caused by reactivation of latent infection rather than primary infection.

Despite the introduction of antiretroviral therapy, approximately 50% of patients with AIDS who are chronically infected with T. gondii develop toxoplasmosis. In a retrospective cohort study of AIDS-defining illnesses in a London clinic population the incidence of cerebral toxoplasmosis remained stable despite the introduction of highly active antiretroviral therapy (Ives et al., 2001). Why the infection does not reactivate in the other 50% of such patients is unknown. Pediatric AIDS and congenital T. gondii infections have been reported in the same infants. Such dual infections, including encephalitis and involvement of other organs (e.g., heart and lungs), usually have been fulminant and rapidly fatal. T. gondii infection has most often been diagnosed at postmortem examination. This infection is emerging as a particular problem in populations with a relatively high prevalence of both T. gondii and HIV infections.

Typical signs and symptoms of toxoplasmic encephalitis in adult AIDS patients include headache, fever, and focal neurologic deficits. Less commonly, meningitis, spinal cord involvement, and signs that reflect involvement of other organs are present. CNS lesions occur throughout the brain, with predilection for involvement of the basal ganglia and corticomedullary junction. Diffuse encephalitis diagnosed only at autopsy also has been reported (Leport, 1991), but most often there are focal lesions that enhance with contrast on brain CT scan or brain magnetic resonance imaging (MRI) scans. MRI scans almost always show multiple lesions (Figure 38-4).

In a recent series of adult AIDS patients with toxoplasmosis (Leport, 1991) the most frequent clinical localization was in the brain, with focal abscesses (83%) and diffuse encephalitis (in the 17% with normal CT scans). Fever occurred in 60% to 70%; 40% to 50% had headaches; 35% to 40% were confused; and 40% to 80% had focal neurologic signs. Specific IgG antibodies are detectable in most (>95%) adult patients with AIDS and toxoplasmosis. Of affected patients with toxoplasmic chorioretinitis, 65% had concomitant cerebral localization. With appropriate treatment there is usually an initial improvement within a few weeks and complete resolution of lesions seen on brain CT scan in 1 to 6 months. Delayed or absent response to this treatment is an indication for brain biopsy. Rupture of thrombosed vessels (secondary to intimal and perivascular inflammatory cell infiltrates) has occurred. At autopsy, 40% to 70% of patients with AIDS and toxoplasmosis have involvement of the heart and lung. Involvement of pancreas, stomach, and intestine has been described.

Opportunistic CNS infections such as toxoplasmosis are less common in children and adolescents than in adults (Mitchell, 2001). When it occurs in older immunocompromised children, toxoplasmosis generally occurs as a result of reactivation of latent infection. However, *T. gondii* may actually be transmitted through organ transplantation and leukocyte transfusion (Figure 38-2). Symptomatic toxoplasmosis has occurred when *T. gondii*–infected hearts or kidneys have been transplanted into seronegative recipients. In cardiac transplant recipients, toxoplasmosis may simulate rejection both clinically and in endomyocardial biopsies if the diagnosis is not suspected. The diagnosis of reactivated or primary toxoplasmosis in recipients of bone-marrow transplants may be particularly difficult because *T. gondii*–specific antibody may be absent or may not increase in titer. Increase in antibody titer without overt disease has occurred when *T. gondii*–infected hearts have been transplanted into seropositive recipients. The incidence of toxoplasmosis is significant when hearts from seropositive donors are given to seronegative recipients. This is not recommended, but when it does occur, prophylaxis with an antimicrobial agent is indicated.

Congenital Toxoplasmosis

Clinical manifestations. Approximately 40% of untreated women who acquire the infection

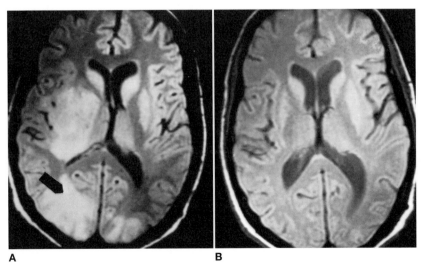

A　　　　　　　　　　　　　**B**

Fig. 38-4 Magnetic resonance image of the brain of a patient with AIDS and toxoplasmic encephalitis before (**A**) and after (**B**) antimicrobial therapy. Note that large areas of necrosis and inflammation in **A** *(arrow)* have resolved in **B**.

during pregnancy transmit *T. gondii* to their fetus. In an otherwise healthy woman, transmission to the fetus occurs only in the setting of primary (not recrudescent) infection. Only 10% to 40% of women who give birth to congenitally infected infants recall any signs or symptoms of acute infection. Rarely, cases of congenital transmission have been reported in women chronically infected with *T. gondii* and immunosuppressed from corticosteroid treatment or AIDS.

Manifestations of congenital infection are protean, varying from a mild or asymptomatic infection to a generalized infection dominated by signs of irreversible CNS damage. Disease may be seen initially in the neonatal period, in the first months of life, or at later ages—up to adulthood. Newborns and young infants are usually detected based on systemic, neurologic, or ophthalmologic signs (Table 38-2). Older children are seen with ophthalmologic and, less frequently, neurologic disease. Couvreur et al. (1984) reported data that indicate the spectrum and frequency of signs and symptoms noted in newborn infants born to mothers whose infections had been diagnosed in a systematic serologic screening program. Only 10% had substantial CNS, ocular, or systemic involvement; 34% had normal clinical examinations, with the exception of retinal scars or isolated calcifications; and 55% had no abnormalities detected. These prospective data from France likely underestimate the true proportion of severe infection because the most severe cases were not referred, therapeutic abortion often eliminated the most severely involved fetuses, and gestational spiramycin therapy may have reduced the severity of infection. Between 33% and 50% of the infants initially thought to have subclinical infection showed signs of infection (most commonly, abnormal CSF) with more detailed evaluation. At face value, however, these data imply that 90% of the infants with congenital toxoplasmosis would have been missed with a routine newborn physical examination.

In infants with generalized or primarily neurologic disease and with no or brief treatment, substantial long-term morbidity can be expected (Table 38-3). For example, of infants with neurologic disease who were reevaluated at 4 years of age (Eichenwald, 1960), 89% had intelligence quotients (IQs) less than 70; 83% had convulsions; 76% had spasticity and palsies; 69% had severely impaired vision; 20% were deaf; and only 9% were normal. Only 16% of the children who initially had generalized disease were normal at follow-up. In a study by Wilson et al. (1980) the outcome for infants who had "subclinical" infection at birth and who were evaluated when they were 9 to 10 years old also revealed substantial sequelae (Table 38-4). Sixteen percent were mentally retarded; 17% had seizures; 27% had unilateral blindness and 20% had bilateral blindness; 25% had hearing impairment; and 86% had sequentially lower IQ scores when tested at 5-year intervals. With 1 year of treatment, outcome apparently is substantially better for most (but not all) such infants (Roizen et al., 1995).

Reported cutaneous manifestations in congenitally infected infants have included thrombocytopenia (e.g., petechiae, hemorrhage, ecchymoses) and rashes (fine punctate; diffuse maculopapular; lenticular deep blue-red; sharply defined and diffuse blue papules). The entire body, including palms and soles, has been involved with macular rashes. Jaundice, cyanosis, and edema secondary to hepatic, pulmonary, myocardial, and renal involvement have been reported.

General and systemic findings have included prematurity, low Apgar scores, intrauterine growth retardation, instability of temperature regulation with hypothermia, lymphadenopathy, hepatosplenomegaly, signs of myocarditis, pneumonitis, nephrotic syndrome, vomiting, diarrhea, and feeding problems. Endocrine abnormalities have also been reported and include hypothyroidism, diabetes insipidus, sexual precocity, and partial anterior hypopituitarism. Neurologic abnormalities have ranged from subtle findings to severe encephalitis. Hydrocephalus may be the only clinical manifestation of congenital toxoplasmosis and may be compensated or may require shunt placement. It may be seen in the perinatal period; later in infancy; or, rarely, up to adulthood. A variety of different seizure patterns may occur in the perinatal period and later in life. Central focal motor deficits have been noted, as have signs of spinal or bulbar involvement. Microcephaly in untreated infants is generally associated with diminished cognitive functioning. Mild and severe sensorineural hearing loss has been reported in approximately 20% of children with no or brief treatment, but this

TABLE 38-2 Numbers and Percentages of 300 Patients with Congenital Toxoplasmosis with Various Clinical Manifestations at Presentation

Clinical manifestations	AGE WHEN FIRST DIAGNOSED								Total
	1-5 mo	6-11 mo	12-23 mo	2-3 yr	4-7 yr	8-14 yr	15-29 yr	30 yr	
Neurologic disorders	42 (58)*	26 (81)	24 (57)	20 (42)	14 (42)	21 (54)	7 (29)	1	155 (52)
Hydrocephalus or microcephalus	40 (55)	12 (38)	14 (33)	6 (13)	—	4 (10)	1 (4)	1	78 (26)
Ocular disorders	52 (71)	27 (84)	32 (76)	26 (54)	31 (94)	35 (90)	24 (100)	1	228 (76)
Intracranial calcification	28 (38)	12 (38)	17 (40)	14 (29)	11 (33)	10 (26)	4 (17)	2	98 (33)
Jaundice	20 (27)	1 (32)	—	—	—	—	—	—	21
Hepatosplenomegaly	13 (18)	—	—	—	—	—	—	—	13

Modified from Couvreur J, Desmonts G: Dev Med Child Neurol 1962,4:519-530.
*Figure outside parentheses, number; figure inside parentheses, percentage of patients diagnosed at that age with this manifestation.

| TABLE 38-3 | Signs and Symptoms Occurring Before Diagnosis or During the Course of Untreated Acute Congenital Toxoplasmosis in 152 Infants and 101 of These Children after Follow-up of 4 or More Years |

	FREQUENCY OF OCCURRENCE (%) IN PATIENTS WITH	
Signs and symptoms	Neurologic disease* (108 patients)	Generalized disease† (44 patients)
Infants		
Chorioretinitis	102 (94)‡	29 (66)
Abnormal spinal fluid	59 (55)	37 (84)
Anemia	55 (51)	34 (77)
Jaundice	31 (29)	35 (80)
Splenomegaly	23 (21)	40 (90)
Convulsions	54 (50)	8 (18)
Fever	27 (25)	34 (77)
Intracranial calcification	54 (50)	2 (4)
Hepatomegaly	18 (17)	34 (77)
Lymphadenopathy	18 (17)	30 (68)
Vomiting	17 (16)	21 (48)
Hydrocephalus	30 (28)	0 (0)
Diarrhea	7 (6)	11 (25)
Pneumonitis	0 (0)	18 (41)
Microcephalus	14 (13)	0 (0)
Eosinophilia	6 (4)	8 (18)
Rash	1 (1)	11 (25)
Abnormal bleeding	3 (3)	8 (18)
Hypothermia	2 (2)	9 (20)
Cataracts	5 (5)	0 (0)
Glaucoma	2 (2)	0 (0)
Optic atrophy	2 (2)	0 (0)
Microphthalmia	2 (2)	0 (0)
	70 Patients	31 Patients
Children 4 Years (or More) Old		
Mental retardation	62 (89)	25 (81)
Convulsions	58 (83)	24 (77)
Spasticity and palsies	53 (76)	18 (58)
Severely impaired vision	48 (69)	13 (42)
Hydrocephalus or microcephalus	31 (44)	2 (6)
Deafness	12 (17)	3 (10)
Normal	6 (9)	5 (16)

Modified from Eichenwald H. In Siim JC (ed). Human toxoplasmosis. Copenhagen: Munksgaard, 1960, pp 41-49. Study was performed in 1947. The most severely involved institutionalized patients were not included in the later study of 101 children.
*Patients with central nervous system disease in the first year of life.
†Patients with nonneurologic diseases during the first 2 months of life.
‡Figure outside parentheses, number; figure inside parentheses, percentage.

was not found in a recent study of treated infants and children (McGhee et al., 1992).

CSF is abnormal in at least one third of congenitally infected infants. Abnormalities include CSF lymphocytic pleocytosis, hypoglycorrhachia, and elevated protein level. Remarkable elevations of CSF protein levels (with values of grams per deciliter when there is aqueductal obstruction and ventricular dilation) are characteristic of this congenital infection. Local production of *T. gondii*–specific antibodies may be present in CSF. Brain CT scan with contrast can determine ventricular size, detect calcifications, and define active inflammatory lesions and porencephalic cystic structures. Skull radiographs and ultrasonography are less sensitive than CT scan for

TABLE 38-4	Development of Adverse Sequelae in Children Born With Subclinical Congenital *Toxoplasma* Infection	
	Group 1*(n = 13)	Group 2†(n = 11)
Ophthalmologic Finding		
No sequelae	2	0
Chorioretinitis		
Bilateral		
Bilateral blindness	0	5
Unilateral blindness	3	3
Moderate unilateral visual loss	0	1
Minimal or no visual loss	5	1
Unilateral		
Minimal or no visual loss	3	0
Mean age at onset (yr)	3.67	0.42
Range	0.08-9.33	0.25-1.00
Recurrences of active chorioretinitis	3	2
Neurologic Finding‡		
No sequelae	8	3
Major sequelae		
Hydrocephalus	0	1
Microcephaly	1	1
Seizures	1	3
Severe psychomotor retardation	1	2
Minor sequelae		
Mild cerebellar dysfunction	2	4
Transiently delayed psychomotor development	2	2
Other Abnormality		
Sensorineural hearing loss		
Moderate unilateral	1 of 10	1 of 9
Mild unilateral	1 of 10	0 of 9
Mild bilateral	1 of 10	1 of 9
Precocious puberty	2	0
Premature thelarche	0	1
Miscellaneous	3	1

Modified from Wilson et al.: Pediatrics 1980;66:767-774.
*No abnormalities found on an extensive newborn evaluation based on awareness of a diagnosis of congenital toxoplasmosis.
†No abnormalities found on a routine newborn physical examination.
‡Of eight children who were tested, 86% had sequentially lower intelligence quotient scores.

detection of calcifications, but ultrasonography may be useful for following ventricular size. Brain MRI and radionuclide scans may be useful to detect active inflammation.

The following case summaries provide examples of infants with subclinical infection; generalized systemic, neurologic, and ophthalmologic disease; and severe neurologic and ophthalmologic disease.

■ **Case 1** *Patient with subclinical disease.* The patient's family lived in a rural area, and two stray cats lived nearby. Although they had no known contact with these cats or with feces from the cats, the family did have a sandbox where the pregnant mother played in the sand with her older children. The mother also prepared a large number of hamburgers for a picnic 2 to 3 weeks before delivery of her son, but she did not recall sampling raw hamburger or eating raw or undercooked meat during her infant's gestation. She had no history of consuming raw milk or raw eggs.

The mother's pregnancy, labor, and delivery were uncomplicated. Her infant was born appropriate for gestational age (AGA) with Apgar scores of 9 and 9 and a birth weight of 3.9 kg, and he had no medical problems in the perinatal period. On the day after delivery the patient's mother noted that she had an enlarged posterior auricular lymph node. She had no other symptoms or signs and an otherwise normal physical examination, which included a retinal examination. The affected lymph node was excised, and microscopic studies of it revealed epithelioid histiocytes and monocytoid cells characteristic of toxoplasmic lymphadenopathy (similar to those shown in Figure 38-3). Serologic tests for the mother and the child were obtained: the infant's serum Sabin-Feldman dye test titer was 1:8,000; his serum IgM ELISA level was 11; the IgM ISAGA level was 12; and the IgA ELISA level was 11. His mother's serum Sabin-Feldman dye test titer was 1:1,024 (300 IU), her IgM ELISA level was 11, and her AC/HS was 1600/>3200.

Results of general ophthalmologic and neurologic examinations, auditory brain stem response testing, and head CT scan with and without contrast were normal. CSF at 5 weeks of age had 30 WBCs/mm³, with 3% PMNs, 91% lymphocytes, 3% monocytes, a protein level of 68 mg/dl, and a glucose level of 39 mg/dl.

The patient was treated with pyrimethamine, sulfadiazine, and leucovorin for 1 year and has had no clinical manifestations (other than slightly elevated CSF protein levels perinatally) of his third-trimester congenital infection.

■ **Case 2** *Patient with generalized systemic, neurologic, and ophthalmologic disease.* This boy was the product of a first pregnancy and unremarkable gestation. During pregnancy his mother occasionally sampled raw hamburger, gardened, and had a pet cat but did not change the litter box.

An emergency cesarean section was performed after 30 hours of labor because of fetal distress (decreased fetal heart rate). The infant's Apgar scores were 2 at 1 minute and 3 at 5 minutes, leading to intubation and mechanical ventilation for his first 24 hours of life. During those 24 hours he had one episode that was considered to be a seizure, and administration of phenobarbital was begun. His birth weight was 3,450 g (fiftieth percentile); length, 19 inches (fiftieth percentile); and head circumference, 36 cm (fiftieth percentile). His platelet count on the first day of life was 44,000/mm³; a platelet transfusion was given and the platelet count subsequently returned to normal. Because of his asphyxial episode, a head CT scan was performed and revealed multiple discrete intracranial calcifications. Because of the presence of calcifications (similar to those in Figure 38-5), the diagnosis of toxoplasmosis was suspected. An ophthalmologic examination revealed bilateral chorioretinitis, which was more prominent on the right side than on the left and involved the right macula. Hepatosplenomegaly was present, but the infant was considered normal otherwise. An examination of his CSF revealed 30 WBCs/mm³, with a predominance of lymphocytes, a protein level of 215 mg/dL, and a glucose level of 86 mg/dL. Serologic test results included a serum dye test titer of 1:1,024; an IgM ELISA level of 2.0; and an IgA ELISA level of 2.5. The mother's serum on the same dates had a dye test titer of 1:8,000; DS IgM ELISA level of 0.2; IgA ELISA level of 0.2; and AC/HS of 400/3,200. The infant was given pyrimethamine, sulfonamides, and leucovorin. His hepatosplenomegaly resolved. He is now 2 years old and has developed completely normally, with strabismus related to his macular scar as his only overt abnormality.

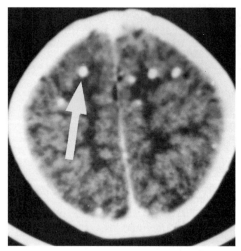

Fig. 38-5 Computed tomographic scan that demonstrates calcifications in the brain of an infant with congenital toxoplasmosis. This infant and other treated infants have developed normally in spite of calcifications *(arrow)* and even microcephaly.

■ **Case 3** *Patient with severe neurologic and ophthalmologic disease.* This boy's mother was a 21-year-old woman of Laotian descent with known hepatitis B surface antigenemia. She had minimal exposure to cats during the third trimester (i.e., she had visited in a house in which cats were present). She did not own a cat, nor did she clean a litter box or get scratched or bitten. She had no gardening or sandbox exposure. On one occasion she ate rare meat during the third trimester; however, she usually consumed well-cooked meat. She denied consumption of raw milk or raw eggs. In the eighth week of gestation a 1-week illness occurred, with swelling of her neck and face and with fever, lymphadenopathy, and night sweats. She was hospitalized, treated with antibiotics for presumed facial cellulitis, and had complete resolution of her symptoms. She also had intermittent headaches throughout her pregnancy. During the twenty-eighth week of gestation, at her request, a fetal ultrasound was performed that demonstrated a fetus with hydrocephalus. From that time on, she routinely underwent ultrasonography every 2 weeks until the thirty-fifth week of gestation.

A male infant was delivered at 35 weeks gestation (34 weeks by Dubowitz) by cesarean section because of increasing ventriculomegaly. The infant's birth weight was 2,325 g (70%); head circumference, 34.5 cm (>90%); and length, 18 inches (70%). Apgar scores were 4 and 9 at 1 and 5 minutes of age, respectively. Hydrocephalus was prominent at birth as demonstrated by CT (similar to that in Figure 38-6). The patient underwent ventriculoperitoneal shunting at 5 days of age, with resolution of increased intracranial pressure and appearance of thicker cortical mantle. Testing of ventricular fluid revealed 870 red blood cells; 43 WBCs; protein level of 1,155 mg/dL; and glucose level of 26 mg/dL. His serum Sabin-Feldman dye test titer was 1:4,096, and DS IgM ELISA level was 4. His IgA ELISA level was 3. His mother's serum Sabin-Feldman dye test titer was 1:2,048; IgM ELISA level was 4; IgA ELISA level was 12; and AC/HS was 800/3,200.

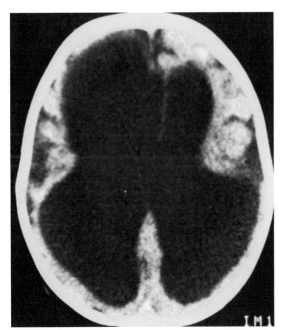

Fig. 38-6 Computed tomographic scan of the brain of an infant with congenital toxoplasmosis and hydrocephalus. Some (but not all) such treated infants with hydrocephalus from congenital toxoplasmosis have developed normally (with normal motor and cognitive function following prompt placement of ventriculoperitoneal shunts and with antimicrobial therapy). Poorer prognosis has been associated with delays in shunt placement or revisions or intercurrent complications such as prolonged hypoxia and hypoglycemia.

Other complications noted during the infant's initial hospitalization included transient anemia, thrombocytopenia, transient hyperbilirubinemia, elevation of liver transaminases, and diabetes insipidus. His examination also documented severe chorioretinitis, microphthalmia, hepatosplenomegaly, an umbilical hernia, and a hydrocele with micropenis. Administration of pyrimethamine, sulfadiazine, and folinic acid was begun at 18 days of age. At 24 days of age, prednisone was added and eventually tapered. He was started on vasopressin therapy.

A repeat CT scan showed worsening hydrocephalus. Another repeat CT scan was performed 4 months later and showed increased cerebral atrophy without clear indication of increased intracranial pressure. The infant is without sight and has substantial delay in development.

Ophthalmologic Disease

Clinical manifestations. In the United States and in Western Europe, *T. gondii* is the most common cause of chorioretinitis, estimated to cause approximately 35% of cases. Toxoplasmic chorioretinitis is most frequently observed as an initial manifestation of or with reactivation

of congenital infection. Almost all untreated congenitally infected individuals develop chorioretinal lesions (Koppe et al., 1986). Chorioretinitis is estimated to occur in 1% of immunologically normal individuals with acute acquired toxoplasmosis.

Chorioretinitis occurs early in gestation, and characteristic lesions have been described as early as 22 weeks gestation (Brezin et al., 1994, Roberts et al., 2001). Infants with active congenital ocular toxoplasmosis may have microphthalmia, impaired vision, cataracts, chorioretinal scars, chorioretinitis, iritis, leukokoria, anisometropia, nystagmus, optic atrophy, microcornea, or strabismus (Mets et al., 1996). Older children may complain of blurred vision, photophobia, epiphora, loss of central vision, or "floaters." Recurrent symptoms occur at irregular intervals. Data from Couvreur et al. (1984) suggest that the appearance of recurrent or new retinal lesions during the first years of life may be prevented by therapy in alternate months with pyrimethamine and sulfadiazine and spiramycin. Longer follow-up is needed for definitive conclusions about whether such therapy reduces symptomatic, progressive ophthalmologic disease.

During an ophthalmoscopic examination, acute focal retinitis is seen as a fluffy white-yellow lesion with surrounding retinal edema and hyperemia (Figure 38-7, *A*). Overlying vitritis may obscure the retina. Active lesions often are adjacent to old inactive lesions. Inactive lesions characteristically are atrophic, white to gray plaques, with distinct borders and choroidal black pigment (Figure 38-7, *B*). The lesions may be single or multiple, large or small, unilateral or bilateral. They are often found at the posterior pole of the retina and commonly involve the macula, but they also occur in the periphery. New lesions are often contiguous with older lesions, suggesting that the pathogenesis of new lesions is associated with cyst rupture and replication of the parasite in adjacent retinal cells. These primary retinal lesions can have secondary effects including papillitis (most often unilateral), optic atrophy, retinal detachment, cortical blindness and nonvascular glaucoma. The following case illustrates some of these findings.

■ **Case 4** *Patient with toxoplasmic chorioretinitis.* During this child's gestation, her mother gardened and sampled uncooked hamburger. The perinatal history was unremarkable except for the birth weight of 2.53 kg at a gestational age of 37 weeks. She had no medical problems

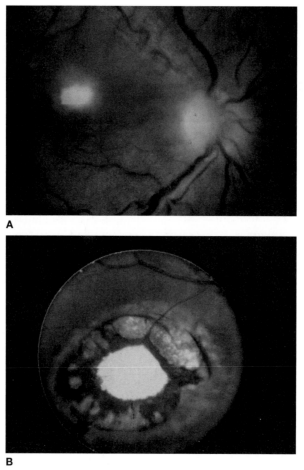

Fig. 38-7 Toxoplasmic chorioretinitis with acute lesion (**A**) and inactive macular scar (**B**). In A there is focal necrotizing retinitis with cottonlike patch in the fundus. Acute lesions (**A**) appear soft and white, have indistinct borders, and may have associated vitritis. Older lesions (**B**) are whitish gray and sharply demarcated and often have areas with choroidal pigment. (Modified from McLeod R, Remington JS. In Behrman RL, Vaughan VC III, Nelson WE [eds]. Nelson's textbook of pediatrics, ed 14. Philadelphia: Saunders, 1990; and Remington JS, Desmonts G. In Remington JS, Klein JO [eds]: Infectious diseases of the fetus and newborn infant, ed 3. Philadelphia: Saunders, 1990.)

identified in the newborn period and did not require hospitalization or treatment for any serious medical illness. Before entering nursery school when she was 4 years old, she had a routine ophthalmologic examination, which revealed decreased vision in her right eye and bilateral macular scars. Her visual acuity was 20/125 OD and 20/25 OS. There were cells in the anterior vitreous of the right eye and a few cells in the anterior vitreous of the left eye. The right vitreous had 1 to 2+ haze caused by the cells. In the right eye there was a one disc diameter foveal scar with a hyperpigmented center surrounded by a deeply pigmented area. A small, one-eighth disc–diameter area of active retinitis was present between the disc and the macular scar. The left fundus had a trace of vitreous haze with macular scarring. The child's serum *Toxoplasma* IgG indirect fluorescent antibody (IFA) titer was 1:4,096, and her *Toxoplasma* IgM IFA titer was 0. The mother's serum contained *Toxoplasma*-specific IgG antibody. The child's active ocular toxoplasmosis was treated with prednisone, pyrimethamine,

triple sulfonamides, and clindamycin. Signs of active retinal disease and vitritis resolved, and therapy was discontinued.

Three years later, her visual acuity was 20/50 OD and 20/30 OS. She had normal discs and vessels in both eyes, with bilateral macular scarring (similar to that shown in Figure 38-7, *B*).

The clinical presentation of acquired toxoplasmic retinochoroiditis differs from congenital ocular disease. These patients are usually older with unilateral ocular disease and a single, active retinochoroidal lesion (Montoya and Remington, 1996). Furthermore, macular involvement is uncommon. This is in contrast to the clustering of lesions, retinochoroidal scars, and macular involvement characteristic of congenital infection. In patients with AIDS, toxoplasmic retinochoroiditis is less common than encephalitis, accounting for between 1% and 3% of retinal infections. Rarely, diffuse toxoplasmic retinochoroiditis may be the initial manifestation of AIDS (Lee et al., 2000).

Holland et al. (1988) described eight patients with presumed toxoplasmic retinochoroiditis and AIDS. Their retinal lesions were frequently bilateral and multifocal. The disease differed from that in immunocompetent patients. Preexisting retinal scars were rare, suggesting that most ocular lesion are the result of newly acquired disease or organisms newly disseminated to the eye from nonocular sites. Histologic examination of two cases, however, showed scant retinal inflammation that is similar to the lesions seen in toxoplasmic encephalitis in AIDS patients. In areas of necrosis, there were numerous *T. gondii* tachyzoites and cysts.

DIAGNOSIS

Multiple serologic tests may be needed to establish the diagnosis of acutely acquired or congenital *Toxoplasma* infection. Each laboratory must establish test values that are diagnostic of infection in particular clinical settings and must provide interpretation of the test results and appropriate quality control. If therapy is based on serologic test results, these results should be confirmed in a reference laboratory (e.g., Palo Alto Research Institute, Palo Alto, California, 650-326-8120; Montoya, 2002). Diagnosis may also be established by microscopic demonstration of tachyzoites in smears prepared from body fluids (e.g., CSF) or tissue sections (e.g., brain biopsy) or by actual isolation of the organism from tissues such as placenta, fetal blood, amniotic fluid, or body fluids that are inoculated into tissue culture or mice. Characteristic histopathologic manifestations may also be noted in a lymph node biopsy.

Isolation

T. gondii can be isolated by inoculation of specimens (from body fluids, leukocytes, fetal blood clots, bone marrow, or homogenates of placenta) into the peritoneum of seronegative mice or into tissue culture. Ideally, material should be processed immediately, although *T. gondii* has been isolated from tissues and blood stored at 4° C overnight. Freezing or treatment of specimens with formalin kills the organism. The peritoneal fluid of inoculated mice is examined microscopically for tachyzoites 6 to 10

days later, or earlier if the mice die. If mice survive 4 to 6 weeks, their sera are then tested for IgG *Toxoplasma* antibody. If their sera contain specific antibody, definitive diagnosis is made by visualization of tissue cysts in the mouse brain. If no cysts are found, homogenates of mouse brain, liver, and spleen are subinoculated into other mice, and the process is repeated.

Tissue cultures (e.g., of fibroblasts) have also been used to isolate *T. gondii*. This apparently is a more convenient but less sensitive method than inoculation into mice. Tissue cultures are inoculated with clinical samples; if the result is positive, plaques generally form as early as 4 days after inoculation. Cultures are stained with Wright's or Giemsa stain and examined for plaques that contain necrotic cells and replicating tachyzoites. Isolation of *T. gondii* from placenta, blood, or body fluids (e.g., CSF or amniotic fluid) is diagnostic for both acute and congenital toxoplasmosis. In contrast, in suspected cases of reactivated disease, isolation of *T. gondii* from tissue homogenates may only reflect the presence of tissue cysts in a chronic, latent infection.

Histology

Tissue sections, smears from brain biopsy, bone marrow aspirates, or cytocentrifuge specimens of body fluids that demonstrate free or intracellular tachyzoites confirm the diagnosis of acute infection. Because tachyzoites are often difficult to see in ordinary stains, immunofluorescent antibody and immunoperoxidase techniques may be useful (Conley et al., 1981). The finding of tissue cysts is diagnostic of infection with *T. gondii* but does not differentiate between acute and chronic infection. Tissue cysts in the placenta or any tissue samples from a newborn do, however, indicate congenital transmission. Toxoplasmic lymphadenitis has characteristic histologic features (see the discussion of pathology), but tachyzoites are generally not demonstrable.

Serologic Testing

Clinical use of serologic tests and representative results in specific clinical settings. Serologic tests to detect *T. gondii*–specific IgG, IgM, or IgA antibodies include the Sabin-Feldman dye test, IFA tests, agglutination tests, and ELISAs. DNA probe methods (e.g., PCR) have been described recently and have been used in France for prenatal diagnosis of congenital infection by amniocentesis. Tables 38-5 and 38-6 list specific tests that may be useful in particular clinical settings. Representative serologic test results from various clinical forms of infection are also listed in Table 38-6.

IgG antibodies. The following serologic tests detect IgG antibodies *to T. gondii*: Sabin-Feldman dye test, IFA, IgG ELISA, direct agglutination, and complement fixation. The Sabin-Feldman dye test and the IgG IFA test measure the same antibodies, and titers are usually of approximately the same magnitude. The Sabin-Feldman dye test is both sensitive and specific. It is generally viewed as the "gold standard" for detection of *T. gondii*–specific IgG. In this test, live tachyzoites incubated with serum that contains antibodies to *Toxoplasma* and an exogenous source of complement will change in shape and no longer take up the vital stain, alkaline methylene blue dye, indicating cell death. The dye test titer is the serum dilution at which half of the tachyzoites are killed. The IgG IFA test measures *Toxoplasma*-specific IgG antibodies, using formalin-fixed tachyzoites, the patient's serum, and antibody to human IgG that is fluorescein conjugated. In both the IgG IFA test and the dye test, antibodies usually appear 1 to 2 weeks after infection and reach high titers (>1:1,000) after 6 to 8 weeks. Low titers of such IgG antibody usually persist for life. Results that demonstrate *T. gondii*–specific IgG using IgG ELISA also correlate well with results of the Sabin-Feldman dye and IgG IFA tests. The complement-fixation test, however, detects IgG antibody that is generated less rapidly than antibody detected by the dye test, IgG IFA test, or IgG ELISA. Antibody detected with the complement-fixation test appears in the serum 3 to 8 weeks after infection, rises over the next 2 to 8 months, and then declines to low levels within a year. This test is not useful for detection of acute infection because of high rates of false-negative results.

Agglutination tests to detect IgG antibody are available commercially in Europe. Formalin-preserved whole parasites are used to detect IgG. Interference of nonspecific IgM antibodies is a problem that can be eliminated with the use of 2-mercaptoethanol. This test is accurate, simple, and relatively inexpensive.

High-avidity IgG antibodies to *T. gondii* appear after 12 to 16 weeks of infection (Jenum et al., 1977).

IgM antibodies. Tests to detect IgM antibodies to *T. gondii* include the IgM IFA; double-sandwich enzyme-linked immunosorbent technique (DS-IgM ELISA); and IgM ISAGA (an agglutination test). Because IgM antibodies usually appear within the first weeks of infection and disappear more rapidly than IgG antibodies, they are used to detect acute infection. IgM does not cross the placenta, so IgM antibodies detected in fetal or neonatal blood samples represent synthesis by an infected fetus or infant. IgM antibodies often are not present in sera of immunodeficient patients with active infection or in normal or immunodeficient patients during recrudescence in the eye. Specific IgM can be detected in sera of approximately 75% of newborns with congenital toxoplasmosis (when sera are tested using the DS-IgM ELISA).

Although the IgM IFA is useful for the diagnosis of acute infection with *T. gondii* in the older child and adult, it is relatively insensitive and therefore not reliable in detection of infection in infants. It detects only 25% of congenital *T. gondii* infections. Moreover, sera containing antinuclear antibodies or rheumatoid factor may yield false-positive reactions in the IgM IFA test.

The DS-IgM ELISA is more specific and sensitive for detecting anti–*T. gondii* IgM antibodies than the IgM IFA (Naot and Remington, 1980). It is useful for detection of both congenital toxoplasmosis in the infant and acute toxoplasmosis in the older child. Values indicative of infection must be determined by each laboratory. In one reference laboratory, levels of 1.7 (ELISA units) or greater usually indicate recently acquired infection in an older child or adult, although presence of specific serum IgM antibody can persist for up to 2 years. In that laboratory a value in serum of greater than 0.2 suggests congenital infection in a fetus or neonate. The DS-IgM ELISA detects 75% of infants with congenital *Toxoplasma* infection compared with detection of 25% of such infants using the IgM IFA. The DS-IgM ELISA avoids false-positive test results caused by rheumatoid factor or antinuclear antibody. The IgM ISAGA combines trapping of the patient's IgM to a solid surface and the use of formalin-fixed organisms or antigen-coated latex particles.

TABLE 38-5 Approach to Serologic Diagnosis of Toxoplasmosis

Patient and specimen	TOXOPLASMA GONDII SPECIFIC IgG*				T. GONDII-SPECIFIC IgM†				T. GONDII-SPECIFIC IgA	T. GONDII-SPECIFIC IgE		OTHER TESTS			
	Dye test	IgG IFA	IgG ELISA	Direct agglutination	DS-IgM ELISA	ISAGA	ELISA for IgM to P30	IFA	ELISA	ELISA	ISAGA	PCR	Isolation	AC/HS	Avidity
Newborn Congenital Toxoplasmosis															
Serum	C	C	C	C	C	C	C	Do not use	C	C	C		C	C	C
CSF	C				C	C							C		
Peripheral blood clot or peripheral blood cells (WBC)									C	C	C	C	C		
Placenta												R	C		
Pregnant Woman															
Maternal serum	C	C	C	C	C	C	C	C	C	C	C			C	C
Amniotic fluid												C	C		
Immunologically Normal Child															
Serum	C	C	C	C	C	C	C	C	C	C				C	
CSF	C				C	C			C						
Immunologically Deficient Child															
Serum	C‡	C	C	C	C‡	C‡	C‡	C‡	C	C	C	C		C	
CSF	C‡				C‡	C‡		C‡	C			C	C		

IgG, Immunoglobulin G; IFA, indirect fluorescent antibody; ELISA, enzyme-linked immunosorbent assay; DS, double sandwich; ISAGA, immunosorbent test for IgM; PCR, polymerase chain reaction; AC/HS, differential agglutination test; C, commercially available; CSF, cerebrospinal fluid; R, research test at present in reference laboratories; WBC, white blood cells.

*When properly standardized, any one of these tests is useful for demonstration of IgG antibody.

†ISAGA is usually most sensitive; IFA is least sensitive (do not use for congenital infection).

‡Rarely positive.

TABLE 38-6   Guidelines for Interpretation of Serologic Tests for Toxoplasmosis*

Test	Positive titer	Titer in congenital infection (infant); acute infection (older child, adult)	Titer in chronic infection	Duration of test elevation of titer
IgG				
Sabin-Feldman dye test	Undiluted	NC, S; OCA, 1:4 to ≥1:1,000 (usual)	1:4 to 1:2,000	Years
Direct agglutination test	≥1:20	NC, S; OCA, rises slowly from negative to low to high titer (1:512)	Stable (≥1:1,000) or slowly decreasing titer	≥1 year
Indirect fluorescent IgG antibody	≥1:10	NC, S; OCA, ≥1:1,000	1:8 to 1:2,000	Years
Indirect hemagglutination test	≥1:16	NC, S; OCA, ≥1:1,000	1:16 to 1:256	Years
Complement fixation	≥1:4	NC, S; OCA, varies among laboratories	Negative to 1:8	Years
IgM				
Indirect fluorescent for IgM	≥1:10, adults	OCA, ≥1:80 (use only for OCA, not NC)	Negative to 1:20	Weeks to months, occasionally years
Double sandwich IgM ELISA	≥0.2, newborns, fetuses ≥1.7, older children, adults	NC, ≥0.2; OCA, ≥1.7	Negative to 1.7 (OCA)	Can be ≥1 year
Immunosorbent test for IgM	≥3, infants; 8, adults	NC, ≥3; OCA, >8	Negative to 1	Unknown, can be ≥1year
IgA				
IgA, ELISA	≥1.0, infants; ≥1.4, adults	NC, ≥1.0; OCA, >1.4	Negative to <1.0 Negative to ≤1.3	Weeks to months, occasionally longer
IgE				
IgE, ELISA	≥1.9 infants and adults	NC and OCA, ≥1.9	Negative	Weeks to months, occasionally longer
Immunosorbent test for IgE	≥4 infants and adults	NC and OCA, ≥4	Negative	Weeks to months, occasionally longer
AC/HS	See Table 38-7	See Table 38-7	See Table 38-7	Usually <9 months
PCR (amniotic fluid; CSF)	Positive	Positive	Negative	Only when Toxoplasma DNA present during active infection
Avidity	Not applicable	Not applicable	High	High test result indicates acquisition of infection occurred more than 12-16 weeks earlier

IgG, Immunoglobulin G; *NC,* titer in newborn with congenital infection; *S,* usually the same as the mother; *OCA,* titer in older child or adult with acute, acquired infection; *ELISA,* enzyme-linked immunosorbent assay; *AC/HS,* differential agglutinin test; *PCR,* polymerase chain reaction; *CSF,* cerebrospinal fluid.

*Values are those of one reference laboratory; each laboratory must provide its own standards and interpretation of results in each clinical setting.

It apparently is more sensitive than the DS-IgM ELISA and, in the same manner, avoids false-positive results from rheumatoid factor or antinuclear antibodies.

IgA and IgE antibodies and AC/HS. Other tests to detect antibody to *T. gondii* include the IgA ELISA; the enzyme-linked immunofiltration assay (for IgA and IgE); the immunosorbent agglutination assay for IgE; and a differential agglutination test, AC/HS (Dannemann et al., 1990). The IgA ELISA apparently is even more sensitive than the IgM ELISA for detection of congenital infection (Decoster et al., 1988; Stepick-Biek et al., 1990). Both *T. gondii*–specific IgM and IgA antibodies demonstrated in ELISA or ISAGA may remain elevated for prolonged times (i.e., many months to years in older children and adults) but more commonly are present only a short time. AC/HS (Dannemann et al., 1990) is useful in differentiating recent acquisition from remote acquisition of infection in older children and adults (Table 38-7). In this test, greater agglutination of acetone-fixed tachyzoites (relative to agglutination of formalin-fixed tachyzoites) is detected in patients with acute infection. This test may be particularly helpful in differentiating recent infection from remote infection in a pregnant woman.

Local antibody production. The amount of *T. gondii*–specific antibody produced locally in CSF or aqueous humor has also been used to establish the presence of *T. gondii* infection. An organism-specific antibody index (OSAI), previously called *antibody coefficient (C)* or Toxoplasma-*specific index*, is calculated as follows:

$$OSAI = \frac{\text{Reciprocal titer in body fluid} \div \text{Concentration of IgG in body fluid}}{\text{Reciprocal titer in serum} \div \text{Concentration of IgG in serum}}$$

Local antibody production is indicated by an OSAI greater than or equal to 8 in aqueous humor for ophthalmologic infection; greater than or equal to 4 in CSF for congenital infection; or greater than or equal to 1 in CSF for AIDS patients. If the serum dye test titer is greater than or equal to 1,000, it is usually not possible to demonstrate local antibody production. IgM may also be present in CSF.

Antibody load. In patients with congenital toxoplasmosis, serum *T. gondii*–specific IgG antibody (present at birth) usually reflects the level of passively transferred maternal IgG antibody. Synthesis of specific antibody by the infected infant often can be detected by serial measurement of the ratio of *T. gondii*–specific IgG to total IgG and comparison to the expected linear decline in this ratio in an uninfected infant (Remington et al., 1995). However, antimicrobial therapy may delay detection of the baby's specific antibody synthesis by this means.

Polymerase chain reaction. PCR is promising for detection of *T. gondii* DNA in amniotic fluid and could potentially be useful for its detection in CSF, intraocular fluid, or peripheral blood. PCR is used to amplify *T. gondii* DNA, which then is identified by hybridization with a labeled probe. A study in France (Hohlfeld et al., 1994) using PCR to test amniotic fluid for the *T. gondii* B1 gene had only one false-negative result and no false-positive

TABLE 38-7 Interpretation of the AC/HS Test

HS result (IU/ml)	AC RESULT (IU/ml)							
	<50	50	100	200	400	800	1600	>1600
<100	NA	NA	A	A	A	A	A	A
100	NA	NA	A	A	A	A	A	A
200	NA	NA	A	A	A	A	A	A
400	NA	NA	A	A	A	A	A	A
800	NA	NA	NA	A	A	A	A	A
1600	NA	NA	NA	NA	A	A	A	A
3200	NA	NA	NA	NA	NA	A	A	A
>3200	NA	NA	NA	NA	NA	NA	A	A

Modified from Thulliez P, Remington JS. J Clin Microbiol 1990;28:1928-1933.
NA, Not acute; *A,* acute.

results, proving PCR more sensitive and specific than conventional methods of testing. This technique, however, has not yet been fully evaluated in the United States.

Diagnosis in Utero

Amniocentesis and fetal ultrasound have been very useful in the diagnosis and treatment of congenital toxoplasmosis (Hohlfeld et al., 1994). These procedures should be performed only by physicians with considerable experience with them and with the processing and interpretation of the data acquired. An example of the use of these techniques and of the need for experience and skill in interpretation of the results follows.

■ **Case 5**   A 19-year-old woman had headaches, malaise, fatigue, and cervical lymphadenopathy 1 month before conception. She did not seek medical care, and her symptoms resolved over a 2-week period. She had cats and kittens that roamed outdoors, but she did not handle their litter box. She denied ingesting any raw or rare meat. On her first prenatal visit at 12 weeks gestation by dates, serologic test results were as follows: Sabin-Feldman dye test, 1:2, 048; IgA ELISA, 10; IgM ELISA, 6; and AC/HS, >1,600/1,600. Results from a fetal ultrasound at 14 weeks gestation were normal. Spiramycin (3 g/day orally) was begun.

PCR to determine whether *T. gondii* DNA (the B1 gene) was present in the cell pellet from 10 ml amniotic fluid was negative. A cell pellet from 19 ml of amniotic fluid was inoculated into mice. Subinoculation studies were negative.

Spiramycin therapy was continued until delivery. Fetal ultrasound examinations were repeated every 2 weeks and were normal. The patient tolerated spiramycin therapy without any ill effects. She delivered a normal, uninfected infant, who was evaluated as described in Box 38-1.

Evaluation of the Infant at Birth

Diagnostic tests (in addition to *T. gondii*–specific serologic tests, attempts to isolate the organism, and histologic tests) that may be useful in evaluation of fetuses and infants with congenital toxoplasmosis are listed in Box 38-1.

THERAPY

Pyrimethamine plus sulfadiazine or trisulfapyrimidines (triple sulfa) act synergistically against *T. gondii*. These antimicrobial agents (plus leucovorin) currently constitute the standard treatment for toxoplasmosis. In addition, spiramycin has been used extensively in France to prevent in utero transmission of infection to fetuses of acutely infected women (Desmonts and Couvreur, 1974) and has been included in treatment regimens for congenital toxoplasmo-

---

BOX 38-1

EVALUATION OF NEONATE WHEN SEROLOGIC TESTS OF MOTHER OR THE ILLNESS OF THE NEONATE INDICATES THAT DIAGNOSIS OF CONGENITAL TOXOPLASMOSIS IS SUSPECTED OR LIKELY

In addition to a careful general examination, when congenital toxoplasmosis is a possible or likely diagnosis, the baby is examined as follows:

Clinical Evaluation and Nonspecific Tests
- By a pediatric ophthalmologist
- By a pediatric neurologist
- CT scan of the brain
- Blood tests
  - Complete blood cell count with differential and platelet counts
  - Serum total of IgM, IgG, IgA, and albumin
- Serum alanine aminotransferase total direct bilirubin
  - CSF, cell count, glucose, protein, and total IgG

***T. gondii*–Specific Tests**
- Serum Sabin-Feldman dye test IgM
  - ELISA, IgM ISAGA, IgA ELISA, IgE
  - ELISA/ISAGA (0.5 ml serum, sent to Serology Laboratory. Palo Alto Medical Foundation, 795 El Camino Real, Palo Alto, CA 94301)
- Lumbar puncture: cerebrospinal fluid (CSF) 0.5 ml CSF sent to Serology Laboratory (see above address) for dye test and IgM ELISA
- Sterile placental tissue (100 g in saline, no formalin from near insertion of cord from the fetal side) and newborn blood obtained for inoculation into mice (2 ml clotted whole blood in red topped tube)
- Maternal serum analyzed for antibody detected by dye test, IgM ELISA, IgA ELISA, IgE ELISA/ISAGA, and AC/HS

AC/HS, Differential agglutination test; *CSF,* cerebrospinal fluid; *CT,* Computed tomography; *ELISA,* enzyme-linked immunosorbent assay; *IgM,* immunoglobulin M; *ISAGA,* immunosorbent agglutination test for IgM.

---

sis after birth (Remington et al., 1995). Clindamycin has been used in conjunction with pyrimethamine to treat toxoplasmosis in AIDS patients who have been unable to tolerate therapy with sulfadiazine.

Pyrimethamine

Pyrimethamine (Daraprim) inhibits dihydrofolate reductase. The plasma half-life is 90 hours in adults and 60 hours in infants (McLeod et al., 1992). Pyrimethamine has caused bone-marrow suppression manifested by thrombocytopenia, granulocytopenia, and megaloblastic anemia. Reversible granulocytopenia is the most frequent adverse effect in treated infants. Seizures have also occurred with overdosage of pyrimethamine. Patients being treated with pyrimethamine should have their neutrophil counts monitored weekly and their platelet counts and hematocrit level monitored monthly. Folinic acid (leucovorin calcium) should always be administered with pyrimethamine to prevent bone-marrow suppression. Folinic acid does not block the inhibitory effect of pyrimethamine and sulfadiazine on *Toxoplasma* replication at dosages used in the treatment of congenital toxoplasmosis.

Zidovudine, on the other hand, appears to antagonize the antitoxoplasmic effect of pyrimethamine and its synergy with sulfadiazine in vitro. Therapy with phenobarbital appears to reduce the half-life of pyrimethamine in infants (McLeod et al., 1992) probably by induction of hepatic enzymes, which degrade pyrimethamine. Pyrimethamine levels in fetal serum when mothers receive 50 mg pyrimethamine daily are in a relatively low, but potentially therapeutic, range (Dorangeon et al., 1990).

Sulfonamides

Sulfadiazine or trisulfapyrimidines (sulfadiazine, sulfamerazine, and sulfamethazine) should be used in combination with pyrimethamine for the treatment of toxoplasmosis. Other sulfonamides are less effective. Sulfadiazine and trisulfapyrimidines antagonize folic acid synthesis by inhibition of dihydrofolate synthetase. Sulfadiazine is rapidly absorbed from the gastrointestinal tract, and peak plasma concentrations are reached within 3 to 6 hours after ingestion of a single dose. Equilibration between maternal and fetal circulation is also established in this time. Sulfonamides readily pass through the placenta and reach the fetus in concentrations sufficient to exhibit both antimicrobial and toxic effects.

The side effects of sulfadiazine or trisulfapyrimidines include bone-marrow suppression, diarrhea, rash, crystalluria with possible stone formation, and acute reversible renal failure. An increase in fluid intake, with maintenance of high urinary flow, is important in patients treated with sulfonamides. Hypersensitivity reactions can also occur, especially in patients with AIDS. Sulfadiazine interferes with the metabolism of hepatic microsomal enzymes and may inhibit metabolism of phenytoin, causing higher serum levels of this antiepileptic agent. Sulfonamides may also potentiate coumarin anticoagulants by displacing them from binding sites.

Spiramycin

Spiramycin is a macrolide and is available to physicians in the United States with individual permission of the Food and Drug Administration (phone 301-827-2335) and can be obtained from the drug manufacturer, Aventis Rhone Poulenc (phone 908-231-3365). It appears to reduce transmission of *T. gondii* from acutely infected pregnant women to their fetuses in utero by 60% (Desmonts and Couvreur, 1979). It is absorbed best without food. Side effects are usually minimal but have included gastrointestinal distress, local vasospasm, dysesthesias, dizziness, flushing, nausea, vomiting, tearing, diarrhea, anorexia, and allergy. There are no known deleterious effects on the fetus.

Clindamycin

Clindamycin is effective against murine toxoplasmosis. However, its effect in human infection is controversial. Despite its lack of penetration into CSF and lack of in vitro activity against *T. gondii* (presumably a metabolite is active in vivo), clindamycin has been used in combination with high dosages of pyrimethamine to treat toxoplasmic encephalitis successfully in patients with AIDS (with efficacy equal to treatment with pyrimethamine and sulfadiazine). It is an alternative therapy in conjunction with pyrimethamine if sulfonamide therapy cannot be tolerated. Uncontrolled studies have reported use of clindamycin to treat ocular toxoplasmosis.

Atovoquone (5-Hydroxy-Naphthoquinone) and Other Antimicrobial Agents

Reactivation of disease resulting from encysted organisms is an increasing problem because of the large numbers of patients with chronic latent infection with *T. gondii* and AIDS. Atovoquone, which appears to inhibit protozoan microbial electron transport enzyme cytochrome b, was felt to be promising as an agent effective against bradyzoites within cysts in vitro (Huskinson-Mark et al., 1991). However, in clinical trials, 40% of patients with AIDS developed relapse of their toxoplasmic encephalitis while being treated with this antimicrobial agent. Other antimicrobial agents with effect on *T. gondii* in vitro or in vivo include new macrolides (roxithromycin, clarithromycin, and azithromycin), cycloguanil, and artether (Holfels et al., 1994).

Therapy in Specific Clinical Settings

Summaries of currently used therapies for toxoplasmosis in specific clinical settings are listed in Tables 38-8 and 38-9.

Congenital toxoplasmosis. Infected newborns should be treated whether or not they have overt clinical signs of infection.

In a study in France mothers received pyrimethamine and sulfonamide therapy to treat their infected fetuses in utero as outlined in Tables 38-8 and 38-9 (Foulon et al., 2000; Remington et al., 2001; Romand et al., 2001). The outcome was considerably better than was found for comparable historic controls who did not receive such treatment in utero (Hohlfeld et al., 1989; Hohlfeld et al., 1994). Subclinical infection was present in 41 treated children, and 12 had only isolated asymptomatic signs (retinal scar with normal vision or cerebral calcifications with normal neurologic status).

Only one had signs of severe congenital infection. Delay in treatment in utero leads to more eye and brain damage in the fetus and infant (Mirlisse et al., cited in Remington et al., 2001).

The most extensive experience in treatment of congenital toxoplasmosis after birth has been with the regimen of Dr. Jacques Couvreur. It uses alternate courses of pyrimethamine, sulfadiazine, and spiramycin (Table 38-9). Couvreur et al. (1984) reported a reduction in early ophthalmologic sequelae with this treatment.

In addition, a U.S. National Collaborative prospective, controlled treatment study with long-term follow-up to determine feasibility, safety, efficacy, and optimal dosage for treatment with pyrimethamine and sulfadiazine is ongoing (McGhee et al., 1992; McLeod et al., 1991a; McLeod et al., 2000; Mets et al., 1992; Remington et al., 2001; Roizen et al., 1992). Preliminary results from this trial indicate that signs of active disease resolve with therapy and suggest that early outcome for most (but not all) treated infants is substantially better than the outcome reported for untreated infants or those treated for only 1 month, as described in the earlier literature (Eichenwald, 1960; Wilson et al., 1980). Neurologic, developmental, auditory, and ophthalmologic outcomes are evaluated. Study of the effect of newer antimicrobial agents that eliminate encysted organisms on ophthalmologic and neurologic sequelae is also planned. Infants can be referred to this

TABLE 38-8	Management of Pregnancies at Risk for Fetal Infection According to Time of Maternal Infection		
Time of maternal infection	Percentages of pregnancies with fetal infection	Prenatal diagnostic tests	Management
Periconception	1% with treatment	Ultrasound every 2 weeks; fetal blood sampling plus amniocentesis	Spiramycin; if fetal infection, termination or possibly antiparasitic treatment
5 to 16 weeks	4% with treatment; 12% without treatment	Ultrasound every 2 weeks; amniocentesis	Spiramycin; if fetal infection, termination or possibly antiparasitic treatment[*]
16 weeks to term	20% to 30%, between 16 and 28 weeks, increasing incidence closer to term with treatment	Ultrasound every 2 weeks; amniocentesis	Spiramycin; if fetal infection, discontinue spiramycin, use antiparasitic treatment[*] or possibly termination

Modified from Daffos F, et al.: N Engl J Med 1988;318:271.
[*]Treatment of the fetus or infant is with pyrimethamine, sulfadiazine, and folinic acid without spiramycin.

TABLE 38-9	Treatment of Toxoplasmosis		
Manifestation of disease	Therapy	Dosage (oral unless specified)	Duration
Congenital toxoplasmosis*	Pyrimethamine*	Loading dose: 2 mg/kg per day for 2 days, then 1 mg/kg/day for 2 or 6 months, then this dose on each Monday, Wednesday, and Friday	1 yr
	Sulfadiazine* and	100 mg/kg/day in two daily divided doses	1 yr
	Leucovorin (folinic acid)*	5-10 mg three times weekly†	1 yr
	Corticosteroids (prednisone)‡	1 mg/kg/day in two daily divided doses	Until resolution of elevated (≥1 g/dl) cerebrospinal fluid protein level or active chorioretinitis that threatens vision
In Immunologically Normal Children			
Lymphadenopathy	No therapy	—	—
Significant organ damage that is life threatening	Pyrimethamine	A = Loading dose: 2 mg/kg/day for 2 days, then maintenance, 1 mg/kg/day	D = Usually 4-6 weeks or 2 weeks beyond time that signs and symptoms have resolved
	and Sulfadiazine	B = 50 mg/kg q12h (maximum 4 g/day)	Same as D
	and Leucovorin	C = 5-20 mg three times weekly†	Same as D
Active chorioretinitis in older children	Pyrimethamine	Same as A	Same as D
	and Sulfadiazine	Same as B	
	and Leucovorin	Same as C	
	Corticosteroid‡	Same as for congenital toxoplasmosis	Same as for congenital toxoplasmosis
In Immunocompromised Children			
Non-AIDS	Pyrimethamine	Same as A	E = 4-6 weeks beyond complete resolution of symptoms and signs
	and Sulfadiazine	Same as B	Same as E
	and Leucovorin	Same as C	Same as E
AIDS	Pyrimethamine	Same as A	May discontinue maintenance treatment when lesions resolved, and CD4 counts are >200 for 4-6 months
	and Sulfadiazine	Same as B	
	and Leucovorin	Same as C	
	Clindamycin may be used instead of sulfadiazine	Reported trials for adults but not infants and children	

Continued

TABLE 38-9   Treatment of Toxoplasmosis—cont'd

Manifestation of disease	Therapy	Dosage (oral unless specified)	Duration
In Pregnant Women with Acute Toxoplasmosis			
First 21 weeks of gestation or until term if fetus not infected	Spiramycin[§]	1 g every 8 h without food	F = Until fetal infection documented or excluded at 21 weeks; if documented, treat with pyrimethamine, leucovorin, and sulfadiazine until term
If fetal infection confirmed after 17th week of gestation or if infection acquired in last few weeks of gestation (after amniocentesis and PCR to determine if fetus is infected with *T. gondii*)	Pyrimethamine	Loading dose: 100 mg/day in divided doses for 2 days followed by 50 mg daily	Same as F
	and Sulfadiazine	100 mg/kg/day in two divided doses (maximum, 4 g/day)	Same as F
	and Leucovorin[†]	5-20 mg daily	Same as F

[*]Optimal dosage, feasibility, toxicity currently being evaluated or planned in ongoing National Collaborative Treatment Trial (phone 773-834-4152).

[†]Adjusted for megaloblastic anemia, granulocytopenia, or thrombocytopenia; blood counts, including platelets, should be monitored as described in text.

[‡]Corticosteroids should be continued until signs of inflammation (high CSF protein ≥1 g/dl) or active chorioretinitis that threatens vision have subsided, dosage then can be tapered and discontinued; use only in conjunction with pyrimethamine, sulfadiazine, and leucovorin.

[§]Available only on request from the Food and Drug Administration (phone 301-827-2335).

National Collaborative study by telephoning 773-834-4152.

A method for preparation of pyrimethamine and sulfadiazine to facilitate their administration to infants, which currently is being used in this National Collaborative study, is shown in Figure 38-8. Dosages of medications being evaluated are outlined in Table 38-9. Therapy with corticosteroids (prednisone, 1 mg/kg/day, divided into two doses) has been recommended when there is elevated CSF protein (≥1 g/dL) or active chorioretinitis that threatens vision (Remington et al., 1995).

Immunologically normal children with lymphadenopathy, severe symptoms, or damage to vital organs. Children with lymphadenopathy alone do not need specific treatment. If severe or persistent symptoms occur or there is evidence of organ damage, therapy with a combination of pyrimethamine, sulfadiazine, and leucovorin is indicated. Patients who are immunologically normal but have severe symptoms or damage to vital organs (e.g., chorioretinitis, myocarditis, or pneumonitis) should be treated until all symptoms and signs resolve, followed by an additional 2 weeks of therapy. The usual course of therapy is approximately 4 to 6 weeks; dosages of medications are listed in Table 38-9. A loading dose of pyrimethamine (2 mg/kg body weight, maximum of 50 mg) is given daily for 2 days, followed by a maintenance dose (1 mg/kg body weight, maximum of 25 mg) daily. The loading dose of sulfadiazine is 75 mg/kg body weight, followed by a maintenance dose of 50 mg/kg body weight every 12 hours. Folinic acid (calcium leucovorin) is administered orally whenever pyrimethamine is given. Dosage is 5 to 20 mg given three to seven times weekly, depending on the results of blood and platelet counts.

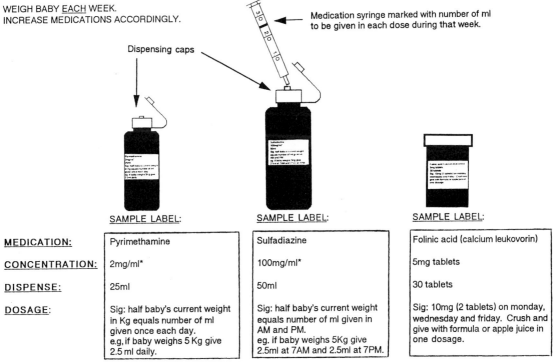

WEIGH BABY <u>EACH</u> WEEK.
INCREASE MEDICATIONS ACCORDINGLY.

Dispensing caps

Medication syringe marked with number of ml
to be given in each dose during that week.

	SAMPLE LABEL:	SAMPLE LABEL:	SAMPLE LABEL:
MEDICATION:	Pyrimethamine	Sulfadiazine	Folinic acid (calcium leukovorin)
CONCENTRATION:	2mg/ml*	100mg/ml*	5mg tablets
DISPENSE:	25ml	50ml	30 tablets
DOSAGE:	Sig: half baby's current weight in Kg equals number of ml given once each day. e.g, if baby weighs 5 Kg give 2.5 ml daily.	Sig: half baby's current weight equals number of ml given in AM and PM. eg. if baby weighs 5Kg give 2.5ml at 7AM and 2.5ml at 7PM.	Sig: 10mg (2 tablets) on monday, wednesday and friday. Crush and give with formula or apple juice in one dosage.

Fig. 38-8 Preparation and administration of medications used to treat congenital toxoplasmosis in a National Collaborative Study. (Modified from McAuley et al., 1994.)

Active chorioretinitis in older children. Chorioretinitis is the most frequent manifestation of congenital disease, but clearly also occurs during acute acquired infection as well (Glasner, 1992; Montoya and Remington, 1996). Relapse may occur throughout childhood and adult life. Although active chorioretinitis may remit spontaneously without specific therapy, treatment with pyrimethamine, sulfadiazine, and leucovorin appears to reduce signs and symptoms. Therapy for active chorioretinitis is outlined in Table 38-9. Therapy should be given in conjunction with care by an ophthalmologist. With treatment, borders of retinal lesions sharpen, and vitreous haze should disappear within approximately 10 days. Corticosteroids should be added if lesions involve the macula, optic nerve head, or papillomacular bundle. Use of clindamycin has been described extensively in the ophthalmologic literature and has been recommended as an alternative to the sulfonamide-pyrimethamine combination. However, definitive studies demonstrating efficacy have not been performed. Surgery may be considered for some secondary sequelae, e.g., cataract, retinal detachment.

Immunocompromised patients. Toxoplasmosis in patients who are immunocompromised by underlying disease (e.g., lymphoma, AIDS) or by therapy (e.g., corticosteroids, cytotoxic drugs) should be treated. Serologic evidence of active infection in an immunocompromised patient, regardless of clinical signs and symptoms, or documentation of the presence of tachyzoites in tissue is an indication for treatment. In patients with AIDS, clinical symptoms with radiologic findings (CT or MRI) that are suggestive of infection may in themselves be indications for treatment. If there is no response to a therapeutic trial of pyrimethamine and sulfadiazine within approximately 10 to 14 days, brain biopsy to exclude other diagnoses should be considered. In 80% of patients with AIDS in whom the diagnosis was made antemortem, there was clear and rapid (<1 month) improvement with antimicrobial treatment. In the same group of patients, more than half of those responding showed complete resolution of clinical and brain CT-scan abnormalities. For immunosuppressed individuals it is imperative to suspect and establish the diagnosis quickly and to begin treatment as soon as possible. In bone marrow–transplant recipients, *T. gondii* infection is often fulminant, undiagnosed, and rapidly fatal (Derouin et al., 1992).

For children whose immunosuppression can be reduced (by discontinuation of chemotherapy or corticosteroids), treatment with sulfadiazine, pyrimethamine, and leucovorin should be continued for 4 to 6 weeks beyond complete resolution of all signs and symptoms of active disease.

In immunocompromised adults with AIDS relapse is frequent if therapy is discontinued when CD4 counts are less than 200 (Liesenfeld et al., 1999). Until agents that can eliminate encysted organisms have demonstrated efficacy in humans, suppressive therapy with pyrimethamine and sulfadiazine should be continued until lesions have resolved and CD4 counts are greater than 200 for 4 to 6 months. Different suppressive regimens are included in Table 38-9. In a recent controlled study the combination of pyrimethamine and sulfadozine, one tablet biweekly, was reported to reduce the occurrence of toxoplasmic encephalitis (Ruf et al., 1991). In this study the incidence of subsequent encephalitis was reduced to 4 of 37 (11%) with prophylaxis and to 8 of 12 (67%) without prophylaxis. When used as primary prophylaxis in seropositive individuals without overt disease, the incidence of subsequent encephalitis was reduced to 2 of 38 (5%) with sulfadoxine and pyrimethamine (Fansidar) and 7 of 28 (25%) without it. It is not known whether suppressive doses of pyrimethamine and sulfonamides are either necessary or effective in preventing relapse in infants with congenital or acute acquired toxoplasmosis and AIDS. Based on data in adults, it is reasonable to treat children with AIDS and toxoplasmic encephalitis with pyrimethamine and sulfadiazine for the remainder of their lives.

Pregnant women with acute acquired T. gondii infection or chronic T. gondii infection and immunocompromise. In general, if *T. gondii* infection is acquired by an immunologically normal mother before conception, the fetus is not at risk for congenital toxoplasmosis. There have been only two reports of a normal woman who acquired *T. gondii* 2 months before conception who transmitted the infection to her fetus in utero (Remington et al., 1995; Vogel et al., 1996). Treatment with spiramycin of an immunologically normal pregnant woman who acquires an acute infection during pregnancy reduces the chance of congenital infection in

her infant by 60% (Desmonts and Couvreur, 1974). Spiramycin (1.5 g every 12 hours without food) is continued throughout pregnancy unless fetal infection is demonstrated by ultrasound or analysis of amniotic fluid (Table 38-8). If evidence of infection is present in the fetus, pyrimethamine, sulfadiazine, and leucovorin therapy (dosages are listed in Table 38-9) have been substituted in alternate months for spiramycin. If no fetal involvement is found, spiramycin alone is continued until term. Such treatment reduces the ability to isolate *T. gondii* from the placenta. In one study, *T. gondii* was isolated from placentas of untreated infected infants 95% of the time, but only 80% of the time from placentas of infected infants whose mothers were treated with spiramycin and only 50% of the time from placentas of infants whose mothers were treated with pyrimethamine and sulfadiazine and spiramycin in alternate months (Couvreur et al., 1988).

Chronically infected women who become immunosuppressed by cytotoxic drugs, corticosteroids, or HIV infection have also transmitted *T. gondii* to the fetus. Most of these women develop toxoplasmosis by recrudescence of latent *T. gondii* rather than from newly acquired infection. Such women, who do not have overt toxoplasmosis, should at least receive spiramycin throughout pregnancy.

PROGNOSIS

Toxoplasmic lymphadenopathy in the immunologically normal individual is self-limited and resolves without antimicrobial therapy. Treatment with pyrimethamine, sulfadiazine, and leucovorin results in resolution of active signs of *T. gondii* infection in most immunologically normal, immunocompromised, and congenitally infected individuals.* The prognosis for infants with congenital toxoplasmosis that is untreated or is treated with 1 month of pyrimethamine and sulfadiazine is poor for those who have neurologic or generalized infection at presentation in their first year of life (Table 38-3). The prognosis also is guarded for those with subclinical infection at birth (Table 38-4). The outcome is substantially better for most (but not all) infants who are treated in utero and/or for 1 year with pyrimethamine

---

*McAuley et al., 1994; McGhee et al., 1992; McLeod et al., 1979; McLeod et al., 1992; Mets et al., 1996; Patel et al., 1996; Roizen et al., 1995; Swisher et al., 1994.

and sulfadiazine (Tables 38-10 and 38-11). Favorable outcomes have been associated with prompt diagnosis and initiation of antimicrobial therapy and with prompt attention to the need for shunting of patients with hydrocephalus or revision of malfunctioning ventriculoperitoneal shunts (McAuley et al., 1994).

PREVENTION

At present, the major component of primary prevention is educating susceptible patients, especially seronegative pregnant or immunodeficient individuals. Health education may decrease the incidence of toxoplasmosis during pregnancy by 60% (Foulon et al., 2000). Given the morbidity, mortality, and expense of the disease in terms of care of affected patients, major attempts to define and initiate better forms of prevention are needed. All physicians responsible for the care of pregnant women, those attempting to conceive, or immunosuppressed patients should inform them of simple measures for prevention. Provision of informational material to pregnant women in France reduced the incidence of congenital infection by 50%. An educational pamphlet and videotape (phone 800-323-9100), as well as information on the Internet at http://www.toxoplasmosis.org, are also available.

The goal of primary prevention is to avoid ingestion of cysts or contact with sporulated oocysts. Methods of prevention are outlined in Figure 38-2. Tissue cysts can be rendered noninfectious by heating meat or eggs to 66° C (150.8° F) or by smoking, curing, or freezing meat to −22° C (−7.6° F). Most home freezers

---

TABLE 38-10 Contrasts of Neurologic and Developmental Outcomes in Eichenwald, Wilson, and Chicago Studies

		PERCENT WITH OUTCOME			
Signs neonatally	Study	Seizures	Abnormal motor/tone	IQ <70	Sequentially lower IQ
Generalized neurologic signs	Eichenwald, 1960 (n = 101)	81	70	86	n/a
	Chicago, 1991a (n = 33)	11	24	32	Not significant[*†]
Subclinical signs	Wilson et al., 1980 (n = 33)	17	21	17	86[*]
	Chicago, 1991a (n = 3)	0	0	0	0[*]

Modified from Boyer KM, McLeod RL. In Long SS, Prober CG, Pickering LK (eds). Principles and practice of infectious diseases. New York: Churchill Livingstone, 1996, pp 645-672. With permission.
[*]In Chicago study: generalized/neurologic, n = 27; subclinical, n = 2. In Wilson study: n = 7.
[†]Three increased, three decreased; thus no significant differences for group; 3/11 (27%).

TABLE 38-11 Fetal Toxoplasmosis: Outcome of Pregnancy and Infant Follow-up After In-Utero Treatment[*]

	TRIMESTER					
	FIRST		SECOND		THIRD	
	1972-1981	1982-1988	1972-1981	1982-1988	1972-1981	1982-1988
Outcome	Number %	Number %	Number %	Number %	Number %	Number
Subclinical	1 10	6 67	23 37	33 77	74 68	2
Benign	5 50	2 22	28 45	10 23	31 29	0
Severe	4 40	1 11	11 18	0	3 3	0
total	10	9	62	43	108	2

Modified from Hohlfeld P, et al. J Pediatr 1989;115:765.
[*]Infants were not treated in utero 1972-1981 and were treated in utero 1982-1988. Trimester indicates time of acquisition of acute infection by the mother. Note in utero treatment was associated with marked diminution of clinical signs or severity of infection.

do not become this cold. Hands should be washed thoroughly after handling raw meat and vegetables. Steak tartare or other foods featuring uncooked meat should be avoided. Eggs should not be ingested raw, and unpasteurized milk (particularly from goats) should not be consumed. Any kitchen surfaces that come in contact with raw meat or vegetables should be washed thoroughly. Patients should also be warned not to touch mucous membranes or eyes while handling raw meat.

To prevent infection with the oocyst, cat feces should be avoided. Cat feces should be disposed of daily (because sporulation occurs 1 to 5 days after excretion) either by incineration or by flushing down the toilet. Cat litter pans should be used with liners and changed by someone other than the pregnant or immunosuppressed individual. The pan can then be rendered free of viable oocysts by pouring boiling water into the pans and letting the water remain for at least 5 minutes before rinsing. Ammonia (7%) can also kill oocysts but requires 3 hours of exposure. Chlorine bleach, dilute ammonia, quaternary ammonia compounds, or other household detergents are not sufficient to destroy oocysts. When working in sand or soil possibly contaminated with cat feces, gloves should be worn. Hands should be thoroughly washed before handling any items that would be ingested or come in contact with mucous membranes. Since the cat is the only animal that is known to produce oocysts, efforts should also be directed toward preventing infection in cats. Feeding cats commercially dried, canned, or cooked food rather than allowing them to hunt possibly infected prey will reduce the likelihood of their infection. These general precautionary measures, rather than serologic testing of cats, are recommended.

Although primary prevention theoretically can be achieved by education about hygienic measures as described previously, secondary prevention consists of identification of acutely infected individuals in high-risk populations and the early institution of specific therapy to prevent or minimize complications. Because approximately 90% of women infected during pregnancy have no clinical illness, sequential serologic testing of seronegative pregnant women is the only way to identify the fetus at risk of congenital infection. Standardized screening, followed by sequential testing, is routinely performed in areas of high incidence, such as

France and Austria. However, there is no universally adopted policy for screening or sequential testing of pregnant women for congenital toxoplasmosis in the United States. Cost-effectiveness has been suggested but not proved (McCabe and Remington, 1988). Problems with the reliability of some commercially available serologic tests have in the past dissuaded certain authors from recommending widespread serologic screening. Before the initiation of therapy in any setting, positive serologic test results should be confirmed in a reference laboratory (e.g., Palo Alto Research Institute; phone 650-326-8120). Some serologic screening programs have involved all women in their childbearing years before and during pregnancy to determine prior exposure (e.g., France), and some have involved screening of all newborns (e.g., the model of the Massachusetts State Screening Program). If women are seronegative, systematic serologic screening at specific intervals during pregnancy is used (Figure 38-9). This is a reasonable approach because it is possible to prevent or modify illness caused by congenital *T. gondii* infection by treatment during gestation and because reliable serologic tests are now commercially available in the United States. The individual suffering and the cost to families and society of caring for children born with congenital toxoplasmosis make increased use of screening tests potentially important (Featherstone, 1981).

THE FUTURE

Major future advances in prevention and treatment of toxoplasmosis are likely. Development of a vaccine to prevent infection in humans and cats remains at an experimental stage, but a number of lines of investigation are promising. Use of educational programs for pregnant and immunocompromised individuals should further reduce infection rates. Paradigms for prevention of congenital infection or its sequelae are being developed and tested. More sensitive and specific serologic and direct (e.g., PCR) tests are being evaluated. Additional reference laboratories to perform serologic testing reliably are needed. Studies to determine optimal means to treat congenital toxoplasmosis and toxoplasmosis in patients with AIDS are in progress. Ongoing development and testing of new antimicrobial agents that eliminate encysted organisms that are the source of recrudescent disease in congenital, ophthalmologic, and disseminated or neurologic

Approach to prenatal prevention, diagnosis, and treatment

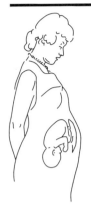

- Dx mother: Systematic serologic screening, before conception and intrapartum

- Rx mother: If acute serology, spiramycin reduces transmission
  Untreated 94 (60%) of 154 versus treated 91 (23%) of 388*

- Dx fetus: Ultrasounds; amniocentesis, PCR at ≥ 18 weeks gestation
  Sensitivity 37 (97%) of 38: specificity 301 of 301[†] Overall
  sensitivity of PCR is 85%. PCR is most sensitive in mid gestation
  and less sensitive early and late in gestation (Romand et.al., 2001).
  Amniocentesis should be performed when suspicion for infection in
  the fetus is high.

- Rx fetus: Pyrimethamine, sulfadiazine or termination
  N=54 livebirths; 34 terminations[§]

- Outcome: All 54 normal development; 19% subtle findings
  7 (13%) intracranical calcifications, 3 (6%) chorioretinal scars[¶]

*Desmonts and Couvreur, 1974.
[†]Hohlfeld et al, 1994.
[§]Daffos et al, 1988.
[¶]Hohlfeld et al, 1989.

Fig. 38-9 Prevention, diagnosis, and treatment of toxoplasmosis.

BOX 38-2
PERTINENT PHONE NUMBERS

Reference laboratory for serology, isolation, and PCR	650-326-8120
FDA for IND number to obtain spiramycin for treatment of a pregnant woman	301-827-2336
Spiramycin (Aventis Rhone Poulenc) for treatment of a pregnant woman	908-231-3365
Congenital toxoplasmosis study	773-834-4152
Educational pamphlet	312-435-4007
Information concerning AIDS and congenital toxoplasmosis	305-547-6676
Educational information on Internet http://www.toxoplasmosis.org	

toxoplasmosis in immunocompromised individuals are promising.

RESOURCES

A variety of resources are available to assist in the prevention and treatment of toxoplasmosis. These resources (with phone numbers) are shown in Box 38-2.

GLOSSARY

AC/HSC: Differential agglutination test using acetone (AC) and formalin (HS) fixed tachyzoites; useful in determining whether infection was acquired in the 6 months before the serum sample was obtained.

Chronic infection with *T. gondii*: Condition of asymptomatic parasite latency that follows primary infection or successful treatment of recrudescence.

Cyst: Contains bradyzoites and is present in chronic infection.

Double sandwich (DS)–IgA ELISA: Measures *T. gondii*–specific IgA; possibly more sensitive than the DS-IgM ELISA for diagnosis of congenital infection.

Double sandwich (DS)–IgE ELISA: Measures *T. gondii*–specific IgE; possibly more sensitive than the IgM ELISA for diagnosis of congenital infection.

Double sandwich (DS)–IgM ELISA: Measures *T. gondii*–specific IgM; positive at birth in approximately 75% of congenitally infected infants.

IgE ISAGA: Measures *T. gondii*–specific IgE; probably more sensitive than the DS-IgM ELISA.

IgM ISAGA: Measures *T. gondii*–specific IgM; usually more sensitive than the DS-IgM ELISA.

Mouse inoculation: Inoculation of body fluid or placental tissue intraperitoneally into mice; mice then are observed for proliferating tachyzoites in their ascitic fluid, brain cyst development, and *T. gondii*–specific serum antibodies.

Oocyst: Contains sporozoites and is excreted by cats.

Sabin-Feldman dye test: "Gold standard" test for measurement of IgG antibody that damages the surface membrane of live tachyzoites in the presence of complement, rendering the tachyzoite unstained by the vital dye methylene blue; performed by reference laboratories.

***Toxoplasma gondii* bradyzoite:** Slowly proliferative form present within tissue cysts in chronic, latent infection; source of infection ingested in undercooked meat.

***T. gondii* sporozoite:** Highly infectious form in oocyst, which sporulates after fecal excretion by cats.

***T. gondii* tachyzoite:** Rapidly proliferative form present in acute and active infection.

Toxoplasmosis: Disease caused by *T. gondii*; may be primary or recrudescent.

BIBLIOGRAPHY

Aspock P. Prevention of congenital toxoplasmosis by serological surveillance during pregnancy: current strategies and future perspectives. In Marget W, Lang W, Gabler-Sandberger E (eds). Parasitic Infections, Immunology, Mycotic Infections, General Topics, vol 3. Munich: MMV Medizin Verlag, 1986.

Boyer KM, McLeod RL. *Toxoplasma gondii* (toxoplasmosis). In Long SS, Prober CG, Pickering LK (eds). Principles and Practice of Infectious Diseases. New York: Churchill Livingstone, 1996.

Brézin AP, Kasner L, Thulliez P, et al. Ocular toxoplasmosis in the fetus: immunohistochemistry analysis and DNA amplification. Retina 1994;14:19-26.

Brown C, McLeod R. Class I MHC genes and CD8+ T cells determine cyst number in *Toxoplasma gondii* infection. J Immunol 1990;145:3438-3441.

Burg JL, Grover CM, Pouletty P, Boothroyd JC. Direct and sensitive detection of a pathogenic protozoan, *Toxoplasma gondii*, by polymerase chain reaction. J Clin Microbiol 1989;27:1787.

Buxton D. Toxoplasmosis: the first commercial vaccine. Parasitol Today 1993;9:335-337.

Buxton D, Innes EA. A commercial vaccine for ovine toxoplasmosis. Parasitology 1995;110(suppl):S11-S16.

Conley JK, Jenkins KA, Remington JS. *Toxoplasma gondii* infection of the central nervous system: use of the peroxidase-antiperoxidase method to demonstrate *Toxoplasma* in formalin-fixed, paraffin-embedded tissue sections. Hum Pathol 1981;12:690.

Couvreur J, Desmonts G. Congenital and maternal toxoplasmosis: a review of 300 congenital cases. Dev Med Child Neurol 1962;4:519-530.

Couvreur J, Desmonts G, Aron-Rosa D. Le pronostic oculaire de la toxoplasmose congenitale: role du traitement. Ann Pediatr 1984;31:855-858.

Couvreur J, Desmonts G, Thulliez P. Prophylaxis of congenital toxoplasmosis: effect of spiramycin on placental infection. J Antimicrob Chemother 1988;22:193-200.

Daffos F, Forestier F, Capella-Pavlovsky M, et al. Prenatal management of 746 pregnancies at risk for congenital toxoplasmosis. N Engl J Med 1988;318:271.

Dannemann BR, Vaughan WC, Thulliez P, et al. The differential agglutination test for diagnosis of recently acquired infection with *Toxoplasma gondii*. J Clin Microbiol 1990; 28:1928.

Darde ML, Bouteille B, Pestre-Alexandre M. Isoenzyme analysis of 35 *Toxoplasma gondii* isolates and the biological and epidemiological implications. J Parasitol 1992;78:786-794.

Decoster A, Darcy F, Caron A, et al. IgA antibodies against P30 as markers of congenital and acute toxoplasmosis. Lancet 1988;2:1104.

Derouin F, Devergie A, Auber P. Toxoplasmosis in bonemarrow transplant recipients: report of seven cases and review. Clin Infect Dis 1992;15:267-270.

Desmonts G, Couvreur J. Congenital toxoplasmosis: a prospective study of 378 pregnancies. N Engl J Med 1974;290:1110-1116.

Desmonts G, Couvreur J. Congenital toxoplasmosis: a prospective study of the offspring of 542 women who acquired toxoplasmosis during pregnancy: pathophysiology of congenital disease. In Thalhammer O, Baumgarten K, Pollak A (eds). Perinatal Medicine: Sixth European Congress. Stuttgart, Germany: Georg Thieme, 1979.

Desmonts G, Couvreur J. Natural history of congenital toxoplasmosis. Ann Pediatr 1984;31:799.

Desmonts G, Remington JS. Direct agglutination test for diagnosis of *Toxoplasma* infection. Method for increasing sensitivity and specificity. J Clin Microbiol 1980;11:562.

Dorangeon PH, Fay R, Marx-Chemla C, et al. Passage transplacentaire de l'association pyrimethamine-sulfadoxine hors du traitement antenatal de la toxoplasmose congenital. Presse Med 1990;2036:22-29.

Dorfman RF, Remington JS. Value of lymph node biopsy in the diagnosis of acute acquired toxoplasmosis. N Engl J Med 1973;289:878.

Duquesne V, Auriault C, Darcy F, et al. Protection of nude rats against *Toxoplasma* infection by excreted-secreted antigen-specific helper T cells. Infect Immun 1990;58: 2120.

Eichenwald HF. A study of congenital toxoplasmosis, with particular emphasis on clinical manifestations, sequelae, and therapy. In Siim JC (ed). Human Toxoplasmosis. Copenhagen: Munksgaard, 1960.

Featherstone H. A Difference in the Family. New York: Penguin, 1981.

Forestier F, Daffos F, Rainant M, Cox WC. The assessment of fetal blood samples. Am J Obstet Gynecol 1988;158:1184-1188.

Foulon W, Naessens A, Ho-Yen D. Prevention of congenital toxoplasmosis. J Perinat Med 2000;28:337-345.

Frenkel JK, Pfefferkorn ER, Smith DD, Fishback JL. Prospective vaccine prepared from a new mutant of *Toxoplasma gondii* for use in cats. Am J Vet Res 1991; 52:759-763.

Glasner PD, Silveira C, Kruszon-Moran D, et al. An unusually high prevalence of ocular toxoplasmosis in Southern Brazil. Am J Ophthalmol 114;136-44, 1992.

Grigg ME, Bonnefoy S, Hehl AB, et al. Success and virulence in *Toxoplasma* as the result of sexual recombination between two distinct ancestries. Science 2001;294: 161-165.

Grover CM, Thulliez P, Remington JS, et al. Rapid prenatal diagnosis of congenital *Toxoplasma* infection by using polymerase chain reaction and amniotic fluid. J Clin Microbiol 1990;28:2297.

Guerina NG, Hsu Ho-Wen, Meissner HC, et al. Neonatal serologic screening and early treatment for congenital *Toxoplasma gondii* infection. N Engl J Med 1994;33: 1858-1863.

Hoff R, Weiblen BJ, Reardon LA, Maguire JH. Screening for congenital toxoplasma infection. In Transplacental Disorders: Perinatal Detection, Treatment, and Management (Including Pediatric AIDS). New York: Alan R Liss, 1990.

Hohlfeld P, Daffos T, Costa JM, et al. Prenatal diagnosis of congenital toxoplasmosis with a polymerase-chain reaction test on amniotic fluid. N Engl J Med 1994; 331:695-699.

Hohlfeld P, Daffos F, Thulliez P, et al. Fetal toxoplasmosis: outcome of pregnancy and infant follow-up after in utero treatment. J Pediatr 1989;115:765-769.

Holfels E, McAuley J, Mack D, et al. In vitro effects of artemisinin ether, cycloguanil hydrochloride (alone and in combination with sulfadiazine), quinine sulfate, mefloquine, primaquine phosphate, trifluoperazine hydrochloride, and verapamil on *Toxoplasma gondii*. Antimicrob Agents Chemother 1994;38:1392-1396.

Holland GN, Engstrom RE Jr, Glasgow BJ, et al. Ocular toxoplasmosis in patients with the acquired immunodeficiency syndrome. Am J Ophthalmol 1988; 106:653-667.

Huskinson-Mark J, Araujo FG, Remington JS. Evaluation of the effect of drugs on the cyst form of *Toxoplasma gondii*. J Infect Dis 1991;164:170-177.

Israelski DM, Remington JS. Toxoplasmic encephalitis in patients with AIDS. In Sande MA, Volberding PA (eds). The Medical Management of AIDS. Philadelphia: Saunders, 1988.

Israelski DM, Tom C, Remington JS. Zidovudine antagonizes the action of pyrimethamine in experimental infection with *Toxoplasma gondii*. Antimicrob Agents Chemother 1989;33:30.

Ives NJ, Gazzard BG, Easterbrook PJ. The changing pattern of AIDS-defining illnesses with the introduction of highly active antiretroviral therapy (HAART) in a London clinic. J Infect 2001;42:138-139.

Jenum PA, Stray-Pedersen B, Gundersen AG. Improved diagnosis of primary *Toxoplasma gondii* infection in early pregnancy by determination of anti-toxoplasma immunoglobulin avidity. J Clin Microbiol 1997;35:1972.

Khan A, Ely K, Kasper L. A purified parasite antigen (p30) mediates CD8 T-cell immunity against fatal *Toxoplasma gondii* infection in mice. J Immunol 1991; 147:3501-3506.

Koppe JG, Kloosterman GJ, deRoever-Bonnet H, et al. Toxoplasmosis and pregnancy, with a long-term follow-up of the children. Eur J Obstet Gynecol Reprod Biol 1974;413:101-110.

Koppe JG, Loewer-Sieger DH, deRoever-Bonnet H. Results of 20-year follow-up of congenital toxoplasmosis. Lancet 1986;1:254-256.

Labadie MD, Hazeman JJ. Apport des bilans de sante de l'efant pour le depistage et l'etude epidemiologique de la toxoplasmose congenitale. Ann Pediatr 1984; 31:823-828.

Lee YF, Chen SJ, Chung YM, et al. Diffuse toxoplasmosis retinochoroiditis as the initial manifestation of acquired immunodeficiency syndrome. J Formos Med Assoc 2000; 99:219-223.

Leport C. Toxoplasmosis in AIDS. 17th International Congress of Chemotherapy, Berlin, Germany, 1991.

Liesenfeld O, Wong SY, Remington JS. Toxoplasmosis in the setting of AIDS. In Bartlett JG, Merrigan TC, Bolognesi D (eds). Textbook of AIDS Medicine. Baltimore: Williams & Wilkins, 1999.

Luft BJ, Naot Y, Araujo FG, et al. Primary and reactivated *Toxoplasma* infection in patients with cardiac transplants: clinical spectrum and problems in diagnosis in a defined population. Ann Intern Med 1983;99:27-31.

Luft BJ, Remington JS. Acute *Toxoplasma* infection among family members of patients with acute lymphadenopathic toxoplasmosis. Arch Intern Med 1984;144:53-56.

Mack D, Johnson J, Roberts F, et al. Murine and human MHC class II genes determine susceptibility to toxoplasmosis. Int J Parasitol 1999;29:1351-1358.

McAuley JB, Boyer KM, Patel D, et al. Early and longitudinal evaluations of treated infants and children and untreated historical patients with congenital toxoplasmosis: the Chicago Collaborative Treatment Trial. Clin Infect Dis 1994b;18:38-72.

McCabe RE, Brooks RG, Dorfman RF, Remington JS. Clinical spectrum in 107 cases of toxoplasmic lymphadenopathy. Rev Infect Dis 1987;9:754.

McCabe RE, Remington JS. Toxoplasmosis: the time has come. N Engl J Med 1988;318:313-315.

McGhee T, Wolters C, Stein L, et al. Absence of sensorineural hearing loss in treated infants and children with congenital toxoplasmosis. Otolaryngol Head Neck Surg 1992;106:75-80.

McLeod R, Boyer K, Roizen N, et al. The child with congenital toxoplasmosis. In Remington JS, Schwartz MN (eds). Curr Clin Top Infect Dis 2000;20:189-208.

McLeod R, Berry PF, Marshall WH, et al. Toxoplasmosis presenting as brain abscesses: diagnosis by computerized tomography and cytology of aspirated purulent material. Am J Med 1979;67:711-714.

McLeod R, Boyer K, Roizen N, et al. Treatment of congenital toxoplasmosis. 17th International Congress of Chemotherapy, Berlin, Germany, 1991a.

McLeod R, Frenkel JK, Estes RG, et al. Subcutaneous and intestinal vaccination with tachyzoites of *Toxoplasma gondii* and acquisition of immunity to peroral and congenital *Toxoplasma* challenge. J Immunol 1988;140: 1632-1637.

McLeod R, Johnson J, Estes R, Mack D. Immunogenetics in pathogenesis of and protection against toxoplasmosis. In Gross U (ed). *Toxoplasma gondii*. Berlin: Springer-Verlag, 1996.

McLeod R, Mack DG, Boyer KM, et al. Phenotypes and functions of lymphocytes in congenital toxoplasmosis. J Lab Clin Med 1990;116:623-635.

McLeod R, Mack D, Brown C. *Toxoplasma gondii*: new advances in cellular and molecular biology. Exp Parasitol 1991b;72:109-121.

McLeod R, Mack D, Foss R, et al. Levels of pyrimethamine in sera and cerebrospinal and ventricular fluids from infants treated for congenital toxoplasmosis. Antimicrob Agents Chemother 1992;36:1040-1048.

McLeod R, Remington JS. Toxoplasmosis. In Behrman RL, Vaughan VC III, Nelson WE (eds). Nelson's Textbook of Pediatrics, ed 14. Philadelphia: Saunders, 1990.

Mets M, Boyer K, McLeod R, et al. Ophthalmic findings in congenital toxoplasmosis. Sarasota, Fla: Association for Research and Vision in Ophthalmology, 1992.

Mets MB, Holfels E, Boyer KM, et al. Eye manifestations of congenital toxoplasmosis. Am J Ophthalmol 1996; 122:309-324.

Mitchell CD, Erlich SS, Mastrucci MT, et al. Congenital toxoplasmosis occurring in infants perinatally infected with human immunodeficiency virus 1. Pediatr Infect Dis 1990;9:512.

Mitchell W. Neurological and developmental effects of IV and AIDS in children and adolescents. Ment Retard Dev Disabil Res Rev 2001;7:211-216

Montoya J, Remington J. Toxoplasmic chorioretinitis in the setting of acute acquired toxoplasmosis. Clin Infect Dis 1996;23:277.

Montoya JG. Laboratory diagnosis of *Toxoplasma gondii* infection and toxoplasmosis. J Infect Dis 2002;1855: S73-S82.

Naot Y, Remington JS. An enzyme-linked immunosorbent assay for detection of IgM antibodies to *Toxoplasma gondii*: use for diagnosis of acute acquired toxoplasmosis. J Infect Dis 1980;142:757.

O'Connor GR. Manifestations and management of ocular toxoplasmosis. Bull NY Acad Med 1974;30:192.

Patel DV, Holfels EM, Vogel NP, et al. Resolution of intracerebral calcifications in children with treated congenital toxoplasmosis. Radiology 1996;199:433-440.

Polis MA. Differential diagnosis of retinal lesions in persons with HIV infection. Opportun Infect Interact 1994;3:1-3.

Prince JB, Araujo FG, Remington JS, et al. Cloning of cDNAs encoding a 28 kilodalton antigen of *Toxoplasma gondii*. Mol Biochem Parasitol 1989;34:3-14.

Remington JS, McLeod R, Desmonts G. In Remington JS, Klein J (eds). Infectious Diseases of the Fetus and Newborn Infant, ed 5. Philadelphia: Saunders, 2001.

Roberts F, McLeod R. Pathogenesis of toxoplasmic retinochoroiditis. Parasitol Today 1999;15:51-57

Roberts F, Mets MB, Ferguson DJP, et al. Histopathological features of ocular toxoplasmosis in the fetus and infant. Arch Ophthalmol 2001;119:51-58.

Roberts T, Frenkel JK. Estimating income losses and other preventable costs caused by congenital toxoplasmosis in people in the United States. J Am Vet Med Assoc 1990; 196:249-256.

Roizen N, Swisher C, Stein M, et al. Neurologic and developmental outcome in treated congenital toxoplasmosis. Pediatrics 1995;95:11-20.

Roizen N, Boyer K, McLeod R, et al. Developmental and neurologic function in treated congenital toxoplasmosis. Baltimore: Society for Pediatric Research, 1992.

Romand S, Wallon M, Franck J, et al. Prenatal diagnosis using polymerase chain reaction on amniotic fluid for congenital toxoplasmosis. Obstet Gynecol 2001;97:296-300.

Roux C, Desmonts G, Molliez N, et al. Toxoplasmose et grossesse. Bilan deux ans de phropylaxie de la toxoplasmose congenitale à la maternité de l'hôpital Saint Antoine (1973-1974). J Gynecol Obstet Biol Reprod 1976;5:249-264.

Ruf B, Schurmann D, Pohle HD. The efficacy of Fansidar in preventing AIDS-associated neurotoxoplasmosis and *Pneumocystis carinii* pneumonia. 17th International Congress of Chemotherapy, Berlin, Germany, 1991.

Ruiz A, Frenkel JK. *Toxoplasma gondii* in Costa Rican cats. Am J Trop Med Hyg 1980;29:1150.

Stepick-Biek P, Thulliez P, Araujo FG, Remington JS. IgA antibodies for diagnosis of acute congenital and acquired toxoplasmosis. J Infect Dis 1990;162:270-273.

Suzuki Y, Wong S-Y, Grumet FC, et al. Evidence for genetic regulation of susceptibility to toxoplasmic encephalitis in AIDS patients. J Infect Dis 1996;173:265-268.

Swisher CN, Boyer K, McLeod R. Clinical toxoplasmosis. Semin Pediatr Neurol 1994;1:4-25.

Townsend JJ, Wolinsky JS, Baringer JR, et al. Acquired toxoplasmosis. Arch Neurol 1975;32:335.

Vogel NP, Patel D, Roizen N, et al. Congenital transmission of *Toxoplasma gondii* from an immunologically normal mother infected prior to pregnancy. Clin Infect Dis 1996;23:1055-1060.

Wilson CB, Remington JS. What can be done to prevent congenital toxoplasmosis? Am J Obstet Gynecol 1980;138:357-363.

Wilson CB, Remington JS, Stagno S, Reynolds DW. Development of adverse sequelae in children born with subclinical congenital *Toxoplasma* infection. Pediatrics 1980;66:767-774.

Wong S-Y, Hajdu MP, Ramirez R, et al. The role of specific immunoglobulin E in the diagnosis of acute *Toxoplasma* infection and toxoplasmosis. J Clin Microbiol 1993;31:2952-2959.

Wong S-Y, Remington JS. Toxoplasmosis in pregnancy. Clin Infect Dis 1994;18:853-861.

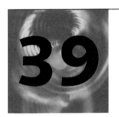

39 TUBERCULOSIS

Jeffrey R. Starke

lthough tuberculosis is an ancient disease that is known to have existed in prehistoric times, it remains one of the most important infectious diseases in the world in terms of morbidity, mortality, and economic impact. Tuberculosis was recognized as a clinical entity in the early nineteenth century but was not determined to be an infectious disease until 1882 when Koch identified *Mycobacterium tuberculosis*. The recognized spread of tuberculosis became a concern of public health authorities, and efforts to control tuberculosis became the cornerstone of modern public health.

Although the cause of tuberculosis is the bacillus *M. tuberculosis*, it has long been recognized that stresses within populations—famine, war, adverse working conditions, population displacements, and crowded living conditions—favor the spread of tuberculosis in human beings and the development of disease from asymptomatic infection. In the mid 1800s the death rate from tuberculosis in large cities in the United States was approximately 400 per 100,000 per year, making it the leading cause of death. Over the next 100 years, despite the lack of specific chemotherapy, the incidence of both disease and death from tuberculosis dropped dramatically as a result of improved health care and living and working conditions, as well as genetic selection within the population.

Tuberculosis currently is in a rapidly shifting position worldwide. After years of steady decline in its incidence in the United States, the Centers for Disease Control and Prevention (CDC) in 1989 developed a plan to eliminate tuberculosis by the year 2010. Unfortunately, the onset of the epidemic as a result of the human immunodeficiency virus (HIV), changes in immigration patterns, and increased transmission of *M. tuberculosis* in congregate settings in urban areas provoked the resurgence of tuberculosis in the United States from the mid-1980s to the mid-1990s. Worldwide, 10 million people develop tuberculosis annually, and one third of the world's population is infected with *M. tuberculosis*. The World Health Organization (WHO) has declared tuberculosis to be a "global health emergency," the first infectious disease to receive this designation (Kochi, 1991). To put it simply, in the early twenty-first century there is more tuberculosis in the world than at any time in the history of mankind.

TERMINOLOGY

The pathophysiology of tuberculosis is complicated, and the time delay between infection and disease makes certain events less distinct. Many experts now divide tuberculosis into three major stages: exposure, infection, and disease (Table 39-1).

Exposure means that the child has had significant contact with an adult or adolescent with suspected or proved infectious pulmonary tuberculosis. The contact investigation—examining those individuals close to a suspected case of tuberculosis with a tuberculin skin test, chest radiograph, and physical examination—is the most important activity to prevent cases of tuberculosis in children (Hsu, 1963). The most frequent setting for exposure of a child is the household, but it can occur in a school, daycare center, or other closed settings (Hoge et al., 1994; Lincoln, 1965). In the exposure stage the tuberculin skin test is negative, the chest radiograph is normal, and the child lacks signs or symptoms of disease. Because development of a reactive tuberculin skin test may take up to 3 months after the child has inhaled droplet nuclei infected with *M. tuberculosis*, some exposed children may be infected but no test can confirm it. Young children in the exposure

731

TABLE 39-1	The Stages of Tuberculosis in Children		
	STAGE		
	Exposure	*Infection*	*Disease*
Skin test	Negative	Positive	Positive (90%)
Physical examination	Normal	Normal	Usually abnormal*
Chest radiograph	Normal	Usually normal†	Usually abnormal‡
Treatment	If <5 years old	Always	Always
Number of drugs	One	One	Three or four

*Up to 50% of older children with pulmonary tuberculosis have a normal physical examination.
†Calcification or a small granuloma are considered infection, not disease.
‡Some children with extrapulmonary tuberculosis have a normal chest radiograph.

stage usually are treated to prevent the rapid development of disseminated or meningeal tuberculosis, which can occur even before the skin test becomes reactive.

Infection occurs when the individual inhales droplet nuclei containing *M. tuberculosis*, which become established intracellularly within the lung and associated lymphoid tissue. The hallmark of tuberculosis infection is a reactive skin test. The child has no signs or symptoms of disease, and the chest radiograph is either normal or reveals only calcifications or granuloma in the lung parenchyma and/or regional lymph nodes. In industrial countries all children with tuberculosis infection should receive treatment, usually with isoniazid, to prevent the development of tuberculosis disease in the near or distant future.

Disease occurs when signs or symptoms or radiographic manifestations caused by *M. tuberculosis* become apparent. Not all infected individuals have the same risk of developing disease. An immunocompetent adult with untreated tuberculosis infection has a 5% to 10% lifetime risk of developing disease. One half of the risk occurs in the first 2 to 3 years after infection. Adults with tuberculosis infection who also have untreated HIV infection have a 5% to 10% annual risk of developing tuberculosis disease. Historic studies show that up to 40% of immunocompetent infants with untreated tuberculosis infection develop disease—often serious, life-threatening forms—within 1 to 2 years.

ETIOLOGY

M. tuberculosis, commonly referred to as the *tubercle bacillus*, is a member of the genus *Mycobacterium*. Mycobacteria are nonmotile,

non–spore forming, pleomorphic, weakly gram-positive rods, 1 to 5 μm long, typically slender, and slightly bent. Some appear beaded and some are clumped under the microscope. The cell wall constituents of mycobacteria determine their most striking biologic properties. The cell walls contain 20% to 60% lipids, largely bound to proteins and carbohydrates. Their growth is slow, with a generation time of 14 to 24 hours on solid media, perhaps because of the slow metabolic exchange through the waxy capsule. Their hydrophobic properties make them difficult to study.

Acid-fastness is the capacity to perform stable mycolate complexes with certain aryl methane dyes—specifically carbolfuchsin, crystal violet, auramine, and rhodamine—which are not removed readily, even by rinsing with 90% ethanol plus hydrochloric acid. The cells appear red when stained with fuchsin (as with the Ziehl-Neelsen or Kinyoun stains), appear purple with crystal violet, or exhibit yellow-green fluorescence under ultraviolet light when stained with auramine and rhodamine, as in Truant stain. Truant stain is considered the best for specimens expected to contain small numbers of organisms.

Identification of various mycobacteria depends on their staining properties and their biochemical and metabolic characteristics. All mycobacteria are obligate aerobes. Their growth requirements are simple. Isolation of *M. tuberculosis* on solid media often takes 3 to 6 weeks, followed by another 2 to 4 weeks for drug susceptibility testing. Identification of specific mycobacterial species often requires a complex set of biochemical tests. Improvements in laboratory methods now permit more rapid culture, identification, and drug susceptibility testing of mycobacteria by automatic radiometric methods, such as BACTEC, in which a decontaminated, concentrated specimen is inoculated into a bottle of medium containing carbon 14–labeled palmitic acid as the substrate. As mycobacteria metabolize the labeled acid, carbon dioxide–14 accumulates in the bottle, where radioactivity can be measured. The addition of appropriate dilutions of antituberculosis drugs permits the evaluation of drug susceptibility. The time for isolation and drug susceptibility testing of mycobacteria can be reduced to 1 to 3 weeks if the radiometric system is used. The use of high-pressure liquid chromatography allows for rapid identification of isolated organisms, usually within 24 hours.

EPIDEMIOLOGY
Incidence and Prevalence

The WHO estimates that during the 1990s there were 90 million new cases of tuberculosis worldwide, with 30 million deaths caused by the disease (Raviglione et al., 1995). About 13 million new cases and 5 million deaths occurred among children younger than 15 years of age. More than 35% of the world's population is infected with *M. tuberculosis*. Without the development of a truly effective vaccine against tuberculosis, it is unlikely that the world's tuberculosis situation will improve in the near future.

The incidence and mortality attributable to tuberculosis in the United States declined steadily during the twentieth century until the year 1985, when the overall case rate was approximately 10 per 100,000, for a total of 22,201 new active cases. Unfortunately, a resurgence of the disease led to the recognition of 26,673 cases in 1992. Although total tuberculosis case numbers rose 20% in the United States from 1985 to 1992, the number of pediatric tuberculosis cases rose 40% (Cantwell et al., 1994b; Starke et al., 1992). Most experts site four causes for these increases: (1) the coepidemic of HIV infection, because immunosuppression from HIV is the most potent risk factor for development of tuberculosis disease in a previously infected adult (Barnes et al., 1991; Selwyn et al., 1989; Whalen et al., 1995); (2) increasing rates of tuberculosis in foreign-born individuals in the United States, caused by an increased number of infected individuals entering the country and more persons developing tuberculosis after arrival; (3) increased

transmission of *M. tuberculosis* in congregate settings, especially jails and prisons, nursing homes, homeless shelters, HIV treatment facilities, certain hospitals, and, rarely, schools (Alland et al., 1994; Bellin et al., 1993; Leggiadro et al., 1989; Small et al., 1994); and (4) a decline in the tuberculosis public health infrastructure in many regions and cities (Brudney and Dobkin, 1991). Fortunately, after much attention and increase in tuberculosis-related budgets, the number of tuberculosis cases in the United States declined again to about 16,000 in 2002.

Decades ago, when tuberculosis was more prevalent in the United States, the risk of exposure to an adult with infectious tuberculosis was high and fairly uniform across the entire population. In most industrialized countries, tuberculosis rates are now highest in some fairly well-defined groups of high-risk persons (Box 39-1). Risk factors can be divided into those that increase the risk of initial infection with *M. tuberculosis* and those that increase the risk of progression from asymptomatic infection to disease. Several recent studies have demonstrated that, in the United States, a questionnaire can be used to identify specific risk factors for a child having a positive tuberculin

---

BOX 39-1

HIGH RISK GROUPS FOR TUBERCULOSIS IN NORTH AMERICA

Increased Risk of Infection

- Foreign-born (or traveled) persons from high-prevalence countries
- Users of illicit drugs
- Residents of jails, prisons, long-term care facilities
- Homeless persons
- Health-care workers who care for high-risk patients
- Children exposed to adults in high-risk groups (except health-care workers)

Increased Rate of Progression of Infection to Disease

- Coinfection with HIV
- Other immunocompromising diseases
- Immunosuppressive therapies
- Malnutrition
- Age less than 4 years

skin test: family history of tuberculosis infection or disease, foreign birth or travel to foreign country with a high incidence of tuberculosis, or contact with adults at increased risk for tuberculosis (Froehlich et al., 2001; Lobato et al., 1998; Ozuah et al., 2001).

Among young adults in the United States, tuberculosis is predominantly a disease of racial and ethnic minorities. Although some studies have indicated that genetic factors may partly control an individual's susceptibility to tuberculosis infection and disease, extrinsic differences in socioeconomic status, nutrition, access to health care, and crowded living conditions undoubtedly contribute heavily to the increased tuberculosis case rates among minority groups. Approximately 85% of childhood tuberculosis cases in the United States occur among African-American, Hispanic, Asian, and Native American children (Ussery et al., 1996).

In 2002 almost 50% of persons with tuberculosis in the United States were foreign born (Talbot et al., 2000). About 20% of tuberculosis cases in children less than 5 years of age and almost 50% of cases among adolescents occur among the foreign born. Children immigrating through established channels to the United States receive neither a chest radiograph nor a tuberculin skin test per normal immigration procedures (Lange et al., 1989; Saiman et al., 2001). In several skin-testing programs in urban areas, between 60% and 90% of the positive tuberculin skin tests occur among foreign-born children (Barry et al., 1990). It is from this pool of infected children that many cases of tuberculosis among adults will arise in the future.

The recent epidemic of HIV infection has had a profound effect on the epidemiology of tuberculosis among children by two major mechanisms (Gutman et al., 1994): (1) HIV-infected adults with tuberculosis may transmit *M. tuberculosis* to children, some of whom will develop tuberculosis disease; and (2) children with HIV infection may be at increased risk of progressing from tuberculosis infection to disease (Hoffman et al., 1996). Several studies of childhood tuberculosis have demonstrated that increased case rates have been associated with a simultaneous increase among HIV-infected adults in the community (Jones et al., 1992). In general, HIV-infected children may be more likely to have contact with HIV-infected adults who are at high risk for tuberculosis.

Tuberculosis may be underdiagnosed among HIV-infected children because of the similarity of its clinical presentation to other opportunistic infections and to conditions related to acquired immunodeficiency syndrome (AIDS), and because of the difficulty in confirming the diagnosis with positive cultures. All children with tuberculosis disease should have HIV serotesting, because the two infections are linked epidemiologically and the recommended treatment for tuberculosis is prolonged for HIV-infected patients.

One of the most important factors determining whether tuberculosis infection will progress to disease is the age of the child. In the United States about 60% to 70% of pediatric cases occur in infants and children less than 5 years of age. The period between 5 and 14 years has often been called the "favored age," because children in this age range may develop infection, but it is much less likely to progress immediately to disease. The gender ratio for tuberculosis disease in children is usually about 1:1, but during adolescence there may be a female predominance (Brailey, 1958). In contrast, in tuberculosis in adults there is a 3:1 male predominance.

Although data on tuberculosis disease in children are readily available, information concerning the incidence and prevalence of tuberculosis infection without disease is lacking. Tuberculosis infection is a reportable condition in only four states, and national surveys were discontinued in 1971. Few other countries have any tuberculin skin test surveillance at all. However, the increased incidence of tuberculosis disease among children in the United States, the results of some skin tests surveys, and the influx of foreign-born children into the United States over the past decade indicate that the pool of infected children and young adults in the United States is probably growing.

Transmission

Transmission of *M. tuberculosis* is from person to person, usually by droplet nuclei that become airborne when the ill individual coughs, sneezes, laughs, sings, or even breathes heavily. These droplet nuclei may remain suspended in the air for hours; long after the infectious person has left the environment. Certain environmental factors such as poor air circulation can enhance transmission. Only particles less than 10 μm in diameter can reach alveoli and establish infection. Rarely, transmission can occur by direct contact with infected body fluids such as urine or purulent sinus tract drainage. Cases of tuberculosis transmitted via lung and liver transplant have been reported. Several patient-related factors are associated with an increased chance of transmission (Blumberg et al., 1995). The most important is a positive acid-fast smear of the sputum, which most closely correlates with the infectivity of the patient. Extensive epidemiologic studies have shown that children with primary tuberculosis rarely infect other children or adults (Starke, 2001; Wallgren, 1937). Tubercle bacilli are relatively sparse in the endobronchial secretions of children with pulmonary tuberculosis, and significant cough is usually lacking. When young children with tuberculosis do cough, they rarely produce sputum, and they lack the tussive force necessary to suspend infectious particles of the correct size. Children with tuberculosis often have been cared for by their families or in hospitals and other institutions without infecting their contacts. When transmission of *M. tuberculosis* has been documented in children's hospitals, it almost invariably has come from an adult with undiagnosed pulmonary tuberculosis (Aznar et al., 1995; George et al., 1986; Weinstein et al., 1995).

Infectivity must be considered in several clinical situations in pediatrics. Children or adolescents with the reactivation form of pulmonary tuberculosis, having cavities or extensive infiltrates in the lungs, should be considered potentially infectious to others (Cardona et al., 1999; Curtis et al., 1999). The CDC has issued guidelines for when children and adolescents with tuberculosis should be considered potentially infectious (Centers for Disease Control and Prevention, 1994). Within a hospital, a child or adolescent with suspected tuberculosis should be isolated if the chest radiograph shows a cavity or extensive infiltrate, if the child has a productive cough, or if a high-risk procedure such as bronchoscopy is being performed. Most experts feel that other children with tuberculosis do not need to be isolated, especially if the adults accompanying the child have received proper evaluation for infectious tuberculosis (Starke, 2001).

It is difficult to determine when a potentially infectious patient with pulmonary tuberculosis is no longer infectious after therapy has begun. The decision must be based on improvement in symptoms, decreased number of acid-fast bacilli in the sputum smear, initial chest radiograph findings, and adherence to treatment. Studies of transmission to animals and retrospective human epidemiology have indicated that most initially infectious patients become noninfectious within 2 weeks or less of starting treatment. However, occasional patients remain infectious for weeks to months after beginning ultimately effective treatment. Many investigations have shown that the vast majority of close contacts of infectious patients are infected before diagnosis and treatment, and that continued exposure to the patient after diagnosis leads to little or no incremental risk of infection.

PATHOGENESIS
Initial Infection

The lung is the most common portal of entry for tubercle bacilli. If the bacilli are ingested, infection in the upper respiratory or intestinal tract may result. This was more common in previous decades when bovine tuberculosis, transmitted in unpasteurized milk, occurred more frequently. Contamination of superficial skin or mucous membrane lesions—such as an abrasion of the sole of the foot or the elbow, an insect bite, or a ritual circumcision—may lead to infection. Infection by inoculation with a sputum-contaminated syringe has been reported. True congenital infection, although rare, occurs either when the mother suffers from lymphohematogenous spread during pregnancy or has smoldering endometritis.

At the site of entry the bacilli multiply and create an area of inflammatory exudate. The bacteria multiply most readily within nonsensitized alveolar macrophages. Almost as soon as the infection occurs, bacilli are carried through the local lymphatic system to the nearest group of lymph nodes that drain the area in which the focus is situated. When the portal of entry is the lung, the bronchopulmonary nodes—either hilar or mediastinal nodes—usually form the complex. Until delayed hypersensitivity develops, the area of infection may expand and remains unencapsulated. These events usually occur at the microscopic level; the patient has no signs or symptoms, and the chest radiograph reveals no lesions. However, occasionally children experience low-grade fever and cough early in the infection, and the chest radiograph may show a localized, nonspecific infiltrate that resolves spontaneously. With the onset of delayed hypersensitivity, the microscopic infiltrate generally increases in size, the regional lymph nodes may enlarge, and the initial lesion becomes caseous and walled-off. Many caseous lesions eventually calcify; most experts estimate at least 6 months are required for calcification to occur. Living tubercle bacilli persist within these walled-off foci for years, perhaps for the life of the individual.

The most common location for the initial infection is subpleural. It appears that virtually any part of the lung has an equal chance of receiving the initial infection. About 70% to 85% of initial infections are initiated by one focus. However, multiple foci are common in children.

Intrathoracic Tuberculosis

In most children the initial infection is walled off, clinical signs and symptoms and radiographic manifestations are absent, and the only manifestation of the initial infection is a reactive tuberculin skin test that develops after the onset of delayed hypersensitivity. The initial lymphadenitis cannot be detected clinically and rarely can be detected on the chest radiograph. However, in some children, particularly infants, the regional lymph nodes increase in size to the point where they cause partial or complete obstruction of the associated bronchus. Acid-fast studies of smears and sections of these enlarged lymph nodes have confirmed that the caseum has few tubercle bacilli; propensity for enlargement of lymph nodes is probably as much a result of the host's immune response as it is of the burden of organisms. At first, the lymph nodes may impinge on the bronchus, compressing it from outside and causing diffuse inflammation of its wall. Eventually, complete obstruction may occur, rarely as a result of external compression, but more often as a result of invasion of the bronchial wall by the caseous lesion, resulting in endobronchial tuberculosis. Other causes of obstruction include (1) damage to the bronchial cartilage that leads to gradual perforation of the bronchus, and (2) formation of plugs of toothpaste-like caseum that partially or completely occlude the bronchus.

There are three possible outcomes of bronchial obstruction. The first is sudden death by asphyxia, which, fortunately, is an extremely rare event. The second is obstructive hyperaer-ation of a lobar segment, an entire lobe, or even an entire lung. This reaction is most common in children younger than 2 years of age. In most cases the obstruction ultimately resolves by itself; however, treatment with corticosteroids and antituberculosis medications may hasten radiographic and clinical recovery. The third possible result is the appearance of a segmental lesion, often appearing fan shaped on the radiograph and almost always involving the segment occupied by the primary pulmonary focus. The radiographic opacity results from a combination of the primary pulmonary focus, the caseous material from an eroded bronchus, the inflammatory response elicited by the caseum, and atelectasis. In some cases, acute secondary bacterial infection plays a part. The younger the child, the more common is the segmental lesion (also known as a *collapse-consolidation lesion*). This lesion is likely to form during the first 3 to 6 months after infection. Multiple segmental lesions can occur simultaneously; up to 25% of children with pulmonary tuberculosis have involvement of more than one lobe.

Other complications may be caused by enlarging thoracic lymph nodes, including stridor and respiratory distress (peritracheal nodes); difficulty swallowing (subcarinal nodes); and bronchoesophageal fistula (subcarinal nodes). Rarely, enlarging nodes may compress the subclavian vein, producing edema of hand and arm, or may erode into major blood vessels including the aorta. Finally, lymph nodes may rupture into the pericardial sac, resulting in pericardial tuberculosis.

Late results of bronchial obstruction include (1) complete reexpansion of the lung and resolution of the radiographic findings; (2) disappearance of the segmental lesion with residual calcification of the primary focus or regional lymph nodes; or (3) scarring and progressive contraction of the lobe or segment, often associated with bronchiectasis (Morrison, 1973). Permanent anatomic sequelae result from untreated segmental lesions in about 60% of cases, even though the abnormality may not be apparent on radiographs. Stenosis of the bronchus and cylindrical bronchiectasis are most common. Fortunately, most of these abnormalities are asymptomatic in the upper lobes. However, secondary infection may occur in the middle and lower lobes, leading to progressive lung damage. Occasionally the chronic vascularity that accompanies bronchiectasis leads to poor oxygen saturation during exercise and to restricted body growth.

Calcification of the primary complex is common, particularly in untreated infection. Calcium usually is deposited as fine particles. creating a stippled effect. However, it may be deposited in large, even enormous masses. Calcification may persist without change or may be reabsorbed within 5 years and eventually disappear completely.

Reactivation pulmonary tuberculosis is the type of disease seen in pulmonary tissue sensitized and immunized by an earlier tuberculosis infection. This type of disease is caused by organisms that were inhaled years or even decades earlier, and which remained dormant within the lung tissue and then became reactivated. Often the stimulus for reactivation (usually involving an insult to the immune system) can be identified, but sometimes there is no obvious predisposing cause. This type of tuberculosis occurs most commonly in the superior segments of the upper lobes. The disease often arises from Assmann and Simon foci, which result from organisms that seeded the upper lobes during the lymphohematogenous spread at the time of initial infection.

Lymphohematogenous Spread

Tubercle bacilli from the lymphadenitis of the primary complex probably are disseminated during the incubation period in all cases of tuberculosis infection. The organisms reach the blood stream either directly from the initial focus or by way of the regional nodes and the thoracic duct. The sporadic dissemination ceases after delayed hypersensitivity develops. Many extrapulmonary lesions regress and heal completely, but some may progress immediately or remain quiescent but contain viable tubercle bacilli. There are three potential clinical outcomes from this dissemination:

1. The lymphohematogenous dissemination may be occult, in which case it produces no signs or symptoms. Again, this is the inciting event for future cases of extrapulmonary tuberculosis and reactivation pulmonary tuberculosis in adolescents and adults.
2. Protracted hematogenous tuberculosis, rarely seen today, is characterized by high spiking fever; hepatomegaly and splenomegaly; and general glandular enlargement, sometimes with repeated evidence of metastatic seeding of the eyes, kidney, and skin. Although this type of tuberculosis in past years often ended tragically in tuberculous meningitis, today it is completely treatable if diagnosed in time.
3. The third form of lymphohematogenous spread is miliary tuberculosis. This arises from a discharge of a caseous focus, often a lymph node, into a blood vessel such as a pulmonary vein. It may be self-propagating, with repeated discharge arising at various sites. It occurs most commonly during the first 2 to 6 months after infection in infancy but can also arise in older children or adults months to years after the initial infection.

RESISTANCE AND IMMUNITY

Natural resistance to tuberculosis infection varies greatly among animal species. The differences between resistant and susceptible animals appears to lie in the ability of the former to produce an effective immune response; this ability may be controlled genetically. Identical twins have shown some concordance in the propensity to develop tuberculosis disease after infection.

Young age appears to predispose to development of tuberculosis disease. However, it is possible that the apparent increased susceptibility is due to genetic factors or to a larger infecting dose of bacteria caused by the more intimate contact between the very young child and the adult source case. Many viral infections depress tuberculin reactivity, but only measles and perhaps influenza have been incriminated in lowering resistance to tuberculosis.

The exact mechanisms by which M. tuberculosis evades host defenses and persists are poorly understood. It appears that a state of intracellular parasitism is established by which the bacilli survive and grow within human cells. The means by which M. tuberculosis resists killing by macrophages has been studied extensively. Viable mycobacteria appear to prevent fusion of phagosomes with lysosomes that contain the toxic substances for killing ingested microbes.

Cell-mediated immunity is regarded as most important in host defense against M. tuberculosis (Dannenberg, 1991). The T cell–mediated immune response involves a variety of cell subsets that are involved in numerous functions, including protection, delayed hypersensitivity, cytolysis, and establishing memory immunity. The functions also involve an array of cytokines, several of which direct cells of the monocyte-macrophage axis to contain and destroy the invading bacilli. The exact role of the individual cytokines is not clear, but an emerging concept is that much of the clinical response to the presence of *M. tuberculosis* is determined by the balance of the cellular-cytokine response, which, to some degree, is under genetic influence (Dannenberg, 1991; Orme et al., 1993). Factors that compromise cell-mediated immunity—such as HIV infection or therapy with corticosteroids or other immunosuppressing agents—often permit the spread or reactivation of infection, leading to tuberculosis disease.

CLINICAL FORMS OF TUBERCULOSIS
Pulmonary Disease

Primary pulmonary tuberculosis. The primary complex includes three elements: the primary pulmonary focus, lymphangitis, and regional lymphadenitis. The hallmark of the initial disease is the relatively large size and importance of the adenitis compared with the relatively insignificant size of the initial focus in the lung. Because lymphatic drainage within the chest occurs predominately from left to right, the nodes in the right upper paratracheal area appear to be the ones most often affected.

Although interpretation of the size of intrathoracic lymph nodes in radiographs can be difficult, they are usually readily apparent when there is adenopathy resulting from tuberculosis (Figure 39-1) (Delacourt et al., 1993b). As the lymph nodes continue to enlarge, partial obstruction of the regional bronchus may lead to hyperinflation and, eventually, to atelectasis (Daly et al., 1952). Figure 39-2 shows an early segmental lesion with hilar adenopathy and atelectasis and, possibly, some infiltrate. The radiographic findings in this type of disease are similar to those caused by aspiration of a foreign body; in essence, the lymph node is acting as the foreign body. Segmental atelectasis and hyperinflation lesions may occur together.

Other radiographic findings occur in some patients (Pineda et al., 1993; Schaaf et al., 1995; Stransberry, 1990). Occasionally children have a picture of lobar pneumonia without adenopathy being readily apparent. In smaller children the radiographic appearance can be that of exudative pneumonia with bowing of the fissure (Figure 39-3). The radiographic picture is similar to that seen with pyogenic pneumonia, particularly when caused by *Klebsiella pneumoniae*. Indeed, secondary

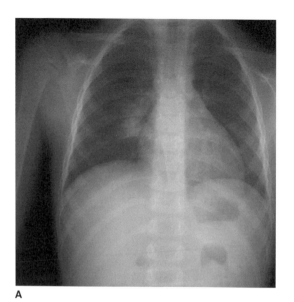

A

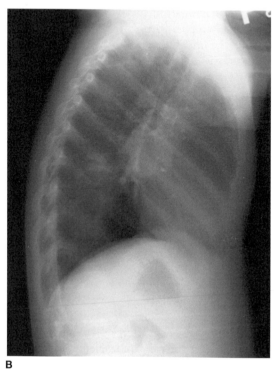

B

Fig. 39-1 A posteroanterior (**A**) and lateral (**B**) chest radiograph of a child with hilar adenopathy caused by *Mycobacterium tuberculosis*.

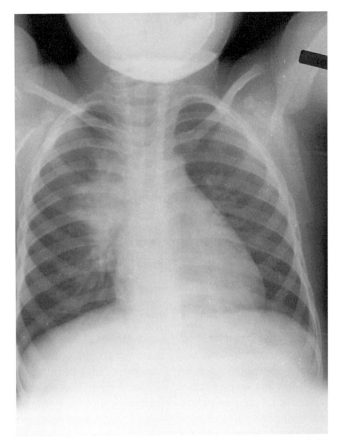

Fig. 39-2 Hilar and mediastinal adenopathy and a partial segmental lesion in a child with tuberculosis.

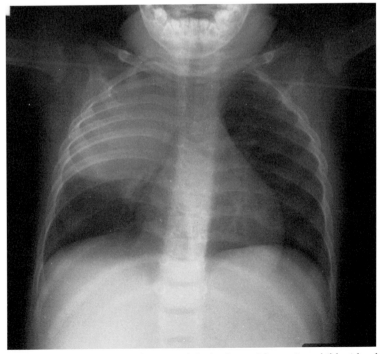

Fig. 39-3 Lobar pneumonia with bowing of the horizontal fissure in a child with tuberculosis. Many of this child's initial symptoms improved after several days of cefuroxime therapy, implying that a secondary bacterial pneumonia may have been present.

bacterial infection of tuberculosis may contribute to this appearance.

The symptoms and physical signs of pulmonary tuberculosis in children are surprisingly meager considering the degree of radiographic changes often seen; the roentgenogram is sicker than the patient (Albisua et al., 2002; Lincoln et al., 1958). The physical manifestations of disease tend to differ by the age of onset. Young infants and adolescents are more likely to have significant signs or symptoms, whereas school-age children usually have clinically silent disease (Schaaf et al., 1993; Vallejo et al., 1994).

In the United States, about one half of infants and children with radiographically moderate to severe pulmonary tuberculosis have no physical findings and are discovered only via contact tracing of an adult with suspected tuberculosis. In developing countries, case finding is passive, and most children diagnosed with pulmonary tuberculosis have more advanced symptomatic disease (Solazar et al., 2001). Infants are more likely to experience signs and symptoms because of their small airway diameters relative to the parenchymal lymph node changes. Nonproductive cough and mild dyspnea are the most common symptoms. Systemic complaints such as fever, night sweats, anorexia, and decreased activity occur less often. Some infants have difficulty gaining weight or develop a true failure-to-thrive presentation. Pulmonary signs are even less common. Some infants and young children with bronchial obstruction show signs of air trapping, such as localized wheezing or decreased breath sounds that may be accompanied by tachypnea or frank respiratory distress. Occasionally these nonspecific symptoms and signs are alleviated by antibiotics, suggesting that bacterial superinfection distal to the focus of tuberculous bronchial obstruction has contributed to the clinical presentation of disease.

Progressive pulmonary tuberculosis. Progressive pulmonary tuberculosis is a serious complication of the primary complex in which the original pulmonary focus, instead of resolving or calcifying, enlarges steadily and develops a large caseous center. The center then liquefies and empties into an adjacent bronchus, creating a primary cavity (Harris et al., 1977; Teeratkulpisarn et al., 1994). This liquefaction is associated with particularly large numbers of tubercle bacilli, resulting in a young child who may be capable of transmitting *M. tuberculosis*

to other individuals. Further dissemination of tubercle bacilli to other parts of the lobe and to the entire lung may occur. On rare occasions, an enlarging primary focus ruptures into the pleural cavity, creating a pneumothorax, bronchopleural fistula, or caseous pyopneumothorax, or into the pericardial sac or mediastinum.

The radiographic and clinical picture of progressive primary tuberculosis is that of bronchial pneumonia with high fever, moderate to severe cough, night sweats, dullness to percussion, rales, and decreased breath sounds. Before chemotherapy the inability to contain the primary focus was associated with a grave outlook; up to 65% of patients died. With appropriate treatment the prognosis is excellent. It may be difficult to distinguish between progressive pulmonary tuberculosis and a simple tuberculous focus with a superimposed acute bacterial pneumonia. Antimicrobial agents effective against common pathogens such as *Staphylococcus* species, *Klebsiella* species, and anaerobes may be indicated in addition to appropriate antituberculosis drugs. During a patient's convalescence from pulmonary tuberculosis, bullous lesions may develop and persist for several months (Matsaniotis et al., 1967). These lesions may be due to bacterial superinfection or to the tuberculosis itself.

Chronic (reactivation) pulmonary tuberculosis. Even before the discovery of antituberculosis drugs, chronic pulmonary tuberculosis was rare in children. It appears more frequently among children in the lower socioeconomic strata of society, among girls, and among patients in whom there has been significant delay in diagnosis. It has been noted that children who survive with a healed, untreated tuberculosis infection acquired before 2 years of age rarely develop chronic pulmonary tuberculosis, but it is a much more frequent complication among children who acquire their initial infection near puberty. In some children, progressive pulmonary tuberculosis cannot be differentiated from chronic tuberculosis unless the approximate date of acquiring the infection is known.

Chronic pulmonary tuberculosis is more common in adolescents than younger children (Lincoln et al., 1960). The radiographic features are typical of those seen in adults—mostly upper lobe infiltrates and, eventually, cavitation (Figure 39-4). Children and adolescents with this type of disease are more likely to experience fever, anorexia, malaise, weight loss, night

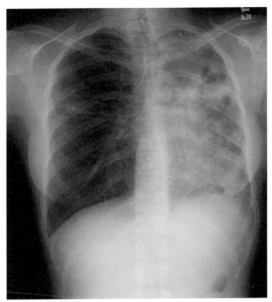

Fig. 39-4 Severe tuberculosis caused by a multidrug resistant strain of *Mycobacterium tuberculosis* in a 15-year-old from Nigeria. There is evidence of early bronchogenic spread from the left to right side.

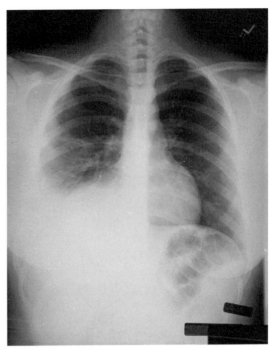

Fig. 39-5 Tuberculous pleural effusion in a teenage girl. The pleural biopsy had caseating granulomas.

sweats, productive cough, chest pain, and hemoptysis than children with primary pulmonary tuberculosis (Burroughs et al., 1999). However, findings on physical examination are usually minor or absent even when cavities or large infiltrates are present. Most signs and symptoms improve within several weeks of starting effective treatment, although cough may last for several months. This form of disease usually remains localized in the lungs because the presensitization of tissue to tuberculin evokes an immune response that prevents further hematogenous spread.

Pleural Effusion

Pleural effusion caused by tuberculosis can be localized or generalized, unilateral or bilateral. Localized pleural effusion so frequently accompanies the primary pulmonary focus that it is practically a component of the primary complex. All tuberculous effusions probably originate as a discharge of bacilli into the pleural space from an adjacent lesion, often a subpleural pulmonary focus. The breakthrough may be small and the pleuritis localized and asymptomatic, or it may occur in the form of a generalized effusion, usually 3 to 6 months after infection (Figure 39-5). Effusions are bilateral in only 5% of cases and probably arise from

bilateral primary infections. Tuberculous pleural effusion is rare in children younger than 2 years of age and uncommon in children younger than 5 years of age. It is more common in boys than in girls but is almost never associated with a segmental lesion.

The onset of pleurisy usually is abrupt, resembling bacterial pneumonia with fever; chest pain; shortness of breath; and, on physical examination, dullness to percussion and diminished breath sounds (Lincoln et al., 1958). Fever may be high and, in untreated cases, last for several weeks.

Thoracentesis is the essential diagnostic procedure. The puncture should be made in the area shown on the radiograph to have the greatest fluid accumulation. The fluid is often a greenish-yellow color, occasionally blood-tinged, with a high protein count and often a low glucose level. There are usually several hundred white cells per mm^3, with a predominance of leukocytes or lymphocytes, depending on the age of the effusion. Tubercle bacilli usually are present in such small numbers that results from direct smears and cultures are disappointing; smears are almost always negative, and pleural fluid cultures are positive in less than 30% of cases. Pleural punch biopsy is a useful diagnostic procedure because the finding of either the typical tubercles on histologic study or culture of the tiny plug from the trocar is more likely to establish the diagnosis. The prognosis for children with tuberculous effusion is generally excellent. Rarely, permanent impairment of pulmonary function occurs secondary to the development of scoliosis.

Pericardial Disease

Tuberculous pericarditis complicates only 0.4% of untreated tuberculosis infections in children. It usually arises by direct invasion or lymphatic drainage from caseous subcarinal nodes, with resulting exudation of hemorrhagic fluids and development of granulation tissue on the visceral and parietal surfaces of the pericardium. The pericardial fluid may be serofibrinous (forming strands upon standing, which may be seen by echocardiography) or hemorrhagic. However, direct acid-fast smear is usually negative. Extensive fibrosis leads to obliteration of the pericardial space, with resulting constrictive pericarditis.

The presenting symptoms usually are nonspecific: low-grade fever; malaise; anorexia; and, more rarely, chest pain (Hugo-Hamman et al., 1994). A pericardial friction rub may be heard, or—if a large effusion is present—tachycardia, distant heart sounds, and a narrow pulse pressure may suggest the diagnosis. The diagnosis is confirmed by radiography; echocardiography; the tuberculin skin test; aspiration of fluid for culture; and, when necessary, biopsy of the pericardium. With appropriate chemotherapy and possibly use of corticosteroids to acutely reduce the size of the effusion, as well as occasional pericardectomy, the prognosis is very good.

Lymphohematogenous Disease

The initial lymphohematogenous spread of tubercle bacilli during the primary infection is usually asymptomatic. Rarely patients experience protracted hematogenous tuberculosis caused by intermittent release of tubercle bacilli as a caseous focus erodes through the wall of a blood vessel. Although the clinical picture may be acute, it is usually indolent and prolonged, with spiking fever accompanying the release of organisms. Multiple organ involvement is common, often leading to hepatosplenomegaly, lymphadenitis in superficial or deep nodes, or

papulonecrotic tuberculids, which appear in crops on the skin. Other organs are involved less commonly. Meningitis, which occurs only late in the course of the disease, may be the cause of death when the disease goes untreated. Early pulmonary involvement is surprisingly mild, but diffuse lung involvement becomes apparent if treatment is not provided promptly.

The most common clinically significant form of disseminated tuberculosis is miliary disease, which occurs when massive numbers of tubercle bacilli are released into the bloodstream, causing disease in two or more organs. This type of disease usually occurs within 2 to 6 months of the primary infection. Although this form of disease is most common in infants and young children, it is also found in older adults as a result of the breakdown of a previously healed or calcified pulmonary lesion that formed years earlier.

The clinical manifestations of miliary tuberculosis are protean and depend on the load of organisms that disseminate and where they lodge (Schuit, 1979). Tissues have different susceptibility to infection; lesions are usually larger and more numerous in the lungs, spleen, liver, and bone marrow than other organs.

The onset of clinical miliary disease is sometimes explosive, with the patient becoming gravely ill in several days. More often the onset is insidious (Hussey et al., 1991). The patient may not be able to pinpoint the exact time of initial symptoms accurately. Early systemic signs include malaise, anorexia, weight loss, and low-grade fever. At this time, abnormal physical signs are usually absent. Within several weeks, hepatosplenomegaly and generalized lymphadenopathy develop in about one half of cases. About this time the fever may become higher and more sustained, although the chest radiograph usually is normal and respiratory symptoms are rare (Optican et al., 1992). Within several more weeks, the lungs become filled with tubercles, and dyspnea, cough, rales, or wheezing occur. As the pulmonary disease progresses, alveolar air block syndrome may result in frank respiratory distress, hypoxia, pneumothorax, or pneumomediastinum. Signs and symptoms of meningitis are found in only 20% to 40% of patients with advanced disease. Chronic or recurrent headache in a patient with miliary tuberculosis usually indicates the presence of meningitis, whereas the onset of abdominal pain or tenderness is usually a sign of tuberculous peritonitis. Cutaneous lesions such as tuberculids, nodules, or purpura may appear in crops. Up to 75% of patients develop choroid tubercles, which are highly specific for miliary tuberculosis.

The diagnosis of miliary tuberculosis is usually established by finding a consistent clinical picture and the typical chest radiograph findings of millet seed–like lesions (Figure 39-6). The tuberculin skin test is nonreactive in up to 50% of patients. Culture confirmation of disease can be extremely difficult and may require a liver, lung, bone marrow, or skin biopsy. In some cases, *M. tuberculosis* can be isolated from sputum, gastric aspirate, blood, or urine.

Central Nervous System

Tubercle bacilli distribute into all parts of the central nervous system (CNS) during lympho-hematogenous spread. They do not multiply as well in nervous tissue as in some other tissues. Tuberculous meningitis rises from caseous foci, often very small ones, situated in the brain or meninges. The caseous foci discharge bacilli directly into the subarachnoid space, resulting in a thick gelatinous exudate that lies in the meshes of the pia-arachnoid, where it infiltrates the walls of meningeal arteries and veins. Inflammation, caseation, and obstruction are produced and extend along small vessels into the cortex, occluding blood vessels and producing infarcts (Leiguarda et al., 1988). The same exudate interferes with the normal flow of the cerebrospinal fluid (CSF) in and out of the ventricular system (Palur et al., 1991). The predilection of the exudate for the base of the brain accounts for the frequent involvement of the third, sixth, and seventh cranial nerves and the optic chiasm. The combination of vascular lesions producing infarcts, interference with CSF flow resulting in hydrocephalus, and direct cranial nerve involvement causes the devastating damage that all too often results from tuberculous meningitis. Profound abnormalities in electrolyte metabolism, especially hyponatremia, also contribute to the pathophysiology. The syndrome of inappropriate antidiuretic hormone secretion is common and may last for weeks after appropriate therapy is started. Salt wasting may make correction of the electrolyte disturbances difficult.

Tuberculous meningitis complicates about 0.3% of untreated tuberculosis infections in children. Meningitis is extremely rare in infants less than 4 months of age because pathologic events usually need that much time to develop. It is most common in children between 6 months and 4 years of age. Because tuberculous

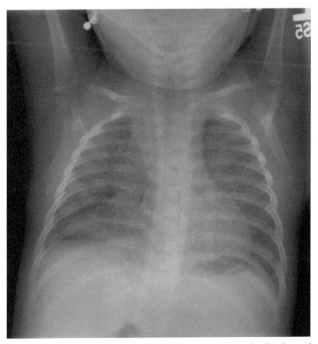

Fig. 39-6 Miliary tuberculosis in an infant whose uncle also had tuberculosis. There is adenopathy in addition to the millet seed–like lesions.

meningitis is an early manifestation of the initial infection, occurring within 2 to 6 months after infection, the adult from whom the child got the infection usually can be identified (Doerr et al., 1995).

Although the onset of tuberculous meningitis may be explosive, it is more often gradual, occurring over a period of several weeks (Curless and Mitchell, 1991; Waeker and Connor, 1990). Rapid progression tends to occur more often in infants and small children, who may experience symptoms for only several days before the onset of acute hydrocephalus, seizures, or cerebral edema (Starke, 1999). The disease is often divided into three stages. The first stage, which typically lasts 1 to 2 weeks, is characterized by nonspecific symptoms such as fever, headache, irritability, drowsiness, and malaise. Focal neurologic signs are absent, but infants may experience a stagnation or loss of developmental milestones. The second stage usually begins abruptly and includes lethargy, nuchal rigidity and Kernig's or Brudzinski's sign, seizures, hypertonia, vomiting, cranial nerve palsies, or other focal neurologic signs. Although some children have no evidence of meningeal irritation at this time, they may have signs of encephalitis such as disorientation, abnormal movements, or speech impairment. The third stage is marked by coma; hemiplegia or paraplegia; hypotension; posturing; deterioration in vital signs; and, eventually, death. Papilledema is noted only late in the clinical course.

One important aid in diagnosis is a history of contact with an adult with tuberculosis; however, the family history for tuberculosis often is falsely negative because the incubation period of meningitis is short and the contagious adult has not yet been discovered (Doerr et al., 1995). The tuberculin skin test is positive in only 50% of cases of tuberculous meningitis. The chest radiograph is often abnormal in children with tuberculous meningitis and reveals changes typical of primary tuberculosis. The most important laboratory test is the evaluation of the CSF. The lumbar spinal fluid usually is clear but under substantially increased pressure. It contains 50 to 500 white blood cells (WBC) per mm³, with polymorphonuclear leukocytes predominant early and lymphocytes predominant later. The spinal fluid glucose level may be at the lower limits of normal if the patient is examined early in the course, but by

the third stage the levels are low. The protein content may be normal at the time of the first spinal tap but rises steadily to very high concentrations. Acid-fast stain of the pellicle of the CSF can be helpful but is positive in less than 10% of cases. Unfortunately, *M. tuberculosis* can be isolated from the CSF in only 50% of cases of tuberculous meningitis in children. Results of culture are more likely to be positive if a larger volume of fluid is obtained. Often the culture confirmation comes from other clinical samples, especially gastric washings in a child who also has pulmonary tuberculosis. Computed tomography (CT) (Wallace et al., 1991) or magnetic resonance imaging (MRI) (Offenbacher et al., 1991) of the brain of patients with tuberculous meningitis may be normal during early stages of disease. With progression, basilar enhancement and communicating hydrocephalus with signs of cerebral edema or early focal ischemia are the most common findings (Ravenscroft et al., 2001). The findings of basilar meningitis, hydrocephalus, or infarct accompanying clinical meningitis in a child should immediately raise the question of tuberculosis as the cause of the meningitis (Lamprecht et al., 2001). In most cases, empiric therapy for tuberculosis should be started while further epidemiologic and laboratory investigations are undertaken.

The prognosis of tuberculous meningitis correlates most closely with the clinical stage at the time chemotherapy has started (Humphries et al., 1990). The vast majority of patients in the first stage have an excellent outcome, whereas most patients in the third stage who survive have permanent disabilities including blindness, deafness, paraplegia, diabetes insipidus, or mental retardation. The prognosis for young infants is also worse.

Tuberculoma is manifested clinically as a brain tumor (Figure 39-7). Tuberculomas account for up to 40% of brain tumors in some areas of the world but are rare in North America. Tuberculomas are more common in children less than 10 years of age. They are usually singular but may be multiple. In adults, lesions are most often supratentorial, but in children they are often infratentorial, located at the base of the brain near the cerebellum. A well-recognized phenomenon is the development of symptomatic intracranial tuberculomas when the child is undergoing therapy for meningeal, miliary, or even pulmonary tuberculosis (Doerr

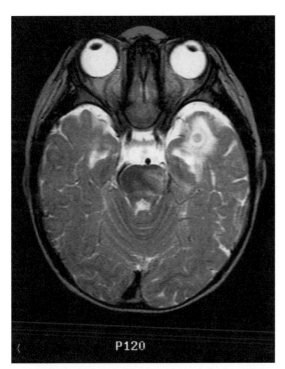

Fig. 39-7 A magnetic resonance image of tuberculoma in a child with culture-positive tuberculous meningitis. The child's presenting signs and symptoms included fever, altered mental status, and hemiparesis.

et al., 1995; Shepard et al., 1986; Teoh et al., 1987). This phenomenon appears to be mediated immunologically; the condition usually responds to corticosteroids and does not necessitate a change in antituberculosis chemotherapy. CT or MRI of the head should be obtained when neurologic signs or symptoms accompany any form of tuberculosis. The most common signs or symptoms accompanying tuberculomas are headaches, convulsions, fever, and other signs and symptoms usually associated with brain abscess or tumor. A tuberculin skin test is usually positive, but the chest radiograph is often normal, because the tuberculoma has developed some time after the initial infection. The major determinant of the specific signs and symptoms is the anatomic location of the tuberculoma. Tuberculous brain abscess is a rare but life-threatening complication of CNS tuberculosis, which usually requires a combination of surgery and medical therapy (Kumar et al., 2002).

Cutaneous Tuberculosis

Cutaneous tuberculosis, which was more common decades ago, arises as an extension of disease from the primary focus, from hematogenous dissemination, or from hypersensitivity to the tubercle bacillus (Kumar et al., 2001). Skin lesions associated with the primary complex may be caused by direct inoculation of bacilli into a traumatized area such as a lesion on the sole of the child's foot or an insect bite. The initial skin focus usually is a small, painless nodule with tiny satellite lesions that turn into indolent ulcers without surrounding inflammation. The most striking feature is regional lymphadenitis, which is what often convinces the patient to see a physician. Fever and other systemic reactions are minimal. A strongly positive tuberculin skin test usually is present. Scrofuloderma represents tuberculosis of the skin overlying a caseous lymph node—most often in the cervical area—that has ruptured to the outside, leaving either a shallow ulcer or a deep sinus tract, sometimes surrounded by nodules.

Manifestations that arise from hematogenous dissemination are papulonecrotic tuberculids and tuberculosis verrucosa cutis. Tuberculids are miliary tubercles in the skin that usually appear as tiny papules with "apple-jelly" centers, most commonly on the trunk, thighs, and face. They are similar to papular urticaria or early varicella lesions. Lupus vulgaris is a rare form of chronic indolent tuberculosis on the face that often seems to evolve from tuberculids. Tuberculosis verrucosa cutis is a condition characterized by a large skin lesion, which usually appears on the arms, legs, or buttocks, suggesting that trauma may play some part in its causation. The lesions often have a warty appearance, but there is no associated regional lymphadenitis. Biopsy and culture of the lesions are often required for correct diagnosis.

Erythema nodosum is a hypersensitivity manifestation of tuberculosis. It occurs most often in young teenage girls. It usually begins with fever and systemic toxicity soon after the initial infection and is characterized by large, deep, and painful indurated nodules on the shins and sometimes on the thighs, elbows, and forearms. The nodules gradually change from a light pink color to a bruiselike appearance. Tuberculin hypersensitivity is pronounced in children with tuberculosis underlying erythema nodosum, and tuberculin skin testing should be performed with extreme caution.

Skeleton

Skeletal tuberculosis usually results from lymphohematogenous seeding of bacilli during the primary infection. The disease also might originate as the result of direct extension from a caseous regional lymph node or by extension from a neighboring infected bone. The time interval between infection and disease can be as short as 1 month in cases of tuberculosis dactylitis or several years or longer for tuberculosis of the hip. The infection usually begins in the metaphysis of the bone. Granulation tissue and caseation—which destroy bone both by direct infection and pressure necrosis—are common. Soft-tissue abscess and extension of the infection through the epiphysis into the nearby joint often complicate bone infection. The infection frequently becomes apparent clinically only after joint involvement progresses.

Weight-bearing bones and joints are affected most commonly by tuberculosis (Bavadekan, 1982; Haygood and Williamson, 1994). Most cases occur in the vertebrae, causing tuberculosis of the spine or Pott's disease. Although any vertebral body can be involved, there is a predilection for the lower thoracic and upper lumbar vertebrae. Involvement of two or more vertebrae is common; these vertebrae are usually contiguous, but there may be skip areas between the lesions. The infection is in the body of the vertebra, leading to bone destruction and collapse. Tuberculous spondylitis progresses from initial narrowing of one or more disk spaces to collapse and wedging of the vertebral body, with subsequent angulation of the spine causing either gibbus or kyphosis. The infection usually extends out from the bone, causing a paraspinal (Pott's), psoas, or retropharyngeal abscess.

The most common clinical signs and symptoms of Pott's disease in children are low-grade fever, irritability, and restlessness, especially at night; back pain without significant tenderness; and abnormal positioning and gait or refusal to walk. Spinal rigidity may be caused by profound muscle spasm, which results from the patient's involuntary effort to immobilize the spine. Neurologic complications most often arise from cervical and lumbar vertebral lesions and include varying degrees of neuroplegia, paraplegia, or quadriplegia. The complications are caused by inflammation of the spinal cord secondary to a neighboring cold abscess, caseum, or granuloma in the extradural area or by spinal vessel thrombosis. Although surgery for spinal tuberculosis was long considered an important adjunct to therapy, most cases are now treated primarily with chemotherapy, surgery being undertaken only if stabilization of the spine is necessary. A surgical procedure may be necessary to obtain clinical material and establish the diagnosis by culture.

Other sites of skeletal tuberculosis, in approximate order of frequency, are the knee, hip, elbow, and ankle (Rasool, 2001). The involvement can range from joint effusion without bone destruction to frank destruction of bone and restriction of the joint caused by chronic fibrosis of the synovial membrane (Vallejo et al., 1994). This more severe type of bone tuberculosis, which usually evolves over months or years, most commonly causes mild pain, stiffness, limp, and restricted joint motion. With tuberculosis of the hip, if the disease is limited at the time of discovery to the acetabulum or the head of the femur, good mobility of the joint usually can be preserved by effective chemotherapy.

The diagnosis of skeletal tuberculosis should be considered in any child who is known to be infected with *M. tuberculosis* and in whom a bone or joint lesion develops, and in any child with a persistent, unexplained bone or joint lesion. The tuberculin skin test is positive in up to 90% of cases. Culture of the joint fluid or bone biopsy usually yields the organism; synovial biopsy often reveals granulomas.

Superficial Lymph Nodes

Tuberculosis of the superficial lymph nodes, often referred to as scrofula, is the most common form of extrapulmonary tuberculosis in children (Dandapat et al., 1990). Historically, scrofula was often caused by drinking unpasteurized cow's milk laden with *Mycobacterium bovis*. Most current cases occur within 6 to 9 months of the initial infection with *M. tuberculosis*, although some cases appear years later. The tonsillar, anterior cervical, and submandibular nodes become involved secondary to extension of the initial lesion from the upper lung field or abdomen. Infected nodes in the inguinal, epitrochlear, or axillary regions result from regional lymphadenitis associated with tuberculosis of the skin or skeletal system.

In the early stages the nodes enlarge gradually. The nodes are firm but not hard, discrete, and nontender. They often feel fixed to underlying or overlying tissues. Disease is most often unilateral, but bilateral involvement may occur because of crossover drainage patterns of lymphatic vessels in the chest and lower neck. As infection progresses, multiple nodes are affected, often resulting in a mass of matted nodes. Systemic signs and symptoms other than low-grade fever are usually absent. The tuberculin skin test is usually reactive. Although a primary pulmonary focus is virtually always present, it is visible radiographically in less than 50% of cases. Occasionally the onset of illness is more acute with rapid enlargement of nodes, high fever, tenderness, and fluctuance simulating pyogenic adenitis. The initial presentation is rarely a fluctuant mass with overlying cellulitis or skin discoloration.

If left untreated, lymph node tuberculosis may resolve, but more often it progresses to caseation and necrosis of the lymph node. The capsule of the node breaks down, resulting in the spread of infection to adjacent nodes and other structures. Rupture results in a draining sinus tract that may require surgical removal.

Infection with pyogenic bacteria may enhance mycobacterial adenitis; it is frequently wise to begin conventional antibacterial therapy while awaiting the results of the tuberculin skin test and other diagnostic maneuvers. Surgical excision of nodes infected with *M. tuberculosis* is usually not necessary; however, because distinguishing between tuberculosis and adenitis caused by nontuberculous mycobacteria can be difficult, and because the treatment of choice for lymph node disease caused by other mycobacteria is complete excision of the nodes, surgical procedures may be undertaken for tuberculous adenitis (Schuit and Powell, 1978). Even with complete surgical removal of the lymph node, however, tuberculous lymphadenitis requires chemotherapy because it is just one part of a systemic infection.

Eye and Ear

Ocular tuberculosis is uncommon in children. When it does occur, the conjunctiva and cornea are the areas most often involved. Unilateral redness and lacrimation are usually associated with the enlargement of the preauricular, submandibular, or cervical lymph nodes. Tuberculosis of the ciliary body or iris and tuberculosis uveitis are exceedingly rare in children. These forms of tuberculosis are very hard to diagnose because there is no material avail-able for culture, the chest radiograph is usually normal, and the adult source of infection often cannot be traced.

Tuberculosis of the middle ear is a relatively rare manifestation (MacAdam and Rubio, 1977). It occurs as a primary focus in the area of the eustachian tube in neonates who have aspirated infected amniotic fluid or older infants who have ingested tuberculous material (Mumtaz et al., 1983). It can occur as a metastatic lesion in older children who have a primary focus elsewhere. Otorrhea is common and painless and may become foul smelling because of the bacterial contamination with enteric organisms. The disease is almost always unilateral. Older patients may complain of tinnitus and "funny noises." The eardrum often is damaged extensively. A large central perforation or several smaller perforations are characteristic. Diagnosis can be difficult for two reasons: (1) stains and cultures are frequently negative, and (2) histology of the affected tissue often shows acute and chronic inflammation without granuloma formation.

Abdomen

Abdominal tuberculosis may occur after ingestion of tubercle bacilli or as part of generalized lymphohematogenous spread (Bhansali, 1977). Tuberculous enteritis always has been uncommon. Tubercle bacilli penetrate the gut wall via the Peyer's patches or the appendix, giving rise to local ulcers followed by mesenteric lymphadenitis and sometimes peritonitis. Occasionally in older children, tuberculous enteritis accompanies extensive pulmonary cavitation as a result of the swallowing of infected secretions. Symptoms and signs include vague abdominal pain, blood in the stools, and sinus formation after a seemingly routine appendectomy. Tuberculous enteritis should be suspected in any child with chronic gastrointestinal complaints and a reactive tuberculin skin test (Saczek et al., 2001). Biopsy, stain, and culture of the lesions are often necessary to confirm the diagnosis.

Tuberculous peritonitis, which occurs most often in young men, is uncommon in adolescents and rare in young children (Chavalittamvong and Talalak, 1982). It arises from direct extension of a primary intestinal focus or from a tuberculous salpingitis. Generalized peritonitis may result from subclinical or miliary hematogenous dissemination. Initially pain and tenderness are often mild. Rarely the lymph nodes, omentum, and peritoneum become matted in children; they can be palpated as a doughy, irregular, nontender mass. Ascites and low-grade fever occur commonly. The tuberculin skin test is usually reactive. The diagnosis usually can be confirmed by paracentesis with appropriate stains and cultures, but this procedure must be performed extremely carefully to avoid bowel intertwined with the matted omentum. Laparoscopy with fine-needle aspiration also may be helpful.

Renal Tuberculosis

Renal tuberculosis is an uncommon complication of pulmonary tuberculosis in children, rarely occurring less than 4 or 5 years after the initial infection (Smith and Lattimer, 1973). However, tubercle bacilli can be recovered from the urine in many cases of miliary tuberculosis and some cases of pulmonary tuberculosis in young children (Ehrlich and Lattimer, 1971). Hematogenous dissemination can give rise to tubercles in the glomeruli, with resultant caseating, sloughing lesions that discharge tubercle bacilli into the tubules. Occasionally an encapsulated caseous mass develops that calcifies or discharges into the pelvis of the kidney in the zone between the renal pyramid and cortex, forming a cavity quite analogous to a pulmonary cavity. Infection can be unilateral or bilateral and can spread downward to involve the bladder. Dysuria with hematuria and/or sterile pyuria are the presenting findings in the urine. They may occur grossly but usually not until late in the course of disease that has strikingly few specific symptoms. Appropriate examination and culture of early morning urine specimens usually reveal tubercle bacilli. A tuberculin skin test is positive in most cases. It should be remembered that urine from patients with renal tuberculosis may be highly infectious and such children should be isolated until their urine is sterile.

Genitourinary System

Tuberculosis of the genital tract is rare in both boys and girls before puberty. The condition originates from lymphohematogenous spread, although it can complicate direct spread from the intestinal tract or bone. Sexual transmission of *M. tuberculosis* has been postulated but never proved. Genital tuberculosis is a particular hazard for adolescent girls with tuberculosis

infection. The fallopian tubes are most often involved, followed in incidence by the endometrium, ovaries, and cervix. The usual symptoms are lower abdominal pain and dysmenorrhea or amenorrhea. Systemic manifestations are often absent, and the chest radiograph is normal in the majority of cases. However, some patients have accompanying pulmonary or pleural tuberculosis. Chronic genital tract infection in women leads to infertility.

Genital tuberculosis in adolescent males can cause epididymitis or orchitis. This condition occurs as a unilateral nodular, painless swelling of the scrotum. Involvement of the glans penis is extremely rare.

Perinatal Tuberculosis

Transmission of tuberculosis infection from mother to infant via the placenta or amniotic fluid has been reported in only about 300 patients. Perinatal tuberculosis can be acquired by the infant via one of several routes. First, transplacental spread via the umbilical vein from a mother with primary hematogenous tuberculosis may occur at the end stages of pregnancy, resulting in true congenital tuberculosis. In these infants the primary infection often is in the liver, although the liver may be bypassed with the primary infection occurring in the lung. Second, aspiration in utero of amniotic fluid infected from endometritis in the mother or from the placenta occurs rarely; this is also a form of true congenital tuberculosis. Third, the infant may ingest infected amniotic fluid or secretions during delivery. Finally, the most common mode of transmission to newborns is inhalation of tubercle bacilli at or soon after birth that originated from the mother or other relatives with infectious pulmonary tuberculosis. It is not always possible to be sure of the type of infection in a particular neonate since only clear-cut evidence of a primary infection in the liver establishes a definite diagnosis of true congenital tuberculosis. However, the presence of early forms of tuberculosis or documentation of endometrial tuberculosis in the mother after delivery is strong evidence of congenital tuberculosis in the infant. When an infant is suspected of having congenital tuberculosis, endometrial biopsy of the mother is an integral part of the evaluation (Vallejo and Starke, 1992).

Diagnosis of perinatal tuberculosis is usually difficult and often delayed (Lee et al., 1998). At least one half of the reported cases have been diagnosed only at autopsy of the baby. Disease in the mother is often overlooked; the mother may have nonspecific symptoms of pulmonary infection or lingering endometritis that are not recognized to be due to tuberculosis (Figueroa-Damian and Arredondo-Garcia, 2001). The early symptoms and signs in the neonate also may be overlooked and may be similar to those caused by other congenital infections. Once the diagnosis is suspected, treatment should be started immediately and diagnostic procedures carried out as rapidly as possible. Tuberculosis in the neonate should be suspected when signs and symptoms consistent with it are present and other causes, especially other congenital infections, have been ruled out.

The clinical manifestations of perinatal tuberculosis vary according to the size of the infecting dose of bacilli and the site and size of the caseous lesions (Hageman et al., 1980; Nemir and O'Hare, 1985). Symptoms and signs usually appear during the second week of life and include loss of appetite and failure to gain weight, fever, discharge from the nose or ear, cough, jaundice, hepatosplenomegaly, and lymph node enlargement (Cantwell et al., 1994a). Respiratory embarrassment may be a late symptom of the disease. Many infants have an initially normal chest radiograph that later becomes abnormal, most often showing a miliary pattern. Hilar and mediastinal lymphadenopathy and lung infiltrates also are common. The most important clue for rapid diagnosis of perinatal tuberculosis is the maternal and family history for tuberculosis. Frequently, however, the mother's disease is discovered only after the neonate's condition is suspected or diagnosed. The infant's tuberculin skin test is negative initially, but it may become positive in 1 to 3 months. A positive acid-fast stain of an early morning gastric washing from a newborn usually indicates tuberculosis. Direct acid-fast stains of middle ear fluid, bone marrow, tracheal aspirates, or biopsy tissue can be useful and should be performed. The CSF should be examined and cultured, although the yield for isolating *M. tuberculosis* is low, because fewer than 25% of infected infants have meningitis.

HIV-Related Disease

In adults infected with both HIV and *M. tuberculosis*, the rate of progression from tuberculosis infection to disease is greatly increased. The clinical manifestations of tuberculosis in HIV-infected patients are typical when the CD4+ cell count is more than 500 per mm^3. Extrapulmonary foci occur in up to 60% of profoundly immunocompromised patients. Pulmonary cavities are rare; lower lobe infiltrates or nodules often accompanied by thoracic adenopathy are common, especially if the patient's tuberculosis infection is recent. Of course, many patients have a nonreactive tuberculin skin test. Sputum is less likely to be produced or to contain visible acid-fast organisms.

When HIV-infected children develop tuberculosis, the clinical features tend to be fairly typical of childhood tuberculosis in immunocompetent patients, although the disease often progresses more rapidly and clinical manifestations are more severe (Blussvan et al., 2002; Chan et al., 1996; Khouri et al., 1992). There is an increased tendency for extrapulmonary disease, especially disseminated disease and meningitis. Diagnosis can be difficult to establish because the yield for cultures is so low in children and because other pulmonary infections or conditions that complicate pediatric AIDS resemble tuberculosis (Kiwanuka et al., 2001). A diligent search for an infectious adult in the child's environment may yield the best clue to the correct diagnosis.

DIAGNOSIS
Tuberculin Skin Test

The Mantoux tuberculin skin test using five tuberculin units of purified protein derivative is the "gold standard" skin test. When administered properly, a wheal 6 to 10 mm in diameter should be raised. It is helpful for the person administering the test to anchor the side of his or her hand against the side of the child's arm and inject the solution in a transverse direction (Figure 39-8). With this technique one can maintain a firm grasp, anticipate the child's tendency to move, and create a fulcrum to guide proper entry of the needle. The amount of induration caused by the test should be measured as accurately as possible by a trained health-care worker (not the parent) 48 to 72 hours after administration (Cheng et al., 1996; Graziani and MacGregor, 1995; Howard and Soloman, 1988). The test should not be interpreted before 48 hours have elapsed, because false-positive results can occur as a result of different immunologic mechanisms. The size of

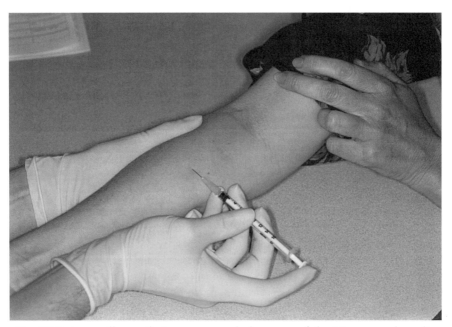

Fig. 39-8 An excellent technique to control placement of the Mantoux tuberculin skin test on an infant or child.

induration should be recorded in the medical record in millimeters even if there is no induration; use of the words *negative* and *positive* should be avoided because interpretation can change as more epidemiologic information becomes available. An occasional patient will have a reaction later than 72 hours after administration; this late induration should be considered the test result (Hsu, 1983). Two recent studies showed that pediatricians tend to misread tuberculin skin tests, interpreting less induration than experts have found in the same reaction (Carter and Lee, 2002; Kendig et al., 1998).

The tuberculin skin test is subject to a variety of factors that can cause false-negative and false-positive results (Huebner et al., 1993). The most common causes of false-negative results are incubation of viral infections such as influenza and varicella; incubation of bacterial infections; overwhelming tuberculosis; recent administration of live viral vaccines; severe malnutrition; diseases and drugs causing anergy; extremes of age (newborns and the elderly); and factors related to the administration of the test. It is acceptable to place the tuberculin skin test at the same time that a live viral vaccine is given or corticosteroids are started, because the test suppression takes several days to weeks to start (Schick and Dolgin,

1963). Approximately 10% of immunocompetent children with culture-documented tuberculosis do not react initially to the tuberculin skin test (Starke and Taylor-Watts, 1989; Steiner et al., 1980). Most become reactive after several months of treatment, suggesting that the disease has caused the anergy. The lack of skin reactivity can be global or specific for tuberculin. Children with tuberculosis and HIV infection more often experience widespread anergy to a variety of skin test antigens, including tuberculin. A negative tuberculin skin test never rules out tuberculosis in a child.

False-positive reactions to the tuberculin skin test most often are attributed to asymptomatic infection by nontuberculous mycobacteria. These cross-reactions are usually small (10 mm) but may be larger. Previous receipt of a bacille Calmette-Guérin (BCG) vaccination can cause increased reactivity to a subsequent tuberculin skin test, but the association is weaker than many clinicians suspect (Comstock et al., 1971; Menzies and Vissandjee, 1992; Mudido et al., 1999). Many studies have shown that fewer than 50% of infants given a BCG vaccination shortly after birth have a reactive tuberculin skin test at 6 to 12 months of age, and virtually all vaccinated infants have a nonreactive skin test by 5 years of age. Older children and adults who receive a BCG vaccination have a higher likelihood of developing a reactive skin test and maintaining it longer, but by 10 to 15 years after vaccination most individuals have lost tuberculin skin test reactivity (Comstock et al., 1971). Many foreign-born individuals who have had BCG vaccination have a reactive tuberculin skin test because they also have been infected with *M. tuberculosis* and are at risk of developing tuberculosis disease in the near or distant future (Carvalho et al., 2002; Lindgren, 1965). In general, the tuberculin skin test reaction should be interpreted in the same manner for persons who have had BCG in the past as it is for those who have not been vaccinated (Almeida et al., 2001; Nemir and Teichner, 1983). Repeated or serial skin testing can cause boosting, an increased response to subsequent tuberculin skin tests in individuals with a waned sensitivity to mycobacterial antigens (Thompson et al., 1979). Children who previously received a BCG vaccine may have a boostable reaction because of the BCG, not tuberculosis infection (Besser et al., 2001; Friedland, 1990; Sepulveda et al., 1988).

There have been several important and significant changes in recommendations by the CDC and the American Academy of Pediatrics (AAP) for the interpretation of a Mantoux tuberculin skin test. The reason for these changes is the inherent difficulty in interpreting a test that has a sensitivity and specificity of only about 95% (Huebner et al., 1993). When a test with these characteristics is applied to a population with a 90% prevalence of tuberculosis infection, the positive predictive value of the skin test is 99%, an excellent result. That is, 99% of the people with positive reactions have true tuberculosis infection. However, if the same test is applied to a population that has only a 1% prevalence of tuberculosis infection, the positive predictive value drops to 15%; 85% of the positive results are falsely positive, mostly caused by biologic variability and infection by nontuberculous mycobacteria. Because the skin test is not only the screening test but also the definitive test, true-positive results cannot be differentiated from false-positive results by further testing. All persons who test positive must therefore be evaluated and treated in the same manner, even though in certain groups the vast majority of those with positive results do not have tuberculosis infection. These false-positive test results lead to unnecessary treatment, cost, and anxiety for the family and clinician. In short, the relatively low sensitivity and specificity of the tuberculin skin test make it useful for persons in high-prevalence groups (at high risk for tuberculosis infection) but undesirable for persons in low-prevalence groups. In general, it is best to avoid tuberculin skin testing for children who do not have a recognized risk factor for acquiring tuberculosis infection.

In recent years the CDC and AAP have recommended varying the size of induration considered positive for different groups and individuals (Box 39-2). This is an attempt to alter the sensitivity and specificity of the test to make it more accurate in very–high-, high-, and low-prevalence groups (American Thoracic Society, 2000). It is crucial to minimize the false-negative results in very–high-risk individuals who are at the highest risk of developing tuberculosis disease in the near future. Similarly, there is great desire to minimize the false-positive results in truly low-risk individuals. For children at the highest risk for tuberculosis infection progressing to disease, a reactive area of 5 mm or more is classified as positive, probably indicating infection by *M. tuberculosis*. For other high-risk groups a reactive area of 10 mm or more is a positive result. For individuals with no risk factors a reaction of 15 mm or more is a positive result. However, even at the 15-mm cut point, the majority of "positive" reactions in truly low-risk individuals is still a false-positive result.

Diagnostic Mycobacteriology

Acid-fast stain and culture. The demonstration of acid-fast bacilli in stained smears of sputum or other body fluids is presumptive evidence of pulmonary tuberculosis in most cases.

BOX 39-2

AMOUNT OF INDURATION TO A MANTOUX TUBERCULIN SKIN TEST CONSIDERED POSITIVE

≥5 mm   Contacts to infectious cases
         HIV-infected or otherwise immunosuppressed
         Abnormal chest radiograph or suspicion of tuberculosis disease
≥10 mm   High-risk individuals listed in Box 39-1
≥15 mm   Individuals without risk factors

However, in children, tubercle bacilli usually are relatively few in number, and sputum cannot be obtained from children younger than 10 years of age (Khan and Starke, 1995). Gastric washings are often obtained in lieu of sputum, although they can be contaminated with acid-fast organisms from the mouth. Fluorescence microscopy of gastric washings has been found useful in settings where malnutrition and tuberculin-negative tuberculosis are rampant. Tubercle bacilli in CSF, pleural fluid, lymph node aspirates, and urine are sparse and only rarely detected on smears. Cultures for tubercle bacilli are of greater importance, not only to confirm the diagnosis but increasingly to permit testing for drug susceptibility. However, if culture and drug susceptibility data are available from the associated adult case and the child has a classic clinical and radiographic presentation of tuberculosis, obtaining cultures from the child adds little to the management because the drug susceptibilities are known and the child will be treated even if his or her cultures are negative.

Painstaking collection of specimens is essential for diagnosis of tuberculosis in children, because fewer organisms are present than in adults. Gastric lavage should be performed in the very early morning, before peristalsis has moved the overnight swallowed respiratory secretions that remain in the stomach. The gastric acidity should be neutralized immediately because acid conditions are poorly tolerated by *M. tuberculosis*. Unfortunately, even with optimal, in-hospital collection of three early morning gastric aspirate samples, *M. tuberculosis* can be isolated from only 30% to 40% of children and 70% of infants with pulmonary tuberculosis. The yield from random outpatient gastric aspirate samples is low, and this practice cannot be recommended. If bronchial secretions can be obtained from a child with suspected tuberculosis by stimulating cough with an aerosol solution (sputum induction), this practice may increase the yield of the culture (Shata et al., 1996). Bronchoscopy also can be an adjunct to culture diagnosis, but, in most studies, the yield of *M. tuberculosis* from bronchoscopy specimens has been lower than from properly obtained gastric washings (Abadco and Steiner, 1992; Chan et al., 1994; de Blic et al., 1991).

Nucleic acid amplification, serologic testing, antigen detection. The main form of nucleic acid amplification studied in children with tuberculosis is the polymerase chain reaction (PCR), which uses specific DNA sequences as markers for the presence of microorganisms (Pastrana et al., 2002). Various PCR techniques, most using the mycobacterial insertion element IS6110 as the DNA marker for *M. tuberculosis* complex organisms, have a sensitivity and specificity of more than 90% compared with sputum culture for detecting pulmonary tuberculosis in adults (Eisenach et al., 1991). However, test performance varies even among reference laboratories, with both false-positive and false-negative results being fairly common. The test is relatively expensive, requires fairly sophisticated equipment, and requires scrupulous technique to avoid cross-contamination of specimens (Dunlap et al., 1995).

Use of PCR in childhood tuberculosis has been limited. Compared with a clinical diagnosis of tuberculosis in children, the sensitivity of PCR has varied from 25% to 83% and the specificity has varied from 80% to 100% (Delacourt et al., 1995; Pierre et al., 1993; Smith et al., 1996). The PCR of gastric aspirates may be positive in a recently infected child even when the chest radiograph is normal, demonstrating the occasional arbitrariness of the distinction between tuberculosis infection and disease in children. PCR may have a useful but limited role in evaluating children with suspected tuberculosis. A negative result on PCR assay never eliminates tuberculosis as a diagnostic possibility, and a positive result does not confirm it. The major use of PCR will be in evaluation of children with significant pulmonary disease when the diagnosis is not established readily by clinical or epidemiologic rounds. PCR may be particularly helpful in evaluating immunocompromised children with pulmonary disease, especially children with HIV infection, although published reports of performance in such children are lacking. PCR also may aid in confirming the diagnosis of extrapulmonary tuberculosis, although only a few case reports involving samples other than sputum or gastric washings have been published (Gomez et al., 2000; Mancao et al., 1994). Currently, in the United States, PCR is approved for use only on acid-fast smear–positive specimens.

Despite hundreds of published studies, serologic testing has found no place in the routine diagnosis of tuberculosis in children.

Studies using a variety of mycobacterial antigens have yielded conflicting results (Delacourt et al., 1993; Turneer et al., 1994). In general, the sensitivity and specificity of the tests are unacceptably low to be of general use. Mycobacterial antigen detection has been evaluated in clinical samples from adults, but rarely from children (Sada et al., 1992). These techniques generally require sophisticated and expensive equipment not available where tuberculosis in children is common (Anderson et al., 2000).

History and Clinical Scoring

In the developing world the only way children with tuberculosis disease are discovered is when they present with a profound illness that is consistent with one presentation of tuberculosis (Harries et al., 2002; Weismuller et al., 2002). Having an ill adult contact is an obvious clue to the correct diagnosis. The only available laboratory test usually is an acid-fast smear of the sputum, which the child rarely produces. In many regions, chest radiographs are not available. To aid in diagnosis, a variety of scoring systems have been devised based on available tests, clinical signs and symptoms, and, most importantly, known exposures to adult cases (Migliori et al., 1992). However, the sensitivity and specificity of these systems can be very low, leading to both overdiagnosis and underdiagnosis.

Even in industrialized countries, epidemiology remains extremely important for the diagnosis of tuberculosis in children. Cases can be culture confirmed in only 40% of children; it is usually the combination of uncovering risk factors for recent tuberculosis infection, a positive tuberculin skin test, and radiographic or clinical evidence of tuberculosis disease that leads to the correct diagnosis. Children with tuberculosis in industrialized countries usually are discovered in one of two ways. One way is the consideration of tuberculosis being the cause of a symptomatic illness. The second way—which may be the method by which half the children are discovered—is during contact investigation of an adult with suspected tuberculosis. Typically, affected children have few signs or symptoms, but investigation reveals a positive tuberculin skin test and an abnormal chest radiograph. In industrialized countries it is rare to find tuberculosis disease in a native-born child as a result of a community- or school-based testing program.

TREATMENT
Antituberculosis Drugs

Over a dozen drugs are used for the treatment of tuberculosis in industrialized countries. Five drugs are used commonly for drug-susceptible tuberculosis (Table 39-2) and eight drugs are used mostly in cases of drug-resistant tuberculosis (Table 39-3).

Isoniazid is the mainstay of treatment of tuberculosis in children. It is inexpensive, readily diffuses into all tissues and body fluids, and produces a very low rate of adverse reactions. It can be administered either orally or intramuscularly. At the usual daily dose of 10 mg/kg, serum concentrations greatly exceed the minimum inhibitory concentration for *M. tuberculosis*. Peak concentrations in blood, sputum, and CSF are reached within a few hours and persist for at least 6 to 8 hours.

Isoniazid is metabolized by acetylation in the liver. Rapid acetylation is more frequent among blacks and Asians than among whites. However, in children there is no known correlation between acetylation rate and efficacy or rate of adverse reactions (Martinez-Roig et al., 1986).

Isoniazid has two principle toxic effects, both of which are rare in children. Peripheral neuritis results from competitive inhibition of pyridoxine utilization. Pyridoxine levels are decreased in children taking isoniazid, but clinical manifestations are rare (Pellock et al., 1985). Routine pyridoxine administration is not recommended except for teenagers with inadequate diets, children from groups with low levels of milk and meat intake, pregnant teenagers and women, and breast-feeding babies (McKenzie et al., 1976). The most common physical manifestation of peripheral neuritis is numbness and tingling in the hands or feet. CNS toxicity from isoniazid is rare, occurring usually when there is significant overdose. Seizures are the most common manifestations (McKenzie et al., 1976; Parish and Brownstein, 1986; Shah et al., 1995).

The major and most feared toxic effect of isoniazid is hepatotoxicity, which is also rare in children but the incidence of which increases with age (Beaudry et al., 1974). Of children taking isoniazid, 3% to 10% experience transient elevated serum transaminase levels. Clinically significant hepatotoxicity is very rare and is more likely to occur in adolescents or children with severe forms of tuberculosis or in

| TABLE 39-2 | Commonly Used Drugs for the Treatment of Tuberculosis in Children |

Drug	Dosage forms	Daily dosage (mg/kg/day)	Twice-weekly dosage (mg/kg/dose)	Maximum daily dose
Ethambutol	Tablets 100 mg 400 mg	15-25	50	2.5 g
Isoniazid*	Scored tablets 100 mg 300 mg Syrup† 10 mg/ml	10-15‡	20-30	Daily, 300 mg; twice weekly, 900 mg
Pyrazinamide	Scored tablets 500 mg	20-40	50	2 g
Rifampin*	Capsules 150 mg 300 mg Syrup Formulated in syrup from capsules	10-20	10-20	Daily, 600 mg; twice weekly, 900 mg
Streptomycin (IM administration)	Vials 1 g 4 g	20-40	20-40	1 g

*Rifamate is a capsule containing 150 mg of isoniazid and 300 mg of rifampin. Two capsules provide the usual adult (>50 kg body weight) daily doses of each drug.
†Most experts advise against the use of isoniazid syrup because of its instability and a high rate of gastrointestinal adverse reaction (diarrhea, cramps).
‡When isoniazid is used in combination with rifampin, the incidence of hepatoxicity increases if the isoniazid dose exceeds 10 mg/kg/day.

| TABLE 39-3 | Drugs for Treatment of Drug-Resistant Tuberculosis in Children |

Drug	Dosage forms	Daily dosage (mg/kg/day)	Maximum daily dose
Capreomycin	Vials 1 g	15-30 (IM)	1 g
Ciprofloxacin	Tablets 250 mg 500 mg 750 mg	Adults 500-1500 mg in 2 divided doses	1.5 g
Clofazamine	Capsules 50 mg 100 mg	50-100 mg/day	200 mg
Cycloserine	Capsules 250 mg	10-20	1 g
Ethionamide	Tablets 250 mg	15-20, given in 2 or 3 divided doses	1 g
Kanamycin	Vials 75 mg/2 ml 500 mg/2 ml 1 g/3 ml	15-30 (IM)	1 g
Levofloxacin	Tablets 250 mg 500 mg 750 mg	Adults 500-750 mg total/day	750 mg
Para-aminosalicylic acid	Packets 4 g	200-300, given in 2 to 4 divided doses	10 g

those who have underlying liver disease or are taking other hepatotoxic medications (Snider and Caras, 1992; Vanderhoof and Ament, 1976). Simultaneous administration of rifampin increases the likelihood of hepatotoxicity, especially if the isoniazid daily dose exceeds 10 mg/kg (Kumar et al., 1991; O'Brien et al., 1983). The possible occurrence of hepatitis raises the issue of routine monitoring of liver enzyme levels in children receiving isoniazid. The advantage of doing so has to be weighed against the expense and the difficulty of ensuring regular physician or clinic visits if the patient and parents know that every clinic visit requires a venipuncture. Most experts prefer to substitute routine questions about appetite and well-being, determination of weight, a check of the appearance of the sclera, and examination of the abdomen for frequent blood drawing. Patients should be counseled to stop the isoniazid and contact the clinician immediately if significant nausea, vomiting, abdominal pain, or jaundice occurs during the use of isoniazid.

Allergic manifestations or hypersensitivity caused by isoniazid are very rare. Isoniazid increases phenytoin levels, which can lead to toxicity by blocking its metabolism level. Occasionally isoniazid reacts with theophylline, requiring modification of its dosage. Rare side effects of isoniazid include pellagra, hemolytic anemia, and a lupuslike reaction with skin rash and arthritis.

Rifampin is a semisynthetic drug that is an important part of the modern management of tuberculosis. It is well absorbed from the gastrointestinal tract during fasting, with peak serum levels occurring within 2 hours. Oral and intravenous forms are available. Like isoniazid, rifampin is distributed widely in tissue and body fluids, including the CSF. Although excretion is mainly via the biliary tract, effective levels are reached in the kidneys and urine. Side effects are more common than with isoniazid and include orange discoloration of urine and tears (with permanent staining of contact lenses); gastrointestinal disturbances; and hepatotoxicity, usually manifested as asymptomatic elevation of serum transaminase levels. Intermittent administration of rifampin over weeks has been associated with thrombocytopenia and an influenza-like syndrome consisting of fever, headache, and malaise. Rifampin can render oral contraceptives ineffective and interacts with several other drugs, including quinidine, warfarin sodium, and corticosteroids.

Pyrazinamide was developed in 1949 but fell into disuse because of hepatotoxicity observed at the then standard dosage of 50 mg/kg/day. In adults a once-daily dosage of 30 mg/kg/day produces adequate serum levels and little liver toxicity. The optimal dosage in children is unknown, but this dosage causes high CSF levels (Donald and Seifart, 1988; Roy et al., 1999), is well tolerated by children (Sanchez-Albisva et al., 1997), and correlates with clinical success in treatment trials of tuberculosis in children. Extensive experience with pyrazinamide in children has verified its safety. Although 10% of adults treated with pyrazinamide develop arthralgias or arthritis resulting from hyperuricemia, and uric acid levels are elevated in children taking pyrazinamide, clinical manifestations of hyperuricemia in children are extremely rare. Hepatotoxicity occurs at high doses but is very rare in children.

Rifamate is a capsule with fixed doses of isoniazid (150 mg) and rifampin (300 mg). Rifater is a pill containing fixed doses of isoniazid, rifampin, and pyrazinamide. These fixed-dose combination capsules and pills should be used whenever possible to ensure that patients on self-supervised therapy are taking all of their tuberculosis medications together.

Streptomycin is used less frequently than in the past for the treatment of childhood tuberculosis but is important for the treatment of drug-resistant disease. It must be given intramuscularly or intravenously. Streptomycin penetrates inflamed meninges fairly well but does not cross uninflamed meninges. Its major current use is in cases where initial isoniazid resistance is suspected or when the child has life-threatening tuberculosis, such as meningitis or disseminated disease. The major toxicity of streptomycin is through the vestibular and auditory portions of the eighth cranial nerve. Renal toxicity is much less frequent. Streptomycin is contraindicated in pregnant women because up to 30% of their infants will suffer severe hearing loss (Snider and Johnson, 1984).

Ethambutol has received limited attention for children. At a dosage of 15 mg/kg/day it is primarily bacteriostatic, and its historic purpose has been to prevent emergence of resistance to other drugs. It is well tolerated by adults and children when given orally once or twice a day. The major potential toxicity is optic neuritis. Review of the world's literature has shown no report of optic toxicity in children, but the drug has not been used widely because of the inability to routinely test visual fields and acuity in children. Ethambutol is not recommended for general use in young children for whom vision cannot be adequately examined, but it can be used safely in children with drug-resistant tuberculosis or who may have been infected with a strain of drug-resistant *M. tuberculosis* when other agents are not available or cannot be used.

Ethionamide is a bacteriostatic drug whose major purpose is treatment of drug-resistant tuberculosis. It penetrates into the CSF very well and may be particularly useful in cases of tuberculous meningitis (Donald and Seifart, 1989). It is generally well tolerated by children but often must be given in two or three divided daily doses because of gastrointestinal disturbance. Ethionamide is chemically similar to isoniazid and can cause significant hepatitis.

Other antituberculosis drugs may be needed for patients with organisms that are resistant to the standard drugs. The aminoglycosides kanamycin, amikacin, and capreomycin have a spectrum of activity that differs from that of streptomycin with respect to individual mycobacterial strains. Cycloserine is an effective antituberculosis drug in adults but has been used infrequently in children because of its major side effects of impairment of thought processes and tendency to cause depression and other psychiatric abnormalities. The drug is usually given in one or two divided doses, and most experts recommend monitoring serum levels during its administration. Pyridoxine supplementation should be given when cycloserine is used. Levofloxacin, ciprofloxacin, and ofloxacin are fluoroquinolones with significant antituberculosis activity that are used commonly for treatment of drug-resistant tuberculosis in adults (Kennedy et al., 1993). These drugs are generally contraindicated for long-term administration in children because they can cause destruction of growing cartilage in some animal models. However, they have been used effectively in cases of drug-resistant tuberculosis in children when other effective agents were not available (Hussey et al., 1992). Para-aminosalicyclic acid is an old tuberculosis drug that was extremely difficult to take because of the need to administer a large number of pills. The drug is now available as granules provided in packets. The major side effect is gastrointestinal intolerance, which is extremely common and necessitates that the drug be given in three or four divided doses. Clofazamine is used to treat leprosy, but many strains of *M. tuberculosis* also are susceptible (Jagannath et al., 1995).

Rationale for Therapy

The tubercle bacillus can be killed only during replication. Environmental conditions for growth are best within lung cavities, leading to a huge bacterial population—up to 10^9 organisms. The caseous lesions that are most common in pediatric tuberculosis contain much smaller numbers of organisms—10^4 to 10^6—than cavitary lesions. Naturally occurring, drug-resistant mutant organisms occur within large populations of tubercle bacilli even before chemotherapy is started. All known genetic loci for drug resistance in *M. tuberculosis* are located on the chromosome; no plasmid-mediated resistance is known. The rate of resistance within large populations of organisms is related to the rate of mutations at these genetic loci. Although a large population of bacilli as a whole may be considered drug-susceptible, a subpopulation of drug-resistant organisms occurs at fairly predictable rates. The estimated frequency of these drug-resistant mutations is about 10^{-6}, but it varies among drugs. Therefore a cavity that contains 10^9 bacilli has thousands of single drug-resistant organisms, whereas a closed caseous lesion contains few, if any, resistant mutants (Swanson and Starke, 1995).

The two microbiologic properties of population size and drug-resistant mutations explain why single antituberculosis drugs cannot cure cavitary tuberculosis in adults (Mitchison and Nunn, 1986). When a single drug is given to these patients, they have some initial improvement in signs and symptoms, but they relapse with organisms that are completely resistant to the administered medication. Fortunately, the occurrence of resistance to one drug is independent of resistance to any other drug because the resistance loci are not linked (Telenti et al., 1993; Zhang, 1993). The chance of having even one organism with mutations causing resistance to two drugs before the start of chemotherapy is on the order of 10^{-13}.

Populations of this size are extremely rare in patients, and organisms naturally resistant to two drugs are essentially nonexistent.

The population size of tubercle bacilli within a patient determines the appropriate therapy. For patients with large bacterial populations (adults with cavities or extensive infiltrates), many single drug-resistant organisms are present, and at least two antituberculosis drugs must be used. Conversely, for patients with tuberculosis infection but no disease, the bacterial population is very small (about 10^3 to 10^4 organisms), drug-resistant organisms are rare, and a single drug can be used. Children with pulmonary tuberculosis and patients of all ages with extrapulmonary tuberculosis have medium-size populations where drug-resistant mutants may or may not be present. In general, these patients are treated with at least two drugs (Biddulph, 1990).

Exposure

Children exposed to potentially infectious adults with pulmonary tuberculosis should be started on treatment, usually isoniazid, if the child is younger than 5 years of age or has other risk factors for the rapid development of tuberculosis disease, such as immunocompromise (Starke and Correa, 1995). Failure to do this may result in development of severe tuberculosis disease even before the tuberculin skin test becomes reactive; the "incubation" period of disease may be shorter than the time it takes for the skin test to become reactive. The child is treated for a minimum of 3 months after contact with the infectious case has been broken by physical separation or effective treatment. After 3 months the tuberculin skin test is repeated. If the second test is positive, infection is documented and isoniazid should be continued for total duration of 9 months; if the second skin test is negative, the treatment can be stopped. If the exposure was to a case with an isoniazid-resistant but rifampin-susceptible isolate, rifampin is the recommended treatment.

Two special circumstances of exposure deserve attention. A difficult situation arises when exposed children are anergic because of HIV infection. These children are particularly vulnerable to rapid progression of tuberculosis, and it will not be possible to tell if infection has occurred. In general, these children should be treated as if they have tuberculosis infection. The second situation is potential exposure of a

newborn to a mother or other adult with a positive tuberculin skin test (Dormer et al., 1959; Steiner and Rao, 1993). The management is based on further evaluation of the adult (Kendig and Rodgers, 1958; Light et al., 1974). If the adult has a normal chest radiograph, no separation of the child from the adult is required. However, the adult should receive treatment for tuberculosis infection and other household members should be evaluated for tuberculosis infection or disease. The infant requires no specific evaluation or treatment unless a case of disease is found. If the mother or other adult has an abnormal chest radiograph, the child should be separated from the adult until evaluation has occurred. If the radiograph, medical and social history, physical examination, and analysis of sputum reveal no evidence of active pulmonary tuberculosis, it is reasonable to assume the infant is at low risk of infection. However, if the adult remains untreated, he or she may develop contagious tuberculosis and expose the infant. If the radiograph and clinical history are suggestive of pulmonary tuberculosis, the child and adult should remain separated until both have begun appropriate chemotherapy. The infant should be evaluated for congenital tuberculosis. The placenta should be examined if at all possible. The infant should receive isoniazid and close follow-up care. The infant should have a tuberculin skin test 3 or 4 months after the adult is judged to be no longer contagious; evaluation of this infant then follows the guidelines for other exposures of children. If no infection is documented during follow-up, it is prudent to repeat a tuberculin skin test in 6 to 12 months.

Infection

Isoniazid is effective in preventing progression of tuberculosis infection in children (Ferrebee, 1969). Before its discovery Brailey (1958) reported a mortality rate of 16% for black children and 8% for white children who were infected with *M. tuberculosis* before 3 years of age. In contrast, other reports have documented no death and no disease in similar children who received isoniazid for 9 to 12 months (Hsu, 1984). Other studies of children of all ages with tuberculosis infection have shown that isoniazid treatment produces a 90% to 100% reduction in tuberculosis disease during the first year after treatment, and the protective effect can last at least 30 years (Comstock et al.,

1979; Hsu, 1983). Although many adults are treated with a 6-month course of isoniazid for tuberculosis infection (International Union Against Tuberculosis Committee on Prophylaxis, 1982; Snider et al., 1986), the CDC and AAP recommend a 9-month duration of isoniazid treatment for adults and children with tuberculosis infection (American Thoracic Society, 2000). If infection is with an isoniazid-resistant but rifampin-susceptible organism, rifampin should be given for 6 months. In general, isoniazid is given on a daily basis. However, patient adherence to treatment is notoriously low, especially if the child's reactive skin test was discovered through a screening program. In situations in which the risk of progression to disease is high and family adherence to taking medication is difficult, isoniazid can be administered twice a week under the direct observation of a third party such as a public health worker or school nurse. This is called directly observed therapy (DOT). Although no studies have been published that document the effectiveness of twice-weekly DOT for tuberculosis infection, there are numerous studies that show its effectiveness in treating tuberculosis disease.

Treatment of tuberculosis infection in children with isoniazid has proved to be very safe (Byrd et al., 1979). Routine testing of blood chemistries and serum liver enzymes is unnecessary unless the child has hepatic disease or dysfunction or is taking other hepatotoxic drugs. It is recommended that the child be evaluated by a clinician every 4 to 6 weeks and that no more than a 6-week supply of medicine be given to avoid the possibility of massive overdose.

Disease

The major importance of the distinction between tuberculosis infection and disease in children is that the treatment regimens for them are different. The bacterial population is much larger in disease, and there is an increased propensity for the emergence of drug resistance with larger mycobacterial populations (British Thoracic Society, 1984). The simple adage to remember is "more bugs, more drugs." Because antituberculosis medications are so well tolerated by children and inadequate treatment can have devastating effects, most experts feel it is safer to overestimate rather than underestimate the extent of disease, particularly in a young child known to be at high risk with recent infection by *M. tuberculosis*. In general, any

radiographic or clinical manifestations that are attributed to the presence of *M. tuberculosis* (except for single granulomas in the lung) are considered disease, and the child is treated with more than one medication. The AAP and CDC currently recommend that standard treatment for pulmonary tuberculosis in children should be a 6-month course of isoniazid and rifampin supplemented during the first 2 months with pyrazinamide (American Thoracic Society, 1994). If the risk for initial isoniazid resistance is significant—particularly if the probable adult source case for infection has risk factors for drug-resistant tuberculosis—a fourth drug, usually ethambutol, should be given until drug susceptibility information is known (Centers for Disease Control and Prevention, 1993). As soon as isoniazid and rifampin susceptibility is established or considered likely, the ethambutol can be discontinued. In many published studies, the overall success rate of this regimen has been greater than 98%, and the incidence of clinically important adverse reactions has been less than 2% (Hong Kong Chest Service/British Medical Research Council, 1991; Tsakalidis et al., 1992). Because of the slow replication time of *M. tuberculosis* and the fairly long half-lives of most antituberculosis medications, they can be administered twice weekly under directly observed therapy after the first 2 to 4 weeks of daily administration (Al-Dossary et al., 2002; Cohn et al., 1990). Studies using twice-weekly therapy have shown results equivalent to those using daily therapy throughout the full 6 months (Kumar et al., 1990; Te Water Naude et al., 2000).

Controlled treatment trials for various forms of extrapulmonary tuberculosis are rare. In most reports, extrapulmonary cases have been combined with pulmonary cases and were not analyzed separately. Several of the 6-month, three- or four-drug trials in children included extrapulmonary cases. Most non–life-threatening forms of drug-susceptible extrapulmonary tuberculosis can be treated with a 6-month regimen of isoniazid, rifampin, and pyrazinamide (Dutt et al., 1986; Jawahar et al., 1990). One exception may be bone and joint tuberculosis, which has a higher failure rate when 6-month chemotherapy regimens are used, especially when surgical intervention has not occurred (Medical Research Council Working Party on Tuberculosis of the Spine, 1993). Most experts recommend 9 to 12 months of therapy for bone and joint tuberculosis. Tuberculous meningitis usually is not included in trials of extrapulmonary tuberculosis therapy because of its serious nature and low incidence. Studies have shown that inclusion of pyrazinamide in the regimen for tuberculous meningitis is extremely important (Donald et al., 1998; Jacobs et al., 1992). The AAP and CDC currently recommend treating tuberculous meningitis for 9 to 12 months, starting with four drugs to guard against initial drug resistance.

Corticosteroids have a place in the treatment of some patients with tuberculosis (Smith, 1958). They never should be used except under the cover of effective antituberculosis drugs. Corticosteroids would be expected to be beneficial in situations when the host inflammatory reaction contributes to tissue damage or impairs function. They should be used in all cases of suspected tuberculous meningitis, especially when increased intracranial pressure is present. Their major actions are to reduce vasculitis; inflammation; and, ultimately, intracranial pressure. Several studies have demonstrated lower rates of mortality and long-term neurologic sequelae among patients with tuberculous meningitis treated with corticosteroids compared with non–steroid-treated control patients (Escobar et al., 1975; Girgis et al., 1991). Corticosteroid treatment also may be considered (1) in cases of acute pericardial effusion when tamponade is occurring; (2) in cases of pleural effusion when there is shift of the mediastinum and acute respiratory embarrassment (Lee et al., 1988); (3) in patients with miliary tuberculosis if the inflammatory reaction is so severe as to produce alveolocapilliary block syndrome; and (4) in patients with enlarged mediastinal lymph nodes that are causing respiratory difficulty or a severe collapse-consolidation lesion, particularly in the lower lobe, where bronchiectasis is likely to be a troublesome sequela (Nemir et al., 1967). The dosage of corticosteroids should be in the anti-inflammatory range—that is, prednisone, 1 to 2 mg/kg every 24 hours for 4 to 6 weeks, with gradual withdrawal. There is no evidence that one corticosteroid is preferable to another.

The major problem with treatment of tuberculosis infection and disease is nonadherence to the drug regimen by patients over the long term (Beyers et al., 1994; Cuneo and Snider, 1989; Snider et al., 1984). In the United States it is almost the standard of care that patients with

tuberculosis disease be treated with DOT (Chaulk et al., 1998; Iseman et al., 1990; Kohn et al., 1996; Weis et al., 1994). Direct observation means that a health-care worker or nonrelated third party (such as a teacher, school nurse, or social worker) is physically present when the patient ingests the medication. Up to 50% of patients taking long-term tuberculosis medications have significant nonadherence without direct observation, and its occurrence is not predictable even by experienced clinicians (Chaulk et al., 1995; Sumartojo, 1993).

Drug Resistance

The incidence of drug-resistant tuberculosis is increasing in the United States and the world as a result of poor adherence by patients, the availability of some antituberculosis drugs in over-the-counter formulations, and poor management of patients by physicians and tuberculosis control programs (Mahmoudi and Iseman, 1993). In the United States about 10% of *M. tuberculosis* isolates are resistant to at least one drug (Bloch et al., 1994; Frieden et al., 1993). The initial drug resistance rate is as high as 40% in adults with pulmonary tuberculosis in some countries, and rates of 20% to 30% are common (Dye et al., 2002). Resistance is most common to streptomycin and isoniazid and is still relatively rare for rifampin. Certain epidemiologic factors—such as disease in an Asian or Hispanic immigrant to the United States, homelessness in some communities, and history of prior antituberculosis therapy—correlate with drug resistance in adult patients (Barnes, 1987; Small et al., 1993). Patterns of drug resistance in children tend to mirror what is found in adult patients in the population (Schaaf et al., 2000; Snider et al., 1985; Steiner et al., 1985). The key to determining drug resistance in childhood tuberculosis usually comes from the drug susceptibility profile of the isolate of the infectious adult contact case.

Therapy for drug-resistant tuberculosis is successful only when at least two bactericidal drugs to which the infecting strain of *M. tuberculosis* is susceptible are given (Passannante et al., 1994). If only one effective drug is given, secondary resistance will develop to it. When isoniazid resistance is considered a possibility on the basis of epidemiologic risk factors or the identification of an isoniazid-resistant source case isolate, a fourth drug, usually ethambutol or streptomycin, should be given initially to the child with tuberculosis disease until the exact susceptibility pattern of the isolate is determined and a more specific regimen can be designed. The exact treatment regimens of drug-resistant tuberculosis must be tailored to the specific pattern of resistance (Goble et al., 1993; Iseman, 1993). Duration of therapy usually is extended to at least 9 to 12 months if either isoniazid or rifampin can be used and to at least 18 to 24 months if resistance to both drugs is present (Park et al., 1996; Telzak et al., 1995). Occasionally, surgical resection of a diseased segment or lobe is required (Iseman et al., 1990). An expert in tuberculosis always should be involved in the management of children with drug-resistant tuberculosis infection and disease (Steiner and Rao, 1993).

PREVENTION
Public Health Measures

Prevention of tuberculosis may involve (1) protection against exposure to the organism; (2) use of antituberculosis drugs in tuberculin-negative individuals with high risk of infection; and (3) immunization of tuberculin-negative individuals. Protection against exposure to disease is the ideal form of prevention. It presupposes thorough pre-employment and ongoing case-finding programs among all who come in contact with children, such as day-care center and school personnel, teachers, health-care workers, babysitters, household workers, and others. The best way to protect a child from acquiring tuberculosis infection is to be sure that the adults in his or her environment do not have active tuberculosis.

It is obvious that the control of tuberculosis—for a community and for individuals—depends on close cooperation between the clinician and the health department. It is critically important that clinicians report suspected cases of tuberculosis to the Public Health Department as soon as possible (Mohle-Boetani and Flood, 2002). The clinician should not wait for microbiologic confirmation of the diagnosis, because it is the reporting of suspicion that leads to the initiation of the contact investigation that may find exposed or infected children and allow them to be treated before disease develops. If the clinician waits for confirmatory laboratory results from the suspected adult case, the child may progress from infection to disease before intervention occurs (Lobato et al., 2000; Mehta and Bentley, 1992; Nolan, 1986).

Since the advent of isoniazid treatment in the 1950s, screening children for tuberculosis infection often has been an integral part of local tuberculosis control programs. The major purpose of finding and treating infected individuals is to prevent future cases of tuberculosis disease (Centers for Disease Control and Prevention, 1994). However, frequent or periodic skin testing of children prevents very few cases of pediatric tuberculosis, especially if the screening is centered on school-age children (Mohle-Boetani et al., 1995). The majority of cases of tuberculosis disease among children occur in preschool-age children, and school-based screenings therefore have little benefit. The major purpose of testing school-age children is to prevent future cases of tuberculosis in adults. Clearly, the best way to prevent tuberculosis disease among children is through prompt contact investigation centered on adults with suspected contagious tuberculosis. These contact investigations not only have the highest yield, because 30% to 50% of household contacts have a positive tuberculin skin test, but they also find the most important individuals—those most recently infected who are in the period of their lives when they are most likely to develop tuberculosis disease. The most important activity in a community to prevent cases of pediatric tuberculosis is the contact investigation performed by the Public Health Department (Kimmerling et al., 1995; Perry and Starke, 1993).

BCG Vaccination

Immunization against tuberculosis would be a tremendous advance for medicine, but in practice it has been fraught with enormous difficulties. The only available vaccines against tuberculosis are the bacille Calmette-Gúerin (or BCG) vaccines, named for the two French investigators responsible for their development. The original vaccine organism was a strain of *M. bovis* attenuated by subculture every 3 weeks for 13 years. The strain was then distributed to dozens of laboratories, each of which continued to subculture the organism under various conditions. The result has been production of many daughter BCG strains that differ widely in morphology, growth characteristics, sensitizing potency, and animal virulence.

The route of administration and dosing schedule for the BCG vaccines are important for determining vaccine efficacies. The preferred route of administration is intradermal injection with a syringe and needle, because it is the only method that permits accurate measurement of an individual dose. The use of this route is relatively expensive, however, and, in developing countries, needles and syringes may be reused, with the resulting danger of transmission of HIV and hepatitis viruses. There are no reported trials comparing various methods of administration, although the complication rates generally are lower with multipuncture devices.

The BCG vaccines are extremely safe in immunocompetent hosts (Gonzalez et al., 1989; Turnbull et al., 2002). Local ulceration and regional suppurative lymphadenitis occur in 0.1% to 1% of vaccine recipients. Local lesions do not suggest underlying immune defects and appear not to affect the level of protection. Rarely, surgical incision of a suppurative draining lymph node is necessary, but this should be avoided if possible. Although osteomyelitis near the inoculation site of BCG has been reported, this effect appears to be related only to certain strains of the vaccine that are no longer in wide use. Systemic complaints such as fever, convulsions, loss of appetite, and irritability are extremely rare after BCG vaccination. There has been great concern recently about the effects of BCG vaccination in HIV-infected children. Currently the World Health Organization recommends BCG vaccination for asymptomatic HIV-infected children (Ryder et al., 1993). However, there is some evidence that local BCG reactions may be more common in HIV-infected children (O'Brien et al., 1995); that disseminated BCG-osis occurs (although rarely); and that complications may occur even decades after the BCG vaccination. In the United States, HIV infection is considered a contraindication to BCG vaccination (Centers for Disease Control and Prevention, 1994).

Accurate assessment of the effectiveness of BCG vaccines is extremely difficult. Recommended vaccine schedules vary widely among countries. The official WHO recommendation is a single dose administered during infancy. However, in some countries, multiple doses are given with or without a reactive tuberculin skin test, or a single dose may be administered later in childhood or during adolescence. The optimal age for administration is completely unknown, since adequate comparative trials never have been performed.

Although dozens of BCG trials on many varied human populations have been reported, the most useful data have come from several controlled trials and several case-control studies. The results of these studies are disparate; some demonstrated a great deal of protection from BCG, but others showed no efficacy at all. A recent metaanalysis of these studies showed the average effectiveness of BCG in preventing pulmonary disease to be about 50% (Colditz et al., 1994); effectiveness was higher for protection against life-threatening forms of tuberculosis in children (Colditz et al., 1995). A variety of explanations for the different apparent responses to BCG vaccines have been proposed, including methodologic and statistical variations among populations, interactions with nontuberculous mycobacteria that either enhance or decrease the protection afforded by BCG, different potencies among the various BCG vaccines, and genetic factors for reaction to BCG within the various study populations. It is apparent that BCG vaccination during infancy has little effect on the ultimate incidence of tuberculosis within a population. However, many experts believe that BCG may be more effective in preventing tuberculosis among infants and young children, particularly the serious forms of tuberculous meningitis and disseminated disease.

In summary, BCG vaccination has worked well in some situations but poorly in others. Clearly, BCG vaccination has had essentially no effect on the control of tuberculosis throughout the world. It does not substantially influence the rate of transmission, because those cases of contagious pulmonary tuberculosis in adults that can be prevented by BCG vaccination constitute a very small fraction of the sources of infection in a population. Any protective effect created by BCG probably wanes over time. The best use of BCG appears to be for prevention of life-threatening forms of tuberculosis in infants and young children.

BCG vaccination never has been adopted as part of the strategy for the control of tuberculosis in the United States. BCG vaccination in the United States is recommended only for tuberculin skin test–negative infants and children who are at high risk of intimate and prolonged exposure to untreated or ineffectively treated patients or to patients with tubercle bacilli that are resistant to both isoniazid and rifampin when other control measures cannot be used (Centers for Disease Control and Prevention, 1996; Kendig, 1969). The only strain of BCG vaccine currently licensed in the United States is the Tice strain, which must be administered with a clumsy multipuncture device.

BIBLIOGRAPHY

Abadco D, Steiner P. Gastric lavage is better than bronchoalveolar lavage for isolation of *Mycobacterium tuberculosis* in childhood pulmonary tuberculosis. Pediatr Infect Dis J 1992;11:738-739.

Albisua I, Artigao FB, Del Castillo F, et al. Twenty years of pulmonary tuberculosis in children: What has changed? Pediatr Infect Dis J 2002;21:49-53.

Al-Dossary FS, Ong LT, Correa AG, Starke JR. Treatment of childhood tuberculosis with a six month directly observed regimen of only two weeks of daily therapy. Pediatr Infect Dis J 2002;21:91-97.

Alland D, Kolkut GE, Moss A, et al. Transmission of tuberculosis in New York City: an analysis by DNA fingerprinting and conventional epidemiologic methods. N Engl J Med 1994;330:1710-1716.

Almeida LMD, Barbieri MA, DaPaixaoAQ, et al. Use of purified protein derivative to assess the risk of infection in children in close contact with adults with tuberculosis in a population with high Calmette-Gúerin bacillus coverage. Pediatr Infect Dis J 2001;20:1061-1065.

American Thoracic Society. Treatment of tuberculosis and tuberculosis infection in adults and children. Am J Respir Crit Care Med 1994;144:1359-1374.

American Thoracic Society and Centers for Disease Control and Prevention. Targeted tuberculin testing and treatment of latent tuberculosis infection. Am J Respir Crit Care Med 2000;161:S221-S247.

Anderson P, Munk ME, Pollock JM, Doherty TM. Specific immune-based diagnosis of tuberculosis. Lancet 2000;356:1099-1104.

Aznar J, Safi H, Romero J, et al. Nosocomial transmission of tuberculosis infection in pediatric wards. Pediatr Infect Dis J 1995;14:44-48.

Barnes PF. The influence of epidemiologic factors on drug resistance rates in tuberculosis. Am Rev Respir Dis 1987;136:325-328.

Barnes PF, Bloch AB, Davidson PT, et al. Tuberculosis in patients with human immunodeficiency virus infection. N Engl J Med 1991;324:1644-1650.

Barry MA, Shirley L, Grady MT, et al. Tuberculosis infection in urban adolescents: results of a school-based testing program. Am J Public Health 1990;80:439-441.

Bavadekan AV. Osteoarticular tuberculosis in children. Prog Pediatr Surg 1982;15:131-151.

Beaudry PH, Brickman HF, Wise MB. Liver enzyme disturbances during isoniazid chemoprophylaxis in children. Am Rev Respir Dis 1974;110:581-584.

Bellin EY, Fletcher DD, Safyer SM. Association of tuberculosis infection with increased time in or admission to the New York City jail system. JAMA 1993;269:2228-2231.

Besser RE, Pakiz B, Schulte J, et al. Risk factors for positive Mantoux tuberculin skin tests in children in San Diego, California: evidence for boosting and possible food borne transmission. Pediatrics 2001;108:305-310.

Beyers N, Gie R, Schaaf H, et al. Delay in the diagnosis, notification, and initiation of treatment and compliance in children with tuberculosis. Tuber Lung Dis 1994;75:260-265.

Bhansali SK. Abdominal tuberculosis: experience with 300 cases. Am J Gastroenterol 1977;67:324-337.

Biddulph J. Short-course chemotherapy for childhood tuberculosis. Pediatr Infect Dis J 1990;9:794-801.

Bloch A, Cauthen G, Onorato I, et al. Nationwide survey of drug-resistant tuberculosis in the United States. JAMA 1994;271:665-671.

Blumberg HM, Watkins DL, Berschling JD, et al. Preventing the nosocomial transmission of tuberculosis. Ann Intern Med 1995;122:658-663.

Blussvan Oud-Alblas HJ, van Vliet ME, Kimpen JL, et al. Human immunodeficiency virus infection in children hospitalized with tuberculosis. Ann Trop Paediatr 2002;22:115-123.

Brailey ME. Tuberculosis in white and Negro children. II. The epidemiologic aspects of the Harriet Lane study. Cambridge, Mass: Harvard University Press, 1958.

British Thoracic Society. A controlled trial of 6 months' therapy in pulmonary tuberculosis, final report: results during the 36 months after the end of chemotherapy and beyond. Br J Dis Chest 1984;78:330-336.

Brudney K, Dobkin J. Resurgent tuberculosis in New York City: human immunodeficiency virus, homelessness, and the decline of tuberculosis control programs. Am Rev Respir Dis 1991;144:745-749.

Burroughs M, Beitel A, Kawamura A, et al. Clinical presentation of tuberculosis in culture-positive children. Pediatr Infect Dis J 1999;18:440-446.

Byrd RB, Horn BR, Solomon DA, et al. Toxic effects of isoniazid in tuberculous chemoprophylaxis: role of biochemical monitoring in 1000 patients. JAMA 1979;241:1239-1241.

Cantwell M, Shehab Z, Costello A, et al. Brief report: congenital tuberculosis. N Engl J Med 1994a;330:1051-1054.

Cantwell M, Snider DE Jr, Cauthern G, et al. Epidemiology of tuberculosis in the United States, 1985 through 1992. JAMA 1994b;272:535-539.

Cardona M, Bek MD, Mills K, et al. Transmission of tuberculosis from a seven-year-old child in a Sydney school. J Pediatr Child Health 1999;35:375-378.

Carter ER, Lee CM. Interpretation of the tuberculin skin test reaction by pediatric providers. Pediatr Infect Dis J 2002;21:200-203.

Carvalho AC, Kritski AL, De Riemer K. Tuberculin skin testing among BCG-vaccinated children who are household contacts. Int J Tuberc Lung Dis 2002;5:297.

Centers for Disease Control and Prevention. Initial therapy for tuberculosis in the era of multidrug resistance. MMWR Recomm Rep 1993;42:1-8.

Centers for Disease Control and Prevention. Guidelines for preventing the transmission of *Mycobacterium tuberculosis* in health-care facilities, 1994. MMWR Recomm Rep 1994;43:1-133.

Centers for Disease Control and Prevention. Screening for tuberculosis and tuberculosis infection in high-risk populations. MMWR Recomm Rep 1995;44:19-34.

Centers for Disease Control and Prevention. The role of BCG vaccine in the prevention and control of tuberculosis in the United States: a joint statement by the Advisory

Council for the Elimination of Tuberculosis and the Advisory Committee on Immunization Practices. MMWR Recomm Rep 1996;45:1-18.

Chan S, Abadco D, Steiner P. Role of flexible fiberoptic bronchoscopy in the diagnosis of childhood endobronchial tuberculosis. Pediatr Infect Dis J 1994;13: 506-509.

Chan SP, Birnbaum J, Rao M. Clinical manifestation and outcome of tuberculosis in children with acquired immunodeficiency syndrome. Pediatr Infect Dis J 1996;15: 443-447.

Chaulk CP, Kazandijian VA. Directly observed therapy for treatment completion of pulmonary tuberculosis. Consensus statement of the Public Health Tuberculosis Guidelines Panel. JAMA 1998;279:943-948.

Chaulk CP, Moore-Rice K, Rizzo R, et al. Eleven years of community-based directly observed therapy for tuberculosis. JAMA 1995;274:945-951.

Chavalittamvong B, Talalak P. Tuberculosis peritonitis in children. Prog Pediatr Surg 1982;15:161-167.

Cheng TL, Ottolin M, Getson P, et al. Poor validity of parent reading of skin test induration in a high-risk population. Pediatr Infect Dis J 1996;15:90-91.

Cohn DL, Catlin BJ, Peterson KC, et al. A 62-dose, 6-month therapy for pulmonary and extrapulmonary tuberculosis. Ann Intern Med 1990;112:407-415.

Colditz G, Berkey CS, Mosteller F, et al. The efficacy of bacillus Calmette-Gúerin vaccination of newborns and infants in the prevention of tuberculosis: meta-analysis of the published literature. Pediatrics 1995;96:29-35.

Colditz G, Brewer T, Berkey C, et al. Efficacy of BCG vaccine in the prevention of tuberculosis: meta-analysis of the published literature. JAMA 1994;271:698-702.

Comstock GW, Baum C, Snider DE Jr. Isoniazid prophylaxis among Alaskan Eskimos: final report of the Bethel isoniazid studies. Am Rev Respir Dis 1979;119:827-830.

Comstock GW, Edwards LB, Nabangxang H. Tuberculin sensitivity eight to fifteen years after BCG vaccination. Am Rev Respir Dis 1971;103:572-575.

Cuneo WD, Snider DE Jr. Enhancing patient compliance with tuberculosis therapy. Clin Chest Med 1989;10: 375-380.

Curless RG, Mitchell CD. Central nervous system tuberculosis in children. Pediatr Neurol 1991;7:270-274.

Curtis A, Ridzon R, Vogel R. Extensive transmission of Mycobacterium tuberculosis from a child. N Engl J Med 1999;341:1491-1495.

Daly JF, Brown DS, Lincoln EM, et al. Endobronchial tuberculosis in children. Dis Chest 1952;22:380-398.

Dandapat MC, Mishra BM, Dash SP, et al. Peripheral lymph node tuberculosis: review of 80 cases. Br J Surg 1990;77:911-912.

Dannenberg AM Jr. Delayed-type hypersensitivity and cell-mediated immunity in the pathogenesis of tuberculosis. Immunol Today 1991;12:228-234.

de Blic J, Azevedo I, Burren C, et al. The value of flexible bronchoscopy in childhood pulmonary tuberculosis. Chest 1991;100:188-192.

Delacourt C, Gobin J, Gaillard J, et al. Value of ELISA using antigen 60 for the diagnosis of tuberculosis in children. Chest 1993a;104:393-398.

Delacourt C, Mani TM, Bonnerot V, et al. Computed tomography with normal chest radiograph in tuberculous infection. Arch Dis Child 1993b;69:430-432.

Delacourt C, Poveda JD, Churean C, et al. Use of polymerase chain reaction for improved diagnosis of tuberculosis in children. J Pediatr 1995;126:703-709.

Doerr CA, Starke JR, Ong LT. Clinical and public health aspects of tuberculous meningitis in children. J Pediatr 1995;127:27-33.

Donald PR, Seifart H. Cerebrospinal fluid pyrazinamide concentrations in children with tuberculous meningitis. Pediatr Infect Dis J 1988;7:469-471.

Donald PR, Seifart HI. Cerebrospinal fluid concentrations of ethionamide in children with tuberculous meningitis. J Pediatr 1989;115:483-486.

Donald PR, Schoeman JF, VanZyl LE, et al. Intensive short course chemotherapy in the management of tuberculous meningitis. Int J Tuberc Lung Dis 1998;2:704-711.

Dormer BA, Harrison I, Swart JA, et al. Prophylactic isoniazid protection of infants in a tuberculosis hospital. Lancet 1959;2:902-903.

Dunlap NE, Harris RH, Benjamin WH Jr, et al. Laboratory contamination of Mycobacterium tuberculosis cultures. Am J Respir Crit Care Med 1995;152:1702-1704.

Dutt AK, Moers D, Stead WW. Short-course chemotherapy for extrapulmonary tuberculosis. Ann Intern Med 1986; 107:7-12.

Dye C, Espinal MA, Watt CJ, et al. Worldwide incidence of multidrug-resistant tuberculosis. J Infect Dis 2002;185: 1197-1202.

Ehrlich RM, Lattimer J. Urogenital tuberculosis in children. J Urol 1971;105:461-465.

Eisenach KD, Sifford MD, Cave MD, et al. Detection of Mycobacterium tuberculosis in sputum samples using a polymerase chain reaction. Am Rev Respir Dis 1991;144: 1160-1163.

Escobar JA, Belsey MA, Dueñas A, et al. Mortality from tuberculous meningitis reduced by steroid therapy. Pediatrics 1975;56:1050-1055.

Ferrebee SH. Controlled chemoprophylaxis trials in tuberculosis: a general review. Adv Tuberc Res 1969;17: 28-106.

Figueroa-Damian R, Arredondo-Garcia JL. Neonatal outcome of children born to women with tuberculosis. Arch Med Res 2001;32:66-69.

Frieden TR, Sterling T, Pablos-Mendez A, et al. The emergence of drug-resistant tuberculosis in New York City. N Engl J Med 1993;328:521-526.

Friedland JR. The booster effect with repeat tuberculin testing in children and its relationship to BCG vaccination. S Afr Med J 1990;77:387-389.

Froehlich H, Ackerson LM, Morozumi PA. Targeted testing of children for tuberculosis: validation of a risk assessment questionnaire. Pediatrics 2001;107:e54.

George RH, Gully PR, Gill ON, et al. An outbreak of tuberculosis in a children's hospital. J Hosp Infect 1986;8:129-142.

Girgis NI, Fariz Z, Kilpatrick ME, et al. Dexamethasone adjunctive treatment for tuberculous meningitis. Pediatr Infect Dis J 1991;10:179-182.

Goble M, Iseman MD, Madsen LA, et al. Treatment of 171 patients with pulmonary tuberculosis resistant to isoniazid and rifampin. N Engl J Med 1993;328:527-532.

Gomez LP, Morris SL, Panduro A. Rapid and efficient detection of extra-pulmonary Mycobacterium tuberculosis by PCR analysis. Int J Tuberc Lung Dis 2000;4: 361-370.

Gonzalez B, Moreno S, Burdach R, et al. Clinical presentation of bacillus Calmette-Guérin infections in patients with immunodeficiency syndromes. Pediatr Infect Dis J 1989;8:201-206.

Graziani AL, MacGregor RR. Self-reading of tuberculin testing vs physician reading. Infect Dis Clin Pract 1995;4:72-74.

Gutman L, Moye J, Zimmer B, et al. Tuberculosis in human immunodeficiency virus–exposed or –infected United States children. Pediatr Infect Dis J 1994;13:963-968.

Hageman J, Shulman S, Schreiber M, et al. Congenital tuberculosis: critical reappraisal of clinical findings and diagnostic procedures. Pediatrics 1980;66:980-984.

Harries AD, Hargreaves NJ, Graham S, et al. Childhood tuberculosis in Malawi: nationwide case-finding and treatment outcomes. Int J Tuberc Lung Dis 2002;6:424-431.

Harris VJ, Dida F, Landers SS, et al. Cavitary tuberculosis in children. J Pediatr 1977;90:660-661.

Haygood T, Williamson S. Radiographic findings of extremity tuberculosis in childhood: back to the future? Radiographics 1994;14:561-570.

Hoffman ND, Kelly C, Futterman D. Tuberculosis infection in human immunodeficiency virus–positive adolescents and young adults: a New York City cohort. Pediatrics 1996;97:198-203.

Hoge C, Fisher L, Donnell D, et al. Risk factors for transmission of Mycobacterium tuberculosis in a primary school outbreak: lack of racial difference in susceptibility to infection. Am J Epidemiol 1994;139:520-530.

Hong Kong Chest Service/British Medical Research Council. Controlled trial of 2, 4, and 6 months of pyrazinamide in 6-month, three-times-weekly regimens for smear-positive pulmonary tuberculosis, including an assessment of a combined preparation of isoniazid, rifampin, and pyrazinamide: results at 30 months. Am Rev Respir Dis 1991;143:700-706.

Howard TP, Soloman DA. Reading the tuberculin skin test: who, when, and how? Arch Intern Med 1988;148:2457-2459.

Hsu KHK. Contact investigation: a practical approach to tuberculosis eradication. Am J Public Health 1963;53:1761-769.

Hsu KHK. Tuberculin reaction in children treated with isoniazid. Am J Dis Child 1983;137:1090-1092.

Hsu KHK. Thirty years after isoniazid: its impact on tuberculosis in children and adolescents. JAMA 1984;251:1283-1285.

Huebner RE, Schein MF, Bass JB. The tuberculin skin test. Clin Infect Dis 1993;17:968-975.

Hugo-Hamman CT, Scher H, DeMoor MMA. Tuberculous pericarditis in children: a review of 44 cases. Pediatr Infect Dis J 1994;13:13-18.

Humphries MJ, Teoh R, Lau J, et al. Factors of prognostic significance in Chinese children with tuberculous meningitis. Tubercle 1990;71:161-168.

Hussey G, Chisolm T, Kibel M. Miliary tuberculosis in children: a review of 94 cases. Pediatr Infect Dis J 1991;10:832-836.

Hussey G, Kibel M, Parker N. Ciprofloxacin treatment of multiply drug-resistant extrapulmonary tuberculosis in a child. Pediatr Infect Dis J 1992;11:408-409.

International Union Against Tuberculosis Committee on Prophylaxis. Efficacy of various durations of isoniazid preventive therapy for tuberculosis: five years of follow-up in the IUAT trial. Bull World Health Organ 1982;160:555-564.

Iseman MD. Treatment of multidrug-resistant tuberculosis. N Engl J Med 1993;329:784-791.

Iseman MD, Cohn DL, Sbarbaro JA. Directly observed treatment of tuberculosis: we can't afford not to try it. N Engl J Med 1993;328:576-578.

Iseman MD, Madsen L, Goble M, et al. Surgical intervention in the treatment of pulmonary disease caused by drug-resistant Mycobacterium tuberculosis. Am Rev Respir Dis 1990;141:623-625.

Jacobs RF, Sunakorn P, Chotpitayasunonah T, et al. Intensive short-course chemotherapy for tuberculous meningitis. Pediatr Infect Dis J 1992;11:194-198.

Jagannath C, Reddy MV, Kailasam S, et al. Chemotherapeutic activity of clofazamine and its analogues against Mycobacterium tuberculosis. Am J Respir Crit Care Med 1995;151:1083-1086.

Jawahar MS, Sivasubramanian S, Vijayan VK, et al. Short-course chemotherapy for tuberculous lymphadenitis in children. BMJ 1990;301:359-362.

Jones D, Malecki J, Bigler W, et al. Pediatric tuberculosis and human immunodeficiency virus infection in Palm Beach County, Florida. Am J Dis Child 1992;146:1166-1170.

Kendig EL Jr. The place of BCG vaccine in the management of infants born to tuberculous mothers. N Engl J Med 1969;281:520-523.

Kendig EL Jr, Kirkpatrick BY, Carter WH, et al. Underreading of the tuberculin skin test reaction. Chest 1998;113:1175-1177.

Kendig EL Jr, Rodgers WL. Tuberculosis in the neonatal period. Am Rev Tuberc Pulm Dis 1958;77:418-422.

Kennedy N, Fox R, Kisyombe GM, et al. Early bactericidal and sterilizing activities of ciprofloxacin in pulmonary tuberculosis. Am Rev Respir Dis 1993; 148:1547-1551.

Khan EA, Starke JR. Diagnosis of tuberculosis in children: increased need for better methods. Emerg Infect Dis 1995;1:115-123.

Khouri Y, Mastrucci M, Hutto C, et al. Mycobacterium tuberculosis in children with human immunodeficiency virus type 1 infection. Pediatr Infect Dis J 1992;11:950-955.

Kimmerling ME, Vaughn ES, Dunlap NE. Childhood tuberculosis in Alabama: epidemiology of disease and indicators of program effectiveness, 1983 to 1993. Pediatr Infect Dis J 1995;14:678-684.

Kiwanuka J, Graham SM, Coulter JB, et al. Diagnosis of pulmonary tuberculosis in children in an HIV-endemic area, Malawi. Ann Trop Paediatr 2001;21:5-14.

Kochi A. The global tuberculosis situation and the new control strategy of the World Health Organization. Tuber Lung Dis 1991;72:1-6.

Kohn MR, Arden MR, Vasilakis J, et al. Directly observed preventive therapy: turning the tide against tuberculosis. Arch Pediatr Adolesc Med 1996;150:727-729.

Kumar A, Misra PK, Mehotra R, et al. Hepatotoxicity of rifampin and isoniazid: is it all drug-induced hepatitis? Am Rev Respir Dis 1991;143:1350-1352.

Kumar B, Rai R, Kaur I, et al. Childhood cutaneous tuberculosis; a study over 25 years from northern India. Int J Dermatol 2001;40:26-32.

Kumar L, Dhand R, Singhi PD, et al. A randomized trial of fully intermittent vs daily followed by intermittent short-course chemotherapy for childhood tuberculosis. Pediatr Infect Dis J 1990;9:802-806.

Kumar R, Pandey CK, Bose N, Sahay S. Tuberculous brain abscess: clinical presentation, pathophysiology and treatment (in children). Childs Nerv Syst 2002;18:118-123.

Lamprecht D, Schoeman J, Donald P, et al. Ventriculoperitoneal shunting in childhood tuberculous meningitis. Br J Neurosurg 2001;15:119-125.

Lange WR, Warnock-Eckhart E, Bean ME. *Mycobacterium tuberculosis* infection in foreign-born adoptees. Pediatr Infect Dis J 1989;8:625-629.

Lee C, Wang W, Lan R, et al. Corticosteroids in the treatment of tuberculous pleurisy: a double-blind, placebo-controlled randomized study. Chest 1988;94:1256-1259.

Lee LH, Le Vea CM, Graman PS. Congenital tuberculosis in a neonatal intensive care unit: case report, epidemiologic investigation and management of exposures. Clin Infect Dis 1998;27:474-477.

Leggiadro RJ, Collery B, Dowdy S. Outbreak of tuberculosis in a family day-care home. Pediatr Infect Dis J 1989;8:52-54.

Leiguarda R, Berthier M, Starkstein S, et al. Ischemic infarction in 25 children with tuberculous meningitis. Stroke 1988;19:200-204.

Light IJ, Saidleman M, Sutherland JM. Management of newborns after nursery exposure to tuberculosis. Am Rev Respir Dis 1974;109:415-419.

Lincoln EM. Epidemics of tuberculosis. Adv Tuberc Res 1965;14:159-197.

Lincoln EM, Davies PA, Bovornkitti S. Tuberculous pleurisy with effusion in children. Am Rev Tuberc 1958;77:271-289.

Lincoln EM, Gilbert L, Morales SM. Chronic pulmonary tuberculosis in individuals with known previous primary tuberculosis. Dis Chest 1960;38:473-482.

Lincoln EM, Harris LC, Bovornkitti S, et al. Endobronchial tuberculosis in children. Am Rev Tuberc Pulm Dis 1958;77:39-61.

Lindgren I. Pathology of tuberculous infection in BCG-vaccinated humans. Adv Tuberc Res 1965;14:203-231.

Lobato M, Hopewell PC: *Mycobacterium tuberculosis* infection after travel to or contact with visitors from countries with a high prevalence of tuberculosis. Am J Respir Crit Care Med 1998;158:1871-1875.

Lobato NM, Mohle-Boetani JC, Royce SE. Missed opportunities for preventing tuberculosis among children younger than five years of age. Pediatrics 2000;106:e75.

MacAdam AM, Rubio T. Tuberculous otomastoiditis in children. Am J Dis Child 1977;131:152-156.

Mahmoudi A, Iseman M. Pitfalls in the care of patients with tuberculosis: common errors and their association with the acquisition of drug resistance. JAMA 1993; 270:65-68.

Mancao MY, Nolte FS, Nahmias AJ, et al. Use of polymerase chain reaction for diagnosis of tuberculous meningitis. Pediatr Infect Dis J 1994;13:154-155.

Martinez-Roig A, Cami J, Llorens-Terol J, et al. Acetylation phenotype and hepatotoxicity in the treatment of tuberculosis in children. Pediatrics 1986;77:912-915.

Matsaniotis N, Kattanis C, Economou-Mavrou C, et al. Bullous emphysema in childhood tuberculosis. J Pediatr 1967;71:703-708.

McKenzie SA, McNab AJ, Katz G. Neonatal pyridoxine responsive convulsions due to isoniazid therapy. Arch Dis Child 1976;51:567-568.

Medical Research Council Working Party on Tuberculosis of the Spine. Twelfth report: controlled trial of short-course regimens of chemotherapy in the ambulatory treatment of spinal tuberculosis. J Bone Joint Surg 1993; 75:240-248.

Mehta JB, Bentley S. Prevention of tuberculosis in children: missed opportunities. Am J Prev Med 1992;8:283-286.

Menzies R, Vissandjee B. Effect of bacille Calmette-Gúerin vaccination on tuberculin reactivity. Am Rev Respir Dis 1992;141:621-625.

Migliori GB, Borghesi A, Rossanigo P, et al. Proposal of an improved score method for the diagnosis of pulmonary tuberculosis in childhood in developing countries. Tuber Lung Dis 1992;73:145-149.

Mitchison DA, Nunn AJ. Influence of initial drug resistance on the response to short-course chemotherapy of pulmonary tuberculosis. Am Rev Respir Dis 1986;133: 423-428.

Mohle-Boetani JC, Flood J. Contact investigations and the continued commitment to control tuberculosis. JAMA 2002;287:1040-1041.

Mohle-Boetani JC, Miller B, Halpern M, et al. School-based screening for tuberculous infection: a cost benefit analysis. JAMA 1995;274:613-619.

Morrison JB. Natural history of segmental lesions in primary pulmonary tuberculosis. Arch Dis Child 1973; 48:90-98.

Mudido PM, Guratudde D, Nakakeeto MK, et al. The effect of bacilli Calmette-Gúerin vaccination at birth on tuberculin skin test reactivity in Ugandan children. Int J Tuberc Lung Dis 1999;3:891-895.

Mumtaz MA, Schwartz RH, Grundfast KM, et al. Tuberculosis of the middle ear and mastoid. Pediatr Infect Dis J 1983;2:234-236.

Nemir RL, Cardona J, Vaziri F, et al. Prednisone as an adjunct in the chemotherapy of lymph node–bronchial tuberculosis in childhood: a double-blind study. II. Further term observation. Am Rev Respir Dis 1967;95:402-410.

Nemir RL, O'Hare D. Congenital tuberculosis. Am J Dis Child 1985;139:284-287.

Nemir RL, Teichner A. Management of tuberculin reactors in children and adolescents previously vaccinated with BCG. Pediatr Infect Dis J 1983;2:446-451.

Nolan R Jr. Childhood tuberculosis in North Carolina: a study of the opportunities for intervention in the transmission of tuberculosis in children. Am J Public Health 1986;76:26-30.

O'Brien K, Ruff A, Louis M, et al. Bacillus Calmette-Gúerin complications in children born to HIV-1–infected women with a review of the literature. Pediatrics 1995;95:414-418.

O'Brien RJ, Long MW, Cross FS, et al. Hepatotoxicity from isoniazid and rifampin among children treated for tuberculosis. Pediatrics 1983;72:491-499.

Offenbacher H, Fazekas F, Schmidt R, et al. MRI in tuberculous meningoencephalitis: report of four cases and review of the neuroimaging literature. J Neurol 1991;238:340-344.

Optican RJ, Ost A, Ravin CE. High-resolution computed tomography in the diagnosis of miliary tuberculosis. Chest 1992;102:941-943.

Orme IM, Anderson P, Boom WH. T-cell response to *Mycobacterium tuberculosis*. J Infect Dis 1993;167:1481-1497.

Ozuah PO, Ozuah TP, Stein REK, et al. Evaluation of a risk assessment questionnaire used to target tuberculin skin testing in children. JAMA 2001;285:451-453.

Palur R, Rajohekhar V, Chandy MJ, et al. Shunt surgery for hydrocephalus in tuberculous meningitis: a long-term follow-up study. J Neurosurg 1991;74:64-69.

Parish RE, Brownstein D. Emergency department management of children with acute isoniazid poisoning. Pediatr Emerg Care 1986;2:88-90.

Park MM, Davis AL, Schluger NW, et al. Outcome of MDR-TB patients, 1983-1993: prolonged survival with appropriate therapy. Am J Respir Crit Care Med 1996;153:317-324.

Passannante M, Gallagher C, Reichman L. Preventive therapy for contacts of multidrug-resistant tuberculosis: a Delphi study. Chest 1994;106:431-434.

Pastrana DG, Torronteras R, Caro P, et al. Comparison of Amplicor, in-house polymerase chain reactions and conventional culture for the diagnosis of tuberculosis in children. Clin Infect Dis 2002;32:17-22. .

Pellock JM, Howell J, Kendig EL Jr, et al. Pyridoxine deficiency in children treated with isoniazid. Chest 1985;87:658-661.

Peloquin CA, MacPhee AA, Berning SE. Malabsorption of antimycobacterial medications. N Engl J Med 1993;329:1122-1123.

Perry S, Starke JR. Adherence to prescribed treatment and public health aspects of tuberculosis in children. Semin Pediatr Infect Dis 1993;4:291-298.

Pierre C, Olivier C, Lecossier D, et al. Diagnosis of primary tuberculosis in children by amplification and detection of mycobacterial DNA. Am Rev Respir Dis 1993;147:420-424.

Pineda P, Leung A, Muller N, et al. Intrathoracic pediatric tuberculosis: a report of 202 cases. Tuber Lung Dis 1993;74:261-266.

Rasool MN. Osseous manifestations of tuberculosis in children. J Pediatr Orthop 2001;21:749-755.

Ravenscroft A, Schoeman JF, Donald PR. Tuberculous granulomas in childhood tuberculous meningitis: radiologic features and course. J Trop Pediatr 2001;47:5-12.

Raviglione MC, Snider D Jr, Kochi A. Global epidemiology of tuberculosis: morbidity and mortality of a worldwide epidemic. JAMA 1995;273:220-226.

Reynes J, Perez C, Lamaury I, et al. Bacille Calmette-Gúerin adenitis 30 years after immunization in a patient with AIDS. J Infect Dis 1989;160:727.

Roy V, Tekur U, Chopra K. Pharmacokinetics of pyrazinamide in children suffering from pulmonary tuberculosis. Int J Tuberc Lung Dis 1999;3:133-137.

Ryder RW, Oxtoby MJ, Mvula M, et al. Safety and immunogenicity of bacille Calmette-Gúerin, diphtheria-tetanus-pertussis, and oral polio vaccines in newborn children in Zaire infected with human immunodeficiency virus type 1. J Pediatr 1993;122:697-702.

Saczek KB, Schaaf HS, Voss M, et al. Diagnostic dilemmas in abdominal tuberculosis in children. Pediatr Surg Int 2001;17:111-115.

Sada E, Aguilar D, Torres M, et al. Detection of lipoarabinomannan as a diagnostic test for tuberculosis. J Clin Microbiol 1992;30:2415-2418.

Saiman L, Aronson J, Zhou J, et al. Prevalence of infectious diseases among internationally adopted children. Pediatrics 2001;108:608-612.

Sanchez-Albisva I, Vidal M, Joya-Verde G, et al. Tolerance of pyrazinamide in short course chemotherapy for pulmonary tuberculosis in children. Pediatr Infect Dis J 1997;16:760-763.

Schaaf HS, Beyers N, Gie RP, et al. Respiratory tuberculosis in childhood: the diagnostic value of clinical features and special investigations. Pediatr Infect Dis J 1995;14:189-194.

Schaaf HS, Gie RP, Beyers N, et al. Tuberculosis in infants less than 3 months of age. Arch Dis Child 1993;69:371-374.

Schaaf HS, Gie RP, Beyers N, et al. Primary drug-resistant tuberculosis in children. Int J Tuberc Lung Dis 2000;4:1-7.

Schick B, Dolgin J. The influence of prednisone on the Mantoux reaction in children. Pediatrics 1963;31:856-859.

Schuit KE. Miliary tuberculosis in children. Am J Dis Child 1979;133:583-585.

Schuit KE, Powell DA. Mycobacterial lymphadenitis in childhood. Am J Dis Child 1978;132:675-677.

Selwyn P, Hartel D, Lewis V, et al. A prospective study of the risk of tuberculosis among intravenous drug users with human immunodeficiency virus infection. N Engl J Med 1989;320:545-550.

Sepulveda RL, Burr C, Ferrer X, et al. Booster effect of tuberculosis testing in healthy 6-year-old schoolchildren vaccinated with bacille Calmette-Gúerin at birth in Santiago, Chile. Pediatr Infect Dis J 1988;7:578-582.

Shah BR, Santucci K, Sinert R, et al. Acute isoniazid neurotoxicity in an urban hospital. Pediatrics 1995;95:700-704.

Shata AMA, Coulter JBS, Parry CM, et al. Sputum induction for the diagnosis of tuberculosis. Arch Dis Child 1996;74:535-537.

Shepard WE, Field ML, James DH, et al. Transient appearance of intracranial tuberculomas during treatment of tuberculous meningitis. Pediatr Infect Dis J 1986;5:599-601.

Small P, Hopewell P, Singh S, et al. The epidemiology of tuberculosis in San Francisco: a population-based study using conventional and molecular methods. N Engl J Med 1994;330:1703-1709.

Small PM, Shafer RW, Hopewell PC, et al. Exogenous reinfection with multidrug-resistant *Mycobacterium tuberculosis* in patients with advanced HIV infection. N Engl J Med 1993;328:1137-1144.

Smith AM, Lattimer JK. Genitourinary tract involvement in children with tuberculosis. NY State J Med 1973;73:2325-2328.

Smith KC, Starke JR, Eisenach K, et al. Detection of *Mycobacterium tuberculosis* in clinical specimens from children using a polymerase chain reaction. Pediatrics 1996;97:155-160.

Smith MHD. The role of adrenal steroids in the treatment of tuberculosis. Pediatrics 1958;22:774-776.

Snider DE Jr, Caras GJ. Isoniazid-associated hepatitis deaths: a review of available information. Am Rev Respir Dis 1992;145:494-497.

Snider DE Jr, Caras GJ, Kaplan JP. Preventive therapy with isoniazid: cost-effectiveness of different durations of therapy. JAMA 1986;255:1579-1583.

Snider DE, Graczyk J, Bek E, et al. Supervised six-months treatment of newly diagnosed pulmonary tuberculosis using isoniazid, rifampin, and pyrazinamide with and without streptomycin. Am Rev Respir Dis 1984;130: 1091-1094.

Snider DE Jr, Johnson KE. Should women taking antituberculosis drugs breastfeed? Arch Intern Med 1984; 144:589-590.

Snider DE Jr, Kelly GD, Cauthen GM, et al. Infection and disease among contacts of tuberculosis cases with drug-resistant and drug-susceptible bacilli. Am Rev Respir Dis 1985;132:125-128.

Solazar GE, Schmitz TL, Cama R, et al. Pulmonary tuberculosis ill children in a developing country. Pediatrics 2001;108:448-453.

Starke JR. Tuberculosis of the central nervous system in children. Semin Pediatr Neurol 1999;6:318-331.

Starke JR. Transmission of *Mycobacterium tuberculosis* to and from children and adolescents. Semin Pediatr Infect Dis 2001;12:115-123.

Starke JR, Correa AG. Management of mycobacterial infection and disease in children. Pediatr Infect Dis J 1995;14:455-470.

Starke JR, Jacobs R, Jereb J. Resurgence of tuberculosis in children. J Pediatr 1992;120:839-855.

Starke JR, Taylor-Watts KT. Tuberculosis in the pediatric population of Houston, Texas. Pediatrics 1989;84:28-35.

Steiner P, Rao M. Drug-resistant tuberculosis in children. Semin Pediatr Infect Dis 1993;4:275-282.

Steiner P, Rao M, Mitchell M. Primary drug-resistant tuberculosis in children: correlation of drug-susceptibility patterns of matched patient and source-case strains of *Mycobacterium tuberculosis*. Am J Dis Child 1985; 139:780-782.

Steiner P, Rao M, Victoria MS, et al. Miliary tuberculosis in two infants after nursery exposure: epidemiologic, clinical, and laboratory findings. Am Rev Respir Dis 1976; 113:267-271.

Steiner P, Rao M, Victoria MS, et al. Persistently negative tuberculin reactions: their presence among children culture-positive for *Mycobacterium tuberculosis*. Am J Dis Child 1980;134:747-750.

Stransberry SD. Tuberculosis in infants and children. J Thorac Imaging 1990;5:17-27.

Sumartojo E. When tuberculosis treatment fails: a social behavior account of patient adherence. Am Rev Respir Dis 1993;147:1311-1320.

Swanson DS, Starke JR. Drug-resistant tuberculosis in pediatrics. Pediatr Clin North Am 1995;42:553-581.

Talbot EA, Moore M, McCray E, et al. Tuberculosis among foreign-born persons in the United States, 1993-1998. JAMA 2000;284:2894-2900.

Te Water Naude JM, Donald PR, Hussey GD, et al. Twice weekly vs. daily chemotherapy for childhood tuberculosis. Pediatr Infect Dis J 2000;19:405-410.

Teeratkulpisarn J, Lumbigagnon P, Pairojkul S, et al. Cavitary tuberculosis in a young infant. Pediatr Infect Dis J 1994;13:545-546.

Telenti A, Imboden P, Marchesi F, et al. Detection of rifampin-resistance mutations in *Mycobacterium tuberculosis*. Lancet 1993;341:647-650.

Telzak EE, Sepkowitz K, Alpert P, et al. Multidrug-resistant tuberculosis in patients without HIV infection. N Engl J Med 1995;333:907-911.

Teoh R, Humphries MJ, O'Mahony G. Symptomatic intracranial tuberculoma developing during treatment of tuberculosis: report of 10 patients and review of the literature. QJM 1987;63:449-460.

Thompson WJ, Glassroth JL, Snider DE Jr, et al. The booster phenomenon in serial tuberculin testing. Am Rev Respir Dis 1979;119:587-597.

Tsakalidis D, Pratsidou P, Hitoglou-Makedou A, et al. Intensive short-course chemotherapy for treatment of Greek children with tuberculosis. Pediatr Infect Dis J 1992;11:1036-1042.

Turnbull PM, McIntyre PB, Achat HM, et al. National study of adverse reactions after vaccination with bacilli Calmette-Gúerin. Clin Infect Dis 2002;34:447-453.

Turneer M, VanNerom E, Nyabenda J, et al. Determination of humoral immunoglobulins M and G directed against mycobacterial antigen 60 failed to diagnose primary tuberculosis and mycobacterial adenitis in children. Am J Respir Crit Care Med 1994;150;1508-1512.

Ussery XT, Valway SE, McKenna M, et al. Epidemiology of tuberculosis among children in the United States. Pediatr Infect Dis J 1996;15:697-704.

Vallejo J, Ong L, Starke JR. Clinical features, diagnosis, and treatment of tuberculosis in infants. Pediatrics 1994; 94:1-7.

Vallejo J, Ong L, Starke JR. Tuberculous osteomyelitis of the long bones in children. Pediatr Infect Dis J 1995; 14:542-546.

Vallejo JG, Starke JR. Tuberculosis and pregnancy. Clin Chest Med 1992;13:693-707.

Vanderhoof JA, Ament ME. Fatal hepatic necrosis due to isoniazid chemoprophylaxis in a 15-year-old girl. J Pediatr 1976;88:867-868.

Waeker NJ Jr, Connor JD. Central nervous system tuberculosis in children: a review of 30 cases. Pediatr Infect Dis J 1990;9:539-543.

Wallace RC, Burton EM, Barrett FF, et al. Intracranial tuberculosis in children: CT appearance and clinical outcome. Pediatr Radiol 1991;21:241-246.

Wallgren A. On contagiousness of childhood tuberculosis. Acta Paediatr 1937;22:229-234.

Weinstein J, Barrett C, Baltimore R, et al. Nosocomial transmission of tuberculosis from a hospital visitor on a pediatrics ward. Pediatr Infect Dis J 1995;14:232-234.

Weis S, Slocum P, Blais F, et al. The effects of directly observed therapy on the rates of drug resistance and relapse in tuberculosis. N Engl J Med 1994;330: 1179-1184.

Weismuller MM, Graham SM, Claessens NJM, et al. Diagnosis of childhood tuberculosis in Malawi: an audit of hospital practice. Int J Tuberc Lung Dis 2002;6: 432-438.

Whalen C, Horsburgh C, Hom D, et al. Accelerated course of human immunodeficiency virus infection after tuberculosis. Am J Respir Crit Care Med 1995;151:129-135.

Zhang Y. Genetic basis of isoniazid resistance of *Mycobacterium tuberculosis*. Rev Microbiol 1993;144: 143-150.

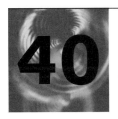

40 URINARY TRACT INFECTIONS

KEITH M. KRASINSKI

The term *urinary tract infection* (UTI) refers to a clinical entity that may involve the urethra and/or bladder (lower urinary tract); and the ureters, renal pelvis, calyces, and/or renal parenchyma (upper urinary tract). Urethritis as a clinical entity is discussed in Chapter 32.

Because it is often impossible to localize the infection to either the lower tract or the upper tract, UTI is a convenient designation. Most bacterial UTIs are characterized by the presence of significant numbers of bacteria in the urine.

The designation *significant bacteriuria* refers to the number of bacteria in excess of the usual bacterial contamination of the anterior urethra. The presence of more than 100,000 bacteria per milliliter of urine in a clean voided specimen probably is the result of infection, not contamination at the time of voiding. Asymptomatic bacteriuria is defined as significant bacteriuria in a patient who has no clinical evidence of active infection.

Lower UTI is usually characterized by dysuria, frequency, urgency, and possibly suprapubic tenderness. The clinical manifestations of acute pyelonephritis may include fever, lumbar pain and tenderness, dysuria, urgency, and frequency associated with significant bacteriuria.

Recurrence of a UTI may be caused by a relapse or a reinfection. A relapse is a recurrence of the infection with the same infecting microorganism, perhaps indicating inadequate therapy. A reinfection is a new infection caused by a bacterium that is different from the one responsible for the previous episode. Specific identification may require serotyping, pyocin typing, phage typing, antibiotic typing, or genetic typing of the bacterium (e.g., *Escherichia coli*), procedures that are not uniformly available to the clinician. These identification tech-niques may also be useful for associating individual incidents with hospital outbreaks of infection. The term *chronic infection* is sometimes used to describe (1) persistence of the UTI associated with the same organism for many months or years, or (2) frequent recurrences over many months or years.

ETIOLOGY

Some of the microorganisms that cause UTIs include the following:

Gram-negative bacteria
- *Escherichia coli*
- *Klebsiella pneumoniae*
- *Proteus mirabilis*
- *Enterobacter aerogenes*
- *Pseudomonas aeruginosa*
- *Serratia marcescens*
- *Salmonella* species
- *Haemophilus influenzae*
- *Gardnerella vaginalis*

Gram-positive bacteria
- *Staphylococcus epidermidis*
- *Enterococcus* species
- *Staphylococcus aureus*
- *Staphylococcus saprophyticus*
- *Streptococcus pneumoniae*

Other agents
- Adenovirus types 11 and 21
- BK virus
- *Candida albicans*
- *Mycoplasma hominis*
- *Ureaplasma urealyticum*
- *Mycobacterium tuberculosis*
- *Schistosoma haematobium*

The most common pathogens are the gram-negative bacilli. Of this group, *E. coli* is responsible for most acute infections. The other gram-negative bacteria—such as *Proteus*, *Pseudomonas*, *Klebsiella*, and *Enterobacter* species—are more likely to be associated with chronic or recurrent infections. *Salmonella* bacteriuria is usually associated with salmonellal sepsis.

Gram-positive bacteria such as *S. epidermidis*, *S. saprophyticus*, and *S. aureus* have been identified as causes of UTIs. Coagulase-negative staphylococci have been detected as urinary tract pathogens in sexually active young women (Bailey, 1973; Vosti, 1975) and newborns (Khan et al., 1975). Coagulase-positive staphylococci may invade the urinary tract through the hematogenous route.

Adenovirus types 11 and 21 and the human papovavirus BK have been reported as causes of acute hemorrhagic cystitis (Hashida et al., 1976; Mufson and Belshe, 1976; Padgett et al., 1987; Rice et al., 1985). Symptomatic and asymptomatic BK viruria is associated with bone marrow transplantation. Fungi such as *C. albicans* may be responsible for UTIs (1) in patients with indwelling catheters during the course of their treatment with antibiotics; (2) in patients immunocompromised as a result of disease, steroids, or cytotoxic chemotherapy; and (3) as a result of renal seeding during fungemia.

PATHOGENESIS

The ascending route is the most common pathway of UTI. Bacteria that colonize the perineum and distal urethra may eventually spread to the bladder. Massage of the urethra such as occurs during masturbation and sexual intercourse forces bacteria into the bladder (Bran et al., 1972; Buckley et al., 1978). Hematogenous spread may occur during the course of neonatal sepsis; however, even in infants, ascending infection leading to bacteremia is more common. Lymphatic spread has been suggested, but it has not been proved (Murphy et al., 1960).

In older children and adolescents with staphylococcal sepsis or endocarditis, hematogenous spread to the kidney may result in abscess formation. Abscesses also result from infection ascending via the collecting system, followed by renal seeding and localized liquefaction. Intense focal edema at the site of kidney infection, which may appear on ultrasonographic exam as a mass effect, has been termed *lobar nephronia*. Intrarenal suppurative necrosis is most evident in the cortex when it occurs; however, abscesses also occur in the medulla. The natural methods of extension include rupture into the renal pelvis and extension through the renal capsule, producing a perinephric (perirenal) abscess. A more chronic destructive process, associated with lipid laden macrophages, and often stone formation, is termed *xanthogranulomatous pyelonephritis*.

The pathogenesis of a UTI is dependent in great part on factors associated with both the microorganism and the host. The following virulence factors of microorganisms are associated with UTIs:
1. Size of inoculum
2. Pili or fimbriae (mucosal cell adherence)
   a. Mannose-sensitive type 1, common
   b. P pili
   c. X pili
3. Surface antigens
4. Motility
5. Urease production

Microorganism

Experimental studies in mice have revealed that the greater the number of organisms delivered to the kidney the greater the chance of inducing pyelonephritis (Gorrill and De Navasquez, 1964). Thus the size of the inoculum is an important factor. Evidence accumulated during the course of studies by Gruneberg et al. (1968) and by Kaijser (1973) indicates that certain organisms apparently are particularly virulent for the urinary tract. Of the 150 or more *E. coli* O serogroups, only a few (01, 02, 04, 06, 07, 075) have been responsible for most UTIs, and these especially include those that possess large quantities of K antigen. *E. coli* K antigen types 11, 24, 36, and 37 account for the majority of isolates from children with pyelonephritis (Kaijser et al., 1977; Marild et al., 1989).

E. coli O antigens are cell-wall lipopolysaccharides that are immunogenic and induce local and systemic antibody responses in patients with pyelonephritis. Strains most often associated with pyelonephritis are representatives of 80 antigen groups. The specific O antigens appear to confer the ability to resist agglutination and bactericidal effects of serum, in contrast to the O serotypes of organisms causing cystitis (Lindberg et al., 1975; Marild et al., 1989; Smith et al., 1977).

A primary pathogenic factor is the presence of carbohydrate-binding proteins (adhesions, lectins, or hemagglutinins) often localized to pili. Pili are important for the attachment of *E. coli* and *P. mirabilis* to the urinary tract epithelium (Silverblatt, 1974). Almost all *E. coli* contain type 1 common pili that bind to mannose-containing receptors (Ofek et al., 1977) on epithelial cells of the urethra and vagina and are thought to be of primary importance in colonizing the lower urinary tract (Iwahi et al., 1983; Svanborg-Eden et al., 1983). *E. coli* isolates from patients with cystitis have a greater avidity and adhere in higher numbers to uroepithelial cells than do *E. coli* fecal isolates (Svanborg-Eden et al., 1976; Svanborg-Eden et al., 1981). Uropathogenic *E. coli* and *P. mirabilis* are capable of altering their surface composition (phase variation) and tend to lose their type 1 pili on arrival in the kidney (Ofek et al., 1981; Silverblatt, 1974). This ability to adapt to the microenvironment constitutes a selective advantage by promoting renal cell attachment and especially because variation of mannose receptors of type 1 pili allows escape from phagocytosis by polymorphonuclear leukocytes (Perry et al., 1983).

P pili bear an adhesin called *PapG* that causes mannose-resistant hemagglutination and binds to specific Galα 1-4 Gal glycolipid receptor sites on human epithelial cells (Kallenius et al., 1981; Leffler and Svanborg-Eden, 1981; Svanborg-Eden et al., 1981; Svanborg-Eden et al., 1983; Stromberg et al., 1990). *E. coli* with P pili have their favored site of attachment on the uroepithelium of the kidneys, where receptors are distributed with greatest density (Svanborg-Eden et al., 1976; Svanborg-Eden et al., 1983). P-fimbriae–expressing organisms elicit higher interleukin (IL)-8, IL-6, and neutrophil responses than P-fimbriae–negative organisms, confirming their virulence characteristics (Wullt et al., 2001). UTIs are more likely to occur in persons who express the P blood group antigen (Lindberg et al., 1983).

A third type of pili, X pili, are also capable of binding to uroepithelium. Their receptor sites have not been identified; however, they also have an affinity for the upper urinary tract.

Motility probably also is an important pathogenic factor. Weyrauch and Bassett (1951) have shown that motile bacteria can ascend in the ureter against the flow of the urine. Moreover, the ascent of these bacteria may be facilitated by the decreased ureteral peristalsis attributed to the endotoxin of gram-negative bacilli.

The production of urease by the infecting bacteria may affect their capacity to cause pyelonephritis. When UTI was induced in experimental animals by the retrograde administration of *P. mirabilis*, a urease-producing organism, there was a high degree of correlation between the number of bacteria in the kidney and the extent of renal damage. However, treatment with a urease inhibitor reduced the extent of renal damage and the number of bacteria in the kidney without a significant decrease in the number of bacteria in the urine (Musher et al., 1975).

Host

The known host defense mechanisms of the urinary tract are as follows:
- Antibacterial activity of urine
- Prostatic secretions of postpubescent males
- Flushing mechanisms of the bladder
- Low vaginal pH
- Estrogen
- Antiadherence effect of uromucoid
- Antiadherence effect of mucopolysaccharide
- Humoral immunity
- Local secretory immunity, IgA
- Lack of P blood group antigen
- Normal flora

The long male urethra, in contrast to the short female urethra, has been implicated as a reason for the disproportionately high female predilection for UTI.

Antibacterial activity of urine against certain bacteria has been described. Kaye (1968) has reported that extremes of osmolality, high urea concentration, low pH, and high concentration of organic acids may inhibit the growth of some bacteria that cause UTIs. However, with the usual range of pH (5.5 to 7.0) and osmolality (300 to 1,200), the rate of growth of *E. coli* has been reported as unaffected (Asscher et al., 1966).

The flushing mechanism of the bladder enhances the spontaneous clearance of bacteria. Voiding and dilution probably play an important role. Overhydration can have the negative effect of diluting and washing out the active antimicrobial substances from the medullary and papillary areas. However, on balance, maintaining urine flow seems prudent.

In adolescents and adults prostatic fluid may inhibit bacterial growth (Stamey et al., 1968). The role of prostatic secretions in prepubescent boys is unknown. The presence of estrogen may enhance the growth of some strains of *E. coli* (Harles et al., 1975). Glucose makes urine a better culture medium, and it inhibits the migrating, adhering, aggregating, and killing functions of polymorphonuclear leukocytes. In addition, the intact mucosal surfaces of animal bladders are resistant to bacterial invasion (Cobbs and Kaye, 1967).

Low vaginal pH apparently is an important factor responsible for lack of colonization (Stamey and Timothy, 1975). For example, serogroups of *E. coli* that usually cause UTIs are more resistant to low pH than serogroups that are less common causes of infection (Stamey and Kaufman, 1975). Similarly, low pH has an inhibitory effect on *P. mirabilis* and *P. aeruginosa* (Stamey and Mihara, 1976). This phenomenon may possibly account for the higher incidence of *E. coli* infection.

Tamm-Horsfall protein is secreted by renal tubular cells and is present in the urine as uromucoid (Orskov et al., 1980). Because uromucoid is rich in mannose residues, it may serve as decoy oligosaccharides that bind, prevent attachment, and allow adequate flushing of bacteria. This hypothesis has been supported by an animal model in which mannose can prevent colonization (Aronson et al., 1979). Tamm-Horsfall protein specifically competes with uroepithelial uroplakin Ia and Ib receptors to bind type 1 fimbriated *E. coli* (Pak et al., 2001). Parsons et al. (1975) have demonstrated that an antiadherence mechanism of the bladder (in rabbits) exists by pretreatment of the bladder with dilute hydrochloric acid. Acid-treated bladders had twentyfold to fiftyfold increases of bacterial adherence over controls. Adherence was enhanced by ablation of mucopolysaccharide and glycosaminoglycan from the surface of bladder epithelium (Parsons et al., 1975; Parsons et al., 1978). This could result from exposure of additional binding sites. The rapid recovery of protection suggests a secretory component that inhibits binding. Increased adherence apparently is species specific (Sobel and Vardi, 1982).

It is possible that antibacterial mechanisms are responsible for the rapid disappearance of bacteria applied to bladder mucosa in an experimental model (Cobbs and Kaye, 1967; Norden et al., 1968; Vivaldi et al., 1965); however, the nature of these mechanisms has not been established. Secretory IgA does decrease adherence and colonization of perineal cells by *E. coli* (Stamey et al., 1978) and is increased in children with UTIs (Uehling and Stiehm, 1971).

The role of humoral immunity as a mechanism of the host's defense against UTI has not been satisfactorily clarified. Hanson et al. (1977) reported that acute *E. coli* pyelonephritis induced serum antibodies to O antigens but rarely to K antigens. In contrast, increased levels of O antibodies were not detected in sera from patients with cystitis or asymptomatic bacteriuria. Using the sensitive enzyme-linked immunosorbent assay (ELISA), Hanson et al. (1977) found high levels of *E. coli* O antibody in the urine of most patients with acute pyelonephritis, lower levels in those with asymptomatic bacteriuria and cystitis, and minimal or no detectable levels in the urine of healthy children. Serum antibodies to O antigen, K antigen, and type 1 pili have been found in patients with pyelonephritis (Hanson et al., 1977; Mattsby-Baltzer et al., 1982; Rene and Silverblatt, 1982), and IgM is the predominant species detected during acute infections. IgG antibody to the lipid A component of gram-negative rods is also detectable and may be a measure of the severity of renal disease and tissue destruction (Mattsby-Baltzer et al., 1981). A secretory IgA response can also be detected in the urine in both upper- and lower-tract disease (Hopkins et al., 1987).

Animal studies suggest that humoral antibody is protective against ascending infection with organisms expressing P pili and O and K antigens (Kaijser et al., 1983; Mattsby-Baltzer et al., 1982; O'Hanley et al., 1983). The protective effect is mediated by blocking attachment to the uroepithelium of the upper urinary tract (Svanborg-Eden and Svennerholm, 1978). The role of the host's normal perineal flora—lactobacilli, *S. epidermidis*, corynebacteria, streptococci, and anaerobes—in preventing colonization with uropathogens is not understood.

A number of factors intrinsic and extrinsic to the host combine to predispose to UTI. They include the following:

Intrinsic factors

- Obstruction
- Stasis
- Reflux
- Pregnancy
- Sexual intercourse (in females)
- Hyperosmolality of renal medulla
- Host cell receptor sites for attachment
- Immunologic cross-reactivity of bacterial antigen and human protein
- Chronic prostatitis
- B or AB blood type
- Genetic predisposition
- Immunodeficiency

Extrinsic factors

- Instrumentation (catheters)
- Antimicrobial agents

Probably the single most important host factor affecting the occurrence of UTIs is urinary stasis resulting from obstruction of urinary flow or bladder dysfunction. This predisposing host condition is more frequently observed in younger patients and should prompt a more timely imaging investigation of the urinary system. The most common causes of stasis include the following:

- Congenital anomalies of ureter or urethra (valves, stenosis, bands)
- Calculi
- Dysfunctional or incomplete voiding
- Extrinsic ureteral or bladder compression
- Neurogenic bladder (functional obstruction)

Stasis is associated with increased susceptibility to infection.

There is a striking correlation between vesicoureteral reflux and the occurrence of UTIs. Reflux, the retrograde flow of urine into the ureter and kidney, is caused by the incompetence of the normal valvular action of the ureterovesicular junction. It may occur when this area is affected by congenital anatomic defects, disease, or distal obstruction. Reflux tends to perpetuate infection by maintaining a residual pool of infected urine in the bladder after voiding. Children with reflux may develop upper UTIs and renal scarring. Smellie and Normand (1975) have reported that reflux can be detected in 30% to 50% of children with symptomatic or asymptomatic bacteriuria and that the scarred kidney associated with reflux is more susceptible to reinfection.

Physiologic alterations of the urinary tract that increase the likelihood of UTI occur as a result of pregnancy. These changes include decreased bladder and ureteral tone, decreased ureteral peristalsis, hydroureter, and increased residual bladder urine, all of which serve to cause or aggravate obstruction, stasis, and reflux.

Sexual intercourse produces transient bacteriuria in females and is associated with an increased risk of UTI. This is substantiated by the studies of Nicolle et al. (1982) and Pfau et al. (1983), which showed that 80% of UTIs begin within 24 hours of intercourse in sexually active women.

Hyperosmolality of the renal medulla inhibits the migration of polymorphonuclear leukocytes to damaged medullary tissue and decreases phagocytosis of bacteria (Rocha and Fekety, 1964).

Several facts suggest a genetic predisposition to UTI, including the association of blood group P antigen (Lindberg et al., 1983) with blood groups B and AB, that is, those lacking anti-B isohemagglutinin (Kinane et al., 1982). Studies on the occurrence of periurethral or vaginal defects in host defenses have been inconclusive. Women with recurrent UTIs who are ABO nonsecretors have vaginal epithelial cells that have substantially more receptors allowing attachment of uropathogenic *E. coli* (Stapleton et al., 1992). Vesicoureteral reflux can also be an inherited trait; therefore, family history is important.

Adult males with chronic prostatitis are at risk for recurrent UTIs because of intermittent seeding of their urinary bladders.

Finally, there is evidence that chronic interactions of the host's immune system with retained bacterial antigens or mimicking host antigens is responsible for chronic progressive renal damage. Bacterial antigen may not be eradicated and may trigger formation of antigen-antibody complexes (Hanson et al., 1977). Tamm-Horsfall protein antigen can permeate the renal interstitial spaces and evoke an aggressive humoral and cellular immune response (Mayrer et al., 1983; Work and Andriole, 1980). The most aggressive response occurs in persons with vesicoureteral reflux independent of bacteriuria. Furthermore, Tamm-Horsfall protein cross-reacts with gram-negative bacilli (Fasth et al., 1980).

Two important extrinsic host factors, instrumentation and antimicrobial agents, predispose to UTI. This is particularly true in hospitalized patients with indwelling catheters and patients with chronic bladder dysfunction. Catheters produce their damage by eroding the slime layer of the urethra and bladder and by serving as a nidus for intraluminal concretions and bacterial colonization (Rubin, 1980). The pericannular space is not subject to mechanical washing out of bacteria, as is the uncatheterized urethra. Suction ulcers of the bladder mucosa develop at the site of the bladder portal when urinary drainage systems are not properly vented (Monson et al., 1977). Additionally, bacteria may find a habitat in the biofilm that develops in catheter lumens. Antimicrobial agents apparently have the effect of altering the host's normal perineal flora, allowing easier colonization with uropathogens. In patients with urinary catheters, antibiotics have the effect of shifting colonization to antibiotic-resistant strains (Britt et al., 1977; Butler and Kunin, 1968; Warren et al., 1982; Warren et al., 1983).

PATHOLOGY

Mucosal and submucosal edema and infiltration of the tissue with leukocytes are the prominent histopathologic changes of cystitis. In patients with acute pyelonephritis and upper UTIs the kidney is usually enlarged; its capsular surface is smooth, and the pelvic mucosa may also be involved. The microscopic findings include edema, congestion, polymorphonuclear infiltration of the interstitium, and abscess formation. Tubules may be distended by exudate consisting of leukocytes, bacteria, and debris, occasionally causing necrosis. The medulla is involved to a greater degree than the cortex.

In patients with chronic pyelonephritis the kidney is usually contracted; its surface is scarred, and its capsule is thickened. The calyces and pelvis are fibrotic, and the thickness of the parenchyma is decreased. The glomeruli show evidence of proliferation, crescents, and hyalinization, and they are surrounded by pericapsular fibrosis. The renal architecture is disrupted by fibrotic bands and collections of lymphocytes, eosinophils, and plasma cells. Tubules are atrophied and dilated.

EPIDEMIOLOGY

UTIs involve all age groups from neonates to geriatric patients. Studies involving routine suprapubic puncture in over 1,000 infants revealed the presence of bacteriuria in 0.1% to more than 1% (Wiswell and Geschke, 1989; Wiswell and Roscelli, 1986; Wiswell et al., 1987). UTI was more common in males, with the majority of these infections occurring in uncircumcised infants. However, circumcision to prevent UTI is not warranted by the low frequency and usually mild nature of the disease. Premature infants have 2 to 3 times this rate of UTI. During preschool years, UTI is more common in girls (4.5%) than in boys (0.5%).

Long-term surveillance studies by Kunin et al. (1962) and Kunin (1970, 1976) of school children revealed persistent bacteriuria in 1.2% of girls and in 0.4% of boys. Each year an additional 0.4% of girls developed bacteriuria. Thus the overall prevalence in school girls was 5%. These studies indicated that the peak incidence of UTI in children occurred between 2 and 6 years of age. White girls tended to have more frequent reinfections than black girls. The incidence of UTI in females of high school and college age is approximately 2%.

CLINICAL MANIFESTATIONS

The clinical manifestations of UTIs are dependent on the age of the patient, as well as the anatomic location and severity of the infection. The following symptoms in newborn infants and in those less than 2 years of age are characteristically nonspecific, such as fever, and some appear to be related to the gastrointestinal tract rather than the urinary tract: failure to thrive, feeding problems, vomiting, diarrhea, abdominal distention, and late-onset jaundice. Infants may have signs of balanitis, prostatitis, and orchitis or overt manifestations of sepsis.

The infection in children more than 2 years of age may be characterized by fever, frequency, and dysuria. Classic signs of cystitis in adults may also result from other causes of urethral irritation in children, such as bubble bath, vaginitis, pinworms, masturbation, or sexual abuse. Abdominal pain, flank pain, and hematuria may be present. The occurrence of enuresis in a child who has been toilet trained could also be a manifestation of a UTI. Young infants and boys may have an obstructive uropathy characterized by dribbling of urine, straining with urination, or a decrease in the force and size of the urinary stream. These findings of obstruction can be aggravated by infection. Other historic elements that should be sought include infrequent voiding, incomplete voiding, and a weak urinary stream.

The manifestations of UTIs in adolescents and adults are fairly specific. Lower urinary tract symptoms include frequency, urgency, dysuria, and painful urination of a small amount of turbid urine that occasionally may be grossly bloody. Fever is usually absent. The differential diagnosis of cystitis includes vaginitis, urethritis, and chemically induced irritation from female hygiene products. In contrast, upper UTI may be characterized by fever, chills, and flank pain or abdominal pain. Upper- and lower-tract symptoms and signs may coexist. Occasionally the lower-tract symptoms may appear 1 to 2 days before the upper-tract symptoms. The clinical manifestations in some patients may be so atypical that they resemble gallbladder disease or acute appendicitis.

Given the appropriate clinical setting, the diagnosis is suggested by the detection of white blood cells (WBCs) and bacteria in the urine. The diagnosis of UTI requires confirmation by quantitative culture of urine and attempts to localize the site of infection.

DIAGNOSIS AND MANAGEMENT

Over the last several years, new data on detection, radiologic assessment, and management have become available and point out the need for well-controlled studies, as well as assessment of long-term outcomes of current strategies. Normal urine is a sterile acellular glomerular filtrate influenced by tubular secretion and absorption.

Presumptive Tests

Pyuria. Pyuria is usually defined as the presence of more than 5 to 8 WBCs per cubic millimeter of uncentrifuged urine. This usually represents more than 1 WBC per high-power field. In centrifuged urine the measurement would be 50 to 100 WBCs/mm^3, that is, more than 5 WBCs per high-power field.

A standardized approach to urinalysis is valuable. Generally, 5 ml of urine is centrifuged at 3,000 rpm for 3 minutes, followed by resuspension of the sediment. The occurrence of more than 20 WBCs per high-power field usually correlates with significant bacteriuria of 100,000 colonies in a clean-catch sample. However, pyuria does not necessarily indicate the presence of a UTI. Patients of all ages with or without pyuria may or may not have an infection. Unfortunately, false-positive result rates of approximately 30% have been reported (Brumfitt, 1965); false-positive results may be caused by vaginal washout, chemical irritation, fever, viral infection, immunization, or glomerulonephritis. It is likely that most patients with symptomatic UTIs will have pyuria.

Microscopic examination of urine for bacteria. A Gram stain of uncentrifuged urine is a useful test for the presumptive diagnosis of UTI. Infection is suggested by the presence of at least 1 bacterium per oil-immersion field in a midstream clean-catch urine specimen, equivalent to approximately 100,000 bacteria per milliliter. On examination of centrifuged sediment, approximately 10 to 100 bacteria per high-power field correlate with significant bacteriuria.

Chemical tests. Nitrite detection in urine is based on the observation that many urinary pathogens convert nitrate to nitrite in the bladder. The nitrite strip for detection of UTI uncommonly yields false-positive results. False-negative results are more common (25% to 30%) as a result of inadequate dietary nitrates; diuresis; an inadequate time for bacterial proliferation; or infections caused by nitrite-negative organisms, including *S. saprophyticus,* *Acinetobacter* species, enterococci, and pseudomonads. The test is best used on concentrated or first-morning samples and may have an important role for outpatient and home monitoring following diagnosis and treatment of a UTI (Todd, 1977).

Leukocyte esterase testing detects enzymes generated by inflammatory cells. This test is neither more sensitive nor more specific than the detection of the cells themselves, but it may be easier to perform in some clinical settings. As with pyuria, a positive test result does not establish the diagnosis of UTI.

Molecular detection of nucleic acids of prokaryotic cells in urine is being developed as a screening test for UTI. Although this method probably will be highly sensitive, it is also relatively expensive and labor intensive; thus its role in clinical-laboratory diagnosis of UTI remains to be determined.

Specific Tests

Culture of carefully collected fresh (less than 30 minutes old, refrigerated or held on ice) urine, minimizing the likelihood of contamination, is the cornerstone of diagnosis of UTI. Overdiagnosis carries the risks of unnecessary treatment and diagnostic work-up, along with their attendant visits and costs, as well as unnecessary worry. Underdiagnosis carries the risks of continued symptoms and chronic progressive renal disease.

Quantitative culture of urine. Urine for culture may be obtained (1) as a midstream clean-catch specimen in adults, adolescents, and older children; (2) by catheterization; or (3) by suprapubic aspiration in young children and infants. Suprapubic aspiration is accomplished by introduction of a needle in the midline 2 to 4 cm above the symphysis pubis, after appropriate disinfection of the skin, with gentle traction applied to the syringe plunger. The needle is advanced through the bladder wall until urine flows into the syringe. Success with this procedure is maximized by ensuring that the patient has not recently voided; by palpating, percussing, or transilluminating the bladder; and by digital compression of the urethra to prevent reflex voiding. Strait catheterization follows gentle cleansing of the anterior urethra with soap and water. The catheter is advanced through the urethra into the bladder until urine flows into the catheter. Because the urethra cannot be sterilized, the first aliquot of urine that flows should be discarded to avoid collecting bacteria that have been pushed into the bladder. A later aliquot should be sent for culture (Todd, 1995). Unfortunately, there are no direct comparative studies of the sensitivity and specificity of these methods in children. A negative culture of a clean-catch specimen would obviate the need for catheterization or suprapubic aspiration. Urine collected as a bag specimen should not be used as a basis for the diagnosis of UTI. Screening for asymptomatic bacteriuria is not usually indicated.

Organisms in any number are considered significant when obtained by suprapubic aspiration. When urine is collected by catheterization, a colony count greater than 1,000 per milliliter of urine is usually considered diagnostic. However, for infants, counts of 10,000 cfu/ml or greater have been obtained from catheterized specimens in the absence of other findings of UTI. Hoberman et al. (1994) propose that for urine obtained by catheter, infections should be defined by a colony count greater than 50,000 cfu/ml and pyuria of at least 10 leukocytes/mm^3. If the quantitative culture from a midstream sample reveals 100,000 bacteria or more per milliliter of urine, it also indicates the presence of significant bacteriuria. A count greater than 10,000 bacteria per milliliter suggests infection in males but is equivocal in females and thus should be repeated if symptoms have persisted. A count of less than 10,000 bacteria per milliliter suggests probable contamination. The specificity of this technique is enhanced from 80% to 95% if significant bacteriuria is demonstrated on repeat testing (Hellerstein, 1982). In the presence of pyuria and symptoms, a single culture indicating significant bacteriuria is considered diagnostic in adolescents and adults.

A false-positive test result may be due to contamination or prolonged incubation of urine before culture. False-negative results may reflect the following: prior antimicrobial therapy, the presence of a fastidious organism that grows slowly or is difficult to culture, rapid flow of urine, inactivation of bacteria by an extremely acid pH, or a break in technique such as spilling soap or other cleansing agents into the urine. Therefore there are clinical situations in which colony counts of less than 100,000 may indicate significant bacteriuria.

Convenient, accurate, inexpensive culture techniques have become available for clinic or office practice. They include the filter-strip, dip-slide, dip-strip, pad culture, and roll tube techniques. Of these techniques the dip-slide apparently is the most sensitive and specific (Eichenwald, 1986). The filter-strip technique does not differentiate gram-negative and gram-positive bacteria. The dip-slide and dip-strip techniques do use discriminating agars that allow differentiation of gram-negative and gram-positive organisms.

The specific bacterium recovered by culture should be identified as a guide to appropriate therapy. Quantitative urine cultures should be performed. Commonly this is done using a 0.001-ml calibrated loop inoculated onto blood agar and MacConkey agar for gram-negative rods and onto chocolate agar for *H. influenzae*. The culture is incubated overnight, counted, and multiplied by 1,000. In certain circumstances, special media (e.g., Sabouraud dextrose agar for fungi and human embryonic kidney, HeLa, or Hep-2 tissue culture for viral isolation) are required. When suprapubic aspiration is performed, 0.1 ml of urine should be spread over the plate, incubated overnight, and counted.

Successful treatment is followed by negative culture results within 24 to 72 hours after institution of therapy. Because of increasing reports of antibiotic resistance and of failure to eradicate the offending organism, antibiotic susceptibilities should also be requested at the time of culture. Subsequent treatment can be tailored to the specific pathogen in neonates and in those with systemic illness, persistent or recurrent symptoms, or persistently positive follow-up cultures. For complicated disease, renal parenchymal disease, and nosocomially acquired organisms, antibiotic susceptibilities on the diagnostic urine specimen are also useful in guiding therapy.

Localization of site of infection. It is important to determine if the infection involves the lower tract (probably cystitis) or the upper tract (probably pyelonephritis). Although pyelonephritis is classically associated with fever, flank pain or tenderness, decreased renal concentrating ability, and an elevated erythrocyte sedimentation rate (ESR), the absence of these findings does not reliably exclude upper-tract disease. Collection of urine by ureteral catheterization for quantitative culture is the most reliable method of localizing the site of infection; however, it is an invasive test and may require general anesthesia. Therefore its role in children is limited to research applications. Stamey et al. (1965) evaluated 95 female adults and 26 male by this method. Their observation that the site of infection was limited to the bladder in 50% of this group could not be predicted by history and physical examination. Localization by bladder washout (Fairley technique) is less invasive and does not require anesthesia; however, this is a cumbersome test and is not routinely performed.

The use of technetium (Tc 99m) dimercaptosuccinic acid (DMSA) or glucoheptonate scanning has gained favor in the early diagnosis of upper–urinary tract infections. DMSA scanning appears to be more sensitive than other easily available methods of localization (Buyan et al., 1993; Majid and Rushton, 1992; Rosenberg et al., 1992). In experimental studies the sensitivity and specificity of scanning were 91% and 99%, respectively, with overall 97% agreement with histopathologic findings (Majid and Rushton, 1992), although there may be substantial interobserver variability in the detection and classification of renal cortical defects (Peng et al., 2001). The detection of antibody coating of bacteria is a sensitive, reliable, noninvasive indicator of renal bacteriuria in adults (Jones et al., 1974; Thomas et al., 1974). After addition of fluorescein-conjugated anti–human globulin to urine, the demonstration of fluorescence of the antibody-coated bacteria indicates upper-tract involvement. Unfortunately, when this immunofluorescence technique has been applied to children with bacteriuria, it has been neither sensitive nor specific (Hellerstein et al., 1978; McCracken et al., 1981). Urinary lactic dehydrogenase (LDH) isoenzyme 5 is more accurate for localizing the site of infection in infants and children. Lorentz and Resnick (1979) have reported that elevations of urinary LDH greater than 150 U/L and elevations of fractions 4 and 5 are good indicators of acute pyelonephritis.

C-reactive protein (CRP) is also useful for distinguishing upper–urinary tract from lower–urinary tract infection and has a sensitivity and specificity of approximately 90% when compared with bladder washout (McCracken et al., 1981). A CRP value greater than 30 µg/ml suggests upper-tract disease.

Finally, response to therapy is a clinical indication of the site of infection in adults. Studies in women indicate that more than 90% of patients with lower-tract UTI but less than 50% of those with upper-tract UTI are cured by a single dose of antibiotic if the organism is susceptible (Fang et al., 1978; Ronald et al., 1976). In children, however, recurrences of infection after short-duration therapy occur in approximately 5% to 30% of those treated (McCracken, 1982; Shapiro, 1982). This does not differ from the frequency of recurrences following conventional therapy.

Attention to other evaluations is also important when considering UTIs. Blood pressure should be measured because hypertension may be caused by chronic renal failure. Abdominal examination may reveal a mass, tenderness, or organomegaly. Genital examination should be conducted to investigate vaginitis and labial adhesions in girls; phimosis in boys; and evidence of irritation, sexual activity, or sexual abuse. Rectal examination allows assessment for lax sphincter tone, which may be associated with neurogenic bladder. Similarly, examination of the back may reveal a dimple or other defect associated with neurogenic bladder as a result of spinal cord involvement.

DIFFERENTIAL DIAGNOSIS

The differential diagnosis of UTI is dependent in great part on the age of the patient. The clinical manifestations in newborn infants and in infants under 2 years of age are nonspecific. The findings of irritability, failure to thrive, vomiting, diarrhea, and jaundice suggest the possibility of bacterial sepsis, acute gastroenteritis, or hepatitis. The appropriate blood, stool, and urine cultures should provide a clue to the correct diagnosis. In older children and adults the various conditions that may simulate cystitis or pyelonephritis should be considered. For example, the symptoms of gonorrheal or chlamydial urethritis may suggest a lower–urinary tract infection. A right-sided pyelonephritis could be confused with acute appendicitis, gallbladder disease, or hepatitis. When the presenting complaint is hematuria and bacterial cultures are negative, viral cultures may reveal the diagnosis. Again, the appropriate cultures and serologic tests should help identify the true diagnosis.

COMPLICATIONS

Failure to recognize and to treat acute UTIs may result in recurrent infections and progression to chronic pyelonephritis. Children with chronic pyelonephritis associated with ureteral reflux and obstructive uropathy may develop consequences of chronic renal failure such as anemia, hypertension, growth failure, and metabolic abnormalities. Nephrolithiasis and stricture formation may also develop and further complicate management. A rare complication is that of renal abscess, which may rupture into the perirenal space.

PROGNOSIS

The prognosis depends on the site of involvement, the presence or absence of obstructive uropathy, and vesicoureteral reflux and is therefore related to the age of the patient. Young patients with obstructive uropathy and infection are much more likely to have serious long-term sequelae. Most single, uncomplicated episodes of infection respond to specific antimicrobial therapy. However, approximately one third of these patients may relapse within 1 year. Relapses decrease in frequency beyond this time; however, 1% of patients may relapse up to 6 years after initial infection. The prognosis is less favorable for patients with obstructive lesions and for those with chronic pyelonephritis. In spite of specific antimicrobial therapy, most of these patients have repeated recurrences, and those with bilateral renal involvement may progress to chronic renal insufficiency.

Reflux can be detected in up to 50% of children with bacteriuria (Boineau and Lewy, 1975; Smellie and Normand, 1975). The confluence of infection and reflux is associated with renal scarring in a subset of these children (Huland and Busch, 1984; McCracken and Eichenwald, 1978; Smellie and Normand, 1975).

TREATMENT

The objectives of treatment of children with UTIs are fourfold: (1) to eliminate the infection, (2) to detect and correct functional or anatomic abnormalities, (3) to prevent recurrences, and (4) to preserve renal function. The achievement of these goals requires successful identification of the causative microorganism, selection of optimal antimicrobial drugs and patient compli-

ance in their use, anatomic and functional evaluation of the urinary tract, screening for recurrent infections with periodic urine cultures, and use of general hygienic measures to prevent reinfections. Surgery is often recommended to correct severe reflux in children with UTIs and especially to correct obstructive lesions.

Antimicrobial Therapy

Parenteral administration of antibiotics is appropriate in patients who are in a toxic state, dehydrated, or incapable of accepting or retaining oral intake or when compliance is not assured. Newborn infants with UTIs and children suspected of having pyelonephritis should be treated empirically at the time of diagnosis because of the frequency of associated bacteremia. Empiric therapy for newborn infants with UTI and suspected sepsis should include cefotaxime (100 mg/kg/day divided q12 hours for infants less than 1 week of age and 150 mg/kg/day divided q8 hours for infants greater than 1 week of age) and ampicillin (100 to 200 mg/kg/day). Table 40-1 provides recommendations for initial therapy of newborn infants without sepsis or meningitis when a specific organism can be predicted or when an organism has been isolated and susceptibilities are not yet available. Alternatively, cefotaxime alone is satisfactory for treatment of enteric gram-negative bacillary UTI.

Older children with suspected pyelonephritis can be treated empirically with ceftriaxone 50 to 75 mg/kg/day given intravenously or intramuscularly, possibly with the addition of an aminoglycoside. Table 40-2 contains recommendations for initial therapy of older children when a specific organism can be predicted or when an organism has been isolated and susceptibilities are not yet available. Recent data indicate that orally administered cephalosporin drugs with activity against gram-negative rods are as effective in the time to defervescence (approximately 25 hours), ability to eradicate the organism from the urine, prevention of recurrences, and prevention of renal scarring at 6 months (Hoberman et al., 1996) as parenterally administered agents. Children with mild symptoms and those with lower UTIs may not require antimicrobial therapy until the results of urine culture are available. If therapy is indicated before the results of culture become available, oral cefixime is suggested because *E. coli* and other gram-negative bacilli are the most common pathogens. Trimethoprim-sulfamethoxazole

TABLE 40-1 Initial Therapy for Predicted Cause of Urinary Tract Infections in Newborn Infants While Awaiting Susceptibility Results

Gram stain	Etiology	Initial therapy
Gram-negative rods	Coliforms (*Escherichia coli, Klebsiella pneumoniae, Enterobacter* spp.)	Cefotaxime 100 mg/kg/day divided q12h <1 week of age, 150 mg/kg/day divided q8h >1 week of age, or Gentamicin 3 mg/kg/day, or Amikacin 10 mg/kg/day
	Pseudomonas aeruginosa	Ceftazidime 100 mg/kg/day divided q12h <1 week of age, 150 mg/kg/day divided q8h >1 week of age (or meropenem or cefipime) AND an aminoglycoside (as above)
Gram-positive cocci in chains	*Enterococcus* spp.	Ampicillin 100 mg/kg/day divided q12h <1 week of age, 150 mg/kg/day divided q8h >1 week of age AND aminoglycoside (as above), Vancomycin 15 mg/kg/dose q24h <26 weeks, q18h 27-34 weeks, q12h 35-42 weeks, q8h >43 weeks gestation
Gram-positive cocci in clusters	*Staphylococcus aureus*	Oxacillin 50-75 mg/kg/day
	S. aureus (methicillin resistant, MRSA)	Vancomycin as above
	Staphylococcus epidermidis	As for *S. aureus*

TABLE 40-2 Initial Therapy for Urinary Tract Infections in Children While Awaiting Susceptibility Results

Condition	Initial therapy
Acute cystitis	Cefixime 8 mg/kg/day q12-24h PO or TMP/SMX 8 mg/kg/day of TMP divided q12h PO or ciprofloxin 500 mg q12h PO for adolescent (not approved for children <18 years of age.)
Acute pyelonephritis Moderately ill (outpatient)	TMP/SMX as above Ciprofloxin as above Amoxicillin clavulanate 7:1 formulation 45 mg amoxicillin component/kg/day divided q12h 4:1 formulation 30 mg amoxicillin component/kg day divided q8h
Severely ill, septic state (hospitalized)	Ceftriaxone 50 mg/kg/day IV/IM q24h or Gentamicin 6 mg/kg/day IV/IM. Fluoroquinolone IV for adolescents (not approved for children <18 years of age)

IM, Intramuscular; *IV*, intravenous; *PO*, by mouth; *SMX*, sulfamethoxazole; *TMP*, trimethoprim.

or amoxicillin may be used as an alternative where resistance is not a problem. Older children and young adults may be treated with ciprofloxacin or another fluoroquinolone. Fluoroquinolone antibiotics are not approved for use in children less than 18 years of age. In selecting antibiotic agents the history of infection (i.e., first versus recurrent), the prior use of antibiotics, and any history of drug allergy should be considered. When the results of urine culture and antibiotic sensitivities are known, the antimicrobial therapy can be changed if necessary. Because many antibiotics are eliminated by glomerular filtration and tubular secretion and achieve high concentrations in the urine, infection may be eradicated even if organisms are resistant. For those treated parenterally a switch to oral therapy can be considered if symptoms have abated and an oral agent to which the pathogen is susceptible is available. For patients who remain symptomatic, repeat culture should be performed and the results of the sensitivity tests should be used as a basis for changing the antimicrobial therapy. A large number of antibiotics have been found useful in the management of UTI. Some antibiotics useful for parenteral administration include ceftriaxone, cefotaxime, ceftazidime, cefazolin, tobramycin, ticarcillin, and ampicillin. Oral agents for therapy of mild to moderate disease and for sequential therapy following initial improvement with parenteral drugs include cefixime, cefpodoxime, cefprozil, cephalexin, loracarbef, trimethoprim-sulfamethoxazole, sulfisoxazole, and ampicillin.

In adolescents with acute obstructive, persistent, or frequently recurrent UTIs and for those with nosocomially acquired organisms, fluoroquinolones, imipenem-cilastatin, ticarcillin-clavulanate, or extended spectrum cephalosporins are acceptable alternative drugs.

For children in whom clinical and laboratory measurements indicate lower-tract infection, the use of single-dose or short-term regimens should be restricted to those beyond the newborn period with their first UTI. However, as a result of the difficulty in localizing infection and cost considerations, it may be more appropriate to complete 10 days of therapy than to risk the need to reevaluate and treat a recurrence. Reexamination of the patient and reculture of the urine after short-term therapy is mandatory. Cefixime, amoxicillin, cefadroxil, nitrofurantoin, and trimethoprim-sulfamethoxazole have all been used in short-term regimens.

A "cure" is defined by clinical improvement and the demonstration of several negative cultures after cessation of therapy. Therapeutic failures after short-course or conventional antibiotic treatment of susceptible organisms suggest upper-tract disease. Consideration should be given to a 6-week regimen in patients who do not respond to conventional therapy.

Follow-up should continue for at least 2 years with a routine culture schema such as monthly urine culture for the first 3 months followed by three cultures 3 months apart and two semiannual cultures. If reinfection occurs, the susceptibility of the organism should be determined, and the appropriate therapy should be instituted. Reinfection is differentiated from recurrence by typing the causative agent.

PREVENTION

Suppressive therapy is used in children after the first UTI while awaiting diagnostic work-up for evidence of obstruction or anatomic abnormalities. Intermediate term (3 to 6 months) suppression is used for children with recurrent but uncomplicated infection. Longer term (1 year or more) suppressive therapy is used in children with recurrent pyelonephritis, as well as in children with functional or anatomic obstruction, dysfunctional voiding, bladder mucosal thickening, reflux, renal abnormalities, and other urinary tract structural abnormalities. All of the following have been used for prophylaxis for UTIs: trimethoprim-sulfamethoxazole (2 mg TMP/10 mg SMX) as a single bedtime dose, or 5 mg TMP/25 mg SMX twice per week; nitrofurantoin (1 to 2 mg/kg as a single daily dose; sulfisoxazole (10 to 20 mg/kg divided q12 hours); nalidixic acid (30 mg/kg divided q12 hours); and methenamine mandelate (75 mg/kg divided q12 hours). Although low-dose ampicillin interferes with adherence of E. coli to bladder mucosa (Redjeb et al., 1982), the clinical relevance of this finding has not been determined. Postcoital UTI may also be reduced by prophylaxis and by voiding after intercourse.

Various other nonspecific general measures may be helpful in preventing recurrences of UTIs. They include adequate fluid intake; frequent voiding, especially before bedtime; proper perineal hygiene, particularly after defecation; and avoidance of chronic constipation, which could produce rectal distention that might distort the bladder. Uncircumcised males with phimosis may benefit from circumcision. Physical and chemical irritants of the urethra should be identified and minimized or eliminated. Persons with functional abnormalities of the bladder benefit from intermittent catheterization programs. Acidification programs and long-term treatment with methenamine are occasionally effective; however, they are difficult to maintain.

RADIOLOGIC EVALUATION

After initial infection in all infants and children less than 2 years of age, radiologic evaluation is indicated. Because anatomic abnormalities are also more common among older boys, radiologic evaluation may also be appropriate for them. In girls older than 2 years, imaging is indicated in the presence of symptomatic infection, physical examination findings suggestive of possible renal or collecting system abnormalities, abnormal voiding, hypertension, or poor physical development (American Academy of Pediatrics, 1999; Eichenwald, 1986). If radiographic studies are not performed in older girls after the primary infection, they are indicated if there is a recurrence. Acute imaging is indicated in children who do not have the expected clinical response to therapy in order to investigate the role of obstruction. Routine radiologic studies need only be delayed until infection and the resultant bladder irritability are resolved.

Information developed by radiologic assessment affects management. Ultrasonography should be performed. Ultrasonography is a rapid, noninvasive method for evaluating the renal parenchyma and renal collecting system and permits imaging of the surrounding retroperitoneum without radiation exposure. Ultrasound has supplanted the intravenous pyelogram and is useful in identifying hydronephrosis, dilation of distal ureters, bladder wall hypertrophy, and the presence of ureteroceles. However, ultrasound may not be able to detect significant reflux or to determine reliably the degree of renal scarring. In one study (Rosenberg et al., 1992), the use of DMSA and ultrasound detected all reflux detected by cystourethrography.

Vesiculoureteral reflux is the most commonly occurring abnormality. Contrast voiding cystourethrogram (VCUG) and radionuclide cystography (RNC), both with observation during voiding, are the currently preferred methods for detecting reflux. VCUG provides more information because it better characterizes reflux and can demonstrate bladder and urethral abnormalities. VCUG is preferred in boys and in girls with evidence of voiding dysfunction while uninfected. RNC has the advantage of less radiation exposure and is the preferred method for following the degree of reflux in those previously diagnosed. Radionuclide cystography may be most useful in older children in whom reflux is considered

unlikely, for screening families, and for follow-up after surgical as well as nonsurgical interventions (Lebowitz, 1992). When imaging studies reveal reflux, they should be repeated in 6 months to follow the course of the finding. When no abnormality is detected, they ordinarily need not be repeated.

Children with no reflux or grade I reflux require only follow-up examination. Children with grade II or III reflux may be candidates for suppressive therapy. If grade III or IV reflux is detected, it probably will be persistent and not be the result of acute infection. Children with grade IV reflux are also candidates for suppressive therapy. However long-term efficacy remains to be determined. Urologic consultation should be obtained for children with high-grade reflux.

Levitt et al. (1977) found that cystograms frequently revealed abnormalities in girls with dysuria and frequency (41%), but pyelograms rarely did (2%). However, if upper-tract disease was suspected, pyelograms detected abnormalities in 40%, and findings included obstruction and hydronephrosis. This usually was true even if a first episode of UTI was being studied. In cases diagnosed as upper-tract disease based on elevations of CRP and ESR and abnormal renal concentrating ability, 7% of children studied by intravenous pyelogram developed renal scarring (Pylkkanen et al., 1981). When diagnostic findings were expanded to include reflux and fever, fever alone had a positive predictive value of 45%, and reflux had a positive predictive value of 40% for children less than 5 years who were likely to have radiographically demonstrable abnormalities (Johnson et al., 1985). In addition to radionuclide Tc 99m DMSA or glucoheptonate scanning for localization, radionuclide scanning appears to have increased sensitivity in detecting renal scars following acute pyelonephritis. Serial observations indicate that approximately two thirds of abnormalities demonstrated acutely resolve over time (Jakobsson et al., 1994; Rosenberg et al., 1992). By contrast, renal scars and associated hypertension may also reflect developmental insults. In the experience of Rushton et al. (1992) all new scarring occurred at sites corresponding to the localization of acute inflammation and appears to be unrelated to vesicoureteral reflux. The long-term clinical consequences of scarring in children with anatomically normal urinary tracts are unknown. Similarly, the clinical importance of the increased sensitivity of DMSA scanning is unknown (Rushton et al., 1992).

When detailed anatomic information is required, computed tomography or magnetic resonance imaging should be performed.

Urologic referrals are appropriate for patients with obstruction, urethral valves, renal scarring, anatomic abnormalities, and dysfunctional voiding.

BIBLIOGRAPHY

American Academy of Pediatrics. Practice parameters: the diagnosis, treatment, and evaluation of the initial urinary tract infection in febrile infants and young children. American Academy of Pediatrics. Committee on Quality Improvement. Subcommittee on Urinary Tract Infection. Pediatrics 1999;103:843-852.

Aronson M, Medalia O, Schori L, et al. Prevention of colonization of the urinary tract of mice with *Escherichia coli* by blocking of bacterial adherence with methyl-a-D-mannopyanoside. J Infect Dis 1979;139:329-332.

Asscher AW. Urine as a medium for bacterial growth. Lancet 1966;2:1037.

Bailey RR. Significance of coagulase-negative *Staphylococcus* in urine. J Infect Dis 1973;127:179.

Boineau FG, Lewy JE. Urinary tract infections in children: an overview. Pediatr Ann 1975;4:515-526.

Bran JL, Levison ME, Kaye D. Entrance of bacteria into the female urinary bladder. N Engl J Med 1972;286:626.

Britt MR, Garibaldi RA, Miller WA, et al. Antimicrobial prophylaxis for catheter-associated bacteriuria. Antimicrob Agents Chemother 1977;11:240-243.

Brumfitt W. Urinary cell counts and their value. J Clin Pathol 1965;18:550.

Buckley RM, McGuckin M, MacGregor RR. Urine bacterial counts following sexual intercourse. N Engl J Med 1978;298:321.

Butler HK, Kunin CM. Evaluation of specific systemic antimicrobial therapy in patients while on closed catheter drainage. J Urol 1968;100:567-572.

Buyan N, Bircan ZE, Asanoglu E, et al. The importance of 99m Tc DMSA scanning in the localization of childhood urinary tract infections. Int Urol Nephrol 1993;25:11-17.

Cobbs CG, Kaye D. Antibacterial mechanisms in the urinary bladder. Yale J Biol Med 1967;40:93.

Eichenwald HF. Some aspects of the diagnosis and management of urinary tract infection in children and adolescents. Pediatr Infect Dis J 1986;5:760-765.

Fang LST, Tolkoff-Rubin NE, Rubin R. Efficacy of single-dose and conventional amoxicillin therapy in urinary tract infection localized by the antibody-coated bacteria technique. N Engl J Med 1978;298:413-416.

Fasth A, Ahlstedt S, Hanson LA, et al. Cross-reaction between Tamm-Horsfall glycoprotein and *Escherichia coli*. Int Arch Allergy Appl Immunol 1980;63:303-311.

Gorrill RH, De Navasquez SJ. Experimental pyelonephritis in the mouse produced by *Escherichia coli, Pseudomonas aeruginosa,* and *Proteus mirabilis.* J Pathol Bacteriol 1964;87:79.

Gruneberg RN, Leigh DA, Brumfitt W. *Escherichia coli* serotypes in urinary tract infection: studies in domicil-

iary, antenatal, and hospital practice. In O'Grady F, Brumfitt W (ed). Urinary tract infection. London: Oxford University Press, 1968.

Hanna BA. The detection of bacteriuria by bioluminescence. Methods Enzymol 1986;311:22-27.

Hanson LA, et al. Antigens of *Escherichia coli,* human immune response, and the pathogenesis of urinary tract infections. J Infect Dis 1977;136:S144.

Hanson LA, Fasth A, Jodal U, et al. Biology and pathology of urinary tract infection. J Clin Pathol 1981;34:695-700.

Harle EMJ, Bullen JJ, Thompson DA. Influence of estrogen on experimental pyelonephritis caused by *Escherichia coli.* Lancet 1975;2:283-286.

Hashida Y, Gaffney PC, Yunis EJ. Acute hemorrhagic cystitis of childhood and papovavirus-like particles. J Pediatr 1976;89:85-87.

Hellerstein S. Recurrent urinary tract infections in children. Pediatric Infect Dis J. 1982;1:271-281.

Hellerstein S, Kennedy E, Nussbaum L, et al. Localization of the site of urinary tract infections by means of antibody-coated bacteria in the urinary sediments. J Pediatr 1978;92:188-193.

Hoberman A, Wald ER, Reynolds EA, et al. Pyuria and bacteriuria in urine specimens obtained by catheter from young children with fever. J Pediatr 1994;124:513-519.

Hoberman A, Wald ER, Reynolds EA, Chanon M. Oral vs. intravenous therapy for acute pyelonephritis in children 1-24 months (abstract 787). Pediatric Research 1996;39:134A.

Hopkins WJ, Uehling DT, Balish E. Local and systemic antibody responses accompanying spontaneous resolution of experimental cystitis in cynomolgus monkeys. Infect Immun 1987;55:1951-1956.

Huland H, Busch R. Pyelonephritic scarring in 213 patients with upper and lower urinary tract infections: long-term follow-up. J Urol 1984;132:940-939.

Iwahi T, Abe Y, Nakao M, et al. Role of type I fimbriae in the pathogenesis of ascending urinary tract infection induced by *Escherichia coli* in mice. Infect Immun 1983;39:1307-1315.

Jakobsson B, Berg U, Svensson L. Renal scarring after acute pyelonephritis. Arch Dis Child 1994;70:111-115.

Johnson CE, Shurin P, Marchant C, et al. Identification of children requiring radiologic evaluation for urinary infection. Pediatr Infect Dis 1985;4:656-663.

Jones SR, Smith JW, Sanford JP. Localization of urinary tract infections by detection of antibody-coated bacteria in urine sediment. N Engl J Med 1974;290:591.

Kaijser B. Immunology of *Escherichia coli*: K antigen and its relation to urinary-tract infection. J Infect Dis 1973;127:670.

Kaijser B, Hanson LA, Jodal U, et al. Frequency of E. coli K antigens in urinary tract infections in children. Lancet 1977;1:663-666.

Kaijser B, Larsson P, Olling S, et al. Protection against acute ascending pyelonephritis caused by *Escherichia coli* in rats, using isolated capsular antigen conjugated to bovine serum albumin. Infect Immun 1983;39:142-146.

Kaijser B, Olling S. Experimental hematogenous pyelonephritis due to *Escherichia coli* in rabbits: the antibody response and its protective capacity. J Infect Dis 1973:128:41.

Kallenius G, Mollby R, Svensson SB, et al. Occurrence of P-fimbriated *Escherichia coli* in urinary tract infection. Lancet 1981;2:1369-1372.

Kaye D. Antibacterial activity of human urine. J Clin Invest 1968;47:2374.

Khan AJ, Evans HE, Bombeck E, et al. Coagulase-negative staphylococcal bacteriuria: a rarity in infants and children. J Pediatr 1975;86:309-313.

Kinane DF, Blackwell CC, Brettle RP, et al. ABO blood group, secretor state and susceptibility to recurrent urinary tract infection in women. BMJ 1982;285:7-9.

Kunin CM. The natural history of recurrent bacteriuria in school girls. N Engl J Med 1970;282:1443.

Kunin CM. Urinary tract infections in children. Hosp Pract 1976;113:91.

Kunin CM, Zacha E, Paquin AJ. Urinary tract infections in school children. I. Prevalence of bacteriuria and associated urologic findings. N Engl J Med 1962;206:1287.

Lebowitz RL. The detection and characterization of vesicoureteral reflux in the child. J Urol 1992;148:1640-1642.

Leffler H, Svanborg-Eden C. Glycolipid receptors for uropathogenic Escherichia coli on human erythrocytes and uroepithelial cells. Infect Immun 1981;34:920-929.

Levitt SB, Bekirov HM, Kogan SJ, et al. Proposed selective approach to radiographic evaluation of children with urinary tract infections. In Birth defects: original article series, vol 13, no 5. New York: The National Foundation—March of Dimes, 1977.

Lindberg H, Hanson LA, Jacobsson B, et al. Correlation of P blood group, vesiculoureteral reflux, and bacterial attachment in patients with recurrent pyelonephritis. N Engl J Med 1983;308:1189-1192.

Lindberg U, Hanson LA, Jodal U, et al. Asymptomatic bacteriuria in school girls. II. Differences in E. coli causing symptomatic and asymptomatic bacteriuria. Acta Pediatr Scand 1975;64:432-436.

Lorentz WB, Resnick MI. Comparison of urinary lactic dehydrogenase with antibody-coated bacteria in the urine sediment as a means of localizing the site of urinary tract infection. Pediatrics 1979;64:672.

Majid M, Rushton HG. Renal cortical scintigraphy in the diagnosis of acute UTI. Semin Nucl Med 1992;22:98-111.

Marild S, Jodal U, Orskov I, et al. Special virulence of the Escherichia coli O1:K1:H7 clone in acute pyelonephritis. J Pediatr 1989;115:40-45.

Mattsby-Baltzer I, Claesson I, Hanson LA, et al. Antibodies to lipid A during urinary tract infection. J Infect Dis 1981;144:319-328.

Mattsby-Baltzer I, Hanson LA, Kaijser B, et al. Experimental Escherichia coli ascending pyelonephritis in rats: changes in bacterial properties and the immune response to surface antigens. Infect Immun 1982;35:639-646.

Maybeck CE. Significance of coagulase-negative staphylococcal bacteriuria. Lancet 1969;2:1150-1152.

Mayrer AR, Miniter P, Andriole VT. Immunopathogenesis of chronic pyelonephritis. Am J Med 1983;75:59-70.

McCracken G, Eichenwald H. Antimicrobial therapy: therapeutic recommendations and a review of new drugs. J Pediatr 1978;93:366.

McCracken GH Jr. Management of urinary tract infections in children. Pediatr Infect Dis J 1982;1(suppl):52-56.

McCracken GH Jr, Ginsburg CM, Namasanthi V, et al. Evaluation of short-term antibiotic therapy in children with uncomplicated urinary tract infections. Pediatrics 1981;67:796-801.

Miller TE, North JD. Host response in urinary tract infections. Kidney Int 1974;5:179.

Monson TP, Macalalad FV, Hamman JW, et al. Evaluation of a vented drainage system in prevention of bacteriuria. J Urol 1977;177:216-219.

Mufson MA, Belshe RB. A review of adenoviruses in the etiology of acute hemorrhagic cystitis. J Urol 1976;115:191.

Murphy JJ. The role of the lymphatic system in pyelonephritis. Surg Forum 1960;10:880.

Musher DM, et al. Role of urease in pyelonephritis resulting from urinary tract infection with Proteus. J Infect Dis 1975;131:177-181.

Nelson JD. Pocketbook of Pediatric Antimicrobial Therapy, ed 14. Baltimore: Williams & Wilkins, 2000.

Nicolle L, Harding GKM, Preiksaitis J, et al. The association of urinary tract infection with sexual intercourse. J Infect Dis 1982;278:635-642.

Norden CW, Green GM, Kass EH. Antibacterial mechanisms of the urinary bladder. J Clin Invest 1968;47:2689-2700.

Ofek I, Mirelman D, Sharon N. Adherence of Escherichia coli to human mucosal cells mediated by mannose receptors. Nature 1977;265:623-625.

Ofek I, Mosek A, Sharon N. Mannose-specific adherence of Escherichia coli freshly extracted in the urine of patients with urinary tract infections and of isolates subcultured from the infected urine. Infect Immun 1981;34:708-711.

O'Hanley PD, Lark D, Falkow S, et al. A globoside-binding Escherichia coli pilus vaccine prevents pyelonephritis (abstract). Clin Res 1983;31:372A.

Orskov I, Ferenez A, Orskov F. Tamm-Horsfall protein or uromucoid is the normal urinary slime that traps type I fimbriated Escherichia coli. Lancet 1980;1:887.

Padgett BL, Walker DL, Desquitado MM, et al. BK virus and non-hemorrhagic cystitis in a child. Lancet 1987;1:770.

Pak J, Pu Y, Zhang ZT, et al. Tamm-Horsfall protein binds to type 1 fimbriated Escherichia coli and prevents E. coli from binding to uroplakin Ia and Ib receptors. J Biol Chem 2001;276:9924-9930.

Parsons CL, Greenspan C, Mulholland SG. The primary antibacterial defense mechanism of the bladder. Invest Urol 1975;13:72-76.

Parsons CL, Schrom SH, Hanno P, et al. Bladder surface mucin: examination of possible mechanisms for its antibacterial effect. Invest Urol 1978;6:196-200.

Peng NJ, Liu RS, Chiou YH, et al. 99Tcm-dimercaptosuccinic acid renal scintigraphy for detection of renal cortical defects in acute pyelonephritis: posterior 180 degrees SPECT versus planar image and 360 degrees SPECT. Nucl Med Commun 2001;4:417-22.

Perry A, Ofek I, Silverblatt JF. Enhancement of mannose-mediated stimulation of human granulocytes by type I fimbriae aggregated with antibodies on Escherichia coli surfaces. Infect Immun 1983;39:1334-1335.

Pfau A, Sacks T, Engtestein D. Recurrent urinary tract infections in premenopausal women: prophylaxis based on an understanding of the pathogenesis. J Urol 1983;129:1152-1157.

Pylkkanen J, Vilska J, Koskimies O. The value of level diagnosis of childhood urinary tract infection in predicting renal injury. Acta Paediatr Scand 1981;70:879-883.

Redjeb SB, Slim A, Horchani A, et al. Effects of ten milligrams of ampicillin per day on urinary tract infections. Antimicrob Agents Chemother 1982;22:1084-1086.

Rene P, Silverblatt FJ. Serological response to *Escherichia coli* pili in pyelonephritis. Infect Immun 1982;37:749-754.

Rice SJ, Bishop JA, Apperly J, et al. BK virus as a case of hemorrhagic cystitis after bone marrow transplant. Lancet 1985;2:844-845.

Rocha H, Fekety FR. Acute inflammation in the renal cortex and medulla following thermal injury. J Exp Med 1964;119:131-138.

Ronald AR, Boutros P, Mourtada H. Bacteriuria localization and response to single-dose therapy in women. JAMA 1976;235:1854-1856.

Rosenberg AR, Rossleigh MA, Brydon MP, et al. Evaluation of acute urinary tract infection in children by dimercaptosuccinic acid scintigraphy: a prospective study. J Urol 1992;148:1746-1749.

Rubin M. Effect of catheter replacement on bacterial counts in urine aspirated from indwelling catheters. J Infect Dis 1980;142:291.

Rushton HG, Majid M, Jantausch B, et al. Renal scanning following reflux and nonreflux pyelonephritis in children: evaluation with 99m Technetium dimercaptosuccinic acid scintigraphy. J Urol 1992;148:898.

Shapiro ED. Short course antimicrobial treatment of urinary tract infections in children: A critical analysis. Pediatr Infect Dis 1982;1:294-297.

Silverblatt FS. Host-parasite interaction in the rat renal pelvis: a possible role of pili in the pathogenesis of pyelonephritis. J Exp Med 1974;140:1696-1711.

Smellie JM, Normand ICS. Bacteriuria, reflux, and renal scarring. Arch Dis Child 1975;50:581.

Smith JW, Jones SR, Kaijser B. Significance of antibody-coated bacteria in urinary sediment in experimental pyelonephritis. J Infect Dis 1977;135:577-581.

Sobel JD, Vardi Y. Scanning electron microscopy study of *Pseudomonas aeruginosa* in vivo adherence to rat bladder epithelium. J Urol 1982;128:414-417.

Stamey TA, et al. Antibacterial nature of prostatic fluid. Nature 1968;218:444-447.

Stamey TA, Govan DE, Palmer JM. The localization and treatment of urinary tract infections: the role of bactericidal urine levels as opposed to serum levels. Medicine 1965;44:1.

Stamey TA, Kaufman MF. Studies of introital colonization in women with recurrent urinary infections. II. A comparison of growth in normal vaginal fluid of common versus uncommon serogroups of E. coli. J Urol 1975; 114:264.

Stamey TA, Mihara G. Studies of introital colonization in women with recurrent urinary infections. V. The inhibitory activity of normal vaginal fluid on *Proteus mirabilis* and *Pseudomonas aeruginosa*. J Urol 1976; 115:416.

Stamey TA, Timothy MM. Studies of introital colonization in women with recurrent urinary infections. I. The role of vaginal pH. J Urol 1975;114:261.

Stamey TA, Wehner N, Mihara G, et al. The immunologic basis of recurrent bacteriuria: role of cervicovaginal antibody in enterobacterial colonization of the introital mucosa. Medicine 1978;57:47-56.

Stapleton A, Nudelman E, Clausen H, et al. Binding of uropathogenic *Escherichia coli* R45 to glycolipids extracted from vaginal epithelial cells is dependent on histo–blood group secretor status. J Clin Invest 1992;90:965-972.

Stromberg N, Marklund B-I, Lund B, et al. Host-specificity of uropathogenic *Escherichia coli* depends on differences in binding specificity to gal 1-4 gal-containing isoreceptors. EMBO J 1990;9:2001-2010.

Svanborg-Eden C, Gotschlich EC, Korhonan TK, et al. Aspects of structure and function of pili of uropathogenic *E. coli*. Prog Allergy 1983;33:189-202.

Svanborg-Eden C, Hagberg L, Hanson LA, et al. Adhesion of *Escherichia coli* in urinary tract infection. CIBA Found Symp 1981;80:161-187.

Svanborg-Eden C, Hanson LA, Jodol U, et al. Variable adherence to normal human urinary tract epithelial cells of *Escherichia coli* strains associated with various forms of urinary tract infection. Lancet 1976;2:490-492.

Svanborg-Eden C, Svennerholm AM. Secretory immunoglobulin A and G antibodies prevent adhesion of *Escherichia coli* to human urinary tract epithelial cells. Infect Immun 1978;22:790-797.

Thomas V, Shelokov A, Forland M. Antibody-coated bacteria in the urine and the site of urinary tract infection. N Engl J Med 1974;290:588.

Todd JK. Management of urinary tract infections: children are different. Pediatr Rev 1995;16:190-196.

Todd JK. Have follow-up of urinary tract infection: comparison of two non-culture techniques. Am J Dis Child. 1977;131:860-861.

Uehling DT, Stiehm ER. Elevated urinary secretory IgA in children with urinary tract infection. Pediatrics 1971;47:40-46.

Vivaldi E, Munoz J, Cotran R, et al. Factors affecting the clearance of bacteria within the urinary tract. In Kass EH (ed). Progress in Pyelonephritis. Philadelphia: FA Davis, 1965.

Vosti KL. Recurrent urinary tract infections: prevention by prophylactic antibiotics after sexual intercourse. JAMA 1975;231:934-940.

Warren JW, Anthony WC, Hoopes JM, et al. Cephalexin for susceptible bacteriuria in afebrile, long-term catheterized patients. JAMA 1982;248:454-458.

Warren JW, Hoopes JM, Muncie HL, et al. Ineffectiveness of cephalexin in treatment of cephalexin-resistant bacteriuria in patients with chronic indwelling urethral catheters. J Urol 1983;129:71-73.

Weyrauch HM, Bassett JB. Ascending infection in an artificial urinary tract. An experimental study. Stanford Med Bull 1951;9:25.

Wiswell TE, Enzenauer RW, Holton ME, et al. Declining frequency of circumcision: implications for changes in the absolute incidence and male to female sex ratio of urinary tract infections in early infancy. Pediatrics 1987;79:338-342.

Wiswell TE, Geschke DW. Risks from circumcision during the first month of life compared with those for uncircumcised boys. Pediatrics 1989;83:1011-1015.

Wiswell TE, Roscelli JD. Corroborative evidence for the decreased incidence of urinary tract infections in circumcised male infants. Pediatrics 1986;78:96-99.

Work J, Andriole VT. Tamm-Horsfall protein antibody in patients with end-stage kidney disease. Yale J Biol Med 1980;53:133-148.

Wullt B, Bergsten G, Connell H, et al. P-fimbriae trigger mucosal responses to *Escherichia coli* in the human urinary tract. Cell Microbiol 2001;3:255-264.

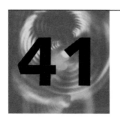

41 VARICELLA-ZOSTER VIRUS INFECTIONS

ANNE A. GERSHON AND PHILIP LARUSSA

Varicella (chickenpox) is a common contagious disease usually of childhood and is the result of primary infection with varicella-zoster virus (VZV). Varicella in children is characterized by a short or absent prodromal period and by a pruritic rash consisting of crops of papules, vesicles, pustules, and eventual crusting, although many skin lesions do not progress to the vesicular stage. In normal children the systemic symptoms are usually mild. Serious complications are the exception but can occur in adults, and in children with deficiencies in cell-mediated immunity (CMI) where the disease may be manifested by an extensive eruption, severe constitutional symptoms, and pneumonia, possibly with a fatal outcome if no antiviral therapy is given.

A live attenuated vaccine (Oka) was licensed for routine use in healthy individuals over the age of 1 year in 1995. Since then, the incidence of varicella and its complications has begun to decrease in the United States. Most states now require that varicella vaccine be administered to children prior to their entry into day care and/or school.

Zoster, which is caused by reactivation of latent VZV acquired during varicella, is characterized by a localized unilateral rash consisting of varicella-like lesions in the distribution of a sensory nerve. Occasionally more than one nerve is involved, and in some patients hematogenous dissemination of virus occurs, leading to a generalized rash developing after the localized eruption. Zoster occurs most often in immunocompromised individuals; it is also more common in the elderly than in the young, and it is more likely to be accompanied by dermatomal pain in adults compared with children.

ETIOLOGY

VZV, a member of the herpesvirus group, is composed of an inner core containing nucleoprotein and DNA, an icosahedral capsid surrounded by a tegument, and an outer lipid-containing envelope. Enveloped VZV particles range in size from 150 to 200 nm (Figure 41-1).

Weller et al. were the first to propagate VZV in vitro and also to show that one virus causes both varicella and zoster. He and his colleagues successfully infected cell cultures of human embryonic lung fibroblasts with vesicular fluid from patients with chickenpox and with zoster, demonstrated the presence of eosinophilic intranuclear inclusion bodies and multinucleated cells typical of VZV in culture, and passed the agent in series, using the cellular components of infected tissue cultures (Weller and Witton, 1958). Using these cultures as the antigen, Weller et al. demonstrated a rise in antibody titer to the agent in convalescent-phase serum from patients with varicella and patients with zoster.

The following body of evidence indicates that the agents that cause varicella and zoster are identical:

1. Varicella was transmitted to susceptible children by inoculating them with vesicular fluid from patients with zoster. The experimental disease was contagious, and it produced chickenpox in other children (Bruusgaard, 1932; Kundratitz, 1925).
2. The cytopathic effect of VZV in tissue cultures was neutralized not only by varicella immune serum but also by zoster immune serum. Both sera also neutralized virus obtained from patients with zoster (Weller and Coons, 1954).
3. Morphologically identical particles were seen in electron microscopic studies of

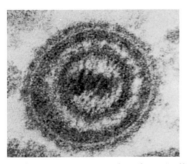

Fig. 41-1 Electron micrograph of varicella-zoster virus. This specimen was obtained from vesicular fluid of a child 1 day after the onset of varicella. The structural elements of the virion are the central DNA core, the protein capsid, the tegument, and the envelope. The last structure contains glycoproteins and is important for infectivity of the virion. (× 175,000). (Courtesy Michael D. Gershon, M.D.)

vesicular fluid from patients with varicella and patients with zoster. Biopsies of skin lesions in both diseases revealed the same type of eosinophilic inclusion bodies, and smears of varicella and zoster lesions showed the same type of multinucleated giant cells. Viruses from both clinical entities were indistinguishable by immunofluorescence assays (Weller and Witton, 1958).

4. Virus obtained from varicella and zoster lesions from the same patient have identical DNA restriction endonuclease digest patterns (Gelb et al., 1987; Hayakawa, et al., 1984; Straus et al., 1984; Williams et al., 1985).

Glycoproteins specified by VZV are present both on the membranes of infected cells and on the envelope of the virus. At least seven glycoproteins, designated gB, gC, gE, gH, gI, gK, and gL have been identified for VZV; they are homologues of glycoproteins of herpes simplex virus (HSV) (reviewed in Arvin and Gershon, 1996). These glycoproteins play important roles in viral pathogenesis and in the generation of cellular and humoral immunity in the infected host. For example, gB and gH are required to facilitate transmission of VZV from one cell to another (Arvin and Gershon, 1996; Edson et al., 1985). In addition to glycoprotein antigens, VZV DNA also encodes for other structural and nonstructural proteins including enzymes and proteins that regulate viral development (Grose, 1987; Straus et al., 1988). VZV

DNA is synthesized in a cascade of immediate early (IE) or α regulatory genes, followed by early (E) or β regulatory and structural genes, followed by late (L) or γ structural genes. Interruption of the cascade, particularly at the IE stage, results in failure to synthesize infectious virus (Hay and Ruyechan, 1994). The linear double-stranded DNA genome of VZV has been fully sequenced (Davison and Scott, 1986). The genome is quite stable, as evidenced by the comparison of viral isolates obtained from patients during primary infection and during subsequent reactivation infection (Gelb et al., 1987; Hayakawa, et al., 1984; Straus et al., 1984; Williams et al., 1985). Genome differences do exist, however, enabling differentiation of vaccine strains of VZV from wild-type strains (Gelb et al., 1987; Hayakawa, et al., 1984; LaRussa et al., 1992; Martin et al., 1982). The Oka vaccine strain has now also been sequenced. There are over 30 mutations present in the vaccine type, but which of these are responsible for attenuation of the vaccine strain has not been determined (Gomi et al., 2000).

VZV does not cause clinical disease in common laboratory animals, although simian forms of varicella have been described. Newborn hairless guinea pigs may be infected with VZV that has been adapted in vitro to guinea pig tissue (Myers and Connelly, 1992).

PATHOLOGY

The following sequence of events is believed to occur when a varicella-susceptible person is infected (Figure 41-2). The virus gains entry at the respiratory mucosa and presumably multiplies in the regional lymphatic tissue. A low-level primary viremia is believed to occur 4 to 6 days after infection, allowing the virus to infect and multiply in the liver, spleen, and possibly other organs. Approximately 10 to 12 days after infection a secondary viremia of greater magnitude occurs, at which time the virus reaches the skin (Grose, 1981). The rash results, on the average, 14 days after infection. Viremia, which has been demonstrated during the early stage of clinical varicella, is more difficult to demonstrate in normal than in immunocompromised children (Asano et al., 1985; Asano et al., 1990, Feldman and Epp, 1976; Feldman and Epp, 1979; Myers, 1979; Ozaki et al., 1986). Viremia has also been reported in some patients with zoster (Feldman

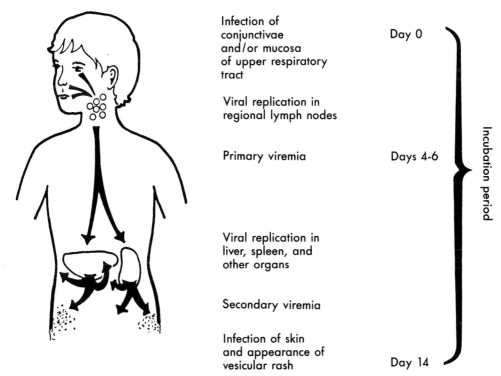

Infection of conjunctivae and/or mucosa of upper respiratory tract — Day 0

Viral replication in regional lymph nodes

Primary viremia — Days 4-6

Viral replication in liver, spleen, and other organs

Secondary viremia

Infection of skin and appearance of vesicular rash — Day 14

Incubation period

Fig. 41-2 Pathogenesis of chickenpox. (From Grose C: Varicella-zoster. Boca Raton, Fla: CRC, 1987).

et al., 1977; Gershon et al., 1978). The skin lesions of varicella begin as macules, the majority of which progress to papules, vesicles, pustules, and crusts over a few days. Some lesions regress after the macular and papular stages. Vesicles are located primarily in the epidermis; the roof is formed by the stratum corneum and stratum lucidum and the floor by the deeper prickle cell layer. Ballooning degeneration of epidermal cells is followed by formation of multinucleated giant cells, many of which contain typical type A intranuclear inclusion bodies. Inclusion bodies are also present in vascular endothelial cells, presumably indicating the mode of spread of virus from the blood to the tissues. Vesicles are formed by accumulation of fluid derived from dermal capillaries, which fills in the space created by degenerating epidermal cells.

As the skin lesions progress, polymorphonuclear leukocytes invade the corium and vesicular fluid (Stevens, et al., 1975), and the fluid changes from clear to cloudy. Interferon has been demonstrated in vesicular fluid and is believed to reflect the CMI response to the virus by the host (Merigan and Stevens, 1978). The resolution of skin lesions leads to the formation of a scab, which is at first adherent but later becomes detached. Mucous membrane lesions develop in the same way but do not progress to scab formation. The vesicles usually rupture and form shallow ulcers, which heal rapidly. Although the most obvious target organ of the virus is the skin, children with benign cases of varicella and transiently elevated aspartate aminotransferase (AST) levels (>50 IU/l) have been described (Myers, 1982; Pitel et al., 1980).

Postmortem examination of infants and adults who died of varicella reveals evidence of involvement of many organs. Areas of focal necrosis and acidophilic inclusion bodies may be present in the esophagus, liver, pancreas, kidney, gastrointestinal tract, ureter, bladder, uterus, and adrenal glands. The lungs show evidence of widely disseminated interstitial pneumonia, with numerous hemorrhagic areas of nodular consolidation. Histologically, the exudate consists chiefly of red blood cells, fibrin, and many mononuclear cells, some containing intranuclear inclusion bodies (Figure 41-3). Encephalitis complicating varicella is pathologically similar to that with measles and to other types of postinfectious encephalitis showing perivascular demyelination in the white matter.

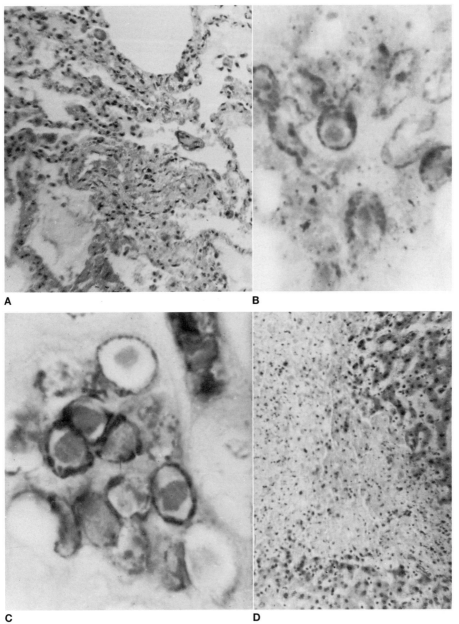

Fig. 41-3 Microscopic sections from a 44-year-old man who died of pulmonary edema after 5 days of hemorrhagic varicella associated with severe right upper quadrant abdominal pain, cough, dyspnea, tachypnea, cyanosis, and hemoptysis. **A,** Interstitial mononuclear cell infiltration and fibrinous exudates in the alveoli of the lung. **B,** Intranuclear inclusion bodies in the lung. **C,** Multinucleated cell with intranuclear inclusions in the skin. **D,** Typical focus of necrosis in the liver. (From Krugman S, et al.: N Engl J Med 1957;257:843-848.)

Latent infection with VZV is believed to develop when sensory nerve endings in the epidermis are invaded by the virus during varicella when the virus is present in its cell-free form on the skin. Virions presumably are transported up the sensory nerves to the ganglia where latency is established. During latency several viral genes are expressed in sensory ganglia; these are mostly IE genes, although some E genes are also expressed. L genes, however, are not expressed, and infectious particles are not formed or released (Croen et al., 1988; Hay and Ruyechan, 1994; Straus and Meier, 1992). Five viral proteins encoded by IE and E genes expressed during latency have been identified in ganglia latently infected with VZV (Annunziato et al., 2001; Lungu et al., 1998; Lungu and Annunziato, 1999; Mahalingham et al., 1996). Reactivation of VZV in human neurons in dorsal root ganglia has been demonstrated, using in situ hybridization in autopsy specimens (Lungu et al., 1995). As shown in Figure 41-4, when viral reactivation occurs, infectious virions are produced, and virions are transported down the sensory nerve to the skin where vesicles appear (Hope-Simpson, 1965; Lungu et al., 1995). Patients with impaired CMI have the highest rate of zoster, which is consistent with the hypothesis that at least some aspects of VZV latency are under immunologic control (Arvin et al., 1978; Gershon et al., 1996; Hardy et al., 1991; Levin, 2001). The incidence of zoster probably increases in the elderly because CMI responses to VZV diminish with advancing age (Burke et al., 1982; Miller, 1980). An increased incidence of zoster with a short latency period has also been observed in children who experienced varicella in prenatal life or early infancy, presumably because of immaturity of the CMI response to VZV during primary infection (Baba et al., 1986; Brunell and Kotchmar, 1981; Dworsky et al., 1980; Guess et al., 1985; Terada et al., 1995). Brunell and Kotchmar (1981) described five infants with zoster, all of whose mothers had varicella between 3 and 7 months gestation. These infants had no evidence of vari-

cella after birth. Presumably all had varicella in utero, because they developed zoster after an average latent period of only 21 months (range, 3 to 41 months). Usually the latent period between varicella and zoster lasts for decades.

Efforts to culture infectious virus from such ganglia have been not been successful. Using in situ hybridization and polymerase chain reaction (PCR), however, VZV DNA and RNA and viral proteins have been demonstrated in human sensory ganglia obtained from autopsy material (Croen et al., 1988; Kennedy et al., 1999; Lungu et al., 1998; Mahalingham et al., 1996). These data indicate that the site of VZV latency is in sensory ganglia.

CLINICAL MANIFESTATIONS OF VARICELLA

After an incubation period of 14 to 16 days, with outside limits of 10 to 21 days, the disease begins with low-grade fever, malaise, and the appearance of rash. In children the exanthem and constitutional symptoms usually occur simultaneously. In adolescents and adults the rash may be preceded by a 1- to 2-day prodromal period of fever, headache, malaise, and anorexia. The typical clinical course of varicella is illustrated in Figure 41-5.

Rash

The typical vesicle of chickenpox is superficially located in the skin. It has thin, fragile

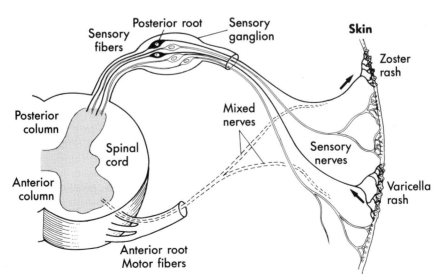

Fig. 41-4 Diagram of proposed pathogenesis of zoster. Latent VZV infection in dorsal root ganglia develops during the rash of varicella. Reactivation of VZV in ganglia may subsequently occur, resulting in zoster. Affected neurons and affected sensory nerves are in black. (Modified from Hope-Simpson RE: Proc R Soc Med 1965;58:9-20.)

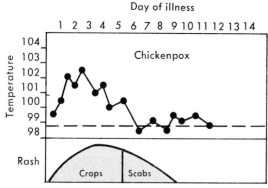

Fig. 41-5 Schematic diagram illustrating clinical course of typical case of chickenpox. Crops of lesions appear, with rapid progression from macules to papules to vesicles to scabs.

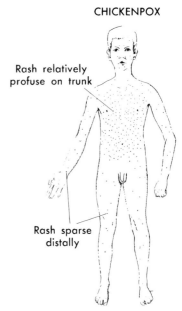

Fig. 41-6 Schematic drawing illustrating typical distribution of rash of chickenpox.

walls that rupture easily. A vesicle resembles a dewdrop in appearance; it usually is elliptical, 2 to 3 mm in diameter, and surrounded by an erythematous area. This red areola is most distinct when the vesicle is fully formed and becomes pustular; it fades as the lesion begins to dry. The drying process, which begins in the center of the vesicle or pustule, produces an umbilicated appearance and eventually a crust. After a variable interval of 5 to 20 days, depending on the depth of skin involvement, the scab falls off, leaving a shallow pink depression. The site of the lesion becomes white, usually with no scar formation. Scarring may follow secondarily infected lesions and prematurely removed scabs.

Skin lesions appear in crops that generally involve the trunk, scalp, face, and extremities. The distribution is typically central, with the greatest concentration of lesions on the trunk and face (Figure 41-6). The rash is more profuse on the proximal parts of the extremities (upper arms and thighs) than on the distal parts (forearms and legs). A distinctive manifestation of the eruption is the presence of lesions in many stages in any one general anatomic area; macules, papules, vesicles, pustules, and crusts are usually located in proximity to each other (Figure 41-7). Many maculopapular lesions progress to the vesicular stage and resolve without crusting.

In the typical case of chickenpox, three successive crops of lesions appear over a 3-day period in the characteristic central distribution just described. The extremes of this picture may range from (1) a single crop of a few scattered lesions to (2) a series of five or more crops

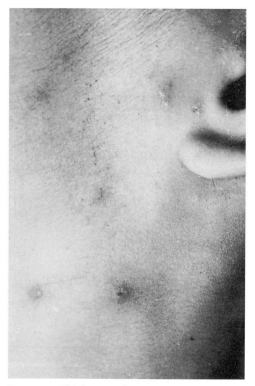

Fig. 41-7 Chickenpox lesions in various stages.

developing over a week, with an uncountable number of lesions covering the entire skin surface of the body. In a study of over 750 cases of chickenpox in otherwise healthy children, the average child developed approximately 300 skin vesicles (Ross et al., 1962). In secondary cases in a household the rash is usually more extensive than in the primary case (Ross et al., 1962).

Vesicles may develop on the mucous membranes of the mouth in addition to the skin. They occur most commonly over the palate and usually rupture so rapidly that the vesicular stage may be missed. They resemble the shallow, white 2- to 3-mm ulcers of herpetic stomatitis. The palpebral conjunctiva, pharynx, larynx, trachea, and rectal and vaginal mucosa may also be involved. Areas of local inflammation such as ammoniacal dermatitis in the diaper area or sunburned skin may have a significant increase in the number of lesions. These vesicles are generally smaller than usual, are usually in the same stage of development, and may become confluent.

In summary, the rash of chickenpox is characterized by (1) a rapid evolution of macule to papule to vesicle to pustule to crust, (2) a central distribution of lesions that appear in crops, (3) intense itching, and (4) the presence of lesions in all stages in any one anatomic area.

Fever

The temperature curve of a typical case of chickenpox is illustrated in Figure 41-5. The height of the fever usually parallels the severity of the rash. When the eruption is sparse, the temperature is usually normal or slightly elevated; an extensive rash more likely will be associated with high and more prolonged fevers. Temperatures up to 40.6° C (105° F) are not unusual in severe cases of chickenpox with involvement of almost the entire skin surface.

Other Symptoms

Headache, malaise, and anorexia usually accompany the fever. In many cases the most distressing symptom is pruritus, which is present during the vesicular stage of the disease.

CLINICAL MANIFESTATIONS OF ZOSTER

A previous clinical or subclinical episode of varicella is a prerequisite. The incubation period of zoster is unknown because it is impossible to determine the time of reactivation of latent VZV. The predilection of the virus for the posterior nerve root areas accounts for the severe pain and tenderness along the involved nerves and the corresponding areas of skin seen in elderly patients. Fever may not be present,

especially in children in whom the disease is often mild.

Zoster occurs only when CMI to VZV is decreased. This depression may be transient, such as when otherwise healthy young persons develop the illness; progressive with increasing age; or secondary to severe immunosuppression induced by diseases such as malignancy, by anticancer chemotherapy or radiotherapy, or after immunosuppression for organ transplantation. Following development of zoster there is a rapid increase in specific CMI in most patients (Berger et al., 1981; Burke et al., 1982).

Zoster is usually characterized by a unilateral rash with a dermatomal distribution. The lesions begin as macules and papules and progress through stages similar to those of varicella. The regional lymph nodes may be enlarged and tender. The rash may appear on the face (involvement of the trigeminal ganglia), the trunk (thoracic ganglia), the shoulders, arms, and/or neck (cervical ganglia), or the perineal area and lower extremities (lumbar or sacral ganglia). When the trigeminal nerve is involved, infection of the maxillary division is associated with lesions of the uvula and tonsillar area; the mandibular division, with lesions of the buccal mucosa or the floor of the mouth and/or anterior part of the tongue; and the ophthalmic division, with scleral and corneal lesions. Infection of the geniculate ganglion of the facial nerve can result in pain, a vesicular eruption in the auditory canal, and facial paralysis, which usually subsides but may be permanent (Ramsay Hunt syndrome). Severe neuralgia, which may persist for many months after convalescence, is much more common in elderly adults than in children. It is also thought that in immunologically normal as well as in immunocompromised hosts, viral reactivation can occur without development of skin lesions; this phenomenon has been termed *zoster sine herpete* (Gershon et al., 1982; Ljungman et al., 1986; Luby et al., 1977; Wilson et al., 1992).

DIAGNOSIS OF VARICELLA
Confirmatory Clinical Factors

The typical case of chickenpox can be recognized clinically with ease. The characteristic diagnostic features include (1) development of a pruritic papulovesicular eruption concentrated on the face, scalp, and trunk and associated with fever and mild constitutional symptoms; (2) the rapid progression of macules to papules, vesicles, pustules, and crusts; (3) the appearance of these lesions in crops; (4) the presence of shallow white ulcers on the mucous membranes of the mouth; and (5) the eventual crusting of the skin lesions. The knowledge of an exposure to a person with either varicella or zoster is always helpful when present.

Detection of the Causative Agent

Laboratory diagnosis by methods such as demonstration of VZV antigens or DNA in, or viral isolation from, skin lesions is indicated for identification of atypical or unusual types of chickenpox. VZV antigens may readily be detected in vesicles by various immunologic means, including direct immunofluorescence with commercially available monoclonal antibodies. Such assays can be performed within an hour's time and can distinguish between VZV and HSV (Gleaves et al., 1988; Olding-Stenkvist and Grandien, 1976; Rawlinson et al., 1989; Zeigler and Halonen, 1985). PCR has proved useful for diagnosis of VZV infection using swabs of lesions or vesicular fluid (Bezold et al., 2001; Espy et al., 2000; LaRussa et al., 1992; LaRussa et al., 1998; Loparev et al., 2000). VZV may be isolated from vesicular fluid obtained within the first 1 to 3 days of rash employing cell cultures such as human embryonic lung fibroblasts, although these assays may not be available in all laboratories and the virus is rather labile.

Detection of the presence of VZV DNA by PCR in cerebrospinal fluid (CSF) has also been used to implicate VZV as causing encephalitis (LaRussa et al., 1994; Puchhammer-Stockl et al., 1991; Quereda et al., 2000).

Serologic Tests

Antibody can be detected in serum within days after onset of varicella and can be expected to increase in titer over the next 1 to 2 weeks. Consequently, a retrospective diagnosis is possible if acute and convalescent serum specimens are available. The first sample of blood should be collected as soon as possible after the onset of disease; the second should be obtained approximately 10 days later. Enzyme-linked immunosorbent assay (ELISA), which is commercially marketed, is the most frequently used serologic test (Gershon and Forghani, 1995). ELISA may also be used to determine immune status to varicella; if a significant amount of antibody is present in serum, it indicates a prior episode of varicella even in the absence of a history of the illness. Unfortunately, however, ELISA assays lack both sensitivity and specificity, which limits their use for evaluating immunity from vaccination (Saiman et al., 2001). The fluorescent antibody to membrane antigen (FAMA) assay, anticomplement immunofluorescence, and radioimmunoassay (RIA) are extremely sensitive but are not commercially available (Gershon and Forghani, 1995). These tests are more sensitive for identification of immunity to varicella than ELISA but are not necessarily any better than ELISA for making a serologic diagnosis of the disease. A latex agglutination (LA) test using latex particles coated with VZV antigen has shown great promise as a sensitive and specific VZV serologic test, especially to document immune status to varicella (Gershon et al., 1994)

A skin test using VZV antigen was developed and used to identify individuals who lack CMI to VZV and may be susceptible to varicella (Kamiya et al., 1977; LaRussa et al., 1985). This test is most accurate in persons under age 40, when there is a good correlation between the presence of specific antibodies and CMI to VZV; however, it is not available in the United States.

Ancillary Laboratory Findings

The white blood cell count is not consistently abnormal, and in most cases it is within the normal range. It is not unusual for adults with primary varicella pneumonia to have leukocytosis with a predominance of polymorphonuclear leukocytes.

DIAGNOSIS OF ZOSTER

Identification of VZV is essential for a definitive diagnosis of zoster. Characteristic zosteriform skin lesions have on occasion been observed in HSV infections; in a study of 47 adults with clinical signs and symptoms compatible with zoster, cultures of skin lesions from six of them (13%) yielded HSV (Kalman and Laskin, 1986). Laboratory diagnosis is made best by demonstration of the virus or viral antigens in vesicular fluid. A fourfold rise in VZV antibody titer 2 to 4 weeks after appearance of lesions provides confirmation of the diagnosis, although increases in VZV antibody titer have been described in HSV infections because of shared antigens between these viruses (Schmidt, 1982; Vafai et al., 1990).

DIFFERENTIAL DIAGNOSIS OF VARICELLA

The differential diagnosis of varicella is also discussed in Chapter 45. Varicella may resemble the following conditions.

Impetigo

The skin lesions of impetigo are vesicular at first but rapidly progress to honey-colored crusts. They differ from chickenpox in appearance and distribution. They do not appear in crops, do not involve the mucous membranes of the mouth, and are not accompanied by constitutional symptoms. The lesions commonly involve the nasolabial area because of the tendency for a child to scratch this area with contaminated fingers. Other areas that are easily scratched also become involved.

Insect Bites, Papular Urticaria, and Urticaria

Insect bites, papular urticaria, and urticaria are not accompanied by constitutional symptoms. They are papular and pruritic but do not have the typical vesicular appearance and distribution. Vesicles, if present, are pinpoint in size. The scalp and mouth are devoid of lesions.

Scabies

The differential points of scabies are the same as those of insect bites. In addition, the observation of burrows between the fingers and toes and the microscopic identification of *Sarcoptes scabiei* help confirm the diagnosis.

Rickettsialpox

Rickettsialpox has the classic triad of signs and symptoms in the following order: (1) the appearance of a primary lesion or eschar on some part of the body, (2) the development of an influenza-like syndrome, and (3) the occurrence of a generalized papulovesicular eruption. The rash of rickettsialpox differs from that of varicella in that the vesicles are much smaller and are superimposed on a firm papule. Crusts do not develop regularly; if they do, they are very small. The diagnosis is confirmed by a specific antibody test.

Eczema Herpeticum and Other Forms of HSV Infection

A patient with eczema herpeticum may have a history of contact with a person who had a fever blister; the rash is caused by either primary or reactivated HSV infection. The vesicular and pustular lesions are most profuse over the sites of eczema. The different type of distribution is the most useful differential point. At times it may be necessary to perform laboratory examinations (e.g., direct immunofluorescence, described previously) to identify the causative agent. Eczema vaccinatum could also be confused with varicella, but because smallpox vaccine is no longer used, this diagnosis is highly unlikely.

In the newborn infant, HSV and varicella may be confused when only a few vesicular skin lesions are present and there is no history of exposure to either virus. In this instance direct immunofluorescence of skin lesions is extremely helpful. Zosteriform lesions in the neonate due to HSV infection have been reported (Music et al., 1971; Rabalais et al., 1991).

Stevens-Johnson Syndrome

With this syndrome there may be a history of use of medications and allergy. Annular skin lesions and extensive involvement of mucous membranes suggest Stevens-Johnson syndrome.

Smallpox

In smallpox the skin lesions are all in one stage of development, there is a concentration of lesions on the hands and feet, and, in general, patients are much sicker than patients with varicella. Smallpox carries a mortality rate of 30%.

COMPLICATIONS OF VZV INFECTION

Complications of varicella are not common; uneventful recovery is the rule except in immunocompromised persons. The following incidence of serious complications in children aged 1 to 14 years per 100,000 cases of varicella has been recorded: encephalitis, 1.7; Reye's syndrome, 3.2; hospitalization, 1.7; and death, 2.0 (Preblud et al., 1984). However, Choo et al. (1995) noted in a retrospective study of varicella in a large health maintenance organization with 250,000 members that the rate of hospitalization ranged from 4 to 11 times higher in children than previously estimated.

Secondary Bacterial Infection

The secondary infection of skin lesions is not common enough to warrant the use of prophylactic antimicrobials. Staphylococci or group A β-hemolytic streptococci may gain entry into the lesions and produce impetigo, furuncles, cellulitis, and erysipelas. Scalded skin syndrome (Melish, 1973; Wald et al., 1973) and toxic shock–like syndrome (Bradley et al., 1991) have both been reported as complications of chickenpox. Although bacterial superinfections can result in septicemia, pneumonia, suppurative arthritis, osteomyelitis, or local gangrene, even in the era before antibiotics were available there was a low incidence of these complications. Bullous impetigo caused by exfoliative toxigenic *Staphylococcus aureus*, phage type II, may be considered a secondary bacterial infection. Neutropenia that occasionally follows varicella may possibly predispose to secondary bacterial infections.

Bullous varicella. Bullous varicella is an unusual manifestation characterized by the simultaneous occurrence of typical varicelliform lesions and bullae. Published reports indicate that the bullous lesions are caused by phage group II staphylococci (Melish, 1973; Wald et al., 1973). These staphylococci produce epidermolytic toxin, the cause of staphylococcal scalded skin syndrome. In this complication, VZV is not present in the bullous fluid.

There is evidence that the incidence of invasive infection with highly virulent group A β-hemolytic streptococci has been increasing in recent years. Following varicella these infections may be superficial or highly invasive, resulting in deep-seated infections such as pneumonia, necrotizing fasciitis, and osteomyelitis (Brogan et al., 1995; Davies et al., 1996; Gonzalez-Ruiz et al., 1995; Mills et al., 1996; Peterson et al., 1996; Vugia et al., 1996; Wilson et al., 1995). Fatalities have been reported. In one epidemiologic study of streptococcal infection, varicella was the most significant risk factor for this infection in children less than 10 years of age, with an attack rate of 4.4 per 100,000 cases and a relative risk of 39 during the 2 weeks following varicella (Davies et al., 1996). Although the issue has been considered controversial, the use of nonsteroidal antiinflammatory drugs (NSAIDs) such as ibuprofen is likely to increase the risk of development of invasive streptococcal infections; consequently, NSAIDs are best avoided in the treatment of fever in varicella (Peterson et al., 1996; Laupland et al., 2000; Lesko et al., 2001).

Second attacks of varicella. It was once generally accepted that varicella could occur only one time during a lifetime. Second attacks of clinical illness are difficult to confirm by laboratory means because most first attacks are diagnosed only clinically. There is a growing body of evidence, however, suggesting that second attacks of varicella may occur. Varicella has been observed in persons shown to have specific antibodies before onset of illness (Gershon et al., 1984a; Gershon et al., 1984b; Junker et al., 1989; Junker et al., 1991; Junker and Tilley, 1994, Weller, 1983). Serologic evidence of subclinical infection of varicella-immune individuals closely exposed to VZV has also been reported (Arvin et al., 1983; Gershon et al., 1984a; Luby et al., 1977). Many second attacks are mild. Second attacks are most common in immunocompromised persons, in those who originally had subclinical infections, and in children who had varicella in early infancy.

Central nervous system involvement. Central nervous system (CNS) involvement is rare but may complicate a mild or a severe infection. Guess et al. (1986) reported an incidence of acute cerebellar ataxia of 1 in 4,000 cases of varicella and of other forms of varicella encephalitis (excluding Reye's syndrome) of 1 in 33,000 cases. According to Peters et al. (1978), cerebellar involvement with ataxia is also the most common form of encephalitis following varicella. If cerebellar ataxia occurs as an isolated phenomenon, the prognosis is excellent. The symptoms usually develop between the third and eighth days after the onset of rash, but at times they may precede the exanthem. It is not yet clear whether CNS involvement represents the direct effect of viral replication or the immune response to the presence of VZV in the CNS. Although VZV is rarely cultured from the spinal fluid in these cases, both VZV specific antibody and DNA have been shown to be present (LaRussa et al., 1993).

The signs of cerebral involvement, which is a more serious complication, include those of meningoencephalitis, with fever, headache, stiff neck, change in sensorium, and occasionally convulsions, stupor, coma, and paralysis. The cerebral form of encephalitis carries a more guarded prognosis. At one time it was difficult to differentiate between varicella encephalitis and Reye's syndrome. In a survey of 59 cases of varicella encephalitis, Applebaum et al. (1953), reported complete recovery in 80%, evidence of brain damage in 15%, and death in 5%. Of

302 cases of varicella encephalitis reported in the United States during 3 years (1963 to 1965), 82 (27.1%) were fatal (McCormick et al., 1969). Other rare CNS complications of VZV infection include transverse myelitis, peripheral neuritis, and optic neuritis (Gilden et al., 2000). In both cerebellar and cerebral types of encephalitis after varicella, CSF changes include pleocytosis with a predominance of lymphocytes, an elevated protein value, and a normal glucose value.

Encephalitis ranging from mild to severe, either accompanying or following zoster, is not uncommon. Other neurologic complications of zoster include motor and autonomic nerve involvement with paralysis and cerebral angiitis (Gilden et al., 2000). These complications of zoster are much more frequent in older adults than in children. Encephalopathy due to reactivation of VZV in the CNS in the absence of rash has been reported in immunocompromised patients (Dueland et al., 1991; Silliman et al., 1993). This form of encephalopathy may be disabling and eventually prove fatal.

Reye's syndrome. Mild to moderate elevations of liver enzyme levels are not infrequent in otherwise healthy children with varicella (Ey and Fulginiti, 1981; Myers, 1982; Pitel et al., 1980). Pitel et al. studied 39 children with varicella; transaminase elevations were greater than normal in 77%. Jaundice is rare, and the condition is almost always self-limited. Until these studies were reported, it was not realized that the liver could be involved in uncomplicated varicella. The relationship, if any, between this asymptomatic form of varicella hepatitis and Reye's syndrome is not known, although some children have experienced severe vomiting episodes during the period of abnormal liver enzyme activity. Lichtenstein et al. (1983) obtained liver biopsies from 19 children who had marked elevation of aminotransferase activity with minimal neurologic symptoms (lethargy) after varicella (8 children) or an upper respiratory infection (11 children). Microscopic evidence suggesting Reye's syndrome was found in 14 (74%). Reye's syndrome as a complication of varicella has now become rare, since the administration of aspirin became contraindicated during chickenpox and because of the widespread use of varicella vaccine.

Varicella in the adult. Varicella, like many other viral infections, is more likely to be severe in adults than in children. The risk of developing severe varicella in persons more than 20 years of age is 25 times greater than it is in children (Preblud et al., 1984). In general, the fever is higher and more prolonged, the constitutional symptoms are more severe, the rash is more profuse, and complications are more frequent in adults compared with children. Primary varicella pneumonia is a significant complication in adults. A prospective evaluation of 114 military personnel with varicella revealed roentgenographic evidence of pulmonary involvement in 16%, although clinical signs were present in only 4% (Weber and Pellecchia, 1965). The severity of varicella in adults may be related to the impaired ability of adults compared with children to mount a CMI response to VZV (Gershon, 1995; Nader et al., 1995).

Varicella pneumonia. Varicella pneumonia has been recognized chiefly in otherwise healthy adults and immunocompromised patients of all ages. It is rare in normal children, but it has been seen in some infants with neonatal varicella (see below). One to 5 days after chickenpox begins, there is an onset of cough, chest pain, dyspnea, tachypnea, and, possibly, cyanosis and hemoptysis. Rales are usually heard over both lung fields. The roentgenogram shows characteristic nodular densities bilaterally (Figure 41-8). The nodular infiltrates vary in size and occasionally coalesce to form larger areas of consolidation. The leukocyte count may be either normal or slightly elevated.

The course of the pneumonia is variable. It may be extremely mild with little or no cough and no respiratory distress, and roentgenographic evidence of the disease may subside within 1 week. On the other hand, respiratory problems may be severe, with chest pain, hemoptysis, cyanosis, a stormy course of 7 to 10 days, and roentgenographic findings that persist for as long as 4 to 6 weeks. Occasionally there is a fatal outcome despite antiviral therapy. Varicella pneumonia may be further complicated by pleural effusion, subcutaneous emphysema, pulmonary edema, and adult respiratory distress syndrome. Some patients with varicella pneumonia show evidence of other visceral involvement such as hepatitis. Mackay and Cairney reported roentgenographic evidence of widespread, evenly distributed 1- to 3-mm nodules of calcific density in seven adults who had severe varicella after the age of 19 years. The roentgenograms were taken 3 to 32

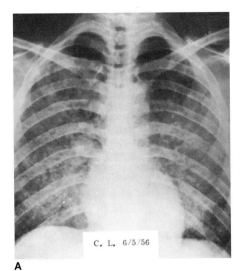

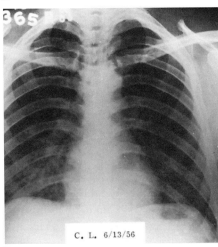

Fig. 41-8 Roentgenograms of the chest of a 24-year-old man with varicella, characterized on the third day by severe cough, dyspnea, tachypnea, cyanosis, and hemoptysis. **A,** Roentgenogram taken on the fourth day of pneumonia, showing extensive nodular infiltrates throughout both lung fields. **B,** Appearance 8 days later; there was considerable clearing. (From Krugman S, Goodrich CH, Ward R: N Engl J Med 1957;257:843-848.)

years after onset of varicella (Mackay and Cairney, 1960). A summary of the epidemiologic and clinical manifestations of primary varicella pneumonia in the pre–antiviral drug era is given in Table 41-1.

Congenital varicella syndrome. The congenital varicella syndrome is rare. Since the 1940s when it was first recognized, less than 100 cases have been recorded in the world literature (Enders et al., 1994; Gershon, 2001a). Frequent manifestations of the syndrome include a hypoplastic extremity, zosteriform skin scarring, microphthalmia, cataracts, chorioretinitis, and abnormalities of the CNS (Table 41-2 and Figure 41-9). There is a spectrum of disease, with most children severely affected but some with only a few stigmata, such as chorioretinitis or vocal cord paralysis (Randel et al., 1996).

The incidence of this syndrome following gestational varicella in the first and second trimesters is approximately 2% (Gershon, 2001a). There have been 10 prospective studies of pregnant women with varicella and their offspring, in which 1,898 pregnancies (maternal varicella in the first 20 weeks in 718) were followed and 13 affected infants resulted (1.8% for first 20 weeks, 0.6% for entire pregnancy). The critical period for development of fetal defects is between the seventh and the twentieth weeks of pregnancy. Fortunately the syndrome is very rare, because there is no practical way to diagnose it in utero. In some patients, congenital defects were identified by fetal ultrasound, but in other affected infants these tests have been normal. There is a high correlation (about 40%) between a hypoplastic extremity and severe brain damage and/or early death (Gershon, 2001a).

The pathogenesis is not understood, but the rarity of the illness and the pattern of cicatricial skin lesions with damage to the nervous system, suggest that the fetus may have experienced varicella secondary to maternal viremia, followed later by viral reactivation, resulting in zoster in utero. It is interesting to note that most infants with the syndrome have also been reported to develop clinical zoster with a short period of viral latency in postnatal life (Gershon, 2001a). This is ascribed to the immature CMI response to VZV in fetal life (Terada et al., 1994). Maternal varicella itself may also be severe during pregnancy, and fatalities have been reported (Gershon, 2001a).

Severe disseminated and fatal varicella in 5- to 10-day-old infants, resembling that in leukemic children, may occur in offspring whose mothers have varicella 5 days or less before delivery. This phenomenon may be related to several factors. In infants who develop the illness between 5 and 10 days of age (an incubation period of approximately 10 days), the cellular immune response to VZV is still immature. In addition, the size of the inoculum introduced into the infant by the mother's viremia may be large, which might

TABLE 41-1 Summary of Epidemiologic and Clinical Manifestations of 30 Cases of Primary Varicella Pneumonia in the Pre–Antiviral Drug Era

Age	Range: 4 to 82 yr			Mean average: 33 yr
	(only two children, 4 and 6 years of age, both with leukemia)			
Sex	Male: 22			Female: 8
Season	January to March: 15 cases	April to June: 14 cases		October to December: 1 case
Day of onset of cough	First: 5	Second: 15	Third: 7	Fourth and fifth: 3
Clinical manifestation	*Severe*	*Moderate*	*Mild*	*None*
Cough	11	8	11	—
Dyspnea	11	7	1	11
Cyanosis	10	0	0	19
Hemoptysis	10	3	1	15
Rales	11	8	1	10
Roentgenographic findings	11	8	11	—
White blood count	Range: 4,000 to 16,200			Mean: 8,600
Complications	Hepatitis (4)			
	Pleural effusion (3)			
	Pulmonary abscesses (2)			
	Subcutaneous emphysema (1)			
	Gastric ulcers (1)			
Deaths	Pulmonary edema (1)			
	Pulmonary abscesses and gastric ulcers (1)			
	Hepatitis (3)			
	Pulmonary abscesses and Hodgkin's disease (1)			
	Leukemia (1)			

TABLE 41-2 Clinical and Laboratory Data of 39 Infants With the Congenital Varicella Syndrome

Occurrence	(%)
After maternal varicella	87
After maternal zoster	13
Time (weeks) of maternal infection	
Median	12
Range	8-28

Major Malformations Described	(%)
Cicatricial skin lesions	72
Ocular abnormalities: cataract, chorioretinitis, Horner's syndrome, microphthalmia, nystagmus	62
Hypoplastic limb	46
Cortical atrophy and/or mental retardation	31
Early death	24

Modified from Gershon A. Chickenpox, measles, and mumps. In Remington JS, Klein JO (eds). Infections of the fetus and newborn infant, ed 3. Philadelphia: Saunders, 1990.

account for the shorter incubation period. Furthermore, when the mother has had varicella for less than 5 days before delivery, she has not made or transferred VZV antibody to her baby; maternally derived antibody may act as a form of passive immunization for the infant born to women who develop varicella a week or longer prior to delivery. The clinical attack rate of varicella in newborn infants born to women with onset of varicella 5 days or less prior to delivery has been reported to range from 20% to 50% (Hanngren et al., 1985; Meyers, 1974; Preblud et al., 1986a). In infected infants who have been neither passively immunized with varicella zoster immune globulin (VZIG) nor treated with an antiviral drug, the mortality rate was approximately 35% (Meyers, 1974). In the United States, prompt administration of passive immunization to newborn infants at risk has made severe varicella of the newborn a rarity (Bakshi et al., 1986).

Disseminated varicella infection in a newborn infant is characterized by hemorrhagic lesions and involvement of the lungs and the liver. Effects on the newborn infant when maternal varicella occurs near term are shown in Table 41-3.

Hemorrhagic, progressive, and disseminated varicella. Varicella in an immunocompromised host may be characterized by a hemorrhagic, progressive, and/or disseminated infection with a potentially fatal outcome. Feldman et al.

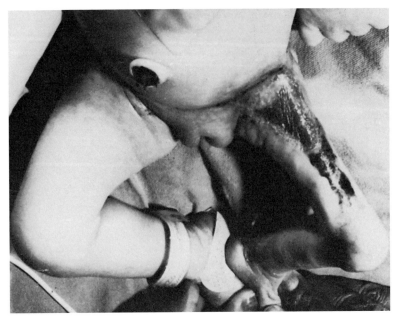

Fig. 41-9 Congenital varicella syndrome illustrating cicatricial skin lesions and hypotrophic left lower limb. (From Srabstein JC et al: J Pediatr 1974;84:239.)

TABLE 41-3	Maternal Varicella Near Term: Effect on the Newborn Infant (50 Cases)	
Onset	Effect
Maternal varicella, 5 or more days before delivery; baby's varicella, age 0-4 days	27 of 27 survived
Maternal varicella, 4 days or less before delivery; baby's varicella, age 5-10 days	10 of 23 survived (7 died of disseminated varicella, 2 had severe disease with survival)

From Gershon AA. In Krugman S, Gershon AA (eds). Infections of the fetus and newborn infant. New York: Alan R. Liss, 1975.

observed 77 children with cancer at St. Jude Children's Research Hospital who contracted varicella in the pre–antiviral therapy era (Feldman et al., 1975). No complications were observed among the 17 children no longer receiving anticancer chemotherapy. In contrast, of the 60 children still receiving anticancer chemotherapy, 19 (32%) had evidence of visceral dissemination, and four (7%) died. Deaths were associated with varicella pneumo-

nia (all four patients) and encephalitis (two of the four patients). Disseminated varicella occurred more frequently in children with absolute lymphopenia who had fewer than 500 lymphocytes/mm³.

A decade later, in an assessment of children with underlying cancer and varicella at the same institution, Feldman and Lott (1987) reported 127 patients observed between 1962 and 1986. They found that despite passive immunization and antiviral therapy, fatalities due to varicella still occurred. Children with leukemia fared more poorly than children with other malignancies, although the incidence of varicella pneumonia was high in each group—32% and 19%, respectively. In children with leukemia who had received passive immunization with VZIG, the incidence of primary viral pneumonia was 15%. Cessation of anticancer chemotherapy during the incubation period did not significantly decrease the incidence of varicella pneumonia.

There are two possible courses of severe varicella in immunocompromised children. In some a fulminant disease with hemorrhagic lesions, pneumonia, and disseminated intravascular coagulation occurs; death usually ensues within a few days, often despite antiviral therapy. In other children a more protracted illness develops, with new crops of vesicles occurring for as long as 2 weeks. At first these children may appear to have mild disease, but as new lesions continue to develop, accompanied by fever, toxicity, abdominal and back pain, and pneumonia, the serious nature of the illness becomes apparent, usually during the second week after onset.

Severe, progressive, fatal varicella infection has also been observed in children treated with high doses of corticosteroids for conditions other than cancer. Gershon et al. (1972) described the development of fulminant varicella in two boys treated with corticosteroids for rheumatic fever; deaths occurred 2 and 4 days after onset of rash. Although children with asthma treated with low doses of steroids apparently are not at risk to develop severe varicella, fatalities have been reported in those receiving high doses (Kasper and Howe, 1991; Silk et al., 1998). Whether the use of inhaled steroids for prophylaxis against asthma predisposes children to varicella is unclear; these children are not considered to be immunocompromised. One anecdotal report of two patients using daily-inhaled steroids to control asthma who developed severe varicella may represent coincidence rather than cause and effect (Choong et al., 1995).

Severe varicella has been described in patients who have undergone renal transplantation (Feldhoff et al., 1981; Lynfield et al., 1992) and bone-marrow transplantation (Koc et al., 2000; Leung et al., 2000; Locksley et al., 1985; Rivera-Vaquerizo et al., 2001) and in children with acquired immunodeficiency syndrome (AIDS) (Acheson et al., 1988; Jura et al., 1989; Pahwa et al., 1988). They and other immunocompromised patients are also at high risk to develop varicella or zoster that may be recurrent and/or chronic, although the frequency of this occurrence is unknown (Acheson et al., 1988; Gershon et al., 1997; Patterson et al., 1989). Although children with HIV infection are at increased risk to develop severe varicella compared to healthy children, their risk is lower than that of children with underlying leukemia (Gershon et al., 1997). Development of zoster in young adults is a sentinel for subsequent development of AIDS (Colebunders et al., 1988; Melbye et al., 1987). Development of zoster at a rate as high as 70% has been reported in children infected with HIV with CD4+ lymphocyte counts under 15% at onset of varicella (Gershon et al., 1997).

It has long been thought that immunocompromised children are predisposed to develop

severe varicella because their CMI response to VZV is deficient. In immunocompromised patients the in vitro lymphocyte response to VZV antigen has been reported to develop more slowly in those with severe disease than in those with an uncomplicated illness (Arvin et al., 1986). Furthermore, lymphocytes from leukemic children with prior varicella show decreased in vitro responses to VZV antigen in comparison to lymphocytes from healthy controls (Giller et al., 1986). This phenomenon is attributed to decreased numbers of circulating lymphocytes rather than to impaired antigen presentation. There is no apparent correlation of poor antibody responses with severe varicella in immunocompromised patients.

Severe and fatal cases of varicella have been observed in children with underlying AIDS in whom a new syndrome of chronic VZV infection has also been described. After recovery from varicella these children may develop scattered, sparse, wartlike lesions from which VZV can be isolated (Jura et al., 1989; Pahwa et al., 1988; Zampogna and Flowers, 2001). Although the natural history of this form of varicella is not yet fully understood, VZV infections seem to smolder in some HIV-infected patients and may eventually result in chronic progressive encephalitis, with a potentially fatal outcome even if treated (Gilden et al., 1988; Pahwa et al., 1988; Silliman et al., 1993). VZV resistant to acyclovir (ACV) has developed in some of these patients who were treated for many months (Jacobson et al., 1990; Linnemann et al., 1990; Pahwa et al., 1988).

Disseminated zoster. Disseminated zoster is not uncommon; it is usually seen in children and adults with marked persistent depression of CMI to VZV. In contrast to what usually appears to occur in the normal host, a viremia develops following the localized dermatomal rash, resulting in an additional generalized rash. Fever is more likely to be present than in localized zoster. The number of skin lesions outside the dermatomal area ranges from a few to thousands; the extent of the rash reflects the seriousness of the infection. Fatalities may occur when there is extensive visceral involvement if no antiviral therapy is given (Feldman and Lott, 1987; Shepp et al., 1986; Whitley et al., 1982).

Patients who have undergone bone-marrow transplantation are at increased risk not only of developing zoster, but also of developing severe symptoms. In a study of 1,394 adults who underwent bone-marrow transplantation, the incidence of zoster after 1 year was approximately 17% (Locksley et al., 1985). Of these adults, 45% developed disseminated disease, and the overall fatality rate in the group was 6% despite antiviral therapy. There was also a high incidence of postherpetic neuralgia, skin scarring, and bacterial superinfections.

Rare Complications

Retinitis due to VZV may be a manifestation of the congenital varicella syndrome, and it may be a complication of zoster in HIV-infected patients (Chambers et al., 1989; Friedman et al., 1994a; Kuppermann et al., 1994). Acute glomerulonephritis has been described in patients either with or without evidence of associated streptococcal infection (Yuceoglu et al., 1967). Myocarditis has also been recorded (Kirk et al., 1987; Lorber et al., 1988; Waagoner and Murphy, 1990), as has orchitis (Liu et al., 1994).

Varicella arthritis is a rare complication that is usually self-limited. The arthritis is usually monoarticular, with swelling, tenderness, pain, and joint effusion, but with no erythema. The synovial fluid contains a predominance of lymphocytes and is free of bacteria (Baird et al., 1991; Mulhern et al., 1971; Priest et al., 1978; Ward and Bishop, 1970). Isolation of VZV from joint fluid obtained from a patient with varicella arthritis has been reported (Priest et al., 1978), and the diagnosis has also been established by PCR (Baird et al., 1991).

A very rare complication of purpura fulminans and gangrene of the extremities and face has been described following varicella (deKoning et al., 1972; Smith, 1967). This complication is thought to be due to a transient autoimmune response with resulting abnormalities in coagulation proteins (Josephson et al., 2001). Another very rare complication of varicella as well as zoster is vasculitis and thrombosis leading to neurologic symptoms (Amlie-Lefond et al., 1995; Bodensteiner et al., 1991; Caekebeke et al., 1990; Fikrig and Barg, 1989; Liu and Holmes, 1990).

PROGNOSIS

Varicella is usually a benign disease of childhood, although some evidence suggests that it may be potentially more serious than previously thought (Choo et al., 1995). The typical case usually clears spontaneously without sequelae or skin scarring. Lesions that are secondarily infected are likely to be followed by permanent scars if the deep layers of the skin are involved. The rare case of sepsis, bacterial pneumonia, or osteomyelitis usually responds to appropriate antibacterial therapy. Preblud et al. (1985) estimated that there are fewer than 10 deaths caused by varicella in infants under 1 year of age in the United States per year, and those occur primarily as a result of pneumonia or encephalitis. Although this represents a risk of death of 8/100,000 cases, four times greater than that of older infants and children with varicella, the risk is obviously very small (Preblud et al., 1985). In the prevaccine era in the United States, there were an estimated 100 deaths annually from varicella and 11,000 hospitalizations (Centers for Disease Control and Prevention, 1999). Because zoster is a secondary infection, the risk of fatalities associated with zoster is lower than that for varicella.

IMMUNITY

An attack of chickenpox usually confers lasting immunity; second attacks are unusual (Gershon et al., 1984a; Junker et al., 1989; Weller, 1983). Varicella-zoster antibody persists for many years after chickenpox. Most immune adults have antibodies detectable by ELISA, FAMA, LA, or RIA.

Transplacental immunity has been examined. In one study 200 mother-infant (cord) serum specimens for VZV antibody were tested by FAMA; 10% of the pairs in this group were seronegative (Gershon et al., 1976b). The maternal and cord blood antibody titers were essentially the same. Women born in the United States were more likely to be immune than those born in Latin American countries. Only 5% of U.S.-born women were seronegative, as compared with 16% of those born in Latin America. A high incidence of susceptibility to varicella in adults from tropical areas also has been noted (Nassar and Touma, 1986). The disappearance of passively acquired antibody in the first year of life is shown in Figure 41-10. By 6 months of age most infants no longer have detectable VZV antibody. Transplacentally acquired VZV antibody has been detected in the blood of low–birth-weight infants, even those weighing less than 1500 g (Raker et al., 1978), but not in infants less than 1000 g at birth (Wang et al., 1983). Development of mild

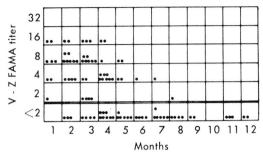

Fig. 41-10 Detection of varicella-zoster antibody in the first year of life in 67 infants. The sensitive fluorescent antibody against membrane antigen (FAMA) test was used for the assay. (From Gershon AA, Raker R, Steinberg S, et al: Pediatrics 1976;58: 692-696.)

varicella in young infants despite the presence of transplacental maternal antibody has been reported (Baba et al., 1982).

The immune correlates of VZV infection remain incompletely understood. During the course of vaccine trials with the live attenuated varicella vaccine it was recognized that the presence of specific serum antibody at the time of exposure to the virus does not necessarily always guarantee protection from clinical varicella, especially in immunocompromised patients. A minority of recipients of varicella vaccine who had underlying leukemia developed mild clinical varicella after an exposure several months after immunization despite serum VZV antibody titers that were predicted as protective (Gershon et al., 1986; Gershon and Steinberg, 1989). In addition, varicella has been reported in persons having detectable VZV antibody after natural infection (Gershon et al., 1984a; Junker et al., 1991; Zaia et al., 1983). These observations led to reexamination of the mechanism by which immunity to varicella is mediated. Serum antibody may not be fully protective; either CMI or secretory immunity may also be important in protection (Arvin and Gershon, 1996; Bogger-Goren et al., 1984; Cooper et al., 1988; Diaz et al., 1989; Giller et al., 1989).

It was recognized many years ago that the prognosis of varicella in children with isolated defects in humoral immunity was excellent. In addition, these children usually developed varicella only once. In contrast, children with congenital defects in CMI were recognized to be at high risk to develop severe infections. Specific CMI to VZV develops after an attack of varicella. Failure to develop a positive cellular

immune response correlates with death from varicella (Arvin et al., 1986; Gershon and Steinberg, 1979; Patel et al., 1979). Various types of CMI to VZV have been described, including T-cell and macrophage cytotoxicity, antibody dependent cellular cytotoxicity (ADCC), and natural killer (NK) cells (Arvin and Gershon, 1996).

The exact roles of humoral and cellular immunity in protection against VZV infection are under continued investigation and are summarized as follows (reviewed in Arvin and Gershon, 1996). Structural and regulatory proteins of VZV are recognized by T-lymphocytes during varicella and play the major role in protection of the host from further VZV infection. This is consistent with the observation that patients with agammaglobulinemia are not subject to bouts of recurrent varicella. Memory immunity mediated by both CD4+ and CD8+ T-lymphocytes is maintained for decades and can be demonstrated by in vitro proliferation and cytokine assays. Memory responses may normally persist because of periodic exogenous re-exposure to others with either varicella or zoster. Immunity may also be maintained by endogenous reexposure to the virus due to subclinical reactivation of latent VZV. Sensitized T-lymphocytes that are exposed to VZV antigens produce cytokines of the Th1 type, such as interleukin 2 (IL-2) and gamma interferon (IFN-γ); these potentiate the clonal expansion of virus-specific T-cells (Arvin and Gershon, 1996). That CMI rather than humoral immunity is required to maintain the balance between the host and latent VZV is demonstrated by the correlation between diminished CMI and the increased risk of zoster in immunocompromised and in elderly individuals. Patients who develop zoster, however, usually have a rapid increase in VZV CMI because of endogenous exposure to viral antigens. This enhanced CMI is usually persistent, which may explain why second episodes of zoster are uncommon. Susceptibility of individuals to VZV reactivation, in contrast, is not related to levels of VZV antibodies. A diagram depicting the summary of the dynamic natural history of VZV infections is shown in Figure 41-11.

EPIDEMIOLOGIC FACTORS

The epidemiology of varicella and zoster has been changing since the licensure of live attenuated varicella vaccine in the United States in

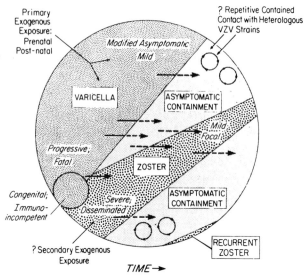

Fig. 41-11 Diagrammatic summary of the natural history of infection with varicella-zoster virus. Two variables are depicted: time and clinical severity. In the competent host the containment period is on the order of decades; however, in the immunocompromised person the two clinical processes may merge without an intervening asymptomatic interval. The containment period after congenital varicella is typically of short duration. During the asymptomatic containment period, episodes of endogenous viral replication probably occur, and contact with heterologous exogenous strains may stimulate host defenses, usually in the absence of overt disease. (From Weller TH: N Engl J Med 1983;309:1362-1368, 1434-1440.)

1995, in Canada in 1999, and in many other countries in the world. The comments that follow are mainly reflective of the prevaccine era.

Chickenpox is worldwide in distribution, being endemic in all large cities. Epidemics do not have the periodicity of measles; they occur at irregular intervals determined chiefly by the size and concentration of new groups of susceptible children. All races and both sexes are equally susceptible. In countries with tropical climates there is decreased spread of VZV among children, and varicella in adults is a common occurrence. Seasonable distribution varies with the particular geographic zone; in temperate areas the incidence rises during the late autumn, winter, and spring. In contrast to varicella, zoster occurs with equal frequency throughout the year.

Varicella is predominantly a disease of childhood, with the highest age incidence between 2 and 10 years. Its occurrence is unusual in adults who have lived in heavily populated urban areas but not uncommon in those who have come from isolated rural areas. Ross et al. observed a group of 641 adults and 501 children who had intimate household exposures to varicella. The overall attack rates were 1.4%

for adults and 78% for children. Of 79 adults with a negative history of varicella, only 8% acquired the disease. In contrast, 87% of 441 children with no history of varicella acquired the disease (Ross et al., 1962).

Studies in New York City have indicated that of 92 consecutive adults with no history of varicella, 23 (25%) were actually susceptible (LaRussa, 1985). Others have noted a similar percentage of susceptibility in adults from throughout the United States (Alter et al., 1986; Steele et al., 1982). In the continental United States, the overall rate of susceptibility to varicella in adults is less than 5%.

Nosocomial varicella is a significant problem, not only because some patients may be at risk to develop a severe infection, but also because of the expense and administrative problems associated with management of a potential hospital outbreak (Krasinski, et al., 1986; Weber et al., 1988). Often physicians, nurses, and other personnel susceptible to varicella must be furloughed after an exposure until the potential incubation period ends. In a study by Weber et al., the cost per year at a university hospital was $56,000 for passive immunization of high-risk susceptible individuals and for furloughs of susceptible personnel (Weber et al., 1988). Similar hospital costs for a year's time were recorded by Krasinski et al. (1986). Transmission of varicella is rare, however, in the setting of the newborn nursery. Only three instances of such nosocomial spread have been recorded (Friedman et al., 1994b; Gershon et al., 1976a; Gustafson et al., 1984).

Although apparent hospital outbreaks of zoster have been described, in many instances they are probably coincidental occurrences because they involve a high proportion of immunocompromised patients (Schimpff et al., 1972). Based on the current understanding of the pathogenesis of zoster as the result of reactivation of latent VZV, hospital outbreaks of zoster would seem to be extremely unlikely to occur. Some apparent cases of zoster are probably second attacks of varicella (Morens et al., 1980).

Zoster is predominately a disease of adults, in contrast to varicella. A study of 108 zoster patients revealed that 69% were 50 years of age or older and less than 10% were children (Miller and Brunell, 1970). In a study of 192 cases the annual incidence of zoster per 1,000 persons was 0.74 in children under 10 years, 2.5 in persons aged 20 to 50, and 10 in those over age 80 (Hope-Simpson, 1965).

Immunocompromised children are at increased risk to develop zoster compared with healthy children. In a study of children with malignant disease the overall rate of zoster was 9% (Feldman et al., 1973). This study involved 1,132 patients over a 10-year period. The rate of zoster in patients with Hodgkin's disease was 22%; it was 10% in children with acute lymphoblast leukemia, and 5% in children with solid tumors. No specific chemotherapy was associated with increased risk of infection. A similar high rate of zoster of about 15% in leukemic children was observed in more recent studies (Brunell et al., 1986; Hardy et al., 1991; Lawrence et al., 1988). Children with HIV infection who develop varicella when they have CD4+ levels of less than 15% have been reported to have a rate of zoster as high as 70% (Gershon et al., 1997).

Chickenpox is one of the most highly contagious diseases, comparable to measles and smallpox in this respect. The infection is spread chiefly by direct contact with a patient with active varicella or zoster. The major source of the virus is probably from skin lesions, although respiratory spread can also occur in varicella (Brunell, 1989; Tsolia et al., 1990). It is virtually impossible to culture VZV from the throat even in the early stages of varicella, but viral isolation from skin vesicles can be easily accomplished. The chances of viral transmission are directly related to the number of skin lesions (Tsolia et al., 1990). Patients are probably most contagious in the early stages of illness when they have the greatest numbers of moist vesicular skin lesions. That the virus is spread by the airborne route has been determined in hospital outbreak studies in which airflow patterns from patient rooms have been examined (Gustafson et al., 1982; Josephson and Gombert, 1988; Leclair et al., 1980). Presumably as a result of scratching the pruritic skin lesions, VZV gains access to the air. Under hospital conditions indirect contact through the medium of a third person has not been documented, and it is not likely that medical personnel carry the infection from one place or patient to another.

A patient with chickenpox can transmit the disease to other susceptible persons from 1 or 2 days before onset of rash until all the vesicles have become dry. A mild case will show complete crusting within 5 days and a severe case within 10 days. Dry scabs do not contain infectious virus, although VZV DNA may still be demonstrable by PCR. Patients with zoster remain infectious to others who have not had varicella as long as new lesions continue to develop and the existing ones remain moist. This may be longer than the interval of contagion for varicella.

TREATMENT

Chickenpox in otherwise healthy children is normally a self-limited disease. Symptomatic therapy includes acetaminophen for high fever and constitutional symptoms. A comparison of the course of varicella in children who did or did not receive acetaminophen revealed minimal differences in the course of the illness, with the children who were treated having a slightly longer course (Josephson and Gombert, 1988). It seems unlikely that the differences in the course of illness are clinically significant, however, and the relief of fever afforded by acetaminophen therapy seems worth the theoretical minimal risk. Aspirin should not be given, because it may lead to development of Reye's syndrome (Mortimer and Lepow, 1962; Starko et al., 1980). Although some reports suggest an association between use of nonsteroidal antinflammatory drugs and severe streptococcal disease in children with varicella, this has not been proved (Peterson et al., 1996). Because it is possible that treatment with nonsteroidal antiinflammatory drugs predisposes to bacterial superinfection, these medications should be avoided in varicella. Oral antihistamines and local applications of calamine lotion may help control the itching of varicella. Fingernails should be kept short and clean in an attempt to minimize secondary skin infections. For the same reason, daily bathing is also recommended during chickenpox.

Treatment of Complications

Bacterial infections. Bacterial infections complicating chickenpox are most often caused by *S. aureus* or group A β-hemolytic streptococci. Infection of local lesions usually responds to simple measures such as warm compresses. Antimicrobial therapy is indicated for cellulitis, sepsis, or pneumonia. The treatment of severe streptococcal and staphylococcal infections is discussed in detail in Chapters 34 and 35, respectively.

Encephalitis. Patients in coma require careful observation and supportive treatment such as parenteral and tube feedings for the maintenance of hydration and adequate nutrition. Corticosteroids have not provided effective therapy for varicella encephalitis. Antiviral therapy may be used but is of no proved value. Cerebellar ataxia is usually a self-limited complication for which specific treatment is unnecessary.

Specific Antiviral Therapy for Varicella and Zoster

The antiviral drug ACV (9,2-hydroxyethoxymethylguanine) has become the drug of choice for specific therapy of VZV infections, but the drug does not prevent or cure latent VZV. ACV is available in topical, oral, and intravenous (IV) formulations, but only the latter two are useful against VZV. Only approximately 15% to 20% of orally administered ACV is absorbed.

ACV is relatively nontoxic because it interferes mainly with synthesis of viral rather than host DNA; it is not antiviral itself. To interfere with DNA synthesis, ACV must be phosphorylated by a virus-induced enzyme: thymidine kinase. This enzyme is present almost exclusively in infected cells; therefore the effect of ACV on uninfected cells is minimal. Because the enzyme is not required for viral synthesis, strains of VZV can become resistant to ACV by either ceasing to produce thymidine kinase or producing a truncated or altered enzyme or altered viral DNA polymerase that will not bind the phosphorylated ACV. A few thymidine kinase-negative, ACV-resistant strains of VZV have been reported in AIDS patients (Jacobson et al., 1990; Linnemann et al., 1990; Pahwa et al., 1988). The clinical relevance of these ACV-resistant viruses remains unknown because resistant strains are less invasive than sensitive strains, and transmission to non-AIDS patients has not been observed. ACV-resistant strains are generally also resistant to drugs like famciclovir and valacyclovir, which have mechanisms of action similar to those of ACV. Foscarnet, a pyrophosphate analogue that exerts its antiviral effect by inhibition of the viral DNA polymerase, has been useful in the treatment of these ACV-resistant strains. Renal toxicity has limited more widespread use of foscarnet.

The dose of ACV used to treat VZV infections is higher than that used to treat HSV infections, because VZV is less sensitive to this drug than is HSV. Usual plasma concentrations necessary for inhibition of VZV are 1 to 2 μg/ml, with a range of roughly 0.5 to 11 μg/ml. Commonly used doses of IV ACV almost always result in plasma levels significantly above maximal inhibitory concentrations for VZV isolates. In contrast, orally administered ACV leads to drug levels (1 1.5 μg/ml) that will inhibit most but not all VZV strains. Toxicity of ACV includes nausea, vomiting, skin rash, phlebitis (if given intravenously), and precipitation of the drug in the renal tubules in poorly hydrated patients. Because ACV is excreted by the kidney, lower doses should be used for patients with abnormalities in renal function (Arvin, 1986).

In a double blind, placebo-controlled study of its efficacy in children with varicella, ACV was administered orally at high dosage in otherwise healthy children (Balfour et al., 1990). An oral dose of 20 mg/kg of ACV four times daily for 5 days was given to 50 children, within 24 hours of onset of the skin rash. A similar group received placebo. The duration of the disease was shortened by approximately 1 day as evidenced by defervescence and healing of rash, but treated children did not return to school any sooner than placebo recipients, and the rate of complications of varicella was not altered by therapy. These studies were confirmed in a larger collaborative controlled study involving about 1,000 children (Dunkel et al., 1991). Treatment with ACV does not appear to interfere with development of immunity to VZV (Englund et al., 1990; Levin et al., 1995). Because the severity of varicella is statistically, but not significantly, clinically altered by ACV, whether or not routinely to treat children with varicella with ACV is problematic. The drug is expensive, and whether there are long-term adverse effects of ACV is not known for certain. Moreover, the possibility that resistance of VZV to ACV may increase with widespread use of this drug must be considered. One possible approach is to give ACV to adolescents, who are at greater risk to develop more significant clinical manifestations of varicella, and to secondary cases of varicella in the household because secondary cases usually are more severe than index cases. Early therapy, administered within the first day of onset of rash, is also important and is potentially easier to implement in secondary cases in a household in which the disease can be quickly recognized. There is positive anecdotal experience in administration of ACV to adults with varicella (Feder, 1990; Haake et al., 1990). A small double blind study suggested that early therapy of adults was worthwhile (Wallace et al., 1992). Widespread use of varicella vaccine will decrease the need to treat patients with varicella.

Orally administered ACV has been used with success to decrease the morbidity of otherwise healthy adults with zoster by relieving acute pain and promoting healing of the skin lesions (Cobo, 1988; Huff et al., 1988; McKendrick et al., 1986; Wood et al., 1988; Wood et al., 1996). A dose of 4 g per day (800 mg five times a day by mouth for 7 days) is used. This same dose may be used to treat adults with varicella. Because otherwise healthy children who develop zoster usually have only a mild illness, ACV is not often given to children with zoster. Newer drugs, valacyclovir and famciclovir, are recommended for treatment of zoster, but have been tested neither in children nor for treatment of varicella. These drugs, referred to as *prodrugs,* are converted in the liver after oral administration to the parent compound. They are well absorbed by the oral route and therefore result in higher drug levels than administration of the parent compound itself, and require less frequent dosing intervals. The parent compound of valacyclovir is ACV; for famciclovir the parent is penciclovir (Spring et al., 1994). These drugs are used at doses of 500 mg (famciclovir) and 1,000 mg (valacyclovir) three times a day orally for 1 to 2 weeks for treatment of zoster in adolescents and adults.

Severe varicella and zoster ACV, administered intravenously, is the drug of choice for treatment of severe varicella or zoster and for varicella that is potentially life threatening. When administered intravenously to immunocompromised children within 3 days of onset of rash, this drug decreases mortality from varicella (Balfour, 1984; Prober et al., 1982) and prevents viral dissemination (Feldman and Lott, 1987; Nyerges et al., 1988). Administering IV ACV also results in more rapid healing of zoster in normal and immunocompromised patients, ameliorates acute pain, and decreases the likelihood of viral dissemination (Balfour, 1984; Balfour et al., 1983; Peterslund, 1988; Shepp et al., 1988). In uncontrolled studies, ACV has been used to treat varicella pneumonia in adults, including pregnant women, with apparent success (Eder et al., 1988; Landsberger et al., 1986; Schlossberg and Littman, 1988). ACV is superior to vidarabine for treatment of VZV infections, mainly because of its lower toxicity (Feldman et al., 1986; Shepp et al., 1988).

For treatment of immunocompromised patients with varicella or zoster, ACV should be administered intravenously at a dose of 1500 mg/m^2 of body surface area per day divided q8 hours, for 7 to 10 days. Reduced doses should be used for patients with impaired renal function. For adolescents a dose of 10 mg/kg of body weight every 8 hours may be used.

Because the dose for newborn infants with severe varicella is not known, use of a dose of 750 mg/m^2/day is suggested. Some investigators have recommended that all infants who develop neonatal varicella, even those who have been passively immunized with VZIG, be treated with ACV (Haddad et al., 1987; Holland et al., 1986; Sills et al., 1987). Another possible approach is to initiate therapy with oral medication, reserving intravenous ACV for those whose infection is progressing. In the United States, most can be expected to recover without antiviral therapy (Hanngren et al., 1985; Preblud et al., 1986a). Very rare fatalities caused by varicella have been recorded in infants who contracted varicella from their mothers near the time of delivery despite administration of VZIG at an appropriate time and dosage (King et al., 1986). The case reported by King et al. is of special interest because the mother developed the rash of varicella on the second postpartum day.

It is recommended that highly immunocompromised children, such as those with leukemia who are still receiving chemotherapy, who have not been actively or passively immunized be treated with intravenous ACV as soon as possible after the diagnosis of varicella has been made, although most patients so treated would be expected to recover on their own. Even if the disease appears mild at first, it is impossible to predict which children will develop severe infections. Once varicella has become severe, ACV may not be effective. There is no consensus as to whether it is preferable to withhold anticancer chemotherapy (including steroids) after an exposure to varicella and/or after the onset of varicella, with the exception that in steroid-dependent children this medication should not be abruptly withdrawn. Decisions about treatment of these patients should be individualized and made in consultation with the oncologist following the child.

It may seem more compelling to treat all highly immunosuppressed patients with varicella, since the mortality rate approaches 10%, than to treat all such patients with zoster, which has a lower mortality rate of perhaps 1 to 2%. Among zoster patients, adults with lymphoproliferative cancers and those who have had bone-marrow transplantation are at greatest risk for severe disease (Whitley et al., 1982). Because ACV is relatively nontoxic, however, an argument can be made to treat most immunocompromised patients with zoster, including children, to decrease morbidity from the illness. In zoster patients who are not especially ill, an attempt to treat with orally administered ACV may be made, using, for children, the doses administered for varicella. (Famciclovir or valacyclovir may be used for adolescents.) The use of antiviral therapy in patients with CNS complications of varicella or zoster is controversial because the underlying pathology is not well understood. Many physicians elect to treat immunocompromised patients with antiviral drugs, but not those who are immunologically normal.

Alternative secondary drugs, vidarabine and interferon, are also effective in treatment of varicella and zoster but have significant toxicity and are rarely used (Arvin et al., 1982; Merigan et al., 1978; Whitley et al., 1982). VZIG is not useful for therapy of VZV infection. Because of issues regarding the long-term persistence of immunity and the availability of varicella vaccine, prophylactic ACV is not usually recommended for those who are susceptible to varicella and have been exposed, although it has been used in research settings (Asano et al., 1993; Huang et al., 1995; Suga et al., 1993; Yoshikawa et al., 1998).

PREVENTIVE MEASURES
Passive Immunization

Preventive measures are not usually recommended for healthy varicella-susceptible children who have been exposed to VZV. On the other hand, exposed susceptible immunocompromised children, and adults proved susceptible, should be passively immunized with VZIG (Centers for Disease Control and Prevention, 1999). Infants whose mothers have the onset of the rash of varicella within 5 days before and 2 days after delivery should be protected with passive immunization. Indications for the use of VZIG, based on the recommendations of the Committee on Infectious Diseases of the American Academy of Pediatrics and the Advisory Committee on Immunization Practices of the Centers for Disease Control and Prevention (CDC) in Atlanta, Georgia, are shown in Box 41-1.

Successful passive immunization against varicella was first accomplished with zoster immune globulin (ZIG). ZIG was prepared from plasma of patients convalescing from zoster. A dose of 5 ml of ZIG, given within 72 hours of a household exposure to children with underlying leukemia, modified chickenpox (Brunell et al., 1969; Gershon et al., 1974; Judelsohn et al., 1974; Orenstein et al., 1981).

ZIG has now been supplanted by VZIG, which is prepared from plasma of healthy donors with high antibody titers against VZV. VZIG is similar to ZIG in its ability to modify varicella in high-risk children (Zaia et al., 1983). The dose of VZIG is 1.25 ml/10 kg of body weight, administered intramuscularly, within 3 days of exposure; the maximal dose is 6.25 ml or 5 vials. VZIG may also be effective up to 5 days after exposure, but it is probably not worthwhile to administer it beyond that interval.

VZIG has been used successfully to modify varicella in approximately 100 newborn infants whose mothers had varicella at delivery (Hanngren et al., 1985; Preblud et al., 1986b). In both studies the attack rate of varicella was approximately 50%, not indicative of a decrease in the attack rate after passive immunization. However, as in immunocompromised children, the illness was clearly modified, with most infants developing mild disease and no fatalities clearly due to varicella. An alternative to VZIG is IV immune globulin (IVIG) (Paryani et al., 1984). Neither VZIG nor IVIG can be expected to prevent or modify zoster in high-risk patients (Groth et al., 1978; Merigan and Stevens, 1978).

Active Immunization

A live attenuated varicella vaccine developed in Japan by Takahashi, the Oka strain, was licensed for routine use in susceptible children and adults in the United States in 1995 (Centers for Disease Control and Prevention, 1996; Takahashi et al., 1974). This vaccine was prepared by serial passage of wild type VZV isolated from an otherwise healthy 3-year-old Japanese boy with varicella whose last name was Oka. After approximately 35 passages in various cell cultures of guinea pig and human origin, the agent remained immunogenic but rarely caused symptoms upon administration by injection.

In clinical studies in the United States in healthy children (Arbeter et al., 1982, Arbeter et al., 1984; Arbeter et al., 1986a; Arbeter et al., 1986b; Brunell et al., 1988; Englund et al., 1989; Johnson et al., 1988; Johnson et al., 1997), healthy adults (Arbeter et al., 1986a; Alter et al., 1985; Gershon et al., 1988; Hardy and Gershon, 1990; Saiman et al., 2001), and children with underlying leukemia (Gershon et al., 1984b; Zaia et al., 1983), the vaccine was demonstrated to be safe and highly effective in preventing severe varicella.

Immunization against varicella in healthy children is associated with minimal adverse effects, mainly a mild rash of about 5 lesions in about 5%, and transient redness, swelling, and rash at the injection site in about 20%. Transmission of vaccine type VZV from healthy vaccinees with a rash to other varicella-susceptible contacts has been recorded only on very rare occasions (Sharrar et al., 2000). Contact cases are mild, indicating the attenuation of the vaccine strain (Sharrar et al., 2000; Tsolia et al., 1990). The vaccine provides approximately 90% protection in prevention of varicella. The few children who develop breakthrough varicella almost always have very mild disease with few skin lesions and little systemic toxicity. In research studies, administering varicella vaccine in combination with measles-mumps-rubella (MMR) vaccine has resulted in excellent antigenic responses to all four viruses (Arbeter et al., 1986b; Arbeter et al., 1988; Brunell et al., 1988; Englund et al., 1989), but the final formulation of this product has not been determined and this combination vaccine is not yet available. However, varicella vaccine and MMR vaccine can be administered simultaneously using separate sites and syringes. As with all live attenuated viral vaccines, an interval of at least 30 days is required before administration of another live virus vaccine, except when vaccines are administered simultaneously.

Varicella vaccine is recommended for healthy varicella-susceptible children and adults. Children between the ages of 12 months and 12 years should be given one dose of vaccine. Adults and children who have reached their thirteenth birthday should be given 2 doses of vaccine at a 4- to 8-week interval. Individuals receiving low or moderate doses of steroids (less than the equivalent of 2 mg/kg/day of prednisone) may be immunized (Centers for Disease Control and Prevention, 1996; Centers for Disease Control and Prevention, 1999; Committee on Infectious Diseases, 1995; Committee on Infectious Diseases, 2000). Contraindications to immunization include severe allergy to any vaccine component, significant immunosuppression, and pregnancy. Because of the association of natural varicella, aspirin use, and Reye's syndrome, the package insert recommends as a precautionary measure that children receiving chronic aspirin therapy not be vaccinated.

The CDC now recommends administration of varicella to healthy susceptible individuals following an exposure to VZV. Data in vaccinated children suggest that the approach will often be effective, although data in adults are more limited (Centers for Disease Control and Prevention, 1999; Watson et al., 2000). Postexposure vaccination may be less effective in adults than children because adults require two doses of vaccine. Varicella vaccine has proved to be effective in prevention of chickenpox in susceptible healthcare workers (Saiman et al., 2001).

Varicella vaccine has been found to be highly effective as it is used in a private practice setting, with an efficacy of 85% in a case control study involving over 200 children with PCR-proved varicella (Vazquez et al., 2001). Varicella vaccine has also been used successfully in day-care settings (Clements et al., 1995; Clements et al., 1999; Clements et al., 2001).

Varicella vaccine has not yet been approved for use in high-risk immunocompromised children in the United States (except for leukemic children who can be immunized on a "compassionate use" basis), despite the demonstrated efficacy of this approach in published studies. Approximately 85% of leukemic children were protected against chickenpox after vaccination, and all were protected from severe disease in studies involving over 500 children. Although 50% of patients with leukemia may develop a vaccine-associated rash in the month after immunization, serious rashes can be prevented by administration of high-dose oral ACV (Gershon et al., 1984b; Gershon et al., 1989; Gershon et al., 1986). Immunocompromised children such as those with leukemia who develop a vaccine-associated rash have greater potential to spread vaccine-type VZV to others than healthy individuals. Contact cases, however, are extremely mild, indicating that the vaccine virus is attenuated (Sharrar et al., 2000; Tsolia et al., 1990). "Breakthrough" cases of wild-type chickenpox in vaccinees with leukemia after exposure to natural VZV have usually been mild (Gershon et al., 1989). Children with chronic renal insufficiency were successfully immunized against chickenpox with few adverse effects except for a mild rash in 5% to 10% (Broyer and Boudailliez, 1985a; Broyer and Boudailliez, 1985b, Broyer et al., 1997).

The incidence of zoster is decreased after vaccination of children with leukemia who are ordinarily at high risk to develop reactivation of VZV (Brunell et al., 1986; Hardy et al., 1991; Lawrence et al., 1988). There is also no evidence of an increased incidence of zoster in vaccinated healthy children or adults (Gershon, 2001; Sharrar et al., 2000). With time, it is anticipated that the incidence of zoster after vaccination will be found to be lower than after natural infection in healthy vaccinees.

Studies thus far indicate that varicella vaccine will provide long-lasting protection from chickenpox, based on persistence of antibodies to VZV after vaccination. Ten- and 20-year follow-up studies from Japan indicated that positive antibody titers and protective immunity were maintained in healthy children for this period (Asano et al., 1983; Asano et al., 1994). Studies in the United States involving over 500 children have indicated persistence of antibodies for as long as 10 years in close to 100% of children (Clements et al., 1995; Johnson et al., 1997; Krause and Klinman, 1995; Kuter et al., 1991; Watson et al., 1994). In some studies, the rate of breakthrough varicella ranged, over an interval of 5 to 10 years after vaccination, between 17% and 34% (Clements et al., 1995; Johnson et al., 1997; Takayama et al., 1997). Nevertheless, breakthrough illnesses were most often mild. These data, however, support arguments for an additional routine dose of vari-cella vaccine even in children less than 13 years old. This seems most likely to be mandated after an effective MMRV is licensed.

With the widespread use of varicella vaccine in the United States, the incidence of chicken-pox is declining in all age groups (Seward et al., 2000a; Seward et al., 2000b). This observation, along with that of the experience in day-care centers (Clements et al., 1999), where the rate of varicella has decreased out of proportion to the numbers of children immunized, indicate that varicella vaccine induces herd immunity.

ISOLATION AND QUARANTINE

Unless there are specific local regulations, isola-tion and quarantine procedures should be indi-vidualized. Most authorities agree that (1) the

patient with chickenpox or zoster should be kept at home until all the vesicles have dried, (2) con-tacts should not be quarantined but merely observed, and (3) efforts to institute isolation precautions within the home to protect siblings are useless and should not be attempted.

On the other hand, rigid isolation precau-tions should be used for the prevention of chickenpox in high-risk children. Appropriate measures should be instituted to prevent con-tact with a definite or potential case of chick-enpox. If exposure has occurred or is inevitable, use of the preventive measures already described are indicated. Widespread use of varicella vaccine may decrease the neces-sity of isolation of cases in the future. An algo-rithm for the management of hospital exposures to varicella is shown in Figure 41-12.

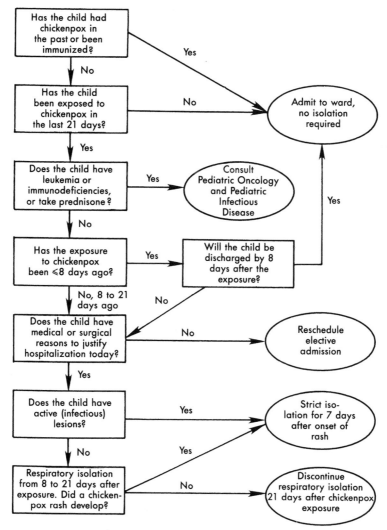

Fig. 41-12 Algorithm for chickenpox exposure. (From Brawley RL, Wenzel RP: An algorithm for chickenpox exposure. Modified from Pediatr Infect Dis J 1984;3: 502-504.)

BIBLIOGRAPHY

Acheson DWK, Leen CL, Tariq WU, et al. Severe and recurrent varicella-zoster virus infection in a patient with the acquired immune deficiency syndrome. J Infect 1988;16:193-197.

Alter SJ, Hammond JA, McVey CJ, et al. Susceptibility to varicella-zoster virus among adults at high risk for exposure. Infect Contr 1986;7:448-451.

Alter SJ, McVey CJ, Jenski L, Myers M. Varicella live virus vaccine in normal susceptible adults at high risk for exposure. Interscience Conference on Antimicrobial Agents and Chemotherapy, 1985.

Amlie-Lefond C, Kleinschmidt-DeMasters BK, Mahlingham R, et al. The vasculopathy of varicella-zoster virus encephalitis. Ann Neurol 1995;37:784-790.

Annunziato PW, Lungu O, Panagiotidis C. Varicella zoster virus in human and rat tissue specimens. Arch Virol Suppl 2001;17:135-142.

Applebaum E, Rachelson MH, Dolgopol VB. Varicella encephalitis. Am J Med 1953;15:523.

Arvin AM, Pollard RB, Rasmussen L, et al. Selective impairment in lymphocyte reactivity to varicella-zoster antigen among untreated lymphoma patients. J Infect Dis 1978;137:531-540.

Arbeter A, Starr S, Weibel RE, et al. Live attenuated varicella vaccine: immunization of healthy children with the Oka strain. J Pediatr 1982;100:886-893.

Arbeter A, Starr SE, Plotkin SA. Varicella vaccine studies in healthy children and adults. Pediatrics 1986a;78 (suppl):748-756.

Arbeter AM, Baker L, Starr SE, et al. Combination measles, mumps, rubella, and varicella vaccine. Pediatrics 1986b;78:742-747.

Arbeter AM, Baker L, Starr SE, et al. Combination measles, mumps, rubella, and varicella vaccine. Pediatrics 1988;78:s742-s747.

Arbeter AM, Starr SE, Preblud S, et al. Varicella vaccine trials in healthy children: a summary of comparative follow-up studies. Am J Dis Child 1984;138:434-438.

Arvin A. Oral therapy with acyclovir in infants and children. Pediatr Infect Dis J 1986;6:56-58.

Arvin A, Gershon A. Live attenuated varicella vaccine. Annu Rev Microbiol 1996;50:59-100.

Arvin A, Koropchak CM, Wittek AE. Immunologic evidence of reinfection with varicella-zoster virus. J Infect Dis 1983; 48:200-205.

Arvin AM, Koropchak CM, Williams BR, et al. Early immune response in healthy and immunocompromised subjects with primary varicella-zoster virus infection. J Infect Dis 1986;154:422-429.

Arvin AM, Kushner JH, Feldman S, et al. Human leukocyte interferon for the treatment of varicella in children with cancer. N Engl J Med 1982;306:761-765.

Arvin AM, Pollard RB, Rasmussen L, Merigan T. Selective impairment in lymphocyte reactivity to varicella-zoster antigen among untreated lymphoma patients. J Infect Dis 1978;137:531-540.

Asano Y, Albrecht P, Vujcic LK, et al. Five-year follow-up study of recipients of live varicella vaccine using enhanced neutralization and fluorescent antibody membrane antigen assays. Pediatrics 1983;72:291-294.

Asano Y, Itakura N, Hiroishi Y, et al. Viremia is present in incubation period in nonimmunocompromised children with varicella. J Pediatr 1985;106:69-71.

Asano Y, Itakura N, Kajita Y, et al. Severity of viremia and clinical findings in children with varicella. J Infect Dis 1990;161:1095-1098.

Asano Y, Suga S, Yoshikawa T, et al. Experience and reason: twenty year follow up of protective immunity of the Oka live varicella vaccine. Pediatrics 1994;94:524-526.

Asano Y, Yoshikawa T, Suga S, et al. Postexposure prophylaxis of varicella in family contact by oral acyclovir. Pediatrics 1993;92:219-222.

Baba K, Yabuuchi H, Takahashi M, et al. Immunologic and epidemiologic aspects of varicella infection acquired during infancy and early childhood. J Pediatr 1982;100:881-885.

Baba K, Yabuuchi H, Takahashi M, et al. Increased incidence of herpes zoster in normal children infected with varicella-zoster virus during infancy: community-based follow up study. J Pediatr 1986;108:372-377.

Baird RE, Daly P, Sawyer M. Varicella arthritis diagnosed by polymerase chain reaction. Pediatr Infect Dis J 1991;12:950-951.

Bakshi S, Miller TC, Gershon A, et al. Failure of VZIG in modification of severe congenital varicella. Pediatr Infect Dis J 1986;5:699-702.

Balfour H. Intravenous acyclovir therapy for varicella in immunocompromised children. J Pediatr 1984;104:134-140.

Balfour H, McMonigal K, Bean B. Acyclovir therapy of varicella-zoster virus infection in immunocompromised patients. J Antimicrob Chemother 1983;12(S):169-179.

Balfour HH, Kelly JM, et al. Acyclovir treatment of varicella in otherwise healthy children. J Pediatr 1990;116:633-639.

Berger R, Florent G, Just M. Decrease of the lymphoproliferative response to varicella-zoster virus antigen in the aged. Infect Immun 1981;32:24-27.

Bezold GD, Lange ME, Gall H, et al. Detection of cutaneous varicella zoster virus infections by immunofluorescence versus PCR. Eur J Dermatol 2001;11:108-111.

Bodensteiner JB, Hille MR, Riggs JE. Clinical features of vascular thrombosis following varicella. Am J Dis Child 1991;146:100-102.

Bogger-Goren S, Bernstein JM, Gershon A, et al. Mucosal cell mediated immunity to varicella zoster virus: role in protection against disease. J Pediatr 1984;105:195-199.

Bradley JS, Schlievert PM, Sample TG. Streptococcal toxic shock–like syndrome as a complication of varicella. Pediatr Infect Dis J 1991;10:77-78.

Brogan TV, Niozet V, Waldhausen JHT, et al. Group A streptococcal necrotizing fasciitis complicating primary varicella: a series of fourteen patients. Pediatr Infect Dis J 1995;14:588-594.

Broyer M, Boudailliez B. Varicella vaccine in children with chronic renal insufficiency. Postgrad Med J 1985a;61 (S4):103-106.

Broyer M, Boudailliez B. Prevention of varicella infection in renal transplanted children by previous immunization with a live attenuated varicella vaccine. Transplant Proc 1985b;17:151-152.

Broyer M, Tete MT, Guest G, et al. Varicella and zoster in children after kidney transplantation: long term results of vaccination. Pediatrics 1997;99:35-39.

Brunell P, Ross A, Miller L, et al. Prevention of varicella by zoster immune globulin. N Engl J Med 1969;280:1191-1194.

Brunell PA. Transmission of chickenpox in a school setting prior to the observed exanthem. Am J Dis Child 1989;143:1451-1452.

Brunell PA, Kotchmar GSJ. Zoster in infancy: failure to maintain virus latency following intrauterine infection. J Pediatr 1981;98:71-73.

Brunell PA, Novelli VM, Lipton SV, et al. Combined vaccine against measles, mumps, rubella, and varicella. Pediatrics 1988;81:779-784.

Brunell PA, Taylor-Wiedeman J, Geiser CF, et al. Risk of herpes zoster in children with leukemia: varicella vaccine compared with history of chickenpox. Pediatrics 1986;77:53-56.

Bruusgaard E. The mutual relation between zoster and varicella. Br J Dermatol Syphilis 1932;44:1-24.

Burke BL, Steele RW, Beard OW, et al. Immune responses to varicella-zoster in the aged. Arch Intern Med 1982;142:291-293.

Caekebeke JFV, Boudewyn P, Peters AC, et al. Cerebral vasculopathy, associated with primary varicella infection. Arch Neurol 1990;47:1033-1035.

Centers for Disease Control and Prevention. Prevention of varicella: Recommendations of the Advisory Committee on Immunization Practices (ACIP). MMWR Morb Mortal Wkly Rep 1996;45:1-36.

Centers for Disease Control and Prevention: Prevention of varicella. MMWR Morb Mortal Wkly Rep 1999;48:1-6.

Chambers RB, Derick RJ, Davidorf FH, et al. Varicella-zoster retinitis in human immunodeficiency virus infection. Arch Ophthalmol 1989;107:960-961.

Choo PW, Donahue JG, Manson JE, et al. The epidemiology of varicella and its complications. J Infect Dis 1995;172:706-712.

Choong K, Zwaignebaum L, Onyett H. Severe varicella after low dose inhaled corticoids. Pediatr Infect Dis J 1995;14:809-811.

Clements D, Moreira SP, Coplan P, et al. Postlicensure study of varicella vaccine effectiveness in a day-care setting. Pediatr Infect Dis J 1999;18:1047-1050.

Clements DA, Armstrong CB, Ursano AM, et al. Over five-year follow-up of Oka/Merck varicella vaccine recipients in 465 infants and adolescents. Pediatr Infect Dis J 1995;14:874-879.

Clements DA, Zaref JI, Bland CL, et al. Partial uptake of varicella vaccine and the epidemiological effect on varicella disease in 11 day-care centers in North Carolina. Arch Pediatr Adolesc Med 2001;155:433-461.

Cobo M. Reduction of the ocular complications of herpes zoster ophthalmicus by oral acyclovir. Am J Med 1988;85:90-93.

Colebunders R, Mann J, Francis H, et al. Herpes zoster in African patients: a clinical predictor of human immunodeficiency virus infection. J Infect Dis 1988;157:314-319.

Committee on Infectious Diseases. Live attenuated varicella vaccine. Pediatrics 1995;95:791-796.

Committee on Infectious Diseases. Varicella vaccine update. Pediatrics 2000;105:136-141.

Cooper E, Vujcic L, Quinnan G. Varicella-zoster virus–specific HLA-restricted cytotoxicity of normal immune adult lymphocytes after in vitro stimulation. J Infect Dis 1988;158:780-788.

Croen KD, Ostrove JM, Dragovic LY, et al. Patterns of gene expression and sites of latency in human ganglia are different for varicella-zoster and herpes simplex viruses. Proc Soc Natl Acad Sci USA 1988;85:9773-9777.

Davies HD, McGeer A, Schwarts B, et al. Invasive group A streptococcal infections in Ontario, Canada. N Engl J Med 1996;335:547-553.

Davison AJ, Scott JE. The complete DNA sequence of varicella-zoster virus. J Gen Virol 1986;67:1759-1816.

deKoning J, Frederiks E, Kerkhoven P. Purpura fulminans following varicella. Helv Paediatr Acta 1972;27:177.

Diaz P, Smith S, Hunter E, et al. T lymphocyte cytotoxicity with natural varicella-zoster virus infection and after immunization with live attenuated varicella vaccine. J Immunol 1989;142:636-641.

Doran TF, DeAngelis C, Baumgardner R, et al. Acetaminophen: more harm than good for chickenpox? J Pediatr 1989;114:1045-1048.

Dueland AN, Devlin M, Martin JR, et al. Fatal varicella-zoster virus meningoradiculitis without skin involvement. Ann Neurol 1991;29:569-572.

Dunkel L, Arvin A, Gershon A, et al. A controlled trial of oral acyclovir for chickenpox in normal children. N Engl J Med 1991;325:1539-1544.

Dworsky M, Whitely R, Alford C. Herpes zoster in early infancy. Am J Dis Child 1980;134:618-619.

Eder SE, Apuzzio JJ, Weiss G. Varicella pneumonia during pregnancy: treatment of two cases with acyclovir. Am J Perinatol 1988;5:16-18.

Edson CM, Hosler BA, Poodry CA, et al. Varicella-zoster virus envelope glycoproteins: biochemical characterization and identification in clinical material. Virology 1985;145:62-71.

Enders G, Miller E, Cradock-Watson J, et al. Consequences of varicella and herpes zoster in pregnancy: prospective study of 1739 cases. Lancet 1994;343:1548-1551.

Englund JA, Arvin A, Balfour H. Acyclovir treatment for varicella does not lower gpI and IE-62 (p170) antibody responses to varicella-zoster virus in normal children. J Clin Virol 1990;28:2327-2330.

Englund JA, Suarez CS, Kelly J, et al. Placebo-controlled trial of varicella vaccine given with or after measles-mumps-rubella vaccine. J Pediatr 1989;114:37-44.

Espy M, Teo R, Ross T, et al. Diagnosis of varicella-zoster virus infections in the clinical laboratory by LightCycler PCR. J Clin Microbiol 2000;38:3187-3189.

Ey JL, Fulginiti VA. Varicella hepatitis without neurologic symptoms or visceral involvement. Pediatrics 1981;67: 285-287.

Feder H. Treatment of adult chickenpox with oral acyclovir. Arch Intern Med 1990;150:2061-2065.

Feldhoff C, Balfour H, Simmons SR, et al. Varicella in children with renal transplants. J Pediatr 1981;98:25-31.

Feldman S, Chaudhary S, Ossi M, et al. A viremic phase for herpes zoster in children with cancer. J Pediatr 1977; 91:597-600.

Feldman S, Epp E. Isolation of varicella-zoster virus from blood. J Pediatr 1976;88:265-267.

Feldman S, Epp E. Detection of viremia during incubation period of varicella. J Pediatr 1979;94:746-748.

Feldman S, Hughes W, Daniel C. Varicella in children with cancer: 77 cases. Pediatrics 1975;80:388-397.

Feldman S, Hughes WT, Kim HY. Herpes zoster in children with cancer. Am J Dis Child 1973;126:178-184.

Feldman S, Lott L. Varicella in children with cancer: impact of antiviral therapy and prophylaxis. Pediatrics 1987;80:465-472.

Feldman S, Robertson PK, Lott L, et al. Neurotoxicity due to adenine arabinoside therapy during varicella-zoster virus infections in immunocompromised children. J Infect Dis 1986;154:889-893.

Fikrig E, Barg NL. Varicella associated intracerebral hemorrhage in the absence of thrombocytopenia. Diagn Microbiol Infect Dis 1989;12:357-359.

Friedman CA, Temple DM, Robbins KK, et al. Outbreak and control of varicella in a neonatal intensive care unit. Pediatr Infect Dis J 1994b;13:152-154.

Friedman SM, Margo CE, Connelly BL. Varicella-zoster virus retinitis as the initial manifestation of the acquired immunodeficiency syndrome. Am J Ophthalmol 1994a; 117:536-538.

Gelb LD, Dohner DE, Gershon AA, et al. Molecular epidemiology of live, attenuated varicella virus vaccine in children and in normal adults. J Infect Dis 1987;155: 633-640.

Gershon A. Varicella vaccine: its past, present, and future. Pediatr Infect Dis J 1995;14:742-744.

Gershon A. Chickenpox, measles, and mumps. In Remington J, Klein J (eds). Infections of the Fetus and Newborn Infant, ed 5. Philadelphia: Saunders, 2001a.

Gershon A, Brunell P, Doyle EF, et al. Steroid therapy and varicella. J Pediatr 1972;81:1034.

Gershon A, Forghani B. Varicella-zoster virus. In Lennette E (ed). Diagnostic Procedures for Viral, Rickettsial, and Chlamydial Infections. Washington, D.C.: American Public Health Association, 1995.

Gershon A, Kalter Z, Steinberg S. Detection of antibody to varicella-zoster virus by immune adherence hemagglutination. Proc Soc Exp Biol Med 1976a;151:762-765.

Gershon A, LaRussa P, Steinberg S, et al. The protective effect of immunologic boosting against zoster: an analysis in leukemic children who were vaccinated against chickenpox. J Infect Dis 1996;173:450-453.

Gershon A, Mervish N, LaRussa P, et al. Varicella-zoster virus infection in children with underlying HIV infection. J Infect Dis 1997;176:1496-1500.

Gershon A, Raker R, Steinberg S, et al. Antibody to varicella-zoster virus in parturient women and their offspring during the first year of life. Pediatrics 1976b;58:692-696.

Gershon A, Steinberg S. Cellular and humoral immune responses to VZV in immunocompromised patients during and after VZV infections. Infect Immun 1979;25:828.

Gershon A, Steinberg S, Borkowsky W, et al. IgM to varicella-zoster virus: demonstration in patients with and without clinical zoster. Pediatr Infect Dis 1982;1: 164-167.

Gershon A, Steinberg S, Brunell P. Zoster immune globulin: a further assessment. N Engl J Med 1974;290:241-245.

Gershon A, Steinberg S, Gelb L, NIAID Collaborative Varicella Vaccine Study Group. Live attenuated varicella vaccine: use in immunocompromised children and adults. Pediatrics 1986;78:757-762.

Gershon A, Steinberg S, LaRussa P. Detection of antibodies to varicella-zoster virus by latex agglutination. Clin Diagn Virol 1994;2:271-277.

Gershon A, Steinberg S, NIAID Collaborative Varicella Vaccine Study Group. Persistence of immunity to varicella in children with leukemia immunized with live attenuated varicella vaccine. N Engl J Med 1989;320: 892-897.

Gershon A, Steinberg S, Silber R. Varicella-zoster viremia. J Pediatr 1978;92:1033-1034.

Gershon AA. The current status of live attenuated varicella vaccine. Arch Virol Suppl 2001b;17:1-6.

Gershon AA, Steinberg S, Gelb L, NIAID Collaborative Varicella Vaccine Study Group. Clinical reinfection with varicella-zoster virus. J Infect Dis 1984a;149:137-142.

Gershon AA, Steinberg S, Gelb L, NIAID Collaborative Varicella Vaccine Study Group. Live attenuated varicella vaccine: efficacy for children with leukemia in remission. JAMA 1984b;252:355-362.

Gershon AA, Steinberg S, Gelb L, NIAID Collaborative Varicella Vaccine Study Group. Live attenuated varicella vaccine: protection in healthy adults in comparison to leukemic children. J Infect Dis 1990;161:661-666.

Gershon AA, Steinberg S, LaRussa P, NIAID Collaborative Varicella Vaccine Study Group. Immunization of healthy adults with live attenuated varicella vaccine. J Infect Dis 1988;158:132-137.

Gilden DH, Kleinschmidt-DeMasters BK, LaGuardia JJ, et al. Neurologic complications of the reactivation of varicella-zoster virus. N Engl J Med 2000;342:635-645.

Gilden DH, Murray RS, Wellish M, et al. Chronic progressive varicella-zoster virus encephalitis in and AIDS patient. Neurology 1988;38:1150-1153.

Giller RH, Bowden RA, Levin M, et al. Reduced cellular immunity to varicella-zoster virus during treatment for acute lymphoblastic leukemia of childhood: in vitro studies of possible mechanisms. J Clin Immunol 1986;6: 472-480.

Giller RH, Winistorfer S, Grose C. Cellular and humoral immunity to varicella zoster virus glycoproteins in immune and susceptible human subjects. J Infect Dis 1989;160:919-928.

Gleaves C, Lee C, Bustamante C, et al. Use of murine monoclonal antibodies for laboratory diagnosis of varicellazoster virus infection. J Clin Microbiol 1988;26: 1623-1625.

Gomi Y, Imagawa T, Takahashi M, et al. Oka varicella vaccine is distinguishable from its parental virus in DNA sequence of open reading frame 62 and its transactivation activity. J Med Virol 2000;61:497-503.

Gonzalez-Ruiz A, Ridgway GL, Cohen SL, et al. Varicella gangrenosa with toxic shock–like syndrome due to group A streptococcus infection in an adult. Clin Infect Dis 1995;20:1058-1060.

Grose C. Varicella-zoster virus: pathogenesis of human diseases, the virus and viral replication, and the major glycoproteins and proteins. In Hyman R (ed). Natural History of Varicella Zoster Virus. Boca Raton, Fla: CRC Press, 1987.

Grose CH. Variation on a theme by Fenner. Pediatrics 1981;68:735-737.

Groth KE, McCullough J, Marker S, et al. Evaluation of zoster immune plasma: treatment of herpes zoster in patients with cancer. JAMA 1978;239:1877-1879.

Guess H, Broughton DD, Melton LJ, et al. Epidemiology of herpes zoster in children and adolescents: a population-based study. Pediatrics 1985;76:512-517.

Guess HA, Broughton DD, Melton LJ, et al. Population-based studies of varicella complications. Pediatrics 1986;78:723-727.

Gustafson TL, Lavely GB, Brauner ER, et al. An outbreak of nosocomial varicella. Pediatrics 1982;70:550-556.

Gustafson TL, Shehab Z, Brunell P. Outbreak of varicella in a newborn intensive care nursery. Am Dis Child 1984;138:548-550.

Haake D, Zakowski PC, Haake DL, et al. Early treatment with acyclovir for varicella pneumonia in otherwise healthy adults: retrospective controlled study and review. Rev Infect Dis 1990;12:788-798.

Haddad J, Simeoni U, Messer J, et al. Acyclovir in prophylaxis and perinatal varicella. Lancet 1987;1:161.

Hanngren K, Grandien M, Granstrom G. Effect of zoster immunoglobulin for varicella prophylaxis in the newborn. Scand J Infect Dis 1985;17:341-347.

Hardy I, Gershon A. Prospects for use of a varicella vaccine in adults. Infect Dis Clin North Am 1990;4:160-173.

Hardy IB, Gershon A, Steinberg S, et al. The incidence of zoster after immunization with live attenuated varicella vaccine. A study in children with leukemia. N Engl J Med 1991;325:1545-1550.

Hay J, Ruyechan WT. Varicella-zoster virus: a different kind of herpesvirus latency? Semin Virol 1994;5:241-248.

Hayakawa Y, Torigoe S, Shiraki K, et al. Biologic and biophysical markers of a live varicella vaccine strain (Oka): identification of clinical isolates from vaccine recipients. J Infect Dis 1984;149:956-963.

Holland P, Isaacs D, Moxon ER. Fatal neonatal varicella infection. Lancet 1986;2:1156.

Hope-Simpson RE. The nature of herpes zoster: a long term study and a new hypothesis. Proc R Soc Med 1965;58:9-20.

Huang Y-C, Lin T-Y, Chiu C-H. Acyclovir prophylaxis of varicella after household exposure. Pediatr Infect Dis J 1995;14:152-154.

Huff C, Bean B, Balfour H, et al. Therapy of herpes zoster with oral acyclovir. Am J Med 1988; 85:84-89.

Jacobson MA, Berger TG, Fikrig S. Acyclovir-resistant varicella-zoster virus infection after chronic oral acyclovir therapy in patients with the acquired immunodeficiency syndrome. Ann Intern Med 1990;112:187-191.

Johnson C, Stancin T, Fattlar D, et al. A long-term prospective study of varicella vaccine in healthy children. Pediatrics 1997;100:761-766.

Johnson CE, Shurin PA, Fattlar D, et al. Live attenuated varicella vaccine in healthy 12- to 24-month old children. Pediatrics 1988;81:512-518.

Josephson A, Gombert ME. Airborne transmission of nosocomial varicella from localized zoster. J Infect Dis 1988;158:238-241.

Josephson C, Nuss R, Jacobson L, et al. The varicella-autoantibody syndrome. Pediatr Res 2001;50:345-352.

Judelsohn RG, Meyers JD, Ellis RJ, et al. Efficacy of zoster immune globulin. Pediatrics 1974;53:476-480.

Junker AK, Angus E, Thomas E. Recurrent varicella-zoster virus infections in apparently immunocompetent children. Pediatr Infect Dis J 1991;10:569-575.

Junker AK, Tilley P. Varicella-zoster virus antibody avidity and IgG-subclass patterns in children with recurrent chickenpox. J Med Virol 1994;43:119-124.

Junker K, Avnstorp C, Nielsen C, Hansen N. Reinfection with varicella-zoster virus in immunocompromised patients. Curr Probl Dermatol 1989;18:152-157.

Jura E, Chadwick E, Gershon A, et al. Varicella-zoster virus infections in children infected with human immunodeficiency virus. Pediatr Infect Dis J 1989;8:586-590.

Kalman CM, Laskin OL. Herpes zoster and zosteriform herpes simplex virus infections in immunocompetent adults. Am J Med 1986; 81:775-778.

Kamiya H, Ihara T, Hattori A, et al. Diagnostic skin test reactions with varicella virus antigen and clinical application of the test. J Infect Dis 1977;136:784-788.

Kasper WJ, Howe P. Fatal varicella after a single course of corticosteroids. Pediatr Infect Dis J 1991;9:729-732.

Kennedy P, Grinfield E, Gow JW. Latent varicella-zoster virus in human dorsal root ganglia. Virology 1999;258:451-454.

King S, Gorensek M, Ford-Jones EL, et al. Fatal varicella-zoster infection in a newborn treated with varicella-zoster immunoglobulin. Pediatr Infect Dis J 1986;5:588-589.

Kirk S, Marlow N, Quershi S. Cardiac tamponade following varicella. Int J Cardiol 1987;17:221-224.

Koc Y, Miller KB, Schenkein DP, et al. Varicella zoster virus infections following allogeneic bone marrow transplantation: frequency, risk factors, and clinical outcome. Biol Blood Marrow Transplant 2000;6:44-49.

Krasinski K, Holzman R, LaCoutre R, et al. Hospital experience with varicella-zoster virus. Infect Control 1986;7:312-316.

Krause P, Klinman DM. Efficacy, immunogenicity, safety, and use of live attenuated chickenpox vaccine. J Pediatr 1995;127:518-525.

Kundratitz K. Experimentelle Ubertragung von Herpes Zoster auf den Mensschen und die Beziehungen von Herpes Zoster zu Varicellen. Monatss fuer Kinder 1925;29:516-523.

Kuppermann BD, Quiceno JI, Wiley C, et al. Clinical and histopathological study of varicella-zoster virus retinitis in patients with the acquired immunodeficiency syndrome. Am J Ophthalmol 1994;118:589-600.

Kuter BJ, Weibel RE, Guess HA, et al. Oka/Merck varicella vaccine in healthy children: final report of a 2-year efficacy study and 7-year follow-up studies. Vaccine 1991;9:641-647.

Landsberger EJ, Hager WD, Grossman JH. Successful management of varicella pneumonia complicating pregnancy. A report of three cases. J Reprod Med 1986;31:311.

LaRussa P, Hughes P, Gershon A, et al. Use of polymerase chain reaction (PCR) assay to identify and type varicella zoster virus. Society for Pediatric Research Annual Meeting, Washington, D.C., May 6, 1993.

LaRussa P, Lungu O, Gershon A, et al. Restriction fragment length polymorphism of polymerase chain reaction products from vaccine and wild-type varicella-zoster virus isolates. J Virol 1992;66:1016-1020.

LaRussa P, Steinberg S, Gershon A. Diagnosis and typing of varicella-zoster virus (VZV) in clinical specimens by polymerase chain reaction (PCR). Presented at thirty-fourth ICAAC, Orlando, Fl, 1994.

LaRussa P, Steinberg S, Gershon A, et al. PCR and RFLP analysis of VZV isolates from the USA and other parts of the world. J Infect Dis 1998;178S:64-66.

LaRussa P, Steinberg S, Seeman MD, Gershon AA. Determination of immunity to varicella by means of an intradermal skin test. J Infect Dis 1985;152:869-875.

Laupland KB, Davies HD, Low DE, et al. Invasive group A streptococcal disease in children and association with varicella-zoster virus infection. Ontario Group A Streptococcal Study Group. Pediatrics 2000;105:E60.

Lawrence R, Gershon A, NIAID Varicella Vaccine Collaborative Study Group, et al. The risk of zoster after varicella vaccination in children with leukemia. N Engl J Med 1988;318:541-548.

Leclair JM, Zaia J, Levin MJ, et al. Airborne transmission of chickenpox in a hospital. N Engl J Med 1980;302:450-453.

Lesko SM, O'Brien KL, Schwartz B, et al. Invasive group A streptococcal infection and nonsteroidal antiinflammatory drug use among children with primary varicella. Pediatrics 2001;107:1108-1115.

Leung TF, Chik KW, Li CK, et al. Incidence, risk factors and outcome of varicella-zoster infection in children after hematopoietic stem cell transplantation. Bone Marrow Transplant 2000;25:167-172.

Levin MJ. Use of varicella vaccines to prevent herpes zoster in older individuals. Arch Virol Suppl 2001;17:151-60.

Levin MJ, Rotbart HA, Hayward AR. Immune response to varicella-zoster virus 5 years after acyclovir therapy of childhood varicella. J Infect Dis 1995;171:1383-1384.

Lichtenstein PK, Heubi JE, Daugherty CC, et al. Grade I Reye's syndrome. A frequent cause of vomiting and live dysfunction after varicella and upper–respiratory-tract infection. N Engl J Med 1983;309:133-139.

Linnemann CC, Biron KK, Hoppenjans WG, et al. Emergence of acyclovir-resistant varicella zoster virus in an AIDS patient on prolonged acyclovir therapy. AIDS 1990;4:577-579.

Liu GT, Holmes GL. Varicella with delayed contralateral hemiparesis detected by MRI. Pediatr Neurol 1990;6:131-134.

Liu H-C, Tsai T-C, Chang P-Y, et al. Varicella orchitis: report of two cases and review of the literature. Pediatr Infect Dis J 1994;13:748-750.

Ljungman P, Lonnqvist B, Gahrton G, et al. Clinical and subclinical reactivations of varicella-zoster virus in immunocompromised patients. J Infect Dis 1986;153:840-847.

Locksley RM, Flournoy N, Sullivan KM, Meyers J. Infection with varicella-zoster virus after marrow transplantation. J Infect Dis 1985;152:1172-1181.

Loparev VN, Argaw T, Krause P, et al. Improved identification and differentiation of varicella-zoster virus (VZV) wild type strains and an attenuated varicella vaccine strain using a VZV open reading frame 62-based PCR. J Clin Microbiol 2000;38:3156-3160.

Lorber A, Zonis Z, Maisuls E, et al. The scale of myocardial involvement in varicella myocarditis. Int J Cardiol 1988;20:257-262.

Luby J, Ramirez-Ronda C, Rinner S, et al. A longitudinal study of varicella zoster virus infections in renal transplant recipients. J Infect Dis 1977;135:659-663.

Lungu O, Annunziato P. VZV: latency and reactivation. In Wolff MH, Schunemann W, Schmidt A (eds). Contributions to Microbiology: Varicella-Zoster Virus: Molecular Biology, Pathogenesis, and Clinical Aspects, vol 3. Basel: Karger, 1999.

Lungu O, Annunziato P, Gershon A, et al. Reactivated and latent varicella-zoster virus in human dorsal root ganglia. Proc Natl Acad Sci USA 1995;92:10980-10984.

Lungu O, Panagiotidis C, Annunziato P, et al. Aberrant intracellular localization of varicella-zoster virus regulatory proteins during latency. Proc Natl Acad Sci USA 1998;95:7080-7085.

Lynfield R, Herrin JT, Rubin RH. Varicella in pediatric renal transplant patients. Pediatrics 1992;90:216-220.

Mackay JB, Cairney P. Pulmonary calcification following varicella. NZ Med J 1960;59:453.

Mahalingham R, Wellish M, Cohrs R, et al. Expression of protein encoded by varicella-zoster virus open reading frame 63 in latently infected human ganglionic neurons. Proc Natl Acad Sci 1996;93:2122-2124.

Martin JH, Dohner D, Wellinghoff WJ, et al. Restriction endonuclease analysis of varicella-zoster vaccine virus and wild type DNAs. J Med Virol 1982;9:69-76.

McCormick WF, Rodnitzky RL, Schochet SSJ, et al. Varicella-zoster encephalomyelitis: a morphologic and virologic study. Arch Neurol 1969;9:251-266.

McKendrick M, McGill J, White J, et al. Oral acyclovir in acute herpes zoster. BMJ 1986;293:1529-1532.

Melbye M, Grossman R, Goedert J, et al. Risk of AIDS after herpes zoster. Lancet 1987;1:728-730.

Melish ME. Bullous varicella: its association with the staphylococcal scalded skin syndrome. J Pediatr 1973;83:1019.

Merigan TC, Rand K, Pollard R, et al. Human leukocyte interferon for the treatment of herpes zoster in patients with cancer. N Engl J Med 1978;298:981-987.

Merigan TC, Stevens DA. The use of zoster immune globulin in the prevention of varicella and treatment of zoster. Fifteenth Congress of the International Blood Transfusion Society, Paris, France, 1978.

Meyers J. Congenital varicella in term infants: risk reconsidered. J Infect Dis 1974;129:215-217.

Miller AE. Selective decline in cellular immune response to varicella-zoster in the elderly. Neurology 1980;30:582-587.

Miller L, Brunell PA. Zoster, reinfection or activation of latent virus? Am J Med 1970; 49:480.

Mills WJ, Mosca VS, Nizet V. Orthopaedic manifestations of invasive group A streptococcal infections complicating primary varicella. J Pediatr Orthop 1996;16:522-528.

Morens DM, Bregman DJ, West M, et al. An outbreak of varicella-zoster virus infection among cancer patients. Ann Intern Med 1980;93:414-419.

Mortimer EA, Lepow ML. Varicella with hypoglycemia possibly due to salicylates. Am J Dis Child 1962;103:583.

Mulhern LM, Friday GA, Perri JA. Arthritis complicating varicella infection. Pediatrics 1971;48:827.

Music SI, Fine EM, Togo Y. Zoster-like disease in the newborn due to herpes-simplex virus. N Engl J Med 1971;284:24-26.

Myers M, Connelly BL. Animal models of varicella. J Infect Dis 1992;166:S48-S50.

Myers MG. Viremia caused by varicella-zoster virus: association with malignant progressive varicella. J Infect Dis 1979;140:229-233.

Myers MG. Hepatic cellular injury during varicella. Arch Dis Child 1982;57:317-319.

Nader S, Bergen R, Sharp M, et al. Comparison of cell-mediated immunity (CMI) to varicella-zoster virus (VZV) in children and adults immunized with live attenuated varicella vaccine. J Infect Dis 1995;171:13-17.

Nassar NT, Touma HC. Brief report: susceptibility of Filipino nurses to the varicella-zoster virus. Infect Control 1986;7:71-72.

Nyerges G, Meszner Z, Gyrmati E, et al. Acyclovir prevents dissemination of varicella in immunocompromised children. J Infect Dis 1988;157:309-313.

Olding-Stenkvist E, Grandien M. Early diagnosis of virus-caused vesicular rashes by immunofluorescence on skin biopsies. I. Varicella, zoster, and herpes simplex. Scand J Infect Dis 1976;8:27-35.

Orenstein W, Heymann D, Ellis R, et al. Prophylaxis of varicella in high risk children: response effect of zoster immune globulin. J Pediatr 1981;98:368-373.

Ozaki T, Ichikawa T, Matsui Y, et al. Lymphocyte-associated viremia in varicella. J Med Virol 1986;19:249-253.

Pahwa S, Biron K, Lim W, et al. Continuous varicella-zoster infection associated with acyclovir resistance in a child with AIDS. JAMA 1988;260:2879-2882.

Paryani SG, Arvin AM, Koropchak C, et al. Varicella zoster antibody titers after the administration of intravenous immune serum globulin or varicella zoster immune globulin. Am J Med 1984;76:124-127.

Patel PA, Yoonessi S, Gershon A, et al. Cell-mediated immunity to varicella zoster virus in subjects with lymphoma or leukemia. J Pediatr 1979;94:223-230.

Patterson L, Butler K, Edwards M. Clinical herpes zoster shortly following primary varicella in two HIV-infected children. Clin Pediatr 1989;28:354.

Peters ACB, Versteeg J, Lindenman J, et al. Varicella and acute cerebellar ataxia. Arch Neurol 1978;35:769.

Peterslund NA. Management of varicella zoster infections in immunocompetent hosts. Am J Med 1988;85:74-78.

Peterson CL, Vugia D, Meyers H, et al. Risk factors for invasive group A streptococcal infections in children with varicella: a case-control study. Pediatr Infect Dis J 1996; 15:151-156.

Pitel PA, McCormick KL, Fitzgerald E, et al. Subclinical hepatic changes in varicella infection. Pediatrics 1980;65:631-633.

Preblud S, Bregman DJ, Vernon LL. Deaths from varicella in infants. Pediatr Infect Dis J 1985;4:503-507.

Preblud S, Cochi S, Orenstein W. Varicella-zoster infection in pregnancy. N Engl J Med 1986a;315:1416-1417.

Preblud S, Nelson WL, Levin M, et al. Modification of congenital varicella infection with VZIG. Interscience Conference on Antimicrobial Agents and Chemotherapy, New Orleans, 1986b.

Preblud S, Orenstein W, Bart K. Varicella: clinical manifestations, epidemiology, and health impact on children. Pediatr Infect Dis 1984;3:505-509.

Priest JR, Groth KE, Balfour HH. Varicella arthritis documented by isolation of virus from joint fluid. J Pediatr 1978;93:990.

Prober C, Kirk LE, Keeney RE. Acyclovir therapy of chickenpox in immunocompromised children—a collaborative study. J Pediatr 1982;101:622-625.

Puchhammer-Stockl E, Popow-Kraupp T, Heinz F, et al. Detection of varicella-zoster virus DNA by polymerase chain reaction in the cerebrospinal fluid of patients suffering from neurological complications associated with chicken pox or herpes zoster. J Clin Microbiol 1991;29:1513-1516.

Quereda C, Corral I, Laguna F, et al. Diagnostic utility of a multiplex herpesvirus PCR assay performed with cerebrospinal fluid from human immunodeficiency virus–infected patients with neurological disorders. J Clin Microbiol 2000;38:3061-3067.

Rabalais GP, Adams G, Yusk J, et al. Zosteriform denuded skin caused by intrauterine herpes simplex virus infection. Pediatr Infect Dis J 1991;10:79-80.

Raker R, Steinberg S, Gershon A, et al. Antibody to varicella-zoster virus in low birth weight infants. J Pediatr 1978;93:505-506.

Randel R, Kearns DB, Sawyer MH. Vocal cord paralysis as a presentation of intrauterine infection with varicella-zoster virus. Pediatrics 1996;97:127-128.

Rawlinson WD, Dwyer DE, Gibbons V, et al. Rapid diagnosis of varicella-zoster virus infection with a monoclonal antibody based direct immunofluorescence technique. J Virol Methods 1989;23:13-18.

Rivera-Vaquerizo PA, Gomez-Garrido J, Vicente-Gutierrez M, et al. Varicella zoster gastritis 3 years after bone marrow transplantation for treatment of acute leukemia. Gastrointest Endosc 2001;53:809-810.

Ross AH, Lencher E, Reitman G. Modification of chickenpox in family contacts by administration of gamma globulin. N Engl J Med 1962;267:369-376.

Saiman L, LaRussa P, Steinberg S, et al. Persistence of immunity to varicella-zoster virus vaccination among health care workers. Infect Control Hosp Epidemiol 2001;22:279-283.

Schimpff S, Serpick A, Stoler B, et al. Varicella-zoster infection in patients with cancer. Ann Intern Med 1972;76:241-254.

Schlossberg D, Littman M. Varicella pneumonia. Arch Intern Med 1988;148:1630-1632.

Schmidt NJ. Further evidence for common antigens in herpes simplex and varicella-zoster virus. J Med Virol 1982;9:27-36.

Seward J, Jumaan A, Schmid S. Varicella vaccine revisited. Nat Med 2000a;6:1298-3000.

Seward JF, Watson BM, et al. Varicella disease after introduction of Varicella vaccine in the United States, 1995-2000. JAMA 287(5):606-611.

Sharrar RG, LaRussa P, Galea S, et al. The postmarketing safety profile of varicella vaccine. Vaccine 2000;19: 916-923.

Shepp D, Dandliker P, Meyers J. Current therapy of varicella zoster virus infection in immunocompromised patients. Am J Med 1988;85:96-98.

Shepp DH, Dandliker PS, Meyers JD. Treatment of varicella-zoster virus infection in severely immunocompromised patients: a randomized comparison of acyclovir and vidarabine. N Engl J Med 1986;314:208-212.

Silk H, Guay-Woodford L, Perez-Atayde A, et al. Fatal varicella in steroid-dependent asthma. J Allergy Clin Immunol 1988;81:47-51.

Silliman CC, Tedder D, Ogle JW, et al. Unsuspected varicella-zoster virus encephalitis in a child with acquired immunodeficiency syndrome. J Pediatr 1993;123: 418-422.

Sills J, Galloway A, Amegavie L, et al. Acyclovir in prophylaxis and perinatal varicella. Lancet 1987; 1:161.

Smith H. Purpura fulminans complicating varicella: recovery with low molecular weight dextran and steroids. Med J Aust 1967;2:685.

Spring S, Laughlin C, Gershon AA, et al. Varicella-zoster virus infection and post-herpetic neuralgia: new insights into pathogenesis and pain management. J Neurol 1994;35:S2-S3.

Starko KM, Ray CG, Dominguez BS, et al. Reye's syndrome and salicylate use. Pediatrics 1980;66:859-864.

Steele R, Coleman MA, Fiser M, et al. Varicella-zoster in hospital personnel: skin test reactivity to monitor susceptibility. Pediatrics 1982;70:604-608.

Stevens D, Ferrington R, Jordan G, et al. Cellular events in zoster vesicles: relation to clinical course and immune parameters. J Infect Dis 1975;131:509-515.

Straus S, Meier JL. Comparative biology of latent varicella-zoster virus and herpes simplex virus infections. J Infect Dis 1992;166:S13-S23.

Straus S, Ostrove J, Inchauspe G, et al. Varicella-zoster virus infections: biology, natural history, treatment, and prevention. Ann Intern Med 1988;108:221-237.

Straus SE, Reinhold W, Smith HA, et al. Endonuclease analysis of viral DNA from varicella and subsequent zoster infections in the same patient. N Engl J Med 1984;311:1362-1364.

Suga S, Yoshikawa T, Ozaki T, et al. Effect of oral acyclovir against primary and secondary viraemia in incubation period of varicella. Arch Dis Child 1993;69:639-643.

Takahashi M, Otsuka T, Okuno Y, et al. Live vaccine used to prevent the spread of varicella in children in hospital. Lancet 1974;2:1288-1290.

Takayama N, Minamitani M, Takayama M. High incidence of breakthrough varicella observed in healthy Japanese children immunized with live varicella vaccine (Oka strain). Acta Paediatr Jpn 1997; 39:663-668.

Terada K, Kawano S, Hiraga Y, et al. Reactivation of chickenpox contracted in infancy. Arch Dis Child 1995;73: 162-163.

Terada K, Kawano S, Yoshihiro K, et al. Varicella-zoster virus (VZV) reactivation is related to the low response of VZV-specific immunity after chickenpox in infancy. J Infect Dis 1994;169:650-652.

Tsolia M, Gershon A, Steinberg S, et al. Live attenuated varicella vaccine: evidence that the virus is attenuated and the importance of skin lesions in transmission of varicella-zoster virus. J Pediatr 1990;116:184-189.

Vafai A, Wroblewska Z, Graf L. Antigenic cross-reaction between a varicella-zoster virus nucleocapsid protein encoded by gene 40 and a herpes simplex virus nucleocapsid protein. Virus Res 1990;15:163-174.

Vazquez M, LaRussa P, Gershon A, et al. The effectiveness of the varicella vaccine in clinical practice. N Engl J Med 2001;344:955-960.

Vugia DJ, Peterson CL, Meyers HB, et al. Invasive group A streptococcal infections in children with varicella in Southern California. Pediatr Infect Dis J 1996;15:146-150.

Waagoner DC, Murphy T. Varicella myocarditis. Pediatr Infect Dis J 1990;9:360-363.

Wald EL, Levine MM, Togo Y. Concomitant varicella and staphylococcal scalded skin syndrome. J Pediatr 1973;83:1017.

Wallace MR, Bowler WA, Murray NB, et al. Treatment of adult varicella with oral acyclovir. A randomized, placebo-controlled trial. Ann Intern Med 1992;117: 358-363.

Wang E, Prober C, Arvin AM. Varicella-zoster virus antibody titers before and after administration of zoster immune globulin to neonates in an intensive care nursery. J Pediatr 1983;103:113-114.

Ward JR, Bishop B. Varicella arthritis. JAMA 1970;212: 1954.

Watson B, Gupta R, Randall T, et al. Persistence of cell-mediated and humoral immune responses in healthy children immunized with live attenuated varicella vaccine. J Infect Dis 1994;169:197-199.

Watson B, Seward J, Yang A, et al. Post exposure effectiveness of varicella vaccine. Pediatrics 2000;105:84-88.

Weber DJ, Rotala WA, Parham C. Impact and costs of varicella prevention in a university hospital. Am J Public Health 1988;78:19-23.

Weber DM, Pellecchia JA. Varicella pneumonia: study of prevalence in adult men. JAMA 1965;192:572.

Weller TH. Varicella and herpes zoster: changing concepts of the natural history, control, and importance of a not-so-benign virus. N Engl J Med 1983;309:1362-1368, 1434-1440.

Weller TH, Coons AH. Fluorescent antibody studies with agents of varicella and herpes zoster propagated in vitro. Proc Soc Exp Biol Med 1954;86:789.

Weller TH, Witton HM. The etiologic agents of varicella and herpes zoster. Serological studies with the viruses as propagated in vitro. J Exp Med 1958;108:869-890.

Whitley R, Soong S, Dolin R, NIAID Collaborative Study Group. Early vidarabine to control the complications of herpes zoster in immunosuppressed patients. N Engl J Med 1982;307:971-975.

Williams DL, Gershon A, Gelb LD, et al. Herpes zoster following varicella vaccine in a child with acute lymphocytic leukemia. J Pediatr 1985;106:259-261.

Wilson A, Sharp M, Koropchak C, et al. Subclinical varicella-zoster virus viremia, herpes zoster, and T lymphocyte immunity to varicella-zoster viral antigens after bone marrow transplantation. J Infect Dis 1992;165: 119-126.

Wilson G, Talkington D, Gruber W, et al. GroupA streptococcal necrotizing fasciitis following varicella in children: case reports and review. Clin Infect Dis 1995;20: 1333-1338.

Winquist AG, Roome A, Hadleer J. Varicella outbreak in a summer camp for HIV-infected children. Pediatrics 2001;107:67-72.

Wood MJ, Kay R, Dworkin RH, et al. Oral acyclovir therapy accelerates pain resolution in patients with herpes zoster: a meta analysis of placebo controlled trials. Clin Infect Dis 1996;22:341-347.

Wood MJ, Ogan P, McKendrick MW, et al. Efficacy of oral acyclovir treatment of acute herpes zoster. Am J Med 1988;85:79-83.

Yoshikawa T, Suga S, Kozawa T, et al. Persistence of protective immunity after postexposure prophylaxis of varicella with oral acyclovir in the family setting. Arch Dis Child 1998;78:61-63.

Yuceoglu AM, Berkovich S, Minkowitz S. Acute glomerular nephritis as a complication of varicella. JAMA 1967;202:113.

Zaia J, Levin M, Preblud S, et al. Evaluation of varicella-zoster immune globulin: protection of immunosuppressed children after household exposure to varicella. J Infect Dis 1983;147:737-743.

Zampogna JC, Flowers FP. Persistent verrucous varicella as the initial manifestation of HIV infection. J Am Acad Dermatol 2001;44:391-394.

Zeigler T, Halonen PE. Rapid detection of herpes simplex and varicella-zoster virus antigens from clinical specimens by enzyme immunoassay. Antiviral Res 1985; 1(suppl):107-110.

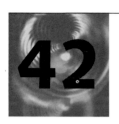

VIRAL HEPATITIS: A, B, C, D, E, AND NEWER HEPATITIS AGENTS

WILLIAM BORKOWSKY AND SAUL KRUGMAN

The term *viral hepatitis* refers to a primary infection of the liver caused by at least five etiologically and immunologically distinct viruses: hepatitis A (HAV), hepatitis B (HBV), hepatitis C (HCV), hepatitis D (HDV), and hepatitis E (HEV). Hepatitis may occur also during the course of disease caused by the following viruses: adenovirus, cytomegalovirus (CMV), Epstein-Barr virus (EBV), herpes simplex virus (HSV), human herpesvirus 6 (HHV-6), human immunodeficiency virus (HIV), and varicella-zoster virus (VZV).

Hepatitis A is synonymous with infectious hepatitis, an ancient disease described by Hippocrates and formerly known as *epidemic jaundice, acute catarrhal jaundice*, and other designations. The fulminant form of the disease was called *acute yellow atrophy of the liver*.

Hepatitis B is synonymous with serum hepatitis, a disease with a more recent history. The first known outbreak occurred in 1883 among a group of shipyard workers who were vaccinated against smallpox with glycerinated lymph of human origin (Lürman, 1885). Later an increased incidence of the disease was observed among patients attending venereal disease clinics, diabetic clinics, and other facilities in which multiple injections were given with inadequately sterilized syringes and needles contaminated with the blood of a carrier. The most extensive outbreak occurred in 1942, when yellow fever vaccine containing human serum caused 28,585 cases of hepatitis B infection with jaundice among U.S. military personnel. It was unknown at the time of vaccination that the human serum component of the vaccine was contaminated with HBV. The additional aliases of hepatitis B recorded in the literature include homologous serum jaundice, transfusion jaundice, syringe jaundice, and postvaccinal jaundice.

Hepatitis C was formerly designated parenterally transmitted non-A, non-B hepatitis (PT-NANB). Non-A, non-B (NANB) hepatitis was recognized as a clinical entity in the 1970s, when specific tests for the identification of HAV and HBV infections became available. The identification of HCV as the most common cause of PT-NANB hepatitis was reported in 1989 (Choo et al., 1989; Kuo et al., 1989).

Hepatitis delta virus is a "defective" RNA virus that can replicate only in the presence of acute or chronic HBV infection. The genome of HDV codes for an internal antigen (HDAg), but the virus is encapsulated by hepatitis B surface antigen (HBsAg) of the helper HBV. The delta antigen was discovered by Rizzetto et al. in 1977.

Hepatitis E was previously called *enterically transmitted NANB* (ET-NANB). Serologic studies of various outbreaks of ET-NANB hepatitis revealed no evidence of HAV or HBV infection (Khuroo, 1980). In retrospect it is clear that these outbreaks were caused by HEV, an agent that was cloned by Reyes et al. in 1990.

Several new hepatitis agents, genetically related to HCV, have been identified and sequenced. These have been designated GB virus A (GBV-A), GB virus B (GBV-B), and GB virus C (GVB-C). Deinhardt (1967) inoculated sera from a surgeon (GB) with non-A, non-B (NANB) hepatitis into primates and induced hepatitis. Decades later, two viruses found in sera from tamarins in which the viruses were propagated were coned, sequenced, and named GB viruses A and B. Simons (1995) subsequently detected and partially sequenced a virus from human serum similar to the A and B viruses and named it GB virus C. In addition, a transfusion-transmissible hepatitis virus closely related to GBV-C, termed *hepatitis G virus*, has also been cloned. These viruses have yet to have an associated illness ascribed to them.

ETIOLOGY
Hepatitis A

Before the mid 1960s knowledge of the properties of HAV was derived from human volunteer studies. The agent survived a temperature of 56° C for 30 minutes (Havens et al., 1944) and was inactivated by heating at 98° C for 1 minute (Krugman et al., 1970). It retained its infectivity after storage at −18° to −70° C for several years. HAV was more resistant to chlorine than many bacteria found in drinking water.

Oral or parenteral administration of the virus caused hepatitis after an incubation period ranging from 15 to 40 days, averaging approximately 30 days. Extensive studies with the MS-1 strain of HAV and the MS-2 strain of HBV confirmed observations by Havens et al. (1944) and Neefe et al. (1946) that hepatitis A and B viruses were immunologically distinct (Krugman et al., 1967).

In 1967 Deinhardt et al. reported the successful transmission of hepatitis A to marmoset monkeys. Later, additional studies by his group (Holmes et al., 1969), Mascoli et al. (1973), Provost et al. (1973), and Maynard (1974) confirmed the successful transmission of human HAV to marmosets. In addition, Dienstag et al. (1975b) successfully transmitted HAV to susceptible chimpanzees.

In 1973 Feinstone et al. reported the identification of 27-nm viruslike particles in the stools of adults who had been infected with the MS-1 strain of HAV. These particles were identified by immune electron microscopy (IEM). These findings were confirmed by Maynard (1974), who induced hepatitis in marmosets by inoculating them with stool filtrates containing the 27-nm particles.

Human HAV was further characterized by Provost et al. (1975b), who reported that the 27-nm particles appeared to have the physical, chemical, and biologic characteristics of an enterovirus. It has been designated enterovirus type 27 (Melnick, 1982). Electron micrographs comparing HAV with HBV are shown in Figure 42-1. Unlike HBV, HAV is a simple,

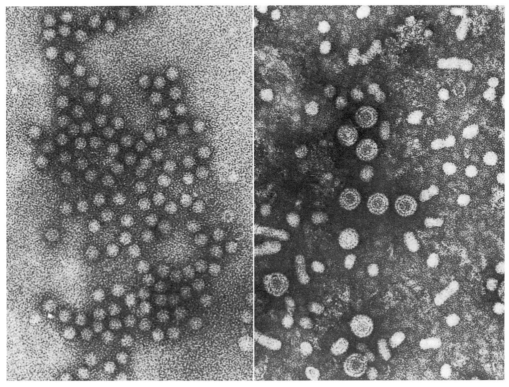

Type A   Type B

Fig. 42-1 Electron micrographs of type A and type B hepatitis viruses. Type A: Note 27-nm particles, uniform in size. Type B: Note 43-nm Dane particles (hepatitis B virus) and spherical and filamentous particles 20 nm in diameter (hepatitis B surface antigen). (From Provost PJ, et al: Am J Med Sci 1975b;270:87.)

nonenveloped RNA virus with a nucleocapsid that has been designated hepatitis A antigen (HA Ag). The HAV capsid consists of 32 capsomeres arranged in icosahedral conformation; it is composed of four virion polypeptides (VP1, VP2, VP3, and VP4). A single-stranded molecule of RNA is present inside the capsid.

Purified HAV is inactivated by formalin, ultraviolet irradiation, heating at 100° C for 5 minutes, or treatment with chlorine (Peterson et al., 1982; Provost et al., 1975b). The purified virus was shown by IEM as specifically aggregated by hepatitis A antibody (anti-HAV).

Miller et al. (1975) prepared HA Ag from infected marmoset liver for use in an immune adherence hemagglutination antibody (IAHA) test. Both HA Ag and anti-HAV can be detected by various established serologic methods, including IEM (Feinstone et al., 1973), radioimmunoassay (RIA) (Hollinger et al., 1975), enzyme immunoassay (EIA) (Duermeyer et al., 1978), and immunofluorescence (IF) (Murphy et al., 1978). The RIA and EIA tests are the most practical for serodiagnosis of acute hepatitis A.

In 1979 Provost and Hilleman reported the propagation of human HAV in primary explant cell cultures of marmoset livers and in the normal fetal rhesus kidney cell line (FRhK6). Provost et al. (1981) subsequently isolated HAV directly from acute-phase human stool specimens by in vitro propagation in an FRhK6 line. Other workers demonstrated that HAV could be cultivated in human diploid fibroblasts (Gauss-Muller et al., 1981), in human amniotic and Vero cells (Kojima et al., 1981), and in African green monkey kidney cell cultures (Daemer et al., 1981). HAV propagates in the cytoplasm and is noncytopathic.

The HAV genome has been cloned by various investigators (Baroudy et al., 1985; Ticehurst et al., 1983). Modern molecular biologic techniques have provided insight into the structure and organization of the virus, thereby revealing similarities to and differences from other enteroviruses.

Hepatitis B

The human volunteer studies of the 1940s indicated that hepatitis B was highly infectious by inoculation. These studies suggested that HBV caused a parenteral infection characterized by a long incubation period of 50 to 180 days and, unlike HAV, was not infectious by mouth.

Studies in the 1960s provided evidence for the existence of two types of viral hepatitis with distinctive clinical, epidemiologic, and immunologic features (Krugman et al., 1967). One type, MS-1, resembled hepatitis A; it was characterized by an incubation period of 30 to 38 days and a high degree of contagion by contact. The other type, MS-2, resembled hepatitis B; it had an incubation period of 41 to 108 days. Contrary to the prevailing concept, the MS-2 strain of HBV was infectious both by mouth and parenterally. The discovery of Australia antigen by Blumberg et al. (1965), and its subsequent association with hepatitis B, had a major impact on the understanding of the etiology and natural history of the disease.

The successful transmission of HBV to chimpanzees was achieved in the early 1970s (Barker et al., 1973; Maynard et al., 1972). The chimpanzee has proved to be a highly sensitive animal model for the study of hepatitis B infection.

By the early 1970s the agent responsible for hepatitis B had been identified and characterized. Electron microscopic examination of serum obtained from patients with acute or chronic type B hepatitis revealed the following types of viruslike particles: (1) spherical particles, 20 nm in diameter (Bayer et al., 1968); (2) filamentous particles, 100 nm or more in length and 20 nm in diameter (Hirschman et al., 1969); and (3) Dane particles, approximately 42 nm in diameter (Dane et al., 1970) (Figure 42-1). The available evidence indicates that the Dane particle is the complete hepatitis B virion and that the 20-nm spherical particles represent excess virus-coat (HBsAg) material. The HBsAg and Dane particles occur free in serum.

Hepatitis B virus (Dane particle). The HBV, a complex 42-nm virion, is a member of a new class of viruses designated *hepadnaviruses*. The precise nomenclature of HBV is hepadnavirus type 1 (Melnick, 1982). Unlike HAV, it has not been propagated successfully in cell culture. Nevertheless, its biophysical and biochemical properties have been well characterized, and the HBV genome has been cloned and sequenced.

A schematic illustration of the structure of HBV and its antigens is shown in Figure 42-2. The virus is a double-shelled particle; its outer surface component, the hepatitis B surface antigen (HBsAg), is immunologically distinct from the inner core component, the hepatitis B core

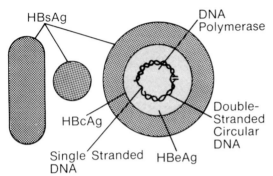

Fig. 42-2 Schematic illustration of the hepatitis B virus and its antigens: hepatitis B surface antigen *(HBsAg)*, hepatitis B core antigen *(HBcAg)*, and hepatitis B e antigen *(HBeAg)*.

antigen (HBcAg). The core contains the genome of HBV, a single molecule of partially double-stranded DNA. One of the strands is incomplete, leaving a single-stranded or gap region. Additional components of the core include DNA-dependent DNA polymerase and hepatitis B e antigen (HBeAg).

A simple, direct molecular hybridization test has been developed to detect HBV DNA in serum. Studies by various investigators have revealed that most HBeAg-positive sera have detectable HBV DNA (Lieberman et al., 1983; Scotto et al., 1983).

Hepatitis B surface antigen. The HBsAg particle contains approximately seven polypeptides. Multiple antigenic specificities of HBsAg are associated with these polypeptides. Serologic analysis of HBsAg particles indicates

that (1) they share a common group-specific determinant, a; and (2) they usually carry at least two mutually exclusive subdeterminants, d or y and w or r (LeBouvier, 1972). The subtypes are the phenotypic expressions of distinct genotype variants of HBV. Four principal phenotypes have been recognized: adw, adr, ayw, and ayr. Other complex permutations of these subdeterminants and new variants are listed in Table 42-1. The subtypes are valuable epidemiologic markers of infection. Protection against infection apparently is conferred by antibody against the a specificity.

Various tests for the detection of HBsAg and anti-HBs have been developed. These techniques have proved very useful for various studies involving (1) the testing of blood donors and blood products, (2) the diagnosis of acute and chronic hepatitis and the hepatitis B carrier state, (3) the epidemiology of hepatitis B infections, (4) various investigations designed to enhance knowledge of the pathogenesis and immunologic aspects of the disease, and (5) the evaluation of active and passive immunization procedures for the prevention of HBV infections.

Hepatitis C

Studies in chimpanzees by Bradley et al. (1987) revealed the presence of a transmissible agent in blood products that caused NANB hepatitis. The agent was sensitive to organic solvents, and it was less than 80 nm in diameter as assessed by filtration. Using large quantities of Bradley's

TABLE 42-1	Nomenclature of Hepatitis B Antigens and Antibodies
HBV	Hepatitis B virus; a 42-nm double shelled virus, originally known as the Dane particle
HBsAg	Hepatitis B surface antigen; the hepatitis B antigen found on the surface of the virus and on the accompanying unattached spherical (22 nm) and tubular particles
HBcAg	Hepatitis B core antigen; the hepatitis B antigen found within the core of the virus
HBeAg	The e antigen, which is closely associated with hepatitis B infection
anti-HBs	Antibody to hepatitis B surface antigen
anti-HBc	Antibody to hepatitis B core antigen
anti-HBc	Antibody to the e antigen

Subdeterminants of HBsAg

ayw1	(a_1y2)	adw$_2$	(a_2^1dw)
ayw2	(a_2^1yw)	adw$_4$	(a_3dw)
ayw3	(a_2^3yw)	adr	
ayw4	(a_3yw)	adyw	
ayr			

From World Health Organization Expert Committee on Viral Hepatitis: Advances in viral hepatitis, WHO Tech Rep Ser No. 602, 1977.

well characterized highly infectious plasma as a source of virus, Choo et al. (1989) cloned the genome of this NANB agent, HCV. It contains a positive single-stranded RNA molecule and consists of about 9,400 bases coding for about 3,100 amino acids. There is about a 40% sequence homology with the family of Flaviviridae in the conserved 5' region, and HCV is now considered a member of this family, most closely resembling pestiviruses. The 5' untranslated region (UTR) extends from the N terminal and probably plays a regulatory role in transcription or translation. Downstream from the UTR are structural sequences encoding the nucleocapsid core and structural regions, called *E1* and E2/NS-1, which code for the glycosylated envelope protein. Further downstream are nonstructural genes, designated sequentially NS-2 to NS-5, which code for a polymerase, replicase, and helicase. There is only one open reading frame (ORF) with splicing performed by viral and cellular enzymes.

Variation in the envelope region is considerable and results in more than 4 strains now classified as genotypes based on genetic relatedness (Okamoto et al., 1992). A change in nomenclature (Simmonds et al., 1993; Simmonds et al., 1994) classifies HCV into "type" (corresponding to major phylogenetic branches for genomic and subgenomic regions) and "subtypes" (divided into more closely related sequences among major groups). The known types are numbered from 1 and the subtypes as a, b, and c. HCV in the United States and Europe is classified as 1a, 1b, 2a, 2b, and 3a. In Japan and China 1b, 2, and 2b predominate. Individuals may be infected with more than one type and subtype, indicating that there is little cross-protection among types. Type 1 HCV appears to be overrepresented among patients with cirrhosis, although all types are capable of producing cirrhosis. Patients with type 1 are also less likely to respond to interferon (IFN) therapy. Although HCV viral load is inversely correlated with potential clearance after IFN therapy, there appears to be no inherent difference in the ability of HCV to replicate and produce unique levels of virus, indicating that viral type and load are independent variables for clinical outcomes.

In addition to infection by HCV types, individuals are usually infected by multiple "quasispecies" within a given classification. These viral swarms represent unique viruses that differ minimally from each other in genetic sequences, produced by both viral mutation and immunologic selection.

HCV can now be quantified using a polymerase chain reaction (PCR)–based assay (Hoffman-La Roche, Nutley, New Jersey) or by a branched chain oligonucleotide technique (Chiron Corporation, Emeryville, California). Although virtually all types can be measured by these two techniques, there may be selective differences in the relative sensitivity of assays for different HCV types, resulting in different measurements.

Hepatitis D

The 35-nm HDV double-shelled particle resembles HBV on electron microscopy. It has an external coat antigen of HBsAg provided by the genome of HBV (the helper virus) and an internal delta antigen (HDAg) provided by the HDV genome. A small, circular RNA molecule is associated with the HDAg; it is single stranded. HDV RNA isolated from infected liver is present in linear or circular forms. The structure and replicative cycle of HDV place it outside of any known family of animal viruses. Three genotypes (I, II, and III) have been described.

Hepatitis E

Viruslike particles, 27 to 30 nm in diameter, were detected by Balayan et al. (1981) in fecal samples from a volunteer who ingested an aqueous extract of feces obtained from patients with enterically transmitted NANB hepatitis. A similar agent was transmitted to marmosets and chimpanzees by Bradley et al. (1987). This cause of ET-NANB hepatitis is the HEV. The genome is a single-stranded positive-sense RNA molecule about 7.5 kilobases long. Three ORFs are present. ORF1 codes for nonstructural regulatory proteins; ORF2 codes for structural protein; ORF3 codes for a protein of undetermined function. The virus is very labile. Its biophysical properties indicate that it is a calicivirus-like agent, although genomic sequences more closely resemble rubella virus.

PATHOLOGY
Acute Viral Hepatitis

The histologic features of acute viral hepatitis caused by various hepatitis viruses (A, B, C, D, and E) may be indistinguishable. The characteristic findings on liver biopsy include necrosis and inflammation of the lobule, architectural consequences of the necrosis, and proliferation of the mesenchymal and bile duct elements. Anicteric hepatitis shows the same histologic appearance as icteric hepatitis but usually with less severity.

The fully developed stage of hepatitis is characterized by degeneration and death of liver cells, proliferation of the Kupffer's cells, mononuclear cell infiltration, and bile duct proliferation. The hepatic cell changes involve the entire lobule, with a concentration of lesions in the centrolobular areas. The cells are usually swollen, but occasionally they are shrunken. As the lesions progress, there may be a variable degree of collapse, condensation of reticulin fibers, and accumulation of ceroid pigment and large phagocytic cells, first within the lobules and later in the portal tracts. In HEV infection the typical changes are focal necrosis with little infiltration and no lobular predilection. The focal lesions resemble those seen in drug-associated toxic hepatitis, with evidence of cholestasis.

During the recovery period the following residual changes may be seen: pleomorphic liver cells around central veins, focal inflammatory infiltration of portal tracts, and a mild degree of fibrosis extending from the portal tracts. Liver cell necrosis is slight or absent, but ceroid pigment may be found in the portal tracts.

Complete resolution is the usual course of all types of viral hepatitis. In most cases complete regeneration of the liver cells is observed after 2 or 3 months. However, other possible consequences include chronic persistent or chronic active hepatitis, resolution of hepatitis with postnecrotic scarring, cirrhosis, or fatal massive necrosis.

Chronic Active Hepatitis

Chronic active hepatitis caused by HBV, HCV, and HDV is characterized histologically by accumulations of lymphocytes and plasma cells that are located in the portal tracts and in foci of necrosis scattered throughout the hepatic lobules. Other findings include disruption of the limiting plate of the hepatic lobule adjacent to the portal tract and extension of the inflammatory reaction out of the portal tract into the hepatic parenchyma. The hepatocytes undergoing necrosis in these areas apparently are entrapped by the inflammatory infiltrate (known as *piecemeal necrosis*). Small clusters of hepatocytes may be surrounded by the inflammatory process, thereby creating a "rosette" appearance. The inflammation may vary in severity and distribution. A predominance of plasma cells may be found in patients with lupoid hepatitis. The pattern of lobular collapse and necrosis bridging portal areas and central veins has been termed *submassive necrosis* or *bridging necrosis* (Boyer and Klatskin, 1970). These findings during a biopsy indicate a poor prognosis.

The presence of portal fibrosis is variable. In more severe cases there is a marked deposition of fibrous tissue in the portal areas, accompanied by collapse of the hepatic lobular architecture and formation of fibrous tissue "bridges" between adjacent portal areas and central veins. In advanced stages the extensive cirrhosis may mask the chronic inflammatory process, resulting in histologic evidence of cryptogenic or macronodular cirrhosis.

Chronic Persistent Hepatitis

In patients with chronic persistent hepatitis the lymphocytic inflammatory infiltration is confined chiefly to the portal tracts. The lobular architecture of the liver is preserved, evidence of hepatocellular damage is minimal or absent, and fibrosis is only slight or absent. Piecemeal necrosis, very typical with chronic active hepatitis, is lacking in chronic persistent hepatitis.

Fulminant Hepatitis

In patients with fulminant hepatitis with death occurring within 10 days, the size of the liver is reduced, and its color is yellow or mottled (acute yellow atrophy). Histologic findings include extensive, diffuse necrosis and loss of hepatocytes, which are replaced by an inflammatory infiltrate composed of both polymorphonuclear and monocytic cells. Because the virus is usually not directly cytotoxic to liver cells, it has been suggested that an exaggerated immune response to a viral antigen is responsible for the cell death. The lobular structure of the liver may be collapsed. Occasionally, however, the architecture of the liver may be well preserved. Kupffer's cells and histiocytes contain phagocytized material from disintegrated liver cells. Bile thrombi may be seen in the canaliculi. Portal triads that usually are retained are filled with monocytes, lymphocytes, and polymorphonuclear cells. Occasionally, surviving liver tissue may be seen in the periphery of the lobules.

Regeneration of liver tissue may begin if patients survive for several days. The regeneration appears as clusters of cells scattered randomly throughout the liver. As regeneration advances, these "pseudolobules" of liver parenchyma appear to form adenoma-like groups of liver cells unrelated to the normal lobular architecture and lacking central veins. Patients who survive fulminant hepatitis usually have a remarkable recovery of liver function. Little or no residual liver damage is seen in biopsy specimens, although occasionally a coarse lobular type of cirrhosis is noted (Karvountzis et al., 1974).

IMMUNOPATHOLOGY
Hepatitis A

Hepatitis A antigen is detected in the cytoplasm of hepatocytes shortly before onset of acute hepatitis. Viral expression decreases rapidly after the appearance of clinical and histologic manifestations and IgM-specific anti-HAV. These findings indicate that hepatocellular damage is caused chiefly by immunologic rather than cytotoxic factors. Propagation of HAV in tissue culture is not associated with a cytopathic effect.

Hepatitis B

The pathologic and clinical consequences of hepatitis B infection is related to at least two factors: (1) HBV is not cytopathogenic, and (2) liver cell necrosis is in great part the result of host defenses. Cell necrosis may be the result of a cellular and immune response to HBV. Acute hepatitis with recovery may be associated with an efficient immune response that eliminates virus-infected cells by means of spotty necrosis. Viral antigens (HBsAg and HBcAg) that may be present in the liver before elicitation of the immune response are eliminated at the height of the acute disease. In contrast, chronic forms of hepatitis B may be the result of a quantitatively or qualitatively ineffective immune response. Under the conditions of high-grade immunosuppression, such as occurs in kidney transplant recipients, HBV may persist in the liver without any substantial liver cell damage. On the other hand, in patients with chronic active hepatitis the occurrence of piecemeal necrosis may be a consequence of a partially deficient immune

state. The available evidence indicates that an immune defect resulting in the incomplete elimination of infected hepatocytes is a cause of chronic HBV infection.

Hepatitis C

Once infection occurs, apoptosis—as well as ballooning degeneration of hepatocytes, damage of bile duct epithelium, microsteatosis and macrosteatosis, and fibrosis—are typical but not pathognomonic of HCV. It remains debatable whether HCV is directly cytopathic. Evidence to support this comes from the rare cases of unusually fulminant hepatitis in immunocompromised liver transplant recipients. It is also unclear whether the exuberance of the immune response or the lack thereof is the principal process resulting in chronic HCV hepatonecrosis. Portal changes (including lymphoid follicular aggregates) are mild and may be due to immunologic mechanisms, including potential autoimmune ones. Histologic events do not appear to reflect simultaneous measurements of serum transaminases. There is also no correlation between histologic activity and the presence of HCV RNA in the liver tissue. It may be difficult to differentiate acute from chronic hepatitis, and it is also difficult to predict clinical outcome based on a single biopsy. HCV RNA sequences may also be found in the lymphocytes of patients with chronic HCV (Zignego et al., 1995). These cells may serve as a source for reinfection of previously infected liver transplant recipients.

CLINICAL MANIFESTATIONS

The similarities and differences between the clinical manifestations of viral hepatitis types A, B, C, D, and E are listed in Table 42-2. The incubation period of hepatitis A ranges between 15 and 40 days, and the onset of symptoms is usually acute. In contrast, the incubation period of hepatitis B is longer (50 to 180 days), and the onset more commonly is insidious. The incubation period of hepatitis C may be the same as that of both type A and type B hepatitis; it may range between 1 and 5 months. In general, the clinical features of hepatitis C resemble type B infection more than type A.

The clinical picture shows great variation. In children the acute disease is generally milder and its course is shorter than in adults. In children or adults, jaundice may be inapparent or

TABLE 42-2   Viral Hepatitis Types A, B, C, D, and E: Comparison of Clinical, Epidemiologic, and Immunologic Features

Features	A	B	C	D	E
Virus	HAV	HBV	HDV	HCV	HEV
Family	Picornavirus	Hepadnavirus	Satellite	Flavivirus	Calicivirus
Genome	RNA	DNA	RNA	RNA	RNA
Incubation period	15-40 days	50-180 days	21-90 days	1-5 months	2-9 weeks
Type of onset	Usually acute	Usually insidious	Usually acute	Usually insidious	Usually acute
Prodrome: arthritis and rash	Not present	May be present	Unknown	May be present	Not present
Mode of transmission					
Oral (fecal)	Usual	No	No	No	Usual
Parenteral	Rare	Usual	Usual	Usual	No
Other	Food- or water-borne	Intimate (sexual) contact, perinatal	Intimate (sexual) contact less common	Intimate (sexual) contact less common	Water-borne transmission in developing countries
Sequelae					
Carrier	No	Yes	Yes	Yes	No
Chronic hepatitis	No cases reported	Yes	Yes	Yes	No cases reported
Mortality	0.1%-0.2%	0.5%-2.0% in uncomplicated cases; may be higher in complicated cases	2%-20%	1%-2% in uncomplicated cases; may be higher in complicated cases	20% in pregnant women; 1% 2% in general population
Immunity					
Homologous	Yes	Yes	Yes	Yes	Yes
Heterologous	No	No	No	No	No

evanescent, or it may persist for many weeks. The course of the disease often may be separated into two phases: preicteric and icteric. However, occasionally jaundice may be the initial symptom.

Preicteric Phase

Fever, when present, appears during the preicteric phase of the disease; often it is absent or fleeting in young children, but in adolescents and adults it may last for 5 days. The temperature ranges from 37.8° to 40° C (100° to 104° F) and generally is accompanied by headache, lassitude, anorexia, nausea, vomiting, and abdominal pain. Urticaria and arthralgia or arthritis occurring during the preicteric phase usually are manifestations of hepatitis B. The liver may be enlarged and tender, and splenomegaly and lymphadenopathy may be present in some patients.

Icteric Phase

Jaundice begins to emerge as the fever subsides; it usually is preceded by the appearance of dark urine (biliuria). In young children the transition to the icteric phase is most often marked by disappearance of symptoms. On the other hand, in adults and older children the icteric phase may be accompanied by an exacerbation of some of the original symptoms, such as anorexia, nausea, vomiting, and abdominal pain. Mental depression, bradycardia, and pruritus—all frequently occurring in adults—are uncommon in children. The stools may be clay colored, but this is an inconstant finding. The icteric phase persists from a few days to as long as a month, with an average duration of 8 to 11 days in children and 3 to 4 weeks in adults. As jaundice fades, the patient's symptoms subside. As a rule, convalescence is rapid and uneventful. Excessive weight loss is more common in adults than in children. In small infants and children less than 3 years of age, hepatitis is usually anicteric. Jaundice is a very rare manifestation of neonatal hepatitis B infection. Most HBV-infected infants born to mothers who are HBV carriers have a chronic asymptomatic infection.

Hepatitis A (HAV)

The course of hepatitis A is shown in Figure 42-3. After an incubation period of approximately 30 days, there is a spiking rise in serum alanine aminotransferase (ALT) levels. The duration of abnormal ALT levels in children is brief, rarely exceeding 2 to 3 weeks. The serum bilirubin value usually becomes abnormal when ALT reaches peak levels. The increased level of serum bilirubin may be transient, and the duration may be as short as 1 day or may persist for more than 1 month. In general, jaundice is transient in children and more prolonged in adults.

The following tests are available for the detection of hepatitis A antibody: IAHA, RIA, and EIA. As indicated in Figure 42-3, RIA anti-HAV is detected very early—at the time of onset of disease. Initially, RIA anti-HAV is predominantly IgM; later it is exclusively IgG. The time

of appearance of EIA anti-HAV is the same for RIA, and the test apparently is equally sensitive.

The duration of illness caused by HAV is variable, ranging from several weeks to several months. The degree of morbidity and the duration of jaundice correlate directly with the patient's age. Even with prolonged acute illness lasting several months, complete resolution of hepatitis usually occurs. Unlike hepatitis B, C, and D, HAV infection does not cause chronic liver disease. Viremia is transient; it is not characterized by a chronic carrier state. Although the outcome of HAV infection is usually favorable, fulminant hepatitis may occur. McNeil et al. (1984) reported three deaths (0.14%) in a series of 2,174 consecutive virologically or serologically confirmed hospitalized cases. Thus the death rate among all hepatitis A cases must be negligible.

Hepatitis B (HBV)

The course of HBV infection is shown in Figures 42-4 and 42-5. The incubation period may range from 2 to 6 months. The detection of HBsAg in the blood of a patient with acute hepatitis is indicative of HBV infection. The characteristic laboratory findings and the profile of abnormal liver function are shown in Table 42-3 and Figure 42-4.

HBsAg may be detected by RIA 6 to 30 days after a parenteral exposure and 56 to 60 days after an oral exposure (Krugman, 1979;

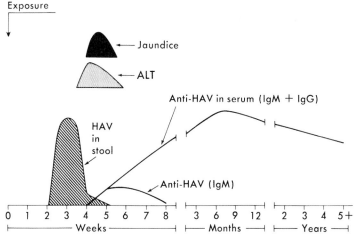

Fig. 42-3 Schematic illustration of serial clinical and laboratory findings in a patient with type A hepatitis. Hepatitis A virus *(HAV)* is detected in stool during the latter part of the incubation period before onset of the disease. Appearance of hepatitis A antibody *(anti-HAV)* coincides with disappearance of HAV in stool. IgM-specific anti-HAV is detected at the time of onset of disease; IgG-specific anti-HAV appears approximately 1 week later. (Modified from Frösner GG: Münch Med Wochenschr 1977;119:825.)

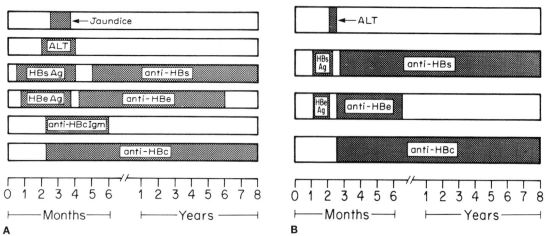

Fig. 42-4 A, Acute hepatitis B followed by recovery, showing results of serial tests for serum alanine aminotransferase *(ALT)*, hepatitis B surface antigen *(HBsAg)* and its antibody *(anti-HBs)*, hepatitis B e antigen *(HBeAg)* and its antibody *(anti-HBe)*, hepatitis B core antibody *(anti-HBc)*, and anti-HBc IgM. **B,** Subclinical hepatitis B infection followed by an immune response. Shaded areas denote "abnormal" or "detectable," and white areas denote "normal" or "not detectable." (From Krugman S: Pediatr Rev 1985;7:3-11.)

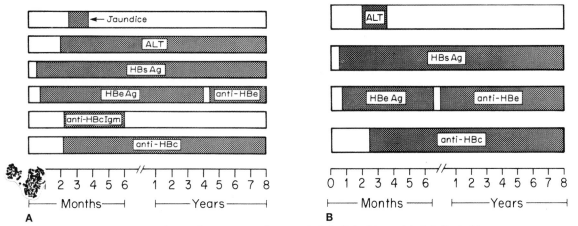

Fig. 42-5 A, Chronic hepatitis B infection. **B,** Subclinical hepatitis B followed by an asymptomatic chronic carrier state. See Figure 42-4 for key. (From Krugman S: Pediatr Rev 1985;7:3-11.)

TABLE 42-3 **Detection of Hepatitis B Surface Antigen and Its Antibody, Antibody to Hepatitis B Core Antigen, and Hepatitis Be Antigen and Its Antibody During the Course of Type B Hepatitis Infection**

Time of hepatitis B infection	HBsAg	Anti-HBs	Anti-HBc	HBeAg	Anti-HBe
Late incubation period	0	0	0	+	0
Early in course of acute hepatitis (<1 week)	+	0	+	+	0
Late in course of acute hepatitis (1 to 4 weeks)	+ or 0	+ or 0	+	+ or 0	0 or +
Convalescence from acute hepatitis					
Early (4 to 8 weeks)	0	+ or 0	+	0	+ or 0
Late (>8 weeks)	0	+	+	0	+ or 0

Anti-HBc, Antibody to hepatitis B core antigen; *anti-HBe,* antibody to HBeAg; *anti-HBs,* antibody to HBsAg; *HBeAg,* hepatitis B e antigen; *HBsAg,* hepatitis B surface antigen; +, Present; 0, not present.

Krugman et al., 1979). The antigen may be detected approximately 1 week to 2 months before the appearance of abnormal levels of ALT and jaundice. In most patients with acute hepatitis B, HBsAg is consistently present during the latter part of the incubation period and during the preicteric phase of the disease. The antigen may become undetectable shortly after onset of jaundice.

The pattern of serum ALT activity is illustrated in Figure 42-4, A. After an incubation period of approximately 50 days, the serum ALT values become abnormal, rising gradually over a period of several weeks. The duration of abnormal ALT activity may be prolonged, usually exceeding 30 to 60 days.

As indicated in Figure 42-4, A, the first antibody that is detectable is anti-HBc. It appears approximately 1 week or more after the onset of hepatitis. The anti-HBc titers, predominantly IgM, are usually high for several months. Thereafter IgM values decline to low or undetectable levels, but anti-HBc persists for many years (Chau et al., 1983). The commercially available test for anti-HBc IgM is a solid-phase immunoassay; its cut-off assay value was established to differentiate high levels of antibody (positive) from low or undetectable levels (negative). The test is negative in healthy HBsAg carriers and in patients with cirrhosis. It may be positive in those with chronic hepatitis characterized by marked inflammatory changes without cirrhosis.

The anti-HBc IgM assay should be useful for differentiating recent from past HBV infections and identifying acute hepatitis B in patients whose HBsAg has declined to undetectable levels before the appearance of anti-HBs (window phase). Antibody to the HBsAg usually appears late, approximately 2 weeks to 2 months after HBsAg is no longer detectable. Anti-HBs is detected in approximately 80% of patients with hepatitis B who eventually become HBsAg negative. In the remainder the antibody levels are too low for detection. Anti-HBs may be detected in approximately 5% to 10% of HBsAg carriers. Up to one third of Chinese and half of Japanese patients with serologic evidence of past HBV infection have detectable HBV DNA in their blood when tested with sensitive detection techniques such as PCR; the loss of HBsAg followed by the emergence of anti-HBsAg antibody does not necessarily indicate the absence of viremia.

The results of tests for HBsAg, HBeAg, anti-HBs, and anti-HBc during the course of hepatitis B are shown in Table 42-3 and in Figures 42-4 and 42-5. Most patients with hepatitis B infection recover completely. However, progression to chronic hepatitis with persistence of HBsAg has been reported in 3% of Taiwanese university students (Beasley et al., 1983), in 8% of homosexual men (Szmuness et al., 1981), and in 13% of Eskimos (McMahon et al., 1985). The risk of chronic hepatitis B infection in infants born to mothers who are HBsAg- and HBeAg-positive carriers may exceed 60%. Other serious consequences of acute HBV infection include fulminant hepatitis, cirrhosis, and hepatocellular carcinoma.

Hepatitis C (HCV)

Most patients with HCV infection are anicteric, especially those who have the contact-acquired sporadic form. The incubation period ranges from 1 to 5 months. The clinical signs and symptoms of the acute illness are milder than those with HAV and HBV infections. However, biochemical evidence of chronic liver disease develops in approximately 50% of patients with posttransfusion hepatitis C (Alter, 1985). HCV infection is found in 0.5% to 8% of blood donors worldwide. As indicated in Figure 42-6, the ALT elevations fluctuate over prolonged periods of time. The interval between exposure to HCV or onset of illness

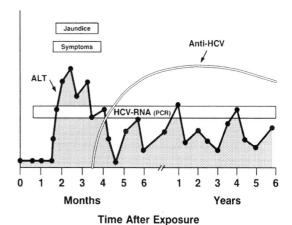

Fig. 42-6 Typical course of a case of acute hepatitis C that progresses to chronic infection and disease. *ALT,* Alanine aminotransferase; *HCV-RNA,* hepatitis C virus ribonucleic acid; *PCR,* polymerase chain reaction; *anti-HCV,* antibody to hepatitis C virus. (From Hoofnagle JH, DiBisceglie AM: Semin Liver Dis 1991;11:78.)

and detection of anti-HCV may be prolonged. In recipients of transfusions the mean interval from onset of hepatitis to anti-HCV detection may be 15 weeks (range 4 to 32 weeks). In general, anti-HCV persists in patients with chronic disease; it may disappear in those with acute resolving hepatitis C (Alter et al., 1989; Farci et al., 1991).

The course of a typical case of posttransfusion hepatitis C is shown in Figure 42-6. Evidence of viremia was detected by the use of PCR technology 2 weeks after a transfusion of HCV-contaminated blood. The first increase in ALT values was detected at 8 weeks, and anti-HCV was detectable at 11 weeks. A 6-year follow-up revealed persistence of positive PCR, detectable anti-HCV, and biopsy evidence of chronic active hepatitis. Long-term prospective studies of patients with posttransfusion (NANB) hepatitis (HCV disease) have revealed evidence of progression to cirrhosis and to hepatocellular carcinoma. In most blood centers, units of blood are screened for antibody to HCV and for elevations of liver transaminases. This should reduce but not completely eliminate HCV transmission, because antibody responses to HCV may be absent for a long time after HCV infection, and liver transaminases may continue to be normal. In the future, HCV RNA screening may be added to decrease the likelihood of HCV infection.

Hepatitis D (HDV)

The clinical manifestations and course of type D hepatitis resemble those of acute or chronic hepatitis B. In general, however, hepatitis D is a more severe disease. The mortality rate of acute HDV hepatitis has ranged from 2% to 20%, compared with less than 1% for acute hepatitis B. In addition, cirrhosis and complications of portal hypertension occur more often and progress more rapidly in patients with hepatitis D. Acute delta hepatitis occurs as either a coinfection or superinfection of hepatitis B (Table 42-2). Coinfection entails a simultaneous onset of acute HBV and HDV infection. In superinfection a chronic HBV carrier is infected with HDV.

The course of acute delta coinfection is shown in Figure 42-7. During the latter part of the incubation period, HBsAg—followed by HDV RNA—appears. Thereafter serum ALT levels begin to rise, followed by the development of clinical symptoms and jaundice. Serum

ALT activity is often biphasic. Resolution of acute liver disease follows clearance of HBsAg and cessation of HDV replication. The antibody to HDV (anti-HDV) that appears shortly after onset of clinical disease is transient. The course of acute delta superinfection followed by the development of chronic delta hepatitis is shown in Figure 42-8. At the time of exposure to HDV this patient was an asymptomatic chronic HBsAg carrier with normal ALT values. At the end of the incubation period there are (1) a rise in serum ALT values; (2) appearance and persistence of HDV RNA; followed

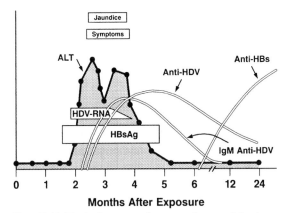

Fig. 42-7 Typical course of a case of acute delta hepatitis coinfection. *ALT*, Alanine aminotransferase; *HBsAg*, hepatitis B surface antigen; *HDV-RNA*, hepatitis delta virus ribonucleic acid; *anti-HDV*, antibody to HDV; *anti-HBs*, antibody to HBsAg. (From Hoofnagle JH, DiBisceglie AM: Semin Liver Dis 1991;11:79.)

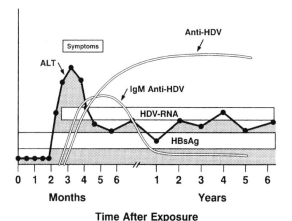

Fig. 42-8 Typical course of a case of acute delta hepatitis superinfection. See Figure 42-7 for key. (From Hoofnagle JH, DiBisceglie AM: Semin Liver Dis 1991;11:80.)

by (3) appearance of IgM anti-HDV, which is transient; and (4) a rise of IgG anti-HDV to high levels that persist.

Hepatitis E (HEV)

The clinical manifestations and course of hepatitis E are essentially the same as those for hepatitis A. However, there are several striking differences. During various epidemics the disease has been rare in children and common in adolescents and young adults. The typical clinical and immunologic correlates of infection are seen in Figure 42-9.

HEV, like HAV, does not cause chronic liver disease. In most patients the illness is self-limiting, and there is no evidence of a chronic carrier state. However, unlike hepatitis A, hepatitis E can be a devastating disease in pregnant women. Whereas the mortality rate from hepatitis A in pregnant women is less than 1%, the rate has ranged from 10% to 20% in outbreaks of hepatitis E. The deaths are caused by fulminant hepatitis and disseminated intravascular coagulation. Mortality is highest during the third trimester and lowest during the first trimester. The mortality rate in nonpregnant women is the same as that among men, less than 1%. Transmission from mother to infant has been reported, with most of the infected infants recovering from their hepatitis. However, one of the infants developed massive hepatic necrosis and died (Khuroo et al., 1995).

At the present time a practical serologic test to confirm a diagnosis of hepatitis E is not available. Immune electron microscopy was the first-generation test used by investigators. Second-generation tests using recombinant proteins in enzyme-linked immunosorbent assay (ELISA) or Western blot format have an 80% to 100% sensitivity. Comparative sensitivity and specificity data are unavailable. Diagnostic tests can also detect HEV antigens using immunofluorescent probes, as well as RNA by PCR.

NEONATAL HEPATITIS INFECTION

HBV is the most common and most important cause of neonatal hepatitis infection, with HCV also assuming increasing importance. To date, perinatal transmission of HDV has not been well documented. It is unlikely that HAV and HEV will prove to be problems, because these infections are not characterized by a carrier state.

Perinatal transmission of HBV from mother to infant during the course of pregnancy or at the time of birth was first reported by Stokes et al. (1954). They observed an infant born by cesarean section to a mother who was a hepatitis B carrier. The infant, who developed hepatitis with jaundice at 2 months of age, later died at age 18 months with advanced fibrosis of the liver.

The availability of tests to detect HBsAg has enabled various investigators to study infants whose mothers had acute hepatitis B or an asymptomatic chronic carrier state during pregnancy (Schweitzer et al., 1972; Stevens et al., 1975). Signs of neonatal hepatitis B infection (antigenemia) are usually not present at the time of birth but may be detected between 2 weeks and 5 months of age. Approximately 5% of infants are infected in utero and approximately 95% at the time of birth. Certain infants escape infection completely; others develop only persistent antigenemia with no liver disease; others may develop severe chronic active hepatitis; and still others may develop fulminant hepatitis (Fawaz et al., 1975).

Perinatal transmission of hepatitis B infection from mother to infant depends in great part on the presence of HBeAg (an indirect marker of viral load that exceeds a million particles per ml of plasma). Infection is most likely to occur if the mother is HBeAg positive (Stevens et al., 1975). Infants born to HBeAg-positive carrier mothers have a 60% to 90% chance of contracting chronic hepatitis B infection and of possible subsequent progression to

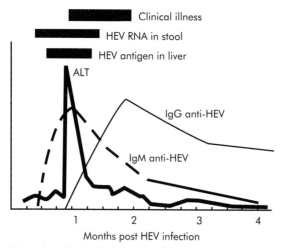

Fig. 42-9 Typical clinical and immunologic correlates of infection.

cirrhosis and hepatocellular carcinoma. In contrast, the attack rate of hepatitis B in infants whose HBsAg-positive mothers are HBeAg negative is less than 20%. These infants usually recover completely, and chronic hepatitis is rare, but occasionally the infection may be fulminant with a fatal outcome (Delaplane et al., 1983). The viruses associated with this rare fulminant course have often been HBV variants with precore mutations (Bahn et al., 1995).

Possible routes of transmission from mother to baby include (1) leakage of virus across the placenta late in pregnancy or during labor; (2) ingestion of amniotic fluid or maternal blood; and (3) breast-feeding, especially if the mother has cracked nipples. Studies by Alter (1980) with HBsAg-positive and HBeAg-positive pregnant chimpanzees revealed that cesarean section and postdelivery isolation did not prevent infection of newborn chimpanzees. They became HBsAg-positive in spite of these precautions.

Infants who inadvertently receive contaminated blood or blood products during the neonatal period may subsequently develop severe hepatitis B. Dupuy et al. (1975) described their experience with 14 infants 2 to 5 months of age who were admitted to the hospital with severe or fulminant hepatitis. Of the 14 infants, 11 had serologic evidence of hepatitis B infection. Of the 11 infants with hepatitis B, 7 received blood derivatives during the neonatal period, and 4 were exposed to their mothers, who were chronic HBsAg carriers. The case fatality rate was very high; 8 of the 14 infants died.

The risk of perinatal transmission of HCV is about 6% to 7% among women without coexistent HIV and three to four times higher in those with HIV infection (Gibb et al. 2000; Nagata et al., 1992; Palomba et al., 1996; Papaevangelou et al, 1998). Transmission from HIV-uninfected mothers appears to be correlated with maternal viremia levels. Vaginal delivery and breast-feeding do not appear to contribute any increased risk.

COURSE AND COMPLICATIONS

Various factors can affect the course of hepatitis infection: age, type of virus, and immunocompetence. In general, hepatitis A and E are mild or inapparent infections in infants and children. However, they are generally more severe in adults. In contrast, infants infected with HBV are more likely to develop chronic

hepatitis B than older children and adults. Compared with hepatitis A infections, hepatitis B, C, and D infections are more likely to progress to chronic liver disease.

Acute Hepatitis

The duration of illness caused by HAV is variable, ranging from several weeks to several months. The degree of morbidity and duration of jaundice correlate directly with age. Even with prolonged acute illness lasting several months, complete resolution of hepatitis usually occurs. Most patients with hepatitis A recover completely. Hepatitis B, C, and D, on the other hand, are associated with more debility and a substantial risk of chronic liver disease. In rare instances, acute hepatitis may progress to a fulminant fatal outcome.

Chronic Persistent Hepatitis

Chronic persistent hepatitis is a pathologic diagnosis based on a liver biopsy. It is an inflammatory process involving only the portal areas. This form of hepatitis usually lasts longer than 6 months, and it is more common and less severe than chronic active hepatitis. In general, the patient is asymptomatic and usually has mild hepatomegaly and moderate elevation of serum aminotransferases without jaundice. Chronic persistent hepatitis may resolve after several years or may progress to chronic active hepatitis. These patients may be HBsAg carriers.

Chronic Active Hepatitis

Chronic active hepatitis, also referred to as *chronic aggressive hepatitis*, is more likely to progress to cirrhosis. The disease is characterized by chronic and recurrent episodes of jaundice, abnormal levels of serum aspartate aminotransferase (AST) and ALT, and evidence of portal hypertension with ascites if the disease progresses to cirrhosis. Severe episodes of hepatic necrosis may terminate in hepatic failure. Most patients with chronic hepatitis (persistent or active) do not have a history of acute illness with jaundice. The disease usually follows mild, anicteric forms of hepatitis.

Fulminant Hepatitis

The occurrence of hepatic failure within the first few days or within 4 weeks after onset of acute hepatitis indicates a fulminant course. When the course is more prolonged and hepatic failure occurs after 1 to 3 months of illness, the term *subacute hepatitis* is used; it is associated with portal hypertension, ascites, and submassive hepatic necrosis. Fulminant hepatitis usually is characterized by mental confusion, emotional instability, restlessness, bleeding manifestations, and coma. The progressive jaundice and coma are associated with a shrinking liver. The Fulminant Hepatic Failure Surveillance Study (Trey, 1972) included 142 patients with fulminant viral hepatitis. The survival rate was influenced by the age of the patient. Of 27 patients less than 15 years of age, 10 (37%) survived; of 73 patients 15 to 44 years of age, 12 (16%) survived; and of 42 patients 45 to more than 75 years of age, 3 (7%) survived. The overall survival rate was 18%.

Each of the hepatitis viruses can cause fulminant hepatitis with similar courses and prognoses, and there are no clinical or prognostic differences among these different forms of fulminant viral hepatitis (Gimson et al., 1983). Fulminant hepatitis B probably occurs more frequently than recognized because HBsAg may be cleared faster in this form of hepatitis than in regular hepatitis B (Tabor et al., 1981). HBV with precore mutations resulting in variants unable to express HBeAg can be associated with fulminant hepatitis (Hasegawa et al., 1991; Liang et al., 1991; Shafritz, 1991).

Simultaneous infection with HBV and HDV seems to increase liver necrosis and to favor the development of fulminant hepatitis B. In a report by Smedile et al. (1982) HDV markers were more common in patients with fulminant hepatitis B (39%) than with ordinary acute hepatitis B (19%), and serologic markers for acute HDV infection (anti-HDV IgM) were positive among 33.8% of patients with fulminant hepatitis B, compared with 4.2% of patients with acute hepatitis B (Govindarajan et al., 1984).

Hepatoma

The striking association between chronic hepatitis B infection and primary hepatocellular carcinoma (PHC) has been well established. The relationship is supported by the following factors: (1) geographic distribution of PHC, (2) presence of HBsAg in serum of patients with PHC, (3) detection of HBV markers in tumor tissue and PHC cell lines, (4) occurrence of PHC in certain animals infected with hepadnaviruses, and (5) integration of the HBV genome in the tumor cell genome.

Worldwide seroepidemiologic studies have revealed a remarkable correlation between the prevalence of HBsAg carriers and the incidence of PHC (Szmuness, 1978). The highest frequency of carrier and PHC rates has been observed in Southeast Asia and sub-Saharan Africa. Various studies have revealed that the prevalence of HBsAg is significantly higher in patients with PHC than in comparable controls (Szmuness, 1978).

Histochemical and immunochemical methods have revealed the presence of HBsAg and HBcAg in the livers of patients with PHC. HBsAg has been detected in both the tumor and the surrounding liver tissue. In addition, cultured cell lines derived from human PHC secrete enormous quantities of HBsAg into supernatant culture media (MacNab et al., 1976). Integration of HBV genome has been demonstrated by molecular hybridization analysis of DNA extracted from human PHC. These studies revealed HBV DNA sequences integrated into the tumor cell genome (Shafritz and Kew, 1981).

The occurrence of PHC in certain animals has provided additional evidence of an association with chronic hepatitis infection. The tumors have been observed in woodchucks infected with woodchuck hepatitis virus, a member of the hepadnavirus group. The inflammatory hepatic lesion caused by active viral infection is associated with a high frequency of hepatoma formation (Popper et al., 1981).

EXTRAHEPATIC MANIFESTATIONS OF VIRAL HEPATITIS

HBV infections may be associated with a variety of extrahepatic manifestations. The following sites may be affected: skin, joints, small arteries and arterioles, and renal glomeruli. The underlying pathology is usually a diffuse and widespread immune complex type of vasculitis. The following syndromes have been identified: (1) serum sickness–like prodrome, (2) polyarteritis nodosa, (3) glomerulonephritis, (4) "essential" mixed cryoglobulinemia, (5) polymyalgia rheumatica, and (6) infantile papular acrodermatitis (Gianotti-Crosti syndrome) (Gocke, 1975).

Serum Sickness–like Prodrome

Serum sickness–like prodrome is characterized by a transient erythematous maculopapular eruption, polyarthralgia, and occasionally actual arthritis and urticaria. These symptoms and signs usually occur during the latter part of the incubation period or early acute phase of the disease, and they last just a few days. During the early phase of the skin and joint manifestations the complement titer and C3 and C4 levels may be transiently suppressed (Alpert et al., 1971). The critical role that the composition of the immune complex plays in the causation of tissue injury has been demonstrated in studies by Wands et al. (1975) on the pathogenesis of arthritis associated with type B (HBsAg-positive) hepatitis.

Polyarteritis Nodosa

The association of polyarteritis nodosa with persistent hepatitis B antigenemia initially was described by Gocke et al. (1970) and Trepo and Thiyolet (1970). The illness usually begins with fever, polyarthralgia, myalgia, rash, and urticaria. The syndrome may evolve over a period of months, and it is characterized by various manifestations of acute vasculitis, including peripheral neuropathies, hypertension, and evidence of renal damage. Biopsy reveals lesions in small arteries characterized by typical fibrinoid necrosis and perivascular infiltration associated with polyarteritis nodosa. Approximately 30% to 40% of patients with polyarteritis nodosa have high titers of HBsAg, but the liver involvement that is present is not the primary problem. Circulating immune complexes composed of HBsAg and anti-HBs are present during the acute phase of the disease. At this time the whole complement titer and C3 levels are decreased. IF studies of biopsy specimens reveal deposition of HBsAg, IgM, IgG, and C3 in a nodular pattern along the elastic membrane of damaged vessels (Gocke et al., 1971). A study of HBsAg-positive and HBsAg-negative patients with polyarteritis nodosa revealed that the fatality rate was essentially equal (42% and 44%, respectively) in the two groups after a 3-year follow-up period (Sergent et al., 1976).

Glomerulonephritis

The association of glomerulonephritis with chronic hepatitis B has been studied by various investigators (Brzosko et al., 1974; Combes et al., 1971; Kohler et al., 1974). They observed typical immune complex deposits along the subepithelial surface of the glomerular basement membrane by electron microscopy. Fluorescent antibody studies showed nodular deposition of HBsAg, immunoglobulin, and C3 in the glomeruli. The glomerulonephritis is usually of the membranous or membranoproliferative type. Most cases of glomerulonephritis in adults have occurred in patients with existing evidence of chronic active hepatitis and a persistent HBsAg carrier state. However, studies by Brzosko et al. (1974) revealed the presence of HBsAg-antibody complex deposits in renal glomeruli in approximately 35% of children with clinical nephrosis or glomerulonephritis. Glomerulonephritis has also been associated with chronic HCV infection.

Other Possible Extrahepatic Syndromes

Mixed cryoglobulinemia. Mixed cryoglobulinemia is an immune complex disease characterized by arthralgias, purpura, weakness, vasculitis, and diffuse glomerulonephritis (Meltzer et al., 1966). Levo et al. (1977) described this syndrome in patients who had evidence of HBV infection and circulating immune complexes composed of HBsAg and anti-HBs. In one study, cryoglobulinemia was found in 36% of patients with chronic HCV infection, and rheumatoid factor was found in the serum of 71% of patients (Pawlotsky et al., 1995).

Autoimmune manifestation. Various autoantibodies have been found in the sera of 40% to 50% of patients with HCV infection, including antinuclear antibodies (ANA), antismooth muscle, and antithyroid antibodies (Pawlotsky et al., 1994). In addition, salivary gland lesions with lymphocytic capillaritis, resembling Sjögren's syndrome, were seen in half of patients with chronic HCV. Autoimmune hepatitis due to HCV appears to be rare in the United States but possibly occurs in Europe (Krawitt, 1996).

Polymyalgia rheumatica. Polymyalgia rheumatica is another distinct connective tissue disorder that has been associated with hepatitis B infection (Bacon et al., 1975; Plouvier et al., 1978).

Papular acrodermatitis. The association of infantile papular acrodermatitis with hepatitis B infection was first described by Gianotti (1973). A striking epidemic of this disease occurred in Japan, involving 153 patients in a pediatric clinic from 1974 to 1977 (Ishimaru et al., 1976; Toda et al., 1978). Of these cases 89% were associated with HBsAg. During the outbreak all of the index cases were 1 year old or younger, but the age ranged from 3 months to 10 years. In approximately 40% of the patients with infantile papular acrodermatitis who were 1 year of age or younger, HBsAg persisted for 1 year.

DIAGNOSIS

The diagnosis of viral hepatitis usually is based on clinical and epidemiologic grounds. The occurrence of jaundice in association with a prior febrile episode and anorexia, nausea, and abdominal pain suggests viral hepatitis. The presence of an elevated serum AST or ALT value provides additional evidence. The diagnostic features of viral hepatitis types A, B, C, D, and E are listed in Table 42-2. The value of specific serologic tests for the diagnosis of various types of hepatitis is dependent on the time the blood is obtained during the course of the disease. The presence of IgM-specific anti-HAV indicates hepatitis A infection. The detection of HBsAg in the serum is indicative of hepatitis B infection. The interpretation of various serologic tests for the diagnosis of hepatitis B infection is shown in Table 42-3. Diagnosis of HCV infection is most easily made serologically using second- and third-generation assays. The first-generation ELISA used a recombinant antigen derived from the NS-4 region but had limited sensitivity. The newer assays include additional antigens derived from the core and NS-3 regions (second generation) and the NS-5 region (third generation). A confirmatory recombinant immunoblot assay (RIBA) is also available for the purpose of determining the specificity of the ELISA. The sensitivity of the later-generation assays is greater than 90%. Because antibodies may appear months after infection or not at all, the use of PCR to detect RNA remains the standard for HCV detection.

DIFFERENTIAL DIAGNOSIS

Before jaundice emerges, the following diseases may be considered in the differential diagnosis: infectious mononucleosis; acute appendicitis; gastroenteritis; influenza; and, in some parts of the world, malaria, dengue, and sandfly fever. The diagnosis of these diseases may be established by the detection of specific etiologic agents, by serologic tests, or by the subsequent course of disease.

In the presence of jaundice the diseases that may be confused with viral hepatitis are congenital or acquired hemolytic jaundice or obstructive jaundice caused by blockage of the bile ducts by stone or tumor or, in infants, congenital atresia; hepatocellular jaundice resulting from chemical poisons, cirrhosis, or neoplasm of the liver (primary or metastatic); spirochetal jaundice (Weil's disease); yellow fever; acute cholangitis; and jaundice associated with various other infections such as infectious mononucleosis, brucellosis, amebiasis, malaria, and syphilis. Before considering these diseases in the differential diagnosis, it would be important to rule out a diagnosis of hepatitis A (absence of IgM anti-HAV) and hepatitis B (absence of HBsAg and IgM anti-HBc). At the present time the test for anti-HVC is not useful for the diagnosis of acute HCV infection. A negative test result does not rule out HCV infection; it may not be detectable for several months after onset of disease. A positive test result may be indicative of a past unrelated infection.

Hemolytic Jaundice

Hemolytic jaundice can be differentiated from obstructive jaundice by the history, the presence of anemia, positive Coombs' test, presence of urobilin in the stools, and absence of bilirubinuria.

Extrahepatic Obstructive Jaundice

Calculi and neoplasms are rare in children. In infancy, congenital obliteration of the bile ducts may present difficulties at first. The distinction should become clear in the course of the illness, because the jaundice progressively deepens and the stools remain chalky or gray. Serum aminotransferase levels are lower than those found in viral hepatitis.

Hepatocellular Jaundice

Hepatocellular jaundice or parenchymal jaundice caused by chemical poisons may be difficult to diagnose in the absence of a history of ingestion of toxic agents. The history is also important in the recognition of cirrhosis or neoplasm, both of which are uncommon in children in the United States.

Drug-Associated Hepatitis

Hepatitis induced by the following drugs may be clinically, biochemically, and morphologically indistinguishable from viral hepatitis: pyrazinamide, isoniazid, zoxazolamine, gold, and cinchophen. A clinical picture similar to the cholestatic form of the disease may be produced by the phenothiazine derivatives (e.g., chlorpromazine), methyltestosterone, ceftriaxone, and contraceptive drugs. Fatal toxic hepatitis has been described in a child receiving indomethacin for rheumatoid arthritis.

Jaundice Associated With Infection

In patients with jaundice associated with infection the diagnosis is established by demonstrating the specific etiologic agent or a rise in the specific antibody in convalescence. Jaundice in the neonatal period should suggest bacterial sepsis, syphilis, CMV infection, toxoplasmosis, congenital rubella, HSV infection, or coxsackie B infection. Neonatal hepatitis associated with these infections is present at the time of birth or several days thereafter. In contrast, hepatitis B is usually detected several weeks to as long as 5 months after birth. The diagnosis is established by detection of HBsAg in the blood.

TREATMENT
Acute Viral Hepatitis

The management of patients with acute hepatitis involves decisions about (1) the duration of bed rest, (2) the choice of a diet, and (3) the value of various nonspecific drugs. At the present time there is no antiviral agent that has been shown to alter the course of either type A or type B hepatitis consistently. Bed rest is recommended for patients who are symptomatic during the acute stage of the disease. Studies by Chalmers et al. (1955) provided the basis for a more liberal attitude toward bed rest during the convalescent period. They observed that ad-lib activity was preferable to rigidly enforced bed rest for prolonged periods of time. The liberal attitude toward bed rest described by Chalmers et al. in the 1950s is just as pertinent in the 1990s. Resumption of normal activity is usually gradual.

Progressively decreasing serum aminotransferase and bilirubin levels are helpful guides to increasing activity. It is not necessary to restrict the activity of an asymptomatic patient for the many weeks and months that the transaminase levels may be elevated. Generally, children return to normal activity much sooner than adults.

Diet is best regulated by the patient's appetite. When the child shows signs of anorexia, liquids such as chicken soup and fruit juices should be given. It is recommended that, with the return of appetite, a normal diet be given that is nutritious, properly balanced, and palatable. There is no contraindication to ingesting fats in moderate amounts.

Corticosteroids and antiviral agents are not recommended for the treatment of acute hepatitis infections caused by HAV, HBV, HCV, HDV, and HEV. However, several case reports indicate that lamivudine therapy (see discussion later in this chapter) may suppress HBV replication in the setting of acute infection following liver transplantation (Andreone et al., 1998).

Chronic Persistent Hepatitis

Because chronic persistent hepatitis is usually a benign, self-limited disorder, normal activity is advised, and dietary restrictions are unnecessary. Corticosteroid or other immunosuppressive forms of therapy are not indicated.

Chronic Active Hepatitis

Patients with chronic active hepatitis may be permitted to carry out normal activities on an ad-lib basis. There is no evidence that bed rest and limitation of activity are of benefit. Alcohol should be avoided. A normal, well-balanced diet is recommended. The effects of various antiviral and immunomodulatory agents has been evaluated for the treatment of chronic hepatitis types B, C, and D. Several studies have revealed that the use of corticosteroids may be detrimental in treating chronic hepatitis B (Hoofnagle, 1987). Adenine arabinoside (Ara-A) and its monophosphate derivative have not been shown effective. To date, the most promising agent has been leukocyte interferon, or IFN-α. Various controlled studies in adults have revealed that it is possible to eliminate HBV replication and to ameliorate liver disease in approximately 40% of patients treated with IFN-α (Hoofnagle et al., 1988). However, it should be noted that (1) the therapy involved a 3- to 6-month course of daily or three-times-per-week subcutaneous inoculations; (2) relapses occurred in approximately 50% of responders after therapy was discontinued; and (3) potential side effects included fever, chills, myalgia, anorexia, irritability, weight loss, and hair loss. Given what is now known, treatment should be considered for patients with >10^6 copies of HBV DNA per ml and when ALT levels are abnormal. When IFN is used to treat chronic hepatitis B for a minimum of 4 months, there is a sustained loss of HBeAg in perhaps a third of individuals (in excess of the 20% per year in controls), a loss of HBsAg in 8% (versus 2% of controls), and HBV DNA loss in 30% to 40% of white individuals versus 17% in controls (Torre et al. 1996). Two products have been used. IFN-α-2a (Roferon-A, Hoffmann-La Roche, Nutley, New Jersey) is usually given as either 5 million units (MU) daily or 10 MU three times a week subcutaneously. IFN-α-2b (Intron A, Schering-Plough, Madison, New Jersey) is also given in this dosage.

In one small trial in Hong Kong the effect of IFN-α-2 on chronic hepatitis B in Asian children was not encouraging (Lai et al., 1987). A subsequent American study suggested that IFN-α therapy was more successful when given to younger children than it was when given to older children (Narkewicz et al., 1995). A multinational trial in children (1 to 17 years of age) using IFN-α-2b for 24 weeks at a dose of 6 MU/m^2 three times a week demonstrated significant benefit (Sokal et al., 1998). Variability in the outcome results may reflect different racial characteristics and ages of the children in the studies. A pilot study of IFN-α (10 MU/m^2 three times a week for 24 weeks) in children who failed therapy with IFN-α demonstrated successful loss of HBV DNA in 41% to 45% and anti-HBeAg conversion in a third of those who were initially eAg positive (Ozen et al., 1999). Intron A is approved by the U.S. Food and Drug Administration (FDA) for use in children with chronic HBV when they are older than 1 year of age. The most desirable of the goals of therapy is to clear HBeAg and demonstrate anti-HBe antibody production. Those who demonstrate both have longer survival and fewer complications of liver disease. Loss of HBsAg occurs in about a third of those who lose eAg.

A very promising preliminary study of the effects of 12 weeks of lamivudine (3TC), a nucleoside analog, found a dose-related clearance of HBV DNA in chronically infected adults. Fifteen percent of treated patients, most of whom had already failed IFN therapy, permanently cleared HBV (Dienstag et al., 1995). It is rapidly absorbed, inhibits reverse transcriptase, and rapidly lowers HBV DNA in the majority of individuals and, when given for 12 months, demonstrates decreases in liver transaminases and improved liver histology in 56%. HBeAg loss with seroconversion can occur in 16% at 1 year versus 4% in controls (Lai et al, 1998). Viral replication may recur when lamivudine is stopped, but HBeAg loss appears durable. In general, there is no particular restriction among patients with regard to selective responses to this therapy. Drug resistance, resulting in YMDD mutants (involving residues 552 to 558 in the polymerase gene), is common (27% at 1 year and up to 58% after 2 years) but usually is not seen before 6 to 12 months of therapy (Liaw et al., 1999). The minimum effective dose is 100 mg/day in adults. On the basis of pharmacokinetic and pharmacodynamic data, a 3-mg/kg/day dose in children (ages 2 to 12 years) with chronic hepatitis B provides levels of exposure and trough concentrations similar to those seen in adults following the administration of doses of 100 mg (Sokal et al., 2000). The optimal duration of therapy is uncertain. Many suggest not stopping therapy until HBeAg conversion has occurred, as the discontinuation may be associated with hepatitis flares. An interim review of a long-term follow-up study involving 58 Chinese patients with chronic hepatitis B shows that nearly half (47%; 27/58) achieved hepatitis e antigen seroconversion after 4 years of treatment with lamivudine (Leung et al., 2001). Seroconversion is defined in this study as the loss of hepatitis B e antigen and gain of antibody to e antigen. In previous annual interim evaluations of this study population, 29% (17/58) of the patients had seroconverted after 2 years of therapy, and 40% (23/58) after 3 years. Two thirds of patients developed YMDD variant hepatitis B virus at some point during treatment. However, 13 of these 39 patients (33%) achieved HBeAg seroconversion despite having a variant strain of hepatitis B with this mutation. In six of these patients, seroconversion occurred after detection of the YMDD variants. Also, 23 of the 39 patients who were determined to have the YMDD variant virus had normal ALT levels at their last clinic visit. The long-term clinical significance of YMDD variant hepatitis B is unknown, but it has been suggested that such mutant viruses may be less likely to cause liver inflammation than the wild type.

Famciclovir, another nucleoside first used to treat herpesvirus infections, also inhibits HBV polymerase. When given at a dose of 500 mg three times a day, HBV DNA was suppressed in all patients, but changes in anti-HBeAg were rare. Although the major mutation producing resistance involves a different residue (i.e., 528) of the polymerase region, there is some cross-resistance between famciclovir and lamivudine, making this combination potentially problematic. Nevertheless, viral breakthrough during famciclovir therapy has responded to a switch to lamivudine (Xiong et al., 1998).

Two other potent inhibitors of HBV polymerase, lobucavir and adefovir dipivoxil, can suppress HBV DNA by three to four orders of magnitude. Small trials suggest that each is likely to be at least as effective as lamivudine. Unfortunately, lobucavir is not currently in clinical development. Therapy with 10 mg of adefovir daily for 1 year resulted in a 39% anti-HBeAg seroconversion, versus 0% in the placebo group (Heathcoat et al., 1998). Resistance to adefovir has not been seen after treatment for as long as 1 year.

The nucleosides mentioned above are relatively free of significant side effects, although higher doses given for a prolonged period may produce toxicity in those treated with adefovir and lobucavir (tumors in rats have been seen with prolonged lobucavir treatment). During treatment ALT increases can be seen in 30% to 40% of patients, but these rates are also seen in recipients of placebo. ALT increases also occur in 20% of patients when therapy is discontinued. These flares often occur prior to HBeAg seroconversion.

Chronic Hepatitis C

Corticosteroid therapy has not been effective against chronic hepatitis C. Recombinant IFN-α therapy was evaluated in a double-blind, placebo-controlled trial (DiBisceglie et al., 1989). Approximately 50% of patients treated with 2 MU of IFN-α three times weekly for 6 months responded with a fall of ALT values to normal and an improvement in liver histologic conditions. However, in about half of responding patients, relapses occurred after cessation of IFN therapy. In fact, the response rate in patients with HCV type 1b is only 40%, whereas those with type 2 have a response rate of almost 80%. A report has described an IFN response gene, located in the NS5A region, that may cause these differences (Enomoto et al., 1995). In addition, the presence of preexisting cirrhosis decreases the likelihood of successful IFN therapy.

The first study of IFN therapy in children was published in 1992, from Spain, and a number of small trials have been reported from Italy, Japan, and the United States since then. The chronically infected children and adolescents were largely derived from transfused groups such as those with hemophilia, thalassemia, and leukemia. Treatments ranged in dose from 1.75 to 10 MU per m² body surface area and in duration from 6 to 12 months. Overall, sustained response rates were seen in 33% to 45% of subjects, suggesting that children responded at least as well as adults. However, one study (Pensati et al., 1999) from Italy suggested that responses were mainly biochemical and not virologic.

Both Roche Laboratories and Schering-Plough have developed a polyethylene-glycol (pegylated) IFN preparation which is time released. Roche's pegylated IFN (Pegysis) requires one administration per week, whereas the IFN treatment currently used is administered three times per week by injection. The very preliminary data on the pegylated IFN is that it may be twice as effective as IFN monotherapy in treating hepatitis C (Lindsay et al., 2001), with long-lasting effects (Swain et al., 2001).

Multiple studies have revealed that adding ribavirin, a synthetic nucleoside analogue that resembles guanosine, as additional primary therapy to IFN or for reinduction of patients who relapse results in diminished liver transaminases and often lower viral RNA levels (McHutchison et al., 1998; Poynard et al., 1998). Pegylated IFN plus ribavirin may be even more beneficial than standard IFN plus ribavirin, particularly in those with type 1 HCV, which is more resistant to therapy (Manns et al., 2001). Ribavirin itself lowers liver transaminases, and serum ALT levels normalize in 40% of patients, but the effects are lost when therapy is continued. Its sole effects on HCV RNA levels are controversial but certainly unimpressive. This suggests that ribavirin may be active by altering the cytokine profile (perhaps from a Th2-like response that favors IL-4 and IL-10 production to a Th1-like response that favors IFN-γ production).

A single oral dose results in a half-life of 44 to 49 hours, with up to sixfold accumulation occurring with chronic dosing. The washout half-life exceeds 11 days. Combination therapy with IFN-α and ribavirin (Rebetron, Schering-Plough) has resulted in sustained responses in more than two thirds of patients chronically infected with HCV genotypes 2 or 3 (in 6 or 12 months of therapy) and in 28% of those with genotype 1 (after 12 months of therapy). Rebetron is FDA approved for the treatment of chronic hepatitis C. A recent study of Rebetron showed that a virologic response at the sixth month after discontinuation of therapy with a combination of IFN-α and ribavirin in patients with chronic hepatitis C is predictive of a 97.8% rate of long-term complete (biochemical and virologic) response. It should be noted that late relapses may be a function of not having fully suppressed plasma HCV, as the sensitivity of the quantitative RNA assay may have not been optimal. Newer assays (HCV SuperQuant or HCV QuantSure by National Genetics Institute, Los Angeles, California; TMA Versant by Bayer, Emeryville, California) have sensitivities that are 2 to 10 times better than those used in these earlier studies. The use of these assays in future trials may better define true responders to therapy.

There is limited experience with this combination in children. In one recent study, 11 patients with persistent HCV viremia who had malignant diseases in remission after treatment were given a 48-week course of combined therapy with IFN-α (5×10^6 U three times weekly) and oral ribavirin (15 mg/kg/day). Seven (64%) of the 11 patients had sustained virologic responses 6 and 12 months after cessation of therapy (Christensson et al., 2000). Side effects were common but generally were mild or moderate.

Ribavirin can induce hemolytic anemia and can be problematic for patients with preexisting anemia, bone-marrow suppression, or renal failure. In these patients, combination therapy should be avoided or attempts should be made to correct the anemia. Hemolytic anemia caused by ribavirin also can be life threatening for patients with ischemic heart disease or cerebral vascular disease. It may also complicate the anemia seen in patients who are on chronic dialysis. Ribavirin is teratogenic, and female patients should avoid becoming pregnant during therapy.

Polyethylene glycol modified interferon or Pegylated IFN-alpha(2a) (PEG-IFN-alpha(2a) [40 kDa]; Pegasys, Hoffman-La Roche) is a new subcutaneous formulation of IFN-alpha(2a), produced by its attachment to a 40 kDa branched polyethylene glycol moiety by a stable amide bond. PEG-IFN-alpha(2a). When it is given as a once weekly 180-microgram dose, it has a markedly increased half life,

which translates into significantly improved efficacy and similar safety and tolerability compared with IFN-alpha in patients with chronic hepatitis C, even with underlying cirrhosis. The combination of PEG-IFN-alpha(2a) (40 kDa) plus ribavirin produces significantly better sustained virological responses than the combination of IFN-alpha(2b) and ribavirin, and it is accompanied by a similar or even lower incidence of adverse events and better quality of life, Hadziyannis SJ, Papatheodoridis GV, 2003). It is fast becoming the treatment of choice for chronic HCV infection.

Thus far, most treatment trials of hepatitis C have involved patients with abnormal ALT levels. It is estimated that a quarter of adults with chronic HCV infection have normal ALTs. This fraction is even higher in children Within this group about a quarter have normal or nonspecific changes in liver histology, and half have chronic persistent hepatitis. Less than a quarter have evidence of chronic active hepatitis or cirrhosis. Despite these relatively mild lesions, a consensus conference recommendation suggested that liver biopsy be done in those with persistently normal ALT levels. It has been estimated that fibrosis progression in this group is about half as rapid as that seen in patients with elevated ALT levels. Several trials of IFN-α in patients with normal ALT levels suggest that sustained virologic responses are comparable to those reported with treatment of patients with elevated ALT levels (i.e., 10% to 15%). Those who cleared virus were noted to develop elevated ALT levels during therapy, with almost half of all treated patients developing elevated ALT levels during or after IFN-α therapy. Whether this group of patients should be offered therapy is controversial and requires an evaluation of relative risk-benefit factors. Perhaps only those with chronic active disease are appropriate candidates.

Chronic Hepatitis D

Corticosteroid therapy has not been beneficial in treating chronic hepatitis D; it is not recommended. A controlled trial with IFN-α revealed transient improvement. Cessation of IFN therapy was followed by a return of viral replication and liver disease (Rizzetto et al., 1986). Another study revealed little impact of IFN therapy (Dalekos et al., 2000). However, it has been suggested that high-dose IFN-α (10 MU, three times weekly) may have efficacy, albeit with a sustained response seen in the minority of patients when treatment was given for 12 months or longer.

Fulminant Hepatitis

Sudden onset of mental confusion, emotional instability, restlessness, coma, and hemorrhagic manifestations in a patient with hepatitis requires prompt therapy. The rationale for the treatment is to combat the deleterious systemic effects of liver failure. The major objective of treatment of fulminant hepatitis is to reduce the load of nitrogenous products entering the portal circulation. Failure of the compromised liver to remove and detoxify these products is probably responsible for the cerebral dysfunction. The following measures are used: (1) restriction of protein intake, (2) removal of protein already in the gastrointestinal tract (use of a laxative and high-colonic irrigations), and (3) suppression of the bacterial population of the bowel (use of neomycin sulfate by mouth or nasogastric tube). The following therapeutic procedures of unproved benefit have been used: (1) corticosteroids; (2) exchange transfusion; (3) cross-perfusion with human, baboon, or pig liver; and (4) total body perfusion. Studies by the Acute Hepatic Failure Study Group (1977) failed to show any difference in survival rates between groups treated with hepatitis B immune serum globulin (HBIG) and those treated with standard immune globulin (IG). There have been isolated reports of dramatic improvement after liver transplantation.

PROGNOSIS

The prognosis of various types of viral hepatitis has been discussed in the sections of this chapter devoted to clinical manifestations and to course and complications. Hepatitis A is a relatively benign disease. Occasionally the illness may be prolonged, but eventually there is complete recovery with no evidence of chronic liver disease. Fatal fulminant hepatitis A may occur, but it is an extraordinarily rare phenomenon.

Most patients with hepatitis B recover completely. However, the risk of chronic infection is extremely variable; it may be low in young healthy adults (approximately 3%) or very high in infants born to HBsAg-and HBeAg-carrier mothers (60% to 90%). The overall risk is near 10%. Chronic hepatitis B infection may progress to cirrhosis of the liver and primary hepatocellular carcinoma. The risk of fatal ful-

minant hepatitis B is low (<2%), except when there is superinfection with HDV. Under these circumstances the mortality rate may be as high as 30% (Hadler et al., 1984).

Observations of patients with posttransfusion and community-acquired hepatitis C have revealed a relatively high incidence of chronic liver disease—approximately 50% (Alter, 1985; Sampliner et al., 1984). Fulminant hepatitis is an occasional outcome. The overall mortality rate is 1% to 2%. Studies in Japan have revealed that HCV infection is associated with the development of hepatocellular carcinoma (Saito et al., 1990). A more recent study (Seeff et al. 2000) suggests that chronic HCV infection may have a more benign course.

Hepatitis E is a relatively benign disease that does not progress to chronic hepatitis. However, it is a highly fatal disease in pregnant women (Kane et al., 1984).

EPIDEMIOLOGIC FACTORS
Hepatitis A

The geographic distribution of hepatitis A is worldwide. It is endemic in parts of the world such as the Mediterranean littoral and parts of Africa, South America, Central America, and the Far East, where its presence creates a danger to susceptible military and civilian persons working or traveling in such areas.

Although no age group is immune, the highest incidence in civilian populations occurs among persons less than 15 years of age. In military groups the youngest persons are the ones chiefly affected. Persons of either sex are equally susceptible to infection.

The well-defined autumn-winter seasonal incidence has changed; no consistent seasonal patterns have been observed. In general, at the present time the incidence of hepatitis is fairly constant throughout the year.

Abundant evidence favors transmission through intestinal-oral pathways. HAV is found in the stools of both naturally and experimentally infected persons. Various studies have revealed that HAV is detectable in blood and stools during the latter part of the incubation period. Viremia is no longer detectable after onset of jaundice when anti-HAV appears. Fecal shedding of HAV persists for approximately 1 week after onset of jaundice (Dienstag et al., 1975a; Krugman et al., 1962). These findings indicate that the infection is usually spread during the preicteric phase of the disease and that it is generally not communicable after the first week of jaundice.

Epidemics have long been known to occur in association with poor sanitation in military camps. Explosive water-, milk-, and food-borne epidemics have been reported. Ingestion of raw shellfish from polluted waters has caused many epidemics. For example, an epidemic of hepatitis A in Shanghai, China, in 1988 involved more than 300,000 persons who had eaten raw hairy clams. HAV was isolated from the gills and digestive tracts of the contaminated clams.

There is evidence also for human association as the principal mode of spread. HAV may be transmitted through the use of blood and blood products or contaminated needles, syringes, and stylets. However, this potential mode of transmission is very rare, chiefly because viremia is transient in hepatitis A infection, and a carrier state does not exist.

When hepatitis A occurs in certain situations—such as in households, day-care centers, orphanages, institutions for mentally handicapped children, military installations, and children's camps—it may smolder for months or years, or it may strike in explosive outbreaks. In families, secondary cases may occur in approximately 20 to 30 days.

Seroepidemiologic surveys by various investigators have provided valuable information about the distribution of anti-HAV in various population groups (Miller et al., 1975; Szmuness et al., 1976; Villarejos et al., 1976). The investigators observed a striking correlation between the presence of anti-HAV and socioeconomic status. Persons from lower socioeconomic groups were more likely to have detectable anti-HAV (past hepatitis A infection) than those from middle and upper socioeconomic groups. The detection of anti-HAV was strongly correlated with age. In New York City the prevalence increased gradually in adults, reaching peak levels in persons 50 years of age or older. In Costa Rica, however, peak levels were reached by 10 years of age. It is clear that the prevalence of anti-HAV (1) varies among different population groups, (2) increases with age, and (3) is independent of sex and race.

It is likely that the continued improvement of environmental and socioeconomic conditions will decrease the probability of exposure to hepatitis A, thereby changing a predominantly childhood infection to one that is more apt to occur in adults. This changing epidemiologic pattern was typical for poliomyelitis during the first half of the twentieth century in the United States. Poliomyelitis, like hepatitis A, is currently a more severe and more disabling disease in adults than in children.

Hepatitis B

Early epidemiologic theories indicated that HBV was transmitted exclusively by the parenteral route. It is now clear, however, that other modes of transmission play an important role in the dissemination of HBV. The experimental demonstration of oral transmission and the demonstration that contact-associated transmission is common have altered previous epidemiologic theories. The term *contact-associated hepatitis* denotes one or more of the following possible modes of transmission: (1) oral-oral, (2) sexual, (3) perinatal, and (4) intimate physical contact of any type. Hepatitis B antigen has been detected in saliva (Ward et al., 1972), in semen (Heathcote et al., 1974), and in many other body fluids.

The major reservoirs of HBV are healthy chronic carriers and patients with acute hepatitis. The infection is transmitted to susceptible persons by transfusion of blood, plasma, or other blood products or by the use of inadequately sterilized needles and syringes. Medical and paramedical personnel may be infected by accidental inoculation or ingestion of contaminated materials. Outbreaks have occurred among drug addicts using unsterilized equipment. Tattooing and acupuncture have been responsible for transmitting the infection. Patients and personnel in the following areas are at high risk: renal dialysis, intensive care, oncology units, and various laboratories in which potentially contaminated blood and tissues are examined.

Seroepidemiologic surveys to detect the presence of HBsAg and anti-HBs have confirmed the worldwide distribution of the disease. The antigen has been detected in all populations, even in those living in the most remote areas devoid of parenteral modes of transmission. The antigen is most prevalent among persons living under crowded conditions and with poor hygienic standards, thus accounting for the endemicity of the disease in institutions for mentally retarded persons and in certain developing countries of the world. The HBsAg carrier rate may range from 0.1% to more than 10%; it is dependent on such factors as geo-

TABLE 42-4	Prevalence of Antibody to Hepatitis B Surface Antigen (anti-HBs) in the Populations Surveyed for HAV Infections		
Country	*Number tested*	*Number anti-HBs–positive*	*Percent positive*
United States	1000	108	10.8
Switzerland	98	3	3.1
Belgium	133	7	5.3
Yugoslavia	97	33	34.0
Israel	112	17	15.2
Taiwan	123	96	78.0
Senegal	96	60	62.5

From Szmuness W, Dienstag JL, Purcell RH, et al: Am J Epidemiol 1977;106:392.

graphic location, age, and sex. The carrier rate is higher in tropical, underdeveloped areas than in temperate, developed countries; it is higher in urban communities than in rural communities and higher among males than among females. As indicated in Table 42-4, the prevalence of anti-HBs in various populations ranges from 3.1% in Switzerland to 78% in Taiwan.

The period of infectivity of patients with hepatitis B is dependent on the presence or absence of a carrier state. HBsAg is detectable in the blood during the latter part of the incubation period and for a variable period after onset of jaundice. Infectivity has also been associated with the presence of HBeAg and a high titer of HBsAg. For example, perinatal transmission of hepatitis B from HBsAg-positive mothers to their infants is highly likely if they are HBeAg positive. On the other hand, HBsAg-positive and anti-HBe–positive mothers are much less likely to transmit infection.

Hepatitis C

The availability of a specific serologic test to detect anti-HCV has clarified the epidemiology of parenterally transmitted and sporadic HCV infection. The distribution of the disease is worldwide, with an estimated 100 million HCV carriers. In the United States, hepatitis C may be the cause of 20% to 40% of all acute hepatitis cases. The largest group of HCV-infected adults has no known risk factor. Persons at high risk of contracting HCV infection include transfusion recipients, intravenous drug users, hemodialysis patients, and health-care workers with frequent blood contact. The risk of transmission from an individual needle stick incident from a known HCV-infected person is about 5% to 10% (Mitsui et al., 1992). Promiscuous homosexual and heterosexual

persons have a low risk of contracting HCV infection, which is not true for HBV. Perinatal transmission of HCV has been well documented and appears to occur at frequencies ranging from 5% to 10%. This rate may rise to levels in excess of 25% in children born to mothers who are HIV infected and may approach 50% if the child also acquires HIV (Papaevangelou et al 1998.).

Hepatitis D

The epidemiology of hepatitis D is characterized by striking similarities to and certain differences from hepatitis B (Table 42-2). The modes of transmission are the same, except that HDV perinatal infection is rare. In general, the prevalence of HDV correlates with the prevalence of HBV in the following high-risk groups: intravenous drug users, persons with hemophilia, and institutionalized mentally retarded patients. In contrast, HDV has not been reported as prevalent in the following HBV high-risk groups: homosexual men and chronic carriers in highly endemic areas such as Southeast Asia, Southern Africa, and Alaska.

Superinfection of chronic HBV carriers has been responsible for epidemics of HDV-associated fulminant hepatitis in Venezuela, Colombia, and Brazil (Buitrago et al., 1986; Hadler et al., 1984). In the United States and in Northern Europe, HDV is most common in drug abusers.

Hepatitis E

The epidemiology of hepatitis E is characterized by certain similarities to and many differences from hepatitis A (Table 42-2). Both hepatitis E and hepatitis A are enterically transmitted diseases that are spread through the fecal-oral route.

Hepatitis A is worldwide in distribution; it is predominantly an infection of children, and the secondary attack rate in household contacts is in excess of 20%. In contrast, hepatitis E has occurred predominantly in certain developing areas of the world during the course of water-borne outbreaks. Hepatitis E is most common in adults but rare in children, and the secondary attack rate in household contacts has been relatively low: less than 3% (Kane et al., 1984).

Hepatitis E epidemics have occurred in China, Southeast and Central Asia, Northern and Western Africa, Mexico, and Central America with periodicity of 5 to 10 years. The epidemics have either been extensive, involving thousands of persons, or smaller focal outbreaks. In endemic areas, HEV accounts for over 50% of acute sporadic hepatitis in adults and children. Seroprevalence studies performed on blood donors from nonendemic countries have found evidence of infection in 1% to 5%. With the exception of a few imported cases, hepatitis E has not occurred in the United States (DeCock et al., 1987). Hepatitis E, unlike hepatitis A, is a highly fatal disease in infected pregnant women, in whom the mortality rate may be 10% to 20%. Few studies have evaluated the efficacy of preexposure and postexposure prophylaxis with immune globulin for the prevention of HEV infection. In studies that compared disease rates of those who received immunoglobulin prepared from individuals (presumably hyperimmune) in endemic areas, no statistical differences were seen when compared with those who received no immunoglobulin.

A detailed discussion of recommendations for prevention of viral hepatitis follows. These recommendations of the Advisory Committee on Immunization Practices (ACIP) were reported in the February 9, 1990 issue of the Public Health Service, Centers for Disease Control Morbidity and Mortality Weekly Report.

IMMUNE GLOBULINS*

Immune globulins are important tools for preventing infection and disease before or after exposure to hepatitis viruses. Immune globulins used in medical practice are sterile solutions of antibodies (immunoglobulins) from human plasma. They are prepared by cold ethanol fractionation of large plasma pools and contain 10% to 18% protein. In the United States, plasma is primarily

obtained from paid donors. Only plasma shown to be free of hepatitis B surface antigen (HBsAg) and antibody to human immunodeficiency virus (HIV) is used to prepare immune globulins.

Immune globulin (IG) (formerly called immune serum globulin, ISG, or gamma globulin) produced in the United States contains antibodies against the hepatitis A virus (anti-HAV) and the HBsAg (anti-HBs). Hepatitis B immune globulin (HBIG) is an IG prepared from plasma containing high titers of anti-HBs.

There is no evidence that hepatitis B virus (HBV), HIV (the causative agent of acquired immunodeficiency syndrome [AIDS]), or other viruses have ever been transmitted by IG or HBIG commercially available in the United States. Since late April 1985 all plasma units for preparation of IGs have been screened for antibody to HIV, and reactive units are discarded. No instances of HIV infection or clinical illness have occurred that can be attributed to receiving IG or HBIG, including lots prepared before April 1985. Laboratory studies have shown that the margin of safety based on the removal of HIV infectivity by the fractionation process is extremely high. Some HBIG lots prepared before April 1985 have detectable HIV antibody. Shortly after being given HBIG, recipients have occasionally been noted to have low levels of passively acquired HIV antibody, but this reactivity does not persist.

Serious adverse effects from IGs administered as recommended have been rare. IGs prepared for intramuscular administration should be used for hepatitis prophylaxis. IGs prepared for intravenous administration to immunodeficient and other selected patients are not intended for hepatitis prophylaxis. IG and HBIG are not contraindicated for pregnant or lactating women.

Preparations of intravenous gamma globulin (IVIG) have been associated with the transmission of HCV (Bjoro et al., 1994). Manufacturers of IVIG and other blood-derived products are currently modifying production routines and screening lots by PCR for HCV RNA to virtually eliminate future HCV transmissions by this route.

HEPATITIS A
Preexposure Prophylaxis*

The major group for whom preexposure prophylaxis is recommended is international travelers. The risk of hepatitis A for

*Abstracted from MMWR 1989:38:388-392. 397-400.

U.S. citizens traveling abroad varies with living conditions, length of stay, and the incidence of hepatitis A infection in areas visited. In general, travelers to developed areas of North America, western Europe, Japan, Australia, and New Zealand are at no greater risk of infection than they would be in the United States. For travelers to developing countries, risk of infection increases with duration of travel and is highest for those who live in or visit rural areas, trek in back country, or frequently eat or drink in settings of poor sanitation. Nevertheless, recent studies have shown that many cases of travel-related hepatitis A occur in travelers with "standard" tourist itineraries, accommodations, and food and beverage consumption behaviors. In developing countries, travelers should minimize their exposure to hepatitis A and other enteric diseases by avoiding potentially contaminated water or food. Travelers should avoid drinking water (or beverages with ice) of unknown purity and eating uncooked shellfish or uncooked fruits or vegetables that they did not prepare.

Hepatitis A vaccines were licensed for use in 1993 and are currently the agent of choice for prophylaxis. Persons should be vaccinated before departure. Both Havrix (GlaxoSmithKline, Research Triangle Park, North Carolina) and Vaqta (Merck and Company, Whitehouse Station, New Jersey) manufacture licensed vaccines in the United States. Havrix can be given to children 2 to 18 years of age in doses of 720 ELISA units (0.5 ml) and 360 ELISA units (0.5 ml). Vaqta dose is 25 units (0.5 ml). Both vaccines, comparable in immunogenicity, have been used to prevent infection and control outbreaks by eliciting antibody levels in excess of that achieved by passive IG therapy, but these levels are 10 to 100 times less than what is seen after natural infection. The level of protection is close to 90% by 2 weeks, >95% one month after the first vaccination, and virtually 100% after a second dose. One approved schedule gives 320 ELISA unit doses at 0, 1, and 6 months. Other studies suggest that a 2-dose schedule of 0 and 6 months using a 720–ELISA unit dose achieves comparable titers. The duration of protection may exceed 7 years after only one dose and 11 years after receiving a booster dose. Models of antibody decline suggest that protection may actually exceed 20 years. A study of vaccination of children as young as 5

months of age showed that immunogenicity was excellent when the mothers were anti-HAV negative, but titers only a tenth as good were seen when the children were born to anti-HAV–positive mothers, suggesting some interference by antibody. In spite of this, hepatitis A vaccine may be given concomitantly with serum IG. One study in adults found that the geometric mean titer of antibody at 8, 12, and 24 weeks in such vaccinees is lower than a group that received vaccine alone (but higher than a group that received only globulin). The overall seropositivity at 24 weeks was also lower (92% vs 97%). However, after a second vaccination at 24 weeks, these differences were no longer seen. Immunocompromised individuals may have less than optimal responses, but that should not preclude vaccination when there is a risk for infection.

Those allergic to a vaccine component in both vaccines should receive IG, which is 80% to 90% effective in preventing clinical hepatitis A and is recommended as preexposure prophylaxis for all susceptible travelers, who have no access to the vaccine, going to developing countries. For travelers a single dose of IG of 0.02 ml/kg of body weight is recommended if travel is for less than 3 months. For those who anticipate a longer stay, 0.06 ml/kg should be used every 5 months.

Postexposure Prophylaxis

Hepatitis A cannot be reliably diagnosed on clinical presentation alone, and serologic confirmation of index patients is recommended before contacts are treated. Serologic screening of contacts for anti-HAV before they are given IG is not recommended because screening is more costly than IG and would delay its administration. For postexposure IG prophylaxis a single intramuscular dose of 0.02 ml/kg is recommended. IG should be given as soon as possible after last exposure; giving IG more than 2 weeks after exposure is not indicated.

Specific recommendations for IG prophylaxis for hepatitis A depend on the nature of the HAV exposure. Candidates for prophylaxis include the following individuals:

1. All household and sexual contacts of persons with hepatitis A.
2. All staff and attendees of day-care centers or homes if (a) one or more children or employees are diagnosed as having hepatitis A, or (b) cases are recognized in two or more households of center attendees.

3. Persons who have close contact with a school- or classroom-centered outbreak.
4. Residents and staff in some institutions, such as prisons and facilities for the developmentally disabled, who have close contact with patients with hepatitis A.
5. Persons exposed to feces of infected patients usually in association with an unsuspected index patient who is fecally incontinent.

IG use might be effective in preventing food-borne or water-borne hepatitis A if exposure is recognized in time. However, IG is not recommended for persons exposed to a common source of hepatitis infection after cases have begun to occur, because the 2-week period during which IG is effective will have been exceeded. If a food handler is diagnosed as having hepatitis A, common-source transmission is possible but uncommon. IG should be administered to other food handlers but is usually not recommended for patrons. However, IG administration to patrons may be considered if all of the following conditions exist: (1) the infected person is directly involved in handling, without gloves, foods that will not be cooked before they are eaten; (2) the hygienic practices of the food handler are deficient, or the food handler has had diarrhea; and (3) patrons can be identified and treated within 2 weeks of exposure. Situations in which repeated exposures may have occurred, such as in institutional cafeterias, may warrant stronger consideration of IG use.

HEPATITIS B
Hepatitis B Prevention Strategies in the United States

The incidence of reported acute hepatitis B cases increased steadily and reached a peak in 1985 (11.50 cases/105/year), despite the introduction of hepatitis B vaccine 3 years previously. Incidence decreased modestly (18%) by 1988 but still remained higher than a decade earlier. This minimal impact of hepatitis B vaccine on disease incidence is attributable to several factors. The sources of infection for most cases include intravenous drug abuse (28%), heterosexual contact with infected persons or multiple partners (22%), and homosexual activity (9%). In addition, 30% of patients with hepatitis B deny any of the recognized risk factors for infection. Finally, adults are not the best vaccination candidates.

The present strategy for hepatitis B prevention is to vaccinate all babies, as well as those individuals at high risk of infection. Most persons receiving vaccine as a result of this strategy are persons at risk of acquiring HBV infection through occupational exposure, a group that accounts for approximately 4% of cases. The major deterrents to vaccinating the other high-risk groups include the lack of knowledge about the risk of disease and its consequences, the lack of public-sector programs, the cost of vaccine, and the inability to access most of the high-risk populations.

For vaccine to have an impact on the incidence of hepatitis B, a comprehensive strategy must be developed that will provide hepatitis B vaccination to persons before they engage in behaviors or occupations that place them at risk of infection. Universal HBsAg screening of pregnant women was recently recommended to prevent perinatal HBV transmission. The previous recommendations for selective screening failed to identify most HBsAg-positive pregnant women. Universal immunization of neonates and adolescents would be expected to successfully prevent infection before these individuals entered into a high-risk group. Immunization between infancy and adolescence is suggested only for those children who were not immunized as infants, particularly in those who are in groups where person-to-person transmission has been documented to be significant. This group includes Alaskan natives, Pacific Islanders, and children of immigrants from countries that experience high rates of HBV infection. Some schools are requiring proof of vaccination for those entering 7th grade.

Hepatitis B Prophylaxis

Three types of products are available for prophylaxis against hepatitis B. Hepatitis B vaccines, first licensed in 1981, provide active immunization against HBV infection, and their use is recommended for both preexposure and postexposure prophylaxis. HBIG provides temporary, passive protection and is indicated only in certain postexposure settings. Lamivudine has been used to prevent reactivation of HBV in patients who are undergoing immunosuppression.

HBIG

HBIG is prepared from plasma preselected to contain a high titer of anti-HBs. In the United

States, HBIG has an anti-HBs titer of >100,000 by RIA. Human plasma from which HBIG is prepared is screened for antibodies to HIV; in addition, the Cohn fractionation process used to prepare this product inactivates and eliminates HIV from the final product. There is no evidence that the causative agent of AIDS (HIV) has been transmitted by HBIG.

Hepatitis B Vaccine

Two types of hepatitis B vaccines are currently licensed in the United States. Plasma-derived vaccine consists of a suspension of inactivated, alum-adsorbed, 22-nm HBsAg particles that have been purified from human plasma by a combination of biophysical (ultracentrifugation) and biochemical procedures. Inactivation is a threefold process using 8 M urea; pepsin at pH 2; and 1:4,000 formalin. These treatment steps have been shown to inactivate representatives of all classes of viruses found in human blood, including HIV. Plasma-derived vaccine is no longer being produced in the United States, and use is now limited to hemodialysis patients, other immunocompromised hosts, and persons with known allergy to yeast.

Currently licensed recombinant hepatitis B vaccines are produced by *Saccharomyces cerevisiae* (common baker's yeast), into which a plasmid containing the gene for the HBsAg has been inserted. Purified HBsAg is obtained by lysing the yeast cells and separating HBsAg from yeast components by biochemical and biophysical techniques. These vaccines contain more than 95% HBsAg protein. Yeast-derived protein constitutes no more than 5% of the final product.

The recommended series of three intramuscular doses of hepatitis B vaccine induces an adequate antibody response in >90% of healthy adults and in >95% of infants, children, and adolescents from birth through 19 years of age. The deltoid (arm) is the recommended site for hepatitis B vaccination of adults and children; immunogenicity of vaccine for adults is substantially lower when injections are given in the buttock. Larger vaccine doses (2 or 4 times normal adult dose) or an increased number of doses (4 doses) are required to induce protective antibody in a high proportion of hemodialysis patients and may also be necessary for other immunocompromised persons (such as those on immunosuppressive drugs or with HIV infection). An adequate antibody response is 10 milli-International Units (mIU)/ml, approxi-

mately equivalent to 10 sample ratio units (SRU) by RIA or positive by EIA, measured 1 to 6 months after completion of the vaccine series.

Field trials of the vaccines licensed in the United States have shown 80% to 95% efficacy in preventing infection or clinical hepatitis among susceptible persons. Protection against illness is virtually complete for persons who develop an adequate antibody response after vaccination. The duration of protection and need for booster doses are not yet fully defined. Between 30% and 50% of persons who develop adequate antibody after three doses of vaccine will lose detectable antibody within 7 years, but protection against viremic infection and clinical disease appears to persist. Immunogenicity and efficacy of the licensed vaccines for hemodialysis patients are much lower than in normal adults. Protection in this group may last only as long as adequate antibody levels persist.

Vaccine Use

Primary vaccination is composed of three intramuscular doses of vaccine, with the second and third doses given 1 and 6 months after the first. Adults and older children should be given a full 1.0-ml dose, whereas children <11 years of age should usually receive half (0.5 ml) this dose. A two-dose regimen has been approved for adolescents and adults. In 2001, the FDA licensed a combined hepatitis b (containing 20 mcg of HbSAg) and hepatitis a (containing 720 ELISA units) vaccine called Twinrix (GlaxoSmithKline Biologics, Rixensart, Belgium) for those over 18 years of age in a schedule of 0, 1, and 6 months. This formulation is attractive for those at high risk for both (e.g., IV drug users) and to those at high risk for liver failure (e.g., transplant recipients). See Table 42-5 for complete information on age-specific dosages of currently available vaccines. An alternative schedule of four doses of vaccine given at 0, 1, 2, and 12 months has been approved for one vaccine for postexposure prophylaxis or for more rapid induction of immunity. However, there is no clear evidence that this regimen provides greater protection than the standard three-dose series. Hepatitis B vaccine should be given only in the deltoid muscle for adults and children or in the anterolateral thigh muscle for infants and neonates. Studies of neonatal vaccinees demonstrate that immunity lasts at least 8 years. Of those immunized at a later date, 13% to 60% may demonstrate a loss of detectable antibody,

TABLE 42-5	Recommended Doses and Schedules of Currently Licensed Hepatitis B Vaccines					
	VACCINE					
	HEPTAVAX-B*,†		RECOMBIVAX HB*		ENGERIX-B*,‡	
Group	Dose (µg)	(ml)	Dose (µg)	(ml)	Dose (µg)	(ml)
Infants of HBV-carrier mothers	10	(0.5)	5	(0.5)	10	(0.5)
Other infants and children <11 years old	10	(0.5)	2.5	(0.25)	10	(0.5)
Children and adolescents 11-19 years old	20	(1.0)	5	(0.5)	20	(1.0)
Adults >19 years old***	20	(1.0)	10	(1.0)	20	(1.0)
Dialysis patients and other immunocompromised persons	40	(2.0)§	40	(1.0)‖	40	(2.0)§,¶

*Usual schedule: three doses at 0, 1, 6 months.
†Available only for hemodialysis and other immunocompromised patients and for persons with known allergy to yeast.
‡Alternative schedule: four doses at 0, 1, 2, 12 months.
§Two 1.0-ml doses given at different sites.
‖Special formulation for dialysis patients.
¶Four-dose schedule recommended at 0, 1, 2, 6 months.
***A combined hepatitis b/hepatitis a vaccine was licensed in 2001 for those older than 18 years.

but immunologic memory (as detected by response to a booster) appears to be present at least 12 years after primary vaccination.

A study in premature children demonstrated that when vaccination was initiated at 1 week of age, antibody responses in excess of 100 mIU were achieved after three immunizations in 90% of those with birth weight >1,500 g but in 70% of those who were lighter (Losonsky et al., 1999). It is advised that premature infants receive a fourth immunization. Another alternative is to delay vaccination in premature infants born to HBsAg negative mothers until they achieve a weight of 2,000 g or greater.

For patients undergoing hemodialysis and for other immunosuppressed patients, higher-vaccine doses or increased numbers of doses are required. A special formulation of one vaccine is available for such persons (Table 42-5). Persons with HIV infection have an impaired response to hepatitis B vaccine. The immunogenicity of higher doses of vaccine is unknown for this group, and firm recommendations on dosage cannot be made at this time.

Vaccine doses administered at longer intervals provide equally satisfactory protection, but optimal protection is not conferred until after the third dose. If the vaccine series is interrupted after the first dose, administration of the second and third doses should be separated by an interval of 3 to 5 months. Persons who are late for the third dose should be given this dose when convenient. Postvaccination testing is not considered necessary in either situation.

In one study the response to vaccination by the standard schedule using one or two doses of one vaccine, followed by the remaining doses of a different vaccine, was comparable to the response to vaccination with a single vaccine. Moreover, because the immunogenicities of the available vaccines are similar, it is likely that responses in such situations will be comparable to those induced by any of the vaccines alone.

The immunogenicity of a series of three low doses (0.1 standard dose) of plasma-derived hepatitis B vaccine administered by the intradermal route has been assessed in several studies. The largest studies of adults show lower rates of developing adequate antibody (80% to 90%) and twofold to fourfold lower antibody titers than with intramuscular vaccination with recommended doses. Nonresponders to three doses of the vaccine may respond when one to three additional doses are given. However, this strategy will continue to fail in about half of the individuals, probably based on HLA-defined inability to present the surface antigen to their T cells. Because these individuals may still respond to core antigens, efforts are in place to develop such vaccines.

Data on immunogenicity of low doses of recombinant vaccines given intradermally are limited. The principal advantages are the lower cost of vaccination with lower concentrations of vaccine antigen, which is a factor in some countries, and the possible enhanced immunogenicity in dialysis patients when it is given repeatedly for many doses. At this time, intradermal vaccination of adults using low doses of vaccine should be done only under research protocol, with appropriate informed consent and with postvaccination testing to identify persons with inadequate response who would be eligible for revaccination. Intradermal vaccination is not recommended for infants or children.

All hepatitis B vaccines are noninfective products, and there is no evidence of interference with other simultaneously administered vaccines.

Data are not available on the safety of hepatitis B vaccines for the developing fetus. Because the vaccines contain only noninfectious HBsAg particles, there should be no risk to the fetus. In contrast, HBV infection of a pregnant woman may result in severe disease for the mother and chronic infection of the newborn. Therefore pregnancy or lactation should not be considered a contraindication to the use of this vaccine for persons who are otherwise eligible.

Vaccine Storage and Shipment

Vaccine should be shipped and stored at 2° C to 8° C but not frozen. Freezing destroys the potency of the vaccine.

Side Effects and Adverse Reactions

The most common side effect observed following vaccination with each of the available vaccines has been soreness at the injection site. Postvaccination surveillance for 3 years after licensure of the plasma-derived vaccine showed an association of borderline significance between Guillain-Barré syndrome and receipt of the first vaccine dose. The rate of this occurrence was very low (0.5 per 100,000 vaccinees) and was more than compensated for by disease prevented by the vaccine, even if Guillain-Barré syndrome is a true side effect. Such postvaccination surveillance information is not available for the recombinant hepatitis B vaccines. Early concerns about safety of plasma-derived vaccine have proven to be unfounded, particularly the concern that infectious agents such as HIV present in the donor plasma pools might contaminate the final product.

Effect of Vaccination on Carriers and Immune Persons

Hepatitis B vaccine produces neither therapeutic nor adverse effects for HBV carriers. Vaccination of individuals who possess antibodies against HBV from a previous infection is not necessary, but it will not cause adverse effects. Such individuals will have a postvaccination increase in their anti-HBs levels. Passively acquired antibody, whether acquired from HBIG or IG administration or from the transplacental route, will not interfere with active immunization.

Prevaccination serologic testing for susceptibility. The decision to test potential vaccine recipients for prior infection rests primarily on cost-effectiveness and should be based on whether the costs of testing balance the costs of vaccine saved by not vaccinating individuals who have already been infected. Estimation of cost-effectiveness of testing depends on three variables: the cost of vaccination, the cost of testing for susceptibility, and the expected prevalence of immune individuals in the group. Testing in groups with the highest risk of HBV infection (HBV marker prevalence of >20%) is usually cost-effective unless testing costs are extremely high. Cost-effectiveness of screening may be marginal for groups at intermediate risk. For groups with a low expected prevalence of HBV serologic markers, such as health professionals in their training years, prevaccination testing is not cost-effective. For routine testing, only one antibody test is necessary (either anti-HBc or anti-HBs). Anti-HBc identifies all previously infected persons, both carriers and noncarriers, but does not differentiate members of the two groups. Anti-HBs identifies persons previously infected, except for carriers. Neither test has a particular advantage for groups expected to have carrier rates of <2%, such as health-care workers. Anti-HBc may be preferred to avoid unnecessary vaccination of carriers for groups with higher carrier rates. If RIA is used to test for anti-HBs, a minimum of 10 sample ratio units should be used to designate immunity (2.1 is the usual designation of a positive test). If EIA is used, the positive level recommended by manufacturers is appropriate.

Postvaccination testing for serologic response and revaccination of nonresponders. Hepatitis B vaccine, when given in the deltoid, produces protective antibody (anti-HBs) in >90% of healthy persons. Testing for immunity after vaccination is not recommended routinely but is advised for persons whose subsequent management depends on knowing their immune status (such as dialysis patients and staff). Testing for immunity is also advised for persons for whom a suboptimal response may be anticipated, such as those who have received vaccine in the buttock, persons >50 years of age, and persons known to have HIV infection. Postvaccination testing should also be considered for persons at occupational risk who may have needle-stick exposures necessitating postexposure prophylaxis. When necessary, postvaccination testing should be done between 1 and 6 months after completion of the vaccine series to provide definitive information on response to the vaccine.

Revaccination of persons who do not respond to the primary series (nonresponders) produces adequate antibody in 15% to 25% after one additional dose and in 30% to 50% after three additional doses when the primary vaccination has been given in the deltoid. Some individuals appear to be nonresponders by virtue of their HLA-DR type (Hsu et al., 1993; Watanabe et al., 1988). Such individuals are not likely to respond when vaccinated with the same antigen. In the future, immunization with a DNA-based vaccine may prove useful in this situation, since studies performed in nonresponder mice suggest that such an approach may extend the spectrum of immunogenic epitopes (Schirmbeck et al., 1995).

For persons who do not respond to a primary vaccine series given in the buttock, data suggest that revaccination in the arm induces adequate antibody in >75%. Revaccination with one or more additional doses should be considered for persons who fail to respond to vaccination in the deltoid and is recommended for those who have failed to respond to vaccination in the buttock.

Need for Vaccine Booster Doses

Available data show that vaccine-induced antibody levels decline steadily with time and that up to 50% of adult vaccinees who respond adequately to vaccine may have low or undetectable antibody levels by 7 years after vaccination. Nevertheless, both adults and children with declining antibody levels are still protected against hepatitis B disease. Current data also suggest excellent protection against disease for 5 years after vaccination among infants born to hepatitis B–carrier mothers. For adults and children with normal immune status, booster doses are not routinely recommended within 7 years after vaccination, nor is routine serologic testing to assess antibody

levels necessary for vaccine recipients during this period. For infants born to hepatitis B–carrier mothers, booster doses are not necessary within 5 years after vaccination. The possible need for booster doses after longer intervals will be assessed as additional information becomes available.

For hemodialysis patients, for whom vaccine-induced protection is less complete and may persist only as long as antibody levels remain above 10 mIU/ml, the need for booster doses should be assessed by annual antibody testing, and booster doses should be given when antibody levels decline to <10 mIU/ml.

Groups Recommended for Preexposure Vaccination

Persons at substantial risk of HBV infection who are demonstrated or judged likely to be susceptible should be vaccinated. They include the following:

1. Persons with occupational risk (e.g., healthcare and public-safety workers)
2. Clients and staff of institutions for the developmentally disabled
3. Staff of nonresidential day-care programs (e.g., schools, sheltered workshops for the developmentally disabled) attended by known HBV carriers
4. Susceptible hemodialysis patients
5. Sexually active homosexual men
6. Users of illicit injectable drugs who are susceptible to HBV
7. Household and sexual contacts of HBV carriers
8. Families accepting orphans or unaccompanied minors from countries of high or intermediate HBV endemicity who prove to be chronic carriers
9. Populations with high endemicity of HBV infection (e.g., Alaskan natives, Pacific Islanders, and refugees from HBV-endemic areas)
10. Inmates (and possibly workers) in long-term correctional facilities
11. Sexually active heterosexual persons with multiple sexual partners
12. Persons who plan to reside for more than 6 months in areas with high levels of endemic HBV and who will have close contact with the local population

Ideally, hepatitis B vaccination of travelers should begin at least 6 months before travel to allow for completion of the full vaccine series.

Nevertheless, a partial series will offer some protection from HBV infection. The alternative four-dose schedule may provide better protection during travel if the first three doses can be delivered before travel (second and third doses given 1 and 2 months, respectively, after the first).

Postexposure Prophylaxis for Hepatitis B

Prophylactic treatment to prevent hepatitis B infection after exposure to HBV should be considered in the following situations: perinatal exposure of an infant born to an HBsAg-positive mother, accidental percutaneous or permucosal exposure to HBsAg-positive blood, sexual exposure to an HBsAg-positive person, and household exposure of an infant <12 months of age to a primary caregiver who has acute hepatitis B.

Various studies have established the relative efficacies of HBIG and hepatitis B vaccine in different exposure situations. For an infant with perinatal exposure to an HBsAg-positive and HBeAg-positive mother, a regimen combining one dose of HBIG at birth with the hepatitis B vaccine series started soon after birth is 85% to 95% effective in preventing development of the HBV carrier state. Regimens involving either multiple doses of HBIG alone or the vaccine series alone have 70% to 85% efficacy.

The risk of HBV infection is primarily related to the degree of contact with blood and to the HBeAg status of the source person. The risk of developing clinical hepatitis if the blood is both HBsAg positive and HBeAg positive is 22% to 31%; the risk of developing serologic evidence of HBV infection is 37% to 62%. By comparison, the risk of developing clinical hepatitis from a needle contaminated with HBsAg-positive, HBeAg-negative blood is 1% to 6%, and the risk of developing serologic evidence of HBV infection, 23% to 37% (Werner and Grady, 1982).

For accidental percutaneous exposure only regimens including HBIG or IG have been studied. Ideally, regimens including either agent should be applied within 24 hours of exposure. The efficacy of HBIG when given >7 days post exposure is unknown. A regimen of two doses of HBIG—one given after exposure and the second given 1 month later—is about 75% effective in preventing hepatitis B in this setting. For sexual exposure a single dose of HBIG is 75% effective if given within 2 weeks of last sexual exposure. The efficacy of IG for postexposure prophylaxis is uncertain. Because of the avail-

ability of HBIG and the wider use of hepatitis B vaccine, IG no longer has a role in postexposure prophylaxis of hepatitis B.

Recommendations on postexposure prophylaxis are based on available efficacy data and on the likelihood of future HBV exposure of the person requiring treatment. In all exposures a regimen combining HBIG with hepatitis B vaccine will provide both short- and long-term protection, will be less costly than the two-dose HBIG treatment alone, and is the treatment of choice.

Perinatal Exposure and Recommendations

Transmission of HBV from mother to infant during the perinatal period represents one of the most efficient modes of HBV infection and often leads to severe long-term sequelae. Infants born to HBsAg-positive and HBeAg-positive mothers have a 70% to 90% chance of acquiring perinatal HBV infection, and 85% to 90% of infected infants will become chronic HBV carriers. Estimates are that >25% of these carriers will die from PHC or cirrhosis of the liver. Infants born to HBsAg-positive and HBeAg-negative mothers have a lower risk of acquiring perinatal infection; however, such infants have had acute disease, and fatal fulminant hepatitis has been reported Prenatal screening of all pregnant women identifies those who are HBsAg positive and allows treatment of their newborns with HBIG and hepatitis B vaccine, a regimen that is 85% to 95% effective in preventing the development of the HBV chronic carrier state.

On February 26, 1991 the ACIP recommended that universal vaccination of infants be incorporated in the routine immunization schedule for infants and children in the United States. The two options proposed by the ACIP committee and the Committee on Infectious Diseases of the American Academy of Pediatrics are as follows:

Option 1. First dose at birth, second dose at 1 to 2 months, and third dose at 6 to 18 months.

Option 2. First dose at 1 to 2 months, second dose at 4 months, and third dose at 6 to 18 months.

The optimal time for immunization of preterm infants has not been determined, but it is suggested that immunization be delayed until the child has achieved a weight of 2 kg or until 2 months of age, when other immunizations are offered.

The ACIP recommendations describing a comprehensive strategy for eliminating transmission of HBV in the United States through universal childhood vaccination are given in the following Morbidity and Mortality Weekly Report from the Centers for Disease Control (1991).

Postexposure Prophylaxis for HCV

The ACIP has offered the following recommendations: "Recent studies indicate that IG does not protect against infection with HCV. Thus, available data do not support the use of IG for prophylaxis of HCV."

Preexposure Prophylaxis of HDV

Prevention of HDV currently depends on preventing chronic HBV infection, as HDV requires HBV for its replication. No products exist that can prevent HDV infection in HBV chronic carriers.

Preexposure Prophylaxis of HEV

No products are available to prevent HEV. IG prepared from plasma of individuals residing in non–HEV-endemic areas is not effective. The efficacy of an IG prepared from plasma of individuals in an endemic area is unclear.

BIBLIOGRAPHY

Acute Hepatic Failure Study Group. Failure of specific immunotherapy in fulminant type B hepatitis. Ann Intern Med 1977;86:272.

Alpert E, Isselbacher KJ, Schur PH. The pathogenesis of arthritis associated with viral hepatitis. N Engl J Med 1971;285:185.

Alter HJ. The infectivity of the healthy hepatitis B surface antigen carrier. In Bianchi L, Gerok W, Sickinger K, Stalder GA (eds). Virus and the Liver. Lancaster, England: MTP Press, 1980.

Alter HJ. Posttransfusion hepatitis: clinical features, risk, and donor testing. In Dodd RY, Barker LF (eds). Infection, Immunity, and Blood Transfusion. New York: Alan R Liss, 1985.

Alter HJ, Purcell RH, Shih JW, et al. Detection of antibody to hepatitis C virus in prospectively followed transfusion recipients with acute and chronic non-A, non-B hepatitis. N Engl J Med 1989;321:1494-1500.

Alter MJ, Margolis H, Krawczynski K, et al. The natural history of community-acquired hepatitis C in the United States. N Engl J Med 1992;327:1899-1905.

Andreone P, Caraceni P, Grazi GL, et al. Lamivudine treatment for acute hepatitis B after liver transplantation. J Hepatol 1998;29:985-989.

Bacon PA, Doherty SM, Zuckerman AJ. Hepatitis B antibody in polymyalgia rheumatics. Lancet 1975;2:476.

Bahn A, Hilbert K, Matine U, et al. Selection of a precore mutant after vertical transmission of different hepatitis B virus mutants is correlated with fulminant hepatitis in infants. J Med Virol 1995;47:336-341.

Balayan MS, Anlzhaparidze AG, Savinskaya SS, et al. Evidence for a virus in non-A, non-B hepatitis transmitted via the fecal-oral route. Intervirology 1981;20:23.

Barker LF, Chisari FV, McGrath PP, et al. Transmission of type B viral hepatitis to chimpanzees. J Infect Dis 1973;127:648.

Baroudy BM, Ticehurse JR, Miele TA, et al. Sequence analysis of hepatitis A virus cDNA coding for capsed proteins and RNA polymerase. Proc Natl Acad Sci USA 1985;82:2143-2147.

Bayer ME, Blumberg BS, Werner B. Particles associated with Australia antigen in the sera of patients with leukemia, Down's syndrome, and hepatitis. Nature 1968;218:1057.

Beasley RP, Hwang L-Y, Lin C-C, et al. Incidence of hepatitis among students at a university in Taiwan. Am J Epidemiol 1983;117:213-222.

Bjoro K, Froland S, Yun Z, et al. Hepatitis C infection in patients with primary hypogammaglobinemia after treatment with contaminated immunoglobulin. N Engl J Med 1994;331:1607-1611.

Blumberg BS, Alter HJ, Visnich S. A "new" antigen in leukemia sera. JAMA 1965;191:541.

Boyer JL, Klatskin G. Pattern of necrosis in acute viral hepatitis: prognostic value of bridging (subacute hepatic necrosis). N Engl J Med 1970;283:1063.

Bradley DW, Krawczynski K, Cook EH, et al. Enterically transmitted non-A, non-B hepatitis: serial passage of disease in cynomologous macaques and tamarins and recovery of disease-associated 27-34 nm viruslike particles. Proc Natl Acad Sci USA 1987;84:6277-6281.

Brzosko WJ, Krawczynski K, Nazarewicz T, et al. Glomerulonephritis associated with hepatitis B surface antigen immune complexes in children. Lancet 1974;2:477.

Buitrago B, Popper H, Hadler SC, et al. Specific histologic features of Santa Marta hepatitis: a severe form of hepatitis D virus infection in northern South America. Hepatology 1986;6:1285-1291.

Centers for Disease Control. Protection against viral hepatitis. MMWR Morb Mortal Wkly Rep 1990;39:1-26.

Centers for Disease Control. Hepatitis B virus: a comprehensive strategy for eliminating transmission in the United States through universal childhood vaccination. MMWR Recomm Rep 1991;40:1-25.

Chalmers TG, et al. Treatment of acute infectious hepatitis. Controlled studies of the effects of diet, rest, and physical reconditioning on the acute course of the disease and on the incidence of relapses and residual abnormalities. J Clin Invest 1955;34:1163.

Chau KH, Hargie MP, Decker RH, et al. Serodiagnosis of recent hepatitis B infection by IgM class anti-HBc. Hepatology 1983;3:141.

Choo QL, Kuo G, Weiner AJ, et al. Isolation of a cDNA derived from blood-borne non-A, non-B viral hepatitis genome. Science 1989;244:359-361.

Christensson B, Wiebe T, Akesson A, Widell A. Interferon-alpha and ribavirin treatment of hepatitis C in children with malignancy in remission. Clin Infect Dis 2000;30:585-586.

Combes B, Shorey J, Barrera et al. Glomerulonephritis with deposition of Australia antigen-antibody complexes in glomerular basement membrane. Lancet 1971;2:234.

Daemer RJ, Feinstone SM, Gust ID, et al. Propagation of human hepatitis A virus in African green monkey kidney cell culture: primary isolation and serial passage. Infect Immun 1981;32:388.

Dalekos GN, Galanakis E, Zervou E, et al. Interferon-alpha treatment of children with chronic hepatitis D virus infection: the Greek experience. Hepatogastroenterology 2000;47:1072-1076.

Dane DS, Cameron CH, Briggs M. Viruslike particles in serum of patients with Australia-antigen–associated hepatitis. Lancet 1970;1:695.

DeCock KMD, Bradley DW, Sanford NL, et al. Epidemic non-A, non-B hepatitis in patients from Pakistan. Ann Intern Med 1987;106:227.

Deinhardt F, Holmes AW, Capps RB, Popper H. Studies on the transmission of human viral hepatitis to marmoset monkeys: I. transmission of disease, serial passages, and description of liver lesions. J Exp Med 1967;125:673.

Delaplane D, Yogev R, Crussi G, Schulman ST. Fatal hepatitis in early infancy. Pediatrics 1983;72:176.

Desmyter J, DeGoote J, Desmet VJ, et al. Administration of human fibroblast interferon in chronic hepatitis-B infection. Lancet 1976;2:645.

DiBisceglie AM, Hoofnagle JH. Antiviral therapy of chronic viral hepatitis. Am J Gastroenterol 1990;85:650-654.

DiBisceglie AM, Martin P, Kassianides C, et al. Recombinant interferon alpha therapy for chronic hepatitis C: a randomized, double-blind, placebo-controlled trial. N Engl J Med 1989;321:1506-1510.

Dienstag JL, Feinstone SM, Kapikian AZ, Purcell RH. Fecal shedding of hepatitis-A antigen. Lancet 1975a;1:765.

Dienstag JL, et al. Experimental infection of chimpanzees with hepatitis A virus. J Infect Dis 1975b;132:532.

Dienstag JL, Perrillo RP, Schiff ER, et al. A preliminary trial of lamivudine for chronic hepatitis B infection. N Engl J Med 1995;333(25):1657-1661.

Duermeyer W, van der Veen J, Koster B. ELISA in hepatitis A. Lancet 1978;1:823.

Dupuy JW, Frommel D, Alagille D. Severe viral hepatitis type B in infants. Lancet 1975;1:191.

Edmondson HA. Needle biopsy in differential diagnosis of acute liver disease. JAMA 1965;191:136.

Enomoto N, Sakuma I, Asahina Y, et al. Comparison of full-length sequences of interferon-sensitive and resistant hepatitis C virus 1b: sensitivity to interferon is conferred by amino acid substitutions in the NS5A region. J Clin Invest 1995;96:224-230.

Farci P, Alter HJ, Wong D, et al. A long-term study of hepatitis C virus replication in non-A, non-B hepatitis. N Engl J Med 1991;325:98-104.

Fawaz KA, Grady GF, Kaplan MM, Gellis SS. Repetitive maternal-fetal transmission of fatal hepatitis B. N Engl J Med 1975;293:1357.

Feinstone SM, Kapikian AZ, Purcell RH. Hepatitis A: detection by immune electron microscopy of a viruslike antigen associated with acute illness. Science 1973;182:1026.

Gauss-Muller V, Frosner GG, Deinhardt F. Propagation of hepatitis A virus in human embryo fibroblasts. J Med Virol 1981;7:233.

Gerber MA, Thung SN. The diagnostic value of immunohistochemical demonstration of hepatitis viral antigens in the liver. Hum Pathol 1987;18:771-774.

Gianotti F. Papular acrodermatitis of childhood: an Australia antigen disease. Arch Dis Child 1973;48:794.

Gibb DM, Goodall RL, Dunn DT, et al. Mother-to-child transmission of hepatitis C virus: evidence for preventable peripartum transmission. Lancet 2000;356:904-907.

Gimson AE, Tedder RS, White YS, et al. Serological markers in fulminant hepatitis B. Gut 1983;24:615-617.

Gocke DJ. Extrahepatic manifestations of viral hepatitis. Am J Med Sci 1975;270:49.

Gocke DJ, et al. Vasculitis in association with Australia antigen. J Exp Med 1971;134:330.

Gocke DJ, Hsv K, Morgan C, et al. Association between polyarteritis and Australia antigen. Lancet 1970;3:1149.

Govindarajan S, Chin KP, Redeker AG, et al. Fulminant B viral hepatitis: role of delta agent. Gastroenterology 1984;86:1417-1420.

Hadler SC, DeMonzon M, Ponzetto A, et al. Delta virus infection and severe hepatitis: an epidemic in Yuepa Indians of Venezuela. Ann Intern Med 1984;100:339-344.

Hadziyannis SJ, Papatheodoridis GV. Peginterferon-alpha2a (40 kDa) for chronic hepatitis C. Expert Opin Pharmacother 2003;4(4):541-551.

Hasewaga K, Hvang JK, Wands JR, et al. Association of hepatitis B viral precore mutations with fulminant hepatitis B in Japan. Virology 1991;185:460-463.

Havens WP Jr, Ward R, Drill VA, Paul JR. Experimental production of hepatitis by feeding icterogenic materials. Proc Soc Exp Biol Med 1944;53:206.

Heathcote J, Cameron CH, Dane DS. Hepatitis-B antigen in saliva and semen. Lancet 1974;1:71.

Heathcote J, Chan R, McHutchison J, et al. A phase 2 multi-center study of oral lobucavir for treatment of chronic hepatitis B. Hepatology 1998;28:318.

Hirschman RJ, et al. Viruslike particles in sera of patients with infectious and serum hepatitis. JAMA 1969;208:1667.

Hollinger FB, Bradley DW, Dreesman GR, et al. Detection of hepatitis A viral antigen by radioimmunoassay. J Immunol 1975;115:1464.

Holmes AW, Wolfe L, Rosenblate H, et al. Hepatitis in marmosets: induction of disease with coded specimens from a human volunteer study. Science 1969;165:816.

Hoofnagle JH. Antiviral treatment of chronic type B hepatitis. Ann Intern Med 1987;107:413-415.

Hoofnagle JH, DiBisceglie AM. Serologic diagnosis of acute and chronic viral hepatitis. Sem Liver Dis 1991;11:78.

Hoofnagle JH, Peters M, Mullen KD, et al. Randomized, controlled trial of recombinant human alpha interferon in patients with chronic hepatitis B. Gastroenterology 1988;95:1318-1325.

Hsu HY, Chang MH, Ho HN, et al. Association of HLA-DR14-DR52 with low responsiveness to hepatitis B vaccine in Chinese residents in Taiwan. Vaccine 1993;11:1437-1440.

Ishimaru Y, Ishimaru H, Toda G, et al. An epidemic of infantile papular acrodermatitic (Gianotti's disease) in Japan associated with hepatitis B surface antigen subtype ayw. Lancet 1976;1:707.

Kane MA, Bradley DW, Shrestha SM, et al. Epidemic non-A, non-B hepatitis in Nepal. JAMA 1984;252:3140-3145.

Karvountzis GD, Redeker AG, Peters RL. Long-term follow-up studies of patients surviving fulminant viral hepatitis. Gastroenterology 1974;67:870.

Khuroo MS. Study of an epidemic of non-A, non-B hepatitis. Am J Med 1980;68:818-824.

Khuroo MS, Kamili S, Jameel S. Vertical transmission of hepatitis E virus. Lancet 1995;345:1025-1026.

Kohler PF, Cronin RE, Hammond WS, et al. Chronic membranous glomerulonephritis caused by hepatitis B antigen-antibody immune complexes. Ann Intern Med 1974;81:488.

Kojima S, Shibayoma T, Sato A, et al. Propagation of human hepatitis A virus in conventional cell lines. J Med Virol 1981;7:273.

Krawitt E. Autoimmune hepatitis. N Engl J Med 1996;334:897-903.

Krugman S. Viral hepatitis, type B: prospects for active immunization. Am J Med Sci 1975;270:391.

Krugman S. Incubation period of type B hepatitis. N Engl J Med 1979;300:625.

Krugman S, et al. Viral hepatitis, type B: studies on natural history and prevention reexamined. N Engl J Med 1979;300:101.

Krugman S, Friedman H, Lattimer C. Viral hepatitis, type A: identification by specific complement fixation and immune adherence tests. N Engl J Med 1975;292:1141.

Krugman S, Giles JP. Viral hepatitis: new light on an old disease. JAMA 1970;212:1019.

Krugman S, Giles JP. Viral hepatitis type B (MS-2 strain): further observations on natural history and prevention. N Engl J Med 1973;288:755.

Krugman S, Giles JP, Hammond J. Infectious hepatitis: evidence for two distinctive clinical, epidemiological, and immunological types of infection. JAMA 1967;200:365.

Krugman S, Giles JP, Hammond J. Hepatitis virus: effect of heat on the infectivity and antigenicity of the MS-1 and MS-2 strains. J Infect Dis 1970;122:432.

Krugman S, Giles JP, Hammond J. Viral hepatitis, type B (MS-2 strain): prevention with specific hepatitis B immune serum globulin. JAMA 1971a;218:1665.

Krugman S, Giles JP, Hammond J. Viral hepatitis, type B (MS-2 strain): studies on active immunization. JAMA 1971b;217:41.

Krugman S, Hoofnagle JH, Gerety RI, et al. Viral hepatitis, type B: DNA polymerase activity and antibody to hepatitis B core antigen. N Engl J Med 1974;290:1331.

Krugman S, Ward R. Infectious hepatitis: current status of prevention with gamma globulin. Yale J Biol Med 1962;34:329.

Krugman S, Ward R, Giles JP. The natural history of infectious hepatitis. Am J Med 1962;32:717.

Krugman S, Ward R, Giles JP, Jacobs AM. Infectious hepatitis: studies on the effect of gamma globulin and on the incidence of inapparent infection. JAMA 1960;174:825.

Kuo G, Choo QL, Alter HJ, et al. An assay for circulating antibodies to a major ecologic virus of human non-A, non-B hepatitis. Science 1989;244:362-364.

Lai CL, Lok ASF, Lin HJ, et al. Placebo-controlled trial of recombinant alpha-2 interferon in Chinese patients with chronic hepatitis B infection. Lancet 1987;2:877-880.

Lai CL, Chien RN, Leung NW, et al. A one-year trial of lamivudine for chronic hepatitis B. Asia Hepatitis Lamivudine Study Group. N Engl J Med 1998; 339(2):61-68.

LeBouvier GL. Subspecificities of the Australia antigen complex. Am J Dis Child 1972;123:420.

Leung NW, Lai CL, Chang TT, et al. On behalf of the Asia Hepatitis Lamivudine Study Group. Extended lamivudine treatment in patients with chronic hepatitis B enhances hepatitis B e antigen seroconversion rates: results after 3 years of therapy. Hepatology 2001;33:1527-1532.

Levo Y, Gorevic PD, Kassab HJ, et al. Association between hepatitis B virus and essential mixed cryoglobulinemia. N Engl J Med 1977;296:1501.

Liang TJ, Hasegawa K, Rimon N, et al. A hepatitis B virus mutant associated with an epidemic of fulminant hepatitis. N Engl J Med 1991;324:1705-1709.

Liaw YF, Chien RN, Yeh CT, et al. Acute exacerbation and hepatitis B virus clearance after emergence of YMDD motif mutation during lamivudine therapy. Hepatology 1999;30:567-572.

Lieberman HM, La Breeque DR, Kew MC, et al. Detection of hepatitis B virus DNA directly in human serum by a simplified molecular hybridization tests: comparison to HBeAg/anti-HBe status in HBsAg carriers. Hepatology 1983;3:285.

Lindsay KL, Trepo C, Heintges T, et al. The Hepatitis Interventional Therapy Group. A randomized, double-blind trial comparing pegylated interferon alpha-2b to interferon alpha-2b as initial treatment for chronic hepatitis C. Hepatology 2001;34:395-403.

Linnen J, Wages J, Zhang-Kack ZY, et al. Molecular cloning and disease association of hepatitis G virus: a transfusion-transmissible agent. Science 1996;271: 505-508.

Lorenz D, et al. Hepatitis in the marmoset: *Saguinus mystax*. Proc Soc Exp Biol Med 1970;135:348.

Losonsky GA, Wasserman SS, Stephens I, et al. Hepatitis B vaccination of premature infants: a reassessment of current recommendations for delayed immunization. Pediatrics 1999;103:E14.

Lürman A. Eine Icterusepidemie. Berl Klin Wochenschr 1885;22:20.

MacNab GM, Alexander JJ, Lecatsas G, et al. Hepatitis B surface antigen produced by a human hepatoma cell line. Br J Cancer 1976;34:509.

Manns MP, McHutchison JG, Gordon SC, et al. Peginterferon alpha-2b plus ribavirin compared with interferon alpha-2b plus ribavirin for initial treatment of chronic hepatitis C: a randomised trial. Lancet 2001;358:958-965.

Martell M, Esteban JI, Quer J, et al. Hepatitis C virus (HCV) circulates as a population of different but closely related genomes: quasispecies nature of HCV genome distribution. J Virol 1992;66:3225-3229.

Mascoli CC, Ittensohn OL, Villarejos VM, et al. Recovery of hepatitis agents in the marmoset from human cases occurring in Costa Rica. Proc Soc Exp Biol Med 1973;143:276.

Maynard JE. Infectivity studies of hepatitis A and B in non-human primates. International Association of Biological Standards Symposium on Viral Hepatitis, Milan, Italy, December 16-19, 1974.

Maynard JE, Berquist KR, Krushak DH, Purcell RH. Experimental infection of chimpanzees with the virus of hepatitis B. Nature 1972;237:514.

McHutchison JG, Gordon SC, Schiff ER, et al. Interferon alpha-2b alone or in combination with ribavirin as initial treatment for chronic hepatitis C. Hepatitis

Interventional Therapy Group. N Engl J Med 1998; 339:1483-1492.

McMahon BJ, Alward WLM, Hall DB, et al. Acute hepatitis B virus infection: relation of age to the clinical expression of disease and subsequent development of the carrier state. J Infect Dis 151:1985;599-603.

McNeil M, Hoy JF, Richards MJ, et al. Etiology of fatal hepatitis in Melbourne. Med J Aust 1984;2:637-640.

Melnick JL. Classification of hepatitis A virus as enterovirus type 72 and of hepatitis B virus as hepadnavirus, type 1. Intervirology 1982;18:105.

Meltzer M, Franklin EC, Elias K, et al. Cryoglobulinemia—a clinical and laboratory study: II. cryoglobulins with rheumatoid factor activity. Am J Med 1966;40:837.

Miller WJ, Prorost PJ, McAleer WJ, et al. Specific immune adherence assay for human hepatitis A antibody. Application of diagnostic and epidemiologic investigations. Proc Soc Exp Biol Med 1975;149:254.

Mitsui T, Iwano K, Masuko K, et al. Hepatitis C infection in medical personnel after needle stick accident. Hepatology 1992;16:1109-1114.

Morrow RH Jr, Smetana HF, Sai FT, et al. Unusual features of viral hepatitis in Accra, Ghana. Ann Intern Med 1968;68:1250-1264.

Murphy BL, Maynard JE, Bradley DW, et al. Immunofluorescence of hepatitis A virus antigen in chimpanzees. Infect Immun 1978;21:663.

Nagata I, Shiraki K, Tanimoto K, et al. Mother-to-infant transmission of hepatitis C virus. J Pediatr 1992;120: 432-434.

Narkewicz, MR, Smith D, Silverman A, et al. Clearance of chronic hepatitis B virus infection in young children after alpha interferon treatment. J Pediatr 1995;127:815-818.

Neefe JR, Gellis SS, Stokes J Jr. Homologous serum hepatitis and infectious (epidemic) hepatitis. Studies in volunteers bearing on immunological and other characteristics of the etiological agents. Am J Med 1946;1:3.

Ohto H, Terazawa S, Sasaki N, et al. Transmission of hepatitis C virus from mother to infants. N Engl J Med 1994;330:744-750.

Okamoto H, Sugiyama Y, Okada S, et al. Typing hepatitis C virus by polymerase chain reaction with type-specific primers: application to clinical surveys and tracing infectious sources. J Gen Virol 1992;73:673-679.

Ozen H, Kocak N, Yuce A, Gurakan F. Retreatment with higher dose interferon alpha in children with chronic hepatitis B infection. Pediatr Infect Dis J 1999;18: 694-697.

Palomba E, Manzini P, Flammengo P, et al. Natural history of perinatal hepatitis C virus infection. Clin Infect Dis 1996;23:47-50.

Papaevangelou V, Pollack H, Borkowsky W, et al. Enhanced transmission of vertical HCV infection to HIV-infected infants of HIV and HCV co-infected women. J Infect Dis 1998;178:1047-1052.

Pawlotsky JM, Ben Yahia M, Andre C, et al. Immunologic disorders in C virus chronic active hepatitis: a prospective case-control serotypes. Hepatology 1994;19:841-848.

Pawlotsky JM, Roudot-Thoraval F, Simmonds P, et al. Extrahepatic immunologic manifestations in chronic hepatitis C and hepatitis C serotypes. Ann Intern Med 1995;122:169-175.

Pensati P, Iorio R, Botta S, et al. Low virologic response to interferon in children with chronic hepatitis C. J Hepatol 1999;31:604-611.

Perillo RP, Schiff ER, Davis GL, et al. A randomized controlled trial of interferon alpha-2b alone and after prednisone withdrawal for the treatment of chronic hepatitis B. N Engl J Med 1990;323:295-301.

Peterson DA, Hurley TR, Hoff JC, et al. Hepatitis A virus infectivity and chlorine treatment. In Szmuness W, Alter HJ, Maynard JE (eds). Proceedings of the 1981 International Symposium on Viral Hepatitis. Philadelphia: Franklin Institute Press, 1982.

Plouvier B, Wattre P, Devulder B. HBsAg in superficial artery of a patient with polymyalgia rheumatica. Lancet 1978;2:932.

Popper H, Shih JW-K, Gerin JL, et al. Woodchuck hepatitis and hepatocellular carcinoma: correlation of histologic with virologic observations. Hepatology 1981;1:91.

Poynard T, Marcellin P, Lee SS, et al. Randomised trial of interferon alpha2b plus ribavirin for 48 weeks or for 24 weeks versus interferon alpha2b plus placebo for 48 weeks for treatment of chronic infection with hepatitis C virus. International Hepatitis Interventional Therapy Group (IHIT). Lancet 1998;352:1426-1432.

Provost PJ, Giesa PA, McAleer WJ, et al. Isolation of hepatitis A virus in vitro in cell culture directly from human specimens. Proc Soc Exp Biol Med 1981;167:201.

Provost PJ, Hilleman MR. Propagation of human hepatitis A virus in cell culture in vitro. Proc Soc Exp Biol Med 1979;160:213.

Provost PJ, Ittensohn OL, Villarejos VM, Hilleman MR. A specific complement fixation test for human hepatitis A employing CR326 virus antigen: diagnosis and epidemiology. Proc Soc Exp Biol Med 1975a;148:961.

Provost PJ, Wolanski BS, Miller WJ, et al. Biophysical and biochemical properties of CR326 human hepatitis virus. Am J Med Sci 1975b; 270:87.

Provost PF, Ittensohn OL, Villarejos VM, et al. Etiologic relationship of marmoset-propagated CR326 hepatitis A virus to hepatitis in man. Proc Soc Exp Biol Med 1973;142:1257-1267.

Reyes GR, Purdy MA, Kim JP. Isolation of cDNA from virus responsible for enterically transmitted non-A, non-B hepatitis. Science 1990;247:1335-1339.

Rizzetto M, Canese MG, Arico S, et al. Immunofluorescence detection of new antigen-antibody system associated to hepatitis B virus in liver and serum of HBsAg carriers. Gut 1977;18:997-1003.

Rizzetto M, Ponzetto A, Borino A. Hepatitis delta virus infection: clinical and epidemiological aspects. In Viral Hepatitis and Liver Disease. New York: Alan R Liss, 1988.

Rizzetto M, Rosina F, Saracco G, et al. Treatment of chronic delta hepatitis with alpha 2 recombinant interferon. J Hepatol 1986;3:S229-S233.

Saito I, Miyamura T, Ohbayashi A, et al. Hepatitis C virus infection is associated with the development of hepatocellular carcinoma. Proc Natl Acad Sci USA 1990;87: 6547-6549.

Sampliner RE, Woronow DI, Alter HJ, et al. Community-acquired non-A, non-B hepatitis. J Med Virol 1984;13:125-130.

Schirmbeck R, Bohm W, Ando K, et al. Nucleic acid vaccination primes hepatitis B surface antigen-specific cytotoxic T lymphocytes in nonresponder mice. J Virol 1995; 69:5929-5934.

Schweitzer IL, Wing A, McPeak C, Spears RL. Hepatitis and hepatitis-associated antigen in 56 mother-infant pairs. JAMA 1972;220:1092.

Scotto J, Hadchouel M, Herej C, et al. Detection of hepatitis B virus DNA in serum by a simple spot hybridization technique. Comparison with results for other viral markers. Hepatology 1983;3:279.

Seeff LB, Miller RN, Rabkin CS, et al. 45-year follow-up of hepatitis C virus infection in healthy young adults. Ann Intern Med 2000;132:105-111.

Sergent I, Lockshin MD, Christian CL, et al. Vasculitis with hepatitis B antigenemia. Long-term observations in nine patients. Medicine 1976;55:1.

Shafritz DA. Variants of hepatitis B virus associated with fulminant liver disease. New Engl J Med 1991;324: 1737-1739.

Shafritz DA, Kew MC. Identification of integrated hepatitis B virus DNA sequences in human hepatocellular carcinoma. Hepatology 1981;1:1.

Shrestha SM, Kane MA. Preliminary report of non-A, non-B hepatitis in Kathmandu Valley. J Inst Med 1983;5:1-10.

Simmonds P, Alberti A, Alter HJ, et al. A proposed system for nomenclature of hepatitis C virus genotypes. Hepatology 1994;19:1321-1324.

Simmonds P, Holmes EC, Cha TA, et al. Classification of hepatitis C virus into 6 major genotypes and a series of subtypes by phylogenetic analysis of the NS-5 region. J Gen Virol 1993;74:2391-2399.

Simons JN, Leary TP, Dawson GJ, et al. Isolation of novel virus-like sequences associated with human hepatitis. Nat Med 1995;1:564-569.

Smedile A, Farci P, Verme G, et al. Influence of delta infection on severity of hepatitis B. Lancet 1982;2:945.

Sokal EM, Conjeevaram HS, Roberts EA, et al. Interferon alpha therapy for chronic hepatitis B in children: a multinational randomized controlled trial. Gastroenterology 1998;114:988-995.

Sokal EM, Roberts EA, Mieli-Vergani G, et al. A dose ranging study of the pharmacokinetics, safety, and preliminary efficacy of lamivudine in children and adolescents with chronic hepatitis B. Antimicrob Agents Chemother 2000;44:590-597.

Stevens CE, Beasley RP, Tsui J, Lee WC. Vertical transmission of hepatitis B antigen in Taiwan. N Engl J Med 1975;292:771.

Stokes J Jr, et al. The carrier-state in viral hepatitis. JAMA 1954;154:1059.

Swain M, Heathcote EJ, Lai MY, et al. Long-lasting sustained virological response in chronic hepatitis C patients previously treated with 40 kda peginterferon alpha-2a (PEGASYS) (abstract 633). Meeting of the American Association for the Study of Liver Diseases, Dallas, November 9-13, 2001.

Szmuness W. Hepatocellular carcinoma and hepatitis B virus: evidence for a causal association. Prog Med Virol 1978;24:40.

Szmuness W, et al. Distribution of antibody to hepatitis A antigen in urban adult population. N Engl J Med 1976;295:755.

Szmuness W, Dienstag JL, Purcell RH, et al. The prevalence of antibody to hepatitis A antigen in various parts of the world: a pilot study. Am J Epidemiol 1977;106:392.

Szmuness W, Stevens CE, Zang EA, et al. A controlled clinical trial of the efficacy of the hepatitis B vaccine (Heptavax B): a final report. Hepatology 1981;1:377-385.

Tabor E, Krugman S, Weiss EC, et al. Disappearance of hepatitis B surface antigen during an unusual case of fulminant hepatitis B. J Med Virol 1981;8:277-282.

Ticehurst JR, Recaniello VR, Baroudy BM, et al. Molecular cloning and characterization of hepatitis A virus with DNA. Proc Natl Acad Sci USA 1983;80:5885.

Toda G, Ishimaru Y, Mayumi M, Oda T. Infantile papular acrodermatitis (Gianotti's disease) and intrafamilial occurrence of acute hepatitis B with jaundice: age dependency of clinical manifestations of hepatitis B virus infection. J Infect Dis 1978;138:211.

Torre D, Tambini R. Interferon-alpha therapy for chronic hepatitis B in children: a meta-analysis. Clin Infect Dis 1996; 23:131-7.

Trepo CH, Thiyolet J. Hepatitis-associated antigen and periarteritis nodosa (PAN). Vox Sang 1970;19:410.

Trey C. The fulminant hepatic surveillance study. CMAJ 1972;106:525.

Villarejos VM, Provost PJ, Ittensohn OL, et al. Seroepidemiologic investigations of human hepatitis caused by A, B, and a possible third virus. Proc Soc Exp Biol Med 1976;152:524.

Wands JR, Mann E, Alpert E, Issel Bacher KJ. The pathogenesis of arthritis associated with acute HB, Ag-positive hepatitis: complement activation and characterization of circulating immune complexes. J Clin Invest 1975;55: 930-936.

Ward R, Borchert B, Wright A, Kline E. Hepatitis B antigen in saliva and mouth washing. Lancet 1972;2:726.

Watanabe H, Matsushita S, Kamikawaji N, et al. Immune suppression gene on HLA-Bw54-DR4-DRw53 haplotype controls nonresponsiveness in humans to hepatitis B surface antigen via CD8+ suppressor T-cells. Hum Immunol 1988;22:9-17.

Werner BG, Grady GF. Accidental hepatitis-B–surface-antigen–positive inoculations: use of e antigen to estimate infectivity. Ann Intern Med 1982;97:367-369.

World Health Organization Expert Committee on Viral Hepatitis. Advances in viral hepatitis. Who Tech Rep Ser No. 602, 1977.

Wu JC, Cho KD, Chen CM, et al. Genotyping of hepatitis D virus by restriction fragment length polymorphism and relation to outcome of hepatitis D. Lancet 1995;346:939-941.

Xiong X, Flores C, Yang H, et al. Mutations in hepatitis B DNA polymerase associated with resistance to lamivudine do not confer resistance to adefovir in vitro. Hepatology 1998; 28:1669-73.

Zignego AL, DeCarli M, Monti M, et al. Hepatitis C virus infection of mononuclear cells from peripheral blood and liver infiltrates in chronically infected patients. J Med Virol 1995;47:58-64.

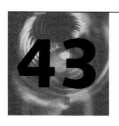

43 VIRAL INFECTIONS OF THE CENTRAL NERVOUS SYSTEM

RICHARD J. WHITLEY

Central nervous system (CNS) symptoms (e.g., headache, lethargy, impaired psychomotor performance) are frequent components of viral infections; however, viral meningitis and encephalitis are unusual manifestations of human disease. Thus, although many individuals develop systemic viral illnesses, disease is usually mild and self-limiting with only a few developing symptomatic involvement of the brain. Viruses vary widely in their potential to produce CNS infection. For some viruses (e.g., mumps), CNS infection is a common but a relatively benign component of the disease syndrome. For others (e.g., Japanese encephalitis), neurologic disease is the most prominent clinical feature of illness. A third group of viruses commonly cause infection, but only rarely cause encephalitis (e.g., herpes simplex virus [HSV]). Finally, there are viruses for which human infection inevitably and exclusively results in CNS disease (e.g., rabies). In addition to acute pathology, other viruses (e.g., measles) can cause syndromes of postinfectious encephalopathy.

When infection involves the CNS, there is potential for neurologic damage and, in some instances, death. Neural tissues are exquisitely sensitive to metabolic derangements, and injured brain tissue recovers slowly and often incompletely (Moorthi et al., 1999; Schlitt et al., 1991). Clinical presentation and patient history, although frequently suggestive of a diagnosis, remain unreliable methods for determining the specific cause of CNS disease (Bale, 1993; Whitley et al., 1989). Tumors, infections, and autoimmune processes in the CNS often produce similar signs and symptoms (Whitley et al., 1989). Different diseases may share a common pathogenic mechanism and, therefore, result in a similar clinical presentation. Furthermore, understanding the pathogenic

mechanism of a disease provides a rational basis for the development of antiviral medications as well as strategies for the prevention of viral CNS infections.

DEFINITIONS

Definitions of CNS viral disease are often based on both virus tropism and disease duration. Inflammation can occur at multiple sites within the brain, accounting for the myriad clinical descriptors of viral neurologic disease. Inflammation of the spinal cord, leptomeninges, dorsal nerve roots, or nerves results in myelitis, meningitis, radiculitis, and neuritis, respectively. *Aseptic meningitis* is a misnomer frequently used to refer to a benign, self-limited, viral infection causing inflammation of the leptomeninges (Hammer and Connolly, 1992; Rotbart, 1997). The term hinders epidemiologic studies because the definition fails to differentiate between infectious (e.g., fungal, tuberculous, viral) and noninfectious causes of meningitis. *Encephalitis* refers to inflammation of brain parenchyma and is usually accompanied by depressed level of consciousness, altered cognition, and/or focal neurologic signs. Acute encephalitis occurs over a relatively short period of time (days), whereas chronic encephalitis manifests over weeks to months. The temporal course of slow infections of the CNS (e.g., kuru, visna, variant Creutzfeldt-Jacob disease [CJD]) overlaps the chronic encephalitides. Slow viral infections of the CNS are distinguished by their long incubation because of a slow replication rate, eventually resulting in death or extreme neurologic disability over months to years (Whitley et al., 2000).

Viral disease in the CNS can also be classified by pathogenesis. Neurologic disease is frequently categorized as either primary or postinfectious. Primary encephalitis results from direct viral entry into the CNS that produces clinically evident cortical or brainstem dysfunction (Johnson, 1987). Subsequent damage results from a combination of virally induced cytopathic effects and the resultant host immune response. Viral invasion, however, remains the initiating event (Johnson, 1987). The parenchyma exhibits neuronophagia and the presence of viral antigens or nucleic acids (Johnson, 1987). A postinfectious encephalitis produces signs and symptoms of encephalitis, temporally associated with a systemic viral infection, without evidence of direct viral invasion in the CNS. Pathologic specimens demonstrate demyelination, perivascular aggregation of immune cells, without evidence of virus or viral antigen, leading some to hypothesize an autoimmune etiology (Johnson, 1987).

Meningitis and encephalitis represent separate clinical entities; however, a continuum exists between these distinct forms of disease. Nevertheless, a discussion of meningitis and encephalitis provides a useful format for this review.

VIRAL MENINGITIS
Epidemiology

Acute viral meningitis and meningoencephalitis represent the majority of viral CNS infections and frequently occur in epidemics with a seasonal distribution (Cassady and Whitley, 1997; Nicolosi et al., 1986). Enteroviruses cause an estimated 90% of cases (in countries that immunize against mumps), and arboviruses constitute the majority of the remaining reported cases in the United States (Hammer and Connolly, 1992; Nigrovic and Chiang, 1986; Pozo et al., 1998; Sawyer, 1999). Mumps is an important cause of viral CNS disease in countries that do not immunize against it. In a Japanese study, mumps was the second leading cause of aseptic meningitis, accounting for approximately 30% of cases (Hosoya et al., 1998). Viral meningitis is not a disease that is reportable to the Centers for Disease Control and Prevention (CDC); however, it is likely that there are over 74,000 cases annually in the United States (Rotbart, 1995; Sawyer, 1999). Most cases occur from late spring to autumn, reflecting the increased incidence of enteroviral and arboviral infections during these seasons (Centers for Disease Control and Prevention, 1994a; Sawyer, 1999). A retrospective survey performed in the 1980s found that the annual incidence of "aseptic meningitis" was

approximately 10.9 per 100,000 persons, or at least four times the incidence passively reported to the CDC during the same period (Nicolosi et al., 1986). Virus was isolated in only 11% of patients in this study, likely reflecting the technologic limits of the period, the infrequency with which viral cultures were performed, and the decreased incidence of viral CNS disease resulting from widespread vaccination against mumps and polio viruses (Nicolosi et al., 1986). Since the advent of molecular based diagnostic techniques (polymerase chain reaction [PCR]), identification rates now approach 50% to 70% (Hosoya et al., 1998; Pozo et al., 1998).

Pathogenesis

The pathogenesis of viral meningitis is not completely understood. Inferences regarding the pathogenesis of viral meningitis are largely derived from data on encephalitis, experimental animal models of meningitis, and clinical observations (Cassady and Whitley, 1997; Hammer and Connolly, 1992). Viruses use two basic pathways to gain access to the CNS—hematogenous and neuronal—regardless of the resulting clinical syndrome (i.e., meningitis or encephalitis). A combination of host and viral factors combined with seasonal, geographic, epidemiologic probabilities influence the probability of CNS infection. For example, arboviral infections occur more frequently in epidemics and show a seasonal variation, reflecting the environmental prevalence of the transmitting vector (Centers for Disease Control and Prevention, 1994). Enteroviral meningitis occurs with greater frequency during the summer and early autumn months, reflecting the seasonal increase in enteroviral infections. The occurrence of enteroviral infections also exemplifies the role played by host physiology in the extent of viral disease. In children less than 2 weeks of age, *Enterovirus* can produce a severe systemic infection, including meningitis or meningoencephalitis (Sawyer, 1999). Of neonates with systemic enteroviral infections, 10% die, and 76% of survivors have permanent sequelae. In children over 2 weeks of age, however, enteroviral infections are rarely associated with severe disease or significant morbidity (Sawyer, 1999).

For hematogenous spread to the CNS, the virus must first either bypass or attach to and enter host epithelial cells to produce infection. Virus then spreads and initially replicates in the regional lymph nodes (e.g., measles, influenza,) or, alternatively, enters the circulatory system where it seeds other tissues (e.g., arboviral infection, enteroviral infection, varicella) (Cassady and Whitley, 1997). Primary viremia allows virus to seed distant locations of the body, especially the reticuloendothelial system, and frequently marks the onset of clinical illness. In rare circumstances, such as disseminated neonatal HSV infection, virus infects the CNS during primary viremia (Kimura et al., 1991; Stanberry et al., 1994). The liver and spleen provide ideal locations for secondary viral replication because of their highly vascular structure and reticuloendothelial network. Secondary viremia results in high titers of virus in the bloodstream, facilitating viral CNS spread. The pathophysiology of viral transport from blood to brain and viral endothelial cell tropism is poorly understood. Virus infects endothelial cells, passively channels through endothelium (pinocytosis or colloidal transport), or bridges the endothelium within migrating leukocytes (Cassady and Whitley, 1997; Wiestler et al., 1992). This transendothelial passage occurs in vessels of the choroid plexus, meninges, and/or cerebrum.

Numerous host defense barriers limit viral dissemination to the CNS. The skin and mucosal surfaces possess mechanical, chemical, and cellular defenses that protect the cells from viral infection (Cassady and Whitley, 1997). Leukocytes and secretory factors (interleukins, interferons, antibodies) further augment these defenses and help eliminate viruses that bridge the epithelial layer. Local immune responses are crucial in limiting systemic viral infection. A prompt inflammatory response can limit viremia and subsequent symptoms of infection. In the liver and spleen, the high degree of parenchymal contact and large number of fixed mononuclear macrophage cells provide an excellent opportunity for host eradication of viremia (Cassady and Whitley, 1997). The blood-brain or cerebrospinal fluid (CSF) barrier, a network of tight endothelial junctions sheathed by glial cells that regulate molecular access to the CNS, further limits virus access to the brain (Bradbury, 1993; Edens and Parkos, 2000; Nagy and Martinez, 1991).

Viral meningitis is a relatively benign, self-limited illness; thus, tissue specimens are rarely available for pathologic study (Sawyer, 1999). The CSF, however, is frequently sampled and demonstrates a mononuclear immune cell response to most viral infections. Certain viral infections, most notably mumps and some enterovirus infections, elicit a polymorphonuclear cell infiltrate in the CSF early during disease. The initial CSF formula mimics bacterial meningitis and later shifts to a mononuclear predominance. Viral antigen presentation by mononuclear histiocytes stimulates the influx of immune cells. Recruited immune cells release soluble factors (interleukins, vasoactive amines) that mobilize other cells and change the permeability of the blood-brain barrier (Abbott, 2000; Becher et al., 2000). Physical and chemical changes in the blood-brain barrier allow the entry of serum proteins (i.e., immunoglobulins and interleukins, further augmenting host immune responses). The cell-mediated immune response is important for eliminating virus from the brain; however, immunoglobulin also has a role in protecting the host in some viral infections. This is best illustrated by the devastating clinical course of enteroviral meningitis in patients with agammaglobulinemia, as well as patients with X-linked hyper-IgM syndrome (Cunningham et al., 1999; Nigrovic and Chiang, 1986; Schmugge et al., 1999). Patients with impaired cell-mediated immunity have a higher incidence of CNS infections with certain viruses such as varicella zoster virus (VZV), cytomegalovirus (CMV), and measles (Cassady and Whitley, 1997).

Clinical Manifestations

Patients' age and immune status and the causative agent influence the clinical manifestations of viral meningitis. Patients with enteroviral meningitis often have nonspecific symptoms such as fever (38° to 40° C) of 3 to 5 days duration, malaise, and headache (Sawyer, 1999; Wilfert et al., 1983). Approximately 50% of patients have nausea or vomiting (Wilfert et al., 1983). Although nuchal rigidity and photophobia are the hallmark sign and symptom for meningitis, 33% of patients with viral meningitis have no evidence of meningismus (Wilfert et al., 1983). Less than 10% of children younger than 2 years of age develop signs of meningeal irritation; they demonstrate fever and irritability (Rorabaugh et al., 1993). Children may also have seizures secondary to fever, electrolyte disturbances, or the infection itself. In the immunocompromised host, enteroviral infection is both a diagnostic quandary and a potentially life-threatening disease. Immunocompromised patients frequently do not mount a brisk immune cell response; therefore, CSF analyses do not necessarily reflect evidence of CNS disease.

Symptoms of meningitis (stiff neck, headache, and photophobia) occur in approximately 11% of men and 36% of women with primary HSV-2 genital infection. In one study, 5% of patients with primary HSV genital infection had meningitis that was severe enough to require hospitalization. All hospitalized patients had evidence of a lymphocytic pleocytosis on CSF analysis (Corey et al., 1983). In another study, HSV-2 was cultured from the CSF of 78% of patients with meningismus during primary genital infection. These patients also exhibited a CSF leukocytosis and subsequent increases in CSF HSV antibody titers (Bergstrom et al., 1990). Recurrent HSV-2 meningitis (with or without genital lesions) occurs, although cases associated with primary infection are more common (Jensenius et al., 1998). HSV meningitis may spread to the CSF neuronally along the sacral nerves. Alternatively, the virus may reach the CSF hematogenously, as virus has been cultured from the blood buffy coat layer (Hammer and Connolly, 1992). Epstein-Barr virus (EBV), VZV, CMV, and parainfluenza virus have all been cultured or detected by PCR in the CSF of patients with meningitis (Arisoy et al., 1993; Echevarria et al., 1994; Echevarria et al., 1997; Hammer and Connolly, 1992; Hosoya et al., 1998).

Laboratory Findings

Initial CSF samples, although frequently suggestive of the diagnosis, are neither sensitive nor specific enough to differentiate viral from bacterial meningitis (Negrini et al., 2000). Instead, epidemiologic trends, patient history, and accompanying laboratory information are important adjuncts in assessing the etiology of meningitis. The CSF in patients with viral meningitis typically exhibits pleocytosis with 10 to 500 leukocytes and a slightly elevated protein level (< 100 mg/dl). The glucose level in the CSF is typically greater than 40% of a simultaneously drawn serum sample. Tremendous variation in CSF formulas exists, with significant overlap between viral and bacterial findings (Negrini et al., 2000). In a retrospective review of over 400 patients with acute viral or bacterial meningitis performed before the *Haemophilus influenzae B* conjugate vac-

cine, investigators found that approximately 20% of the CSF samples that grew bacteria exhibited a CSF pleocytosis <250 white blood cells (WBC) per mm^3 (Hammer and Connolly, 1992). Of the patients with bacterial meningitis, 15% had a CSF lymphocytosis, whereas 40% of the patients with viral meningitis had a predominance of polymorphonuclear cells. Some investigators recommend repeating the lumbar puncture 6 to 12 hours later, as the CSF profile of patients with viral meningitis will shift from a polymorphonuclear to a lymphocytic pleocytosis over this period (Feigin and Shackelford, 1973). However, in one study performed during an echovirus epidemic, eight of nine children with presumed enteroviral meningitis had failed to develop CSF lymphocyte predominance when a lumbar puncture was repeated 5 to 8 hours later. A retrospective study found that during an enterovirus outbreak, 51% of patients demonstrated polymorphonuclear predominance in the CSF profile, despite symptoms of greater than 24 hours' duration, but the cause of meningitis could not be confirmed in most cases (Negrini et al., 2000). Other investigators have confirmed that the change to a lymphocytic CSF profile occurs 18 to 36 hours into the illness (Varki and Puthuran, 1979). Most clinicians do not obtain CSF viral cultures (Ahmed et al., 1997; Ramers et al., 2000; van Vliet et al., 1998).

Diagnosis

Historically, the techniques for identifying viral meningitis were insensitive and often impractical. Although virus can be cultured from CSF during the early stages of the infection, this has little utility in the acute management of a patient with CNS disease (Bergstrom et al., 1990). Depending on the study cited and diagnostic methods used, investigators identify a causative agent in only 25% to 67% of presumed CNS infections (Ahmed et al., 1997; Whitley et al., 1989). Now, however, molecular techniques have advanced identification of agents. Recently, PCR and reverse transcriptase (RT)–PCR have been used to diagnose enteroviral meningitis in both immune competent patients and in those with agammaglobulinemia, indicating both sensitivity and specificity (Ahmed et al., 1997; van Vliet et al., 1998). PCR provides a rapid and reliable test for verifying the cause of certain types of meningitis. These techniques provide results within 24 to 36 hours and therefore may limit the duration of hospitalization, antibiotic use, and excessive diagnostic procedures (Ramers et al., 2000). As it relates to the diagnosis of arboviral disease, the use of molecular techniques is fraught with greater variability (Bergstrom et al., 1990; Ramers et al., 2000; Sawyer, 1999). Because of the diverse viral causes of arboviral infection, the development of specific primers that can hybridize across multiple viral families (Alphaviradae, Flaviviridae, Bunyaviridae) has been difficult. Currently there is an emphasis on the development of improved "universal group primers" to perform an initial group screening, followed by RT-PCR using higher specificity primers as a second viral diagnostic test (Kuno, 1998). For other infections, molecular techniques are the standard for diagnosing viral meningitis (Pozo et al., 1998; Rotbart, 1995).

Differential Diagnosis

Unusual but treatable infections should always be considered and investigated in patients with a CSF pleocytosis and negative conventional bacterial cultures. Spirochetes (*Treponema*, *Borrelia*, *Leptospira*), *Mycoplasma*, *Bartonella*, and mycobacteria can produce a pleocytosis with negative gram stain and negative bacterial cultures. Fastidious bacteria (*Listeria*) may fail to grow in culture and occasionally may produce a mononuclear pleocytosis similar to that caused by viral meningitis, as can occur in infants, the elderly, and immunocompromised patients. Some bacteria do not directly infect the CNS but can release toxins that create a change in the level of consciousness; for example *Staphylococcus aureus* and *Streptococcus pyogenes* produce exotoxin-mediated toxic shock syndrome. Parameningeal infections, especially from infected sinuses, produce a pleocytosis and CNS symptoms; however, these infections more frequently have encephalitis with focal neurologic changes and altered mental status as the presenting sign. Similarly, partially treated bacterial infections can have CSF findings resembling viral meningitis. Fungal and parasitic infections can produce CNS infections, although they uncommonly produce only meningitis. The exceptions to this rule are coccidiomycosis and *Cryptococcus* infection, which characteristically produce meningitis rather than any focal CNS disease. *Cryptococcus*, for example, produces subacute meningitis in both normal and immunosuppressed

patients and remains the leading cause of fungal meningitis (Rotbart, 1997). *Candida* infection, *Aspergillus* infection, histoplasmosis, and blastomycosis frequently cause focal parenchymal disease of the CNS. These fungal infections, although often considered in the differential diagnosis for an immunocompromised host, also cause disease in the normal host. Parasites like *Naeglaeria fowleri* produce meningoencephalitis with purulent CSF findings. A history of recent summertime swimming in a stagnant pond raises suspicion for this infection.

Noninfectious processes that can produce true aseptic meningitis include hematologic malignancies, medications, autoimmune diseases, and foreign material and proteins. Leukemia produces a CSF pleocytosis with cancerous cells and occurs most frequently with acute lymphocytic leukemia, although subarachnoid involvement can also occur in acute myelogenous leukemia. Immunomodulatory drugs such as intravenous immunoglobulin or antilymphocyte globulin (OKT-3) can cause aseptic meningitis. Of the medications associated with meningitis, nonsteroidal antiinflammatory agents, sulfa-containing drugs, and cytosine arabinoside are the most common offenders. Drug-induced aseptic meningitis frequently occurs in patients with underlying connective tissue or rheumatologic diseases (Hammer and Connolly, 1992; Rotbart, 1997). Epithelial or endothelial cysts can rupture and spill their contents (keratin, protein), producing a brisk inflammatory response that mimics meningitis.

Treatment and Prognosis

The fundamental principle of therapy for viral meningitis lies in the identification of potentially treatable diseases. Until recently, no therapy existed for most cases of viral meningitis. Efforts instead focused on preventive strategies (largely through vaccination), as well as identification of treatable meningitis due to nonviral causes. Antiviral therapies are emerging for the treatment of enteroviral meningitis (Pevear et al., 1999; Rotbart, 1999). Despite recent chemotherapeutic and diagnostic advances in the diagnosis of enteroviral infection, the presence of meningitis warrants careful assessment of patients for a treatable, nonviral cause. The clinician must also anticipate and treat the complications of viral CNS disease (seizures, syndrome of inappropriate antidiuretic hormone, hydrocephalus, raised intracranial pressure). Supportive therapy includes hydration and administration of antipyretics and analgesics.

As noted above, in the normal host, viral meningitis is a relatively benign self-limited disease. A prospective study in children less than 2 years of age, for example, found that even in the 9% of children who develop evidence of acute neurologic disease (complex seizures, increased intracerebral pressure, or coma) long-term prognosis is excellent. During follow-up (42 months), children with acute CNS complications performed neurodevelopmental tasks and achieved developmental milestones as well as children with an uncomplicated course (Rorabaugh et al., 1993).

Currently antibody preparations and an antiviral agent, pleconaril (see below), have shown activity against enterovirus infection in case reports and animal studies. Randomized, controlled trials, however, have not supported their routine use in enteroviral meningitis. In case reports, immunoglobulin preparations given systemically or intrathecally retarded mortality and morbidity in agammaglobulinemic patients with enteroviral meningitis. Despite the administration of immunoglobulin, patients do not eliminate virus from the CSF and in turn develop chronic enteroviral meningitis (Dwyer and Erlendsson, 1988; McKinney and Katz, 1987). As noted previously, enteroviral infections in neonates frequently produce overwhelming viremia and CNS disease. A blinded, randomized, controlled trial did not demonstrate clinical benefit for enterovirus-infected neonates with severe life-threatening disease who received intravenous immunoglobulin (Abzug et al., 1995).

A recently developed antiviral agent, pleconaril (3-[3,5-Dimethyl-4-[[3-(3-methyl-5-isoxazolyl)propyl]oxy]phenyl]-5-trifluoromethyl-1,2,4-oxadiazole) (ViroPharma Inc., Exton, Pennsylvania), is a bioavailable, small-molecule inhibitor of picornavirus replication that binds the capsid and prevents uncoating of viral RNA. Because of homology among picornavirus, enterovirus, and rhinovirus capsid structure, the drug has activity against these viruses as well (Pape et al., 1999). Randomized, controlled, double-blind clinical trials, although demonstrating slight improvements in adults with enteroviral meningitis, have not had the substantial efficacy initially anticipated, and

the results have not been published in peer-reviewed literature. In the 32 adults with aseptic meningitis, duration of headache in the pleconaril group was decreased to an average 6.5 days, versus 18.3 days for placebo recipients (Rotbart, 1999). The duration of headache in the placebo control group was greater than previously reported. Similarly, if one uses the objective measurement of duration of analgesic use (historical average control = 5 days) versus that reported in the pleconaril study (placebo group = 11.5 days), the statistically significant 5.3 days of analgesic use by the pleconaril group is less dramatic (Rotbart, 1999; Rotbart et al., 1998). Pleconaril may yet prove beneficial in the treatment of severe life-threatening disease (neonatal sepsis, disease in the immunocompromised patient, encephalomyelitis). An ongoing multicenter randomized controlled trial is evaluating pleconaril in severe neonatal infection, but preliminary information is unavailable at this time.

Specific antiviral agents are available for treatment of meningitis due to several other viral causes. Although no definitive clinical trials have been conducted, most authors recommend the use of intravenous acyclovir for HSV meningitis, as it decreases the duration of primary disease and may limit meningeal involvement (Whitley et al., 1992). There are no data on benefit of antiviral treatment or on suppressive therapy for recurrent HSV CNS disease (Conway et al., 1997; Jensenius et al., 1998). Antiviral therapy exists for VZV infections of the CNS and should be instituted in these patients (De La et al., 2000; de Silva et al., 1996; Gilden et al., 2000), although there have been no controlled clinical trials to prove efficacy of such therapy. The issue of therapy for CMV CNS infection in the immunocompromised host is more problematic, and therapy should be tailored based on the clinical likelihood of infection.

VIRAL ENCEPHALITIS
Epidemiology

As with viral meningitis, the incidence of viral encephalitis is underestimated by passive reporting systems (Nicolosi et al., 1986; reviewed by Whitley and Gnann, 2002). An estimated 20,000 cases of encephalitis occur annually in the United States; however, from 1990 to 1994 the CDC received only 740 to 1,340 (0.3 to 0.54 per 100,000) annual reports of persons with encephalitis (Centers for Disease Control and Prevention, 1999b; Johnson, 1987). A review of the cases in Olmsted County, Minnesota from 1950 to 1980 reported the incidence of viral encephalitis to be twice that reported by the CDC (Nicolosi et al., 1986). A prospective multicenter study in Finland reported results similar to the Olmsted County study, showing an incidence of encephalitis of 10.5 per 100,000 (Koskiniemi et al., 1997). HSV CNS infections occur without seasonal variation, affect all ages, and constitute the majority of fatal cases of endemic encephalitis in the United States (Cassady and Whitley, 1997). Arboviruses, a group of over 500 arthropod-transmitted RNA viruses, are the leading cause of encephalitis worldwide and in the United States (Ho and Hirsch, 1985). Arboviral infections occur in epidemics and show a seasonal predilection, reflecting the prevalence of the transmitting vector (Centers for Disease Control and Prevention, 1998a). Asymptomatic infections vastly out-number symptomatic infections. Patients with disease may develop a mild systemic febrile illness or viral meningitis (Tsai, 1991). Encephalitis occurs in a minority of persons with arboviral infections, but the case fatality rate varies from 5% to 70%, depending on causative organism and patient age. La Crosse encephalitis is the most commonly reported arboviral disease in the United States, and St. Louis encephalitis (SLE) is the most frequent cause of epidemic encephalitis (Centers for Disease Control and Prevention, 1998).

Japanese B encephalitis (JE) and rabies constitute the majority of cases of encephalitis outside of North America. JE, a member of the Flavivirus genus, occurs throughout Asia and causes epidemics in China despite routine immunization (Cassady and Whitley, 1997). In warmer locations, virus occurs endemically. As with the other arboviral infections, asymptomatic infections occur more frequently than symptomatic infections. However, the disease has a high case fatality rate and leaves half of the survivors with significant neurologic morbidity (Cassady and Whitley, 1997). Rabies is endemic around much of the world. Because of the immunization of domesticated animals, human infections in the United States have decreased over the last decades to one to three cases per year. In areas outside the United States, human cases of rabies number in the

thousands and are caused by bites from unvaccinated domestic animals following contact with infected wild animals.

Postinfectious encephalitis, an acute demyelinating process, has also been referred to as *acute disseminated encephalomyelitis* (ADEM) or *autoimmune encephalitis* and accounts for approximately 100 to 200 additional cases of encephalitis annually (Centers for Disease Control and Prevention, 1999). The disease historically produced approximately one third of the encephalitis cases in the United States and was associated with measles, mumps, and other exanthematous viral infections (Cassady and Whitley, 1997; Stuve and Zamvil, 1999). Postinfectious encephalitis is now associated with antecedent upper respiratory virus (notably influenza virus) and varicella infections in the United States (Cassady and Whitley, 1997; Johnson, 1987). Measles continues to be the leading cause of postinfectious encephalitis worldwide and complicates 1 of every 1,000 measles infections (Johnson, 1987).

Slow infections of the CNS or transmissible spongiform encephalopathies (TSEs) occur sporadically worldwide. Although not caused by a classic infectious agent, brief consideration is warranted. The prototypical TSE is CJD, occurring at high rates within families and having an estimated incidence of 0.5 to 1.5 cases per million population (Whitley et al., 2000). Other TSEs are listed in Box 43-1 (Whitley et al., 2000). In 1986, cases of a TSE in cattle—bovine spongiform encephalopathy (BSE)—were reported in the United Kingdom. Throughout Europe, other livestock that were fed supplements containing meat and bone meal were affected, and cross-species transmission of BSE has been documented, leading to a ban in the use of bovine offal in fertilizers, pet food, and other animal feed (Whitley et al., 2000). A decrease in the recognized cases of BSE has occurred since the institution of these restrictions. Concomitant with the increase in incidence of BSE in Europe, an increase in cases of an atypical CJD also occurred, suggesting animal-to-human transmission. The report of atypical CJD (unique clinical and histopathologic findings) affecting young adults (an age at which CJD rarely has been diagnosed) led to the designation of a new disease, variant CJD (vCJD). According to the World Health Organization fact sheet, there have been 129 confirmed cases of

---

vCJD reported in the United Kingdom, six in France, and one each in Ireland, Italy, Canada, and the United States (WHO, 2001).

Pathogenesis

The pathogenesis of encephalitis is similar to that of viral meningitis and requires that viruses reach the CNS by hematogenous or neuronal spread. Viruses most frequently gain access to the CNS after a high-titer secondary viremia and cell-free or cell-associated CNS entry (Hammer and Connolly, 1992; Stanberry et al., 1994). Other than direct entry via cerebral vessels, virus can initially infect the meninges and, then, enter the parenchyma across either ependymal cells or the pial linings. Viruses exhibit differences in neurotropism and neurovirulence (Sharpe and Fields, 1985). For example, enteroviruses with similar receptors produce very different diseases. Five coxsackie B viruses (B1 through B5) readily produce CNS infections, whereas type B6 rarely produces

neurologic infection (Rotbart, 1997). Similarly, viral genes have been discovered that influence the neurovirulence of HSV-1 (Whitley et al., 1993). Compared with wild type virus, mutant HSV-1 viruses in the $\gamma_1 34.5$ gene have a decreased ability to cause encephalitis and death following intracerebral inoculation in mice (Whitley et al., 1993).

In addition to viral factors, host physiology is also important in determining the extent and location of viral CNS disease. Age, sex, and genetic differences among hosts influence viral infections and clinical course (Griffin et al., 1994; Sawyer, 1999). Host age influences the clinical manifestations and sequelae. Variations in macrophage function between individuals can result in clinically distinct infections and disease. Moreover, macrophage-antigen response can change with age and is important in limiting spread of infection within a patient (Goldsmith et al., 1998; Johnson, 1964). In addition to age, physical activity may be another important host factor that determines the severity of infection. Exercise has been associated with increased risk for paralytic poliomyelitis and may result in an increased incidence of enteroviral myocarditis and aseptic meningitis (Gatmaitan et al., 1970; Russell, 1947). Increasingly, host differences are being recognized as equally important determinants of disease at the cellular and molecular level.

In addition to blood-borne spread of virus to the brain, neuronal transmission plays an important role in pathogenesis; HSV and rabies are the best examples. Sensory and motor neurons contain transport systems that carry materials along the axon to (retrograde) and from (anterograde) the nucleus. Peripheral or cranial nerves provide access to the CNS and shield the virus from immune regulation.

Rabies classically infects by the myoneural route and provides a prototype for peripheral neuronal spread (Mrak and Young, 1994). Rabies virus replicates locally in soft tissue following a bite from a rabid animal. After primary replication, the virus enters the peripheral nerve by acetylcholine receptor binding. Once in the muscle, virus buds from the plasma membrane and crosses myoneural spindles or enters across the motor end plate (Lentz, 1990; Mrak and Young, 1994). The virus travels by anterograde and retrograde axonal transport to infect neurons in the brainstem and limbic system. Virus spreads from the diencephalic and hippocampal structure to the remainder of the brain, killing the animal (Mrak and Young, 1994). Virus also infects the CNS through cranial nerves, as suggested from animal studies but without supporting data in humans (Barnett et al., 1993; Barnett et al., 1994).

The pathologic findings of encephalitis are unique for each virus and reflect differences in pathogenesis and virulence. In the case of typical HSV encephalitis, a hemorrhagic necrosis (Johnson, 1987) occurs in the inferomedial temporal lobe, with evidence of perivascular cuffing, lymphocytic infiltration, and neuronophagia (Nahmias et al., 1982). Pathologic specimens with rabies encephalitis demonstrate microglial proliferation, perivascular infiltrates, and neuronal destruction. The location of the pathologic findings can be limited to the brainstem areas (dumb rabies) or the diencephalic, hippocampal, and hypothalamic areas (furious rabies) based on the immune response mounted against the infection (Mrak and Young, 1994).

Some viruses do not directly infect the CNS but produce immune system changes that result in parenchymal damage. Patients with postinfectious encephalitis exhibit focal neurologic deficits and altered consciousness associated temporally with a recent (1 to 2 weeks) viral infection or immunization (Stuve and Zamvil, 1999). Pathologic specimens, while they show evidence of demyelination by histologic or radiographic analysis, do not demonstrate evidence of viral infection in the CNS by culture or antigen tests. Patients with postinfectious encephalitis have subtle differences in their immune systems, and some authors have proposed an autoimmune reaction as the pathogenic mechanism of disease (Cassady and Whitley, 1997).

The TSEs are noninflammatory CNS diseases involving the accumulation of an abnormal form of a normal glycoprotein, the prion protein (PrP) (Pruisner, 1982). These encephalopathies differ in mode of transmission. Although most of the TSEs are experimentally transmissible by direct inoculation in the CNS, such transmission rarely occurs except for iatrogenic transmissions (Whitley et al., 2000). The scrapie agent spreads by cell-to-cell contact. There is no evidence for lateral transmission in the case of BSE or vCJD, and all cases appear to have occurred following parenteral administration or ingestion of affected materials. The transmissible agents remain infectious after treatments that normally inactivate viruses or nucleic acids (detergent formalin, ionizing radiation, nucleases) (Pruisner, 1982). Most of the experimental work on TSEs has involved analysis of the scrapie agent. The current working theory is that posttranslational alteration of the normally α-helical form of the PrP protein results in a protease-resistant β-pleated sheet structure that accumulates in neurons, leading to progressive dysfunction, cell death, and subsequent astrocytosis. In studies on the scrapie agent, gastrointestinal tract involvement with infection of abdominal lymph nodes occurs first, followed by brain involvement a year or more later (Cassady and Whitley, 1997). Experimental subcutaneous inoculation in mice and goats also leads to local lymph node involvement followed by splenic spread and, then, CNS involvement. The mode of transmission to the CNS (direct vs. hematogenous) and the infectivity of body fluids at different stages of infection are not known.

Clinical Manifestations

Although physical examination of the patient usually does not suggest the cause of disease, a few considerations are essential. For patients with acute viral encephalitis, the distinction between generalized and focal neurologic findings is important. In a nonepidemic setting, the most common viral cause of focal encephalopathic findings is HSV (Whitley et al., 1982; Whitley et al., 1989). However, when signs and symptoms of patients with biopsy-proved herpes simplex encephalitis (HSE) are compared with those of patients who did not have HSV CNS infection, there were no distinguishing clinical characteristics. Viruses that usually cause diffuse encephalitic diseases can, on occasion, localize to one area of the brain and mimic HSE (Whitley et al., 1989), as summarized in Table 43-1.

A distinction must be made clinically between viral encephalitis and postinfectious encephalomyelitis. Postinfectious encephalomyelitis generally follows a vague viral syndrome, usually of the respiratory tract, and is most common in children. Neurologic findings vary and reflect the areas of the brain involved. Demyelination is a prominent pathologic finding. The distinction between postinfectious encephalomyelitis and acute viral encephalitis is crucial, because the management and prognosis are often quite different.

TABLE 43-1	Diseases That Mimic Herpes Simplex Encephalitis

Diseases	Number of patients
Treatable (n = 46)	
Infection	
Abscess or subdural empyema	
• Bacterial	5
• Listeria	1
• Fungal	2
• Mycoplasma	2
Tuberculosis	6
Cryptococcal infection	3
Rickettsial infection	2
Toxoplasmosis	1
Mucormycosis	1
Meningococcal meningitis	1
Other viruses	
• Cytomegalovirus	1
• Influenza A*	4
• Echovirus infection*	3
Tumor	5
Subdural hematoma	2
Systemic lupus erythematosus	1
Adrenal leukodystrophy	6
Nontreatable (n = 49)	
Vascular disease	11
Toxic encephalopathy	5
Reye's syndrome	1
Viral (n = 40)	
Arbovirus infection	
• St. Louis encephalitis	7
• Western equine encephalitis	3
• California encephalitis	4
Eastern equine encephalitis	2
Other herpesviruses	
Epstein-Barr virus	8
Other viruses	
Mumps virus	3
Adenovirus	1
Progressive multifocal leukoencephalopathy (JC virus)	1
Lymphocytic choriomeningitis virus	1
Subacute sclerosing panencephalitis (measles virus)	2

Modified from Whitley RJ, Cobbs CG, Alford CA, Jr., et al: JAMA 1989;262:234-239.
*Investigational drug therapy.

Most patients have a prodromal illness with myalgias, fever, and anorexia reflecting the systemic viremia. The clinical hallmark of acute viral encephalitis is a triad of fever, headache, and altered level of consciousness. Other common clinical findings include disorientation, behavioral and speech disturbances, and focal or diffuse neurologic signs, such as hemiparesis or seizures. These clinical findings distinguish a patient with encephalitis from one with viral meningitis, who can have headache, nuchal rigidity, and fever, but not altered sensorium or focal neurologic findings. Clinical findings reflect the specific areas of CNS involvement, which is determined, in large part, by the tropism of different viruses for different cell types. For example, polioviruses preferentially infect motor neurons; rabies selectively infects neurons of the limbic system; and mumps can infect epithelial cells of the choroid plexus. Infection of cortical neurons results in abnormal electrical activity and can be associated with seizures or focal deficits. Demyelination may follow destruction of oligodendroglial cells, whereas involvement of ependymal cells can result in hydranencephaly. The predilection of HSV for temporal lobe involvement, as illustrated in Figure 43-1, leads to clinical findings of aphasia, anosmia, temporal lobe seizures, and other focal abnormalities. Only two viruses—rabies and B virus—produce encephalitis without significant meningeal involvement; however, most patients with encephalitis have a concomitant meningitis.

Laboratory Findings and Diagnosis

Establishing an etiologic diagnosis of encephalitis is just as difficult as for viral meningitis. As with the latter, epidemiologic features such as the season of year, prevalent diseases within the community, travel, recreational activities (e.g., caving or hiking), occupational exposures, and animal contacts (e.g., insect or animal bite) may provide helpful clues to the diagnosis. Late summer and early fall are seasons when enteroviral infections are encountered in temperate climates. Similarly, during warm summer months, mosquito propagation may enhance the likelihood of transmission of arthropod-borne viruses.

A CSF pleocytosis usually occurs in encephalitis but is not necessary for the diagnosis. WBC counts typically number in the 10s to 100s per cubic mm in viral encephalitis, although higher counts occur (Ho and Hirsch, 1985). The CSF glucose levels are usually normal, although some viral infections (Eastern equine encephalitis

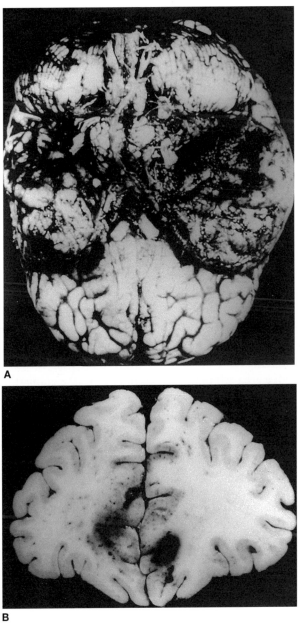

Fig. 43-1 Coronal section of brain from patient with herpes simplex encephalitis.

[EEE]) produce studies consistent with acute bacterial meningitis (Cassady and Whitley, 1997). Some viruses (HSV) produce a hemorrhagic necrosis, and the CSF exhibits this with moderately high protein levels and evidence of red blood cells. Supratentorial and cerebellar tumors can produce increased intracranial pressure and can mimic encephalitis. A careful fundoscopic examination should be performed to rule out any evidence of papilledema and increased intracranial pressure before CSF is obtained.

Unlike meningitis, encephalitis often requires additional laboratory and radiologic tests to establish the diagnosis. The clinical circumstances of the patient and the likely causative agent dictate specific laboratory and radiologic evaluations. Historically, the standard for diagnosis has been brain biopsy and viral culture. However, PCR has, for the most part, replaced this approach. For some viruses [HSV, enterovirus, VZV, Jamestown Canyon (JC) virus], PCR detection of viral nucleic acids from the CSF has replaced culture and brain biopsy as the standard for diagnosing encephalitis (D'Arminio et al., 1997; Fujimoto et al., 1998; Hosoya et al., 1998; Jeffery et al., 1997;

Poggio et al., 2000; Pozo et al., 1998; Read and Kurtz, 1999; van Vliet et al., 1998). Radiographic studies that support the diagnosis of focal encephalitis are computerized tomography (CT) scan and magnetic resonance imaging (MRI). The increased sensitivity of MRI to alterations in brain water content and the lack of bone artifacts make this the neuroradiologic modality of choice for CNS infections (Smith, 1992). MRI detects parenchymal changes earlier than CT and better defines the extent of a lesion (Smith, 1992). Furthermore, MRI is more sensitive for detecting evidence of demyelinating lesions in the periventricular and deep white matter, thus allowing the differentiation of parainfectious from acute viral encephalitis (Smith, 1992). Patients with viral encephalitis frequently have diffuse or focal epileptiform discharges with background slowing (Bale, 1993). These changes, seen on electroencephalogram (EEG), precede CT or MRI evidence of encephalitis and provide a sensitive, although nonspecific, diagnostic test. EEG changes in the temporal lobe area strongly suggests a diagnosis of HSE, but absence of these changes does not rule out HSE.

Historically, patients with viral encephalitis required a battery of different diagnostic tests. HSE, for example, could be diagnosed acutely by brain biopsy and viral culture or retrospectively by CSF antibody and convalescent serologic tests (Nahmias et al., 1982). Routine evaluation of acute and convalescence sera to demonstrate either seroconversion or seroboosting is of no practical value in the decision to institute treatment, but remains useful for retrospective diagnosis of some infections (e.g., arboviral encephalitis). New diagnostic assays have simplified the diagnosis of viral infections of the brain. For example, an enzyme-linked immunosorbent assay (ELISA) that detects IgM antibodies in the CSF from patients with presumed JE is both sensitive and specific, as most patients have antibodies at the time of hospitalization and virtually all patients have acquired them by the third day of illness.

A CSF PCR is used to diagnosis infection with enteroviruses, HSV, VZV, HHV-6, EBV, and CMV (Casas et al., 1999) as well as a few arboviruses (California encephalitis group, JE, West Nile virus [WNV], SLE, dengue fever virus types 1 to 4, and yellow fever virus); however, the development of universal arboviral primers has been difficult (Kuno, 1998; Pozo

et al., 1998; Read and Kurtz, 1999; van Vliet et al., 1998). The successful detection of viral DNA in the CSF is influenced by the duration, extent, and cause of disease. Application of PCR is rapid and sensitive and provides a less invasive means to diagnose encephalitis. For example, only 4% of CSF cultures are positive in patients with sporadic HSE; however, 53 of 54 patients with biopsy-proved HSE have evidence of HSV DNA in the CSF by PCR. Cerebrospinal fluid PCR has a sensitivity of >95% and a specificity approaching 100% in patients with HSE (Lakeman et al., 1995). In the three cases where the CSF PCR was positive but the brain biopsy negative, biopsy samples were improperly prepared before viral culture or the biopsy site was suboptimal (Lakeman et al., 1995). Efforts now focus on correlating viral nucleic acid copy number with clinical outcome (Domingues et al., 1997).

The TSEs are currently diagnosed only by histologic examination of brain tissue, characteristic EEG, MRI changes, and clinical correlation. A CSF examination shows normal values or slightly elevated protein levels. The EEG in classic CJD reveals generalized slowing early in the disease, punctuated by biphasic or triphasic peaks late in the disease with the onset of myoclonus. MRI changes late in the illness reveal global atrophy with hyperintense signal from the basal ganglia (Whitley et al., 2000). Fluid attenuation inversion recovery (FLAIR) MRI provides greater sensitivity and demonstrates signal intensity changes in the cortex that T2-weighted spin-echo MRI cannot detect (Vrancken et al., 2000). Histopathologic examination of the brain using a specific antibody to the PrP-res protein confirms the presence of the disease. In addition, evidence of gliosis, neuronal loss, and spongiform changes supports the diagnosis. In cases of vCJD, characteristic amyloid plaques (so-called florid plaques) microscopically define the disease. The florid plaques are not seen in other TSEs and consist of flowerlike amyloid deposits surrounded by vacuolar halos. The detection of PrP-res in the tonsillar tissue by immunohistochemical staining is also strongly supportive of the diagnosis of vCJD (Whitley et al., 2000).

Differential Diagnosis

Identifying treatable disease expeditiously is a priority in patients presenting with neurologic changes. In patients with suspected HSE undergoing brain biopsy for confirmation of disease, alternate diagnoses are frequently found. Of the 432 patients, only 45% had biopsy-confirmed HSE, and in 22% brain biopsy established another cause of the encephalitis (Whitley, 1989). Of these, 40% had a treatable disease (9% of the biopsy group), including bacterial abscess, tuberculosis, fungal infection, tumor, subdural hematoma, and autoimmune disease. Of the remaining 60%, the majority had identifiable but nontreatable encephalitis of viral origin. A third group of 142 patients (33%) went undiagnosed even after brain biopsy and the conventional diagnostic tests (Whitley et al., 1989), as summarized in Table 43-1.

More specifically, mass lesions in the CNS (tumor, abscess, or blood) can cause focal neurologic changes, fever, and seizures resembling the signs and symptoms of encephalitis. Metabolic disorders (e.g., hypoglycemia, uremia, inborn errors of metabolism) and toxin-mediated disorders (e.g., ingestions, tick paralysis, or Reye's syndrome) can cause decreased consciousness, seizures, and evidence of background slowing on EEG. Limbic encephalitis can produce protracted encephalitis and is caused by paraneoplastic phenomena. Treatable infectious causes of encephalitis must be vigorously investigated. *Mycoplasma* infection produces demyelinating brainstem encephalitis in approximately 0.1% of infections.

SELECTED CLINICAL SYNDROMES
Herpes Simplex Encephalitis

Human infection caused by HSV is ubiquitous, but encephalitis caused by this virus is, fortunately, uncommon. Nonetheless, HSE has played an important role in our understanding of viral infections of the CNS. HSE was one of the first human infections to be routinely diagnosed using methods of molecular biology (e.g., PCR for detection of HSV DNA in CSF), as noted previously (Boerman et al., 1989; Lakeman et al., 1995; Powell et al., 1990; Puchhammer-Stockl et al., 1990; Rowley et al., 1990). Furthermore, HSE is one of the first viral infections to be successfully treated with antiviral chemotherapy (Longson et al., 1983; Whitley et al., 1986).

HSV is the most common cause of nonepidemic, acute focal encephalitis in the United States (Whitley and Lakeman, 1995). The estimated frequency of occurrence is one case per 250,000 to 500,000 population annually. HSE occurs throughout the year; approximately one third of the cases of HSE develop in patients less than 20 years of age and one half in individuals over the age of 50. In the absence of effective antiviral therapy, the mortality for HSE is >70%, with only 2.5% of individuals returning to normal function.

Acyclovir is the treatment of choice for HSE, but morbidity and mortality remain high; mortality is 28% at 18 months after acyclovir treatment (Longson et al., 1983; McGrath et al., 1997). Age of the patient level of consciousness at presentation, and duration of encephalitis all influence the outcome in patients receiving acyclovir therapy. If the level of consciousness as measured by the Glasgow coma score was six or less, a poor outcome was uniform, irrespective of the age of the patient (Whitley, 1989). If disease was present for 4 or fewer days, the likelihood of survival increased from 65% to 100% among acyclovir recipients. At 2 years after treatment, 30% of acyclovir recipients were judged to be normal or mildly impaired, 9% had moderate sequelae, and 53% of the patients were dead or severely impaired. Relapse of HSV infection of the CNS following therapy occurs. From studies of neonatal HSE, approximately 8% of babies who received acyclovir had a documented virologic relapse if treated for 10 days at a dosage of 10 mg/kg every 8 hours. Relapse has not been documented when higher doses are administered for 21 days. The exact percentage of adults and older children who suffer relapse is unknown, but reports have suggested that relapse can occur following therapy and may be as high as 5% (Ito et al., 2000).

A distinction must be made between HSV infections of the CNS that occur during the neonatal period and infections in older children and adults. Beyond the neonatal period, the overwhelming majority of cases of HSV encephalitis are attributable to HSV-1. On the basis of serologic studies, approximately one third of these cases are caused by primary HSV-1 infection, and two thirds result from viral reactivation (Whitley, 1996). Studies in animal models have demonstrated reactivation of latent HSV from the trigeminal ganglia with transport of virus along nerves of the olfactory tract to the brain. The pathogenesis of HSV encephalitis in humans is not known. The possibility of reactivation of latent virus in brain tissue has not been excluded.

In contrast, neonates most often acquire HSV infection from virus shed in the maternal genital tract at the time of vaginal delivery. HSV-2 infection of the brain in newborns with multiorgan disseminated infection is likely blood borne and associated with a diffuse encephalitic process, resulting in generalized encephalomalacia. However, when disease involves only the CNS of the newborn, neuronal transmission of virus to the CNS initially results in unitemporal involvement that extends to bitemporal disease, as occurs in older children and adults. Babies with HSV type 1 infection of the CNS have a significantly better neurologic outcome than those with HSV type 2 infection. Recently, the use of a higher dose of acyclovir (20 mg/kg every 8 hours) for 21 days has decreased mortality to 5% for newborns with HSV encephalitis; approximately 40% of survivors develop normally. The reasons for the differences in the pathogenesis and tropism of HSV-1 and HSV-2 CNS infections are not well understood (Gerber et al., 1995; Vahlne et al., 1980).

B Virus

B virus (cercopithecine herpesvirus) causes enzootic infection of macaque monkeys that usually results in little or no disease in the animal (Jainkittivong et al., 1998). However, B virus can cause severe and fatal encephalitis in humans when transmitted by the bite or scratch of an infected macaque (Centers for Disease Control and Prevention, 1998b; Ostrowski et al., 1998). Human disease is characterized by a nonspecific prodrome of fever and malaise (possibly with herpetic blisters at the inoculation site), progressing to a rapidly ascending encephalomyelitis. The mortality rate for human encephalitis caused by B virus encephalitis is 50% to 70%. No evidence suggests that B virus can cause a subclinical infection in humans (Freifeld et al., 1995). Persons who experience a bite, scratch, or mucosal exposure from a potentially infected macaque should thoroughly decontaminate the wound. Prophylactic antiviral therapy is recommended for persons who have a high-risk exposure (Holmes et al., 1995). Because of the high mortality rate associated with B virus encephalitis, patients should be treated with intravenous acyclovir or ganciclovir, although the therapeutic experience with this disease is limited.

Rabies

Rabies, a zoonotic disease caused by a rhabdovirus, remains one of the very few human

infections with a mortality rate near 100%. Conversely, rabies can be readily prevented by judicious use of passive and active immunization, even after infection has occurred (Moran et al., 2000). In the developing world, infected dogs remain the primary vector for human rabies (Anonymous, 1997). In the United States and Western Europe, human infection is more likely due to exposure to bats or wild terrestrial mammals (Krebs et al., 2000). The incubation period for rabies in humans can range from 5 days to longer than 6 months, although the usual period is 20 to 60 days (Plotkin, 2000). After a prodromal period of fever, malaise, anxiety, and pain or itching at the site of the bite wound, patients with rabies develop overt CNS findings, which may be predominately encephalopathic or paralytic (Plotkin, 2000). The patient progresses to coma, cardiorespiratory failure, and ultimately to death. Other than supportive care, no therapy for human rabies is available. The best diagnostic method for laboratory confirmation is detection of rabies virus RNA in saliva by RT-PCR, which has high sensitivity and specificity (Hanlon et al., 1999; Noah et al., 1998). Alternative diagnostic methods include demonstration of virus antigens in biopsies of brain, nuchal skin, or corneal impressions. Medical management of rabies is focused on prevention. Veterinarians and other individuals who are at high-risk for exposure to rabies should be vaccinated. Unimmunized persons who have a risky exposure to a potentially rabid animal should receive postexposure vaccination with both human rabies immune globulin and rabies vaccine. Modern rabies vaccines produced in human tissue culture cell lines or avian embryo cultures are more efficacious and much better tolerated than older vaccines produced in animal nervous tissues (Benda and Polomik, 1969).

Since 1996, several deaths have been reported in Queensland, Australia from a rabieslike disease caused by Australian bat lyssavirus (ABL), which causes enzootic infection of flying foxes and other bats (Hanna et al., 2000; Samaratunga et al., 1998). Preexposure or postexposure administration of standard rabies vaccine appears to be protective against human infection with ABL.

Arthropod-Borne Encephalitis Viruses

Viruses transmitted to humans by the bites of arthropods (especially mosquitoes and ticks) are major causes of encephalitis worldwide, as illustrated in Table 43-2 (Griffin, 1990). These encephalitides are predominately caused by viruses from the Togavirus (e.g., EEE), Flavivirus (e.g., JE) and Bunyavirus (e.g., La Crosse encephalitis) families. An antigenically related group of Flaviviruses accounts for hundreds of thousands of cases of human infection around the globe each year. These include mosquito-borne diseases such as SLE (North America), Murray Valley encephalitis (Australia), WNV encephalitis (Africa and the Middle-East), and JE (Asia), as well as Far Eastern tick-borne encephalitis (Russia) and Western tick-borne encephalitis (Europe) (Whitley, 1990).

JE virus, transmitted by *Culex* mosquitoes, probably causes more cases of acute encephalitis than the other arthropod-borne viruses combined. Over the last 75 years, from its focus in China and Southeast Asia, JE has expanded westward to India and Pakistan, northward to eastern Russia, eastward to the Philippines, and

TABLE 43-2	**Arboviruses That Cause Encephalitis**	
Virus	*Vector*	*Geographic location*
Togaviridae		
Alphavirus		
Eastern equine	Mosquitoes *(Culiseta, Aedes)*	Eastern and Gulf coasts of United States, Caribbean, and South America
Western equine	Mosquitoes *(Culiseta, Culex)*	Western United States and Canada
Venezuelan equine	Mosquitoes *(Aedes, Culex, and others)*	South and Central America, Florida and Southwest United States
Flaviviridae		
West Nile complex		
St. Louis	Mosquitoes *(Culex)*	Widespread in United States
Japanese	Mosquitoes *(Culex)*	Japan, China, Southeast Asia, and India
Murray Valley	Mosquitoes *(Culex)*	Australia and New Guinea
West Nile	Mosquitoes *(Culex)*	United States, Africa, Europe, Middle East, and Asia
Ilheus	Mosquitoes *(Psorophora)*	South and Central America
Rocio	Mosquitoes (?)	Brazil
Tick-borne-complex		
Far Eastern	Ticks *(Ixodes)*	Eastern USSR
Central European	Ticks *(Ixodes)*	Central Europe
Kyasanur Forest	Ticks *(Haemophysalis)*	India
Louping-Ill	Ticks *(Ixodes)*	England, Scotland, and Northern Ireland
Powassan	Ticks *(Ixodes)*	Canada and Northern United States
Negishi	Ticks (?)	Japan
Bunyaviridae		
Bunyavirus		
California	Mosquitoes *(Aedes)*	Western United States
La Crosse	Mosquitoes *(Aedes)*	Mid and Eastern United States
Jamestown Canyon	Mosquitoes *(Culiseta)*	United States and Alaska
Snowshoe hare	Mosquitoes *(Culiseta)*	Canada, Alaska, and Northern United States
Tahyna	Mosquitoes *(Aedes, Culiseta)*	Czechoslovakia and Yugoslavia, Italy and Southern France
Inkoo	Mosquitoes (?)	Finland
Phlebovirus		
Rift Valley	Mosquitoes *(Culex, Aedes)*	East Africa
Reoviridae		
Orbivirus		
Colorado tick fever	Ticks *(Dermacentor)*	Rocky Mountains of United States

Modified from Griffin DE. In Galasso GJ, Whitley RJ, Merigan TC (eds). Antiviral agents and viral diseases of man. New York: Raven Press, 1990; 461-495.

southward to Australia. In the northern range, epidemics of JE can occur during the warm summer months, whereas in the warmer southern areas disease occurs throughout the year (Solomon et al., 2000). In China alone, at least 20,000 symptomatic cases of JE are reported annually (Vaughn and Hoke, 1992). The ratio of symptomatic to asymptomatic infections with JE virus is estimated to be 1:25 to 1:1,000 (Solomon et al., 2000). In areas where JE is common, it is primarily a disease of children, but more cases are seen in adults when the virus moves into a previously unexposed population. After a few days of nonspecific symptoms, patients with JE present with headache, vomiting, and altered mentation; seizures are reported in 85% of children and 10% of adults. Other characteristic findings include coarse tremor, dystonia, rigidity, and a characteristic masklike facies. A variant of JE that is associated with poliomyelitis-like acute flaccid paralysis has recently been reported (Solomon et al., 1998a). MRI reveals a characteristic pattern of mixed intensity or hypodense lesions, especially in the thalamus but also in basal ganglia and midbrain (Kalita and Mista, 2000). Diagnosis is facilitated by detection of IgM in CSF (Solomon et al., 1998b). The mortality rate for patients hospitalized with JE is about 30%. Approximately 50% of survivors have severe neurologic sequelae, including motor weakness, intellectual impairment, and seizure disorders. Therapy for JE is limited to intensive supportive care. An effective formalin-inactivated vaccine against JE is available and is recommended for inhabitants of endemic areas as well as travelers entering rural endemic areas (Centers for Disease Control and Prevention, 1993). An attenuated live virus vaccine for JE has been developed in China, but is less widely available than the inactivated vaccine (Tsai et al., 1998b).

In the United States, most cases of arthropod-borne encephalitis in recent years have been attributed to La Crosse virus, EEE, and SLE (Table 43-3). La Crosse virus, a bunyavirus in the California encephalitis serogroup, causes aseptic meningitis and encephalitis, primarily in school-aged children. Although the mortality rate associated with La Crosse encephalitis is low, 10% to 15% of survivors have significant neurologic deficits (McJunkin et al., 1998; McJunkin et al., 2001). EEE occurs during the summer months along the eastern and Gulf coasts of the United States. In contrast to La Crosse encephalitis, EEE frequently occurs among older adults. Patients with EEE experience a short prodromal illness, then fever, headache, and generalized seizures; the illness may progress to include stupor or coma (Deresiewicz et al., 1997). MRI reveals focal lesions in the basal ganglia, thalami, and brain stem. The mortality rate is 30% to 40%, and at least one third of survivors have significant neurologic sequelae. High CSF white count ($>500/mm^3$) and low serum sodium (≤130 mmol/l) are associated with poor outcome (Deresiewicz et al., 1997).

Beginning in August 1999, an epidemic of viral encephalitis occurred in and around New York City that ultimately resulted in 62 cases and 7 deaths. On the basis of positive serologic results, the outbreak was initially attributed to SLE. However, a simultaneous epidemic of deaths among wild and exotic captive birds suggested that SLE virus (which does not ordinarily kill the avian host) might not be the correct pathogen. Ultimately, the etiologic agent was identified as WNV (Centers for Disease Control and Prevention, 1999a). WNV encephalitis is a well-described disease in Africa and the Middle East but had not previously been encountered in the western hemisphere. As a harbinger of the appearance of WNV in North America, the first major WNV epidemic in Europe occurred in Romania in 1996 and was characterized by a high rate of neurologic complications (Tsai et al., 1998a). Using hospital-based surveillance, 393 confirmed cases of WNV infection were identified in Romania; most of these patients had meningoencephalitis. The mortality rate clearly increased with age; the overall fatality/case ratio was 4.3%, with all deaths occurring in patients over 50 years of age. The number of mild cases occurring in the Romanian population could not be calculated, but the overall seroprevalence rate was 4.1%. Clinical findings were similar in the Romanian and New York outbreaks. Patients typically had abrupt onset of fever, headache, neck stiffness, and vomiting. Patients who progressed to encephalitis demonstrated depressed consciousness, disorientation, and generalized weakness. In both Romania and the United States, additional cases of WNV infection appeared during the following summer, with geographic expansion of human and animal infections proving successful over-wintering of WNV and estab-

TABLE 43-3 Characteristics of Selected Mosquito-Borne Arbovirus Encephalitides in the United States

Characteristic	Western equine	Eastern equine	Venezuelan	St. Louis	La Crosse	West Nile
Geographic distribution	Western, Midwest U.S.	Eastern, Gulf Coast, Southern U.S.	South America, Southern U.S.	Central, Western, Southern U.S.	Central, Eastern U.S.	East Coast U.S., Africa, Middle East, Europe
Age group affected	Infants and adults >50 yr old	Children and adults	Adults	Adults >50 yr old	Children	Adults
Mortality (%)	5-15	30-40	1	2-20	<1	<5
Sequelae	Moderate in infants; low in others	>30% of survivors	Rare	20% of survivors	10%-15%	Low
Symptoms	Headache, altered consciousness, seizures	Headache, altered consciousness, seizures	Headache, myalgia, pharyngitis	Headache, nausea, vomiting, disorientation, stupor, irritability	Seizures, paralysis, focal weakness	Seizures, myelitis, optic neuritis

Modified from Whitley RJ: N Engl J Med 1990;323:242-250.

lishment of an enzootic cycle of transmission involving birds and mosquitoes (Centers for Disease control and Prevention, 2001; Cernescu et al., 2000). The pattern of recent epidemics of WNV in Europe and North America indicates that migratory birds contribute to dispersion of the virus, suggesting that WNV has the potential to cause new outbreaks (Hubalek and Halouzka, 1999). In the summer of 2000, an unexpectedly large outbreak of WNV encephalitis occurred in Israel, with more than 250 confirmed cases and 19 deaths, all in patients over the age of 50 years (Siegel-Itzkovich, 2000). There is currently no vaccine to prevent WNV infection. Preventive measures include vector avoidance and mosquito-control programs (Centers for Disease Control and Prevention, 2000).

Enteroviral Infections

Enteroviruses (including polioviruses, coxsackieviruses, and echoviruses) cause a wide spectrum of human diseases, including myocarditis and pericarditis, exanthems and enanthems, conjunctivitis, and meningitis, most of which are mild and self-limited. However, certain of the enteroviruses have the potential to cause severe and even fatal neurologic disease, the best known of which is poliomyelitis. Other enteroviruses are frequent causes of seasonal aseptic meningitis and (less commonly) meningoencephalitis, especially in young infants. In 1998, a large outbreak of enteroviral infection (hand-foot-and-mouth disease and herpangina) occurred in Taiwan, with over 60% of the cases attributed to enterovirus 71 (Ho et al., 1999). What distinguished this enteroviral epidemic was the high rate of neurologic complications among children infected with enterovirus 71 (Huang et al., 1999). A total of 405 patients with serious enteroviral infection were identified. Most were under 5 years of age, and the mortality rate in this group was 19.3%. Among patients with positive viral cultures, enterovirus 71 was isolated from 75% of the hospitalized patients and from 92% of the patients who died (Ho et al., 1999). The typical clinical presentation was rhombencephalitis, characterized by myoclonus, tremors, ataxia, and cranial nerve involvement (Huang et al., 1999). The most severely affected children presented with evidence of brain stem involvement (including neurogenic shock and pulmonary edema), which indicated a poor prognosis (Wang et al.,

1999). MRI demonstrated distinctive high-intensity lesions localized to the midbrain, pons, and medulla (Wang et al., 1999). Long-term neurologic sequelae were frequent among the children with rhombencephalitis who survived. Although other outbreaks of enterovirus 71 disease have been reported, none have had the level of serious neurologic involvement seen in the Taiwanese epidemic. There is currently no vaccine (other than for polio) or approved antiviral treatment for enteroviral infections, although the antiviral drug pleconaril shows promise and is currently undergoing clinical evaluation (Pevear et al., 1999).

New Paramyxoviruses: Nipah and Hendra Viruses

In 1997, an outbreak of encephalitis was noted among pig farm workers in Malaysia but was attributed to JE. Encephalitis recurred in September 1998, and both clinical and epidemiologic characteristics made it clear that JE was not the correct diagnosis. A paramyxovirus isolated from a Malaysian patient with encephalitis demonstrated in vitro characteristics similar to Hendra virus, a new morbillivirus previously isolated from horses and humans in Australia in 1995 (Selvey et al., 1995). Subsequent virologic studies have shown that the Malaysian pathogen, now named *Nipah virus*, is closely related to but distinct from Hendra virus and that the two belong to a new genus within the family Paramyxoviridae (Chua et al., 2000). Epidemiologic investigations demonstrated that Nipah virus is transmitted to humans by close contact with infected pigs, probably via the respiratory route (Goh et al., 2000). The infection does not require an insect vector and is not readily transmitted from person-to-person. Presenting signs and symptoms of patients with Nipah virus encephalitis include fever, headache, dizziness, vomiting, and altered mental status (Goh et al., 2000; Paton et al., 1999). Clinical features such as hypertension, tachycardia, areflexia, and hypotonia suggest brain stem involvement. MRI scanning shows a distinctive picture of discrete 2- to 7-mm lesions disseminated throughout the brain but occurring mainly in the subcortical and deep white matter of the cerebral hemispheres (Sarji et al., 2000). Pathologic correlation suggests that the lesions seen on MRI are due to widespread microinfarctions resulting from small vessel vasculitis (Chua et al., 1999). Among 94 patients hospitalized with Nipah virus encephalitis in Malaysia from February to June 1999, 32% died, 53% had full recovery, and 15% of survivors had persistent neurologic deficits (Goh et al., 2000). Aggressive culling of all infected or exposed pigs terminated the epidemic. As with Hendra, the natural reservoir for Nipah virus appears to be pteropid bats, with pigs serving as hosts for viral amplification (Enserink, 2000).

PREVENTION

Prevention remains the mainstay of therapy. Historically the most frequent cause of viral CNS disease, mumps, has largely been eliminated through vaccination. Live attenuated vaccines against measles, mumps, and rubella have resulted in a dramatic decrease in the incidence of encephalitis in industrialized countries. Measles continues to be the leading cause of postinfectious encephalitis in developing countries, however, and complicates 1 of every 1,000 measles infection (Johnson, 1987). Vaccination has also changed the incidence of previously common viral CNS disease. In 1952, poliomyelitis affected 57,879 Americans. Widespread vaccination has eradicated the disease currently from the western hemisphere (Centers for Disease Control and Prevention, 1994b). Vaccines exist for some arboviral infections. Vaccination against JE virus has reduced the incidence of encephalitis in Asia; however, in China where 70 million children are immunized for JE, 10,000 cases still occur annually (Rosen, 1986).

Vaccination is not cost effective for preventing all viral infections. For example, vector avoidance, the use of mosquito deterrents, and mosquito abatement programs provide less costly strategies for preventing arboviral encephalitides in the United States (Bale, 1993; Centers for Disease Control and Prevention, 1998a). Preexposure and immediate postexposure prophylaxis are the only ways known to prevent death in rabies-exposed individuals (Mrak and Young, 1994). Case reports exist of patients surviving symptomatic rabies, but all of these patients had some prior immunity or received postexposure prophylaxis prior to developing symptoms, as discussed above. The U.S. Food and Drug Administration has implemented guidelines eliminating whole blood or blood components

prepared from individuals who later developed CJD or vCJD. Changes in the agricultural practices in Europe and bans on infected cattle have led to a decline in cases of vCJD. In North America one case of vCJD has been reported in the United States and one in Canada. The U.S. Department of Agriculture has programs in place to monitor for TSEs in livestock.

TREATMENT

Patients with encephalitis, depending on the cause and the extent of CNS involvement, require treatment tailored to their clinical situation. Currently few antiviral medications are available to treat CNS infections. Antiviral therapy exists for HSV-1, HSV-2, VZV, CMV, and HIV infections. The introduction of acyclovir and vidarabine has resulted in a sharp decline in mortality and morbidity from herpes infections. Neonatal mortality from disseminated HSV disease and HSE has declined from 70% to 40% since the development of acyclovir and vidarabine (Kimberlin et al., 2001a; Kimberlin et al., 2001b). Varicella immunoglobulin (VZIG) and acyclovir have reduced the complications from primary VZV infection and zoster in the neonate and immunocompromised patient. Although controlled trials have not evaluated the efficacy of acyclovir in VZV encephalitis, the medication is routinely used to treat this complication (Balfour, 1993; Cinque et al., 1997). With the increase of HIV infection, diseases previously limited to the neonatal and postnatal period now occur with increasing frequency in the adult population. Ganciclovir and foscarnet are used for the treatment of CMV encephalitis, although controlled clinical trials have not confirmed the efficacy of treatment (Maschke et al., 2000; Soontornniyomkij et al., 1998). In cases of postinfectious encephalitis, no randomized controlled trial has confirmed the benefit of immunomodulatory drugs. In practice clinicians often treat postinfectious encephalitis with different immunomodulators in an attempt to limit T-cell–mediated destruction of the CNS (Balestri et al., 2000; Pradhan et al., 1999; Stuve and Zamvil, 1999). It is important to note that no placebo-controlled studies have been performed, and immunomodulatory therapy is based simply on isolated case reports. As with most case reports, clinical failures and iatrogenic morbidity from a therapeutic modality are rarely ever reported.

CONCLUSION

Numerous factors influence the clinical manifestations of viral CNS infections. An individual's age, immune history, cultural practices, and genetic make-up can influence the clinical expression of viral infection as readily as the viral serotype, receptor preference, viral load, and cell tropism (Cassady and Whitley, 1997). Changes in behavior, in cultural beliefs, increased travel, and the modification of environment alter disease patterns and expose individuals to new infectious agents. Infections of the CNS, therefore, must be examined in a geographic, cultural, and environmental context as well as at the cellular, molecular, and genetic levels (Briese et al., 1999; Lanciotti et al., 1999). Contemporary disease changes are relevant. The last 5 years have seen an outbreak of a deadly and previously unknown encephalitis virus (Nipah), dramatic extension of the range of a well-known arbovirus (WNV), and unexpected neurovirulence from a common pediatric pathogen (enterovirus 71). Each of these outbreaks suggests the high probability of future epidemics of encephalitis caused by previously unknown pathogens or novel manifestations of known agents. The Nipah virus epidemic highlights the potential for amplification of zoonotic viruses when agricultural practices force huge numbers of animals into close quarters, creating an ideal environment for exchange of pathogens. The WNV outbreak in the United States demonstrates how a pathogen can suddenly appear on the other side of the world. Although WNV is naturally spread to new regions by migratory birds, there is at least the suspicion that the New York outbreak could have originated with illegal importation of infected birds. These scenarios suggest the need for clinicians to develop a broad differential diagnosis when evaluating a new patient with viral encephalitis of acute onset. Improvements in our ability to diagnose CNS infections will produce a better understanding of the pathogenesis and true extent of CNS viral disease.

BIBLIOGRAPHY

Abbott NJ. Inflammatory mediators and modulation of blood-brain barrier permeability. Cell Mol Neurobiol 2000;20:131-147.

Abzug M, Keyserling HL, Lee ML, et al. Neonatal enterovirus infection: virology, serology, and effects of intravenous immunoglobulin. Clin Infect Dis 1995;20:1201-1206.

Ahmed A, Brito F, Goto C, et al. Clinical utility of the polymerase chain reaction for diagnosis of enteroviral meningitis in infancy. J Pediatr 1997;131:393-397.

Anonymous. World survey of rabies, 1997. Wkly Epidemiol Rec 1999;74:381-384.

Arisoy ES, Demmler GJ, Thaker S, Doerr C. Meningitis due to parainfluenza virus type 3: report of two cases and review. Clin Infect Dis 1993;17:995-997.

Bale JF, Jr. Viral encephalitis. Med Clin North Am 1993;77:25-42.

Balestri P, Grosso S, Acquaviva A, Bernini M. Plasmapheresis in a child affected by acute disseminated encephalomyelitis. Brain Dev 2000;22:123-126.

Balfour HH, Jr. Current management of varicella zoster virus infections. J Med Virol 1993;suppl(1):74-81.

Barnett EM, Cassell D, Perlman S. Two neurotropic viruses, herpes simplex virus type 1 and mouse hepatitis virus, spread along different neural pathways from the main olfactory bulb. Neuroscience 1993;57:1007-1025.

Barnett EM, Jacobsen G, Evans G, et al. Herpes simplex encephalitis in the temporal cortex and limbic system after trigeminal nerve inoculation. J Infect Dis 1994;169:782-786.

Becher B, Prat A, Antel JP. Brain-immune connection: immunoregulatory properties of CNS-resident cells. Glia 2000;29:293-304.

Benda R, Polomik F. Course of air-borne infection caused by B virus (Herpesvirus simiae). I. Lethal inhalation dose of B virus for rabbits. J Hyg Epidemiol Microbiol Immunol 1969;13:24-30.

Bergstrom T, Vahlne A, Alestig K, et al. Primary and recurrent herpes simplex virus type 2 induced meningitis. J Infect Dis 1990;162:322-330.

Boerman RH, Arnoldus EP, Raap AK. Polymerase chain reaction and viral culture techniques to detect HSV in small volumes of cerebrospinal fluid; an experimental mouse encephalitis study. J Virol Methods 1989;25:189-197.

Bradbury MW. The blood-brain barrier. Exp Physiol 1993;78:453-472.

Briese T, Jia XY, Huang C, et al. Identification of a Kunjin/West Nile-like flavivirus in brains of patients with New York encephalitis. Lancet 1999;354:1261-1262.

Casas I, Pozo F, Trallero G, et al. Viral diagnosis of neurological infection by RT multiplex PCR: a search for entero- and herpesviruses in a prospective study. J Med Virol 1999;57:145-151.

Cassady KA, Whitley KJ. Pathogenesis and pathophysiology of viral central nervous system infections. In Scheld WM, Whitley RJ, Durack DT (eds). Infections of the Central Nervous System. New York: Raven Press, 1997.

Centers for Disease Control and Prevention. Inactivated Japanese encephalitis virus vaccine. Recommendations of the Advisory Committee on Immunization Practices (ACIP). MMWR Morb Mortal Wkly Rep 1993;42:1-15.

Centers for Disease Control and Prevention. Summary of notifiable diseases, United States, 1994. MMWR Morb Mortal Wkly Rep 1994a;43:1-98.

Centers for Disease Control and Prevention. Expanded program on immunization. Certification of poliomyelitis eradication—the Americas. MMWR Morb Mortal Wkly Rep 1994b;43:720-722.

Centers for Disease Control and Prevention. Arboviral infections of the central nervous system—United States, 1996-1997. MMWR Morb Mortal Wkly Rep 1998a;47:517-522.

Centers for Disease Control and Prevention. Fatal cercopithecine herpesvirus 1 (B virus) infection following a mucocutaneous exposure and interim recommendations for worker protection. MMWR Morb Mortal Wkly Rep 1998b;47:1073-1076.

Centers for Disease Control and Prevention. Outbreak of West Nile–like viral encephalitis—New York, 1999. MMWR Morb Mortal Wkly Rep 1999a;48:845-849.

Centers for Disease Control and Prevention. Summary of notifiable diseases, United States, 1998. MMWR Morb Mortal Wkly Rep 1999b;47:1-116.

Centers for Disease Control and Prevention. Guidelines for surveillance, prevention, and control of West Nile virus infection—United States. MMWR Morb Mortal Wkly Rep 2000;49:25-28.

Centers for Disease Control and Prevention. Human West Nile virus surveillance—Connecticut, New Jersey, and New York, 2000. MMWR Morb Mortal Wkly Rep 2001;50:265-268.

Cernescu C, Nedelcu NI, Tardei G, et al. Continued transmission of West Nile virus to humans in southeastern Romania, 1997-1998. J Infect Dis 2000;181:710-712.

Chua KB, Bellini WJ, Rota PA, et al. Nipah virus: a recently emergent deadly paramyxovirus. Science 2000;288: 1432-1435.

Chua KB, Goh KJ, Wong KT, et al. Fatal encephalitis due to Nipah virus among pig-farmers in Malaysia. Lancet 1999;354:1257-1259.

Cinque P, Bossolasco S, Vago L, et al. Varicella-zoster virus (VZV) DNA in cerebrospinal fluid of patients infected with human immunodeficiency virus: VZV disease of the central nervous system or subclinical reactivation of VZV infection. Clin Infect Dis 1997;25:634-639.

Conway JH, Weinberg A, Ashley RL, et al. Viral meningitis in a preadolescent child caused by reactivation of latent herpes simplex (type 1). Pediatr Infect Dis J 1997;16:627-629.

Corey L, Adams HG, Brown ZA, Holmes KK. Genital herpes simplex virus infections: clinical manifestations, course and complications. Ann Intern Med 1983;98: 958-972.

Cunningham CK, Bonville CA, Ochs HD, et al. Enteroviral meningoencephalitis as a complication of X-linked hyper IgM syndrome. J Pediatr 1999;134:584-588.

D'Arminio MA, Cinque P, Vago L, et al. A comparison of brain biopsy and CSF-PCR in the diagnosis of CNS lesions in AIDS patients. J Neurol 1997;244:35-39.

De La BA, Rozenberg F, Caumes E, et al. Neurological complications of varicella-zoster virus infection in adults with human immunodeficiency virus infection. Scand J Infect Dis 2000;32:263-269.

Deresiewicz RL, Thaler SJ, Hsu L, Zamani AA. Clinical and neuroradiographic manifestations of eastern equine encephalitis. N Engl J Med 1997;336:1867-1874.

de Silva SM, Mark AS, Gilden DH, et al. Zoster myelitis: improvement with antiviral therapy in two cases. Neurology 1996;47:929-931.

Domingues RB, Lakeman FD, Pannuti CS, et al. Advantage of polymerase chain reaction in the diagnosis of herpes simplex encephalitis: presentation of 5 atypical cases. Scand J Infect Dis 1997;29:229-231.

Dwyer JM, Erlendsson K. Intraventricular gamma-globulin for the management of enterovirus encephalitis. Pediatr Infect Dis J 1988;7:S30-S33.

Echevarria JM, Casas I, Martinez-Martin P. Infections of the nervous system caused by varicella-zoster virus: a review. Intervirology 1997;40:72-84.

Echevarria JM, Casas I, Tenorio A, et al. Detection of varicella-zoster virus-specific DNA sequences in cerebrospinal fluid from patients with acute aseptic meningitis and no cutaneous lesions. J Med Virol 1994;43:331-335.

Edens HA, Parkos CA. Modulation of epithelial and endothelial paracellular permeability by leukocytes. Adv Drug Deliv Rev 2000;41:315-328.

Enserink M. Emerging diseases. Malaysian researchers trace Nipah virus outbreak to bats. Science 2000;289: 518-519.

Feigin RD, Shackelford PG. Value of repeat lumbar puncture in the differential diagnosis of meningitis. N Engl J Med 1973;289:571-574.

Freifeld AG, Hilliard J, Southers J, et al. A controlled seroprevalence survey of primate handlers for evidence of asymptomatic herpes B virus infection. J Infect Dis 1995;171:1031-1034.

Fujimoto S, Kobayashi M, Uemura O, et al. PCR on cerebrospinal fluid to show influenza-associated acute encephalopathy or encephalitis. Lancet 1998;352:873-875.

Gatmaitan BG, Chason JL, Lerner AM. Augmentation of the virulence of murine coxsackie-virus B-3 myocardiopathy by exercise. J Exp Med 1970;131:1121-36.

Gerber SI, Belval BJ, Herold BC. Differences in the role of glycoprotein C of HSV-1 and HSV-2 in viral binding may contribute to serotype differences in cell tropism. Virology 1995;214:29-39.

Gilden DH, Kleinschmidt-DeMasters BK, LaGuardia JJ, et al. Neurologic complications of the reactivation of varicella-zoster virus. N Engl J Med 2000;342:635-645.

Goh KJ, Tan CT, Chew NK, et al. Clinical features of Nipah virus encephalitis among pig farmers in Malaysia. N Engl J Med 2000;342:1229-1235.

Goldsmith K, Chen W, Johnson DC, Hendricks RL. Infected cell protein (ICP) 47 enhances herpes simplex virus neurovirulence by blocking the CD8+ T cell response. J Exp Med 1998;187:341-348.

Griffin DE. Viral infections of the central nervous system. In Galasso GJ, Whitley RJ, Merigan TC (eds). Antiviral Agents and Viral Diseases of Man. New York: Raven Press, 1990.

Griffin DE, Levine B, Tyor WR, et al. Age-dependent susceptibility to fatal encephalitis: alphavirus infection of neurons. Arch Virol 1994;9(suppl):31-39.

Hammer SM, Connolly KJ. Viral aseptic meningitis in the United States: clinical features, viral etiologies, and differential diagnosis. Curr Clin Top Infect Dis 1992;12:1-25.

Hanlon CA, Smith JS, Anderson GR. Recommendation of a national working group on prevention and control of rabies in the United States. Article II: Laboratory diagnosis of rabies. The National Working Group on Rabies Prevention and Control. J Am Vet Med Assoc 1999;215: 1444-1446.

Hanna JN, Carney IK, Smith GA, et al. Australian bat lyssavirus infection: a second human case with a long incubation period. Med J Aust 2000;172:597-599.

Ho DD, Hirsch MS. Acute viral encephalitis. Med Clin North Am 1985;69:415-429.

Ho M, Chen ER, Hsu KH, et al. An epidemic of enterovirus 71 infection in Taiwan. Taiwan Enterovirus Epidemic Working Group. N Engl J Med 1999;341:929-935.

Holmes GP, Chapman LE, Stewart JE, et al. Guidelines for preventing and treating B virus infections in exposed persons. Clin Infect Dis 1995;20:421-439.

Hosoya M, Honzumi K, Sato M, et al. Application of PCR for various neurotropic viruses on the diagnosis of viral meningitis. J Clin Virol 1998;11:117-124.

Huang CC, Liu CC, Chang YC, et al. Neurologic complications in children with enterovirus 71 infection. N Engl J Med 1999;341:936-942.

Hubalek Z, Halouzka J. West Nile fever—a reemerging mosquito-borne viral disease in Europe. Emerg Infect Dis 1999;5:643-650.

Ito Y, Kimura H, Yabuta Y, et al. Exacerbation of herpes simplex encephalitis after successful treatment with acyclovir. Clin Infect Dis 2000;30:185-187.

Jainkittivong A, Langlais RP. Herpes B virus infection. Oral Surg Oral Med Oral Pathol Oral Radiol Endod 1998;85:399-403.

Jeffery KJ, Read SJ, Peto TE, et al. Diagnosis of viral infections of the central nervous system: clinical interpretation of PCR results. Lancet 1997;349:313-317.

Jensenius M, Myrvang B, Storvold G, et al. Herpes simplex virus type 2 DNA detected in cerebrospinal fluid of 9 patients with Mollaret's meningitis. Acta Neurol Scand 1998;98:209-212.

Johnson R. The pathogenesis of herpes virus encephalitis. II. A cellular basis for the development of resistance with age. J Exp Med 1964;120:359-374.

Johnson RT. The pathogenesis of acute viral encephalitis and postinfectious encephalitis. J Infect Dis 1987;155:359-364.

Kalita J, Mista UK. Comparison of CT scan and MRI findings in the diagnosis of Japanese encephalitis. J Neurol Sci 2000;174:3-8.

Kimberlin DW, Lin C-Y, Jacobs RF, et al. The safety and efficacy of high-dose intravenous acyclovir in the management of neonatal herpes simplex virus infections. Pediatrics 2001a;108:230-238.

Kimberlin DW, Lin C-Y, Jacobs RF, et al. Natural history of neonatal herpes simplex virus infections in the acyclovir era. Pediatrics 2001b;108:223-229.

Kimura H, Futamura M, Kito H, et al. Detection of viral DNA in neonatal herpes simplex virus infections: Frequent and prolonged presence in serum and cerebrospinal fluid. J Infect Dis 1991;164:289-293.

Koskiniemi M, Korppi M, Mustonen K, et al. Epidemiology of encephalitis in children. A prospective multicenter study. Eur J Pediatr 1997;156:541-545.

Krebs JW, Smith JS, Rupprecht CE, et al. Rabies surveillance in the United States during 1998. J Am Vet Med Assoc 2000;215:1786-1798.

Kuno G. Universal diagnostic RT-PCR protocol for arboviruses. J Virol Methods 1998;72:27-41.

Lakeman FD, Whitley RJ, National Institute of Allergy and Infectious Diseases Collaborative Antiviral Study Group. Diagnosis of herpes simplex encephalitis: application of polymerase chain reaction to cerebrospinal fluid from brain biopsied patients and correlation with disease. J Infect Dis 1995;172:857-863.

Lanciotti RW, Roehrig JT, Deubel V, et al. Origin of West Nile virus responsible for an outbreak on encephalitis in the northeastern United States. Science 1999;286:2333-2337.

Lentz TL. The recognition event between virus and host cell receptor: a target for antiviral agents. J Gen Virol 1990;71:751-766.

Longson M, Klapper PE, Cleator GM. The treatment of herpes encephalitis. J Infect 1983;6:15-16.

Maschke M, Kastrup O, Esser S, et al. Incidence and prevalence of neurological disorders associated with HIV since the introduction of highly active antiretroviral therapy (HAART). Neurol Neurosurg Psychiatry 2000;69:376-380.

McGrath N, Anderson NE, Croxson MC, et al. Herpes simplex encephalitis treated with acyclovir: diagnosis and long term outcome. J Neurol Neurosurg Psychiatry 1997;63:321-326.

McJunkin JE, de los Reyes EC, Irazuzta JE, et al. La Crosse encephalitis in children. N Engl J Med 2001;344:801-807.

McJunkin JE, Khan RR, ,Tsai TF. California-La Crosse encephalitis. Infect Dis Clin North Am 1998;12:83-93.

McKinney RE, Katz SL. Chronic enteroviral meningoencephalitis in agammaglobulinemic patients. Rev Infect Dis 1987;9:334-356.

Moorthi S, Schneider WN, Dombovy ML. Rehabilitation outcomes in encephalitis—a retrospective study, 1990-1997. Brain Inj 1999;13:139-145.

Moran GJ, Talan DA, Mower W, et al. Appropriateness of rabies postexposure prophylaxis treatment for animal exposures. Emergency ID Net Study Group. JAMA 2000;284:1001-1007.

Mrak RE, Young L. Rabies encephalitis in humans: pathology, pathogenesis and pathophysiology. J Neuropathol Exp Neurol 1994;53:1-10.

Nagy Z, Martinez K. Astrocytic induction of endothelial tight junctions. Ann NY Acad Sci 1991;633:395-404.

Nahmias AJ, Whitley RJ, Visintine AN, et al. National Institute of Allergy and Infectious Diseases Collaborative Antiviral Study Group. Herpes simplex encephalitis: laboratory evaluations and their diagnostic significance. J Infect Dis 1982;145:829-836.

Negrini B, Kelleher KJ, Wald ER. Cerebrospinal fluid findings in aseptic versus bacterial meningitis. Pediatrics 2000;105:316-319.

Nicolosi A, Hauser WA, Beghi E, Kurland LT. Epidemiology of central nervous system infections in Olmsted County, Minnesota, 1950-1981. J Infect Dis 1986;154:399-408.

Nigrovic LE, Chiang VW. Cost analysis of enteroviral polymerase chain reaction in infants with fever and cerebrospinal fluid pleocytosis. Arch Pediatr Adolesc Med 1986;154:817-821.

Noah DL, Drenzek CL, Smith JS, et al. Epidemiology of human rabies in the United States, 1980 to 1996. Ann Intern Med 1998;128:922-930.

Ostrowski SR, Leslie MJ, Parrott T, et al. B virus from pet macaque monkeys: an emerging threat in the United States? Emerg Infect Dis 1998;4:117-121.

Pape WJ, Fitzsimmons TD, Hoffman RE. Risk for rabies transmission from encounters with bats, Colorado, 1977-1996. Emerg Infect Dis 1999;5:433-437.

Paton NI, Leo YS, Zaki SR, et al. Outbreak of Nipah-virus infection among abattoir workers in Singapore. Lancet 1999;354:1253-1256.

Pevear DC, Tull TM, Seipel ME, Groarke JM. Activity of pleconaril against enteroviruses. Antimicrob Agents Chemother 1999;43:2109-2115.

Plotkin SA. Rabies. Clin Infect Dis 2000;30:4-12.

Poggio GP, Rodriguez C, Cisterna D, et al. Nested PCR for rapid detection of mumps virus in cerebrospinal fluid from patients with neurological diseases. J Clin Microbiol 2000;38:274-278.

Powell KF, Anderson NE, Frith RW, et al. Non-invasive diagnosis of herpes simplex encephalitis. Lancet 1990;335:357-358.

Pozo F, Casas I, Tenorio A, et al. Evaluation of a commercially available reverse transcription-PCR assay for diagnosis of enteroviral infection in archival and prospectively collected cerebrospinal fluid specimens. J Clin Microbiol 1998;36:1741-1745.

Pradhan S, Gupta RP, Shashank S, et al. Intravenous immunoglobulin therapy in acute disseminated encephalomyelitis. J Neurol Sci 1999;165:56-61.

Pruisner SB. Novel proteinaceous infectious particles cause scrapie. Science 1982;216:136-144.

Puchhammer-Stockl E, Popow-Kraupp T, Heinz FX, et al. Establishment of PCR for the early diagnosis of herpes simplex encephalitis. J Med Virol 1990;32:77-82.

Ramers C, Billman G, Hartin M, et al. Impact of a diagnostic cerebrospinal fluid enterovirus polymerase chain reaction test on patient management. JAMA 2000;283:2680-2685.

Rappole JH, Derrickson SR, Hubalek Z. Migratory birds and spread of West Nile virus in the Western Hemisphere. Emerg Infect Dis 2000;6:319-328.

Read SJ, Kurtz JB. Laboratory diagnosis of common viral infections of the central nervous system by using a single multiplex PCR screening assay. J Clin Microbiol 1999;37:1352-1355.

Rorabaugh ML, Berlin LE, Heldrich F, et al. Aseptic meningitis in infants younger than 2 years of age: acute illness and neurologic complications. Pediatrics 1993;92:206-211.

Rosen L. The natural history of Japanese encephalitis virus. Annu Rev Microbiol 1986;40:395-414.

Rotbart HA. Enteroviral infections of the central nervous system. Clin Infect Dis 1995;20:971-981.

Rotbart HA. Antiviral therapy for enteroviral infections. Pediatr Infect Dis J 1999;18:632-633.

Rotbart HA. Viral meningitis and the aseptic meningitis syndrome. In Scheld WM, Whitley RJ, Durack DT (eds). Infections of the Central Nervous System. Philadelphia: Lippincott-Raven, 1997.

Rotbart HA, Brennan PJ, Fife KH, et al. Enterovirus meningitis in adults. Clin Infect Dis 1998;27:896-898.

Rowley A, Lakeman F, Whitley, et al. Rapid detection of herpes simplex virus DNA in cerebrospinal fluid of patients with herpes simplex encephalitis. Lancet 1990;335:440-441.

Russell WR. Poliomyelitis: pre-paralytic stage and the effect of physical activity on the severity of paralysis. Br Med J 1947;2:1023-1028.

Samaratunga H, Searle JW, Hudson N. Non-rabies Lyssavirus human encephalitis from fruit bats: Australian bat Lyssavirus (pteropid Lyssavirus) infection. Neuropathol Appl Neurobiol 1998;24:331-335.

Sarji SA, Abdullah BJ, Goh KJ, et al. MR imaging features of Nipah encephalitis. Am J Roentgenol 2000;175:437-442.

Sawyer MH. Enterovirus infections: diagnosis and treatment. Pediatr Infect Dis J 1999;18:1033-1039.

Schlitt M, Chronister RB, Whitley RJ. Pathogenesis and pathophysiology of viral infections of the central nervous system. In Scheld WM, Whitley RJ, Durack DT (eds). Infections of the Central Nervous System. New York: Raven Press, 1991.

Schmugge M, Lauener R, Seger RA, et al. Chronic enteroviral meningo-encephalitis in X-linked agammaglobulinaemia: favorable response to anti-enteroviral treatment. Eur J Pediatr 1999;158:1010-1011.

Selvey LA, Wells RM, McCormack JG, et al. Infection of humans and horses by a newly described morbillivirus. Med J Aust 1995;162:642-645.

Sharpe AH, Fields BN. Pathogenesis of viral infections. Basic concepts derived from the reovirus model. N Engl J Med 1985;312:486-497.

Siegel-Itzkovich J. Twelve die of West Nile virus in Israel. BMJ 2000;321:724.

Smith RR. Neuroradiology of intracranial infection. Pediatr Neurosurg 1992;18:92-104.

Solomon T, Dung NM, Kneen R, et al. Japanese encephalitis. J Neurol Neurosurg Psychiatry 2000;68:405-415.

Solomon T, Kneen R, Dung NM, et al. Poliomyelitis-like illness due to Japanese encephalitis virus. Lancet 1998a;351:1094-1097.

Solomon T, Thao LT, Dung NM, et al. Rapid diagnosis of Japanese encephalitis by using an immunoglobulin M dot enzyme immunoassay. J Clin Microbiol 1998b;36:2030-2034.

Soontornniyomkij V, Nieto-Rodriguez JA, Martinez AJ, et al. Brain HIV burden and length of survival after AIDS diagnosis. Clin Neuropathol 1998;17:95-99.

Stanberry LR, Floyd-Reising SA, Connelly BL, et al. Herpes simplex viremia: report of eight pediatric cases and review of the literature. Clin Infect Dis 1994;18:401-407.

Stuve O, Zamvil SS. Pathogenesis, diagnosis, and treatment of acute disseminated encephalomyelitis. Curr Opin Neurol 1999;12:395-401.

Tsai TF. Arboviral infections in the United States. Infect Dis Clin North Am 1991;5:73-102.

Tsai TF, Popovici F, Cernescu C, et al. West Nile encephalitis epidemic in southeastern Romania. The Lancet 1998a;352:767-771.

Tsai TF, Yu YX, Jia LL, et al. Immunogenicity of live attenuated SA14-14-2 Japanese encephalitis vaccine—a comparison of 1- and 3-month immunization schedules. J Infect Dis 1998b;177:221-223.

Vahlne A, Svennerholm B, Sandberg M, et al. Differences in attachment between herpes simplex type 1 and type 2 viruses to neurons and glial cells. Infect Immun 1980;28:675-680.

van Vliet KE, Glimaker M, Lebon P, et al. Multicenter evaluation of the Amplicor Enterovirus PCR test with cerebrospinal fluid from patients with aseptic meningitis. The European Union Concerted Action on Viral Meningitis and Encephalitis. J Clin Microbiol 1998;36:2652-2657.

Varki B, Puthuran P. Value of second lumbar puncture in confirming the diagnosis of aseptic meningitis. Arch Neurol 1979;36:581-582.

Vaughn DW, Hoke CH Jr. The epidemiology of Japanese encephalitis: prospects for prevention. Epidemiol Rev 1992;14:197-221.

Vrancken AF, Frijns CJ, Ramos LM. FLAIR MRI in sporadic Creutzfeldt-Jakob disease. Neurology 2000;55:147-148.

Wang SM, Liu CC, Tseng HW, et al. Clinical spectrum of enterovirus 71 infection in children in southern Taiwan, with an emphasis on neurological complications. Clin Infect Dis 1999;29:184-190.

Whitley RJ. Viral encephalitis. N Engl J Med 1990;323:242-250.

Whitley RJ. Herpes simplex virus. In Scheld WM, Whitley RJ, Durack DT (eds). Infections of the Central Nervous System. Philadelphia: Lippincott-Raven, 1996.

Whitley RJ, Alford CA Jr, Hirsch MS, et al. Vidarabine versus acyclovir therapy in herpes simplex encephalitis. N Engl J Med 1986;314:144-149.

Whitley RJ, Cobbs CG, Alford CA Jr, et al. Diseases that mimic herpes simplex encephalitis: diagnosis, presentation and outcome. JAMA 1989;262:234-239.

Whitley RJ, Gnann JW. Acyclovir: a decade later. N Engl J Med 1992;327:782-789.

Whitley RJ, Gnann JW. Viral encephalitis: familiar infections and emerging pathogens. Lancet 2002;359:507-513.

Whitley RJ, Kern ER, Chatterjee S, et al. Replication, establishment of latency, and induced reactivation of herpes simplex virus g1 34.5 deletion mutants in rodent models. J Clin Invest 1993;91:2837-2843.

Whitley RJ, Lakeman F. Herpes simplex infections of the central nervous system: therapeutic and diagnostic considerations. Clin Infect Dis 1995;20:414-420.

Whitley RJ, MacDonald N, Asher DM, Committee on Infectious Diseases. Technical report: transmissible spongiform encephalopathies: a review for pediatricians. Pediatrics 2000;106:1160-1165.

Whitley RJ, Soong S-J, Linneman C Jr, et al. Herpes simplex encephalitis: clinical assessment. JAMA 1982;247:317-320.

Wiestler OD, Leib SL, Brustle O. Neuropathology and pathogenesis of HIV encephalopathies. Acta Histochem Suppl 1992;42:107-114.

Wilfert CM, Lehrman SN, Katz SL. Enteroviruses and meningitis. Pediatr Infect Dis J 1983;2:333-341.

World Health Organization. WHO Fact Sheet. Bovine Spongiform encephalopathy 2002;113.

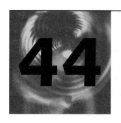

44

WOUNDS, ABSCESSES, AND OTHER INFECTIONS CAUSED BY ANAEROBIC BACTERIA

SHIRLEY JANKELEVICH

GENERAL PRINCIPLES OF ANAEROBIC INFECTIONS

Infections caused by anaerobic bacteria are an important cause of morbidity and mortality in the pediatric population, although the incidence of these infections is lower in the pediatric than in the adult population (Citron et al., 1995). Anaerobic bacteria are the predominate bacteria at all mucosal sites, and although many different anaerobic bacteria exist in each site, only a subset is responsible for causing disease. Anaerobes may be present in pure culture or as part of a mixed infection with other anaerobic and aerobic bacteria and may cause serious and life-threatening infection at any site in the body, from the intracranium to muscle and bone. The ability of certain anaerobes to cause disease is determined by factors at the site of infection, inoculum size, virulence factors of the organisms, and the health of the individual.

Identification of anaerobic bacteria from an infected site is dependent on an understanding of the normal distribution of anaerobic bacterial species that are present at sites involved in infection, as well as proper handling techniques of clinical specimens for anaerobic bacteriology. Knowledge of antimicrobial susceptibility of anaerobic and aerobic bacteria in mixed infections is necessary in making appropriate treatment choices. Finally, the importance of surgical drainage and débridement in the treatment of many anaerobic infections cannot be overemphasized.

Epidemiology

A decrease in anaerobic infections has been reported over the past 10 years, probably because of improved surgical prophylaxis and diagnosis and treatment of infections caused by anaerobic bacteria as well as the use of broad-spectrum antibiotics that have activity against anaerobes in the appropriate clinical setting (Olsen et al., 1999). Children have a decreased incidence of anaerobic infection than adults, most likely because of the lower frequency of debilitating diseases in children that predispose to anaerobic infections, such as lung abscesses and gynecologic infections. However, certain children may be at higher risk of anaerobic infection. These include neonates and children with neurologic impairments, chronic renal insufficiency, leukemia and other malignant neoplasms, and immunologically comprising conditions (Brook, 1995; Citron et al., 1995; Dunkle et al., 1976; Thirmuoothi et al., 1976). Anaerobic bacteria isolated from children revealed that infections in the abdomen were the source of 50% of anaerobic isolates. The head and neck, soft tissue below the waist, blood, respiratory system, cerebrospinal fluid (CSF), and unknown infections accounted for the remaining isolates (Citron et al., 1995).

Etiology

Anaerobic bacteria are defined as those bacteria that do not require oxygen for growth and replication. For simplicity, anaerobic bacteria can be classified into two groups based on tolerance to oxygen: the aerotolerant bacteria and the strict (obligate) anaerobic bacteria (Loesche, 1969). Aerotolerant bacteria, such as *Prevotella* (formerly *Bacteroides*) *melaninogenicus* and *Fusobacterium nucleatum,* can grow in the presence of low concentration of oxygen (0.1% to 4%), depending on the isolate. Although strict anaerobes, such as *Clostridium haemolyticum* and some *Treponema* species, generally cannot grow in the presence of greater than 0.5% oxygen and will die after a brief exposure to air, most anaerobic bacterial pathogens are aerotolerant and will remain viable if exposed to air for several hours.

Anaerobic pathogens may be from an endogenous or exogenous source. The vast majority of pathogens are from an endogenous origin. These bacteria normally colonize mucosal surfaces and may cause disease after damage to the mucosal barrier or skin allows bacterial invasion. The most common endogenous pathogenic bacteria causing human disease are (1) the gram-negative bacilli, *Bacteroides* species, *Prevotella* species, *Fusobacterium* species, and *Porphyromonas* species; (2) the gram-positive cocci, *Peptostreptococcus* species, and microaerophilic streptococci; (3) a subset of the spore-forming gram-positive bacilli, *Clostridium* species; and (4) the non–spore-forming gram-positive bacilli *Actinomyces*, *Propionibacterium* species, *Eubacterium lentum* and *Bifidobacterium* species. The most common exogenous anaerobic bacterial pathogens are *Clostridium botulinum* and *Clostridium tetani* (Olsen et al., 1999). These spore-forming bacteria are found in soil or contaminated food. The spores gain entry through the gastrointestinal (GI) tract or through soil-contaminated wounds, germinate, multiply, and elaborate a variety of toxins with different pathogenic effects. *Clostridium difficile,* an anaerobic pathogen that also produces toxins, is often endogenous but may be acquired from the environment or other colonized persons.

Pathogenesis

Every surface of the body, including skin, mouth, and GI, respiratory, and genitourinary tracts, has numerous microenvironments that provide ideal growth conditions (i.e., decreased oxygen tension and low oxidation-reduction potential) for endogenous aerobic and anaerobic microflora.

A balanced ecologic system found in each microenvironment is relatively stable over time but can be changed by factors such as antibiotics, chemotherapeutic agents, obstruction, and various diseases. Undesirable consequences may occur when the balance is changed, leading to proliferation of endogenous anaerobes that are normally kept in check. Alteration in the normal GI flora with administration of antibiotics can allow unrestrained growth of *C. difficile,* resulting in sufficient toxin production to cause pseudomembranous colitis. Obstruction, stasis, tissue destruction, aerobic infection, and decreases in normal blood flow may allow aerobic and anaerobic bacteria to gain access into normally sterile sites and act synergistically to produce infection. Examples of pathogenic conditions that promote anaerobic infections are GI obstruction, trauma or surgery, aspiration of vomitus into lungs, human and animal bites, and wounds that become contaminated with soil containing clostridial spores. These pathogenic processes result in lowered oxygen tension and accumulation of reducing products, leading to conditions that favor infection with endogenous anaerobes, usually in combination with facultative aerobic bacteria. In addition, numerous virulence factors produced by anaerobes, such as toxins and enzymes that can destroy host tissue, neutrophils and macrophages, polysaccharide capsules that promote formation of abscesses and protect bacteria from phagocytosis, and adherence factors that promote the invasion and growth of anaerobes, result in abscess formation. Once infection is established and an abscess is formed, the microenvironment within the abscess sustains the infectious processes. Continued growth of bacteria and destruction of tissue maintain a favorable reducing environment for anaerobic bacteria and abscess enlargement.

Immunity

Experimental evidence suggests that several arms of the immune system may function in the control of anaerobic infections. Cellular immunity may play a role in protection against abscess formation by *Bacteroides fragilis* (Onderdonk et al., 1982; Powell et al., 1985). Phagocytic activity may also be important in controlling anaerobic infections (Klempner, 1984), although the response may be compromised in mixed or pure anaerobic infections (Styrt and Gorbach, 1989). *B. fragilis* and *P. melaninogenicus* may be protected from opsonophagocytosis by capsule formation (Zaleznik and Kasper, 1982). Neutrophilic chemotaxis may be suppressed by *Bacteroides* species (Styrt and Gorbach, 1989). Factors produced by anaerobes may protect other bacteria from host defenses, as exemplified by the inhibition of phagocytosis of *Proteus mirabilis* and *Escherichia coli* by *B. fragilis* and *P. melaninogenicus* (Rotstein, 1993). In addition, virulence factors may directly destroy host leukocytes. Although there is extensive experimental evidence demonstrating a role for phagocytosis and host humoral and cellular immunity in controlling anaerobic infections, the contribution of each host defense in vivo is not yet known.

Diagnosis

An important part of the diagnosis of anaerobic infection is an understanding of the pathogenic processes that lead to anaerobic infection and proper collection, transport, and culture of the organisms from the infected site. Anaerobes are the predominant bacterial species on mucosal surfaces. Therefore, both anaerobic and aerobic infection should be suspected when infections occur near oral, GI, or genital mucosa. The presence of gas and foul odor may point to an anaerobic infection but also may occur with infections caused by aerobic bacteria. It is imperative that samples of blood, infected fluid, and tissue be collected properly and handled carefully to permit the growth and identification of anaerobes. All specimens should be kept in a low-oxygen, moist, warm environment and should be transported to the microbiology laboratory soon after collection. Blood should be collected in both anaerobic (unvented) and aerobic (vented) bottles. Aspirates should be collected, whenever possible, by needle and syringe. Air should be expelled from the syringe, and the contents of the syringe should be injected into an anaerobic transport tube or vial containing, if possible, a prereduced transport medium. If a specimen must be collected with a swab, an oxygen-free swab obtained from the microbiology laboratory should be used. The oxygen-free swab should then be transported to the microbiology laboratory in an oxygen-free transport container. Clinical specimens obtained by swab from superficial lesions; from vaginal, cervical, and urethral sites; from sites in the respiratory tract that have contacted the oral mucosa; and from stool or the rectal area will be contaminated with the normal anaerobes that colonize those sites. Such specimens should not be sent for anaerobic culture. Tissue from the infected site should be should be placed in oxygen-free transport tubes or vials containing a prereduced transport medium. Consultation with the microbiology laboratory before sample collection is strongly recommended and will provide guidance on the proper collection and transport of these specimens.

The need for susceptibility testing of anaerobic bacteria isolated from clinical infections is controversial, although the clinical outcome in certain situations may be improved if drug susceptibility tests lead to the use of appropriate antibiotics. These include (1) serious or life-threatening infections such as central nervous system (CNS) infection, bacteremia, or endocarditis; (2) infections that require prolonged therapy such as osteomyelitis and septic arthritis; (3) infections that do not respond to the initial regimen chosen; (4) infections that recur; and (5) infections with bacteria with variable resistance patterns or high virulence, those that have been isolated in pure culture, or those whose susceptibility patterns have not been established (Olsen et al., 1999).

Treatment

The initial treatment of infections involving anaerobic bacteria requires that the clinician be familiar with the pathogens expected at the site of infection, the antibiotic susceptibility patterns of the pathogens in that geographic area, the ability of the antibiotics to penetrate the structures involved in the infection, the toxicity of the antibiotics, and the effect of the antibiotics on the normal bacterial flora (Falagas and Siakavellas, 2000). Table 44-1 provides information on important bacterial causes of the most common anaerobic infections and suggests empiric regimens that can be used to treat an infection until the bacterial pathogens have been identified. Once the empiric antibiotic regimen is administered, the patient must be assessed frequently, and if there is lack of improvement 48 to 72 hours after appropriate surgical intervention, a different antibiotic regimen may need to be instituted. The decision should be based, in part, on the types and susceptibility patterns of the isolated pathogens. Table 44-2 lists antibiotics that may be used to treat anaerobic infections in children. Consultation with a specialist in infectious diseases should be strongly considered.

Many factors associated with anaerobic infections may alter effectiveness of antibiotic therapy. Properties of the anaerobic environment within the abscess and enzymes produced by anaerobic bacteria may decrease or eliminate antibiotic activity. Tissue necrosis with resultant decreased blood flow to the site of infection may prevent many antibiotics from gaining entry into an abscess. Aminoglycosides cannot be used to treat anaerobic infections, because this group of antibiotics requires oxygen transport to penetrate the bacterial cell envelope. In addition, aminoglycosides become inactivated by purulent

TABLE 44-1 Bacterial etiologies of common pediatric anaerobic infections and suggested empiric treatment

Site	Types of infection	Mild to moderate infection	Severe infection	Predominant anaerobic bacteria	Predominant aerobic or facultative anaerobic bacteria
Superficial and subcutaneous soft tissue (lesions near head and neck usually associated with respiratory bacteria; those near abdomen and pelvis usually associated with enteric flora)	Non-necrotizing infections: Infected gastrostomy site Pilonidal abscess Infected decubitus ulcer		Ampicillin/sulbactam or Clindamycin plus cefotaxime (or ceftriaxone) plus aminoglycoside or Imipenem/cilastatin or Meropenem or Metronidazole, oxacillin, cefotaxime (or ceftriaxone) plus aminoglycoside	*Bacteroides* spp. (including *Bacteroides fragilis*) *Clostridium* spp. *Fusobacterium* spp. *Peptostreptococcus* spp. *Porphyromonas* spp. *Prevotella* spp.	*Staphylococcus aureus* *Streptococcus pyogenes* *Escherichia coli* and other enteric gram-negative bacilli *Enterococcus* spp.
Subcutaneous tissue	Necrotizing infections: Bacterial synergistic gangrene		Oxacillin or vancomycin plus gentamicin or third-generation cephalosporin	Anaerobic streptococci	*S. aureus* Gram-negative enteric bacteria or microaerophilic or gram-negative enteric bacteria
	Anaerobic cellulites Synergistic Nonclostridial Anaerobic Myonecrosis Necrotizing fasciitis Clostridial myonecrosis	Clostridial and nonclostridial anaerobic cellulitis	Penicillin plus clindamycin plus aminoglycoside or third-generation cephalosporin	*Clostridium* spp. *Bacteroides* spp. Anaerobic streptococci	
Fascia and muscle	Necrotizing infections: Necrotizing fasciitis Synergistic nonclostridial anaerobic myonecrosis		Penicillin plus clindamycin plus aminoglycoside or third-generation cephalosporin or Imipenem or	*Bacteroides* spp. (including *B. fragilis*) *Clostridium* spp. *Peptostreptococcus* spp. *Prevotella* spp.	*S. pyogenes* *S. aureus* Gram-negative enteric bacilli

Site/Condition	Antibiotic therapy	Usual pathogens	Anaerobic pathogens
	meropenem or ticarcillin plus aminoglycoside / or / Clindamycin plus cefotaxime (or ceftriaxone) with or without aminoglycoside / or / Chloramphenicol plus aminoglycoside (if patient is penicillin allergic)	*S. aureus* / Gram-negative enteric bacilli	
Umbilicus / Omphalitis	Clindamycin plus cefotaxime / or / Metronidazole plus oxacillin plus aminoglycoside		*Bacteroides* spp. / *Clostridium* spp. / *Peptostreptococcus* spp.
Human, dog, or cat bite or clenched fist injury	Amoxicillin/clavulanate / or / Cefuroxime	*Streptococcus* spp. / *S. aureus* / *Staphylococcus epidermidis* / *Corynebacterium* spp. / *Eikenella corrodens* / *Pasteurella* spp. (dog and cat) / *Capnocytophaga canimorsus* (dog)	*Bacteroides* spp. (including *B. fragilis*) / *Clostridium* spp. / *Fusobacterium* spp. / *Peptostreptococcus* spp. / *Porphyromonas* spp. / *Prevotella* spp.
Intracranial (only antibiotics that can penetrate the blood-brain barrier should be used) / Intracranial abscess or subdural empyema secondary to extension of infection in head or neck	Metronidazole plus oxacillin plus cefotaxime (or ceftriaxone) / or / (if patient is allergic to penicillin) vancomycin plus metronidazole plus aztreonam or gentamicin	*S. aureus* / Gram-negative enteric bacilli / *Streptococcus* spp. / *Haemophilus* spp.	*Actinomyces* / *Bacteroides* spp. (including *B. fragilis*) / *Fusobacterium* spp. / *Peptostreptococcus* spp. / *Porphyromonas* spp. / *Prevotella* spp.

Continued

TABLE 44-1 Bacterial etiologies of common pediatric anaerobic infections and suggested empiric treatment—cont'd

Site	Types of infection	Mild to moderate infection	Severe infection	Predominant anaerobic bacteria	Predominant aerobic or facultative anaerobic bacteria
Blood	Anaerobic bacteremia		Metronidazole plus aminoglycoside plus ampicillin or Ampicillin and sulbactam plus aminogylcoside or Imipenem/cilastatin or Meropenem	*Bacteroides* spp. *Clostridium* spp. *Fusobacterium* spp. *Propionibacterium acnes*	
	Intraabdominal infection or peritonitis secondary to gastrointestinal pathology (neonate)		Vancomycin plus gentamicin (or cefotoxime) plus clindamycin (or metronidazole)	*Bacteroides* spp. (including *B. fragilis*) *Clostridium* spp. (including *Clostridium difficile*)	*Klebsiella pneumoniae* *Enterobacter* spp. Other gram-negative enteric bacilli *Streptococcus* spp. *S. epidermidis* *Candida albicans*
	Intraabdominal infection or peritonitis secondary to gastrointestinal pathology (see text for details for primary peritonitis and peritonitis due to peritoneal dialysis)	Intraabdominal abscess Peritonitis Ruptured appendix or appendiceal abscess Postoperative wound infection following bowel or female genital tract surgery	Metronidazole plus cefotaxime (or ceftriaxone) or aminoglycoside or aztreonam or Ampicillin/sulbactam plus aminoglycoside or Ticarcillin/clavulanate or Imipenem/cilastatin or Meropenem	*Bacteroides* spp. (including *B. fragilis*) *Clostridium* spp. *Fusobacterium* spp. *Peptostreptococcus* spp. *Porphyromonas* spp. *Prevotella* spp.	*Streptococcus* spp. *E. coli* *K. pneumoniae* *Pseudomonas aeruginosa* Other gram-negative bacilli
Liver	Liver abscess		Metronidazole plus cefotaxime (or	*Bacteroides* spp. (including *B. fragilis*)	*S. aureus* *E. coli*

884

Site	Condition	Antimicrobial therapy	Anaerobes	Aerobes/other
		ceftriaxone) or ticarcillin/clavulanate or Ampicillin/sulbactam or Metronidazole plus imipenem/cilastatin or meropenem or Metronidazole plus oxacillin plus aminoglycoside or Clindamycin plus aminoglycoside	*Fusobacterium* spp. *Peptostreptococcus* spp. *Clostridium* spp. *Prevotella* spp.	*Klebsiella* spp. *Enterobacter* spp. *Pseudomonas* spp. *Proteus* spp. *Streptococcus* group D Less common: *Candida* spp. *Entamoeba histolytica* *Echinococcus*
Spleen	Splenic abscess	Metronidazole plus cefotaxime (or ceftriaxone) or ticarcillin/clavulanate or ampicillin/sulbactam or Metronidazole plus imipenem/cilastatin or meropenem or Metronidazole plus oxacillin plus aminoglycoside or Clindamycin plus aminoglycoside	*Bacteroides* spp (including *fragilis*) *Fusobacterium* spp. *Peptostreptococcus* spp. *Clostridium* spp.	*S. aureus* *Streptococcus* spp. *E. coli* *Proteus mirabilis* *Streptococcus* group D *K. pneumoniae* Viridans streptococci *Citrobacter freundii* Less common: *Salmonella* spp. *M tuberculosis* *Candida* spp. *Aspergillus* spp. *Brucella* spp.
Retroperitoneum and psoas muscle	Retroperitoneal and psoas abscess		*Bacteroides* spp. (including *B. fragilis*) *Clostridium* spp. *Fusobacterium* spp. *Peptostreptococcus* spp. *Porphyromonas* spp. *Prevotella* spp.	*S. aureus* *Streptococcus* spp. *E. coli* *P. mirabilis*

Continued

TABLE 44-1 Bacterial etiologies of common pediatric anaerobic infections and suggested empiric treatment—cont'd

Site	Types of infection	Mild to moderate infection	Severe infection	Predominant anaerobic bacteria	Predominant aerobic or facultative anaerobic bacteria
Anus or rectum	Anorectal abscess		Metronidazole plus oxacillin plus aminoglycoside or Clindamycin plus aminoglycoside	*Bacteroides* spp. (including *B. fragilis*) *Clostridium* spp. *Fusobacterium* spp. *Peptostreptococcus* spp. *Porphyromonas* spp. *Prevotella* spp.	*S. aureus* *Streptococcus* spp. *E. coli* and other gram-negative enteric bacilli
Bone	Anaerobic osteomyelitis		Clindamycin or Ticarcillin/clavulanate	*Bacterioides* spp. Anaerobic gram-positive cocci *Fusobacterium* spp.	*S. aureus* *Streptococcus* spp. Gram-negative bacilli

TABLE 44-2   **Antibiotics for the treatment of anaerobic infections in children**

Antibiotic	Active against (in vitro)*	Precautions, restrictions on use, conditions requiring dose adjustment, and comments†	Tissue distribution and uses in anaerobic infections
Amoxicillin/clavulanate‡, §	*Actinomyces* *Bacteroides* spp. *Clostridium* spp. *Fusobacterium* spp. (+/−) *Prevotella* spp. *Porphyromonas* spp. (+/−) *Peptostreptococcus* spp. *Propionibacterium* spp.	Should not be used for serious or severe infections Resistant to inactivation by many β-lactamases Renal insufficiency Approved for use in neonates and children	Lungs, pleural and peritoneal fluid; poor penetration into CSF
Ampicillin‡	*Clostridium* spp. *Peptostreptococcus* spp. *Propionibacterium* spp.	Inactivated by β-lactamases produced by bacteria resistant to penicillins and cephalosporins Renal insufficiency	Wide distribution into tissue, moderate CSF penetration if inflammation present
Ampicillin/sulbactam‡	*Actinomyces* *Bacteroides* spp. *Clostridium* spp. *Fusobacterium* spp. *Prevotella* spp. *Porphyromonas* spp. *Peptostreptococcus* spp. *Propionibacterium* spp	Resistant to a wide range of β-lactamases Renal insufficiency Approved for skin and skin structure infections for children ≥1 year old Safety and effectiveness have not been established for children <12 years old for intraabdominal infections	Wide distribution into tissue, moderate CSF penetration if inflammation present
Cefoxitin‡, §	(+/−) *Actinomyces* (+/−) *Bacteroides* spp. *Clostridium* spp. *Fusobacterium* spp. *Prevotella* spp. *Porphyromonas* spp. (+/−) *Peptostreptococcus* spp. *Propionibacterium* spp.	Resistant to a wide range of β-lactamases Renal insufficiency Not approved for use in children <3 months old	Wide distribution including urine, pleural fluid, joints, bile; little in CSF even if meningeal inflammation present
Chloramphenicol	*Actinomyces* *Bacteroides* spp. *Clostridium* spp. *Fusobacterium* spp. *Prevotella* spp. *Porphyromonas* spp. *Peptostreptococcus* spp. *Propionibacterium* spp.	Serious and fatal blood dyscrasias (aplastic anemia, hypoplastic anemia, thrombocytopenia, granulocytopenia) Gray baby syndrome can occur in neonates (also seen in neonates born to mothers receiving chloramphenicol) Hepatic insufficiency MUST measure serum levels for all patients	Wide distribution including liver; kidney; pleural fluid, ascitic fluid; CSF (even in the absence of meningeal inflammation); brain

Continued

TABLE 44-2 Antibiotics for the treatment of anaerobic infections in children—cont'd

Antibiotic	Active against (in vitro)*	Precautions, restrictions on use, conditions requiring dose adjustment, and comments†	Tissue distribution and uses in anerobic infections
Clindamycin	(+/−) *Clostridium* spp. *Fusobacterium* spp. (+/−) *Peptostreptococcus* spp. (+/−) *Porphyromonas* spp. (+/−) *Prevotella* spp. *Propionibacterium* spp.	May be associated with pseudomembranous colitis	Wide distribution including ascites, pleural and synovial fluid, bone, bile; little in CSF even if meningeal inflammation present
Imipenem/cilastatin‡,§	*Actinomyces* *Bacteroides* spp. *Clostridium* spp. *Fusobacterium* spp. *Peptostreptococcus* spp. *Porphyromonas* spp. *Prevotella* spp. *Propionibacterium* spp.	Highly resistant to most β-lactamases; Should not be used in children with CNS infection (increases risk of seizures) Renal insufficiency Approved for use in neonates and children	Widely distributed, including pleural fluid, bone, bile, intestine, peritoneal fluid, interstitial fluid, and wound fluids; low concentration in CSF Clinical uses as monotherapy: • Intraabdominal infection • Gynecologic infections
Meropenem§	*Bacteroides* spp. *Clostridium* spp. *Fusobacterium* spp. *Peptostreptococcus* spp. *Prevotella* spp. *Porphyromonas* spp. *Propionibacterium* spp.	Highly resistant to most β-lactamases Renal insufficiency Not approved for use in children <3 months old	Widely distributed throughout the body Clinical uses as monotherapy: • Intraabdominal infection • Gynecologic infections
Metronidazole	*Bacteroides* spp. *Clostridium* spp. *Fusobacterium* spp. (+/−) *Peptostreptococcus* spp. *Prevotella* spp.	Use with caution if severe hepatic or renal disease	Widely distributed to all tissues and fluids including CSF
Penicillin G‡	(+/−) *Actinomyces* *Clostridium* spp. *Fusobacterium* spp. (+/−) *Peptostreptococcus* spp. *Propionibacterium* spp.	Renal insufficiency	Wide distribution including urine, tissue fluid, peritoneal fluid, gallbladder, other; moderate CSF penetration if inflammation present

Piperacillin‡	(+/–) *Actinomyces* *Clostridium* spp. *Fusobacterium* spp. *Peptostreptococcus* spp. *Porphyromonas* spp. *Prevotella* spp. *Propionibacterium* spp.	Renal insufficiency Safety and efficacy not established for children <12 years old	Poor distribution into CSF through uninflamed meninges
Piperacillin/tazobactam‡	(+/–) *Actinomyces* *Bacteroides* spp. *Clostridium* spp. *Fusobacterium* spp. *Prevotella* spp. *Porphyromonas* spp. *Peptostreptococcus* spp. *Propionibacterium* spp.	Renal insufficiency Safety and efficacy not established for children <12 years old	Poor distribution into CSF through uninflamed meninges
Ticarcillin/clavulanate‡	(+/–) *Actinomyces* (+/–) *Bacteroides* spp. *Clostridium* spp. *Fusobacterium* spp. *Prevotella* spp. (+/–) *Peptostreptococcus* spp. *Propionibacterium* spp.	Renal and hepatic insufficiency Approved for children ≥3 months old	Distribution into CSF unknown

CNS, Central nervous system; CSF, cerebrospinal fluid.
(+/–) >80% but < 90% of isolates tested in vitro were inhibited by the antibiotic.
Clostridium difficile not included in evaluation of antimicrobial efficacy.
†Consult appropriate pharmaceutical resources for further discussion of other precautions, as well as drug interactions.
‡Hypersensitivity reactions may occur in patients with penicillin hypersensitivity.
§Induces β-lactamase production by many gram-negative enteric bacteria, and may cause inactivation of β-lactam antibiotics that are used concurrently.

material and the low pH found in abscesses. β-Lactam antibiotics, which work by preventing cell wall formation in actively growing bacteria, cannot kill bacteria within an abscess because abscesses contain large numbers of organisms that are usually in the stationary phase of growth. β-Lactam antibiotics may also be inactivated by the production of β-lactamases produced by anaerobic organisms such as *B. fragilis.* Therefore, in a mixed anaerobic and aerobic infection, a β-lactam antibiotic determined to be active in vitro against a bacterial isolate from the infected site may be inactive against the isolate within the abscess (O'Keefe et al., 1978).

Although antibiotics are essential in the treatment of anaerobic infection, the difficulty in eradicating anaerobes from an infected site with antibiotics alone most often necessitates the use of surgical débridement of necrotic tissue and removal of infected material from an abscess. Fortunately, drainage of certain abscesses may be achieved percutaneously if guided by ultrasound or computed tomography (CT).

Several classes of antibiotics, each with its own spectrum of activity against anaerobes, are available. However, the frequency of antibiotic resistance continues to increase in some organisms, especially in multiply-resistant *B. fragilis,* which now limits the use of some antibiotics that were previously the mainstay of therapy for anaerobic bacterial infections. The mechanisms by which anaerobic bacteria become resistant to antibiotics are numerous and complex. The mechanisms of bacterial resistance to β-lactam antibiotics include (1) production of β-lactamases that inactivate β-lactam antibiotics such as penicillin G, ampicillin, and piperacillin (seen in *Bacteroides* species, especially *B. fragilis, Prevotella* species, especially *Prevotella melaninogenicus, Porphyromonas* species, *Fusobacterium* species, and, less commonly, *Clostridium* species); (2) decreased penetration of antibiotic through the bacterial cell wall; and (3) alteration of penicillin binding proteins (PBPs), so that the β-lactam antibiotics can no longer kill the bacteria by preventing cell wall synthesis (seen in *Bacteroides* species, especially *B. fragilis*).

Antibiotics for Anaerobic Infections

Antibiotics with the greatest activity against anaerobes include metronidazole, β-lactam antibiotics with β-lactamase inhibitors, β-lactam antibiotics with decreased susceptibility to inactivation by β-lactamases, and chloramphenicol.

Metronidazole is a very active bactericidal antibiotic with excellent activity against a broad range of strict anaerobic bacteria. Metronidazole has excellent penetration into tissues, abscess cavities, and fluids, including the CNS. Metronidazole may also be able to suppress the production of toxin by clostridia (Finegold and Wexler, 1996). Because it has decreased activity against some anaerobic gram-positive cocci and lack of activity against non–spore-forming, anaerobic, gram-positive bacilli (*Propionibacterium acnes, Actinomyces,* and *Eubacterium)* and aerobic bacteria, it cannot be used as a single agent in a mixed aerobic and anaerobic infection. Metronidazole in combination with antibiotics active against gram-positive anaerobes and aerobic bacteria is recommended for the treatment of polymicrobial anaerobic infections and as a single agent for the treatment of *C. difficile* infection (Kasten, 1999).

β-lactam antibiotics with β-lactamases inhibitors are agents that are combined with an inhibitor that inactivates β-lactamases produced by bacteria. These agents include amoxicillin/clavulanate, ampicillin/sulbactam, piperacillin/tazobactam, and ticarcillin/clavulanate. They have broad activity against many types of aerobic and anaerobic bacteria and may be used as a single agent in certain mixed aerobic and anaerobic infections.

β-Lactam antibiotics with decreased susceptibility to inactivation by β-lactamases include imipenem/cilastatin, meropenem, and cefoxitin. The β-lactam ring of these antibiotics has increased resistance to inactivation by β-lactamases. Both imipenem/cilastatin and meropenem are potent broad-spectrum antibiotics with excellent activity against many aerobic bacteria (including *Pseudomonas aeruginosa*) and anaerobic bacteria and excellent tissue penetration. Meropenem has better CNS penetration than imipenem/cilastatin and does not induce seizures in patients who are predisposed to developing seizures (e.g., history of seizures or current CNS pathology). Meropenem has been shown to safe and effective for the treatment of intraabdominal infections in infants and children (Arrieta, 1997). Cefoxitin is a cephalosporin with good activity against many aerobic and anaerobic bacteria. However, because approximately 20% of *B. fragilis* strains and *Clostridium* species are now resistant to cefoxitin, this antibiotic is not recommended as a single agent for the treatment of serious anaerobic infections.

Of note is that both cefoxitin and imipenem/cilastatin are potent inducers of β-lactamase production from gram-negative bacilli that may be present in a mixed infection. Therefore, a β-lactamase–susceptible antibiotic that is used in conjunction with cefoxitin or imipenem/cilastatin will most likely be rendered inactive.

Chloramphenicol is a broad-spectrum antibiotic with excellent activity against both aerobic bacteria and anaerobic bacteria, including *B. fragilis*. It also has excellent tissue distribution and penetrates well into abscesses and the CNS. However, because of its association with irreversible fatal aplastic anemia that is not dose related, chloramphenicol should be used only in specific situations in which no alternative antibiotic is appropriate (e.g., CNS infections in patients with β-lactam allergy) (Kasten, 1999).

β-Lactamase–susceptible β-lactam antibiotics have limited activity against anaerobic bacteria because of increasing resistance. The β-lactam rings of penicillin G, ampicillin, and piperacillin are easily hydrolyzed by β-lactamases, and therefore these agents should not be used to treat infections with bacteria that produce β-lactamases, such as *B. fragilis*, *Prevotella*, or *Poryphyromonas* (Finegold and Wexler, 1996).

Clindamycin has been a key antianaerobic antibiotic for many years, although increased resistance in 10% to 20% of *Peptostreptococcus* species, 88% of *B. fragilis* strains (Kasten, 1999), and some *Clostridium* species has been observed. Clindamycin may be used as a substitute for penicillin in cases of penicillin allergy. Clindamycin may be advantageous in the treatment of infections caused by clindamycin-susceptible *Clostridium* species because it has the ability to suppress the production of toxin (Finegold and Wexler, 1996). Although clindamycin has excellent penetration into many tissues, it is poorly distributed into the CNS and should not be used for the treatment of CNS infections. Clindamycin has been associated with the development of *C. difficile* colitis.

In summary, when choosing the initial antibiotic regimen for treatment of an anaerobic infection, several principles should guide the clinician. These principles are (1) β-lactam antibiotics that are hydrolyzed by β-lactamases, such as penicillin and ampicillin, should not be used to treat infections with *B. fragilis*, *Prevotella* species, or *Porphyromonas* species;

(2) antibiotic resistance patterns at the hospital or institution should be factored into the decision regarding the choice of regimens; and (3) therapy should be directed against the bacterial species that are most virulent, most prevalent, and most resistant to antimicrobial agents (Finegold, 1997).

WOUND AND SOFT-TISSUE INFECTIONS

Wound and soft-tissue infections include superficial infections of the skin and skin structures, subcutaneous infections, and deeper infections of the fascia or muscle. The type of bacteria infecting the wound, the level of tissue infected, and the absence or presence of tissue necrosis generally classifies them. The categorization of some soft-tissue infections, however, is complicated by the variable involvement of several layers of tissue.

The most common superficial infections that may involve anaerobes include furuncles, paronychia, infected ulcers and cysts, infected gastrostomy tube site wound (Brook, 1995), infected tracheostomy site wound (Brook, 1995), and hidradenitis suppurativa. Subcutaneous tissue infections include cutaneous and subcutaneous abscesses (Brook and Frazier, 1990), pilonidal abscess (Sondenaa et al., 1995), infected decubitus ulcers (Brook, 1995), infected bite wounds (Griego et al., 1995), and the superficial necrotizing soft-tissue infections (nonclostridial anaerobic cellulitis, clostridial anaerobic cellulitis, and bacterial synergistic gangrene). The deeper necrotizing soft-tissue infections are necrotizing fasciitis and clostridial and nonclostridial myonecrosis.

Pathogenesis

Soft-tissue infections most often occur after introduction of endogenous or exogenous bacteria into soft tissue due to minor or major trauma, surgery, ischemia, obstruction of drainage, presence of foreign body or blood, and vascular stasis. Once infection is established, virulence factors elaborated by the infecting pathogens and synergy between the infecting bacteria often determine the extent and severity of infection.

Etiology

Either aerobic or anaerobic bacteria may cause infections of soft tissue, and both may be present simultaneously. Synergism may occur between anaerobic and aerobic bacteria within a wound, causing more severe infection than that caused by either organism alone. The method of wound acquisition and the site of infection in part determine the types of pathogens found. For example, in postsurgical wound infections, bacteria from exogenous sources include hospital-acquired organisms, such as methicillin-resistant *Staphylococcus aureus* and various gram-negative bacteria, especially *P. aeruginosa*, whereas those from endogenous sources include *S. aureus,* group A β-hemolytic streptococci, and aerobic and anaerobic bacteria normally found in the gut.

Epidemiology

A variety of conditions lead to soft-tissue and wound infections. Surgical wounds may become infected during or after an operative procedure. Wounds acquired from an animal or human bite may become infected, depending on the source, type, and location of the bite. Traumatic wounds are more likely to become infected if either exogenous or endogenous bacteria are introduced into the wound. In addition, certain children, such as those with neurologic impairment, are at increased risk of certain types of wound infections.

Postoperative wound infections are a major cause of soft-tissue infections in children. Several factors appear to increase the incidence of these infections (Cruse and Foord, 1976; Dineen, 1961; Leigh et al., 1974; Nichols, 1980). Increased length of stay in the hospital before surgery and longer duration of surgery are associated with a higher incidence of wound infection. Neonates have a higher rate of wound infection than older children. Contaminated wounds become infected more often than clean wounds. Administration of perioperative antibiotics also influences the incidence of postoperative infections. A higher incidence of abdominal wound infections was noted for patients given perioperative antibiotics for clean (uncontaminated) surgery, whereas infection was decreased with administration of perioperative antibiotics for contaminated surgery. An increased risk of postsurgical infection is also present in penetrating trauma (Nichols et al., 1984), emergent surgery, and repeat surgical procedures. In children, appendicitis was the condition most frequently associated with postsurgical abdominal infection, probably because of the frequency of this surgical condition in this age population. The risk of developing a wound infection after removal of a normal or an inflamed appendix without suppuration (clean-contaminated surgery) is approximately 10% in patients without preoperative or perioperative antibiotic prophylaxis (Forster et al., 1986), whereas the presence of a gangrenous or perforated appendix (dirty surgery) was associated with an infection rate of about 35%.

Children with increased risk of decubitus ulcers, gastrostomy, and tracheostomy wound site infections (Brook, 1995) are those with neurologic impairments. Paronychia is more common in children who nail bite or finger suck. Pilonidal abscesses are more common in pubescent children, possibly because of plugging and secondary infection of hair follicles in the pilonidal sinus (Sondenaa et al., 1995). Neonates may rarely develop two life-threatening infections—omphalitis and periumbilical necrotizing fasciitis.

Animal and human bites often become infected. Although dogs cause the majority of these bites, cat bites more often become infected. Location of bites may alter the risk of infection. Bites located on the hands are twice as likely to become infected as those located elsewhere.

Superficial Soft-Tissue Infections

Furuncles and carbuncles. Furuncles are localized pyogenic infections that originate from hair follicles. Carbuncles result from the coalescence of several furuncles. They usually occur in areas exposed to friction and perspiration. Although *S. aureus* is most commonly found in these lesions, less commonly anaerobic bacteria, such as *Peptococcus, Peptostreptococcus,* and *Bacteroides* species have been associated with furuncles that develop in the groin area. Therapy requires drainage, either by application of moist heat locally or, if unsuccessful, by surgical incision. If surrounding cellulitis is present, administration of systemic antibiotics with an antistaphylococcal antibiotic such as dicloxacillin is required. If the lesion is present in an area associated with anaerobic bacteria, clindamycin can be used.

Infected cysts. Epidermal cysts may become infected with aerobic and/or anaerobic bacteria. Isolates most frequently encountered are *S. aureus,* streptococci, *Peptostreptococcus,* and *Bacteroides* species. These cysts can be found about the head, trunk, extremities, perineum, and vulvovaginal and scrotal areas. Surgical drainage and antimicrobial agents directed at the organisms isolated are required (Brook, 1989a).

Hidradenitis suppurativa. Hidradenitis suppurativa is a chronic, recurrent infection of apocrine glands that become plugged with keratinous material (Olafsson and Khan, 1992). Lesions usually develop in plugged, inflamed glands in the axilla, groin, and buttocks. This condition is more common in adults but may occur at the time of puberty as well. Bacteria associated with these lesions are staphylococci, non-hemolytic streptococci, gram-negative bacilli, *Bacteroides* species, and anaerobic gram-positive cocci. Antibiotic treatment may not be successful, because the precipitating condition is chronic plugging of apocrine gland ducts, inflammation, formation of sinus tracts, and scarring, creating conditions that may not allow entry of antibiotics to the sites of infection. Local care to promote drainage and antibiotic therapy directed at the bacteria isolated from the lesion should be instituted initially. Occasionally, in very severe disease, radical excision of the area with skin grafting is required.

Infected gastrostomy tube sites. Gastrostomy site infection may occur in patients who require prolonged gastrostomy tube feeding (Brook, 1995). The infection manifests as an area of induration and erythema, with exudate formation in and around the gastrostomy wound site. Leakage of gastric contents from the wounds may be present and may contribute to the presence of anaerobes in the wound. A mixed bacterial population is usually found with anaerobes predominating. The most common isolates found in these wounds are *Peptostreptococcus* species, *B. fragilis* group, *E. coli*, and *Enterococcus* species (Brook, 1995), although other aerobic bacteria, such as *S. aureus*, and anaerobic bacterial species may be present. Bacteremia may be present in a minority of patients. After wound cultures are obtained, local wound care should be instituted. In cases of more severe infection, blood cultures should be obtained and empiric systemic therapy should be directed against the most frequent isolates, as well as *S. aureus* (Table 44-1). The therapy should then be directed at the organisms isolated from the wound and blood.

Subcutaneous Tissue Infections

Pilonidal abscess. Pilonidal abscesses occur when a pilonidal sinus, a midline closure defect in the sacral region, becomes infected, probably after the sinus becomes plugged with debris (Sondenaa et al., 1995). Occasionally, infection may be chronic, resulting in chronic pilonidal sinus disease. Anaerobes and enteric gram-negative bacilli usually cause infection.

S. aureus is less commonly isolated. Treatment consists of incision and drainage and may be followed by systemic antibiotics directed at anaerobes and enteric gram-negative bacilli. Postoperative wound infections and recurrences of disease are not uncommon in this condition.

Infected decubitus ulcers. Decubitus ulcers may develop in immobilized or bedridden children (Brook, 1995). Pressure on tissue that exceeds vascular perfusion pressure results in tissue ischemia. Tissue breakdown is further aggravated by moisture and friction, resulting in tissue maceration. Endogenous bacteria, aerobic and anaerobic, find easy entrance into the wound and can penetrate layers of tissues, resulting in further necrosis of the ulcer, bacteremia, sepsis, osteomyelitis, and infection of joints. Regions most often affected by decubitus ulcers are those that overlie bony prominences such as the sacrum, greater trochanter, and heels. Ulcers located in regions such as the sacrum are more likely to become infected with fecal flora. Polymicrobial infection of these ulcers is most common. *S. aureus*, *Peptostreptococcus* species, *Bacteroides* species, and gram-negative enteric bacteria are most commonly isolated. Cultures should be obtained from decubitus ulcers by collecting material from deep within the wound. Treatment consists of surgical débridement of necrotic tissue, antimicrobial treatment, and local wound care. If the ulcer is deep and wide, skin grafting is sometimes necessary. Recommended empiric antibiotic regimens are listed in Table 44-1.

Infected bite wounds. Over 300,000 persons with a median age of 15 years seek medical attention in an emergency room annually in the United States for bite wounds (Talan et al., 1999). The three most common sources of bite wounds are dogs, cats, and humans, in order of decreasing frequency. Approximately 3% to 8% of dog bites and 28% to 90% of cat bites become infected, with many requiring hospitalization for intensive antibiotic treatment (Talan et al., 1999). Dog bites often cause crush injury but may also result in punctures, avulsions, tears, and abrasions (Goldstein, 1992; Zook et al., 1980). However, with cat bites, small diameter puncture wounds occur, allowing bacteria to enter deep into tissue. Development of infection occurs rapidly, with median time to infection of 12 hours for cat bites and 24 hours for dog bites (Talan et al., 1999).

Infection of bite wounds is most often polymicrobial, although certain infecting microorganisms are unique to the source of the bite. Anaerobic bacteria are present in about 40% to 75% of dog, cat, and human bites. The most common aerobic pathogens isolated from dog and cat bite wounds are *Pasteurella* species, followed by isolates of streptococci, staphylococci, *Moraxella, Corynebacterium,* and *Neisseria* (Talan et al., 1999). Anaerobic bacteria isolated are *B. fragilis, Prevotella, Porphyromonas, Peptostreptococcus,* and *Fusobacterium* species. Fortunately, most anaerobes from animals do not produce β-lactamases. A much less commonly encountered bacterium from infected wound bites is *Capnocytophaga canimorsus* (formerly DF-2). Infection with this organism has been reported to result in fatal infections in patients with certain predisposing conditions such as splenectomy and steroid therapy.

Human bites that occur as a clenched fist injury can result in a very serious infection with major complications. Such injuries usually result to a hand that has made forceful contact with another individual's mouth. A puncture or laceration of the skin may occur, inoculating bacteria into the deep tissue of the hand. If injury occurs over the metacarpophalangeal joint, infection can enter the joint, resulting in inoculation of human oral bacteria into the tendon sheath. Complications of this injury include septic arthritis, osteomyelitis, spread of infection into the compartments of the hand, laceration of tendons and nerves, and fractures of the phalangeal or metacarpal bones. Often, multiple bacterial isolates are found in infected human bites, usually with a predominance of anaerobic bacteria. The most frequently encountered aerobes are streptococci, *S. aureus, Staphylococcus epidermidis, Corynebacterium* species, and *E. corrodens.* The most common anaerobic isolates seen are *B. fragilis, Prevotella, Porphyromonas, Peptostreptococcus, Fusobacterium,* and *Clostridium* species. Anaerobes found in human bites, unlike those found in animal bites, often produce β-lactamases.

Other infectious agents can also be transmitted through animal bites. Cat bites may transmit *Bartonella henselae* (cat scratch bacillus), and both cat and dog bites may introduce *C. tetani* or rabies virus into the bite. Human bites may be associated with transmission of herpesvirus types 1 and 2, hepatitis B and C, *Actinomyces* species, *C. tetani, Mycobacterium*

tuberculosis, and *Treponema pallidum.* The transmission of human immunodeficiency virus (HIV) via human bites appears unlikely, although not improbable.

Treatment of a bite wound includes extensive irrigation. Although débridement should be performed to remove devitalized or crushed tissue and contaminating material, puncture wounds usually cannot be débrided without causing more extensive trauma. If signs of infection are present, aerobic and anaerobic cultures should be obtained before irrigation and débridement. Care must be taken so that cultures represent bacteria within the wound. Primary closure of bite wounds is controversial. Primary closure should not be performed on deep puncture wounds, wounds present for greater than 24 hours, infected wounds, and bites to the hands. Antibiotic therapy should be directed against *Pasteurella,* streptococci, staphylococci, and anaerobes (Table 44-1) (Talan et al., 1999). The risk of tetanus and rabies needs to be considered when treating a bite wound. Information regarding the patient's last tetanus immunization should be obtained. A fully immunized child with a minor bite wound that is carefully irrigated needs no further tetanus prophylaxis. The need for administration of tetanus immunization and immunoglobulin for bites resulting in complicated wound is determined by the patient's immunization status. Rabies immune globulin and rabies immunization may be required for certain animal bites.

Necrotizing Soft-Tissue Infections

Anatomy and pathogenesis. Knowledge of the structure of the skin is important for an understanding of the pathophysiology of these life-threatening soft-tissue infections. The skin consists of two layers: the stratified squamous keratinizing epithelium, and the deeper layer of connective tissue called the *dermis.* The epithelial layer contains no blood vessels and is therefore dependent on the diffusion of interstitial fluid from the well-vascularized dermis. The dermis rests on the superficial fascia, a layer of subcutaneous tissue that is superficial to muscle. The blood supply to both the overlying skin and the underlying adipose tissue is derived from arteries that lie in the superficial fascia. Therefore, any infectious process that causes thrombosis of these blood vessels will result in necrosis of the overlying soft tissue.

Necrotizing soft-tissue infections are caused by growth of bacteria, most often anaerobes, which elaborate various toxins that result in liquefaction necrosis of the infected tissues. *S. aureus,* some *Clostridium* species, and streptococci can elaborate hyaluronidase, an enzyme that digests hyaluronic acid, the ground substance of connective tissue, whereas *Clostridium perfringens* produces collagenase, a proteolytic enzyme that digests collagen. Synergism between different species of bacteria that coexist in an infected site permits increased growth and greater tissue destruction, increasing the severity of necrotizing soft-tissue infections. Bacteria that often exhibit this phenomenon are *Bacteroides* species; anaerobic streptococci; and *Clostridium* species, in combination with such aerobic bacteria as coliforms, streptococci, and staphylococci.

Inoculation of bacteria into a wound that contains necrotic debris, old hematoma, or foreign material such as sutures, that is already infected with aerobic or facultative bacteria, or that has had its blood supply disrupted because of the surgical procedure provides an ideal reducing environment for growth of bacteria that cause necrotizing infections. Pathogenic anaerobes associated with necrotizing infections are, to varying degrees, tolerant of low amounts of oxygen. Thus, these bacteria, once introduced into the wound, can remain viable until conditions result in decreased oxygen tension and exponential growth. The proliferation of these anaerobes results in the accumulation of by-products of anaerobic metabolism, which further reduces the local environment, enhancing bacterial growth and extension of the infection.

As the infection extends along the fascial planes, edema and necrosis of the superficial fascia and the deeper layer of the dermis occur. Compression or destruction of the nerves innervating the skin and thrombosis of the small blood vessels result in anesthesia. Initially, the overlying skin may show only mild signs of pathology, such as edema, and may not exhibit the classic signs of local tissue inflammation. Because of the paucity of symptoms, early diagnosis of such processes may be very difficult. As the underlying disease progresses and the deep tissues become necrotic, the overlying skin also becomes visibly necrotic. Pressure caused by edema and exudation into the infected underlying soft tissue may result in the formation of large bullae in the skin that rupture, releasing the foul-smelling serosanguineous exudate. However, by the time this occurs, the infectious process is already life threatening, and intervention at this stage often does not prevent death.

Superficial Necrotizing Soft-Tissue Infections

Bacterial synergistic gangrene. Bacterial synergistic gangrene (progressive bacterial synergistic gangrene) is a slowly progressing infection involving the dermis and, less commonly, the fascia (Baxter, 1972; Meleny, 1933). Coinfection of tissue with *S. aureus* or gram-negative bacilli and microaerophilic or anaerobic streptococci results in a synergistic infection. Local tissue destruction and decreased oxidation-reduction potential resulting from infection with aerobic bacteria enable entry of anaerobic or microaerophilic streptococci into the tissue. Infection can then extend beyond the site of the initial wound. Although any area can be affected, abdominal wounds and tissue around ileostomies or colostomies, surgical drains, or retention sutures may be more likely to develop such an infection because of contamination with the offending bacteria during or after abdominal surgery.

Predominant early signs of infection are local exquisite pain, tenderness, edema, and erythema. Subsequently, the central portion of the wound develops a purplish coloration surrounded by a margin of erythema and eventually ulcerates and becomes undermined. If left untreated, the infection spreads from the zone of gangrenous skin at the periphery of the lesion to involve the fascia. Because fever and signs of systemic illness often appear later in the course of infection, the serious nature of the infection may not be realized early in the disease course.

Once the diagnosis is entertained, culturing two separate sites should identify the infecting bacteria. One sample should be taken from the central portion of the wound to identify aerobic bacteria. A second specimen obtained from the undermined margins should be cultured anaerobically. This infection has a poor response to antibiotic therapy alone because of the presence of extensive necrosis, and wide surgical excision of the lesion is often required. Treatment with empiric intravenous antibiotics, directed against anaerobic and microaerophilic streptococci, *S. aureus,* and a wide range of gramnegative enteric organisms, should be instituted promptly. Table 44-1 provides two empiric antibiotic regimens. Once bacterial isolates are identified, antibiotic therapy should then be directed against bacteria isolated from the wound. Full recovery can be achieved with early treatment. Treatment delays may necessitate wide excision of the infected area, leading to prolonged hospital stay and skin grafting.

Anaerobic Cellulitis (Clostridial and Nonclostridial Anaerobic Cellulitis)

Anaerobic cellulitis is a necrotizing infection of devitalized subcutaneous tissue. The infection is usually superficial to the fascia (Bessman and Wagner, 1975; Bornstein et al., 1964; MacLennan, 1962).

Clostridia are the usual cause of these infections, although other non–spore-forming anaerobes in combination with gram-negative enteric bacteria have also been implicated. Anaerobic cellulitis develops within 3 days after bacterial contamination of subcutaneous tissue and spreads rapidly through adjacent tissue. Early in the course, mild pain, erythema, and edema of the skin around the wound are present. As the infection progresses, the skin overlying the infected area becomes erythematous and tender, and skin necrosis and small flat blebs that discharge a serous, foul-smelling liquid may be present. Crepitance is often present because of subcutaneous gas. The patient is usually not systemically ill. Aerobic and anaerobic blood culture, as well as Gram stain and aerobic and anaerobic cultures of the exudate from either the wound or from the blebs on the skin should be obtained. Plain radiographs will reveal abundant gas in the superficial soft tissues. A frozen-section biopsy may reveal the level of soft tissue affected by the necrotic process. Anaerobic cellulitis is treated by antibiotic therapy and local débridement to remove the infected necrotic tissue. Empiric antibiotic treatment should have activity against *Clostridium* species, *Bacteroides* species, anaerobic streptococci, and gram-negative enteric organisms (Table 44-1). Full recovery is expected with early treatment.

Infections That Extend to the Fascia

Necrotizing fasciitis. Necrotizing fasciitis, also known as *hospital gangrene* and *hemolytic streptococcal gangrene,* is a life-threatening, rapidly progressive necrotizing infection that has been, fortunately, relatively uncommon in the pediatric population. Necrotizing fasciitis has been classified into three distinct groups

based on the pathogens that cause the disease (Adams et al., 1990). Type I is a polymicrobial infection, usually on the trunk, and is caused by aerobic and anaerobic bacteria. Type II is due to group A *Streptococcus,* sometimes in combination with *S. aureus,* and usually involves the extremities. Type III is caused by pathogenic marine *Vibrio* species that enter skin through a lesion that has been exposed to seawater or marine animals.

Necrotizing fasciitis may involve any area of the body, including the perineum, scrotum, and penis (Fournier's gangrene) in children (Adams et al., 1990). It often manifests within 1 to 4 days after trauma, contamination of a surgical wound, or infection of skin vesicles following chickenpox (Falcone et al., 1988), but it may also occur without known antecedent trauma in patients with neutropenia or diabetes mellitus. In neonates, most cases of necrotizing fasciitis involve the periumbilical area, and to a much lesser degree, the thorax, back, extremities, and scalp (Hsieh et al., 1999). Periumbilical necrotizing fasciitis in the neonate usually occurs within the first 2 weeks of life, and, although it has been considered a complication of omphalitis, a recent study suggests that this relationship may not always be present (Brook, 1998; Weber et al., 2001). Predisposing conditions associated with necrotizing fasciitis at other sites in neonates include mammitis, balanitis, and fetal scalp monitoring (Hsieh et al., 1999).

The infection is frequently polymicrobial, usually involving aerobic bacteria, including enteric gram-negative bacilli, enterococci, streptococci, and *S. aureus,* as well as anaerobic bacteria, including *Bacteroides, Peptostreptococcus,* and *Clostridium* species. In monomicrobial infections, *S. aureus* is the most common bacteria isolated (Barker et al., 1987; Guiliano et al., 1977; Hsieh et al., 1999).

Pain and swelling around the site of infection are the initial symptoms. Induration and erythema occur within 24 hours. A purple discoloration and hypesthesia of the overlying skin develop, along with extensive tissue edema. Within 3 to 5 days after initial infection, skin necrosis occurs and bullae that elaborate thick, foul-smelling purple fluid appear. Crepitance may be present over the affected area. Severe systemic toxicity occurs, with decreased myocardial contractility, oliguria, adult respiratory distress syndrome, and extensive extravasation of intravascular fluid into tissue. Electrolyte abnormalities, bone marrow suppression, hemolysis, and hypocalcemia caused by saponification of the necrotic subcutaneous fat are often observed.

Because the early external signs may be only pain, mild swelling, and erythema, it may be very difficult to distinguish necrotizing fasciitis from other, less serious soft-tissue infections. A very important diagnostic feature of necrotizing fasciitis is the lack of response to antibiotics appropriate for the suspected skin infection (Fontes et al., 2000). Frozen-section biopsy, a procedure that allows evaluation of the pathology and organisms underlying the intact skin, is a rapid and very helpful test that can be performed by the surgeon to make an early diagnosis of necrotizing fasciitis (Stamenkovic and Lew, 1984). Ultrasonography, CT scanning, and magnetic resonance imaging (MRI) may be helpful in making the diagnosis of necrotizing fasciitis (Chao et al., 1999; Weber et al., 2001). Plain radiographs may occasionally show subcutaneous gas. A key to the diagnosis at a later stage of this infection is the ability to pass a sterile instrument along a plane superficial to the deep fascia without resistance. This phenomenon is observed because necrosis of the overlying dermis and epidermis undermines the overlying skin. Aerobic and anaerobic cultures of blood and wound exudate, along with Gram stain, should be obtained.

Because of the systemic toxicity that results from this infection, patients require correction of fluid, electrolyte, hematologic, renal, cardiac, and pulmonary abnormalities. For necrotizing fasciitis not associated with a marine injury, empiric therapy should cover group A *Streptococcus*, *S. aureus*, gram-negative enteric bacteria, and anaerobes that include *Bacteroides*, *Peptostreptococcus*, and *Clostridium* species. Several empiric regimens have been suggested and are shown in Table 44-1. Antibiotic treatment can be tailored to cover the pathogens isolated from blood and surgical specimens.

Emergent widespread surgical débridement of all necrotic tissue must be performed to decrease mortality from this disease. Repeat débridement within 24 to 48 hours may be necessary because of continued dissection of the infection into surrounding tissue. Investigational treatment modalities of hyperbaric oxygen for necrotizing fasciitis and intravenous immune globulin for necrotizing fasciitis associated with

streptococcal toxic shock syndrome have been explored and may decrease the mortality due to these infections (Fontes et al., 2000).

Patients who survive the infection often require an extensive hospital stay. Disfigurement often results from the radical débridement required to treat this disease. This infection has a high mortality. Even with appropriate and early surgical débridement, the mortality may not be reduced to less than 30%.

Synergistic nonclostridial anaerobic myonecrosis. Synergistic nonclostridial anaerobic myonecrosis (Baxter, 1972), also called *synergistic necrotizing cellulitis, cutaneous gangrene, necrotizing cutaneous myositis,* and *gram-negative anaerobic cutaneous gangrene,* is an uncommon, aggressive, life-threatening necrotizing infection that affects the skin, dermis, fascia, and muscle. It is a polymicrobial infection. Anaerobic streptococci, *Bacteroides* species, and several species of gram-negative enteric bacilli are most frequently isolated.

The infection occurs within 3 to 14 days after contamination of a wound. Exquisite tenderness around the wound that is out of proportion to the physical findings is often the first symptom. The area around the wound is initially only erythematous. Unfortunately, by the time edema and a characteristic blue-gray discoloration occur, there is already extensive muscle necrosis. Bullae form in the overlying skin and drain a foul-smelling liquid described as "dishwater pus," and occasionally crepitance can be felt. Systemic toxicity develops rapidly.

Aerobic and anaerobic blood cultures and cultures of the exudate, present only in the later stages of this disease, should be obtained. Frozen-section biopsy may be helpful in determining the presence of tissue necrosis underlying the relatively normal appearing skin early in the disease course and will provide material for bacterial culture. Biopsy will also help distinguish myonecrosis from necrotizing fasciitis, which leaves the underlying muscle intact.

Hypovolemia, acidosis, clotting disturbances, anemia, septic shock, renal failure, disorientation, and adult respiratory distress syndrome can occur early in this infection. Correction of these disturbances and intensive cardiovascular support must be provided in preparation for the emergent radical surgical débridement that is required to treat this disease. Débridement may need to be repeated to ensure removal of all necrotic tissue. Antibiotics can control the extension of infection only if removal of all necrotic and infected tissue is complete. Empiric antibiotics should cover anaerobic and gram-negative enteric organisms. Because this disease may be clinically indistinguishable from clostridial myonecrosis, an antibiotic active against *Clostridium* species should initially be used, as shown in Table 44-1. Radical débridement, necessary for the treatment of this disease, is associated with severe disfigurement. Irreversible multisystem organ failure may occur. Untreated, the mortality of this disease is about 75%. Treated early, the mortality still reaches 10%.

Clostridial myonecrosis (gas gangrene). Clostridial myonecrosis is an uncommon but virulent life-threatening necrotizing infection of all the soft tissues, including the muscle (Darke et al., 1977; Fromm and Silen, 1969; Hart et al., 1983). It may occur in any tissue that has been devitalized by trauma, surgery, or the normal process of umbilical cord necrosis after delivery. Once devitalized tissue is infected with clostridia, elaboration of clostridial exotoxins and enzymes that cause necrosis of adjacent muscle allows the infection to spread extensively and rapidly into healthy, untraumatized muscle. *C. perfringens,* the most virulent of these organisms, is most often responsible for this disease. Toxins released from the organisms are absorbed into the systemic circulation and cause massive hemolysis, cardiotoxicity, renal failure, and CNS dysfunction. The massive hemolysis, in turn, leads to hemoglobinuria, jaundice, and renal failure.

Aside from sudden and severe pain in the wound, which spreads along the path of the infection, there is a paucity of physical findings initially. With progression of disease, skin overlying the affected area becomes pale and tense because of the underlying edema caused by massive myonecrosis. Occasionally the underlying muscle may be so edematous that herniation through an incision site may occur. Anaerobic metabolism by clostridia results in gas accumulation within the infected tissues. Serous, nonpurulent exudate, described as having a sickly sweet odor, emanates from the wound, and the skin overlying the affected area takes on a bronze or purple coloration. The disease is so rapidly progressive that these changes in the skin can occasionally progress over a period of hours. Changes in mental status and rapid onset of severe systemic toxicity occur,

notably with tachycardia out of proportion to the moderate rise in temperature. Within a short time, hypotension and renal failure occur, and, if untreated, this infection leads to death rapidly, sometimes within 12 hours.

As soon as this disease is suspected, anaerobic and aerobic cultures from blood should be obtained and Gram stain should be performed immediately on material from the wound and skin bullae. If gram-positive bacilli are seen, surgical débridement should be planned immediately. In the early stages of infection, it may be very difficult to distinguish clostridial myonecrosis from anaerobic cellulitis and necrotizing fasciitis. Although CT may be helpful in detecting gas in muscle, surgical examination of the wound may be the only way to distinguish clostridial myonecrosis from the other necrotizing infections. The dermis, fascia, and muscle must be carefully examined for signs of necrosis and for the presence and types of bacteria. Once the diagnosis is entertained, surgery should never be delayed while awaiting scheduling of CT scan or results of wound culture. Full critical care support is required before and during immediate surgical débridement of all compromised subcutaneous tissue and muscle, as well as necrotic debris and hematomata. Although treatment with antibiotics alone will not alter the course of this disease, it may play a role in limiting infection once full débridement is achieved. The antibiotic choice for *Clostridium* species is penicillin, given intravenously in high doses as the sodium salt (hyperkalemia caused by renal failure and muscle and erythrocyte destruction are often present). A patient who has a penicillin allergy can be treated with chloramphenicol or clindamycin, although some strains of clostridia have become resistant to clindamycin. Additional antibiotic coverage may be needed if other bacterial species are seen on Gram stain. Hyperbaric oxygen therapy, in combination with surgical débridement and antibiotic therapy, may decrease mortality from this disease (Hart et al., 1983). Children who survive have prolonged hospital courses with slow recovery and require reconstructive surgery because of the extensive surgical débridement that is required to arrest the infection. Mortality for clostridial myonecrosis is about 60%.

ANAEROBIC BACTEREMIA

Anaerobes are infrequent but clinically important causes of bacteremia. Because delay or failure to administer antibiotics directed against these pathogens can often lead to death, it is essential that the clinician be aware of the clinical conditions associated with anaerobic bacteremia.

Epidemiology

Anaerobes are a minor but important contributor to bacteremia in neonates and children (Brook, 1989b; Thirmuoothi et al., 1976); 1% to 3% of pathogens isolated from blood are identified as anaerobes (Berner et al., 1998; Kellogg et al., 2000; Ronnestad et al., 1998; Zaidi et al., 1995). This incidence is similar to that found in adults (Bartlett and Dick, 2000). The low frequency of anaerobic bacteremia has led to the proposal that anaerobic blood cultures be obtained only for patients with predisposing clinical conditions (Berner et al., 1998; Ortiz and Sande, 2000). Although this proposal has great merit, reports of unexpected cases of anaerobic bacteremia should be taken into consideration (Brook, 1980c; Templeton et al., 1983; Thompson et al., 2001).

Clinical conditions that predispose neonates to anaerobic bacteremia included premature rupture of membranes, maternal chorioamnionitis, necrotizing enterocolitis (NEC), prematurity, immune deficiencies, and anatomic congenital anomalies that allow bacteria to gain access to sterile sites (Brook, 1998). The most common infections associated with anaerobic bacteremia in neonates were NEC, meningitis, pneumonia, and omphalitis (Brook, 1998). Conditions that predisposed children beyond the neonatal period to anaerobic bacteremia include Crohn's disease, cancer, neurologic impairment, immunodeficiencies, and postanginal sepsis (Lemierre's syndrome) (Brook, 1989b; Brook, 1995; Citron et al., 1995).

Etiology

Anaerobic bacteremia, as in the case of many other infections due to anaerobic bacteria, may be polymicrobial and often involves both anaerobic and aerobic bacteria. Bacterial isolates from cases of neonatal anaerobic bacteremia include *Fusobacterium* species, *Bacteroides* species, *Propionibacterium* species, *Peptostreptococcus* species, *Veillonella* species, *Eubacterium* species, and *Lactobacillus acidophilus* (Brook, 1990; Thompson et al., 2001). In children beyond the neonatal period, the most common isolates found in cases of anaerobic bac-

teremia are *B. fragilis,* other *Bacteroides* species, *Clostridium* species, *Peptostreptococcus* and *Fusobacterium* species, and *P. acnes* (Berner et al., 1998; Brook, 1980a; Brook, 1989b; Citron et al., 1995). The species of bacteria isolated from the blood often reflects the primary portal of entry and give clues that may help identify the source of infection. The isolation of fecal anaerobes such as *B. fragilis* and *Clostridium* species suggests a GI source of infection, whereas *Peptostreptococcus* species and *Fusobacterium* species are often associated with sinusitis, oropharyngeal infection, and chronic otitis media (Brook, 1980a). Bacteremia with *P. acnes* may indicate that a CSF or cardiovascular shunt is infected (Brook, 1980a). In all cases of bacteremia, a careful search for the source of infection should be made.

Clinical Manifestations

Bacteremia due to most species of anaerobic bacteria has no features that distinguish it from bacteremia due to aerobic bacteria. The symptoms often reflect the anatomic source of infection. Bacteremic infections with *Clostridium septicum,* however, are notable for the devastating and rapidly fatal clinical course due to bacterial toxins that cause severe hemolysis, shock, and sepsis.

Diagnosis

A high degree of clinical suspicion is often needed to make the diagnosis of anaerobic bacteremia. The diagnosis of anaerobic bacteremia is often made empirically, because isolation of anaerobic bacteria takes a week or longer owing to their slow growth. The presence of a pathologic process or condition that predisposes the child to infection with anaerobic bacteria often suggests the primary source of infection, although secondary sites of infection may occur. The secondary sites may be adjacent to the original site (meningitis or subdural abscess after direct extension of infection in sinuses) (Brook, 1989b) or distant from the primary source (osteomyelitis after hematogenous spread of bacteria from an oropharyngeal source). Therefore, appropriate diagnostic procedures such as plain radiographs, radionuclide scans, ultrasound, CT scans, or MRI must be undertaken to identify these sites.

Complications

The mortality rate for anaerobic bacteremia in children varies between 18% and 37% (Brook, 1980a; Brook, 1990; Dunkle et al., 1976). In neonates, the highest mortality occurs in those with *Bacteroides* bacteremia (Brook, 1990). The mortality often reflects the child's age, severity of the underlying disease, location of primary and secondary sites of infection, pathogen(s), rapidity of diagnosis, and institution of appropriate antibacterial agents.

Treatment

Anaerobic bacteremia is often polymicrobial, and identification of anaerobic organisms requires considerable time. Initial treatment, therefore, is often empirical and should cover suspected anaerobic and aerobic bacteria. The antibiotics chosen should be based on the source of infection, if one has been identified (e.g., abdominal, oropharyngeal process), and the prevalence of bacterial resistance in the geographic locale (Citron et al., 1995). Recommendations for empiric therapy are given in Table 44-1. Once pathogens are identified and their susceptibility determined, the narrowest spectrum antibiotic(s) that covers the isolated organisms should be used. The source of infection, if not obvious, should be identified, and surgical débridement or drainage should be performed if a collection of pus is found.

INTRACRANIAL ABSCESSES

In children, bacterial infections of the CNS associated with anaerobic bacteria include brain abscess, subdural and epidural empyema, suppurative intracranial thrombophlebitis, and, less commonly, spinal subdural and epidural abscess. Most of these infections occur as a complication of infection outside the CNS, with the type, location, and microbiology of the intracranial lesions reflecting the source of infection. Because these infections are life threatening, they require rapid therapeutic intervention.

Epidemiology

Brain abscess and subdural empyema secondary to sinus infections are the most common intracranial infections associated with anaerobic bacteria in children and primarily occur in older children (Gallagher et al., 1998; Giannoni et al., 1998). A well reported phenomenon that occurs predominantly in adolescent males is the development of subdural empyema after frontal sinusitis without history of chronicity (Kaufman et al., 1983). Otogenic infections and dental abscesses may also cause

intracranial infections, but less frequently than infection of the sinuses. Before the age of antibiotics, chronic otitis media (OM) and mastoiditis were major causes of intracranial suppurative infection. Other conditions that put children at risk for intracranial complications are cyanotic congenital heart disease (CCHD) and pulmonary arteriovenous fistulas. Of children with CCHD—including those with tetralogy of Fallot, dextroposition of the great arteries, complete atrioventricular canal, tricuspid atresia, double outlet right ventricle, and truncus arteriosis—2% to 6% develop brain abscesses because of the presence of right-to-left intracardiac shunts (Fischbein et al., 1981; Spires et al., 1985; Theophilo et al., 1985). Children who have had intracranial trauma such as fractures of the paranasal sinuses, neurosurgical procedures, or congenital malformations such as dermal sinuses and encephaloceles are at increased risk for brain or subdural infection (Chen et al., 1999).

Pathogenesis

Intracranial infections can occur following direct extension of infection intracranially through the cranial bones or via the valveless diploic or emissary veins. Infection in the frontal sinuses can readily spread intracranially through the thin frontal bones and via the diploic veins to cause subdural and extradural empyema, frontal brain abscess, subgaleal abscess, and septic thrombophlebitis of cortical veins and intracranial venous sinuses (Fairbanks and Milmoe, 1985). Subdural and extradural empyema can be present simultaneously (Hlavin et al., 1994). Ethmoid sinus infection can also result in subdural empyema. Abscesses from infected mastoids are most likely spread contiguously to the temporal lobe or cerebellum, possibly through the internal auditory canal or cochlear and vestibular aqueducts, or between temporal suture lines (Gower and McGuirt, 1983; Spires et al., 1985). Sphenoid sinusitis, although relatively uncommon, can spread to the temporal lobe or sella turcica (Lew et al., 1983). Dental abscesses, especially those involving the molar teeth, can lead to brain abscesses (usually in the frontal but occasionally in the temporal lobes) (Hollin et al., 1967), as well as subdural empyema (Brook, 1992).

Brain abscesses from a distant infected site often occur when pathologic conditions cause decreased brain capillary blood flow, leading to microinfarction and reduced tissue oxygenation. Such conditions may occur in patients with CCHD because of increased blood viscosity secondary to polycythemia or in patients with septic emboli released from a distal infected site (endocarditis, osteomyelitis) (Wispelwey and Scheld, 1995). Hematogenously spread abscesses usually occur along the distribution of the middle cerebral artery in the frontal and parietal lobes. Occasionally, subdural empyema can occur via hematogenous spread (Wispelwey and Scheld, 1995). Penetrating head trauma may result in the formation of brain abscess or subdural empyema after introduction of bacteria through a break in the dura (Foy and Skarr, 1980; Tay and Garland, 1987).

Pathology

Brain abscesses are thought to evolve through several stages that can be distinguished by differences in contrast enhancement on pre- and post-contrast CT scan (Britt et al., 1981; Britt and Enzmann, 1983) and by MRI (Smith and Arvin, 1992). In the early stages, referred to as *cerebritis,* the site of infection is localized but unencapsulated, whereas in the later stage the mature abscess has a fibrous, collagenized capsule encasing the necrotic center. In all stages, edema may surround the abscess. The significance in distinguishing the stages of the abscess is that the response to antibiotic therapy without surgical drainage may differ according to stage. Abscesses in very early stages may respond to prolonged antibiotic therapy alone, whereas those with established capsule formation require either aspiration or drainage or excision of the abscess (Keren, 1984; Smith and Arvin, 1992; Wispelwey and Scheld, 1995).

Subdural empyema is a collection of pus within the potential space between the dura and arachnoid, the two outer layers of the meninges (Greenlee, 1995a; Smith and Hendrick, 1983). In contrast to collections in the epidural space that remain small because of tethering of the dura to the suture lines of the skull, subdural space collections of pus can spread unimpeded over both cerebral hemispheres and also collect at the base of the brain and along the falx cerebri. Septic thrombosis of bridging veins crossing the subdural space may result, causing hemorrhagic infarction. Life-threatening transtentorial herniation caused by subdural mass effect and cerebral edema may eventually occur (Greenlee, 1995a; LeBeau et al., 1973).

Intracranial epidural (extradural) abscesses are located between the cranial bone and dura, which forms the innermost layer of the cranial periosteum (Greenlee, 1995b; Smith and Hendrick, 1983). They occur most often as a complication of frontal sinusitis but can also be secondary to mastoiditis, craniotomy, or head trauma (Greenlee, 1995b). After extension of bacteria within the frontal sinus through the frontal bone, the pus collects between the osteomyelitic bone and dura and remains relatively confined within this space. Further complications occur, however, when the infection spreads via bridging veins into the subdural space.

Etiology

Anaerobic and aerobic bacterial pathogens found in intracranial infections are often a subset of those found in the primary source of infection (Chun et al., 1986; Jadavji et al., 1985). The role of anaerobic bacteria in these infections has probably been underestimated (Brook, 1992), especially in those patients who have developed brain abscesses or empyemas secondary to spread from a contiguous focus of infection (e.g., paranasal sinusitis, mastoiditis, or odontogenic infection). Predominant anaerobic organisms due to infection at a contiguous site are *Peptostreptococcus* species, *Fusobacterium* species, *Bacteroides* species, (including *B. fragilis*) and *Prevotella* species. Aerobic bacteria associated with these infections are *S. aureus,* Enterobacteriaceae, α- and β-hemolytic streptococci, and *Haemophilus* species. Hematogenous brain abscesses in children with CCHD are most frequently caused by anaerobic and microaerophilic streptococci and viridans streptococci (Brook, 1989b). Bacteria associated with posttraumatic brain abscesses include *S. aureus,* Enterobacteriaceae, and *Clostridium* species, whereas *S. aureus* and *P. acnes* may be associated with abscess after neurosurgical procedures. Infections associated solely with aerobic bacteria include subdural empyemas and brain abscesses secondary to meningitis.

Clinical Manifestations

Brain abscesses are space-occupying lesions. Headache and fever are often present. Depending on the location, there may be progressive focal neurologic deficits, as well as general signs of increased intracranial pressure. Nausea, vomiting, seizures, meningismus, and papilledema are variably present. The primary focus of infection may be apparent based on the history and physical examination.

Patients with subdural empyema are usually acutely ill with fever, headache, and meningismus. If enlargement occurs, signs of an intracranial mass lesion will be present. Signs and symptoms attributable to the primary source of infection may be noted. Epidural abscess often has an indolent course, unless accompanied by a subdural collection. If the abscess is secondary to frontal sinusitis, frontal bone osteomyelitis (Pott's puffy tumor) may be seen.

Intracranial abscess or empyema may be associated with venous sinus thrombosis. In addition to clinical findings caused by abscess or empyema, characteristic signs and symptoms associated with thrombosis of each different venous sinus may be observed (Greenlee, 1995b).

Diagnosis

An intracranial lesion should be suspected in a child with fever and focal neurologic signs. A lumbar puncture is often not helpful in making the diagnosis of an intracranial lesion and, because of the risk of herniation, is contraindicated in these cases until studies determine that an intracranial mass lesion is not present. A radiologic imaging procedure should be performed as rapidly as possible. CT scan with contrast is extremely sensitive in showing the presence of an established brain abscess but may be less sensitive in the detection of a subdural empyema and epidural abscess. Furthermore, contrast-enhanced CT scanning cannot distinguish between brain abscess and neoplasms, granuloma, cerebral infarction, and resolving hematoma (Wispelwey and Scheld, 1995). CT is also less helpful in the early stages of abscess formation or if abscess rupture into the ventricles has occurred. Contrast-enhanced MRI scan is superior to contrast-enhanced CT for the diagnosis of brain abscess, especially in the early stage of abscess formation and determination of the success of therapy. MRI is often preferred for the diagnosis of subdural empyema and epidural abscess because of its increased specificity and sensitivity in determining the presence of these infections and in distinguishing them from other CNS lesions (Haimes et al., 1989; Wispelwey and Scheld, 1995). MRI also permits the diagnosis of venous sinus thrombosis. Technetium brain scan is also a very sensitive test in the diagnosis of brain abscess, but it will not distinguish abscess from necrotic tumor or infarction. In neonates, ultrasonography is often useful in the diagnosis of brain abscess. If there is a delay in obtaining a CT or MRI and a distinction between bacterial meningitis and a mass lesion cannot be made, blood cultures should be obtained and antibiotics started while awaiting scheduling and results of the imaging procedure.

Differential Diagnosis

Although there are many potential causes of intracranial lesions, the differential diagnosis can be narrowed by the history, physical examination, and presence of factors that may predispose the patient to different types of intracranial lesions. The presence of sinusitis, otitis, mastoiditis, recent periodontal or neurosurgical procedures, head trauma, CCHD, or meningitis should alert the physician to the possibility of a CNS infection. A history of travel may suggest a parasitic infection. Other CNS lesions that must be considered in the diagnosis are herpes simplex encephalitis, CNS vasculitis, cerebral infarction, and tumor. In children with AIDS, intracranial lesions that must be considered include toxoplasmosis, CNS lymphoma, and cryptococcal and other fungal lesions.

Treatment

Treatment of intracranial abscesses most often consists of medical and surgical treatment. In addition to supportive care that includes control of intracranial pressure and seizures, empiric antibiotics that have been shown to penetrate into intracranial sites of infection must be used (Kramer et al., 1969). Until the microbial agents are identified, an antibiotic regimen that provides coverage against streptococci, staphylococci, anaerobes, and gram-negative bacilli (Donald, 1990; Sjoln et al., 1993) should be initiated (Table 44-1). The initial regimen may be altered once the primary source and bacteria are identified.

For brain abscess, surgical aspiration through a burr hole or by stereotatic CT guidance (Lunsford and Nelson, 1984; Wispelwey and Scheld, 1995) or craniotomy with complete abscess excision is often required (Stepanov, 1988; Wispelwey and Scheld, 1995). In early stages of abscess development, it may be possible to treat unencapsulated abscesses (cerebritis) with prolonged antibiotic treatment (Wispelwey and Scheld, 1995). Although the appropriate length of antibiotic treatment is unknown, a generally accepted course of therapy is 4 to 8 weeks, with at least 3 weeks of therapy administered intravenously. Early abscesses not drained may require a longer duration of therapy.

Treatment of subdural empyema and epidural abscess includes prompt institution of empiric antibiotic therapy (Table 44-1) and urgent surgical drainage. For all intracranial infections, the primary source of infection as well as other structures involved in the infection (e.g., frontal bone osteomyelitis) should be identified and treatment administered.

Complications and Prognosis

Brain abscesses and subdural empyemas can result in a mass effect, causing midline shifts, necrosis, and herniation, all of which can result in permanent and severe neurologic impairment, seizure disorder, and/or death. Brain abscesses can also rupture into ventricles, resulting in ventriculitis, meningitis, and septic thrombosis. Subdural empyemas can enlarge rapidly and extend over a large area of the brain; severe neurologic sequelae can result if rapid intervention does not occur. Because of the often insidious nature of epidural abscesses, neurologic sequelae and a mass lesion effect may not be seen until the abscess becomes sufficiently large or until it extends into the subdural space.

The advent of antibiotics and the use of radio imaging, which now allow early intervention, have decreased complications and lowered mortality from 40% to 60% to between 0% and 24%.

INTRAABDOMINAL INFECTIONS

Intraabdominal infections are a major cause of morbidity and mortality in the pediatric population. In children, most intraabdominal infections follow perforation of the appendix, which, unfortunately, remains common, with an estimated incidence of 23% to 88%. Intraabdominal infections can also occur if the bowel wall integrity is compromised by bowel wall ischemia or necrosis, as in necrotizing enterocolitis, intussusception, volvulus, incarcerated hernia; by perforation of the bowel, as in rupture of an inflamed appendix or Meckel's diverticulum, Crohn's disease, and ulcerative colitis; trauma to the bowel; after surgery on the GI tract, with resulting contamination of the peritoneal cavity with bowel flora (Brook, 1989b); and, in female

patients, by rupture of a tuboovarian abscess. Microorganisms can also enter the intraabdominal cavity during episodes of bacteremia or can be spread from adjacent infected organs such as the uterine cavity and fallopian tubes. Most infections remain localized, occurring as single or multiple abscesses that occur within different anatomic spaces or within solid viscera, such as liver and spleen, although they can also become generalized.

The difficulty in diagnosing localized intraabdominal infections in the infant and toddler may lead to a delay in treatment and result in extension of infection throughout the peritoneal cavity. In the older child, the history and physical examination often enable the physician to determine the location and extent of infection. Diagnostic radiologic studies are often necessary to ascertain the site and extent of infection. A decision, in consultation with the surgical service, must be made about the need and method of surgical drainage. Microbiologic specimens, aerobic and anaerobic, should be obtained. The patient's medical history and age, the location of the infection, and the results of microbiologic specimens should guide the physician in the use of antimicrobial agents and other facets of appropriate medical management.

Anatomy

The relationships between the spaces and organs within the abdomen dictate the localization or spread of intraabdominal infections (Meyers, 1987). The abdomen is anatomically divided into three compartments—the peritoneal cavity, the retroperitoneum, and the abdominal wall—and infection can spread among these compartments.

The peritoneal cavity is enclosed by a serous membrane, the peritoneum, which forms a sac within the abdominal cavity and covers most of the abdominal organs. During embryogenesis, the abdominal viscera undergo complex rotation, and the simple peritoneal sac becomes compartmentalized. Recesses and pathways develop within the peritoneal cavity that have the potential to collect and sequester infected fluid or allow movement of infected fluid from one area of the abdomen to another.

The intraperitoneal organs are suspended within the peritoneal sac by folds of peritoneum, called mesenteries and ligaments. Several abdominal structures are only partially encased by peritoneum. These are the liver, spleen, ascending and descending colon, and rectum. The bare area of the liver comes in direct contact with the diaphragm. The pancreas and duodenum are overlaid with peritoneum but are located within the retroperitoneal area. In the male, the peritoneum is a closed sac. However, in the female, the peritoneum has continuity with the mucous membranes of the fallopian tubes. This communication allows the spread of infection of the female genital tract to the intraperitoneal cavity.

The lesser peritoneal sac is separated from the greater peritoneal cavity by the lesser omentum. These two peritoneal cavities communicate through a small opening called the *epiploic foramen (Winslow's foramen)*. Infected fluid in the lesser sac lies between the stomach and pancreas and can enter the right subhepatic space through Winslow's foramen, resulting in an abscess that overlies the right kidney. However, collections of infected material in the lesser sac may become sequestered if closure of Winslow's foramen due to inflammation occurs, resulting in a lack of symptoms normally seen when infection involving the greater sac occurs.

The normal flow of peritoneal fluid via distinct pathways within the peritoneal cavity determines the spread of infection within the peritoneal space (Meyers, 1987). Infected fluid collections originating from distal intraperitoneal foci can form in areas where fluid normally collects. Fluid in the left upper peritoneal space collects in the left subphrenic space and does not travel caudally, because flow is limited anatomically. However, the right paracolic gutter provides a freely communicating pathway between right subhepatic and subphrenic spaces and the pelvis, making these three spaces the most common sites of abscess formation within the intraperitoneal cavity.

Intraabdominal Abscesses

Epidemiology. In children, intraperitoneal abscesses are most commonly caused by appendicitis with perforation (Janik and Firor, 1979). Abscesses also result from abdominal surgical procedures and trauma, especially those involving the colon.

Pathogenesis. An abscess is a collection of bacteria, pus, and necrotic material that has been localized but not resolved by the body's defense system. Viable bacteria within the abscess cavity may continue multiplying, resulting in increased abscess size. In early stages of

abscess formation or in the neutropenic host, localization of infection may not occur, resulting in a phlegmon, or inflammatory mass, that can serve as a continued source of infection with seeding of other areas of the body. It is important to make a distinction between a phlegmon and an abscess, because drainage is usually required for abscess resolution, whereas a phlegmon cannot be drained but will respond to appropriate antibiotic therapy.

Abscesses form within the abdomen when bacteria enter the normally sterile peritoneal space and cannot be cleared by the defense mechanisms of the peritoneum. Such situations occur when there is incomplete resolution of diffuse peritonitis or localization of a GI perforation without complete clearing of the contaminating material. An abscess can also occur after contamination of a preexisting hematoma with bacteria or from spread of infected CSF at the peritoneal tip of a ventriculoperitoneal (VP) shunt.

The location of abscess formation is dependent on the source of the contaminating bacteria and flow of peritoneal fluid (Levison and Bush, 1995; Wilson, 1982a). Most abscesses from appendiceal rupture remain in the right lower quadrant, although the infecting material may be distributed within the peritoneal cavity to the pelvic area and to the subphrenic and subhepatic spaces via the right paracolic gutter (Mackenzie and Young, 1975). Abscesses can form in the spaces between the loops and mesentery of the small bowel or paracolic gutters (Wilson, 1982a). Abscesses secondary to direct spread from the liver and spleen will be located in the subphrenic space. Many left-sided subphrenic abscesses occur after colonic surgery (Wang and Wilson, 1977). Abscesses in the lesser peritoneal sac occur infrequently but are very important clinically because of the difficulty in diagnosing them. Although many abscesses are solitary, multiple abscesses are found in approximately 15% of cases of intraabdominal abscesses.

Etiology. The microorganisms found within an intraabdominal abscess are determined by the age of the child and source of the abscess. Intraabdominal abscesses in neonates after perforation of the bowel reflect normal bowel colonization, as well as changes in the GI flora caused by nosocomially transmitted bacteria and the use of antibiotics. A greater predominance of aerobic bacteria including *K. pneumoniae*,

Enterobacter *species,* Streptococcus *species,* and *S. epidermidis* (Bradley, 1985) have been seen in neonatal abscesses, although anaerobes, including *C. difficile,* also have been isolated (Brook, 1989a).

Abscesses arising from the stomach, liver, and biliary tract have a predominance of coliform bacteria, although anaerobes are also present. Abscesses arising from the ileum and colon have a predominance of anaerobes. Most abscesses are polymicrobial and contain both anaerobic and aerobic bacteria. The anaerobic bacteria usually found in these abscesses are *B. fragilis, P. melaninogenicus,* and *Peptococcus, Peptostreptococcus, Fusobacterium,* and *Clostridium* species. The aerobic and facultative organisms most commonly cultured are *E. coli,* α- and γ-hemolytic streptococci, enterococci, *K. pneumoniae,* and *P. aeruginosa* (Brook, 1980b; Brook, 1987). Most of the *B. fragilis* species and many enteric gram-negative isolates produce β-lactamases. Abscesses that result from infected CSF at the peritoneal tip of a VP shunt often involve *S. epidermidis* as well as other bacteria such as *E. coli.*

Clinical manifestations. Abscesses may form within several days after a perforation of a viscus or may occur several weeks after diffuse peritonitis (Wilson, 1982a). Fever, usually low grade initially, becomes persistent, rising and often spiking in nature. There is usually anorexia, nausea, and vomiting. The presence of chills implies either concomitant bacteremia or impending perforation or extension of the abscess to adjacent organs.

The clinical presentation of intraabdominal abscesses depends to a great extent on their location (Wilson, 1982a). Abscesses located in the subphrenic and intermesenteric spaces often have few localizing signs, whereas abscesses in the pelvis often are associated with nonspecific lower abdominal pain, diarrhea caused by irritation of the rectum, rectal pain, and urinary urgency caused by pressure on the bladder. It is important to remember that children who are receiving steroids or antibiotics or are neutropenic may have minimal symptoms attributable to an intraabdominal abscess.

Diagnosis. An intraabdominal abscess should be suspected in a patient who has recently undergone abdominal surgery for a condition such as appendicitis or one with a history of bowel disease or trauma who now has abdominal pain, diaphragmatic symptoms, and fever.

Leukocytosis will be present in nonimmunosuppressed patients.

The location of intraabdominal abscesses is often determined by history, symptoms, and localizing peritoneal signs. Subphrenic, intermesenteric, and pelvic abscess may be difficult to diagnose because of their location, although certain signs may be helpful in determining their presence (Wilson, 1982a). Subphrenic abscesses produce dyspnea; chest pain; and short, shallow breathing caused by pain on motion of the diaphragm. Decreased breath sounds and dullness to percussion at the lung base because of pleural effusion, atelectasis, pneumonitis, or empyema will often be present. Unfortunately, prominence of signs attributable to the chest often confuses the diagnosis in such cases. If the abscess is located between the liver and the diaphragm, referred shoulder pain may be present. An anteriorly located subphrenic abscess will produce upper abdominal tenderness and peritoneal signs. However, if the subphrenic abscess is in the lesser sac, it is posterior to the liver and, therefore, separated from the anterior abdominal wall. Affected patients have upper and midabdominal pain that radiates to the back and no peritoneal signs until the abscess is very large. Patients with intermesenteric abscesses may have fever but often do not have localizing signs, although most of the patients have a paralytic ileus with decreased bowel sounds and abdominal distention. Pelvic abscesses do not produce lower abdominal rigidity, because the pelvic parietal peritoneum is supplied by the obturator nerve (L2, 3, and 4), which does not innervate the overlying pelvic abdominal musculature. Therefore, on examination of the lower abdomen, there are few signs, although tenderness to deep palpation may be found. The most important part of the physical examination in a child with suspected pelvic infection is the rectal (or vaginal) examination. A bimanual examination permits palpation of a mass in the pelvis through the anterior abdominal wall and the rectum. A tender, bulging mass may be felt through the anterior rectal wall.

Abscesses should be distinguished from other pathologic conditions that cause fever and vague abdominal pain. These include appendicitis, tumor or hematoma, salpingitis, and tuboovarian abscess.

Aerobic and anaerobic blood cultures should be performed for any child with a suspected intraabdominal abscess and fever. Culture samples obtained at the time of abscess drainage should be placed in a syringe that is tightly capped after removal of air and transported to the microbiology laboratory for anaerobic and aerobic culturing within 2 hours. Culture for fungus should also be done, because *Candida* species can overgrow in the gut of a patient who has recently been receiving broad-spectrum antibiotics.

CT is a radiologic procedure that is highly accurate in determining the presence of an abscess (Knochel et al., 1980; Kuhn and Berger, 1980). Opacification of the bowel with oral contrast agent is important for distinguishing air-fluid levels in the GI tract from that in an abscess cavity. Water-soluble contrast agent should be used in cases of suspected leakage of intraluminal contents. Intravenous contrast helps distinguish abscess from hematoma by enhancing the abscess capsule. CT scanning has an added advantage in percutaneous drainage of an accessible abscess because of its excellent visualization of the abscess and the surrounding anatomy. MRI also gives exquisite anatomic detail without the requirement of contrast (Baker et al., 1985; Cammoun et al., 1985), but it may not be available at all health-care facilities and is more costly. Young children often require sedation for either procedure.

The chest radiographs, anterior-posterior and lateral views, may be helpful in determining the presence of a subphrenic abscess, because a basal pneumonic process, pleural effusion, and fixed elevation of the diaphragm may be seen. Unfortunately, plain chest radiographs may lead to the misdiagnosis of a primary pneumonic process. In advanced cases of subphrenic abscess, an air-fluid level below the diaphragm not attributable to the stomach air bubble may be present.

Ultrasonography at the bedside is useful in those patients too ill to be transported to a CT scanner or in those who require emergent diagnosis. Problems with ultrasonography include the requirement that the transducing probe make contact with the skin (which may not be possible in patients who have recently undergone abdominal surgery); decreased resolution of the images because of the presence of bowel gas; and accuracy that to a great degree depends on the skill of the radiologist. For visualization of a pelvic abscess, the bladder must be filled to displace bowel loops from the pelvis.

Radionuclide scanning with gallium citrate or indium-111–labeled leukocytes is useful in determining the presence and location of an intraabdominal abscess. These tests, however, are not useful within the first 2 weeks after either a peritoneal infection or surgery, because the isotopes will localize to inflamed peritoneal and incisional areas. Problems with gallium citrate imaging are excretion by the colon, potentially masking the presence of abscesses, and uptake of the isotope by certain tumors. Patients must be able to wait 48 to 72 hours for completion and interpretation of the images. Indium-111 has the advantages of reduced time for interpretation and not being excreted into the colon. However, labeled leukocytes must be able to retain their ability to accumulate at sites of inflammation.

Treatment. In addition to supportive therapy and antibiotic therapy, abscess drainage should be performed as soon as possible because most abscesses will not resolve with antibiotic treatment alone (Levison and Bush, 1995). The drainage procedure depends on the location and number of abscesses. Surgical exploration may be required if several abscesses are suspected or if they are inaccessible to percutaneous catheter drainage. Percutaneous drainage of intraabdominal abscesses may be possible in certain patients (Levison and Bush, 1995; Pruitt and Simmons, 1988; Stanley et al., 1984). The criteria for percutaneous drainage are precise definition of the abscess location and accessibility. Patients with ongoing signs of intraabdominal sepsis may require exploration of the abdomen to determine whether several abscesses or a continued source of bacterial contamination is present. Pelvic abscesses can be drained percutaneously through the anterior rectal wall or posterior vaginal vault. All septa within the abscess cavity must be disrupted and a drain placed in the abscess cavity so that complete drainage is achieved.

An empiric antibiotic regimen that will adequately cover aerobic and anaerobic bowel flora in the abscess should be administered (Levison and Bush, 1995; Solomkin et al., 1984). Several antibiotic regimens are presented in Table 44-1. Recent hospitalization and antibiotic treatment increase the risk of infection with multiply resistant bacteria, as well as fungal pathogens, most often *Candida* species. The organisms isolated from blood and abscess material and their antibiotic susceptibilities should determine the choice of antibiotics after abscess drainage.

Complications and prognosis. Early diagnosis and treatment have improved the outcome of intraabdominal abscesses (Saini et al., 1983). However, life-threatening complications of untreated abscesses still occur. Extension of the abscess into an adjacent structure or perforation of a hollow viscus by an abscess can result in serious complications. Subphrenic abscesses can rupture through the diaphragm into the pleural space or bronchus. Abscesses located in the pelvis can spread along various fascial planes, resulting in retroperitoneal and ischiorectal abscesses, as well as necrotizing infections in the buttocks, hips, and thighs. An abscess can serve as a source of ongoing intraabdominal sepsis, leading to septic shock, multiple system failure, and death. Infertility from adhesion formation may result from pelvic abscesses involving uterine tubes or ovaries.

Prolonged hospitalizations and antibiotic therapy, occasionally greater than a month, are often required for the treatment of intraabdominal abscesses (Altemeier et al., 1973). Rapid diagnosis, adequate drainage, and appropriate antibiotic therapy usually result in a favorable prognosis. Abscesses located in the subphrenic space, lesser sac, or pelvis carry a higher mortality because of delayed recognition and treatment.

Peritonitis

Anatomy and physiology. The peritoneum encases the largest cavity in the body, with a surface area of about 1.7 m² in an adult, which is equivalent to that of the skin (Wilson et al., 1982). The peritoneum acts as a passive, semipermeable barrier to bidirectional diffusion of water and solutes and is well equipped to eliminate contaminated fluids from the peritoneal cavity. Normally the peritoneal membrane secretes several milliliters of sterile fluid, which lubricates the surface, allowing the intraperitoneal structures to slide past each other. Normal peritoneal fluid is serous in appearance with a solute concentration similar to that of plasma, a specific gravity of less than 1.016, protein content of less than 3 gm/dl, and few leukocytes.

Fluid and small contaminating particles within the peritoneal cavity are removed through stomata located in the peritoneal surface of the diaphragm (Wilson et al., 1982).

These openings lead to lymphatics within the diaphragm that drain into substernal lymph nodes and ultimately into the thoracic duct. The flow of intraperitoneal fluid to the diaphragmatic lymphatics depends on flow of fluid upward toward the subphrenic spaces, movement of the diaphragm, and intraabdominal pressure. Diaphragmatic contraction and relaxation increase flow to the lymphatics, while general anesthesia and paralytic ileus decrease clearance of fluids.

The large surface area of the peritoneum and its ability to allow bidirectional diffusion of water and solutes has great physiologic implications in diffuse peritonitis. Injury to such a large, permeable surface area is comparable to that of an extensive burn to the skin and can lead to severe fluid losses with potentially fatal hemodynamic consequences.

Epidemiology. In the neonate, most cases of peritonitis are caused by perforation of the gut from a variety of conditions that cause bowel ischemia and/or perforation (Lister, 1991). These conditions include necrotizing enterocolitis, bowel obstruction caused by atresia or stenosis, meconium ileus, or Hirschsprung's disease, and gastric or duodenal perforation. In the older child, peritonitis becomes more frequent because of the increased incidence of appendicitis. The adolescent girl with gonococcal pelvic inflammatory disease may develop gonococcal peritonitis if direct extension to the peritoneum occurs.

An increased frequency of peritonitis occurs in patients undergoing peritoneal dialysis and in patients such as those with nephrotic syndrome or cirrhosis, who have decreased opsonic activity in preexisting ascitic fluid (Levison and Bush, 1995). Primary (spontaneous) peritonitis in children may occur in both immunocompetent and immunocompromised children, although immunocompromised children are at greater risk. Splenectomized children are at risk for the development of peritonitis with encapsulated bacteria.

Pathogenesis and pathophysiology. Processes that introduce bacteria, foreign material, and fluid into the peritoneal cavity (bowel perforation) and prevent its clearing (diaphragmatic paralysis caused by general anesthesia) predispose to the development of peritonitis (Maddaus et al., 1988). Early responses of the peritoneum to infection include nonspecific inflammation that results in vasodilation, increased capillary permeability, edema, fluid transudation into the peritoneal cavity, and influx of neutrophils. Bacteria and their toxins are often absorbed via the lymphatics and capillaries, causing bacteremia and toxemia. Accumulation of products such as complement, immunoglobulins, clotting factors, and fibrin occurs. The fibrin results in the eventual formation of adhesions, an attempt to localize infection.

As infection continues, massive fluid loss into the peritoneal cavity occurs because of extensive transudation of fluid from the plasma into the layer of peritoneal connective tissue, peritoneal cavity, and lumen of the paralytic bowel (third-space effect). An adult with untreated peritonitis can lose several liters of fluid in 24 hours, resulting in hemodynamic and electrolyte abnormalities that, if not corrected, can result in death.

Etiology. Infection of the peritoneal cavity secondary to rupture of an abdominal viscus most often involves aerobic and anaerobic bacteria found in the GI tract.

Peritonitis in the neonate caused by rupture of an abdominal viscus involves those organisms that colonize the gut of the neonate— *E. coli, K. pneumoniae, Enterobacter* species, *S. aureus,* and *Candida* species, as well as anaerobic bacteria, such as *Clostridium* species and *B. fragilis* (Bell, 1985). In addition, *S. epidermidis* has been found in the peritoneal fluid in some infants with peritonitis associated with necrotizing enterocolitis (Mollitt et al., 1988). Peritonitis due to extension of omphalitis through the clotted umbilical vessels is predominantly caused by *S. aureus,* group A streptococci, *E. coli, K. pneumoniae,* and *P. mirabilis* (Brook, 1980a), although these infections can also be mixed aerobic and anaerobic infections and, less commonly, anaerobic infections alone. In neonates, the peritoneum can also be seeded during bacteremia with organisms such as group B streptococci (Chadwick et al., 1983).

Primary (spontaneous) peritonitis results from hematogenous spread of bacteria to the peritoneal cavity (Fowler, 1971; McDougal et al., 1975). In young girls it is monomicrobial, associated most often with *S. pneumoniae* and group A streptococci. Children with nephrotic syndrome develop peritonitis with staphylococci, streptococci, and gram-negative bacteria (Speck et al., 1974). Patients with cirrhosis may develop peritoneal infections with bowel flora, such as *E. coli* and *Bacteroides* and *Clostridium*

species. Splenectomized children may develop peritonitis with encapsulated bacteria such as *H. influenzae* and pneumococci. Immunosuppressed patients with lymphomas and leukemias and children who receive high-dose steroid treatment may develop peritonitis caused by gram-negative enteric bacteria, which include *Klebsiella, Enterobacter, Serratia,* and *Pseudomonas* species, as well as streptococci, enterococci, *Candida* species, and other fungi. Gonococcal peritonitis can occur in adolescent girls if direct extension of gonococcal pelvic inflammatory disease to the peritoneum occurs.

Peritonitis occurring in the setting of peritoneal dialysis is often caused by skin flora, enteric bacteria, or environmental organisms (Powell et al., 1985; Rubin et al., 1980). Most often *S. aureus,* coagulase-negative staphylococci, and streptococci are isolated from the dialysate fluid. Gram-negative bacteria such as *E. coli, Candida* species, and, less commonly, atypical mycobacteria may also be found.

Clinical manifestations. Peritonitis in the newborn usually occurs within the first few days of life, because most of the predisposing conditions, such as bowel obstruction, are present at birth. Signs and symptoms attributable to the underlying condition will be present; however, the diagnosis of peritonitis may be difficult to make because of the paucity of localizing signs. The neonate will appear ill, often with hypothermia, vomiting, and abdominal distention, and, if gross contamination of the peritoneal cavity has occurred, inflammation of the abdominal wall may be present. As the infection progresses, shock develops.

In the older child, diffuse abdominal guarding, rigidity and rebound tenderness, tympanitic abdomen, and decreased bowel sounds will be detected on physical examination early in the disease process. Rectal or vaginal examination will reveal signs of pelvic tenderness. The child with normal immune function will have leukocytosis, often greater than 20,000 cells/mm^3, with a predominance of neutrophils. Patients who are receiving high-dose steroid treatment or who have severe neutropenia may not be febrile and may have little or no abdominal tenderness and rebound. These patients, however, will have decreased bowel activity. With disease progression, nausea and vomiting, distention, high fever, and toxemia will be evident; as septic shock ensues, low white blood cell count, anemia, and signs of disseminated intravascular coagulation develop. Fluid and electrolyte abnormalities and decreased urine output due to "third spacing" also occur. If untreated, metabolic acidosis caused by depression of cardiac function and vasoconstriction develops, followed eventually by capillary leak syndrome, leading to pulmonary edema, decreased ventilatory ability and, eventually, acute respiratory distress syndrome.

In girls with gonococcal peritonitis, right upper quadrant tenderness caused by gonococcal perihepatitis (Fitz-Hugh–Curtis syndrome) will be present. Peritonitis caused by contamination of the dialysis catheter will be accompanied by cloudy peritoneal dialysate fluid and tachycardia, hyperventilation, and fever.

Diagnosis. Diagnosis of peritonitis is made by assessing clinical manifestations and physical findings, taking into account any special concomitant medical conditions of the patient. Plain radiographs, which should include upright, supine, and left lateral decubitus positions of the abdomen, may be helpful in demonstrating free air in the peritoneal cavity if perforation of the GI tract has occurred. In such cases, free air will be evident under the diaphragm in the upright film and between the right lobe of the liver and the right diaphragm in the left lateral decubitus film. A paralytic ileus, as well as fluid between bowel loops, may also be seen. CT and ultrasonography are helpful in determining the presence of increased peritoneal fluid.

Peritoneal fluid, obtained during paracentesis, laparotomy, or from the dialysis catheter in the patient undergoing continuous ambulatory peritoneal dialysis will be cloudy fluid and contain bacteria and an abundance of neutrophils, if normal immune function is present (Schumer et al., 1964). Aerobic and anaerobic cultures of blood and peritoneal fluid should be obtained. Gram stain, stains for fungus, and acid-fast bacilli of peritoneal fluid are very helpful in choosing empiric antibiotics. Mycobacteria cultures should be done if the patient is receiving peritoneal dialysis or has had exposure to an individual with tuberculosis. If tuberculous peritonitis is suspected, a peritoneal biopsy to search for granulomas and tuberculous organisms may be necessary if the peritoneal fluid does not yield the organism by special stain or culture. All organisms isolated should be tested for antimicrobial sensitivities.

Differential diagnosis. In the neonate, abdominal processes, such as necrotizing enterocolitis or meconium peritonitis, may be indistinguishable from bacterial peritonitis. In the older child, noninfectious processes that cause peritoneal irritation and abdominal pain can mimic peritonitis. These include familial Mediterranean fever, porphyria, lead toxicity, and chylous ascites.

Treatment. Treatment consists of prompt and aggressive correction of hemodynamic and respiratory abnormalities, determination of the source of peritoneal contamination, removal of contaminating intraperitoneal material and foreign bodies, débridement of necrotic tissue, and institution of empiric antibiotics. Intraoperative peritoneal irrigation may be helpful in decreasing the intraperitoneal bacterial burden (Wilson, 1982b).

Peritonitis caused by bowel contamination should be treated with antibiotics active against bowel flora (Table 44-1). Previously hospitalized children who have developed peritonitis because of a ruptured abdominal viscus, however, may be colonized with highly drug-resistant nosocomial pathogens, such as *Pseudomonas* species or *Enterococcus* species. The antibiotic resistance patterns for these pathogens at the medical institution should be obtained from the hospital epidemiology service, and children should be treated appropriately with agents active against these bacteria, in consultation with the infectious diseases service. For the neonate with necrotizing enterocolitis and peritonitis, vancomycin, in addition to gentamicin and clindamycin or cefotaxime and metronidazole, should be considered for empiric therapy to provide coverage of *S. epidermidis*. Adjustments in the antimicrobial regimen should be made in all cases as soon as the identification and antibiotic sensitivities of the isolated organisms are known.

The treatment of the immunocompetent child with primary peritonitis should include an antimicrobial regimen active against staphylococci, streptococci, and gram-negative enteric organisms. Because peritonitis in children with nephrotic syndrome, cirrhosis, peritoneal dialysis, lymphoma, or leukemia may involve bacteria with high levels of antibiotic resistance, fungi, or unusual mycobacteria, assistance from the infectious diseases consultation in choosing the appropriate antimicrobial regimen is recommended.

Complications and prognosis. Peritonitis is a life-threatening condition that rapidly leads to septic shock, multiorgan system failure, intraabdominal abscesses requiring reoperation and repeat drainage procedures, postsurgical abdominal wound infection, and adhesions as well as prolonged hospitalization (Machiedo et al., 1985). The rapid institution of antibiotic administration, supportive therapy, and surgery for secondary bacterial peritonitis after bowel perforation has lead to a decrease in mortality from 70% to about 30%.

Acute Appendicitis

Epidemiology. Acute appendicitis is the most common acute surgical disease of the abdomen in pediatric patients (Janik and Firor, 1979), with an estimate incidence of 60,000 to 80,000 cases annually (Sivit et al., 2001), and is one of the most frequent causes of pediatric hospitalizations. Although it is found in children of all ages, it is rare during the first year of life. Approximately 4% of cases of appendicitis in children occur before the age of 3 years. The highest frequency of appendicitis is between ages 12 and 20 years.

Pathogenesis and etiology. Obstruction of the appendiceal lumen is a major contributor to the development of appendicitis. Obstruction may be caused by fecaliths, concretions of fecal material, hypertrophy of lymphoid tissue within the appendix because of a concurrent viral infection such as measles and adenovirus, ingested foreign material such as seeds of vegetables and fruits, and intestinal parasites such as *Ascaris,* pinworm *(Enterobius vermicularis),* and whipworm *(Trichuris trichiura).* Luminal obstruction results in the accumulation of mucosal secretions, which causes a rapid rise in intraluminal pressure, venous congestion, and compression of blood vessels that supply the distal appendix. Conditions that favor multiplication of bacteria in the lumen and subsequent bacterial invasion result and may lead to rupture of the ischemic wall of the appendix. Appendiceal rupture and release of its intraluminal contents into the intraperitoneal cavity occur in 10% of patients with acute appendicitis within the first 24 hours and in 50% within the first 48 hours after the onset of symptoms.

The infection may be localized through the formation of adhesions between the cecum and the ileum and by migration of part of the greater omentum to the inflamed appendix, which wraps itself around the organ. If appendicitis develops over a longer period of time, an inflammatory appendiceal phlegmon, which subsequently develops into an abscess, results. Because the greater omentum is poorly developed in children less than 2 years of age, localization of infection may not occur. If appendiceal rupture occurs, infection can spread to the pelvic recess and the right subhepatic space via the normal flow of peritoneal fluid.

Bacteria reflecting normal bowel flora are usually found within in the inflamed appendix and in surrounding areas after appendiceal rupture. The organisms include *B. fragilis, Peptococcus* species, *Peptostreptococcus* species, *Fusobacterium* species, *P. melaninogenicus, Clostridium* species, *E. coli,* α- and γ-hemolytic streptococci, enterococci, and *P. aeruginosa* (Brook, 1980a). *Streptococcus pneumoniae* has also been isolated from several cases of appendicitis (Heltber et al., 1984).

Clinical manifestations. The presentation of appendicitis is influenced by the age of the child and the position of the appendix. The atypical clinical presentation that occurs in approximately one third of children (Sivit et al., 2001) and the difficulty in distinguishing appendicitis from other intraabdominal processes results in either delay in diagnosis or unnecessary surgical procedures. The presentation in infants and toddlers is nonspecific or is suggestive of acute infectious gastroenteritis (Murch, 2000), and the diagnosis is often not entertained because of infrequency of appendicitis in these age groups (Snyder and Chaffin, 1952). Infants usually have an acute abdominal process that is accompanied by abdominal distention, fever, bilious vomiting, and diarrhea. A tender abdomen with guarding and, less commonly, erythema, edema, or cellulitis over the right lower quadrant with a palpable mass in that region will be found.

In the older child, colicky or diffuse abdominal pain is the most constant symptom of acute appendicitis. In the classical presentation, in which the appendix is in the retrocecal position, appendicular distention results in pain that usually begins in the periumbilical or epigastric region, then shifts to McBurney's point in the right lower quadrant within several hours, becoming constant and severe. In some of these patients, pain may begin in the right lower quadrant. Loss of appetite, nausea, and vomiting are common. Diarrhea or constipation and diarrhea are less common. Fever usually appears within 24 hours after the onset of pain. Shallow, rapid breathing may be present because of pain on diaphragmatic movement during respiration. Physical examination reveals tenderness and guarding in the right iliac fossa. Because the iliopsoas muscle also becomes irritated, the child may experience pain on extension of the right thigh when he or she is lying on the left side (psoas test). A tender, palpable mass in the right lower quadrant may be present if a localized abscess is forming around the appendix. Rebound tenderness is a reliable test to use if the diagnosis of appendicitis is unclear. If the appendix ruptures, a sudden decrease in abdominal pain that lasts about an hour may occur. If diffuse peritonitis results from rupture, generalized tenderness with guarding will be found.

Atypical presentations of appendicitis may occur if the inflamed appendix is directed downward to the pelvis or behind the ileum because the inflamed appendix does not contact the parietal peritoneum. Thus, early symptoms of appendiceal distention are present, but because the pain does not localize typically, a delay in diagnosis occurs frequently. In these cases, laparotomy may need to be performed to confirm the diagnosis and avoid perforation of the appendix.

Diagnosis. Because the diagnosis of appendicitis is complicated by the nonspecific presentations of young children; atypical presentations in the older child; the wide variety of nonsurgical conditions that mimic appendicitis; and the lack of a definitive, diagnostic laboratory test, all children with abdominal pain lasting longer than 6 hours should be carefully observed by the pediatrician for continued or worsening abdominal pain. Preliminary laboratory studies, such as white blood cell count and urinalysis, can be done in the physician's office, and frequent contact with the patient should be made. Leukocytosis may not be helpful because it is present in only two thirds of cases of appendicitis. Pathologic conditions that need to be considered in the differential diagnosis of acute appendicitis (Knight and Vassy, 1981) include acute mesenteric adenitis, respiratory infections, renal disease, psoas abscess, hepatitis A and B, diseases of the terminal ileum, a variety of other abdominal surgical conditions, and diseases of the female genital tract. In the granulocytopenic child, necrotizing enterocolitis of the cecum (typhlitis or neutropenic enterocolitis) may present a picture similar to that seen with acute appendicitis.

Radiographic studies in select cases may aid in the diagnosis of appendicitis. However, general use of these modalities for diagnosis from 1987 to 1998 did not result in a decrease in misdiagnosis of appendicitis (Flum et al., 2001). Furthermore, while CT and ultrasonography often aid in the diagnosis of appendicitis in certain hospital settings, a recent study showed that the general use of CT and ultrasonography did not improve the overall accuracy of diagnosis or decrease the negative appendectomy rate, but instead delayed surgical consultation (Lee et al., 2001). It is important to remember that when one is diagnosing appendicitis, no radiologic procedure should replace careful and repeated examination of the patient (Ang et al., 2001; Wilson et al., 2001). CT imaging with oral soluble contrast can reveal appendiceal thickening and dilation with surrounding inflammation, allow differentiation of an appendiceal abscess from a phlegmon, and provide accurate information on the location and extent of disease. The use of CT imaging for the detection of appendicitis, however, requires that the child be able to ingest contrast material so that the GI tract is adequately opacified. High-resolution ultrasonography with graded compression may be helpful, but the accuracy of diagnosis is operator dependent and the sensitivity and specificity in various studies ranges from approximately 40% to 95% (Sivit et al., 2001). Ultrasonography also allows visualization of only a limited field. Other radiologic studies are less helpful. Plain abdominal radiographs may show a calcified appendicolith or a mass displacing the intestine, but they are usually nondiagnostic. Although a barium enema may show nonfilling of the appendix and extrinsic mass effect on the cecum, terminal ileum, and ascending colon, other pathologic processes involving the right side of the abdomen may cause these findings. Once appendiceal rupture has occurred and intraabdominal abscesses are suspected, both CT and ultrasonography may provide high accuracy and sensitivity in the detection of abscesses, although bowel gas and mesenteric fat decrease the ability of ultrasound to detect midabdominal abscesses (Medelson and Lindsell, 1987).

Treatment. Once the diagnosis of appendicitis is entertained, a surgical evaluation should take place as soon as possible. Treatment with an appropriate antibiotic regimen as indicated in Table 44-1 should begin immediately if perforation is suspected. Appendectomy should be performed without delay for unruptured appendicitis or ruptured appendicitis with peritonitis. In certain cases of uncomplicated appendicitis, laparoscopic appendectomy may be performed (Krisher et al., 2001), permitting a shorter recovery period and less postoperative pain (Lintula et al., 2001). Aerobic and anaerobic culture results from specimens taken from the inflamed appendix, periappendiceal area, and peritoneal fluid obtained during surgery should guide the final choice of antibiotics.

To prevent wound infection, perioperative prophylactic antibiotics (Busuttil et al., 1981; Winslow et al., 1983) such as clindamycin plus an aminoglycoside or third-generation cephalosporin or cefoxitin alone (Bauer et al., 1989) should be administered approximately 30 minutes before surgery (Bates et al., 1989) and discontinued in 24 hours in cases of unruptured appendicitis.

Consensus recommendations for duration of antibiotic treatment following appendectomy for complicated appendicitis are 3 to 14 days (Hoelzer et al., 1999) postoperatively. Recently, it was proposed that antibiotics be discontinued based on normalization of the white blood cell count with ≤3% immature neutrophils, normal temperature for >24 hours, and no difficulty eating. Such an approach was taken in 32 children with appendicitis complicated by perforation or gangrenous appendix after the children had appendectomy. Of the 32 children, only one who did not meet all criteria developed recurrent infection (Hoelzer et al., 1999). For some children with complicated appendicitis who are clinically stable, piperacillin-tazobactam (Fishman et al., 2000) or meropenem (Bradley et al., 2001) administered intravenously on an outpatient basis may be an alternative to continued in-hospital antibiotic treatment.

Children with an appendiceal phlegmon are managed conservatively (Skoubo-Kristensen and Hvid, 1982). These children are observed carefully, treated with intravenous antibiotic therapy until resolution of infection is achieved, and are given an interval appendectomy 2 to 3 months later.

Management of appendiceal abscess in children is controversial, however. The conventional approach has been urgent surgical drainage, with or without appendectomy (Oliak et al.,

2001). However, surgical removal of an appendiceal abscess results in a complication rate of 30% because of wound infection, fecal fistula, small bowel obstruction, prolonged ileus, and recurrent abscess (Bradley and Isaacs, 1978). Therefore, if infection is localized and there are no signs of peritonitis, conservative management consisting of intravenous fluids, antibiotic therapy, and careful observation for signs of spread of infection is often practiced (Bagi et al., 1987; Oliak et al., 2001; Skoubo-Kristensen and Hvid, 1982; Yamini et al., 1998). Conservative management may have a substantially lower complication rate than urgent surgical abscess drainage and appendectomy. A potential complication of this approach is recurrent appendicitis, which may occur at a rate of 10% to 20% (Oliak et al., 2001) if interval appendectomy is not performed 4 to 12 weeks later. Unfortunately, interval appendectomy also has complications with rates that range from 3% to 19% (Oliak et al., 2001). A third safe and effective alternative to surgery or conservative management of appendiceal abscess is percutaneous catheter drainage under ultrasound or CT guidance (Bagi et al., 1987; Jamieson et al., 1997; Shapiro et al., 1989).

Complications and prognosis. Very few complications occur from unruptured appendicitis when surgical removal is performed without delay following the onset of symptoms. The mortality for acute appendicitis with prompt diagnosis and removal of the unruptured appendix is about 0.1% (Luckmann, 1989).

Unrecognized appendicitis, however, leads to appendiceal perforation in 15% to 37% of children, resulting in diffuse peritonitis and intraperitoneal abscess (Janik and Firor, 1979) and adhesion formation. Bacteremia and fistula formation between the appendix and the bladder may occur if the appendix perforates. Portal vein thrombophlebitis with subsequent development of pyogenic liver abscesses and cholangitis may occur if appendicitis remains untreated. This complication, which carries a high mortality, is now very rare. Postoperative wound infections complicate surgical treatment of appendicitis with rates of 5% in cases of uncomplicated appendicitis, rising to 30% if rupture has occurred.

PYOGENIC LIVER ABSCESS
Epidemiology

Pyogenic liver abscess is a potentially life-threatening infection (Dehner and Kissane, 1969)

that is, fortunately, uncommon. A recent study has shown an incidence in children of 25 per 100,000 hospital admissions (Pineiro-Carrero and Andres, 1989). Although children with immunosuppressive states (Pineiro-Carrero and Andres, 1989) such as chronic granulomatous disease, leukemia, and immunosuppression associated with liver transplantation (Kusne et al., 1988) and those who have had procedures such as hepaticojejunostomy or choledochojejunostomy (Ecoffey et al., 1987) for correction of biliary atresia or choledochal cysts are at higher risk of hepatic infection, many cases are cryptogenic (Ecoffey et al., 1987).

Pathogenesis

Bacteria may reach the liver by several different routes. Hematogenous spread of bacteria to the liver through the hepatic artery occurs during episodes of bacteremia (Dehner and Kissane, 1969). Bacteria can travel to the liver via the portal veins in children with infectious or inflammatory diseases of the bowel such as appendicitis or Crohn's disease. Liver abscess may occur in neonates who develop infection of the umbilical vein after omphalitis or umbilical vein catheterization (Brook, 1989b). Liver abscesses may also occur from contiguous spread of infection, via transport of bacteria through lymphatics from pathologic processes such as appendicitis, or after penetrating or blunt trauma to the liver.

Etiology

Liver abscesses are most frequently mixed polymicrobial infections of aerobic and anaerobic bacteria but may also be caused by aerobes or anaerobes alone. Anaerobic bacteria frequently isolated include *Peptostreptococcus* species, *Bacteroides* species, *Fusobacterium* species, *Clostridium* species, and *Prevotella* species (Brook and Frazier, 1998). Aerobic and facultative bacteria include *E. coli, Streptococcus* group D, *Klebsiella* species, *Enterobacter* species, *Pseudomonas* species, and *Proteus* species, as well as *S. aureus* (Brook, 1989b; Brook and Frazier, 1998). Immunosuppressed patients may have multiple *Candida* microabscesses (Sobel, 1988). Amebic liver abscess should also be considered, because, worldwide, liver abscess is more frequently caused by infection with *Entamoeba histolytica* than bacteria. Although uncommon, hydatid cysts in liver caused by infection with *Echinococcus* may also be responsible for nonpyogenic hepatic abscesses in the appropriate clinical setting.

Clinical Manifestations

Patients often present with nonspecific signs and symptoms, making the diagnosis of liver abscess difficult. Children with solitary liver abscesses may have a subacute course, whereas those with multiple hepatic abscesses often have spiking fevers, chills, nausea, vomiting, anorexia, malaise, and weakness. Hepatomegaly and liver tenderness may be present. Abscesses located in the right lobe may cause pleuritic pain.

Diagnosis

Blood cultures may be positive in patients with liver abscesses. Usually alkaline phosphatase and, less commonly, liver transaminase levels are elevated. Nonspecific laboratory abnormalities include leukocytosis, anemia, and an elevated erythrocyte sedimentation rate. Sensitive radiologic imaging techniques that can be employed are CT or MRI scanning, ultrasonography, and radioisotopic scanning (Pineiro-Carrero and Andres, 1989). Crohn's disease should be considered in any nonimmunosuppressed child with liver abscess (Teague et al., 1988).

Treatment

Antimicrobial therapy and drainage of pyogenic liver abscesses are required for a good outcome (Gerzof et al., 1985; McCorkell and Niles, 1985). Drainage may be achieved by ultrasound- or CT-guided percutaneous catheter placement (Do et al., 1991), although a poor clinical response after percutaneous drainage will require an open drainage procedure (Barnes et al., 1987).

Empiric antibiotics should be directed at the expected organisms as indicated in Table 44-1. Extended antibiotic treatment of 4 to 6 weeks is often necessary (Barnes et al., 1987). Ultrasonography, CT, or MRI scanning should be used to monitor response. Antifungal therapy should be considered in immunosuppressed patients.

Complications and Prognosis

Improved diagnostic techniques and percutaneous drainage procedures have markedly decreased mortality from pyogenic liver abscesses. Morbidity and mortality, however, remain high in neonates (Brook, 1989b), in children who have serious underlying disease, and in those whose diagnosis has been delayed.

SPLENIC ABSCESS
Epidemiology

Splenic abscesses are very uncommon in healthy children. Children who are at risk for developing splenic abscesses include those with sickle-cell anemia in whom bland infarcts form within the spleen; children with endocarditis or sepsis originating in a distant site from which infected emboli are sent to the spleen (Chun et al., 1980); children with an enlarged spleen who develop subcapsular infarcts; and children with immunodeficiency states that prevent the spleen from performing its normal role of clearing organisms.

Pathogenesis and Etiology

Conditions that predispose to splenic abscess formation are necrosis, infarcts, and hematoma within the spleen. These splenic lesions may be infected with bacteria that reach the spleen by several different routes. The most common route is by hematogenous seeding of organisms from a remote site via the splenic artery. In about 75% of patients with infection of the spleen, multiple abscesses are found in other organs (Simson, 1980), including the liver, brain, and kidneys. Splenic abscess can also occur by direct invasion of bacteria from a subphrenic abscess.

Splenic abscesses are often polymicrobial and may be caused by aerobic or anaerobic bacteria alone or by a mixture of aerobic and anaerobic bacteria. Anaerobic bacteria isolated from splenic abscess include *Peptostreptococcus* species, *Bacteroides* species, *Fusobacterium* species, and *Clostridium* species; aerobic and facultative bacteria include *E. coli, P. mirabilis, Streptococcus* group D, *K. pneumoniae, S. aureus,* viridans streptococci, and *Citrobacter freundii* (Brook and Frazier, 1998; Green, 2001). *Salmonella* species can cause splenic abscesses in patients with diseases that predispose to splenic infarction (such as sickle-cell anemia) and decreased phagocytic and opsonizing ability. *M. tuberculosis* reaches the spleen during the initial lymphohematogenous spread. In children with hematologic malignancies, fungi such as *Candida* and *Aspergillus* species may enter the spleen during periods of fungemia, resulting in microabscesses. Bacteria in splenic abscesses that result from extension of a subphrenic abscess will reflect the aerobic and anaerobic organisms found in that abscess. Rarely, splenic abscesses can be caused by *Brucella* species

Clinical Manifestations

Splenic microabscesses that are deep within the spleen often have few manifestations directly attributable to infection of the spleen. Localizing signs such as left-sided pleuritic pain in the lower chest, upper abdomen, or costovertebral angle may occur. Following splenic abscess enlargement, splenomegaly, splenic capsule irritation, and pain that radiates to the left shoulder often occur.

Most patients will be febrile and may have left upper quadrant tenderness. In advanced disease, cachexia, tachycardia, and constant pain may be present. In many cases, differentiating symptoms caused by splenic abscess from those of the underlying disease state may be difficult.

Diagnosis

The diagnosis of splenic abscess should be considered in any patient with a history of fever and pain in the left side of the chest, the upper abdomen, the flank, or the shoulder, especially in the setting of splenic trauma (Sands et al., 1986), abnormal heart valves, sickle-cell anemia, or any other conditions that predispose to splenic infection.

Leukocytosis is often present, unless there is neutropenia from an underlying disease. Blood cultures for aerobic and anaerobic bacteria or fungi may yield organisms if the splenic abscess is serving as a source of continued bacteremia or fungemia. A rise in *Brucella* serum antibody titers suggests brucellosis. Aerobic, anaerobic, acid-fast bacilli, *Brucella,* and fungal cultures of samples from splenic abscesses may reveal the cause and suggest the primary source of infection.

Ultrasonography, CT, and MRI are the most sensitive radiologic procedures for the detection of splenic abscesses. On CT scan, splenic abscesses can be seen as focal lesions with lower density than the surrounding tissue. Splenic lesions caused by fungi, tuberculosis, and brucellosis have characteristic appearances on CT (Berlow et al., 1984). In addition, CT can be used to determine the presence of other intraabdominal foci of infection.

Treatment

Until the infecting organism(s), the source, and extrasplenic foci of infection have been determined, empiric intravenous antibiotics should be started promptly after blood cultures are obtained. The patient's clinical history and presenting signs and symptoms will be helpful in determining which antibiotics to use. Splenic abscess that occurs after development of an intraabdominal abscess should be treated with antibiotics that are active against bowel flora (Table 44-1), whereas those occurring after trauma should be treated with an agent that provides coverage against *S. aureus* and streptococci. Once the microbial cause has been determined, antimicrobial treatment should be directed against these organisms. For patients with a hematologic malignancy, fungal disease and antifungal therapy should be considered.

CT-guided catheter drainage of splenic abscesses may be an effective method of treatment, although splenectomy has been the treatment of choice for isolated splenic abscess (Berkman et al., 1983; Lerner and Spataro, 1984; Stepanov, 1988).

Complications and Prognosis

Although most splenic abscesses remain localized in the spleen, intermittent bacteremia caused by release of the organisms from infected splenic foci can occur, leading to seeding of distant sites. Rupture of abscesses into the pleural space through the diaphragm, causing a thoracic empyema, or into the abdomen, causing a subphrenic abscess or generalized peritonitis, can occur. Hemorrhage into an abscess cavity may also occur. Untreated splenic abscesses carry a grave mortality because of the underlying disease and the many serious complications of splenic infection (Linos et al., 1983). Solitary splenic abscess carries a more favorable prognosis, because two thirds of these patients have lesions confined to the spleen.

RETROPERITONEAL ABSCESS
Epidemiology

Retroperitoneal abscesses are uncommon in both the adult and pediatric population but carry a high mortality because of the difficulty in diagnosis and delay in treatment (Altemeier and Alexander, 1961; Neuhof and Arheim, 1944).

Anatomy and Pathogenesis

The retroperitoneum is a complex anatomic region consisting of potential spaces located between the posterior parietal peritoneum and

the posterior part transversalis fascia (Simons et al., 1983). This space extends superiorly to the undersurface of the diaphragm and inferiorly to the pelvic rim. The retroperitoneum is anatomically divided into three potential spaces: the space anterior to the kidneys (the anterior retroperitoneal or pararenal space), the perirenal space, and the space posterior to the kidneys (the posterior retroperitoneal or pararenal space).

The anterior retroperitoneal space is located between the posterior peritoneum and the fascia that surrounds the kidney anteriorly. Because this space contains the retroperitoneal portions of the duodenum, ascending and descending colon, pancreas, and the appendix, which is retrocecally located, infection involving any of these organs and viscera may cause retroperitoneal abscesses (Altemeier and Alexander, 1961, Evans et al., 1971; Sheinfeld et al., 1987). In addition, anatomic communications between the perirenal space and the psoas space, between the posterior retroperitoneal space and the lateral abdominal wall, and between adjacent retroperitoneal compartments allow the spread of infection to and from the retroperitoneal space.

Etiology

Retroperitoneal abscesses following appendiceal perforation contain anaerobic and aerobic bowel flora. Abscesses resulting from perinephric infection may be caused by *S. aureus* or gram-negative organisms, such as *E. coli* and *Proteus* species (Altemeier and Alexander, 1961).

Clinical Manifestations

Patients with retroperitoneal infections have few localizing symptoms and are often ill out of proportion to the physical findings. Fever; chills; nonlocalized abdominal pain; flank pain; abdominal distention; weakness and pain in the ipsilateral hip, thigh, or knee; and psoas spasm may be present (Altemeier and Alexander, 1961). Symptoms may be present for weeks before a diagnosis is made. The chronicity of illness often results in anorexia, weight loss, and malaise.

Diagnosis

On physical examination, a tender mass, representing the abscess if sufficiently large, as well as flank tenderness, may be present. If the psoas space is involved, the child may have pain on extension of the ipsilateral thigh (psoas sign). Leukocytosis with a left shift is usually present, along with anemia of chronic disease if the disease has been long standing. If a perinephric abscess is present, proteinuria, pyuria, and bacteriuria may be seen (Altemeier and Alexander, 1961). Anaerobic and aerobic blood cultures may be positive if the abscess is seeding the blood.

CT (Gerzof and Gale, 1982; Simons et al., 1983) and MRI provide precise anatomic localization of retroperitoneal abscesses. If not available, other less helpful imaging studies may be used. Plain x-ray films may show an abnormal psoas shadow, scoliosis, and, if present, gas within the abscess. An abnormal intravenous pyelogram may demonstrate kidney involvement. Radioisotopic imaging allows localization of an infectious process but entails a delay in the diagnosis (Simons et al., 1983). Ultrasonography is useful in establishing the presence of an abscess, especially in a child who is too ill to be taken to a CT or MRI scanner (Gerzof and Gale, 1982).

Treatment

An antibiotic regimen as indicated in Table 44-1 that has activity against *S. aureus*, gram-negative organisms, and anaerobic bowel flora should be instituted as soon as the diagnosis is made. Surgical (Altemeier and Alexander, 1961) or CT-guided drainage (Gerzof and Gale, 1982) should be performed, and abscess material should be cultured for aerobic and anaerobic organisms. The parenteral antibiotic regimen should be altered to provide coverage against the isolated organisms and should be continued for 2 to 3 weeks after drainage. The underlying conditions leading to abscess should be determined and corrected.

Complications and Prognosis

Abscesses can rupture into the intraperitoneal space and can extend long distances along the fascial plane superiorly to the subdiaphragmatic space, mediastinum, and thoracic cavity; laterally to the anterior abdominal wall and subcutaneous tissue of the flank; and inferiorly to the thigh, hip, and psoas muscle (Altemeier and Alexander, 1961). These complications are now rarely seen because of improved diagnostic techniques and earlier intervention. The prognosis is favorable in those retroperitoneal infections that are treated early. Diagnostic delays often result in complications that confer higher morbidity and mortality.

PSOAS ABSCESS
Epidemiology

Psoas abscesses are life-threatening but uncommon infections in children. Primary infection of the psoas muscle is due to hematogenous spread of bacteria from a focus of infection. It occurs more often in children younger than age 15 years (Stephenson et al., 1991) and is the most common form of psoas abscess in developing countries (de Jesus Lopes Filho et al., 2000). Secondary psoas abscesses occur following direct extension from an adjacent focus of infection and are most commonly due to abdominal infections. Secondary psoas abscesses are more prevalent in the United States and Europe than are those due to hematogenous spread (de Jesus Lopes Filho et al., 2000). Because the diagnosis of psoas abscess is often very difficult to make, delays in the institution of therapy are substantial, leading to increases in morbidity and mortality.

Anatomy

The psoas muscle is the major muscle of the anterior wall of the back (Gordin et al., 1983). It is invested in fascia and contains fibers that originate from the transverse processes of the twelfth thoracic vertebra and the five lumbar vertebrae and courses inferiorly through the crura of the diaphragm on either side of the vertebral column to merge with the iliac muscle (Bresee and Edwards, 1990; Simons et al., 1983). The iliopsoas muscle then crosses the sacroiliac joint and passes beneath the inguinal ligament and inserts into the lesser trochanter of the femur. Over its long course from the mediastinum to the femur, it makes contact with or is in close proximity to several key anatomic structures, including the posterior perirenal fascia, ureters, iliac muscle, sacroiliac joint, inguinal ligament, inguinal lymph nodes, hip joint, and trochanteric bursa. Thus the psoas muscle can provide a pathway for and be involved in inflammatory processes of mediastinum, the thigh, and the posterior retroperitoneal space (van Dyke et al., 1987).

Pathogenesis

In children with primary infection of psoas muscle, often no source of infection can be found, suggesting that the abscess may have resulted from hematogenous seeding of the muscle from a relatively minor skin or upper respiratory infection (Firor, 1972; Stephenson et al., 1991). Secondary infection of the psoas muscle may occur following retrocecal appendiceal rupture, Crohn's disease, or a perirenal abscess. In addition, infectious processes such as vertebral osteomyelitis and discitis involving the twelfth thoracic and the five lumbar vertebrae, septic arthritis of the sacroiliac joint, and osteomyelitis of the ileum can perforate the psoas fascia and cause a psoas abscess (van Dyke et al., 1987). Suppurating bacterial infection of the inguinal nodes has also been reported to extend to the underlying psoas muscle (Maull and Sachatello, 1974).

Etiology

Before the decreasing incidence of tuberculous infection of the spine (Pott's disease) psoas abscesses were often caused by *M. tuberculosis* (Schwaitzberg et al., 1985). Currently, *S. aureus* is the most commonly isolated pathogen from primary psoas abscesses (Firor, 1972; Stephenson et al., 1991) and secondary abscesses originating from vertebral, sacroileal, and perirenal infections. However, if the primary source of the psoas abscess is from a perirenal infection caused by obstructive pyelonephritis, gram-negative bacteria, such as *E. coli* and *Proteus species,* may be isolated. Aerobic and anaerobic bowel flora may be found in psoas abscesses that occur following perforations of retroperitoneal abdominal structures (Bresee and Edwards, 1990).

Clinical Manifestations

The symptoms of psoas abscess are often vague because of the posterior location of the psoas muscle. The most common symptoms are limp and pain in the hip. Fever may be present, and if the infection is chronic, a history of anorexia and weight loss is often found. Other clinical findings include pain in the abdomen, flank, back, and iliac fossa, over the groin, and in the thigh (Song et al., 2001). On examination, the child often keeps the ipsilateral hip in flexion and externally rotated, as this position releases tension of the psoas muscle. Scoliosis, caused by the child leaning toward the side of the infected psoas muscle in an attempt to relieve the pain, is also often seen. Pain on straight–leg-raising may be elicited, and a tender mass may often be felt in the iliac fossa (Bresee and Edwards, 1990).

Diagnosis

Delays in the diagnosis of psoas abscess occur, in part because of the lack of unique clinical and laboratory tests that point to the diagnosis and also because the condition can mimic disorders of several nearby anatomic structures. The psoas muscle cannot easily be examined and often elicits sympathetic responses in adjacent structures. Thus, the differential diagnosis includes septic hip; osteomyelitis of the femoral head, ileum, sacrum, and vertebrae; discitis; paraspinal and retroperitoneal abscess; and noninfectious diseases, such as Perthes' disease, hip dislocation, and tumor. Septic arthritis of the hip is the most frequently misdiagnosed entity, in part because of clinical findings and also because of the presence of a sympathetic sterile effusion in the hip secondary to an ipsilateral psoas abscess (Song et al., 2001). Should septic hip be entertained in the diagnosis, however, it must always be ruled out by hip aspiration. The neutrophil count and erythrocyte sedimentation rate are often nonspecifically elevated. Sterile pyuria may be seen occasionally because the ureter, which lies over the psoas muscle, becomes inflamed. In cases of primary psoas abscess, blood cultures are often positive. A history of tuberculosis exposure should be elicited, and if positive, skin testing with purified protein derivative (PPD) and an anergy control panel should be placed and a chest x-ray should be obtained.

Plain radiographs of the abdomen may show nonspecific signs of infection that include a bulging or obliterated psoas shadow and scoliosis. If the infection has originated from the vertebral column, bony changes may be seen. An intravenous pyelogram (IVP) may show medial deviation of the lower third of the ureter on the affected side. Radioisotopic scanning with gallium or indium-labeled white blood cells are helpful in localizing the lesion, but there is a delay in obtaining results, especially with gallium scanning. Ultrasonography is very helpful in showing changes in the psoas muscle consistent with abscess. It should be noted that CT with intravenous contrast (Lee and Glaser, 1986) and MRI (Gordin et al., 198; Stephenson et al., 1991) are the most powerful radiographic tools available for detection of psoas abscesses. Both of these radiographic modalities provide the clearest anatomic details of the psoas muscle and surrounding tissues and allow detection of infection from an adjacent organ.

Treatment

Febrile and ill-appearing children with psoas abscess should be treated with antibiotics that are active against the most common organisms associated with these abscesses. The antibiotics should provide coverage against *S. aureus,* gram-negative bacilli, and anaerobic bowel flora until further microbiologic data and information on the possible source of infection are available (Table 44-1). Drainage of the psoas muscle abscess, either surgically or by ultrasound or CT-guided percutaneous aspiration (Gordin et al., 1983; Mueller et al., 1984) may be necessary for microbiologic diagnosis or if the patient does not respond to conservative, empiric antibiotic treatment. Parenteral antibiotics directed against the organisms isolated from the blood and abscess should be continued for 2 to 3 weeks after defervescence (Gordin et al., 1983). The underlying source of secondary psoas abscesses should always be sought and corrected.

Complications and Prognosis

Infection from psoas abscess may rarely extend anteriorly into the retrofascial space or spread within the fascial plane of the psoas muscle, resulting in vertebral or hip osteomyelitis. With early diagnosis and treatment, a favorable outcome of uncomplicated psoas abscesses is expected. However, prolonged delay in detection and treatment or psoas disease that has been caused by extension of infection at another site may have a less favorable prognosis.

ANORECTAL ABSCESSES
Epidemiology

Anorectal abscesses occur most frequently in neonates and infants (Arminski and Mclean, 1965), with a large male preponderance. Although the incidence of anorectal abscesses in children is not known, one large study showed that 2.5% of children with proctologic disease had an anorectal abscess (Mentzer, 1956). Immunosuppression and neutropenia increase the risk of developing anorectal abscesses (Arditi and Yogev, 1990). Children with ulcerative colitis and Crohn's disease, diabetes mellitus, chronic granulomatous disease, and recent rectal surgery and those receiving high-dose steroids are also at risk for this disease (Arditi and Yogev, 1990).

Pathogenesis

Anorectal abscesses may occur by extension of bacteria through the normally intact anal mucosal barrier (Arditi and Yogev, 1990). Small tears, abrasions, or fissures in the anal mucosa that may occur during bouts of diarrhea or constipation result in the invasion of bowel organisms through the anal mucosa. Congenital abnormalities of the anal glands may also play a role in the formation of some perianal abscesses (Nix and Stringer, 1997). Infection within the anal canals can lead to abscess formation anywhere along the path of the anal ducts, from the anal mucosa to the intersphincteric space. Disease can extend laterally through the external sphincter muscle into the fat contained within the ischiorectal fossa (Howard, 1987) or inferiorly to form a perianal abscess, which may exit via a fistula in ano at the anal skin (Arditi and Yogev, 1990). Infection can also spread superiorly to the space between the internal sphincter and the levator ani, a space that lies just inferior to the pelvic peritoneum.

Etiology

The majority of anorectal abscesses contain multiple organisms, with a predominance of anaerobic bacteria. The most frequently isolated bacteria include *Bacteroides* species, *P. melaninogenicus, Peptostreptococcus* species, *E. coli, K. pneumoniae,* and *S. aureus* (Arditi and Yogev, 1990; Brook and Martin, 1980).

Clinical Manifestations

Abscess location influences the clinical presentation of anorectal abscesses. The older child with a superficial abscess (perianal abscess) usually complains of pain when sitting and walking, may refuse to walk or may have an abnormal gait, and will have redness and swelling in the perianal area. An enlarging perianal abscess may produce pain with defecation, coughing, and sneezing. However, abscesses located in the deeper anorectal tissue, such as those in the ischiorectal fossa or in the pelvirectal region, often have poorly localized, deep, throbbing pain and are often associated with rigors, fever, malaise, decreased appetite, and lower abdominal pain.

Diagnosis

On physical examination, perianal abscesses are erythematous, tender, indurated regions near the anus. Digital examination reveals no pain in the anal canal beyond the superficial lesion. It is important to distinguish early perianal abscess formation from cellulitis of the perianal skin caused by group A β-hemolytic streptococci and hidradenitis suppurativa, because these diseases do not require surgical treatment. Perianal abscesses should also be distinguished from an anorectal fistula that extends from the anorectal abscess. These fistulous tracts, located in the perianal region, discharge pus or mucus into the anorectal canal and are important clues to the presence of a deeper abscess. Often, deep abscesses are difficult to detect. Aside from a fistulous tract, often the only evidence of these abscesses is brawny edema of the perianal area on the affected side and a tender mass deep to the rectal wall on rectal examination. Because of delay in diagnosis and treatment, affected patients are often febrile and ill appearing by the time the diagnosis is made.

Elevation of the white blood cell count is usually present unless the child is neutropenic. Bacteremia may be present in children who have signs of systemic toxicity. Imaging studies are usually not indicated in children with abscesses detectable by rectal examination. However, in systemically ill children who are thought to have deep abscesses, CT or MRI will be helpful in the diagnosis.

Treatment

Patients should be treated empirically with antibiotics that are active against aerobic and anaerobic bowel flora and *S. aureus* (Table 44-1).

The standard of care in the immunocompetent child for these abscesses has been prompt surgical drainage or aspiration of the abscess, even if local fluctuance is not palpable (Arditi and Yogev, 1990). Material obtained from drainage or aspiration of the abscesses should be sent for Gram stain and aerobic and anaerobic culture. Culture results should guide further antibiotic therapy. Recently, conservative management of perianal abscess and fistula in healthy infants, with neither surgical intervention nor administration of antibiotics, has also been studied (Rosen et al., 2000). Complete resolution occurred within 12 months from initial onset of symptoms in the 12 male infants with perianal abscess and fistula managed with this conservative approach (Rosen et al., 2000).

Treatment of anorectal abscesses in the immunocompromised host remains controversial. Parenteral antibiotics should be given initially to those immunocompromised patients who do not have fluctuance, extensive infection, or sepsis. Incision and drainage, however, may be necessary if there is disease progression (Arditi and Yogev, 1990; Shaked et al., 1986).

Complications and Prognosis

A 40% complication rate from anorectal abscesses has been reported but is much higher in immunocompromised children because of their underlying disease and inability to localize infection (Glenn et al., 1988). Complications include development of anorectal fistulae, recurrence of the abscess, and bacteremia (Arditi and Yogev, 1990). Fistulae may develop even with appropriate surgical and antibiotic treatment. Less commonly, life-threatening septicemia and necrotizing fasciitis can occur (Howard, 1987) especially in the immunocompromised host (Glenn et al., 1988).

ANAEROBIC OSTEOMYELITIS

Anaerobic osteomyelitis, either hematogenous or secondary to an infected adjacent structure, occurs infrequently. However, since 1978, several publications have presented over 40 cases of anaerobic osteomyelitis in children (Beauchamp and Cimolai, 1991; Brook, 1980c; Chazan et al., 2001; Templeton et al., 1983; Thisted et al., 1987). Involved bones included temporal bone, ethmoid bone, frontal bone, maxillae, mandible, occipital bone, metacarpals, femur, tibia, humerus, ulna, and vertebrae. In some cases, osteomyelitis occurred in previously normal bone. Predisposing conditions included trauma, sickle-cell anemia (Templeton et al., 1983), and infection in an adjacent structure—including the mastoid, sinuses, teeth, and scalp. Polymicrobial infections of anaerobes alone or in combination with aerobes were commonly found, although cultures yielding a single anaerobic isolate also occurred. The most common anaerobic bacteria were *Bacteroides* species, anaerobic gram-positive cocci, and *Fusobacterium* species A rare case of actinomycosis of the mandible has also been reported (Thisted et al., 1987). Coinfecting aerobic bacteria include *S. aureus,* streptococci, and gram-negative bacilli.

Treatment includes surgical débridement and prolonged administration of antibiotics that are active against the isolated bacteria and have adequate penetration of the bone. Empiric therapeutic recommendations are indicated in Table 44-1 (Falagas and Siakavellas, 2000). Consultation with a specialist in infectious diseases may be necessary to help interpret the culture results and chose the most appropriate antibiotic regimen. Duration of therapy ranges from 4 to 8 weeks.

BIBLIOGRAPHY

Adams J, et al. Fournier's gangrene in children. Urology 1990;35:439.

Altemeier W, Alexander J. Retroperitoneal abscess. Arch Surg 1961;83:512-524.

Altemeier W, Culbertson W, Fuller W, et al. Intra-abdominal abscesses. Am J Surg 1973;125:70-79.

Ang A, Chong NK, Daneman A. Pediatric appendicitis in "real-time": the value of sonography in diagnosis and treatment. Pediatr Emerg Care 2001;17:334-340.

Arditi M, Yogev R. Perirectal abscess in infants and children: report of 52 cases and review of literature. Pediatr Infect Dis J 1990;9:411-415.

Arminski T, Mclean D. Proctologic problems in children. JAMA 1965;194:137-139.

Arrieta A. Use of meropenem in the treatment of serious infections in children: review of the current literature. Clin Infect Dis 1997;24(suppl 2):S207-S212.

Bagi P, Dueholm S, Karstrup S. Percutaneous drainage of appendiceal abscess. Dis Colon Rectum 1987;30:352.

Baker H, Berquist T, Kispert D, et al. Magnetic resonance imaging in a routine clinical setting. Mayo Clin Proc 1985;60:75-90.

Barker F, et al. Streptococcal necrotizing fasciitis: comparison between histological and clinical features. J Clin Pathol 1987;40:335-341.

Barnes P, DeLock K, Reynolds T, et al. A comparison of amebic and pyogenic abscess of the liver. Medicine 1987;66:472-483.

Bartlett JG, Dick J. The controversy regarding routine anaerobic blood cultures. Am J Med 2000;108:505-506.

Bates T, et al. Timing of prophylactic antibiotics in abdominal surgery. Br J Surg 1989;76:52-56.

Bauer T, et al. Antibiotic prophylaxis in acute nonperforated appendicitis. Ann Surg 1989;209:307-311.

Baxter C. Surgical management of soft tissue infections. Surg Clin North Am 1972;52:1483-1499.

Beauchamp RD, Cimolai N. Osteomyelitis of the pelvis due to *Fusobacterium nucleatum*. Can J Surg 1991;34:618-620.

Bell M. Peritonitis in the newborn—current concepts. Pediatr Clin North Am 1985;32:1181-1201.

Berkman W, Harris SA, Bernadina MER. Nonsurgical drainage of splenic abscesses. AJR Am J Roentgenol 1983;141:395-396.

Berlow M, Spirt B, Weil J. CT follow-up of hepatic and splenic fungal microabscesses. J Comput Assist Tomogr 1984;8:42-45.

Berner R, Schumacher RF, Bartelt S, et al. Predisposing conditions and pathogens in bacteremia in hospitalized children. Eur J Clin Microbiol Infect Dis 1998;17: 337-340.

Bessman A, Wagner W. Nonclostridial gas gangrene. JAMA 1975;233:958.

Bornstein D, Weinberg A, Swartz M, et al. Anaerobic infections: a review of current experience. Medicine 1964; 43:207.

Bradley E, Isaacs J. Appendiceal abscess revisited. Arch Surg 1978;113:130.

Bradley J. Neonatal infections. Pediatr Infect Dis 1985;4: 315-320.

Bradley JS, Behrendt CE, Arrieta AC, et al. Convalescent phase outpatient parenteral antiinfective therapy for children with complicated appendicitis. Pediatr Infect Dis J 2001;20: 19-24.

Bresee J, Edwards M. Psoas abscess in children. Pediatr Infect Dis J 1990;9:201-206.

Britt R, Enzmann D. Clinical stages of human brain abscesses on serial CT scans after contrast infusion. Computerized tomographic, neuropathological, and clinical correlations. J Neurosurg 1983;59:972-989.

Britt R, Enzmann D, Yeager A. Neuropathological and computerized tomographic findings in experimental brain abscess. J Neurosurg 1981;55:590-603.

Brook I. Anaerobic bacteremia in children. Am J Dis Child 1980a;143:1052.

Brook I. Bacterial studies of peritoneal cavity and postoperative wound drainage following perforated appendix in children. Ann Surg 1980b;192:208-212.

Brook I. Osteomyelitis and bacteremia caused by *Bacteroides fragilis:* a complication of fetal monitoring. Clin Pediatr (Phila) 1980c;19:639-640.

Brook I. Microbiology of intraabdominal abscesses in children. Am J Dis Child 1987;141:1148.

Brook I. Microbiology of infected epidermal cysts. Arch Dermatol 1989a;125:1658.

Brook I. Pediatric Anaerobic Infection, ed 2. St. Louis: Mosby, 1989b.

Brook I. Bacteremia due to anaerobic bacteria in newborns. J Perinatol 1990;10:351-356.

Brook I. Aerobic and anaerobic bacteriology of intracranial abscesses. Pediatr Neurol 1992;8:210-214.

Brook I. Anaerobic infections in children with neurological impairments. Am J Ment Retard 1995;99:579-594.

Brook I. Microbiology of necrotizing fasciitis associated with omphalitis in the newborn infant. J Perinatol 1998; 18:28-30.

Brook I, Frazier E. Aerobic and anaerobic bacteriology of wounds and cutaneous abscesses. Arch Surg 1990;125: 1445-1451.

Brook I, Frazier EH. Microbiology of liver and spleen abscesses. J Med Microbiol 1998;47: 1075-1080.

Brook I, Martin W. Aerobic and anaerobic bacteriology of perirectal abscess in children. Pediatrics 1980;66: 282-284.

Busuttil R, et al. Effect of prophylactic antibiotics in acute nonperforated appendicitis: a prospective, randomized, double-blind clinical study. Ann Surg 1981;194:502.

Cammoun D, Hendee W, Davis K. Clinical application of magnetic resonance imaging—current status. West J Med 1985;143:793-803.

Chadwick E, Shulman S, Yogev R. Peritonitis as a late manifestation of group B streptococcal disease in newborns. J Pediatr Infect Dis 1983;142-143.

Chao HC, Kong MS, Lin TY. Diagnosis of necrotizing fasciitis in children. J Ultrasound Med 1999;18:277-281.

Chazan B, Strahilevitz J, Millgram MA, et al. *Bacteroides fragilis* vertebral osteomyelitis secondary to anal dilatation. Spine 2001;26:E377-E378.

Chen CY, Lin KL, Wang HS, Lui TN. Dermoid cyst with dermal sinus tract complicated with spinal subdural abscess. Pediatr Neurol 1999;20:157-160.

Chun C, Johnson J, Hofstetter M, Raff M. Brain abscess, a study of 45 consecutive cases. Medicine 1986;65:415-431.

Chun C, Raff L, Contreras L, et al. Splenic abscess. Medicine 1980;59:50.

Citron D, Goldstein E, Kenner M, et al. Activity of ampicillin/sulbactam, ticarcillin/clavulanate, clarithromycin, and eleven other antimicrobial agents against anaerobic bacteria isolated from infections in children. Clin Infect Dis 1995;20(suppl 2):S356-S360.

Cruse P, Foord R. A five-year prospective study of 23,649 surgical wounds. Arch Surg 1976;107:206.

Darke S, King A, Slack W. Gas gangrene and related infection: classification, clinical features and aetiology, management and mortality. A report of 88 cases. Br J Surg 1977;64:104-112.

Dehner L, Kissane J. Pyogenic hepatic abscesses in infancy and childhood. J Pediatr 1969;74:763-773.

de Jesus Lopes Filho G, Matone J, Arasaki CH, et al. Psoas abscess: diagnostic and therapeutic considerations in six patients. Int Surg 2000;85:339-343.

Dineen P. A critical study of 100 consecutive wound infections. Surg Gynecol Obstet 1961;113:91-96.

Do H, Lambiase R, Deyoe L, et al. Percutaneous drainage of hepatic abscesses: comparison of results in abscesses with and without intrahepatic biliary communication. Am J Roentgenol 1991;157:1209-1212.

Donald F. Treatment of brain abscess. J Antimicrob Chemother 1990;25:310.

Dunkle L, Brotherton M, Feigin R. Anaerobic infections in children: a prospective study. Pediatrics 1976;57:311.

Ecoffey C, Rothman E, Bernard O, et al. Bacterial cholangitis after surgery for biliary atresia. J Pediatr 1987;111:824-829.

Evans J, Meyers M, Bosniak M. Acute renal and perirenal infections. Semin Roentgenol 1971;6:274-291.

Fairbanks P, Milmoe G. The diagnosis and management of sinusitis in children. Complications and sequelae: an otolaryngologist's perspective. Pediatr Infect Dis J 1985; 4 (suppl 6):375-379.

Falagas ME, Siakavellas E. *Bacteroides, Prevotella*, and *Porphyromonas* species: a review of antibiotic resistance and therapeutic options. Int J Antimicrob Agents 2000; 15:1-9.

Falcone P, Pricolo V, Edstrom L. Necrotizing fasciitis as a complication of chicken pox. Clin Pediatr 1988;27:339.

Finegold SM. Perspective on susceptibility testing of anaerobic bacteria. Clin Infect Dis 1997;25(suppl 2):S251-S253.

Finegold SM, Wexler HM. Present studies of therapy for anaerobic infections. Clin Infect Dis 1996;23(suppl 1): S9-S14.

Firor H. Acute psoas abscess in children. Clin Pediatr 1972; 11:228-231.

Fischbein C, Rosenthal A, Fischer E, et al. Risk factors for brain abscess in patients with congenital heart disease. Am J Cardiol 1981;34:97-102.

Fishman S, Pelosi L, Klavon S, O'Rourke E. Perforated appendicitis: prospective outcome analysis for 150 children. J Pediatr Surg 2000;35:923-926.

Flum DR, Morris A, Koepsell T, Dellinger EP. Has misdiagnosis of appendicitis decreased over time? A population-based analysis. JAMA 2001;286:1748-1753.

Fontes RA Jr, Ogilvie CM, Miclau T. Necrotizing soft-tissue infections. J Am Acad Orthop Surg 2000;8: 151-158.

Forster M, et al. A randomized comparative study of sulbactam plus ampicillin vs metronidazole plus cefotaxime in the management of acute appendicitis in children. Rev Infect Dis 1986;8(suppl 5):S634-S638.

Fowler R. Primary peritonitis: changing aspects 1956-1970. Aust Paediatr J 1971;7:73-83.

Foy P, Skarr M. Cerebral abscesses in children after pencil-tip injuries. Lancet 1980;2:662-663.

Fromm D, Silen W. Postoperative clostridial sepsis of the abdominal wall. Am J Surgery 1969;118:517-520.

Gallagher RM, Gross CW, Phillips CD. Suppurative intracranial complications of sinusitis. Laryngoscope 1998;108: 1635-1642.

Gerzof S, Gale M. Computed tomography and ultrasonography for diagnosis and treatment of renal and retroperitoneal abscesses. Urol Clin North Am 1982;9:185-193.

Gerzof S, Johnson W, Robbins A, et al. Intrahepatic pyogenic abscesses: treatment by percutaneous drainage. Am J Surg 1985;149:487-494.

Giannoni C, Sulek M, Friedman EM. Intracranial complications of sinusitis: a pediatric series. Am J Rhinol 1998;12:173-178.

Glenn J, Cotton D, Wesley R, Pizzo P. Anorectal infections in patients with malignant diseases. Rev Infect Dis 1988;10:42-52.

Goldstein E. Bite wounds and infection. Clin Infect Dis 1992;14:633-640.

Gordin F, Stamler C, Mills J. Pyogenic psoas abscesses: noninvasive diagnostic techniques and review of the literature. Rev Infect Dis 1983;5:1003-1011.

Gower D, McGuirt W. Intracranial complication of acute and chronic infectious ear disease: a problem still with us. Laryngoscope 1983;93:1028-1033.

Green BT. Splenic abscess: report of six cases and review of the literature. Am Surg 2001;67: 80-85.

Greenlee J. Subdural empyema. In Mandell G, Bennett J, Dolin R (eds). Principal and Practice of Infectious Disease. New York: Churchill Livingstone, 1995a.

Greenlee J. Epidural abscess. In Mandell G, Bennett J, Dolin R (eds): Principal and Practice of Infectious Diseases. New York: Churchill Livingstone, 1995b.

Griego R, et al. Dog, cat, and human bites: a review. J Am Acad Dermatol 1995;33:1019-1029.

Guiliano A, Lewis F, Hadley K, Blaisdell F. Bacteriology of necrotizing fasciitis. Am J Surg 1977;134:5256.

Haimes A, et al. MR imaging of brain abscesses. AJNR Am J Neuroradiol 1989;10:279.

Hart G, Lamb R, Strauss M. Gas gangrene: I. A collective review. J Trauma 1983;23:991-1000.

Heltber O, Korner B, Schouenborg P. Six cases of acute appendicitis with secondary peritonitis caused by *Streptococcus pneumoniae*. Eur J Clin Microbiol 1984;3:141-143.

Hlavin M, et al. Intracranial suppuration: a modern decade of postoperative subdural empyema and epidural abscess. Neurosurgery 1994;34:974-981.

Hoelzer DJ, Zabel DD, Zern JT. Determining duration of antibiotic use in children with complicated appendicitis. Pediatr Infect Dis J 1999;18:979-982.

Hollin S, Hayashi H, Gross S. Intracranial abscesses of odontogenic origin. Oral Surg 1967;23:277-293.

Howard R. Anal and perianal infections. In Howard R, Simmons R (eds). Surgical Infectious Diseases. Norwalk, Conn: Appleton and Lange, 1987.

Hsieh WS, Yang PH, Chao HC, Lai JY. Neonatal necrotizing fasciitis: a report of three cases and review of the literature. Pediatrics 1999;103:e53.

Jadavji T, Humphreys R, Prober C. Brain abscess in infants and children. Pediatr Infect Dis J 1985;4:394-398.

Jamieson D, Chait P, Filler R. Interventional drainage of appendiceal abscess in children. AJR Am J Roentgenol 1997;169:1619-1622.

Janik J, Firor H. A 20-year study of 1,640 children at Cook County (Illinois) Hospital. Arch Surg 1979;114:717.

Kasten MJ. Clindamycin, metronidazole, and chloramphenicol. Mayo Clin Proc 1999;74:825-833.

Kaufman D, Litman N, Miller M. Sinusitis: induced subdural empyema. Neurology 1983;33:123-132.

Kellogg JA, Manzella JP, Bankert DA. Frequency of low-level bacteremia in children from birth to fifteen years of age. J Clin Microbiol 2000;38:2181-2185.

Keren G. Nonsurgical treatment of brain abscesses: report of two cases. Pediatr Infect Dis J 1984;3:331-334.

Klempner M. Interactions of polymorphonuclear leukocytes with anaerobic bacteria. Rev Infect Dis 1984;6:S40-S44.

Knight P, Vassy L. Specific diseases mimicking appendicitis in childhood. J Pediatr Surg 1981;116:744.

Knochel J, Koehler P, Lee T, et al. Diagnosis of abdominal abscesses with computed tomography, ultrasound, and 111-indium-leukocyte scans. Radiology 1980;137: 25.

Kramer P, Griffith R, Campbell R. Antibiotic penetration of the brain: a comparative study. J Neurosurg 1969; 31:295.

Krisher S, Browne A, Dibbins A, et al. Intra-abdominal abscess after laparoscopic appendectomy for perforated appendicitis. Arch Surg 2001;136:438-441.

Kuhn J, Berger P. Computed tomographic diagnosis of abdominal abscesses in children. Ann Radiol (Paris) 1980;23:153-158.

Kusne S, Dummer J, Singh N, et al. Infections after liver transplantation. An analysis of 101 consecutive cases. Medicine 1988;67:132-143.

LeBeau J, Creissard P, Harispe L, et al. Surgical treatment of brain abscess and subdural empyema. J Neurosurg 1973;38:198-203.

Lee J, Glaser H. Psoas muscle disorder: magnetic resonance imaging. Radiology 1986;160:683-687.

Lee SL, Walsh AJ, Ho HS. Computed tomography and ultrasonography do not improve and may delay the diagnosis and treatment of acute appendicitis. Arch Surg 2001;136:556-562.

Leigh D, Simmons K, Norman E. Bacterial flora of the appendix fossa in appendicitis and postoperative wound infection. J Clin Pathol 1974;27:997-1000.

Lerner R, Spataro RF. Splenic abscesses: percutaneous drainage. Radiology 1984;153:643-645.

Levison M, Bush L. Peritonitis and other intra-abdominal infections. In Mandell G, Bennett J, Dolin R (eds). Principles and Practice of Infectious Disease. New York: Churchill Livingston, 1995.

Lew D, Mongomery W, et al. Sphenoid sinusitis: a review of 30 cases. N Engl J Med 1983;309:1149-1154.

Linos D, Nogarney D, Mcilrath D. Splenic abscess—the importance of early diagnosis. Mayo Clin Proc 1983;58: 261-264.

Lintula H, Kokki H, Vanamo K. Single-blind randomized clinical trial of laparoscopic versus open appendectomy in children. Br J Surg 2001;88:510-514.

Lister J. Meconium and bacterial peritonitis. In Lister J (ed). Neonatal Surgery, ed 3. London: Butterworths, 1991.

Loesche W. Oxygen sensitivity of various anaerobic bacteria. Appl Microbiol 1969;18:723-727.

Luckmann R. Incidence and case fatality rates for acute appendicitis in California: a population-based study of the effects of age. Am J Epidemiol 1989;129:905-918.

Lunsford L, Nelson P. Stereotactic exploration of the brain in the era of computed tomography. Surg Neurol 1984;22:222-230.

Machiedo G, Tikellis J, Suval W, et al. Reoperation for sepsis. Am Surg 1985;51:149.

Mackenzie M, Young D. Subphrenic abscess in children. Br J Surg 1975;62:305-308.

MacLennan J. The histotoxic clostridial infections of man. Bact Rev 1962;26:177.

Maddaus M, Ahrenholz D, Simmons R. The biology of peritonitis and implications for treatment. Surg Clin North Am 1988;68:431-443.

Maull K, Sachatello C. Retroperitoneal iliac fossa abscess. A complication of suppurative lymphadenitis. Am J Surg 1974;127:270-274.

McCorkell S, Niles N. Pyogenic liver abscess: another look at medical management. Lancet 1985;1:803-806.

McDougal W, Izant RJ, Zollinger RJ. Primary peritonitis in infancy and childhood. Ann Surg 1975;181:310.

Meleny F. A differential diagnosis between certain types of infectious gangrene of the skin with particular reference to hemolytic streptococcus gangrene and bacterial synergistic gangrene. Surg Gynecol Obstet 1933;56:847.

Mendelson R, Lindsell D. Ultrasound examination of the paediatric acute abdomen. Br J Radiol 1987;60:414-416.

Mentzer C. Anorectal disease. Pediatr Clin North Am 1956;3:113-125.

Meyers M. Dynamic radiology of the abdomen: normal and pathologic anatomy, ed 2. New York: Springer-Verlag, 1987.

Mollitt D, Tepas J, Talbert J. The role of coagulase-negative staphylococcus in neonatal necrotizing enterocolitis. J Pediatr Surg 1988;23:60-63.

Mueller P, Ferrucci J, Wittenberg J, et al. Iliopsoas abscess: treatment by CT-guided percutaneous catheter drainage. AJR AM J Roentgenol 1984;142:359-362.

Murch SH. Diarrhoea, diagnostic delay, and appendicitis. Lancet 2000;356:787.

Neuhof H, Arheim E. Acute retroperitoneal abscess and phlegmon: a study of sixty-five cases. Ann Surg 1944;119:741-758.

Nichols R. Infections following gastrointestinal surgery: intraabdominal abscess. Surg Clin North Am 1980;60: 197-212.

Nichols R, et al. Risk of infection after penetrating abdominal trauma. N Engl J Med 1984;311:1065.

Nix P, Stringer MD. Perianal sepsis in children. Br J Surg 1997;84:819-821.

O'Keefe J, Tally F, Barza M, et al. Inactivation of penicillin G during experimental infection with *Bacteroides fragilis*. J Infect Dis 1978;137:437.

Olafsson S, Khan M. Musculoskeletal features of acne, hidradenitis suppurativa, and dissecting cellulitis of the scalp. Rheum Dis Clin North Am 1992;18:215.

Oliak D, Yamini D, Udani VM, et al. Initial nonoperative management for periappendiceal abscess. Dis Colon Rectum 2001;44:936-941.

Olsen I, Solberg CO, Finegold SM. A primer on anaerobic bacteria and anaerobic infections for the uninitiated. Infection 1999;27:159-165.

Onderdonk A, Markham R, Zaleznik D, et al. Evidence for T cell-dependent immunity to *Bacteroides fragilis* in an intraabdominal abscess model. J Clin Invest 1982;69:9-16.

Ortiz E, Sande MA. Routine use of anaerobic blood cultures: are they still indicated? Am J Med 2000;108:445-447.

Pineiro-Carrero V, Andres J. Morbidity and mortality in children with pyogenic liver abscess. Am J Dis Child 1989;143:1424-1427.

Powell D, san Luis E, Calvin S, et al. Peritonitis in children undergoing continuous ambulatory peritoneal dialysis. Am J Dis Child 1985;139:29-32.

Pruitt T, Simmons R. Status of percutaneous catheter drainage of abscesses. Surg Clin North Am 1988;68:89-105.

Ronnestad A, Abrahamsen TG, Gaustad P, Finne PH. Blood culture isolates during 6 years in a tertiary neonatal intensive care unit. Scand J Infect Dis 1998;30:245-251.

Rosen NG, Gibbs DL, Soffer SZ, et al. The nonoperative management of fistula-in-ano. J Pediatr Surg 2000;35:938-939.

Rotstein O. Interactions between leukocytes and anaerobic bacteria in polymicrobial surgical infections. Clin Infect Dis 1993;16:S190-S194.

Rubin J, Rogers W, Taylor H, et al. Peritonitis during continuous ambulatory peritoneal dialysis. Ann Intern Med 1980;92:7-13.

Saini S, Kellum J, O'Leary M, et al. Improved localization and survival in patients with intra-abdominal abscesses. Am J Surg 1983;145:136.

Sands M, Page D, Brown R. Splenic abscess following nonoperative management of splenic rupture. J Pediatr Surg 1986;21:900-901.

Schumer W, Lee D, Jones B. Peritoneal lavage in postoperative therapy of late peritoneal sepsis. Surgery 1964;55:841.

Schwaitzberg S, Porkorny W, Thurston R, et al. Psoas abscess in children. J Pediatr Surg 1985;(20):339.

Shaked A, Shinar E, Fruend H. Managing the granulocytopenic patient with acute perianal inflammatory disease. Am J Surg 1986;152:510-512.

Shapiro M, Gale M, Gerzof S. CT of appendicitis. Radiol Clin North Am 1989;27:753-762.

Sheinfeld J, Erturk E, Spatoro R, Cockett A. Perinephric abscess: current concepts. J Urol 1987;137:191-194.

Simons G, Sty J, Starshak R. Retroperitoneal and retrofascial abscess: a review. J Bone Joint Surg Am 1983;65:1041-1057.

Simson J. Solitary abscess of the spleen. Br J Surg 1980;67:106-110.

Sivit CJ, Siegel MJ, Applegate KE, Newman KD. When appendicitis is suspected in children. Radiographics 2001;21:247-262; questionnaire 288-294.

Sjoln J, Lilja A, Ericsson N, et al. Treatment of brain abscess with cefotaxime and metronidazole: prospective study on 15 consecutive patients. Clin Infect Dis 1993;17:857-863.

Skoubo-Kristensen E, Hvid I. The appendiceal mass. Results of conservative management. Ann Surg 1982;196:584-587.

Smith H, Hendrick E. Subdural empyema and epidural abscess in children. J Neurosurg 1983;58:392.

Smith RR, Arvin MC. Neuroradiology of intracranial infection. Semin Neurol 1992;12:248-262.

Snyder W, Chaffin L. Appendicitis during the first two years of life: report on twenty-one cases and review of four hundred forty-seven cases from the literature. Arch Surg 1952;64:549.

Sobel J. Candida infections in the intensive care unit. Crit Care Clin North Am 1988;4:325-344.

Solomkin J, et al. Antibiotic trials in intraabdominal infections: a critical evaluation of study design and outcome reporting. Ann Surg 1984;200:29.

Sondenaa K, et al. Bacteriology and complications of chronic pilonidal sinus treated with excision and primary suture. Int J Colorect Dis 1995;10:161-166.

Song J, Letts M, Monson R. Differentiation of psoas muscle abscess from septic arthritis of the hip in children. Clin Orthop 2001:258-265.

Speck W, Dresdale S, McMillan R. Primary peritonitis and the nephrotic syndrome. Am J Surg 1974;127:267.

Spires J, Smith R, Catlin F. Brain abscesses in the young. Otolaryngol Head Neck Surg 1985;93:468-474.

Stamenkovic M, Lew P. Early recognition of potentially fatal necrotizing fasciitis. The use of frozen-section biopsy. N Engl J Med 1984;310:1689-1693.

Stanley P, Atkinson J, Reid B, Gilsanz V. Percutaneous drainage of abdominal fluid collections in children. AJR Am J Roentgenol 1984;142:813-816.

Stepanov S. Surgical treatment of brain abscess. Neurosurg 1988;22:724-730.

Stephenson C, Seibert J, Golladay E, et al. Abscess of the iliopsoas muscle diagnosed by magnetic resonance imaging and ultrasonography. South Med J 1991;84:509-511.

Styrt B, Gorbach S. Recent developments in the understanding of the pathogenesis and treatment of anaerobic infections. N Engl J Med 1989;321:240-246.

Talan D, Citron D, et al. Bacteriological analysis of infected dog and cat bites. Emergency Medicine Animal Bite Infection Study Group. N Engl J Med 1999;340:85-92.

Tay J, Garland J. Serious head injuries from lawn darts. Pediatrics 1987;79:261-263.

Teague M, Baddour L, Wruble L. Liver abscess: a harbinger of Crohn's disease. Am J Gastroenterol 1988;83:1412.

Templeton WC 3rd, Wawrukiewicz A, Melo JC, et al. Anaerobic osteomyelitis of long bones. Rev Infect Dis 1983;5:692-712.

Theophilo F, Markikis E, Theophilo L, et al. Brain abscess in childhood. Child Nerv Syst 1985;1:324-328.

Thirmuoothi M, Keen B, Dajani A. Anaerobic infections in children: a prospective study. J Clin Microbiol 1976;3:318.

Thisted E, Poulsen P, Christensen PO. Actinomycotic osteomyelitis in a child. J Laryngol Otol 1987;101:746-748.

Thompson C, McCarter YS, Krause PJ, Herson VC. *Lactobacillus acidophilus* sepsis in a neonate. J Perinatol 2001;21:258-260.

van Dyke J, Holley H, Anderson D. Review of iliopsoas anatomy and pathology. Radiographics 1987;7:53-84.

Wang D, Wilson S. Subphrenic abscess. The new epidemiology. Arch Surg 1977;112:934.

Weber DM, Freeman NV, Elhag KM. Periumbilical necrotizing fasciitis in the newborn. Eur J Pediatr Surg 2001;11:86-91.

Wilson EB, Cole JC, Nipper ML, et al. Computed tomography and ultrasonography in the diagnosis of appendicitis: when are they indicated? Arch Surg 2001;136:670-675.

Wilson S. Intraabdominal abscess: subphrenic, lesser sac, intermesenteric, and pelvic. In Wilson S, Finegold S, Williams R (eds). Intra-Abdominal Infection. New York: McGraw-Hill, 1982a.

Wilson S. Secondary bacterial peritonitis. In Wilson S, Finegold S, Williams R (eds). Intra-Abdominal Infections. New York: McGraw-Hill, 1982b.

Wilson S, Serota A, Williams R. Anatomy and physiology of the peritoneum. In Wilson SE, Finegold SM, Williams RA (eds). Intra-abdominal infection. New York, McGraw-Hill, 1982.

Winslow R, Dean R, Harley J. Acute nonperforation appendicitis. Efficacy of brief antibiotic prophylaxis. Arch Surg 1983;118:651-655.

Wispelwey B, Scheld W. Brain abscess. In Mandell G, Bennett J, Dolin R (eds). Principles and Practice of Infectious Diseases. New York: Churchill Livingstone, 1995.

Yamini D, Vargas H, Bongard F, et al. Perforated appendicitis: is it truly a surgical urgency? Am Surg 1998;64: 970-975.

Zaidi AK, Knaut AL, Mirrett S, Reller LB. Value of routine anaerobic blood cultures for pediatric patients. J Pediatr 1995;127:263-268.

Zaleznik D, Kasper D. The role of anaerobic bacteria in abscess formation. Ann Rev Med 1982;33:217-229.

Zook E, et al. Successful treatment protocol for canine fang injuries. J Trauma 1980;20:243-246.

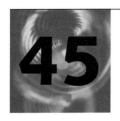

45 DIAGNOSIS OF ACUTE EXANTHEMATOUS DISEASES

SAUL KRUGMAN

EFFECTS OF DIAGNOSIS

Under certain circumstances a physician who examines a patient with a rash is charged with a grave responsibility. An error in diagnosis may have a profound effect on the patient, the contacts, and the community. The following examples (effect on the patient, effect on contacts, and effect on the community) will serve as illustrations.

Effect on the Patient

The disease of a patient with meningococcemia was mistakenly diagnosed as measles. Specific therapy was not started early; however, a potential fatality was averted when the disease was finally recognized and treated. Another patient with scarlet fever was said to have rubella. Complicating otitis media could have been prevented if the correct diagnosis had been made and appropriate treatment had been instituted.

Effect on Contacts

A classic clinical picture of exanthem subitum in an infant was erroneously labeled as rubella. Under normal circumstances this mistake would have been of little consequence. In this instance, however, the patient's mother was 2 months pregnant and had never had rubella. The error in diagnosis created an unnecessary period of anxiety for the parents, who had visions of the future birth of a congenitally malformed infant.

A child with mild measles was said to have rubella. A young sibling contact developed severe measles complicated by pneumonia. This situation could have been prevented by a correct diagnosis, which would have dictated the immediate administration of measles vaccine or prophylactic immune globulin to abort or attenuate the sibling's disease.

Effect on the Community

On March 5, 1947, a 47-year-old businessman was admitted to Bellevue Hospital in New York City because of fever and rash. The initial diagnosis was toxic eruption, and the patient was admitted to a dermatology ward. On March 8 he was transferred to a communicable disease hospital, where he subsequently died. The proved cause of his death was smallpox. A small outbreak of the disease was initiated in the general hospital, spreading out from this focus. In the end there were twelve cases of smallpox and two deaths. There were several additional deaths among the 5 million persons who were vaccinated in New York City. The cost in time, effort, and money was incalculable, and the affairs of the entire city and its inhabitants were seriously disrupted. Concerns regarding a bioterrorism introduction of smallpox raise the possibility of a similar future episode. An adult with severe hemorrhagic varicella might be erroneously diagnosed as having smallpox.

DIFFERENTIAL DIAGNOSIS

The rashes of various exanthematous diseases are so similar in appearance that they may be clinically indistinguishable. On the other hand, each disease has a characteristic total clinical picture that is distinctive. The differential diagnosis of the acute exanthems is based on a number of factors, including (1) the past history of infectious disease and immunization, (2) type of prodromal period, (3) features of the rash, (4) presence of pathognomonic or other diagnostic signs, and (5) laboratory diagnostic tests.

An attack of many of the exanthematous diseases is followed by permanent immunity. Consequently, a history of measles, for example, might preclude that diagnosis. However, the history is only as reliable as the memory of the patient or the parent or the accuracy of the original diagnosis.

The character and duration of the prodromal period are also important. Some diseases have a prolonged (4 or more days) prodromal period before the rash appears; in others it may be short or absent. In certain diseases the prodrome is characterized by respiratory tract symptoms; in others, influenza-like symptoms predominate.

The character, distribution, and duration of the rash require evaluation. An eruption may be discrete or confluent and central or peripheral in distribution, and it may persist for 1 to 2 weeks or disappear within 1 day.

Pathognomonic and other signs are always helpful diagnostic clues. Koplik's spots, for example, simplify the recognition of measles.

The final diagnosis in many instances, especially involving those illnesses with which physicians and parents are unfamiliar, cannot be made on clinical grounds alone. Laboratory diagnostic tests must be used for identification of the causative agent or for demonstration of the development of specific antibodies.

CLASSIFICATION OF ACUTE EXANTHEMATOUS DISEASES

The acute exanthematous diseases may be conveniently separated into two categories: those characterized by an erythematous maculopapular or punctiform eruption and those characterized by a papulovesicular eruption. These two types of rash are associated with many conditions other than the acute exanthematous diseases. These diseases and other conditions are given in the accompanying lists.

The following diseases and conditions are characterized by a maculopapular eruption:
• Measles
• Atypical measles
• Rubella
• Scarlet fever
• Staphylococcal scalded skin syndrome
• Staphylococcal toxic shock syndrome
• Meningococcemia
• Typhus and tick fevers
• Toxoplasmosis
• Cytomegalovirus infection
• Erythema infectiosum (Parvovirus)
• Roseola infantum (HHV-6)
• Enteroviral infections
• Infectious mononucleosis
• Toxic erythemas
• Drug eruptions
• Sunburn

• Miliaria
• Kawasaki disease

The following diseases and conditions are characterized by a papulovesicular eruption:
• Varicella-zoster infections
• Smallpox
• Eczema herpeticum
• Eczema vaccinatum
• Coxsackievirus and other enterovirus infections
• Atypical measles
• Rickettsialpox
• Impetigo
• Insect bites
• Papular urticaria
• Drug eruptions
• Molluscum contagiosum
• Dermatitis herpetiformis

The preceding lists do not include all the conditions associated with a rash.

DIFFERENTIAL DIAGNOSIS OF MACULOPAPULAR ERUPTIONS

The acute exanthems and other conditions listed previously are frequently or occasionally characterized by a maculopapular eruption. These diseases may be differentiated by a complete evaluation of four of the categories described in this discussion of differential diagnosis: (1) prodromal period, (2) rash, (3) presence of pathognomonic or other diagnostic signs, and (4) laboratory diagnostic tests.

Prodromal Period

Measles. As indicated in Figure 45-1, the rash of measles is preceded by a 3- or 4-day prodromal period of fever, conjunctivitis, coryza, and cough.

Atypical measles. The prodromal period of atypical measles is usually characterized by fever, cough, headache, myalgia, and occasionally pleuritic chest pain preceding the onset of rash by 2 to 4 days.

Rubella. In rubella in children there is usually no prodromal period (Figure 45-1). The appearance of the rash may be the first obvious sign of illness. Lymphadenopathy that precedes the rash is usually asymptomatic in children. Adolescents and adults may have a variable 1- to 4-day period of malaise and low-grade fever before the rash appears. The temperature may be normal.

Scarlet fever. The rash of scarlet fever occurs within 12 hours of the onset of fever, sore throat, and vomiting. Occasionally the prodromal period may be prolonged to 2 days (Figure 45-1).

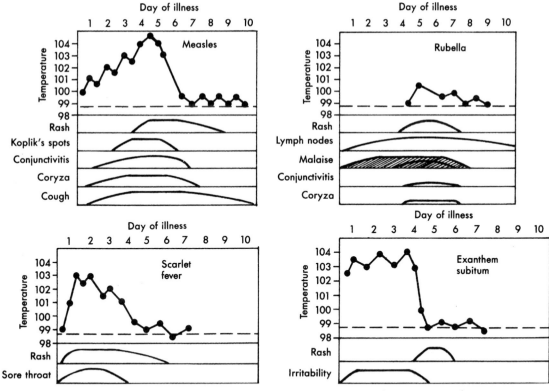

Fig. 45-1 Schematic diagrams illustrating differences between four acute exanthems characterized by maculopapular eruptions.

Staphylococcal scalded skin syndrome. Fever and irritability occur at the time of onset of rash in patients with staphylococcal scalded skin syndrome; there is no prodromal period.

Staphylococcal toxic shock syndrome. High fever, headache, confusion, sore throat, vomiting, diarrhea, and shock may precede or may be associated with the rash of staphylococcal toxic shock syndrome.

Meningococcemia with or without meningitis. The prodrome of meningococcemia with or without meningitis is variable. Usually the rash appears within 24 hours. The initial symptoms are fever, vomiting, malaise, irritability, and possibly a stiff neck.

Epidemic and murine typhus. A 4- to 6-day prodromal period precedes the appearance of the rash of epidemic and murine typhus. It is characterized by high fever, chills, headache, and generalized aches and pains.

Rocky Mountain spotted fever. In patients with Rocky Mountain spotted fever the onset of rash is preceded by a 3- to 4-day period of fever, chills, headache, malaise, and anorexia.

Erythema infectiosum. In patients with erythema infectiosum no prodromal period is typ-

ically present. Usually the first sign of the illness is the appearance of the rash.

Roseola infantum. A 3- or 4-day prodromal period of high fever and irritability precedes the rash of exanthem subitum, which appears as the temperature falls to normal by crisis (Figure 45-1).

Enteroviral infections. Echovirus type 16 infection (Boston exanthem) may have a prodromal period resembling that of exanthem subitum, but the fever tends to be lower. Fever and constitutional symptoms in echovirus types 4, 6, and 9 and in coxsackievirus infections may precede but usually coincide with the appearance of the rash.

Kawasaki disease. A nonspecific febrile illness with sore throat precedes the rash of mucocutaneous lymph node syndrome by 2 to 5 days.

Toxic erythemas, drug eruptions, sunburn, and miliaria. Toxic erythemas, drug eruptions, sunburn, miliaria, and other noninfectious conditions with a maculopapular eruption do not have prodromal periods.

Rash

Measles. The rash of measles is reddish brown, appears on the face and neck first, and progresses downward to involve the trunk and extremities in sequence. As indicated in Figure 45-2, the eruption is generalized by the third day. The lesions on the face, neck, and upper trunk tend to be confluent; those on the lower trunk and extremities are usually discrete. The eruption fades by the fifth or sixth day, with brownish staining first, followed by branny desquamation. The hands and feet do not desquamate.

Atypical measles. The rash of atypical measles associated with previous immunization with killed measles vaccine resembles Rocky Mountain spotted fever more than typical measles. The eruption is characterized by erythematous, urticarial, papular, petechial, and purpuric lesions with a predilection for the extremities, especially the hands, wrists, feet, and ankles; occasionally the lesions may be vesicular.

Rubella. The rash of rubella is pink, begins on the face and neck, and progresses downward to the trunk and extremities more rapidly than in measles; it becomes generalized within 24 to 48 hours. The lesions are usually discrete rather than confluent, and those that develop first are the earliest to fade. Consequently, on the third day the face is usually clear, and only the extremities may be involved. The eruption usually disappears by the end of the third day, and as a rule it does not desquamate. The striking contrast between the distribution of measles and rubella rashes on the third day of eruption is illustrated in Figure 45-2.

Scarlet fever. The rash of scarlet fever is an erythematous punctiform eruption that blanches on pressure. It appears first on the flexor surfaces and rapidly becomes generalized, usually within 24 hours. The forehead and cheeks are smooth, red, and flushed, but the area around the mouth is pale (circumoral pallor). The lesions are most intense and prominent in the neck, axillary, inguinal, and popliteal skin folds (Figure 45-2). Desquamation is characteristic, and, in contrast to measles, it involves the hands and feet.

Staphylococcal scalded skin syndrome. In staphylococcal scalded skin syndrome the rash is a generalized, erythematous, scarlatiniform eruption; it has a sandpaper-like texture. The erythema is accentuated in the skin folds, simulating Pastia's lines. The skin is tender. The course of the rash is different from that of scarlet fever. Within 1 to 2 days bullae may appear, and the epidermis may separate into large sheets, revealing a moist, red, shiny surface beneath. In contrast, the pattern of desquamation is different in scarlet fever; it occurs 1 to 2 weeks later and is characterized by fine, branny flakes or thin sheets of skin.

Staphylococcal toxic shock syndrome. The rash of staphylococcal toxic shock syndrome is

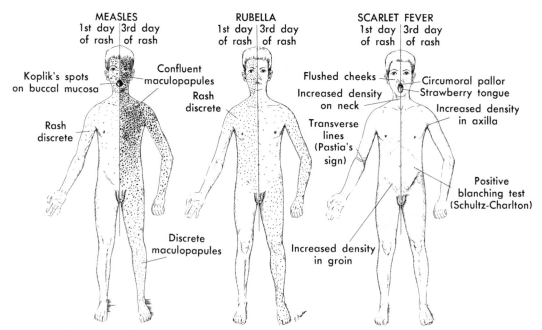

Fig. 45-2 Schematic drawings illustrating differences in appearance, distribution, and progression of rashes of measles, rubella, and scarlet fever.

scarlatiniform in appearance; it occurs most prominently on the trunk and extremities and is associated with edema of the face and limbs and desquamation.

Meningococcemia. In patients with meningococcemia an early, transient maculopapular eruption may precede the petechial, purpuric rash, which often is present when the patient seeks medical attention. In contrast to measles, this early exanthem has no regular, predictable distribution.

Epidemic and murine typhus. The characteristic rash of epidemic and murine typhus is a maculopapular and petechial eruption that has a central distribution. The face, palms, and soles are not involved as a rule.

Rocky Mountain spotted fever. The eruption of Rocky Mountain spotted fever is maculopapular and petechial, with a peripheral distribution. The palms and soles usually are involved, and occasionally the face also may be affected.

Erythema infectiosum. The afebrile patient with asymptomatic erythema infectiosum develops a characteristic rash that erupts in three stages, in the following sequence: (1) red, flushed cheeks with circumoral pallor (slapped-cheek appearance); (2) maculopapular eruption over upper and lower extremities (the rash assumes a lacelike appearance as it fades); and (3) an evanescent stage characterized by subsidence of the eruption, followed by a recurrence precipitated by a variety of skin irritants.

Roseola infantum. The lesions of exanthem subitum are typically discrete rose-red maculopapules that frequently appear on the chest and trunk first and then spread to involve the face and extremities. The eruption usually disappears within 2 days. Occasionally it fades within several hours.

Enteroviral infections. The rashes of echovirus and coxsackievirus infections are often rubella-like in appearance. The lesions are usually maculopapular, discrete, nonpruritic, and generalized. Unlike in measles, desquamation and staining do not occur. Petechial lesions suggesting meningococcemia may rarely be noted in echovirus type 9 and coxsackievirus A type 9 infections.

Kawasaki disease. In patients with Kawasaki disease there is a generalized erythematous rash with elements of macules and papules. The palms and soles are swollen and reddened, eventually peeling after several days or weeks. Dryness with erythema of the lips, mouth, and tongue accompanies bilateral conjunctival injection (see Chapter 18).

Drug eruptions and toxic erythemas. Drug eruptions and toxic erythemas may be characterized by maculopapular eruptions that may simulate any of the diseases listed previously.

Sunburn. Sunburn may be confused with the rash of scarlet fever, particularly if there is a coincident sore throat. The eruption is confined to the area not protected by a bathing suit.

Miliaria. The fine punctiform lesions of miliaria are chiefly confined to the flexor areas. The rash is usually not generalized, and it does not desquamate as a rule.

Presence of Pathognomonic or Other Diagnostic Signs

Measles. Koplik's spots are pathognomonic for measles.

Atypical measles. Atypical measles is frequently associated with radiographic evidence of pneumonia and occasionally with pleural effusion.

Rubella. In patients with rubella, lymphadenopathy (particularly postauricular and occipital) is a common manifestation, but it also may occur in other diseases.

Scarlet fever. A strawberry tongue and exudative or membranous tonsillitis are typical of scarlet fever.

Staphylococcal scalded skin syndrome. An associated staphylococcal infection such as impetigo or purulent conjunctivitis may be present with staphylococcal scalded skin syndrome. Nikolsky's sign is present.

Staphylococcal toxic shock syndrome. The scarlatiniform eruption of staphylococcal toxic shock syndrome is associated with high fever, toxicity, and a shocklike state.

Meningococcemia. A petechial purpuric eruption associated with meningeal signs would point to meningococcemia.

Epidemic and murine typhus. A maculopapular petechial eruption centrally distributed in a person living in an area where epidemic typhus is endemic is suggestive of the disease.

Rocky Mountain spotted fever. A history of a recent tick bite in a person with a maculopapular, petechial, peripherally distributed eruption is characteristic of Rocky Mountain spotted fever.

Toxoplasmosis. The acquired infection of toxoplasmosis may be characterized by one or more of the following syndromes: (1) fever, pneumonitis, and rash; (2) lymphadenopathy; (3) encephalitis; and (4) chorioretinitis. (See Chapter 38.)

Erythema infectiosum. Erythema infectiosum is suggested by the slapped-face appearance in an otherwise well child.

Enteroviral infections. The rash of enteroviral infections may be associated with aseptic meningitis. The infections occur most commonly during the summer and fall months.

Infectious mononucleosis. A triad of membranous tonsillitis, lymphadenopathy, and splenomegaly suggests infectious mononucleosis as a possibility.

Laboratory Diagnostic Tests

Measles. The measles enzyme-linked immunosorbent assay (ELISA) and hemagglutination-inhibition (HI) test are the most readily available. The pattern of appearance of antibody is shown in Figure 20-4. A fourfold or greater rise in measles antibody is detected during convalescence; the peak HI titer usually ranges between 1:256 and 1:1024. The blood picture typically shows leukopenia.

Atypical measles. Extraordinary rises in measles HI antibody have been detected within 2 weeks after onset of atypical measles. The titers may exceed 1:100,000.

Rubella. As indicated in Figure 30-3 a positive throat culture for rubella virus and evidence of a rise in antibody level are helpful diagnostic aids. The blood picture shows either a normal or low white blood cell count.

Scarlet fever. Group A hemolytic streptococci may be cultured from the nasopharynx. There is usually a rise in antistreptolysin O titer.

Staphylococcal scalded skin syndrome. A culture of skin or other sites of infection is positive for phage group II staphylococci in staphylococcal scalded skin syndrome.

Staphylococcal toxic shock syndrome. Cultures of various mucosal surfaces or purulent lesions should be positive for *Staphylococcus aureus.*

Meningococcemia. The microorganism causing meningococcemia may be observed on Gram stain and recovered from the blood, spinal fluid, or petechiae.

Epidemic and murine typhus. The Weil-Felix agglutination reaction with *Proteus* OX-19 is positive. Specific antibody tests are available for epidemic and murine typhus.

Rocky Mountain spotted fever. The Weil-Felix agglutination reaction with *Proteus* OX-19 and OX-2 is positive. Thrombocytopenia, hyponatremia, and hypoalbuminemia are common. Specific Rocky Mountain spotted fever antibody tests are available.

Toxoplasmosis. A rise in *Toxoplasma* antibody titer during convalescence indicates acute toxoplasmosis.

Erythema infectiosum. Diagnostic testing for erythema infectiosum is discussed in Chapter 25. Standardized serologic tests to confirm parvovirus B-19 infection are increasingly available.

Roseola infantum. There is no diagnostic test for roseola infantum at present. Specific virologic and serologic tests to detect human herpesvirus type 6 are not readily available commercially (see Chapter 16). The blood picture shows leukopenia when the rash appears.

Enteroviral infections. Echoviruses and coxsackieviruses may be recovered from stools, throat, blood, or cerebrospinal fluid (CSF). The diagnosis is confirmed by demonstrating a rise in neutralizing antibody titer to the specific virus.

Infectious mononucleosis. In patients with infectious mononucleosis the blood smear is positive for abnormal lymphocytes. The monospot test and heterophil agglutination test are positive. Results of liver function tests such as for aminotransferases are abnormal. Epstein-Barr virus antibody appears during convalescence (Chapter 9).

DIFFERENTIAL DIAGNOSIS OF PAPULOVESICULAR ERUPTIONS

The acute exanthems and other conditions usually characterized by a papulovesicular eruption comprise a separate group. The following differential criteria are similar to those used for the maculopapular eruptions.

Prodromal Period

Varicella. As indicated in Figure 45-3, a prodromal period is usually absent in patients with chickenpox. The rash and constitutional symptoms, particularly in children, occur simultaneously. In adolescents and adults, however, there may be a 1- or 2-day prodromal period of fever, headache, malaise, and anorexia.

Smallpox. The smallpox rash is preceded by a 3-day period of chills, headache, backache, and severe malaise (Figure 45-3). A transient rash with bathing-trunk distribution may occur during the prodrome.

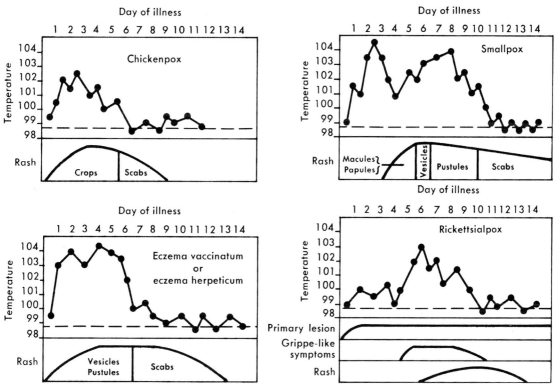

Fig. 45-3 Schematic diagrams illustrating differences between four acute exanthems characterized by papulovesicular eruptions.

Herpes simplex, herpes zoster, and vaccinia. Herpes simplex, herpes zoster, and vaccinia occur without any prodromal period (eczema vaccinatum and herpeticum; see Figure 45-3).

Rickettsialpox. In patients with rickettsialpox a generalized papulovesicular eruption is preceded by the development of (1) an initial lesion (an eschar), and (2) an influenza-like syndrome (see Figure 45-3).

Rash

Varicella. The rash of chickenpox is characterized by (1) rapid evolution of macules to papules to vesicles to crusts; (2) central distribution of lesions, which appear in crops (Figure 45-4); (3) presence of lesions in all stages in any one anatomic area; (4) presence of scalp and mucous membrane lesions; and (5) eventual crusting of nearly all the skin lesions.

Smallpox. The rash of smallpox is characterized by (1) slow evolution of macules to papules to vesicles to pustules to crusts; (2) peripheral distribution of lesions, which are most prominent on the exposed skin surfaces (Figure 45-4); (3) presence of lesions in the same stage in any one anatomic area; and (4) skin lesions that are more deep seated than those of varicella.

Eczema herpeticum and vaccinatum. In patients with eczema herpeticum and vaccinatum the vesicular and pustular lesions are most profuse on the sites of eczema. Mouth and scalp lesions are generally absent.

Herpes Zoster. The lesions of herpes zoster are unilateral and distributed along the line of the affected nerves; vesicles are grouped together and tend to become confluent.

Atypical measles. The papulovesicular lesions of atypical measles may appear on the face and the trunk. During the crusting phase they resemble varicella. This eruption may or may not be associated with the characteristic maculopapular eruption that resembles Rocky Mountain spotted fever in its peripheral distribution.

Rickettsialpox. The primary lesion of rickettsialpox is an eschar that measures 1.5 cm or more in diameter. The generalized papulovesicular eruption is composed of tiny vesicles superimposed on a firm papule. The vesicles are much smaller than those of chickenpox. Many lesions do not crust.

Impetigo. The lesions of impetigo, at first vesicular, become confluent and rapidly progress to the pustular and crusting stage. They do not appear in crops, they commonly involve the

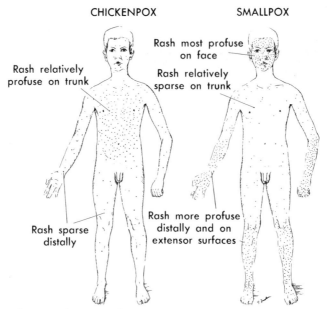

Fig. 45-4 Schematic drawings illustrating differences in distribution of rashes of chickenpox and smallpox.

nasolabial area and other sites available for scratching, and they do not involve the oral mucous membranes.

Insect bites and papular urticaria. Insect bites and papular urticaria do not have a typical vesicular appearance and do not involve the scalp or mucous membranes.

Molluscum contagiosum. The lesions of molluscum contagiosum are scattered, discrete, firm, small nodular elevations without any surrounding red areolae.

Dermatitis herpetiformis. Dermatitis herpetiformis is characterized by erythematous papulovesicular lesions that are symmetrical in distribution, by a chronic course, and by healing with residual pigmentation.

Laboratory Diagnostic Tests

Varicella. The virus of varicella is isolated from vesicular fluid or may be identified on smears by indirect immunofluorescence. Detection of specific varicella-zoster antibody during convalescence is accomplished by means of one of the following tests: fluorescent antibody to membrane antigen (FAMA), ELISA, and latex agglutination (LA) (see Chapter 4).

Smallpox. The virus of smallpox may be identified by electron microscopy or gel diffusion.

Eczema herpeticum. Herpes simplex virus may be isolated in tissue culture, and the viral antigen may be identified in smears by indirect immunofluorescence. In eczema herpeticum, a rise in the level of antibodies during convalescence may be demonstrated.

Eczema vaccinatum. The laboratory tests for eczema vaccinatum are the same as those for smallpox.

Herpes zoster. The laboratory tests for herpes zoster are the same as those for chickenpox.

Rickettsialpox. The isolation of *Rickettsia akari* from the blood can be achieved by inoculation of the yolk sac of embryonated eggs. The rise in the level of rickettsialpox and Rocky Mountain spotted fever antibodies occurs during convalescence.

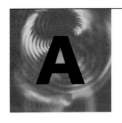

ANTIMICROBIAL DRUGS*

DRUGS FOR TREATMENT OF PARASITIC INFECTIONS

Parasitic infections are found throughout the world. With increasing travel, immigration, use of immunosuppressive drugs and the spread of AIDS, physicians anywhere may see infections caused by previously unfamiliar parasites. The following table lists first-choice and alternative drugs for most parasitic infections. The manufacturers of the drugs are listed on page 949.

*From the Medical Letter Handbook of Antimicrobial Therapy, 2000, The Medical Letter, Inc, New Rochelle, New York.

Infection	Drug	Adult dosage	Pediatric dosage
Acanthamoeba Keratitis			
Drug of choice:	See footnote 1		
Amebiasis (Entamoeba Histolytica)			
Asymptomatic			
Drug of choice:	Iodoquinol	650 mg tid × 20 days	30-40 mg/kg/day (max 2 g) in 3 doses × 20 days
	OR		
	Paromomycin	25-35 mg/kg/d in 3 doses × 7 days	25-35 mg/kg/day in 3 doses × 7 days
Alternative:	Diloxanide furoate*	500 mg tid × 10 days	20 mg/kg/d in 3 doses × 10 days
Mild to moderate intestinal disease[2]			
Drug of choice:	Metronidazole	500-750 mg tid × 10 days	35-50 mg/kg/day in 3 doses × 10 days
	OR Tinidazole[3]*	2 g/day divided tid × 3 days	50 mg/kg (max 2 g) qd × 3 days
Severe intestinal and extraintestinal disease			
Drug of choice[2]:	Metronidazole	750 mg tid × 7 days	35-50 mg/kg/day in 3 doses × 7 days
	OR Tinidazole[3]*	600 mg bid to 800 mg tid × 5 days	50-60 mg/kg/day (max 2 g) × 5 days

*Availability problems. See pp. 949-950.

[1]For treatment of keratitis caused by *Acanthamoeba*, concurrent topical use of 0.1% propamidine isethionate (Brolene) plus neomycin-polymyxin B-gramicidin ophthalmic solution has been successful (Hargrave et al., Ophthalmology 1999;106:952). In addition, 0.02% topical polyhexamethylene biguanide (PHMB) and/or chlorhexadine has been used successfully in a large number of patients (Radford et al., Br J Ophthalmol 1998;82:1387). PHMB is available as Baquacil (ICI America), a swimming pool disinfectant (Yee and Winarko, Am J Hosp Pharm 1993;50: 2523).

[2]Treatment should be followed by a course of iodoquinol or paromomycin in the dosage used to treat asymptomatic amebiasis.

[3]A nitro-imidazole similar to metronidazole, but not marketed in the United States, tinidazole appears to be at least as effective as metronidazole and better tolerated. Ornidazole, a similar drug, is also used outside the United States. Higher dosage is for hepatic abscess.

Continued

Infection	Drug	Adult dosage	Pediatric dosage
Amebic Meningoencephalitis, Primary			
Naegleria			
Drug of choice:	Amphotericin B[4,5]	1 mg/kg/day IV, uncertain duration	1 mg/kg/day IV, uncertain duration
Acanthamoeba			
Drug of choice:	See footnote 6		
Balamuthia mandrillaris			
Drug of choice:	See footnote 7		
Ancylostoma Caninum (Eosinophilic Enterocolitis)			
Drug of choice:	Albendazole[5] OR	400 mg once	400 mg once
	Mebendazole OR	100 mg bid × 3 days	100 mg bid × 3 days
	Pyrantel pamoate[5]	11 mg/kg (max 1g) × 3 days	11 mg/kg (max 1g) × 3 days
Ancylostoma Duodenale, see Hookworm			
Angiostrongyliasis			
Angiostrongylus cantonensis			
Drug of choice[8]:	Mebendazole[5]	100 mg bid × 5 days	100 mg bid × 5 days
Angiostrongylus costaricensis			
Drug of choice:	Mebendazole[5]	200-400 mg tid × 10 days	200-400 mg tid × 10 days
Alternative:	Thiabendazole[5]	75 mg/kg/day in 3 doses × 3 days (max 3 g/day)[9]	75 mg/kg/day in 3 doses × 3 days (max 3 g/day)[9]
Anisakiasis *(Anisakis)*			
Treatment of choice:	Surgical or endoscopic removal		
Ascariasis (Ascaris Lumbricoides, Roundworm)			
Drug of choice:	Albendazole[5] OR	400 mg once	400 mg once
	Mebendazole	100 mg bid × 3 days or 500 mg once	100 mg bid × 3 days or 500 mg once
	OR		
	Pyrantel pamoate[5]	11 mg/kg once (max 1 g)	11 mg/kg once (max 1 g)

[4]A *Naeglaeria* infection was treated successfully with intravenous and intrathecal use of both amphotericin B and miconazole, plus rifampin (Seidel et al., N Engl J Med 1982;306:346). Other reports of successful therapy are questionable.

[5]An approved drug, but considered investigational for this condition by the U.S. Food and Drug Administration

[6]Strains of *Acanthamoeba* isolated from fatal granulomatous amebic encephalitis are usually susceptible in vitro to pentamidine, ketoconazole (Nizoral), flucytosine (Ancobon) and (less so) to amphotericin B. One patient with disseminated cutaneous infection was treated successfully with intravenous pentamidine isethionate, topical chlorhexidine, and 2% ketoconazole cream, followed by oral itraconazole (Slater et al., N Engl J Med 1994; 331:85).

[7]A recently described free-living leptomyxid ameba that causes subacute to chronic granulomatous disease of the CNS. In vitro pentamidine isethionate 10 µg/ml is amebastatic (Denney et al., Clin Infect Dis 1997;25: 1354). One patient, according to *Medical Letter* consultants, was successfully treated with clarithromycin (Biaxin) 500 mg tid, fluconazole (Diflucan) 400 mg once daily, sulfadiazine 1.5 g q6h, and flucytosine (Ancobon) 1.5 g q6h.

[8]Antiparasitic drugs can provoke neurologic symptoms, and most patients recover spontaneously without them. Analgesics, corticosteroids, and careful removal of CSF at frequent intervals can relieve symptoms (Pien and Pien, Int J Infect Dis 1999;3: 161). Albendazole, levamisole (Ergamisol), or ivermectin have been used successfully in animals.

[9]This dose is likely to be toxic and may have to be decreased.

Infection	Drug	Adult dosage	Pediatric dosage
Babesiosis (Babesia Microti)			
Drugs of choice[10]:	Clindamycin[5]	1.2 g bid IV or 600 mg tid PO × 7 days	20-40 mg/kg/day PO in 3 doses × 7 days
	plus quinine	650 mg tid PO × 7 days	25 mg/kg/day PO in 3 doses × 7 days
	OR		
	Atovaquone[5]	750 mg bid PO × 7-10 days	20 mg/kg bid PO × 7-10 days
	plus azithromycin[5]	1,000 mg daily PO × 3 days, then 500 mg daily × 7 days	12 mg/kg daily PO × 7-10 days

Balamuthuia Mandrillaris, *see* Amebiq Meningoencephalitis Primary

Infection	Drug	Adult dosage	Pediatric dosage
Balantidiasis (Balantidium coli)			
Drug of choice:	Tetracycline[5,11]	500 mg qid × 10 days	40 mg/kg/day (max 2 g) in 4 doses × 10 days
Alternatives:	Iodoquinol[5]	650 mg tid × 20 days	40 mg/kg/day in 3 doses × 20 days
	Metronidazole[5]	750 mg tid × 5 days	35-50 mg/kg/day in 3 doses × 5 days

Infection	Drug	Adult dosage	Pediatric dosage
Baylisascariasis (Baylisascaris Procyonis)			
Drug of choice:	See footnote[12]		

Infection	Drug	Adult dosage	Pediatric dosage
Blastocystis Hominis			
Drug of choice:	See footnote[13]		

Infection	Drug	Adult dosage	Pediatric dosage
Capillariasis (Capillaria Philippinensis)			
Drug of choice:	Mebendazole[5]	200 mg bid × 20 days	200 mg bid × 20 days
Alternatives:	Albendazole[5]	400 mg daily × 10 days	400 mg daily × 10 days

Chagas' Disease, see Trypanosomiasis

Clonorchis Sinensis, see Fluke

Infection	Drug	Adult dosage	Pediatric dosage
Cryptosporidiosis (Cryptosporidium)			
Drug of choice[14]:	Paromomycin[5]	25-35 mg/kg/day in 2 or 4 doses	25-35 mg/kg/day in 2 or 4 doses

[10]Exchange transfusion has been used in severely ill patients with high (>10%) parasitemia (Boustani and Gelfard, Clin Infect Dis 1996;22:611). Combination therapy with atovaquone and azithromycin may be better tolerated (Krause et al., American Society of Tropical Medicine and Hygiene Annual Meeting, 46:247, 1997, abstract 430). Concurrent use of pentamidine and trimethoprim-sulfamethoxazole has been reported to cure an infection with B. *divergens* (Raoult et al., Ann Intern Med 1987;107:944).

[11]Use of tetracyclines is contraindicated in pregnancy and in children less than 8 years old.

[12]No drugs have been demonstrated to be effective. However, albendazole, mebendazole, thiabendazole, levamisole (Ergamisol) and ivermectin could be tried. Steroid therapy may be helpful, especially in eye and CNS infections. Ocular baylisascariasis has been treated successfully using laser photocoagulation therapy to destroy the intraretinal larvae.

[13]Clinical significance of these organisms is controversial, but metronidazole 750 mg tid × 10 days or iodoquinol 650 mg tid × 20 days has been reported to be effective (Stenzel and Borenam, Clin Microbiol Rev 1996;9:563). Metronidazole resistance may be common (Haresh et al., Trop Med Int Health 1999;4:274). Trimethoprim-sulfamethoxazole is an alternative regimen (Ok et al., Am J Gastroenterol 1999;94: 3245).

[14]Treatment is not curative in immunocompromised patients, and infection is self-limited in immunocompetent patients. Combination therapy with azithromycin 600 mg daily has been effective in some patients (Smith et al., J Infect Dis 1998; 178:900). Nitazoxanide (an investigational drug in the United States manufactured by Romark Laboratories, Tampa, Florida, 813-282-8544, www.romarklaboratories.com), 500-1000 mg PO bid, may be used as an alternative (Rossignol et al., Trans R Soc Trop Med Hyg 1998;92:663). Duration of therapy is uncertain.

Continued

Infection	Drug	Adult dosage	Pediatric dosage
Cutaneous Larva Migrans (Creeping Eruption, Dog and Cat Hookworm)			
Drug of choice:	Albendazole[5] OR	400 mg daily × 3 days	400 mg daily × 3 days
	Ivermectin[5] OR	200 μg/kg daily × 1-2 days	200 μg/kg daily × 1-2 days
	Thiabendazole[15]	Topically	Topically
Cyclospora			
Drug of choice:	Trimethoprim-sulfamethoxazole[5,16]	TMP 160 mg, SMX 800 mg bid × 7 days	TMP 5 mg/kg, SMX 25 mg/kg bid × 7 days
Cysticercosis, see Tapeworm			
Dientamoeba fragilis			
Drug of choice:	Iodoquinol	650 mg tid × 20 days	30-40 mg/kg/day (max 2 g) in 3 doses × 20 days
	OR Paromomycin[5]	25-35 mg/kg/day in 3 doses × 7 days	25-30 mg/kg/day in 3 doses × 7 days
	OR Tetracycline[5,11]	500 mg qid × 10 days	40 mg/kg/day (max 2g) in 4 doses × 10 days
Diphyllobothrium Latum, see Tapeworm			
Dracunculus Medinensis (Guinea Worm)			
Drug of choice:	Metronidazole[5,17]	250 mg tid × 10 days	25 mg/kg/day (max 750 mg) in 3 doses × 10 days
Echinococcus, see Tapeworm			
Entamoeba Histolytica, see Amebiasis			
Entamoeba Polecki			
Drug of choice:	Metronidazole[5]	750 mg tid × 10 days	35-50 mg/kg/day in 3 doses × 10 days
Enterobius Vermicularis (Pinworm)			
Drug of choice:	Pyrantel pamoate	11 mg/kg base once (max 1 g); repeat in 2 weeks	11 mg/kg once (max 1 g); repeat in 2 weeks
	OR Mebendazole	100 mg once; repeat in 2 weeks	100 mg once; repeat in 2 weeks
	OR Albendazole[5]	400 mg once; repeat in 2 weeks	400 mg once; repeat in 2 weeks

[15]Davis et al., Arch Dermatol 1993;129:588.
[16]HIV-infected patients may need higher dosage and long-term maintenance.
[17]Not curative, but decreases inflammation and facilitates removing the worm. Mebendazole 400-800 mg/day for 6 days has been reported to kill the worm directly.

Infection	Drug	Adult dosage	Pediatric dosage

Fasciola Hepatica, see Fluke

Filariasis

Wuchereria bancrofti, Brugia malayi

Drug of choice:[18,19]	Diethylcarbamazine[20]*	Day 1: 50 mg PC
		Day 2: 50 mg tid
		Day 3: 100 mg tid
		Days 4 through 14:
		  6 mg/kg/day in
		  3 doses
			Day 1: 1 mg/kg PC
			Day 2: 1 mg/kg tid
			Day 3: 1-2 mg/kg tid
			Days 4 through 14:
			  6 mg/kg/day in
			  3 doses

Loa loa

Drug of choice[19,21]:	Diethylcarbamazine[20]*	Day 1: 50 mg PC
		Day 2: 50 mg tid
		Day 3: 100 mg tid
		Days 4 through 21:
		  9 mg/kg/day in
		  3 doses
			Day 1: 1 mg/kg PC
			Day 2: 1 mg/kg tid
			Day 3: 1-2 mg/kg
			Days 4 through 21:
			  9 mg/kg/day in
			  3 doses

Mansonella ozzardi

Drug of choice:	See footnote[22]		

Mansonella perstans

Drug of choice:	Mebendazole[5] OR Albendazole[5]	100 mg bid × 30 days 400 mg bid × 10 days	100 mg bid × 30 days 400 mg bid × 10 days

Mansonella streptocerca

Drug of choice[23]:	Diethylcarbamazine* Ivermectin[5]	6 mg/kg/day × 14 days 150 µg/kg once	6 mg/kg/day × 14 days 150 µg/kg once

Tropical pulmonary eosinophilia (TPE)

Drug of choice:	Diethylcarbamazine*	6 mg/kg/day in 3
		  doses × 14 days
			6 mg/kg/day in 3
			  doses × 14 days

Onchocerca volvulus (River blindness)

Drug of choice:	Ivermectin[24]	150 µg/kg once,
		  repeated every
		  6-12 months until
		  asymptomatic
			150 µg/kg once,
			  repeated every
			  6-12 months until
			  asymptomatic

Fluke, Hermaphroditic

Clonorchis sinensis (Chinese liver fluke)

Drug of choice:	Praziquantel	75 mg/kg/day in 3
		  doses × 1 day
			75 mg/kg/day in 3
			  doses × 1 day

---

[18]A single dose of ivermectin, 200 µg/kg, is effective for treatment of microfilaremia but does not kill the adult worm. In a limited study, single-dose diethylcarbamazine (6 mg/kg) was as macrofilaricidal as a multidose regimen against *W. bancrofti* (Norões et al., Trans R Soc Trop Med Hyg 1997;91:78).

[19]Antihistamines or corticosteroids may be required to decrease allergic reactions due to disintegration of microfilariae in treatment of filarial infections, especially those caused by *Loa loa.*

[20]For patients with no microfilariae in the blood, full doses can be given from day 1.

[21]In heavy infections with *Loa loa*, rapid killing of microfilariae can provoke an encephalopathy. Apheresis has been reported to be effective in lowering microfilarial counts in patients heavily infected with *Loa loa* (Ottesen, Infect Dis Clin North Am 1993;7:619). Albendazole and ivermectin have also been used to reduce microfilaremia, but because of slower onset of action, albendazole is preferred (Klion et al., J Infect Dis 1993;168:202; Kombila et al., Am J Trop Med Hyg 1998;58:458). Albendazole may be useful for treatment of loiasis when diethylcarbamazine is ineffective or cannot be used, but repeated courses may be necessary (Klion et al., Clin Infect Dis 1999;29:680). Diethylcarbamazine, 300 mg once weekly, has been recommended for prevention of loiasis (Nutman et al., N Engl J Med 1988;319:752).

[22]Diethylcarbamazine has no effect. Ivermectin, 200 µg/kg once, has been effective.

[23]Diethylcarbamazine is potentially curative because of activity against both adult worms and microfilariae but is not available in the United States for this indication from the CDC. Ivermectin is active only against microfilariae.

[24]Annual treatment with ivermectin, 150 µg/kg, can prevent blindness due to ocular onchocerciasis (Mabey et al., Ophthalmology 1996;103:1001).

Continued

Infection	Drug	Adult dosage	Pediatric dosage
	OR		
	Albendazole[5]	10 mg/kg × 7 days	10 mg/kg × 7 days
Fasciola hepatica (Sheep liver fluke)			
Drug of choice[25]:	Triclabendazole*	10 mg/kg once	10 mg/kg once
Alternative:	Bithionol*	30-50 mg/kg on alternate days × 10-15 doses	30-50 mg/kg on alternate days × 10-15 doses
Fasciolopsis buski, Heterophyes heterophyes, Metagonimus yokogawai (Intestinal flukes)			
Drug of choice:	Praziquantel[5]	75 mg/kg/day in 3 doses × 1 day	75 mg/kg/day in 3 doses × 1 day
Metorchis conjunctus (North American liver fluke)[26]			
Drug of choice:	Praziquantel[5]	75 mg/kg/day in 3 doses × 1 day	75 mg/kg/day in 3 doses × 1 day
Nanophyetus salmincola			
Drug of choice:	Praziquantel[5]	60 mg/kg/day in 3 doses × 1 day	60 mg/kg/day in 3 doses × 1 day
Opisthorchis viverrini (Southeast Asian liver fluke)			
Drug of choice:	Praziquantel	75 mg/kg/day in 3 doses × 1 day	75 mg/kg/day in 3 doses × 1 day
Paragonimus westermani (Lung fluke)			
Drug of choice:	Praziquantel[5]	75 mg/kg/day in 3 doses × 2 days	75 mg/kg/day in 3 doses × 2 days
Alternative[27]:	Bithionol*	30-50 mg/kg on alternate days × 10-15 doses	30-50 mg/kg on alternate days × 10-15 doses
Giardiasis *(Giardia Lamblia)*			
Drug of choice:	Metronidazole[5]	250 mg tid × 5 days	15 mg/kg/day in 3 doses × 5 days
Alternatives[28]:	Quinacrine[29]	100 mg PO tid × 5 days (max 300 mg/day)	2 mg/kg PO tid × 5 days (max 300 mg/day)
	Tinidazole[2]*	2 g once	50 mg/kg once (max 2 g)
	Furazolidone	100 mg qid × 7-10 days	6 mg/kg/day in 4 doses × 7-10 days
	Paromomycin[5,30]	25-35 mg/kg/day in 3 doses × 7 days	25-35 mg/kg/day in 3 doses × 7 days
Gnathostomiasis *(Gnathostoma Spinigerum)*			
Treatment of choice[31]:	Surgical removal		
	OR		
	Albendazole[5]	400 mg bid × 21 days	

[25]Unlike infections with other flukes, *Fasciola hepatica* infections may not respond to praziquantel. Triclabendazole (Fasinex-Novartis), a veterinary fasciolide, may be safe and effective, but data are limited (López-Vélez et al., Eur J Clin Microbiol 1999;18:525). It should be given with food for better absorption.

[26]MacLean et al., Lancet 1996;347:154.

[27]Triclabendazole may be effective in a dosage of 5 mg/kg once daily for 3 days or 10 mg/kg twice in 1 day (Calvopiña et al., Trans R Soc Trop Med Hyg 1998;92:566).

[28]Albendazole 400 mg daily × 5 days may be effective (Hall and Nahar, Trans R Soc Trop Med Hyg 1993;87:84). Bacitracin zinc or bacitracin 120,000 U bid for 10 days may also be effective (Andrews et al., Am J Trop Med Hyg 1995;52:318).

[29]Quinacrine is not available commercially, but as a service can be compounded by Medical Center Pharmacy, New Haven, Connecticut (203-785-6818) or Panorama Compounding Pharmacy, 6744 Balboa Blvd, Van Nuys, CA 91406 (800-247-9767).

[30]Not absorbed; may be useful for treatment of giardiasis in pregnancy.

[31]Ivermectin has been reported to be effective in animals, but there are few data regarding use in humans (Anantaphruti et al., Trop Med Parasitol 1992;43:65; Ruiz-Maldonado and Mosqueda-Cabrera, Int J Dermatol 1999;38:52).

Infection	Drug	Adult dosage	Pediatric dosage
Gongylonemiasis (*Gongylonema Spp.*)			
Treatment of choice[32]:	Surgical removal OR		
	Albendazole[5]	10 mg/kg/day × 3 days	10 mg/kg/day × 3 days
Hookworm (*Ancylostoma Duodenale, Necator Americanus*)			
Drug of choice:	Albendazole[5] OR	400 mg once	400 mg once
	Mebendazole OR	100 mg bid × 3 days or 500 mg once	100 mg bid × 3 days or 500 mg once
	Pyrantel pamoate[5]	11 mg/kg (max 1 g) × 3 days	11 mg/kg (max 1 g) × 3 days
Hydatid Cyst, see Tapeworm			
Hymenolepis Nana, see Tapeworm			
Isosporiasis (*Isospora Belli*)			
Drug of choice:	Trimethoprim-sulfamethoxazole[5,33]	160 mg TMP, 800 mg SMX qid × 10 days, then bid × 3 weeks	
Leishmaniasis (Cutaneous due to *L. Mexicana, L. Tropica, L. Major, L. Braziliensis*; mucocutaneous mostly due to *L. Braziliensis*; visceral due to *L. Donovani* [Kala-azar], *L. Infantum, L. Chagasi*)			
Drug of choice[34]:	Sodium stibogluconate* OR	20 mg Sb/kg/day IV or IM × 20-28 days[35]	20 mg Sb/kg/day IV or IM × 20-28 days[35]
	Meglumine antimonate*	20 mg Sb/kg/day IV or IM × 20-28 days[35]	20 mg Sb/kg/day IV or IM × 20-28 days[35]
	OR Amphotericin B[5]	0.5-1 mg/kg IV daily or every 2 days for up to 8 weeks	0.5-1 mg/kg IV daily or every 2 days for up to 8 weeks
	OR Liposomal Amphotericin B[36]	3 mg/kg/day days 1-5, and 3 mg/kg/day days 14, 21[37]	3 mg/kg/day days 1-5, and 3 mg/kg/day days 14, 21[37]
Alternatives:	Pentamidine	2-4 mg/kg daily or every 2 days IV or IM for up to 15 doses[38]	2-4 mg/kg daily or every 2 days IV or IM for up to 15 doses[38]

[32]Eberhard et al., Am J Trop Med Hyg 1999;61:51.

[33]In sulfonamide-sensitive patients, pyrimethamine 50-75 mg daily in divided doses has been effective (Ackers, Semin Gastrointest Dis 1997;8:33).

[34]For treatment of kala-azar, oral miltefosine 100-150 mg daily for 4 weeks was 97% effective after 6 months. Gastrointestinal adverse effects are common, and the drug is contraindicated in pregnancy (Jha et al., N Engl J Med 1999;341:1795).

[35]May be repeated or continued. A longer duration may be needed for some forms of visceral leishmaniasis (Herwaldt, Lancet, 1999;354:1191).

[36]Three preparations of lipid-encapsulated amphotericin B have been used for treatment of visceral leishmaniasis. Largely based on clinical trials in patients infected with *L. infantum*, the FDA approved liposomal amphotericin B (AmBisome) for treatment of visceral leishmaniasis (Meyerhoff, Clin Infect Dis 1999;28:42; Berman, Clin Infect Dis 1999;28:49). Amphotericin B lipid complex (Abelcet) and amphotericin B cholesteryl sulfate (Amphotec) have also been used with good results. Some studies indicate that *L. donovani* resistant to pentavalent antimonial agents may respond to lipid-encapsulated amphotericin B (Sundar et al. Ann Trop Med Parasitol 1998;92: 755).

[37]The dose for immunocompromised patients with HIV is 4 mg/kg/day on days 1-5 and 4 mg/kg/day on days 10, 17, 24, 31, 38. The relapse rate is high, suggesting that maintenance therapy may be indicated.

[38]4 mg/kg qod × 15 doses for *L. donovani*; 2 mg/kg qod × 7 or 3 mg/kg qod × 4 doses for cutaneous disease.

Continued

Infection	Drug	Adult dosage	Pediatric dosage
Leishmaniasis—cont'd			
	OR		
	Paromomycin[39*]	Topically twice daily × 10-20 days	
Lice (Pediculus Humanus, P. Capitis, Phthirus Pubis)[40]			
Drug of choice:	1% Permethrin[41]	Topically	Topically
	OR		
	0.5% Malathion[42]	Topically	Topically
Alternative:	Pyrethrins with piperonyl butoxide[41]	Topically	Topically
	OR		
	Ivermectin[5, 43]	200 µg/kg once	200 µg/kg once
Loa Loa, see Filariasis			
Malaria (Plasmodium Falciparum, P. Ovale, P. Vivax, and P. Malariae) Chloroquine-resistant P. falciparum[44] ORAL			
Drugs of choice:	Quinine sulfate	650 mg q8h × 3-7 days[45]	25 mg/kg/day in 3 doses × 3-7 days[45]
	plus doxycycline[5,11]	100 mg bid × 7 days	2 mg/kg/d × 7 days
	or plus tetracycline[5,11]	250 mg qid × 7 days	6.25 mg/kg qid × 7 days
	or plus pyrimethamine-sulfadoxine[46]	3 tablets at once on last day of quinine	<1 yr: ¼ tablet 1-3 yr: ½ tablet 4-8 yr: 1 tablet 9-14 yr: 2 tablets
	or plus clindamycin[5,47]	900 mg tid × 5 days	20-40 mg/kg/day in 3 doses × 5 days

[39]Two preparations of paromomycin have been studied. The first, a formulation of 15% paromomycin and 12% methylbenzethonium chloride in soft white paraffin for topical use, has been reported to be effective in some patients against cutaneous leishmaniasis due to *L. major* (Ozgoztasi and Baydar, Int J Dermatol 1997;36:61). The second, injectable paromomycin (aminosidine, not available in the United States), has been used successfully for the treatment of kala-azar in India, where antimony resistance is common (Jha et al., BMJ 1998;316:1200).

[40]For infestation of eyelashes with crab lice, use petrolatum. For pubic lice, treat with 5% permethrin or ivermectin as for scabies (see p. 946).

[41]A second application is recommended 1 week later to kill hatching progeny. Some lice are resistant to pyrethrins and permethrin (Pollack, Arch Pediatr Adolesc Med 1999;153:969).

[42]Medical Letter 1999;41:73.

[43]Ivermectin is effective against adult lice but has no effect on nits (Bell, Pediatr Infect Dis J 1998;17:923).

[44]Chloroquine-resistant *P. falciparum* occurs in all malarious areas except Central America west of the Panama Canal Zone, Mexico, Haiti, the Dominican Republic, and most of the Middle East (chloroquine resistance has been reported in Yemen, Oman, Saudi Arabia, and Iran).

[45]In Southeast Asia, relative resistance to quinine has increased, and the treatment should be continued for 7 days.

[46]Fansidar tablets contain 25 mg of pyrimethamine and 500 mg of sulfadoxine. Resistance to pyrimethamine-sulfadoxine has been reported from Southeast Asia, the Amazon basin, sub-Saharan Africa, Bangladesh, and Oceania.

[47]For use in pregnancy.

Infection	Drug	Adult dosage	Pediatric dosage
Alternatives[48]:	Mefloquine[49,50]	750 mg followed by 500 mg 12 h later	15 mg/kg PO followed by 10 mg/kg PO 8-12 h later (<45 kg)
	Halofantrine[51*]	500 mg q6h × 3 doses; repeat in 1 week[52]	8 mg/kg q6h × 3 doses (<40 kg); repeat in 1 week[52]
	Atovaquone[53]	500 mg bid × 3 days	11-20 kg: 125 mg bid × 3 days 21-30 kg: 250 mg bid × 3 days 31-40 kg: 375 mg bid × 3 days
	plus proguanil	200 mg bid × 3 days	11-20 kg: 50 mg bid × 3 days 21-30 kg: 100 mg bid × 3 days 31-40 kg: 150 mg bid × 3 days
	or plus doxycycline[5,11] Artesunate[*] **plus**	100 mg bid × 3 days 4 mg/kg/day × 3 days	2 mg/kg/day × 3 days
	mefloquine[49,50]	750 mg followed by 500 mg 12 h later	15 mg/kg followed 8-12 h later by 10 mg/kg
Chloroquine-resistant P. vivax[54] Drug of choice:	Quinine sulfate	650 mg q8h × 3-7 days[45]	25 mg/kg/day in 3 doses × 3-7 days[45]

[48]For treatment of multiple-drug–resistant *P. falciparum* in Southeast Asia, especially Thailand, where resistance to mefloquine and halofantrine is frequent, a 7-day course of quinine and tetracycline is recommended (Watt et al., Am J Trop Med Hyg 1992;47:108). Artesunate plus mefloquine (Luxemburger et al., Trans R Soc Trop Med Hyg 1994;88:213), artemether plus mefloquine (Karbwang et al., Trans R Soc Trop Med Hyg 1995;89:296), and mefloquine plus doxycycline are also used to treat multiple-drug–resistant *P. falciparum*.

[49]At this dosage, adverse effects including nausea, vomiting, diarrhea, dizziness, disturbed sense of balance, toxic psychosis, and seizures can occur. Mefloquine is teratogenic in animals and should not be used for treatment of malaria in pregnancy. It should not be given together with quinine, quinidine or halofantrine, and caution is required in using quinine, quinidine, or halofantrine to treat patients with malaria who have taken mefloquine for prophylaxis. The pediatric dosage has not been approved by the FDA. Resistance to mefloquine has been reported in some areas, such as the Thailand-Myanmar and Thailand-Cambodia borders and in the Amazon basin, where 25 mg/kg should be used.

[50]In the United States, a 250-mg tablet of mefloquine contains 228 mg mefloquine base. Outside the United States, each 275-mg tablet contains 250 mg base.

[51]May be effective in multiple-drug–resistant *P. falciparum* malaria, but treatment failures and resistance have been reported, and the drug has caused lengthening of the PR and QTc intervals and fatal cardiac arrhythmias. It should not be used for patients with cardiac conduction defects or with other drugs that may affect the QT interval, such as quinine, quinidine and mefloquine. Cardiac monitoring is recommended. Variability in absorption is a problem; halofantrine should not be taken 1 hour before to 2 hours after meals because food increases its absorption. It should not be used in pregnancy.

[52]A single 250-mg dose can be used for repeat treatment in mild to moderate infections (Touze et al., Lancet 1997;349:255).

[53]Atovaquone plus proguanil is marketed as a combination tablet in many countries and will soon be available in the United States (250 mg atovaquone/100 mg proguanil as Malarone and 62.5 mg atovaquone/25 mg proguanil as Malarone Pediatric [Glaxo Wellcome]). The combination should be used only for acute uncomplicated malaria caused by *P. falciparum*. The dose of Malarone for 3-day treatment of malaria is 4 tablets daily in adults; 3 adult tablets daily for children 31-40 kg; 2 adult tablets daily for children 21-30 kg; and 1 adult tablet daily for children 11-20 kg. To enhance absorption, it should be taken within 45 minutes after eating (Looareesuwan et al., Am J Trop Med Hyg 1999;60:533). Although approved for once daily dosing, to decrease nausea and vomiting the dose can be divided in two.

[54]*P. vivax* with decreased susceptibility to chloroquine is a significant problem in Papua-New Guinea and Indonesia. There are also a few reports of resistance from Myanmar, India, Thailand, the Solomon Islands, Vanuatu, Guyana, Brazil, and Peru.

Continued

Infection	Drug	Adult dosage	Pediatric dosage
	plus doxycycline[5,11]	100 mg bid × 7 days	2 mg/kg/day × 7 days
	or plus pyrimethamine-sulfadoxine[46]	3 tablets at once on last day of quinine	<1 yr: ¼ tablet
			1-3 yr: ½ tablet
			4-8 yr: 1 tablet
			9-14 yr: 2 tablets
	OR Mefloquine	750 mg followed by 500 mg 12 h later	15 mg/kg followed 8-12 h later by 10 mg/kg
Alternatives:	Halofantrine[51,55*] Chloroquine	500 mg q6h × 3 doses 25 mg base/kg in 3 doses over 48 h	8 mg/kg q6h × 3 doses
	plus primaquine[56]	2.5 mg base/kg in 3 doses over 48 h	

All Plasmodium except Chloroquine-resistant P. falciparum[44] and Chloroquine-resistant P. vivax[54]
ORAL

Drug of choice:	Chloroquine phosphate[57]	1 g (600 mg base), then 500 mg (300 mg base) 6 h later, then 500 mg (300 mg base) at 24 and 48 h	10 mg base/kg (max 600 mg base), then 5 mg base/kg 6 h later, then 5 mg base/kg at 24 and 48 h

All Plasmodium
PARENTERAL

Drug of choice[58]:	Quinidine gluconate[59,60]	10 mg/kg loading dose (max 600 mg) in normal saline slowly over 1-2 h, followed by continuous infusion of 0.02 mg/kg/min until oral therapy can be started	Same as adult dose
	OR Quinine dihydrochloride[59,60]	20 mg/kg loading dose IV in 5% dextrose over 4 h, followed by 10 mg/kg over 2-4 h q8h	Same as adult dose

[55]Baird et al., J Infect Dis 1995;171:1678.

[56]Primaquine phosphate can cause hemolytic anemia, especially in patients whose red cells are deficient in glucose-6-phosphate dehydrogenase. This deficiency is most common in African, Asian, and Mediterranean peoples. Patients should be screened for G-6-PD deficiency before treatment. Primaquine should not be used during pregnancy.

[57]If chloroquine phosphate is not available, hydroxychloroquine sulfate is as effective; 400 mg of hydroxychloroquine sulfate is equivalent to 500 mg of chloroquine phosphate.

[58]Exchange transfusion has been helpful for some patients with high-density (>10%) parasitemia, altered mental status, pulmonary edema, or renal complications (Miller et al., N Engl J Med 1989;321:65).

[59]Continuous EKG, blood pressure, and glucose monitoring are recommended, especially in pregnant women and young children.

[60]Quinidine may have greater antimalarial activity than quinine. The loading dose should be decreased or omitted in those patients who have received quinine or mefloquine. If more than 48 hours of parenteral treatment is required, the quinine or quinidine dose should be reduced by ⅓ to ½.

Infection	Drug	Adult dosage	Pediatric dosage
		(max 1,800 mg/day) until oral therapy can be started	
Alternative:	Artemether[61*]	3.2 mg/kg IM, then 1.6 mg/kg daily × 5-7 days	Same as adult dose
Prevention of relapses: P. vivax and P. ovale only			
Drug of choice:	Primaquine phosphate[56,62]	26.3 mg (15 mg base)/ day × 14 days or 79 mg (45 mg base)/ week × 8 weeks	0.3 mg base/kg/day × 14 days

Malaria, Prevention of[63]

Chloroquine-sensitive areas[44]

Infection	Drug	Adult dosage	Pediatric dosage
Drug of choice:	Chloroquine phosphate[64,65]	500 mg (300 mg base), once/week[66]	5 mg/kg base once/week, up to adult dose of 300 mg base[66]

Chloroquine-resistant areas[44]

Infection	Drug	Adult dosage	Pediatric dosage
Drug of choice:	Mefloquine[50,65,67]	250 mg once/week[66]	<15 kg: 5 mg/kg[66] 15-19 kg: ¼ tablet[66] 20-30 kg: ½ tablet[66] 31-45 kg: ¾ tablet[66] >45 kg: 1 tablet[66]
	OR Doxycycline[5,65]	100 mg daily[68]	2 mg/kg/day, up to 100 mg/day[68]
	OR Atovaquone/Proguanil[53]	250 mg/100 mg (1 tablet) daily[69]	11-20 kg: 62.5 mg/25 mg[69] 21-30 kg: 125 mg/50 mg[69] 31-40 kg: 187.5 mg/75 mg[69]

[61]White, N Engl J Med 1996;335:800. Not available in the United States.

[62]Relapses have been reported with this regimen and should be treated with a second 14-day course of 30 mg base/day.

[63]No drug regimen guarantees protection against malaria. If fever develops within a year (particularly within the first 2 months) after travel to malarious areas, travelers should be advised to seek medical attention. Insect repellents, insecticide-impregnated bed nets and proper clothing are important adjuncts for malaria prophylaxis.

[64]In pregnancy, chloroquine prophylaxis has been used extensively and safely.

[65]For prevention of attack after departure from areas where *P. vivax* and *P. ovale* are endemic, which includes almost all areas where malaria is found (except Haiti), some experts prescribe in addition primaquine phosphate 15 mg base (26.3 mg)/day or, for children, 0.3 mg base/kg/day during the last 2 weeks of prophylaxis. Others prefer to avoid the toxicity of primaquine and rely on surveillance to detect cases when they occur, particularly when exposure was limited or doubtful. See also footnotes 56 and 62.

[66]Beginning 1-2 weeks before travel and continuing weekly for the duration of stay and for 4 weeks after leaving.

[67]The pediatric dosage has not been approved by the FDA, and the drug has not been approved for use during pregnancy. However, it has been reported to be safe for prophylactic use during the second or third trimester of pregnancy and possibly during early pregnancy as well (CDC Health Information for International Travel, 1999-2000, page 120; Smoak et al., J Infect Dis 1997;176:831). Mefloquine is not recommended for patients with cardiac conduction abnormalities. Patients with a history of seizures or psychiatric disorders should avoid mefloquine (Medical Letter 1990;32:13). Resistance to mefloquine has been reported in some areas, such as Thailand; in these areas, doxycycline should be used for prophylaxis. In children less than 8 years old, proguanil plus sulfisoxazole has been used (Suh and Keystone, Infect Dis Clin Pract 1996;5:541).

[68]Beginning 1-2 days before travel and continuing for the duration of stay and for 4 weeks after leaving. Use of tetracyclines is contraindicated in pregnancy and in children less than 8 years old. Doxycycline can cause gastrointestinal disturbances, vaginal moniliasis, and photosensitivity reactions.

[69]Shanks et al., Clin Infect Dis 1998;27:494; Lell et al., Lancet 1998;351:709. Beginning 1-2 days before travel and continuing for the duration of stay and for 1 week after leaving.

Continued

Infection	Drug	Adult dosage	Pediatric dosage
Alternatives:	Primaquine[5,56,70]	30-mg base daily	0.5-mg/kg base daily
	Chloroquine phosphate[65]	Same as chloroquine-sensitive	Same as chloroquine-sensitive
	plus pyrimethamine-sulfadoxine[46] for presumptive treatment[71]	Carry a single dose (3 tablets) for self-treatment of febrile illness when medical care is not immediately available	<1 yr: ¼ tablet
			1-3 yr: ½ tablet
			4-8 yr: 1 tablet
			9-14 yr: 2 tablets
	or plus proguanil[72]	200 mg daily	<2 yr: 50 mg daily
			2-6 yr: 100 mg
			7-10 yr: 150 mg
			>10 yr: 200 mg

Microsporidiosis

Ocular (Encephalitozoon hellem, Encephalitozoon cuniculi, Vittaforma corneae [Nosema corneum])

Drug of choice:	Albendazole[5] plus fumagillin[73]	400 mg bid	

Intestinal (Enterocytozoon bieneusi, Encephalitozoon [Septata] intestinalis)

Drug of choice[74]:	Albendazole[5]	400 mg bid	

Disseminated (E. hellem, E. cuniculi, E. intestinalis, Pleistophora spp., Trachipleistophora spp., and Brachiola vesicularum)

Drug of choice[75]:	Albendazole[5]	400 mg bid	

Mites, *see Scabies*

Moniliformis Moniliformis

Drug of choice:	Pyrantel pamoate[5]	11 mg/kg once, repeat twice, 2 weeks apart	11 mg/kg once, repeat twice, 2 weeks apart

Naegleria Species, see Amebic Meningoencephalitis, Primary

Necator Americanus, see Hookworm

Oesophagostomum Bifurcum

Drug of choice:	See footnote[76]		

---

[70]Several studies have shown that daily primaquine beginning 1 day before departure and continued until 2 days after leaving the malaria area provides effective prophylaxis against chloroquine-resistant *P. falciparum* (Schwartz and Regev-Yochay, Clin Infect Dis 1999;29:1502). Some studies have shown less efficacy against *P. vivax*.

[71]In areas with strains resistant to pyrimethamine-sulfadoxine, atovaquone/proguanil or atovaquone plus doxycycline can also be used for presumptive treatment. See p. 941 for dosage.

[72]Proguanil (Paludrine Wyeth Ayerst, Canada; Zeneca, United Kingdom), which is not available alone in the United States but is widely available in Canada and overseas, is recommended mainly for use in Africa south of the Sahara. Prophylaxis is recommended during exposure and for 4 weeks afterward. Proguanil has been used in pregnancy without evidence of toxicity (Phillips-Howard and Wood, Drug Saf 1996;14:131).

[73]Ocular lesions due to *E. hellem* in HIV-infected patients have responded to fumagillin eyedrops prepared from Fumidil-B, a commercial product (Mid-Continent Agrimarketing, Inc., Olathe, Kansas, 1-800-547-1392) used to control a microsporidial disease of honey bees (Diesenhouse, Am J Ophthalmol 1993;115:293). For lesions due to *V. corneae*, topical therapy is generally not effective and keratoplasty may be required (Davis et al., Ophthalmology 1990;97:953).

[74]Octreotide (Sandostatin) has provided symptomatic relief in some patients with large volume diarrhea. Oral fumagillin (see footnote 73) has been effective in treating *E. bieneusi* (Molina et al., AIDS 1997;11:1603) but has been associated with thrombocytopenia. Highly active antiretroviral therapy may lead to microbiologic and clinical response in HIV-infected patients with microsporidial diarrhea (Foudraine et al., AIDS 1998;12:35; Carr et al., Lancet 1998;351:256).

[75]Molina et al., J Infect Dis 1995;171:245. There is no established treatment for *Pleistophora*.

[76]Albendazole or pyrantel pamoate may be effective (Krepel et al., Trans R Soc Trop Med Hyg 1993;87:87).

Infection	Drug	Adult dosage	Pediatric dosage
Onchocerca Volvulus, see Filariasis			
Opisthorchis Viverrini, see Fluke			
Paragonimus Westermani, see Fluke			
Pediculus Capitis, Humanus, Phthirus Pubis, see Lice			
Pinworm, see Enterobius			
***Pneumocystis* Carinii Pneumonia (PCP)**[77]			
Drug of choice:	Trimethoprim-sulfamethoxazole	TMP 15 mg/kg/day, SMX 75 mg/kg/day, oral or IV in 3 or 4 doses × 14-21 days	Same as adult dose
Alternatives:	Pentamidine	3-4 mg/kg IV daily × 14-21 days	Same as adult dose
	OR		
	Trimetrexate	45 mg/m² IV daily × 21 days	
	plus folinic acid	20 mg/m² PO or IV q6h × 24 days	
	OR		
	Trimethoprim[5]	5 mg/kg PO tid × 21 days	
	plus dapsone[5]	100 mg PO daily × 21 days	
	OR		
	Atovaquone	750 mg bid PO × 21 days	
	OR		
	Primaquine[5,56]	30 mg base PO daily × 21 days	
	plus clindamycin[5]	600 mg IV q6h × 21 days, or 300-450 mg PO q6h × 21 days	
Primary and secondary prophylaxis			
Drug of Choice:	Trimethoprim-sulfamethoxazole	1 tab (single or double strength) PO daily or 1 DS tab 3 times per week	TMP 150 mg/m², SMX 750 mg/m² in 2 doses PO on 3 consecutive days per week
Alternatives[78]:	Dapsone[5]	50 mg PO bid, or 100 mg PO daily	2 mg/kg (max 100 mg) PO daily
	OR		
	Dapsone[5]	50 mg PO daily or 200 mg each week	
	plus pyrimethamine[79]	50 mg or 75 mg PO each week	
	OR		
	Pentamidine aerosol	300 mg inhaled monthly via *Respirgard II* nebulizer	>5 yr: same as adult dose

[77]In severe disease with room air PO$_2$ ≤ 70 mm Hg or Aa gradient ≥ 35 mm Hg, prednisone should also be used (Gagnon et al., N Engl J Med 1990;323:1444; Caumes et al., Clin Infect Dis 1994;18:319).

[78]Weekly therapy with sulfadoxine 500 mg/pyrimethamine 25 mg/leucovorin 25 mg was effective PCP prophylaxis in liver transplant patients (Torre-Cisneros et al., Clin Infect Dis 1999;29:771).

[79]Plus leucovorin 25 mg with each dose of pyrimethamine.   *Continued*

Infection	Drug	Adult dosage	Pediatric dosage
	OR Atovaquone[5]	1,500 mg daily PO	

Roundworm, see Ascariasis

Scabies *(Sarcoptes Scabiei)*

Drug of choice:	5% Permethrin	Topically	Topically
Alternatives:	Ivermectin[5,80] 10% Crotamiton	200 µg/kg PO once Topically	200 µg/kg PO once

Schistosomiasis *(Bilharziasis)*

S. haematobium

Drug of choice:	Praziquantel	40 mg/kg/day in 2 doses × 1 day	40 mg/kg/day in 2 doses × 1 day

S. japonicum

Drug of choice:	Praziquantel	60 mg/kg/day in 3 doses × 1 day	60 mg/kg/day in 3 doses × 1 day

S. mansoni

Drug of choice:	Praziquantel	40 mg/kg/day in 2 doses × 1 day	40 mg/kg/day in 2 doses × 1 day
Alternative:	Oxamniquine[81]	15 mg/kg once[82]	20 mg/kg/day in 2 doses × 1 day[82]

S. mekongi

Drug of choice:	Praziquantel	60 mg/kg/day in 3 doses × 1 day	60 mg/kg/day in 3 doses × 1 day

Sleeping Sickness, see Trypanosomiasis

Strongyloidiasis *(Strongyloides Stercoralis)*

Drug of choice[83]:	Ivermectin	200 µg/kg/day × 1-2 days	200 µg/kg/day × 1-2 days
Alternative:	Thiabendazole	50 mg/kg/day in 2 doses (max 3 g/day) × 2 days[9]	50 mg/kg/day in 2 doses (max 3 g/day) × 2 days[9]

Tapeworm—Adult (Intestinal Stage)

Diphyllobothrium latum (fish), Taenia saginata (beef), Taenia solium (pork), Dipylidium caninum (dog)

Drug of choice:	Praziquantel[5]	5-10 mg/kg once	5-10 mg/kg once
Alternative:	Niclosamide	2 g once	50 mg/kg once

Hymenolepis nana (dwarf tapeworm)

Drug of choice:	Praziquantel[5]	25 mg/kg once	25 mg/kg once

Tapeworm—Larval (Tissue Stage)

Echinococcus granulosus (hydatid cyst)

Drug of choice[84]:	Albendazole	400 mg bid × 1-6 months	15 mg/kg/day (max 800 mg) × 1-6 months

[80]Effective for crusted scabies in immunocompromised patients (Larralde et al., Pediatr Dermatol 1999;16:69; Patel et al., Aust J Dermatol 1999;40:37).

[81]Oxamniquine has been effective in some areas in which praziquantel is less effective (Stelma et al., J Infect Dis 1997;176:304). Oxamniquine is contraindicated in pregnancy.

[82]In East Africa, the dose should be increased to 30 mg/kg, and in Egypt and South Africa, 30 mg/kg/day × 2 days. Some experts recommend 40-60 mg/kg over 2-3 days in all of Africa (Shekhar, Drugs 1991;42:379).

[83]In immunocompromised patients or disseminated disease, it may be necessary to prolong or repeat therapy or use other agents. A veterinary parenteral formulation of ivermectin was used in one patient (Chiodini et al., Lancet 2000;355:43).

[84]Patients may benefit from or require surgical resection of cysts. Praziquantel is useful preoperatively or in case of spill during surgery. Percutaneous drainage with ultrasound guidance plus albendazole therapy has been effective for management of hepatic hydatid cyst disease (Khuroo et al., N Engl J Med 1997;337:881).

Infection	Drug	Adult dosage	Pediatric dosage
Echinococcus multilocularis			
Treatment of choice:	See footnote[85]		
Cysticercus cellulosae (cysticercosis)			
Treatment of choice:	See footnote[86]		
Alternative:	Albendazole	400 mg bid × 8-30 days; can be repeated as necessary	15 mg/kg/day (max 800 mg) in 2 doses × 8-30 days; can be repeated as necessary
	OR		
	Praziquantel[5]	50-100 mg/kg/day in 3 doses × 30 days	50-100 mg/kg/day in 3 doses × 30 days
Toxocariasis, see Visceral Larva Migrans			
Toxoplasmosis *(Toxoplasma Gondii)*[87]			
Drugs of choice[88]:	Pyrimethamine[89]	25-100 mg/day × 3-4 weeks	2 mg/kg/day × 3 days, then 1 mg/kg/day (max 25 mg/day) × 4 weeks[90]
	plus sulfadiazine	1-1.5 g qid × 3-4 weeks	100-200 mg/kg/day × 3-4 weeks
Alternative[91]:	Spiramycin*	3-4 g/day × 3-4 weeks	50-100 mg/kg/day × 3-4 weeks
Trichinosis *(Trichinella Spiralis)*			
Drugs of choice:	Steroids for severe symptoms **plus** mebendazole[5]	200-400 mg tid × 3 days, then 400-500 mg tid × 10 days	200-400 mg tid × 3 days, then 400-500 mg tid × 10 days

[85]Surgical excision is the only reliable means of treatment. Some reports have suggested use of albendazole or mebendazole (Hao et al., Trans R Soc Trop Med Hyg 1994;88:340; WHO Group, Bull WHO 1996;74:231).

[86]Initial therapy of parenchymal disease with seizures should focus on symptomatic treatment with anticonvulsant drugs. Treatment of parenchymal disease with albendazole and praziquantel is controversial, and randomized trials have not shown a benefit. Obstructive hydrocephalus is treated with surgical removal of the obstructing cyst or CSF diversion. Prednisone 40 mg PO may be given in conjunction with surgery. Arachnoiditis, vasculitis or cerebral edema is treated with prednisone 60 mg daily or dexamethasone 4-16 mg/day combined with albendazole or praziquantel (White, Annu Rev Med 2000;51:187). Any cysticercocidal drug may cause irreparable damage when used to treat ocular or spinal cysts, even when corticosteroids are used. An ophthalmic exam should always be done before treatment to rule out intraocular cysts.

[87]In ocular toxoplasmosis with macular involvement, corticosteroids are recommended for an anti-inflammatory effect on the eyes.

[88]To treat CNS toxoplasmosis in HIV-infected patients, some clinicians have used pyrimethamine 50-100 mg daily (after a loading dose of 200 mg) with a sulfonamide and, when sulfonamide sensitivity developed, have given clindamycin 1.8-2.4 g/day in divided doses instead of the sulfonamide (Remington et al., Lancet 1991;338:1142; Luft et al., N Engl J Med 1993;329:995). Atovaquone plus pyrimethamine appears to be an effective alternative in sulfa-intolerant patients (Kovacs et al., Lancet 1992;340:637). Treatment is followed by chronic suppression with lower dosage regimens of the same drugs. For primary prophylaxis in HIV patients with <100 CD4 cells, either trimethoprim-sulfamethoxazole, pyrimethamine with dapsone or atovaquone with or without pyrimethamine can be used (USPHS/IDSA, MMWR Recomm Rep 1999;48:41, 1999). See also footnote 89.

[89]Plus leucovorin 10-25 mg with each dose of pyrimethamine.

[90]Congenitally infected newborns should be treated with pyrimethamine every 2 or 3 days and sulfonamide daily for about 1 year (Remington and Desmonts in Remington and Klein [eds], Infectious Disease of the Fetus and Newborn Infant, ed 4, Philadelphia: Saunders, 1995, p 140).

[91]For prophylactic use during pregnancy. If it is determined that transmission has occurred in utero, therapy with pyrimethamine and sulfadiazine should be started.

Continued

Infection	Drug	Adult dosage	Pediatric dosage
Trichinosis—cont'd			
Alternative:	Albendazole[5]	400 mg PO bid × 8-14 days	400 mg PO bid × 8-14 days
Trichomoniasis (*Trichomonas Vaginalis*)			
Drug of choice[92]:	Metronidazole	2 g once; or 250 mg tid or 375 mg bid PO × 7 days	15 mg/kg/day orally in 3 doses × 7 days
	OR Tinidazole[3]*	2 g once	50 mg/kg once (max 2 g)
Trichostrongylus			
Drug of choice:	Pyrantel pamoate[5]	11 mg/kg base once (max 1 g)	11 mg/kg once (max 1 g)
Alternative:	Mebendazole[5] OR	100 mg bid × 3 days	100 mg bid × 3 days
	Albendazole[5]	400 mg once	400 mg once
Trichuriasis (*Trichuris Trichiura, Whipworm*)			
Drug of choice:	Mebendazole	100 mg bid × 3 days or 500 mg once	100 mg bid × 3 days or 500 mg once
Alternative:	Albendazole[5]	400 mg once[93]	400 mg once[93]
Trypanosomiasis			
T. cruzi (American trypanosomiasis, Chagas' disease)			
Drug of choice:	Benznidazole*	5-7 mg/kg/day in 2 divided doses × 30-90 days	Up to 12 yr: 10 mg/kg/day in 2 doses × 30-90 days
	OR Nifurtimox[94]*	8-10 mg/kg/day in 3-4 doses × 90-120 days	1-10 yr: 15-20 mg/kg/day in 4 doses × 90 days; 11-16 yr: 12.5-15 mg/kg/day in 4 doses × 90 days
T. brucei gambiense (West African trypanosomiasis, sleeping sickness)—hemolymphatic stage			
Drug of choice[95]:	Pentamidine isethionate[5]	4 mg/kg/day IM × 10 days	4 mg/kg/day IM × 10 days
Alternative:	Suramin*	100-200 mg (test dose) IV, then 1 g IV on days 1, 3, 7, 14, and 21	20 mg/kg on days 1, 3, 7, 14, and 21
	OR Eflornithine*	See footnote[96]	

[92]Sexual partners should be treated simultaneously. Metronidazole-resistant strains have been reported and should be treated with metronidazole 2-4 g/day × 7-14 days. Desensitization has been recommended for patients allergic to metronidazole (Pearlman et al., Am J Obstet Gynecol 1996;174:934).

[93]In heavy infection, it may be necessary to extend therapy to 3 days.

[94]No longer manufactured, but available from CDC in selected cases. The addition of gamma interferon to nifurtimox for 20 days in a limited number of patients and in experimental animals appears to have shortened the acute phase of Chagas' disease (McCabe et al., J Infect Dis 1991;163:912).

[95]Suramin is the drug of choice for treatment of *T. b. rhodesiense*. For treatment of *T. b. gambiense*, pentamidine and suramin have equal efficacy but pentamidine is better tolerated.

[96]Eflornithine is highly effective in *T. b. gambiense* and variably effective in *T. b. rhodesiense* infections. It is available in limited supply only from the WHO and is given 400 mg/kg/day IV in four divided doses for 14 days.

Infection	Drug	Adult dosage	Pediatric dosage

T. brucei rhodesiense (East African trypanosomiasis, sleeping sickness)—hemolymphatic stage

Drug of choice:	Suramin[*]	100-200 mg (test dose) IV, then 1 g IV on days 1, 3, 7, 14, and 21	20 mg/kg on days 1, 3, 7, 14, and 21
	OR		
	Eflornithine[*]	See footnote[96]	

Trypanosomiasis late disease with CNS involvement (T. brucei gambiense or T. brucei rhodesiense)

Drug of choice:	Melarsoprol[97][*]	2-3.6 mg/kg/days IV × 3 days; after 1 wk 3.6 mg/kg per day IV × 3 days; repeat again after 10-21 days	18-25 mg/kg total over 1 month; initial dose of 0.36 mg/kg IV, increasing gradually to max 3.6 mg/kg at intervals of 1-5 days for total of 9-10 doses
	OR		
	Eflornithine	See footnote[96]	

Visceral Larva Migrans[98] (Toxocariasis)

Drug of choice:	Albendazole[5]	400 mg bid × 5 days	400 mg bid × 5 days
	Mebendazole[5]	100-200 mg bid × 5 days	100-200 mg bid × 5 days

Whipworm, see Trichuriasis

Wuchereria bancrofti, see Filariasis

---

[97]In frail patients, begin with as little as 18 mg and increase the dose progressively. Pretreatment with suramin has been advocated for debilitated patients. Corticosteroids have been used to prevent arsenical encephalopathy (Pepin et al., Trans R Soc Trop Med Hyg 1995;89:92). Up to 20% of patients fail to respond to melarsoprol (Barrett, Lancet 1999;353:1113).

[98]For severe symptoms or eye involvement, corticosteroids can be used in addition.

MANUFACTURERS OF SOME ANTIPARASITIC DRUGS

albendazole—Albenza (SmithKline Beecham)

[*]aminosidine, see paromomycin

[*]artemether—Artenam (Arenco, Belgium)

[*]artesunate—(Guilin No. 1 Factory, People's Republic of China)

atovaquone—Mepron (Glaxo Wellcome)

atovaquone/proguanil—Malarone (Glaxo Wellcome)

bacitracin—many manufacturers

[*]bacitracin-zinc—(Apothekernes Laboratorium A.S., Oslo, Norway)

[*]benznidazole—Rochagan (Roche, Brazil)

[†]bithionol—Bitin (Tanabe, Japan)

chloroquine HCl and chloroquine phosphate —Aralen (Sanofi), others

crotamiton—Eurax (Westwood-Squibb)

dapsone—(Jacobus)

[†]diethylcarbamazine citrate USP—(University of Iowa School of Pharmacy)

[*]diloxanide furoate—Furamide (Boots, United Kingdom)

[*]eflornithine (difluoromethylornithine, DFMO) —Ornidyl (Ilex-Oncology)

furazolidone—Furoxone (Roberts)

[*]halofantrine—Halfan (SmithKline Beecham)

iodoquinol—Yodoxin (Glenwood), others

ivermectin—Stromectol (Merck)

malathion—Ovide (Medicis)

mebendazole—Vermox (McNeil)

mefloquine—Lariam (Roche)

[*]meglumine antimonate—Glucantime (Aventis, France)

---

[*]Not available in the United States.

[†]Available under an Investigational New Drug (IND) protocol from the CDC Drug Service, Centers for Disease Control and Prevention, Atlanta, GA 30333; 404-639-3670 (evenings, weekends, or holidays: 404-639-2888).

[*]Not available in the United States.

[†]Available under an Investigational New Drug (IND) protocol from the CDC Drug Service, Centers for Disease Control and Prevention, Atlanta, GA 30333; 404-639-3670 (evenings, weekends, or holidays: 404-639-2888).

*melarsoprol—Arsobal (Aventis)

metronidazole—Flagyl (Searle), others

*miltefosine—(Asta Medica, Germany)

*niclosamide—Yomesan (Bayer, Germany)

†nifurtimox—Lampit (Bayer, Germany)

*nitazoxanide—Cryptaz (Romark)

*ornidazole—Tiberal   (Hoffman-LaRoche, Switzerland)

oxamniquine—Vansil (Pfizer)

paromomycin—Humatin (Parke-Davis); aminosidine (topical and parenteral formulations not available in United States)

pentamidine isethionate—Pentam 300, NebuPent (Fujisawa)

permethrin—Nix (Glaxo Wellcome), Elimite (Allergan)

praziquantel—Biltricide (Bayer)

primaquine phosphate USP

*proguanil—Paludrine (Wyeth Ayerst, Canada; Zeneca, United Kingdom)

*propamidine isethionate—Brolene (Aventis, Canada)

pyrantel pamoate—Antiminth (Pfizer)

pyrethrins and piperonyl butoxide—RID (Pfizer), others

pyrimethamine   USP—Daraprim   (Glaxo Wellcome)

quinine sulfate—many manufacturers

*quinine dihydrochloride

†sodium stibogluconate—Pentostam (Glaxo Wellcome, United Kingdom)

‡spiramycin—Rovamycine (Aventis)

†suramin sodium—(Bayer, Germany)

thiabendazole—Mintezol (Merck)

*tinidazole—Fasigyn (Pfizer)

*triclabendazole—Fasinex (Novartis Agribusiness)

trimetrexate—Neutrexin (US Bioscience)

DRUGS FOR HIV INFECTION

Highly active antiretroviral therapy (HAART) combining three or four drugs has become the standard of care for treatment of human immunodeficiency virus (HIV) infection. Since the last *Medical Letter* article on this subject, several new drugs have become available, and new clinical trials have broadened the range of acceptable combinations. None of the drugs currently available can eradicate HIV infection, but used in combination they can decrease viral replication, improve immunologic status and prolong life.

---

*Not available in the United States.

†Available under an Investigational New Drug (IND) protocol from the CDC Drug Service, Centers for Disease Control and Prevention, Atlanta, GA 30333; 404-639-3670 (evenings, weekends, or holidays: 404-639-2888).

---

*Not available in the United States.

†Available under an Investigational New Drug (IND) protocol from the CDC Drug Service, Centers for Disease Control and Prevention, Atlanta, GA 30333; 404-639-3670 (evenings, weekends, or holidays: 404-639-2888).

‡Available in the United States only from the manufacturer.

Dosage and Cost of Drugs for Treatment of HIV Infection

Drug	Usual oral adult dosage	Cost[1]
Nucleoside Reverse Transcriptase Inhibitors		
Abacavir (ABC; *Ziagen*—Glaxo Wellcome)*	300 mg bid	$366.31
Didanosine (ddl; *Videx*—Bristol-Myers Squibb)*	200 mg bid or	
	400 mg once/day[2]	227.43
Lamivudine (3TC; *Epivir*—Glaxo Wellcome)*	150 mg bid[3]	272.59
Stavudine (d4T; *Zerit*—Bristol-Myers Squibb)*	40 mg bid[4]	286.02
Zalcitabine (ddC; *Hivid*—Roche)	0.75 mg tid	218.48
Zidovudine (ZDV; *Retrovir*—Glaxo Wellcome)*	200 mg tid or 300 mg bid	318.52
Zidovudine plus lamivudine (*Combivir*—Glaxo Wellcome)	1 tablet bid[5]	591.07

*Available in a liquid or oral powder formulation.

[1]Cost to the pharmacist for 30 days' treatment, based on wholesale price (AWP) listings in *Drug Topics Red Book Update*, February 2000.

[2]With tablets: for patients <60 kg, 125 mg PO bid; >60 kg, 200 mg PO bid. With powder, dosage varies from 167 mg (<60 kg) to 250 mg (>60 kg) bid. Doses should be taken at least 30 minutes before meals or at least 2 hours afterward.

[3]For patients less than 50 kg, 2 mg/kg bid.

[4]For patients less than 60 kg, 30 mg bid.

[5]Each tablet contains 300 mg of zidovudine and 150 mg of lamivudine.

Dosage and Cost of Drugs for Treatment of HIV Infection—cont'd

Drug	Usual oral adult dosage	Cost[1]
Nonnucleoside Reverse Transcriptase Inhibitors		
Delavirdine (*Rescriptor*—Agouron)	400 mg tid	$282.96
Efavirenz (EFV; *Sustiva*—Dupont)	600 mg once/day[6]	394.20
Nevirapine (*Viramune*—Roxane)*	200 mg bid[7]	278.64
Protease Inhibitors		
Amprenavir (*Agenerase*—Glaxo Wellcome)*	1,200 mg bid[8]	$634.44
Indinavir (*Crixivan*—Merck)	800 mg tid[9]	463.50
Nelfinavir (*Viracept*—Agouron)*	750 mg tid or	609.12
	1,250 mg bid[10]	676.80
Ritonavir (*Norvir*—Abbott)*	600 mg bid[11] or 100-400 mg bid[12]	667.80
Saquinavir (*Invirase*—Roche)[13]	600 mg tid[14]	603.95
(*Fortovase*—Roche)[15]	1,200 mg tid[14]	623.13

[6]At bedtime for at least the first 2-4 weeks. The drug, which is marketed in 50-, 100- and 200-mg capsules, may be taken with or without food, but not with a fatty meal.

[7]Patients should take 200 mg once/day for the first 2 weeks of treatment to decrease the risk of rash.

[8]Can be taken with or without food, but not with a fatty meal.

[9]With water or other liquids, 1 hour before or 2 hours after a meal, or with a light meal. Patients should drink at least 48 ounces (1.5 L) of water daily.

[10]Nelfinavir should be taken with food.

[11]With food. The drug is available as a soft gelatin capsule. The liquid formulation has an unpleasant taste; the manufacturer suggests taking it with chocolate milk or a liquid nutritional supplement.

[12]When used in combination with other protease inhibitors.

[13]Hard gelatin capsules.

[14]Saquinavir should be taken with or within 2 hours after a full meal.

[15]Soft gelatin capsules.

Concerns about patients' adherence to the regimen, adequate serum concentrations, and prevention of drug resistance have led to increased use of drugs that can be taken once or twice daily and dual protease inhibitor combinations (Lucas et al., Ann Intern Med 1999;131:2). Drug regimens recommended by *Medical Letter* consultants are listed in the table on p. 955. Adult regimens and dosages may not be applicable to children (*Guidelines for Use of Antiretroviral Agents in Pediatric HIV Infection*, HIV/AIDS Treatment Information Service, www.hivatis.org).

NUCLEOSIDE REVERSE TRANSCRIPTASE INHIBITORS (nRTIs)

Nucleoside analogs inhibit HIV reverse transcriptase and slow or prevent HIV replication in infected cells.

Class-Specific Characteristics

All nRTIs except for didanosine are taken in two to three doses per day without regard to meals and generally do not interact with other drugs. Didanosine can be taken once daily and must be taken on an empty stomach. It may decrease the absorption of other anti-HIV drugs if taken simultaneously. All nRTIs can cause a rare but potentially fatal syndrome of lactic acidosis with hepatic steatosis (Boxwell and Styrt, Intersci Conf Antimicrob Agents Chemother [ICAAC] 1999;39:496, abstract 1284).

Zidovudine (AZT)

Zidovudine can be given in combination with any other nRTI except for stavudine. Using zidovudine plus stavudine causes antagonism both in vitro and in vivo. Zidovudine plus lamivudine with or without a protease inhibitor has been recommended for prevention of HIV infection after needlestick or sexual exposures (MMWR Recomm Rep 1998;47:1). Zidovudine is available in 100-mg capsules and 300-mg tablets, and in a fixed-dose combination with lamivudine as Combivir. Resistance to zidovudine is increasingly common in newly infected patients and those previously treated with the drug (Boden et al., JAMA 1999;282:1135). Adverse effects of zidovudine include anemia, neutropenia, nausea, vomiting, headache, fatigue, confusion, malaise, myopathy, and hepatitis.

Stavudine (d4T)

Stavudine is used both in initial combination therapy and after failure of zidovudine-containing regimens. One study in patients with <4 weeks' previous treatment, CD4 counts over 200 cells/ml and low baseline HIV RNA levels found that stavudine/didanosine/indinavir lead to lower HIV RNA levels and higher CD4 counts than zidovudine/lamivudine/indinavir at 48 weeks (Eron et al., Clin Infect Dis 1999;22:962, abstract 14). Stavudine is well tolerated but may cause dose-related peripheral sensory neuropathy, which often disappears when the drug is stopped and may not recur when it is restarted at a lower dose. Serum aminotransferase activity may increase, and pancreatitis has occurred rarely, but may be more common with combined use of didanosine.

Didanosine (ddI)

Didanosine is used in combination with zidovudine or stavudine, plus a protease inhibitor or non-nucleoside reverse transcriptase inhibitor. The combination of didanosine and zalcitabine is not recommended because of overlapping toxicities. Treatment-limiting toxicities of didanosine have been painful dose-related peripheral neuropathy, pancreatitis, and gastrointestinal disturbances. The risk of pancreatitis may be increased with concomitant use of stavudine. Didanosine can interfere with absorption of drugs that require gastric acidity such as dapsone, ketoconazole, doxycycline, fluoroquinolones, delavirdine, indinavir and others; they should be taken at least 1 to 2 hours apart. Didanosine tablets must be chewed or crushed into water. Using didanosine twice daily, as a buffered powder in water or by preparing the pediatric powder in water plus liquid antacid (final concentration 10 mg/ml) may improve gastrointestinal tolerance.

Lamivudine (3TC)

Lamivudine is the best tolerated of the nRTIs, but even in combination therapy, HIV strains may become resistant to lamivudine in vitro. An increase in HIV viral load early during treatment with a lamivudine-containing regimen is often an indication of resistance to the drug. Lamivudine-resistant strains may be cross-resistant to zalcitabine, didanosine, and abacavir. Because lamivudine is also active against hepatitis B virus (HBV), HIV-positive patients with chronic HBV infection may experience a flare of hepatitis if lamivudine is withdrawn or if their HBV strain becomes resistant to the drug (Bessesen et al., Clin Infect Dis 1999;28:1032). Adverse effects are uncommon; pancreatitis has been reported

rarely in children (Lewis et al., J Infect Dis 1996;174:6).

Zalcitabine (ddC)

Zalcitabine appears to be the least effective of the nucleoside analogs and is infrequently used. Dose-related peripheral neuropathy can be severe and persistent and is more likely in those with diabetes mellitus or didanosine treatment. Other adverse effects include rash, stomatitis, esophageal ulceration, pancreatitis, and fever.

Abacavir

In previously untreated patients, abacavir plus zidovudine and lamivudine raised CD4 counts and lowered plasma HIV RNA to undetectable levels in about three quarters of patients (Fischl et al., Conf Retrovir Opportun Infect 1999;6: 70, abstract 19). A second study in previously untreated patients found that 48 weeks of either abacavir or indinavir combined with zidovudine and lamivudine were similarly effective overall, but the indinavir combination was more effective in patients with high baseline viral loads (>100,000 copies/ml) and in lowering viral loads to undetectable levels (<50 copies/ml) (Staszewski et al., ICAAC 1999;39: 472, abstract 505). HIV strains resistant to zidovudine and lamivudine may also be resistant to abacavir. Patients with extensive prior anti-HIV nucleoside therapy are less likely to respond to treatment with abacavir.

In 5% of patients, a severe hypersensitivity reaction with fever, respiratory or gastrointestinal symptoms, malaise, and rash develops after a mean of 11 days' treatment. Symptoms resolve after the drug is stopped, but if patients take abacavir again after this reaction, it recurs rapidly and tends to be more severe; hypotension, respiratory distress, and death have been reported (Saag et al., AIDS 1998;12:F203). When rash occurs without systemic symptoms associated with hypersensitivity, the drug can sometimes be continued.

NUCLEOTIDE REVERSE TRANSCRIPTASE INHIBITOR
Adefovir (Preveon—Gilead)

Nucleotides are phosphorylated nucleosides; nucleoside and nucleotide RTIs have a similar mechanism of action. In vitro adefovir, which is available only through an expanded access protocol, is active against HIV, herpes simplex, cytomegalovirus, HHV-6, and hepatitis B. The main adverse effect of adefovir has been dose-related proximal renal tubular dysfunction occurring in up to 30% of patients, usually at least 20 weeks after starting the drug and resolving slowly (median time 11 weeks) after dose reduction or discontinuation. The FDA refused to approve the drug for treatment of HIV infections, and the manufacturer no longer plans to use the drug in HIV clinical trials.

NONNUCLEOSIDE REVERSE TRANSCRIPTASE INHIBITORS (nnRTIs)

Like the nucleoside analogs, these drugs inhibit reverse transcriptase, but by a different mechanism.

Class-Specific Characteristics

Combinations of nnRTIs with nRTIs or protease inhibitors tend to be at least additive in reducing HIV replication in vitro. In patients without previous anti-HIV treatment, an nnRTI combined with two nRTIs can reduce HIV RNA levels and increase CD4 counts. HIV isolates resistant to nRTIs and protease inhibitors remain sensitive to nnRTIs, but cross-resistance is common within the nnRTI class. Resistance to the nnRTIs develops rapidly if they are used alone or with only one nRTI. All nnRTIs can cause rash that can sometimes be severe. Nevirapine has been associated with Stevens-Johnson syndrome. All nnRTIs are metabolized by hepatic cytochrome P450 enzymes, so drug interactions can occur with protease inhibitors and many other drugs (Merry et al., AIDS 1998;12:1163; Barry et al., Clin Pharmacokinet 1999;36:289); concurrent use of delavirdine or nevirapine with rifampin is not recommended.

Efavirenz

Efavirenz is the only nnRTI that can be taken once a day. One study in previously untreated patients found that 72 weeks of efavirenz/zidovudine/lamivudine was more effective than indinavir/zidovudine/lamivudine in lowering HIV RNA levels, even among patients with high baseline RNA levels (>100,000 copies/ml), and the efavirenz combination was better tolerated (Staszewski et al., N Engl J Med 1999;341:1865). Brief studies in treatment-experienced patients or those failing other regimens have shown that efavirenz in combination with at least two other new agents can be effective in suppressing plasma HIV RNA levels and raising CD4 counts. The most common adverse effects have been dizziness, headache, insomnia, inability to concentrate, and rash. Vivid dreams, nightmares and hallucinations can occur. Central nervous system effects tend to occur between 1 and 3 hours after each dose, and usually stop occurring within a few days or weeks. Fetal abnormalities occurred in pregnant monkeys exposed to efavirenz. Dosage of methadone and other opiates often needs to be increased if efavirenz is used concurrently.

Nevirapine

In one 48-week study, nevirapine/didanosine/stavudine was as effective as indinavir/didanosine/stavudine in decreasing viral load and more effective than lamivudine/didanosine/stavudine in patients with high baseline viral loads (Murphy et al., ICAAC 1999;39 addendum:8, abstract LB-22). Rash is common early in treatment with nevirapine and can be more frequent and more severe than with other nnRTIs. Fever, nausea, and headache can also occur. To decrease the incidence of rash, nevirapine should be given in a single 200-mg dose for the first 2 weeks, followed by 200 mg twice per day. In one study 400 mg once daily was as effective as bid dosing (Raffi et al., ICAAC 1999;39:519, abstract 1978). As with efavirenz, dosage of methadone and other opiates often need to be increased if nevirapine is used concurrently.

Delavirdine

A study comparing delavirdine/zidovudine/didanosine, delavirdine plus either zidovudine or didanosine, and zidovudine plus didanosine in patients with mean CD4 counts of 295 cells/mm^3 and <6 months prior HIV treatment showed modest benefit from the triple combination (Friedland et al., J AIDS 1999;21:281). Unlike other nnRTIs, delavirdine raises protease inhibitor levels. Rash may be less frequent and less severe with delavirdine than with other nnRTIs; the drug can be continued or restarted in most cases.

PROTEASE INHIBITORS

Protease inhibitors prevent cleavage of protein precursors essential for HIV maturation, infection of new cells and replication.

Class-Specific Characteristics

In patients with advanced HIV infection, use of a protease inhibitor in combination with other drugs has led to marked clinical improvement and prolonged survival. Most protease inhibitors potently suppress HIV in vivo. An exception is the Invirase formulation of saquinavir, which is poorly absorbed. Although viral isolates resistant to one protease inhibitor may appear susceptible to others in vitro, the clinical effectiveness of changing from one protease inhibitor to another after resistance has developed is not clear. Many clinicians would consider using two new protease inhibitors in combination with other drugs when resistance to multiple other drugs including protease inhibitors has occurred. All protease inhibitors can cause gastrointestinal intolerance and increased aminotransferase activity. Use of these drugs has been associated with increased bleeding in hemophiliacs, hyperglycemia, new onset or worsening diabetes, insulin resistance, fat wasting and redistribution, and hyperlipidemia (Walli et al., AIDS 1998;12:F167; Carr et al., Lancet 1999;353:2093). All protease inhibitors are metabolized by hepatic cytochrome P450 enzymes; drug interactions are common and can be severe. Rifampin, which decreases the effect of protease inhibitors, should generally be avoided.

Saquinavir

A soft-gel preparation (Fortovase) with improved bioavailability and potency has largely replaced the older formulation (Invirase). In one study, Fortovase 1,600 mg bid or 1,200 mg tid plus two nucleosides produced similar lowering of HIV RNA levels (Cohen et al., ICAAC 1999;39:473, abstract 508). Saquinavir is usually well tolerated.

Ritonavir

Ritonavir is well absorbed and at full doses produces high concentrations that potently inhibit HIV in serum and lymph nodes. The drug is available as a poorly tolerated liquid or in 100-mg capsules. Ritonavir is now mainly used in low doses (100 to 400 mg bid) with minimal intrinsic antiviral activity to increase the serum concentrations and decrease the dosage frequency of other protease inhibitors (Hsu et al., Clin Pharmacokinet 1998;35:275). Adverse reactions are common but less likely with low doses. In addition to the protease class-specific adverse effects, ritonavir causes circumoral and peripheral paresthesias, altered taste, nausea and vomiting, and frequent drug interactions.

Indinavir

Indinavir is also a potent protease inhibitor with good oral bioavailability. Studies using the drug in dosage of 1,200 mg bid were stopped because

it was less effective than the standard dosage of 800 mg tid. In addition to class-specific adverse effects, indinavir causes asymptomatic elevation of indirect bilirubin, dermatologic changes including alopecia, dry skin and mucous membranes, paronychia and ingrown toenails, kidney stones, and renal insufficiency (Kopp et al., Ann Intern Med 1997;127:119; Bouscarat et al., N Engl J Med 1999;341:618). Patients should drink 1 to 2 liters of water daily to minimize renal adverse effects.

Nelfinavir

Nelfinavir is probably the most commonly used protease inhibitor because it is generally well tolerated. Diarrhea, which usually resolves with continued use, is its main adverse effect. Dosages of 1,250 mg bid or 750 mg tid are equally effective (Post et al., Clin Infect Dis 1999;22:1029, abstract 334).

Amprenavir

Amprenavir is the newest protease inhibitor for HIV infection. It can be taken with or without food, but a high-fat meal can decrease its absorption. It is available in large capsules (150 mg and 50 mg) and an oral solution (15 mg/ml). Both contain amounts of vitamin E that exceed the recommended daily allowance (RDA), so patients should be advised not to take vitamin E supplements concurrently. Cross-resistance with other protease inhibitors is still undetermined. In a small 24-week study, amprenavir/zidovudine/lamivudine lowered viral loads to under 500 copies/ml (Murphy et al., J Infect Dis 1999; 179:808). The most common adverse effects have been nausea, diarrhea, perioral paresthesias, vomiting and rash (Pedneault et al., Conf Retrovir Opportun Infect 1999;6:140, abstract 386). Many patients with rash can continue or restart amprenavir if the rash is mild or moderate, but about 1% of patients have developed severe rashes, including Stevens-Johnson syndrome.

Lopinavir (ABT-378)

A new protease inhibitor available through an expanded access trial (1-888-711-7193), lopinavir is highly potent in vitro, especially when combined with low doses of ritonavir. Early clinical results appear to be encouraging (Eron et al., ICAAC 1999;39 addendum:18, abstract LB-20). Lopinavir/ritonavir appears to be well tolerated, causing only mild gastrointestinal adverse effects and headache.

USE OF ANTIRETROVIRALS IN PREGNANCY

Ideally, to prevent transmission of HIV from any infected woman to her offspring, most clinicians would give full doses of two nucleosides plus a protease inhibitor, started as early in the pregnancy as possible. Zidovudine alone, started after the fourteenth to thirty-fourth week of gestation and given to the infant for the first 6 weeks of life, reduced HIV transmission from 26% to 8% (Connor et al., N Engl J Med 1994;331:1173). One study found that zidovudine alone taken orally for just 3 to 4 weeks before delivery and during labor decreased the risk of transmission by 50% (Shaffer et al., Lancet 1999;353:773). Surveillance data suggest that zidovudine given to the mother only during labor and to the infant within 48 hours after birth may also decrease HIV transmission (Wade et al., N Engl J Med 1998;339:1409). Unpublished data suggest that a combination of zidovudine plus lamivudine started at the onset of labor and given to the infant for 1 week after delivery may be more effective than zidovudine alone (www.unaids.org; UNAIDS study, 1999). Use of zidovudine during pregnancy has not been associated with fetal malformations, but mitochondrial dysfunction has been reported in eight children exposed to zidovudine or zidovudine combined with lamivudine, including 2 fatalities (Blanche et al., Lancet 1999;354:1084). A recent study in Uganda found that one dose of nevirapine given to the mother at the onset of labor and one to the infant 24 to 72 hours after delivery decreased the rate of neonatal HIV transmission, was easier to administer, and was much less expensive than zidovudine (Guay et al., Lancet 1999; 354:795).

Drugs of Choice for Treatment of HIV Infection in Adults

Drugs of Choice

2 nucleosides[1] + 1 protease inhibitor[2]
2 nucleosides[1] + 1 nonnucleoside[3]
2 nucleosides[1] + ritonavir[4] + another protease inhibitor[5]

Alternatives

1 protease inhibitor[2] + 1 nucleoside + 1 nonnucleoside[3]
2 protease inhibitors (each in low doses)[5] + 1 nucleoside + 1 nonnucleoside[3]
abacavir + 2 other nucleosides[1]
2 protease inhibitors (each full dose)

---

[1]One of the following: zidovudine + lamivudine; zidovudine + didanosine; stavudine + lamivudine; stavudine + didanosine; zidovudine + zalcitabine

[2]Nelfinavir, indinavir, saquinavir soft gel capsules, amprenavir or ritonavir. Ritonavir is used less frequently because of troublesome adverse effects. The Invirase formulation of saquinavir generally should not be used.

[3]Efavirenz is often preferred. Nevirapine causes more adverse effects. Nevirapine and delavirdine require more doses, and have had shorter follow-up in reported studies. Combinations of efavirenz and nevirapine with protease inhibitors require increasing the dosage of the protease inhibitor.

[4]Ritonavir is usually given in dosage of 100 to 400 mg bid when used with another protease inhibitor.

[5]Protease inhibitors that have been combined with ritonavir 100 to 400 mg bid include indinavir 400 to 800 mg bid, amprenavir 600 to 800 mg bid, saquinavir 400 to 600 mg bid and nelfinavir 500 to 750 mg bid.

Some Drugs Interactions

Interacting drugs	Adverse effects (probable mechanism)	Comments and recommendations
Zidovudine, with:		
Amprenavir	Possible zidovudine toxicity (decreased metabolism)	Monitor clinical status
Methadone	Increased zidovudine toxicity (mechanism unknown)	Based on study in 9 HIV positive patients; monitor clinical status
Rifampin	Possible decreased zidovudine effect (increased metabolism)	Monitor clinical status

Continued

Some Drugs Interactions—cont'd

Interacting drugs	Adverse effects (probable mechanism)	Comments and recommendations
Ribavirin	Antagonism in vitro	Avoid concurrent use
Stavudine	Antagonistic in vitro and in vivo	Avoid concurrent use
Didanosine, with:		
Amprenavir	Decreased amprenavir absorption	Give at least 1 hour apart
Dapsone	Decreased dapsone absorption	Give at least 2 hours apart
Delavirdine	Decreased absorption of both drugs	Give at least 1 hour apart
Fluoroquinolones	Decreased absorption of ciprofloxacin and probably other fluoroquinolones	Avoid concurrent use or give quinolone 2 hours before or 6 hours after
Ganciclovir	Possible didanosine toxicity (decreased renal excretion)	Monitor clinical status
Indinavir	Decreased indinavir absorption	Give 1 hour apart
Itraconazole	Decreased itraconazole absorption	Relapse of cryptococcal meningitis in HIV patients treated with itraconazole
Ketoconazole	Decreased absorption of both drugs	Give 2 hours apart
Stavudine	Increased risk of pancreatitis	Monitor for clinical and laboratory signs of pancreatitis

Nonnucleoside Reverse Transcriptase Inhibitors

Efavirenz, with:

Amprenavir	Possible decreased amprenavir effect (increased metabolism)	Monitor clinical status, amprenavir dose may need to be increased
Benzodiazipines, cisapride	Possible increased toxicity (decreased metabolism)	Theoretical*; high concentration of cisapride may lead to dangerous arrhythmias
Clarithromycin	Possible decreased clarithromycin effect; increased risk of skin rash (increased metabolism)	Monitor clinical status
Indinavir	Decreased indinavir effect (increased metabolism)	Manufacturer recommends increased indinavir dosage from 800 mg to 1,000 mg q8h
Methadone	Decreased methadone concentrations (increased metabolism)	Possible withdrawal symptoms; monitor clinical status and increase methadone dose as needed
Rifampin	Possible decreased efavirenz effect (increased metabolism)	Monitor clinical status
Ritonavir	Possible increased toxicity of both drugs (decreased metabolism)	Monitor clinical status and liver enzymes
Saquinavir	Decreased saquinavir effect (increased metabolism)	Add additional protease inhibitor
Nevirapine with:		
Contraceptives, oral	Possible decreased contraceptive effect (increased metabolism)	Theoretical; use alternate contraceptive method
Indinavir, nelfinavir, ritonavir, saquinavir or amprenavir	Possible decreased protease inhibitor effect (increased metabolism)	One clinical and pharmacokinetic study found no adverse interaction with nelfinavir. Indinavir manufacturer recommends dosage increase to 1,000 mg q8h
Methadone	Decreased methadone effect (increased metabolism)	Several case reports of methadone withdrawal when starting nevirapine; monitor clinical status and increase methadone dose as needed

*Manufacturer recommends avoiding concurrent use if possible.

Some Drugs Interactions—cont'd

Interacting drugs	Adverse effects (probable mechanism)	Comments and recommendations
Rifampin	Possible decreased nevirapine effect (increased metabolism)	Monitor clinical status; nevirapine dose may need to be increased
Delavirdine, with:		
Benzodiazepines, cisapride or clarithromycin	Delavirdine decreases metabolism and may increase toxicity	Theoretical*; high concentrations of cisapride may lead to dangerous cardiac arrhythmias
Didanosine	Decreased absorption of both drugs	Give at least 1 hour apart
Indinavir, amprenavir	Possible toxicity (decreased metabolism)	Monitor clinical status
Nelfinavir	Possible nelfinavir toxicity (decreased metabolism); possible decreased delavirdine effect (mechanism unknown); neutropenia has occurred	Monitor clinical status and neutrophil counts
Rifabutin	Possible rifabutin toxicity (decreased metabolism) and decreased delavirdine effect (increased metabolism)	Avoid concurrent use
Rifampin	Decreased delavirdine effect (increased metabolism)	Avoid concurrent use
Ritonavir	Possible ritonavir toxicity (decreased metabolism)	In one study ritonavir concentration increased by 70%; dose of ritonavir may need to be lowered
Saquinavir	Possible saquinavir toxicity (decreased metabolism); may cause hepatotoxicity	Monitor clinical status

Protease Inhibitors
Saquinavir, with:

Amprenavir	Decreased amprenavir effect (increased metabolism)	Monitor clinical status
Cisapride	Possible ventricular arrhythmia (saquinavir decreases metabolism)	Theoretical*
Delavirdine	Possible saquinavir toxicity (decreased metabolism); may cause hepatotoxicity	Monitor clinical status
Efavirenz	Decreased saquinavir effect (increased metabolism)	Add additional protease inhibitor
Indinavir, nelfinavir	Possible saquinavir toxicity (decreased metabolism)	Interaction may be therapeutically useful, but adverse effects may increase
Nevirapine	Decreased saquinavir effect (increased metabolism)	Theoretical*
Rifabutin, rifampin	Decreased saquinavir effect (increased metabolism)	Avoid concurrent use of rifampin and rifabutin
Ritonavir	Marked increase in saquinavir concentration with old formulation	Interaction may be therapeutically useful, but adverse effects may increase

Ritonavir, with

Amiodarone, benzodiazepines, bepridil, bupropion, cisapride, clozapine, flecainide, piroxicam, propafenone, quinidine, tricyclic antidepressants or zolpidem	Ritonavir decreases metabolism and may increase toxicity	Theoretical*; high concentrations of cisapride may lead to dangerous cardiac arrhythmias

Continued

Some Drugs Interactions—cont'd

Interacting drugs	Adverse effects (probable mechanism)	Comments and recommendations
Amprenavir	Increased amprenavir toxicity (decreased metabolism)	Ritonavir and amprenavir doses may both need to be decreased
Clarithromycin	Possible clarithromycin toxicity (probably decreased metabolism)	May need to reduce clarithromycin dosage in patients with renal impairment
Contraceptives, oral	Possible decreased contraceptive effect of ethinyl estradiol (mechanism not established)	Use alternative contraceptive
Efavirenz	Possible increased toxicity of both drugs (decreased metabolism)	Monitor clinical status and liver enzymes
Itraconazole, ketoconazole	Possible toxicity of both drugs (mutual decreased metabolism)	Monitor clinical status
Ergot alkaloids	Ergotism (decreased metabolism)	Avoid concurrent use
Meperidine	Decreased meperidine effect (increased metabolism with chronic ritonavir therapy)	Avoid long-term use
Methadone	Decreased methadone effect (increased metabolism)	Possible withdrawal symptoms, monitor clinical status
Nelfinavir	Possible nelfinavir toxicity (decreased metabolism)	Clinical significance unclear
Rifabutin	Rifabutin toxicity (decreased metabolism)	Manufacturer recommends decreased rifabutin dose by at least ¾. Further dosage reduction may be necessary
Rifampin	Possible decreased ritonavir effect (probably increased metabolism)	Avoid concurrent use; alternative agents should be considered
Saquinavir	Marked increase in saquinavir concentration; less with new formulation	Interaction may be therapeutically useful, but adverse effects may increase if dose is not adjusted
Sildenafil	Possible increased sildenafil toxicity (decreased metabolism)	Single fatal case in patient taking ritonavir and saquinavir; avoid concurrent use
Indinavir, with:		
Amprenavir	Possible decreased indinavir effect (increased metabolism) and increased amprenavir toxicity (decreased metabolism)	Monitor clinical status
Benzodiazepines, or cisapride	Indinavir decreases metabolism and may increase toxicity	Theoretical*; high concentrations of cisapride may lead to dangerous cardiac arrhythmias
Delavirdine	Possible indinavir toxicity (decreased metabolism)	Monitor clinical status
Didanosine	Decreased indinavir absorption	Give 1 hour apart
Efavirenz	Decreased indinavir effect (increased metabolism)	Manufacturer recommends increasing indinavir dose from 800 mg to 1,000 q8h
Ketoconazole	Possible indinavir toxicity (mechanism not established)	Consider reduction of indinavir dosage
Nelfinavir	Possible toxicity of both drugs (decreased metabolism)	Monitor clinical status
Nevirapine	Possible decreased indinavir effect (increased metabolism)	Indinavir's manufacturer recommends dosage increase
Rifabutin	Possible rifabutin toxicity (mechanism not established) and decreased indinavir concentration (increased metabolism)	Consider decreasing dosage of rifabutin and increasing dosage of indinavir

Some Drugs Interactions—cont'd

Interacting drugs	Adverse effects (probable mechanism)	Comments and recommendations
Rifampin	Possible decreased indinavir effect (increased metabolism)	Avoid concurrent use
Saquinavir	Possible saquinavir toxicity (decreased metabolism)	Interaction may be therapeutically useful, but adverse effects may increase
Nelfinavir, with:		
Benzodiazepines, or cisapride	Nelfinavir decreases metabolism and may increase toxicity	Theoretical*; high concentrations of cisapride may lead to dangerous cardiac arrhythmias
Contraceptives, oral	Possible decreased contraceptive effect (increased metabolism)	Use alternative contraceptive method
Delavirdine	Possible nelfinavir toxicity (decreased metabolism); decreased delavirdine effect (mechanism unknown); neutropenia has occurred	Monitor clinical status and neutrophil counts
Indinavir	Possible toxicity of both drugs (decreased metabolism)	Monitor clinical status
Methadone	Decreased methadone effect (increased metabolism)	Several case reports; monitor clinical status
Nevirapine	Possible decreased nelfinavir effect (increased metabolism)	One clinical and pharmacokinetic study found no adverse interaction
Rifabutin	Possible rifabutin toxicity (decreased metabolism)	Manufacturer recommends decreasing rifabutin dosage by half
Rifampin	Possible decreased nelfinavir effect (increased metabolism)	Avoid concurrent use
Ritonavir	Possible nelfinavir toxicity (decreased metabolism)	Clinical significance unclear
Saquinavir	Possible saquinavir toxicity (decreased metabolism)	Interaction may be therapeutically useful, but adverse effects may increase
Amprenavir, with:		
Amiodarone, bepridil, cisapride, benzo-diazepines, ergot alkaloids, lidocaine, tricyclic antide-pressants, quinidine	Amprenavir decreases metabolism and may increase toxicity	Theoretical*; high concentrations of cisapride may lead to dangerous cardiac arrhythmias
Abacavir	Possible increased amprenavir toxicity (decreased metabolism)	Monitor clinical status
Antacids	Possible decreased amprenavir effect (decreased absorption)	Give at least 1 hour apart
Didanosine	Possible decreased amprenavir effect (decreased absorption)	Give at least 1 hour apart
Efavirenz	Possible decreased amprenavir effect (increased metabolism)	Monitor clinical status, amprenavir dose may need to be increased
Indinavir	Possible decreased indinavir effect (increased metabolism) and increased amprenavir toxicity (decreased metabolism)	Monitor clinical status
Ketoconazole, itraconazole	Possible antifungal and amprenavir toxicity (decreased metabolism)	Monitor clinical status
Rifabutin	Possible increased rifabutin toxicity (decreased metabolism)	Rifabutin dosage should be decreased

Continued

Some Drugs Interactions—cont'd

Interacting drugs	Adverse effects (probable mechanism)	Comments and recommendations
Rifampin	Decreased amprenavir effect (increased metabolism)	Amprenavir concentration decreased 90% in one study; avoid concurrent use
Ritonavir	Increased amprenavir toxicity (decreased metabolism)	Ritonavir and amprenavir doses may both need to be decreased
Saquinavir	Decreased amprenavir effect (increased metabolism)	Monitor clinical status
Sildenafil	Possible sildenafil toxicity (decreased metabolism)	Amprenavir manufacturer suggest lowering sildenafil dosage
Warfarin	Possible increased anticoagulant effect	Monitor INR
Zidovudine	Possible zidovudine toxicity (decreased metabolism)	Monitor clinical status

PRINCIPAL ADVERSE EFFECTS OF ANTIMICROBIAL DRUGS

Adverse effects of antimicrobial drugs vary with dosage, duration of administration, concomitant therapy, renal and hepatic function, immune competence, and the age of the patient. The principal adverse effects of antimicrobial agents are listed in the following table. The designation of adverse effects as "frequent," "occasional" or "rare" is based on published reports and on the experience of *Medical Letter* consultants. Information about adverse interactions between drugs, including probable mechanisms and recommendations for clinical management, are available in the current edition of *The Medical Letter Handbook of Adverse Drug Interactions* and in the *Medical Letter Drug Interactions Program.*

Abacavir

Ziagen

   Frequent. Hypersensitivity reaction with fever, GI or respiratory symptoms and rash

   Occasional. Arthralgias; anemia
   Rare. Anaphylaxis; pancreatitis

Acyclovir

Zovirax; others

   Frequent. Local irritation at infusion site
   Occasional. Local reactions with topical use; headache, rash, nausea, diarrhea, vertigo, and arthralgias with oral use; decreased renal function sometimes progressing to renal failure; metabolic encephalopathy; bone marrow depression; abnormal hepatic function in immunocompromised patients
   Rare. Lethargy or agitation; tremor; disorientation; hallucinations; transient hemiparesthesia

Albendazole

Albenza

   Occasional. Abdominal pain; reversible alopecia; increased serum transaminase activity; migration of ascaris through mouth and nose
   Rare. Leukopenia; rash; renal toxicity

Amantadine

Symmetrel; others

Frequent. Livedo reticularis and ankle edema; insomnia; dizziness; lethargy

Occasional. Depression; psychosis; confusion; slurred speech; congestive heart failure; orthostatic hypotension; urinary retention; GI disturbance; rash; visual disturbance; sudden loss of vision; increased seizures in epilepsy

Rare. Convulsions; leukopenia; neutropenia; eczematoid dermatitis; oculogyric episodes; photosensitivity

Amikacin

Amikin

Occasional. Vestibular damage; renal damage; fever; rash

Rare. Auditory damage; CNS reactions; blurred vision; nausea; vomiting; neuromuscular blockade and apnea, may be reversible with calcium salts; paresthesias; hypotension

Aminosalicylic Acid

Paser

Frequent. GI disturbance

Occasional. Allergic reactions; liver damage; renal irritation; blood dyscrasias; thyroid enlargement; malabsorption syndrome

Rare. Acidosis; hypokalemia; encephalopathy; vasculitis; hypoglycemia in diabetics

Aminosidine

See Paromomycin

Amoxicillin

See Penicillins

Amoxicillin/Clavulanic Acid

See Penicillins

Amphotericin B Deoxycholate

Fungizone; others

Frequent. Renal damage; hypokalemia; thrombophlebitis at site of peripheral vein infusion; anorexia; headache; nausea; weight loss; bone marrow suppression with reversible decline in hematocrit; chills, fever, vomiting during infusion, possibly with delirium, hypotension or hypertension, wheezing, and hypoxemia, especially in cardiac or pulmonary disease

Occasional. Hypomagnesemia; normocytic, normochromic anemia

Rare. Hemorrhagic gastroenteritis; blood dyscrasias; rash; blurred vision; peripheral neuropathy; convulsions; anaphylaxis; arrhythmias; acute liver failure; reversible nephrogenic diabetes insipidus; hearing loss; acute pulmonary edema; spinal cord damage with intrathecal use

Amphotericin B Lipid Formulations

Ambisone; Abelcet; Amphotec

Ampicillin

See Penicillins

Ampicillin/Sulbactam

See Penicillins

Amprenavir

Agenerase

Frequent. GI upset; oral and perioral paresthesis; rash

Occasional. Hyperglycemia; increased aminotransferase activity; abnormal fat distribution

Rare. Severe rash including Stevens-Johnson syndrome; hemolytic anemia

Artemether

Artenam

Occasional. Neurologic toxicity; possible increase in length of coma; increased convulsions; prolongation of QTc interval

Artesunate

Occasional. Ataxia; slurred speech; neurologic toxicity; possible increase in length of coma; increased convulsions; prolongation of QTc interval

Atovaquone

Mepron; Malarone (with proguanil)

Frequent. Rash; nausea

Occasional. Diarrhea; increased aminotransferase activity; cholestasis

Azithromycin

Zithromax

Occasional. Nausea; diarrhea; abdominal pain; headache; dizziness; vaginitis

Rare. Angioedema; cholestatic jaundice; photosensitivity; reversible dose-related hearing loss

AZT

See Zidovudine

Aztreonam

Azactam

Occasional. Local reaction at injection site; rash; diarrhea; nausea; vomiting; increased aminotransferase activity

Rare. Thrombocytopenia; pseudomembranous colitis

Bacitracin

Many manufacturers
Frequent. Nephrotoxicity; GI disturbance
Occasional. Rash; blood dyscrasias
Rare. Anaphylaxis

Benznidazole

Rochagan
Frequent. Allergic rash; dose-dependent polyneuropathy; GI disturbances; psychic disturbances

Bithionole

Bitin
Frequent. Photosensitivity reactions; votmiting; diarrhea; abdominal pain; urticaria
Rare. Leukopenia; toxic hepatitis

Capreomycin

Capastat
Occasional. Renal damage; eighth-nerve damage; hypokalemia and other electrolyte abnormalities; pain, induration, excessive bleeding, sterile abscess at injection site
Rare. Allergic reactions; leukocytosis, leukopenia; neuromuscular blockade and apnea with large IV doses, reversed by neostigmine

Carbenicillin

See Penicillins

Cephalosporins

cefaclor—*Ceclor*; cefadroxil—*Duricef*, others; cefamandole—*Mandol*; cefazolin—*Ancef*, others; cefdinir—*Omnicef*; cefepime—*Maxipime*; cefixime—*Suprax*; cefonicid—*Monocid*; cefoperazone—*Cefobid*; cefotaxime—*Claforan*; cefotetan—*Cefotan*; cefoxitin—*Mefoxin*; cefpodoxime—*Vantin*; cefprozil—*Cefzil*; ceftazidime—*Fortaz, Tazidime, Tazicef, Ceptaz*; ceftibuten—*Cedax*; ceftizoxime—*Cefizox*; ceftriaxone—*Rocephin*; cefuroxime—*Kefurox, Zinacef*; cefuroxime axetil—*Ceftin*; cephalexin—*Keflex*, others; cephapirin—*Cefadyl*, others; cephradin—*Velosef*, others; loracarbef—*Lorabid*
Frequent. Thrombophlebitis with IV use; serum-sickness–like reaction with prolonged parenteral administration; moderate to severe diarrhea, especially with cefoperazone and cefixime

Occasional. Allergic reactions, rarely anaphylactic; pain at injection site; GI disturbance; hypoprothrombinemia, hemorrhage with cefamandole, cefoperazone or cefotetan; rash and arthritis ("serum-sickness") with cefaclor or cefprozil, especially in children; cholelithiasis with ceftriaxone; vaginal candidiasis (especially with cefdinir)

Rare. Hemolytic anemia; hepatic dysfunction; blood dyscrasias; renal damage; acute interstitial nephritis; pseudomembranous colitis; seizures; toxic epidermal necrolysis

Chloramphenicol

Chloromycetin; others
Occasional. Blood dyscrasias; gray syndrome (cardiovascular collapse); GI disturbance
Rare. Fatal aplastic anemia, even with eye drops or ointment, possibly leukemia; allergic and febrile reactions; peripheral neuropathy; optic neuritis and other CNS injury; pseudomembranous colitis

Chloroquine HCL and Chloroquine Phosphate

Aralen; others
Occasional. Pruritus; vomiting; headache; confusion; depigmentation of hair; skin eruptions; corneal opacity; weight loss; partial alopecia; extraocular muscle palsies; exacerbation of psoriasis, eczema, and other exfoliative dermatoses; myalgias; photophobia
Rare. Irreversible retinal injury (especially when total dosage exceeds 100 g); discoloration of nails and mucous membranes; nerve-type deafness; peripheral neuropathy and myopathy; heart block; blood dyscrasias; hematemesis

Cidofovir

Vistide
Frequent. Nephrotoxicity; ocular hypotony; neutropenia
Occasional. Metabolic acidosis; uveitis; Fanconi syndrome

Cinoxacin

Cinobac; others—Probably same as nalidixic acid

Ciprofloxacin

Cipro—See Fluoroquinolones

Clarithromycin

Biaxin

Occasional. Nausea; diarrhea; abdominal pain; abnormal taste; headache; dizziness

Rare. Reversible dose-related hearing loss; pseudomembranous colitis; pancreatitis

Clindamycin

Cleocin; others

Frequent. Diarrhea; allergic reactions

Occasional. Pseudomembranous colitis, sometimes severe, can occur even with topical use

Rare. Blood dyscrasias; esophageal ulceration; hepatotoxicity; arrhythmia due to QTC prolongation

Clofazimine

Lamprene

Frequent. Ichthyosis; pigmentation of skin, cornea, retina and urine discoloration; dryness and irritation of eyes; GI disturbance

Occasional. Epigastric distress; headache; retinal degeneration

Rare. Splenic infarction, bowel obstruction, and GI bleeding with high doses

Cloxacillin

See Penicillins

Colistimethate

See Polymyxins

Crotamiton

Eurax

Occasional. Rash

Cycloserine

Seromycin; others

Frequent. Anxiety; depression; confusion; disorientation; paranoia; hallucinations; somnolence; headache

Occasional. Peripheral neuropathy; liver damage; malabsorption syndrome; folate deficiency

Rare. Suicide; seizures; coma

Dapsone

Frequent. Rash; transient headache; GI irritation; anorexia; infectious mononucleosis-like syndrome

Occasional. Cyanosis due to methemoglobinemia and sulfhemoglobinemia; other blood dyscrasias, including hemolytic anemia; nephrotic syndrome; liver damage; peripheral neuropathy; hypersensitivity reactions; increased risk of

lepra reactions; insomnia; irritability; uncoordinated speech; agitation; acute psychosis

Rare. Renal papillary necrosis; severe hypoalbuminemia; epidermal necrolysis; optic atrophy; agranulocytosis; neonatal hyperbilirubinemia after use in pregnancy

Delavirdine

Rescriptor—Similar to nevirapine, but rash may be less severe

Demeclocycline

See Tetracyclines

Dicloxacillin

See Penicillins

Didanosine

ddI; *Videx*

Frequent. Peripheral neuropathy; diarrhea; nausea; vomiting; abdominal pain

Occasional. Pancreatitis; hyperuricemia; increased aminotransferase activity; hypokalemia; headache; insomnia; constipation; loss of taste; fever; rash; convulsions and other cerebral symptoms; glucose imbalance; severe lactic acidosis; retinal depigmentation

Rare. Hepatic failure; retinal atrophy in children

Diethylcarbamazine Citrate

Hetrazan

Frequent. Severe allergic or febrile reactions in patients with microfilaria in the blood or the skin; GI disturbances

Rare. Encephalopathy

Diloxanide Furoate

Furamide

Frequent. Flatulence

Occasional. Nausea; vomiting; diarrhea

Rare. Diplopia; dizziness; urticaria; pruritus

Dirithromycin

Dynabac—Similar to erythromycin

Doxycycline

See Tetracyclines

Efavirenz

Sustiva

Frequent. Dizziness; headache; inability to concentrate; insomnia and somnolence; rash

Occasional. Vivid dreams; nightmares; hallucinations; fever; Stevens-Johnson syndrome in children
Rare. Pancreatitis; peripheral neuropathy

Eflornithine

Difluoromethylornithine, DFMO, *Ornidyl*
Frequent. Anemia; leukopenia
Occasional. Diarrhea; thrombocytopenia; seizures
Rare. Hearing loss

Enoxacin

See Fluoroquinolones

Erythromycin

Ery-Tab; others
Frequent. GI disturbance
Occasional. Stomatitis; cholestatic hepatitis especially with erythromycin estolate in adults
Rare. Allergic reactions, including severe respiratory distress; pseudomembranous colitis; hemolytic anemia; hepatotoxicity; transient hearing loss with high doses, prolonged use, or in patients with renal insufficiency; ventricular arrhythmias including torsades de pointes with IV infusion; aggravation of myasthenia gravis; hypothermia; pancreatitis; hypertrophic pyloric stenosis following treatment of infants

Ethambutol

Myambutol
Occasional. Optic neuritis; allergic reactions; GI disturbance; mental confusion; precipitation of acute gout
Rare. Peripheral neuritis; possible renal damage; thrombocytopenia; toxic epidermal necrolysis; lichenoid skin eruption

Ethionamide

Trecator-SC
Frequent. GI disturbance
Occasional. Liver damage; CNS disturbance, including peripheral neuropathy; allergic reactions; gynecomastia; depression; myalgias; hypotension
Rare. Hypothyroidism; optic neuritis; arthritis; impotence

Famciclovir

Famvir
Occasional. Headache; nausea; diarrhea

Fluconazole

Diflucan
Occasional. Nausea; vomiting; diarrhea; abdominal pain; headache; rash; increased hepatic enzyme concentrations
Rare. Severe hepatic toxicity; exfoliative dermatitis; anaphylaxis; Stevens-Johnson syndrome; toxic epidermal necrolysis; hair loss

Flucytosine

Ancobon
Frequent. GI disturbance, including severe diarrhea and ulcerative colitis; rash; hepatic dysfunction; blood dyscrasias, including pancytopenia and fatal agranulocytosis
Occasional. Confusion; hallucinations
Rare. Anaphylaxis

Fluoroquinolones

ciprofloxacin—*Cipro;* enoxacin—*Penetrex;* gatifloxacin—*Tequin;* levofloxacin—*Levaquin;* lome-floxacin—*Maxaquin;* moxifloxacin—*Avelox;* norfloxacin—*Noroxin;* ofloxacin—*Floxin;* sparfloxacin—*Zagam;* trovafloxacin—*Trovan*
Occasional. Nausea; vomiting; abdominal pain; dizziness; headache; tremors; restlessness; confusion; rash; *Candida* infections of the pharynx and vagina; eosinophilia; neutropenia; increased hepatic enzyme activity; increased serum creatinine concentration; insomnia; diarrhea; leukopenia; photosensitivity reactions, especially with lomefloxacin and sparfloxacin; prolongation of QTc interval with sparfloxacin
Rare. Hallucinations; delirium; psychosis; vertigo; paresthesias; blurred vision and photophobia; severe hepatitis; seizures; pseudomembranous colitis; interstitial nephritis; vasculitis; possible exacerbation of myasthenia gravis; serum-sickness–like reaction; anaphylaxis; toxic epidermal necrolysis; anemia; tendinitis or tendon rupture; torsades de pointes; fatal hepatic necrosis with eosinophilic infiltrates with trovaflaxacin; pancreatitis; rhabdomyolysis with ofloxacin

Foscarnet

Foscavir
Frequent. Renal dysfunction; anemia; nausea; disturbances of Ca, P, Mg, and K metabolism
Occasional. Headache; vomiting; fatigue; genital ulceration; seizures; neuropathy
Rare. Nephrogenic diabetes insipidus; cardiac arrhythmias; hypertension

Fosfomycin

Monurol
  Frequent. Diarrhea
  Occasional. Vaginitis

Furazolidone

Furoxone
  Frequent. Nausea; vomiting
  Occasional. Allergic reactions, including pulmonary infiltration; hypotension; urticaria; fever; vesicular rash; hypoglycemia; headache
  Rare. Hemolytic anemia in G-6-PD deficiency and neonates; disulfiram-like reaction with alcohol; MAO-inhibitor interactions; polyneuritis

Ganciclovir

Cytovene
  Frequent. Neutropenia; thrombocytopenia
  Occasional. Anemia; fever; rash; abnormal liver function; neurologic toxicity; phlebitis
  Rare. Hypertension; cardiac arrhythmias; nausea; vomiting; abdominal pain; diarrhea; eosinophilia; hypoglycemia; alopecia; pruritus; urticaria; renal toxicity; psychiatric disturbances; seizures

Gatifloxacin

Tequin—See Fluoroquinolones

Gentamicin

Garamycin; others
  Occasional. Vestibular damage; renal damage; rash
  Rare. Auditory damage; neuromuscular blockade and apnea, reversible with calcium or neostigmine; disturbed mental function; polyneuropathy; anaphylaxis

Griseofulvin

Fulvicin-U/F; others
  Occasional. GI disturbance; allergic and photosensitivity reactions
  Rare. Proteinuria; blood dyscrasias; mental confusion; paresthesias; exacerbation of lupus erythematosus; fixed-drug eruption; reversible liver damage; lymphadenopathy; exacerbation of leprosy

Halofantrine

Halfan
  Occasional. Diarrhea; abdominal pain; pruritus; prolongation of QTc and PR interval

Imipenem-Cilastatin

Primaxin
  Occasional. Phlebitis; pain at injection site; drug fever; urticaria; other rashes; pruritus; nausea and vomiting, transient hypotension during intravenous infusion; diarrhea
  Rare. Seizures; pseudomembranous colitis

Imiquimod

Aldara
  Frequent. Local erythema, erosion, and excoriation
  Occasional. Itching, burning, and pain

Indinavir

Crixivan
  Frequent. Hyperbilirubinemia; dysuria; kidney stones; flank pain; hematuria; crystalluria
  Occasional. Hemolytic anemia; increased aminotransferase activity; gastrointestinal disturbances; glucose intolerance; abnormal fat distribution; increased bleeding in hemophiliacs; paronychia
  Rare. Rash

Interferon-α

Alferon N; Infergen; Intron A; Roferon-A; Rebetron with ribavirin
  Frequent. Transient flu-like syndrome; fatigue; anorexia; nausea; diarrhea; rash; dry skin or pruritus; weight loss; change in taste; bone marrow suppression; increased aminotransferase activity; depression; anxiety; insomnia
  Occasional. Paresthesias; alopecia; diaphoresis; reactivation of herpes labialis; hypothyroidism and hyperthyroidism; tinnitus; activation of autoimmune diseases, including diabetes
  Rare. Visual disturbance and retinopathy; hypertension; cardiac arrhythmias; renal failure; nephrotic syndrome; hearing loss

Iodoquinol

Yodoxin; others
  Occasional. Rash; acne; slight enlargement of the thyroid gland; nausea; diarrhea; cramps; anal pruritus
  Rare. Optic neuritis; optic atrophy; loss of vision; peripheral neuropathy after prolonged use in high dosage (for months); iodine sensitivity

Isoniazid

Nydrazid; others

Occasional. Peripheral neuropathy; liver damage, potentially fatal, particularly in patients more than 35 years old; glossitis and GI disturbance; allergic reactions; fever

Rare. Blood dyscrasias; red cell aplasia; depression; agitation; auditory and visual hallucinations; paranoia; optic neuritis; hyperglycemia; folate and vitamin B_6 deficiency; pellagra-like rash; keratitis; lupus erythematosus–like syndrome; chronic liver injury; cirrhosis; Stevens-Johnson syndrome

Itraconazole

Sporanox
Occasional. Nausea; epigastric pain; headache; dizziness; edema; hypokalemia; rash; hepatic toxicity

Ivermectin

Stromectol
Occasional. Mazzotti-type reaction seen in onchocerciasis, including fever, pruritus, tender lymph nodes, headache, and joint and bone pain
Rare. Hypotension

Kanamycin

Kantrex; others
Occasional. Eighth-nerve damage affecting mainly hearing that may be irreversible and may not be detected until after therapy has been stopped (most likely with renal impairment); renal damage
Rare. Rash; fever; peripheral neuritis; parenteral or intraperitoneal administration may produce neuromuscular blockade and apnea, not reversed by neostigmine or calcium gluconate

Ketoconazole

Nizoral
Frequent. Nausea; vomiting
Occasional. Decreased testosterone synthesis; gynecomastia; oligospermia and impotence in men; abdominal pain; rash; hepatitis; pruritus; dizziness; constipation; diarrhea; fever and chills; photophobia; headache
Rare. Fatal hepatic necrosis; liver injury with jaundice; transient elevated transaminase; severe epigastric burning and pain; may interfere with adrenal function; anaphylaxis

Lamivudine

3TC; *Epivir*

Rare. Headache; nausea; dizziness; nasal symptoms; rash; pancreatitis in children; neuropathy; lactic acidosis

Levofloxacin

Levoquin—See Fluoroquinolones

Lincomycin

Lincocin; others
Frequent. Diarrhea, sometimes progressing to severe pseudomembranous colitis
Occasional. Allergic reactions, rarely anaphylactic
Rare. Blood dyscrasias; hypotension with rapid IV injection

Lomefloxacin

See Fluoroquinolones

Loracarbef

See Cephalosporins

Malathion

Ovide
Occasional. Local irritation

Mebendazole

Vermox
Occasional. Diarrhea; abdominal pain; migration of ascaris through mouth and nose
Rare. Leukopenia; agranulocytosis; hypospermia

Mefloquine

Lariam
Frequent. Vertigo; lightheadedness; nausea; other GI disturbances; nightmares; visual disturbances; headache; insomnia
Occasional. Confusion
Rare. Psychosis; hypotension; convulsions; coma; paresthesias

Meglumine Antimoniate

Glucantime—Similar to sodium stibogluconate

Melarsoprol

Arsobal
Frequent. Myocardial damage; albuminuria; hypertension; colic; Herxheimer-type reaction; encephalopathy; vomiting; peripheral neuropathy
Rare. Shock

Meropenem

Merrem—Similar to imipenem, but may be less likely to cause seizures

Methenamine Hippurate

Hiprex, Urex
    Occasional. GI disturbance; dysuria; allergic reactions

Methenamine Mandelate

Mandelamine; others
    Occasional. GI disturbance; dysuria; allergic reactions

Methicillin

See Penicillins

Metronidazole

Flagyl; others
    Frequent. Nausea; headache; anorexia; metallic taste
    Occasional. Vomiting; diarrhea; insomnia; weakness; dry mouth; stomatitis; vertigo; tinnitus; paresthesia; rash; dark urine; urethral burning; disulfiram-like reaction with alcohol; candidiasis
    Rare. Seizures; pseudomembranous colitis; ataxia; leukopenia; peripheral neuropathy; pancreatitis; encephalopathy

Mezlocillin

See Penicillins

Miconazole *(Monistat)*

    Occasional. Phlebitis; thrombocytosis; chills; intense, persistent pruritus; rash; vomiting; hyperlipidemia; dizziness; blurred vision; local burning and irritation with topical use
    Rare. Anemia; thrombocytopenia; hyponatremia; renal insufficiency; anaphylaxis; cardiac and respiratory arrest with initial dose

Minocycline

See Tetracyclines

Moxifloxacin

Avelox—See Fluoroquinolones

Nafcillin

See Penicillins

Nalidixic Acid

NegGram; others
    Frequent. GI disturbance; rash; visual disturbance

    Occasional. CNS disturbance; acute intracranial hypertension in young children and rarely in adults; photosensitivity reactions, sometimes persistent; convulsions; hyperglycemia
    Rare. Cholestatic jaundice; blood dyscrasias; fatal immune hemolytic anemia; arthralgia or arthritis; lupus-like syndrome; confusion, depression, excitement, visual hallucinations

Natamycin

Natacyn
    Rare. Conjunctival chemosis, hyperemia

Nelfinavir

Viracept
    Frequent. Mild to moderate diarrhea
    Occasional. Increased aminotransferase activity; rash; nausea; glucose intolerance; increased bleeding in patients with hemophilia; abnormal fat distribuation

Neomycin

    Occasional. Eighth-nerve and renal damage, same as with kanamycin but hearing loss may be more frequent and severe and may occur with oral, intraarticular, irrigant, or topical use; GI disturbance; malabsorption with oral use; contact dermatitis with topical use
    Rare. Neuromuscular blockade and apnea that may be reversed by IV neostigmine or calcium gluconate; pseudomembranous colitis

Netilmicin

Netromycin—Probably similar to gentamicin; thrombocytosis, prolonged prothrombin time, drug fever have also been reported

Nevirapine

Viramune
    Frequent. Rash, can progress to Stevens-Johnson syndrome
    Occasional. Fever; nausea; headache

Niclosamide

Niclocide
    Occasional. Nausea; abdominal pain

Nifurtimox

Lampit
    Frequent. Anorexia; vomiting; weight loss; loss of memory; sleep disorders; tremor; paresthesias; weakness; polyneuritis
    Rare. Convulsions; fever; pulmonary infiltrates and pleural effusion

Nitrofurantoin

Macrodantin; others
   Frequent. GI disturbance; allergic reactions, including pulmonary infiltration
   Occasional. Lupus-like syndrome; blood dyscrasias; hemolytic anemia; peripheral neuropathy, sometimes severe; pulmonary fibrosis
   Rare. Cholestatic jaundice; chronic active hepatitis, sometimes fatal; focal nodular hyperplasia of liver; pancreatitis; trigeminal neuralgia; crystalluria; increased intracranial pressure; lactic acidosis; parotitis; severe hemolytic anemia in G-6-PD deficiency

Norfloxacin

See Fluoroquinolones

Novobiocin

Albamycin
   Frequent. Cholestatic jaundice; allergic reactions; GI disturbance; neonatal hyperbilirubinemia
   Occasional. Severe blood dyscrasias

Nystatin

Mycostatin; others
   Occasional. Allergic reactions; fixed drug eruption; GI disturbance

Ofloxacin

See Fluoroquinolones

Ornidazole

Tiberal
   Occasional. Dizziness; headache; gastrointestinal disturbances
   Rare. Reversible peripheral neuropathy

Oseltamivir Phosphate

TamiFlu
   Occasional. Nausea; vomiting; headache

Oxacillin

See Penicillins

Oxamniquine

Vansil
   Occasional. Headache; fever; dizziness; somnolence and insomnia; nausea; diarrhea; rash; hepatic enzyme changes; ECG changes; EEG changes; orange-red discoloration of urine
   Rare. Seizures; neuropsychiatric disturbances

Oxytetracycline

See Tetracyclines

Para-aminosalicylic Acid

See Aminosalicylic Acid

Paramomycin

aminosidine; *Humatin*
   Frequent. GI disturbances with oral use
   Rare. Eighth-nerve damage (mainly auditory) and renal damage when aminosidine is given IV; vertigo; pancreatitis

Penicillins

amoxicillin—*Amoxil*, others; amoxicillin/ clavulanic acid—*Augmentin*; ampicillin—*Principen*, others; ampicillin/sulbactam—*Unasyn*; carbenicillin indanyl—*Geocillin*; cloxacillin; dicloxacillin—*Dycill*, others; methicillin; mezlocillin—*Mezlin*; nafcillin—*Nafcil*, others; oxacillin; penicillin G; penicillin V; piperacillin—*Pipracil*; piperacillin/tazobactam—*Zosyn*; ticarcillin—*Ticar*; ticarcillin/clavulanic acid—*Timentin*
   Frequent. Allergic reactions, rarely anaphylactic; rash (more common with ampicillin and amoxicillin than with other penicillins); diarrhea (most common with ampicillin and amoxicillin/clavulanic acid); nausea and vomiting with amoxicillin/clavulanic acid in children
   Occasional. Hemolytic anemia; neutropenia; pseudomembranous colitis; platelet dysfunction with high doses of piperacillin, ticarcillin, nafcillin, or methicillin; cholestatic heptiis with amoxicillin/clavulanic acid
   Rare. Hepatic damage with semisynthetic penicillins; granulocytopenia or agranulocytosis with semisynthetic penicillins; renal damage with semisynthetic penicillins and penicillin G; muscle irritability and seizures, usually after high doses in patients with impaired renal function; hyperkalemia and arrhythmias with IV potassium penicillin G given rapidly; bleeding diathesis; Henoch-Schönlein purpura with ampicillin; thrombocytopenia with methicillin and mezlocillin; terror, hallucinations, disorientation, agitation, bizarre behavior and neurologic reactions with high doses of procaine penicillin G, oxacillin, or ticarcillin; hypokalemic alkalosis and/or sodium overload with high doses of ticarcillin or nafcillin; hemorrhagic cystitis with methicillin; GI bleeding with dicloxacillin; tissue damage with extravasation of nafcillin

Pentamidine Isethionate

Pentam 300; NebuPent; others

Frequent. Hypotension; hypoglycemia often followed by diabetes mellitus; vomiting; blood dyscrasias; renal damage; pain at injection site; GI disturbances

Occasional. May aggravate diabetes; shock; hypocalcemia; liver damage; cardiotoxicity; delirium; rash

Rare. Herxheimer-type reaction; anaphylaxis; acute pancreatitis; hyperkalemia and vomiting with amoxicillin/clavulanic acid in children

Permethrin

Nix; others

Occasional. Burning; stinging; numbness; increased pruritus; pain; edema; erythema; rash

Piperacillin

See Penicillins

Piperacillin/Tazobactam

See Penicillins

Polymyxins

colistimethate—*Coly-Mycin*, polymyxin B—generic

Occasional. Renal damage; peripheral neuropathy; thrombophlebitis at IV injection site with polymyxin B

Rare. Allergic reactions; neuromuscular blockade and apnea with parenteral administration, not reversed by neostigmine but may be by IV calcium chloride

Praziquantel

Biltricide

Frequent. Abdominal pain; diarrhea; malaise; headache; dizziness

Occasional. Sedation; fever; sweating; nausea; eosinophilia

Rare. Pruritus; rash; edema; hiccups

Primaquine Phosphate

Frequent. Hemolytic anemia in G-6-PD deficiency

Occasional. Neutropenia; GI disturbances; methemoglobinemia

Rare. CNS symptoms; hypertension; arrhythmias

Proguanil

Paludrine; Malarone (with atovaquone)

Occasional. Oral ulceration; hair loss; scaling of palms and soles; urticaria

Rare. Hematuria (with large doses); vomiting; abdominal pain; diarrhea (with large doses); thrombocytopenia

Pyrantel Pamoate

Antiminth, others

Occasional. GI disturbances; headache; dizziness; rash; fever

Pyrazinamide

Frequent. Arthralgia; hyperuricemia

Occasional. Liver damage; GI disturbance; acute gouty arthritis; rash

Rare. Photosensitivity reactions; acute hypertension

Pyrethrins with Piperonyl Butoxide (*RID*, others)

Occasional. Allergic reactions

Pyrimethamine (*Daraprim*)

Occasional. Blood dyscrasias; folic acid deficiency

Rare. Rash; vomiting; convulsions; shock; possibly pulmonary eosinophilia; fatal cutaneous reactions with **pyrimethamine-sulfadoxine** (*Fansidar*)

Quinacrine

Frequent. Disulfiram-like reaction with alcohol; nausea and vomiting; colors skin and urine yellow

Occasional. Headache; dizziness

Rare. Rash; fever; psychosis; extensive exfoliative dermatitis in patients with psoriasis

Quinine Dihydrochloride

Frequent. Cinchonism (tinnitus, headache, nausea, abdominal pain, visual disturbance)

Occasional. Deafness; hemolytic anemia; other blood dyscrasias; photosensitivity reactions; hypoglycemia; arrhythmias; hypotension; drug fever

Rare. Blindness; sudden death if injected too rapidly

Quinine Sulfate

See Quinine Dihydrochloride

Quinupristin/Dalfopristin

Synercid

Frequent. Local irritation and thrombophlebitis with peripheral IV administration; arthralgias; myalgias; increase in conjugated bilirubin

Occasional. Nausea; rash; increased aminotransferase activity

Ribavirin

Virazole, Rebetron with interferon-α

Occasional. Anemia; headache; abdominal cramps and nausea; fatigue; elevation of bilirubin; teratogenic and embryolethal in animals and mutagenic in mammalian cells; rash; conjunctivitis; bronchospasm with aerosol use; hyperuricemia; depression

Rifabutin

Mycobutin—Similar to rifampin; also iritis, uveitis, leukopenia, arthralgia

Rifampin

Rifadin, Rimactane

Frequent. Colors urine, tears, saliva, CSF, contact lenses, and lens implants red-orange

Occasional. Liver damage; GI disturbance; allergic reactions

Rare. Flulike syndrome, sometimes with thrombocytopenia, hemolytic anemia, shock, and renal failure, particularly with intermittent therapy; acute organic brain syndrome; acute adrenal crisis in patients with adrenal insufficiency; renal damage; severe proximal myopathy

Rifampin-Isoniazid

Rifamate—See individual drugs

Rifampin-Isoniazid-Pyrazinamide

Rifater—See individual drugs

Rifapentine

Priftin—Similar to rifampin; higher rate of hyperuricemia

Rimantadine

(Flumadin)—Similar to amantadine, but lower risk of CNS effects

Ritonavir

Norvir

Frequent. Nausea; diarrhea; vomiting; asthenia

Occasional. Abdominal pain; anorexia; dyspepsia; circumoral and peripheral paresthesias; rash; altered taste; elevated serum triglycerides, cholesterol; increased aminotransferase activity; cholestasis; glucose intolerance; abnormal fat distribution; increased bleeding in hemophiliacs

Rare. Nephrotoxicity

Saquinavir

Invirase; Fortovase

Occasional. Diarrhea; abdominal discomfort; nausea; glucose intolerance; abnormal fat distribution; increased aminotransferase activity; increased bleeding in hemophiliacs

Rare. Rash

Sodium Stibogluconate

Pentostam

Frequent. Muscle and joint pain; fatigue; nausea; increased aminotransferase activity; T-wave flattening or inversion; pancreatitis

Occasional. Weakness; abdominal pain; liver damage; bradycardia; leukopenia; thrombocytopenia; rash; vomiting

Rare. Diarrhea; pruritus; myocardial damage; hemolytic anemia; renal damage; shock; sudden death

Sparfloxacin

Zagam—See Fluoroquinolones

Spectinomycin

Trobicin

Occasional. Soreness at injection site; urticaria; dizziness; nausea; chills; fever; insomnia; decreased urine output; allergic reactions

Spiramycin

Rovamycine

Occasional. GI disturbances

Rare. Allergic reactions

Stavudine

D4T; *Zerit*

Frequent. Peripheral neuropathy

Occasional. Increased aminotransferase activity

Rare. Rash; pancreatitis

Streptomycin

Frequent. Eighth-nerve damage (mainly vestibular), sometimes permanent; paresthesias; rash; fever; eosinophilia

Occasional. Pruritus; anaphylaxis; renal damage

Rare. Blood dyscrasias; neuromuscular blockade and apnea with parenteral administration, usually reversed by neostigmine; optic neuritis; hepatic necrosis; myocarditis; hemolytic anemia and renal failure; pseudomembranous colitis; toxic erythema; Stevens-Johnson syndrome

Sulfonamides

Frequent. Allergic reactions (rash, photosensitivity, drug fever)

Occasional. Kernicterus in newborn; renal damage; liver damage; Stevens-Johnson syndrome (particularly with long-acting sulfonamides); hemolytic anemia; other blood dyscrasias; vasculitis

Rare. Transient acute myopia; pseudomembranous colitis; reversible infertility in men with sulfasalazine; CNS toxicity with trimethoprim-sulfamethoxazole in patients with AIDS

Suramin Sodium

Frequent. Vomiting; pruritus; urticaria; paresthesias; hyperesthesia of hands and feet; photophobia; peripheral neuropathy

Occasional. Kidney damage; blood dyscrasias; shock; optic atrophy

Terbinafine

Lamisil

Frequent. Headache; GI disturbance

Occasional. Taste disturbance; rash; pruritus; urticaria; toxic epidermal necrolysis; erythema multiforme; increased aminotransferase activity

Rare. Serious hepatic injury; anaphylaxis; pancytopenia; agranulocytosis; severe neutropenia; changes in ocular lens and retina; parotid swelling

Tetracyclines

demeclocycline—*Declomycin*; doxycycline—*Vibramycin*, others; minocycline—*Minocin*, others; oxytetracycline—*Terramycin*, others; tetracycline hydrochloride—*Sumycin*, others

Frequent. GI disturbance; bone lesions and staining and deformity of teeth in children up to 8 years old, and in the newborn when given to pregnant women after the fourth month of pregnancy

Occasional. Malabsorption; enterocolitis; photosensitivity reactions (most frequent with demeclocycline); vestibular toxicity with minocycline; increased azotemia with renal insufficiency (except doxycycline, but exacerbation of renal failure with doxycycline has

been reported); renal insufficiency with demeclocycline in cirrhotic patients; hepatic injury; parenteral doses may cause serious liver damage, especially in pregnant women and patients with renal disease receiving 1 g or more daily; esophageal ulcerations; cutaneous and mucosal hyperpigmentation, tooth discoloration in adults with minocycline

Rare. Allergic reactions, including serum sickness and anaphylaxis; pseudomembranous colitis; blood dyscrasias; drug-induced lupus with minocycline; autoimmune hepatitis; increased intracranial pressure; fixed-drug eruptions; diabetes insipidus with demeclocycline; transient acute myopia; blurred vision, diplopia, papilledema; photoonycholysis and onycholysis; acute interstitial nephritis with minocycline; aggravation of myasthenic symptoms with IV injection, reversed with calcium; possibly transient neuropathy; hemolytic anemia

Thiabendazole

Mintezol

Frequent. Nausea; vomiting; vertigo; headache; drowsiness, pruritus

Occasional. Leukopenia; crystalluria; rash; hallucinations and other psychiatric reactions; visual and olfactory disturbance; erythema multiforme

Rare. Shock; tinnitus; intrahepatic cholestasis; convulsions; angioneurotic edema; Stevens-Johnson syndrome

Ticarcillin

See Penicillins

Ticarcillin/Clavulanic Acid

See Penicillins

Tinidazole

Fasigyn

Occasional. Metallic taste; nausea; vomiting; rash

Tobramycin

Nebcin; others—Probably same as with gentamicin; possible delirium

Trifluridine

Viroptic

Occasional. Burning or stinging; palpebral edema

Rare. Epithelial keratopathy; hypersensitivity reactions

Trimethoprim

Proloprim; others
> *Frequent.* Nausea, vomiting with high doses
> *Occasional.* Megaloblastic anemia; thrombocytopenia; neutropenia; rash; fixed drug eruption
> *Rare.* Pancytopenia; hyperkalemia

Trimethoprim-Sulfamethoxazole

Bactrim; Septra; others
> *Frequent.* Rash; fever; nausea and vomiting
> *Occasional.* Hemolysis in G-6-PD deficiency; acute megaloblasticanemia; granulocytopenia; thrombocytopenia; pseudomembranous colitis; kernicterus in newborn; hyperkalemia
> *Rare.* Agranulocytosis; aplastic anemia; hepatotoxicity; Stevens-Johnson syndrome; aseptic meningitis; fever; confusion; depression; hallucinations; deterioration in renal disease; intrahepatic cholestasis; methemoglobinemia; pancreatitis; ataxia; CNS toxicity in patients with AIDS; renal tubular acidosis; hyperkalemia

Trimetrexate

Neutrexin, with "leucovorin rescue"
> *Occasional.* Rash; peripheral neuropathy; bone marrow depression; increased serum aminotransferase activity

Troleandomycin

TAO
> *Occasional.* Stomatitis; GI disturbance; cholestatic jaundice
> *Rare.* Allergic reactions

Trovafloxacin

See Fluoroquinolones

Valacyclovir

Valtrex—Generally same as acyclovir
> *Rare.* Thrombotic thrombocytopenic purpura (hemolytic uremic syndrome in severely immunocompromised patients treated with high doses)

Vancomycin

Vancocin; others
> *Frequent.* Thrombophlebitis; fever, chills
> *Occasional.* Eighth-nerve damage (mainly hearing) especially with large or continued doses (more than 10 days), in presence of renal damage, and in the elderly; neutropenia; renal damage; allergic reactions; rash; "redman" syndrome

> *Rare.* Peripheral neuropathy; hypotension with rapid IV administration; exfoliative dermatitis

Zalcitabine

ddC; *Hivid*
> *Frequent.* Peripheral neuropathy
> *Occasional.* Stomatitis; esophageal ulceration; nausea; headache; fever; fatigue; abdominal pain; diarrhea; rash
> *Rare.* Pancreatitis

Zanamivir

Relenza
> *Occasional.* Nasal and throat discomfort; headache; cough; broncospasm in patients with asthma

Zidovudine

Retrovir
> *Frequent.* Anemia; granulocytopenia; nail pigment changes; nausea; fatigue
> *Occasional.* Thrombocytosis; headache; insomnia; confusion; diarrhea; rash; fever; myalgias; myopathy; light-headedness
> *Rare.* Seizures; lactic acidosis; Wernicke's encephalopathy; cholestatic hepatitis; transient ataxia and nystagmus with acute large overdosage

DOSAGE OF ANTIMICROBIAL AGENTS

In choosing the dosage of an antimicrobial drug, the physician must consider the site of infection, the identity and antimicrobial susceptibility of the infecting organism, the possible toxicity of the drug of choice, and the condition of the patient, with special attention to renal function. This article and the table that follows on p. 974 offer some guidelines for determining antimicrobial dosage, but dosage recommendations taken out of context of the clinical situation may be misleading.

Renal Insufficiency

Antimicrobial drugs excreted through the urinary tract may be toxic for patients with renal insufficiency if they are given in usual therapeutic doses, because serum concentrations in these patients may become dangerously high. Nephrotoxic and ototoxic drugs such as gentamicin or other aminoglycosides may damage the kidney, further decreasing the excretion of these drugs, leading to higher blood concentrations that may be ototoxic and may cause additional renal damage. In patients with renal insufficiency, therefore, an antimicrobial drug with minimal nephrotoxicity, such as a penicillin, is preferred. When nephrotoxic drugs must be used, renal function should be monitored. Measurements of serum creatinine or blood urea nitrogen (BUN) concentrations are useful as indices of renal function, but are not as accurate as measurements of creatinine clearance; serum creatinine and BUN concentrations may be normal even with significant loss of renal function.

In renal insufficiency, control of serum concentrations of potentially toxic drugs can be achieved either by varying the dose or by varying the interval between doses. Serum antimicrobial concentrations should be measured whenever possible; rigid adherence to any dosage regimen can result in either inadequate or toxic serum concentrations in patients with renal insufficiency, particularly when renal function is changing rapidly.

Children's Dosage

Many antimicrobial drugs have such a broad therapeutic index that it makes no difference in practice if children's dosage is based on weight or on surface area. Where dosage considerations are important in preventing severe toxic effects, as with the aminoglycosides, recommendations for safe usage are derived primarily from experience with dosage based on weight.

Once-Daily Aminoglycosides

Current data suggest that once-daily doses of gentamicin, tobramycin, and amikacin are as effective for most indications as multiple daily doses and are equally or less nephrotoxic (Bailey et al., Clin Infect Dis 1997;24:786). Monitoring 24-hour trough drug levels is recommended to minimize the risk of toxicity. Once-daily doses of aminoglycosides are not recommended for treatment of endocarditis.

The Table

Dosage

The recommendations in the table that follows are based on the judgment of *Medical Letter* consultants. In some cases they differ from the manufacturer's recommendations, partly because clinical experience reported after the labeling is approved is not always reflected by an appropriate change in the manufacturer's recommendations. The range of dosage specified for some drugs may not include relatively rare indications. In general, lower doses are sufficient for treatment of urinary tract infection, and higher doses are recommended for such severe infections as meningitis, endocarditis, and the sepsis syndrome.

Interval

More than one interval between doses is recommended for some drugs. In general, the longer intervals should be used for infections of the urinary tract and for intramuscular administration. Recommendations are made in hours throughout, but many oral drugs can be given three or four times during the daytime for convenience. For maximum absorption, which is often not necessary, most oral antibiotics should be given at least 30 minutes before or 2 hours after a meal.

Antimicrobial Drug Dosage[*]

	ADULTS		CHILDREN	
	Oral	*Parenteral*	*Oral*	*Parenteral*
Abacavir	300 mg q12h		8 mg/kg q12h	
Acyclovir	200 mg q4h × 5 or 400 mg q8h[1]	5-15 mg/kg q8h	20 mg/kg q6h	5-20 mg/kg q8h
Amantadine	100 mg q12-24h		4.4 mg/kg q12-24h	
Amikacin		5 mg/kg q8h, 7.5 mg/kg q12h or 15 mg/kg q24h		5 mg/kg q8h or 7.5 mg/kg q12h
Amoxicillin	250-500 mg q8h or 500-875 mg q12h		6.6-13.3 mg/kg q8h or 15 mg/kg q12h	
Amoxicillin/ clavulanic acid	250-500 mg[3] q8h or 500-875 mg[3] q12h		6.6-13.3 mg/kg[3] q8h or 15 mg/kg[3] q12h	
Amphotericin B		0.3-1.5 mg/kg[4] q24h		0.3-1.5 mg/kg[4] q24h
Amphotericin B cholesteryl sulfate complex		3-4 mg/kg q24h		3-4 mg/kg q24h
Amphotericin B lipid complex		5 mg/kg q24h		5 mg/kg q24h
Amphotericin B liposomal		3-5 mg/kg q24h		3-5 mg/kg q24h
Ampicillin	500 mg q6h	1-2 g q4-6h	12.5-25 mg/kg q6h	25-50 mg/kg q6h[7]
Ampicillin/ sulbactam		1-2 g[8] q6h		50 mg/kg[8] q6h
Amprenavir[9]	1,200 mg q12h		20 mg/kg q12h[10] or 15 mg/kg q8h[10]	
Azithromycin	250-1,000 mg[11] q24h	500 mg q24h	5-12 mg/kg[11] q24h	
Aztreonam[9]		1-2 g q6-8h		30 mg/kg q6-8h
Carbenicillin indanyl sodium	1-2 tablets[†] q6h		7.5-12.5 mg/kg q12h	

[†]Tablets contain 382 mg of carbenicillin.

[*]Antiparasitic drug dosages are found in the article on this subject. The articles on antiviral and antifungal drugs, prophylaxis, sexually transmitted diseases, and HIV infection also include dosage recommendations.

[1]For treatment of initial genital herpes. For suppression of genital herpes, 400 mg q12h is used. For treatment of varicella, 800 mg q6h and for zoster 800 mg q4h × 5 are recommended.

[2]Give full dose once, then monitor levels.

[3]Dosage based on amoxicillin content. For doses of 500 or 875 mg, 500-mg or 875-mg tablets should be used, because multiple smaller tablets would contain too much clavulanic acid. The 875-mg, 500-mg and 250-mg tablets each contain 125 mg clavulanic acid. 125-mg chewable tablets and 125 mg/5 ml oral suspension both contain 31.25 mg clavulanic acid; 250-mg chewable tablets and 250-mg/5-ml oral suspension both contain 62.5 mg clavulanic acid.

[4]Given intravenously once a day, over a period of 2 to 4 hours.

[5]Or up to 1.5 mg/kg given every other day.

Usual maximum dose/day	Dose	ADULT DOSAGE IN RENAL FAILURE FOR CREATININE CLEARANCE (ml/min)			Extra dose after hemodialysis
		80-50	50-10	<10	
600 mg		Not recommended			
4 g oral 45 mg/kg IV	10 mg/kg	q8h	q12-24h	2.5 mg/kg q24h	yes
200 mg	100 mg	q24h	100-200 mg/d q24-48h	200 mg q7d	no
1.5 g	5 mg/kg	q12h	q24-36h	See footnote 2	yes
3 g	500 mg	q8h	q12h	q24h	yes
1.5 g	500 mg	Q8h	q12h	q24h	yes
1 mg/kg[5]		Change not required[6]			no
4 mg/kg		Not known			
5 mg/kg		Not known			
5 mg/kg		Not known			
14 g	2 g	q8h	q8h	q12h	yes
8g	2 g	q6-8h	q8-12h	q24h	yes
2,400 mg/day		Change not required			
500 mg		Change not required			Unknown
8 g	1 g q6-8h	500-1,000 mg q8h	500-750 mg q8h	250-500 mg q8h	yes
3 g		See package insert			

[6]Amphotericin B is potentially nephrotoxic. A pre- and post-dose IV bolus of 500 ml normal saline may decrease toxicity. Temporary interruption of therapy may be required when the serum creatinine exceeds 3 mg/dl.

[7]For meningitis in children caused by ampicillin-sensitive H. influenzae type b, Medical Letter consultants recommend up to 400 mg/kg/day. Meningitis should be treated q4h.

[8]Dosage based on ampicillin content.

[9]Dosage adjustment may be necessary in patients with hepatic dysfunction.

[10]Using capsules. Also available in solution: 22.5 mg/kg q12h or 17 mg/kg q8h (max 2,800 mg/day).

[11]For adults: 500 mg on day 1 and 250 mg/day on days 2-5. 1 g once for C. trachomatis urethritis. For children: 10 mg/kg on day 1 and 5 mg/kg on days 2 to 5 for acute otitis media and 12 mg/kg for 5 days for pharyngitis/tonsillitis.

Continued

Antimicrobial Drug Dosage*—cont'd

	ADULTS		CHILDREN	
	Oral	*Parenteral*	*Oral*	*Parenteral*
Cefaclor	250-500 mg q8h or 375-500 mg q12h		6.6-13.3 mg/kg q8h	
Cefadroxil	1 g q2-24h		15 mg/kg q12h	
Cefamandole		500 mg-2 g q4-8h		50-150 mg/kg/day, divided q4-8h
Cefazolin		500 mg-1.5 g q6-8h		25-100 mg/kg/day, divided q6-8h
Cefdinir	300 mg q12h or 600 mg q24h		7 mg/kg q12h or 14 mg/kg q24h	
Cefepime		1-2 g q8-12h		50 mg/kg q8-12h
Cefixime	200 mg q12h or 400 mg q24h		4 mg/kg q12h or 8 mg/kg q24h	
Cefonicid		500 mg-2 g q24h		
Cefoperazone[9]		500 mg-4 g q6-12h		25-100 mg/kg q12h
Cefotaxime		1-2 g q4-12h		50-180 mg/kg/day divided q4-6h
Cefotetan		500 mg-3 g q12h		
Cefoxitin		1-3 g q4-6h		80-160 mg/kg/day, divided q4-6h
Cefpodoxime	100-400 mg q12h		10 mg/kg q24h or 5 mg/kg q12h	
Cefprozil	250-500 mg q12h		15 mg/kg q12h	
Ceftazidime		250 mg-2 g q8-12h		30-50 mg/kg q8h
Ceftibuten	400 mg q24h		9 mg/kg q24h	
Ceftizoxime		500 mg-4 g q8-12h		50 mg/kg q6-8h
Ceftriaxone		1-2 g q12-24h		50-100 mg/kg/day, divided q12-24h
Cefuroxime		750 mg-1.5 g q8h		50-150 mg/kg/day, divided q6-8h
Cefuroxime axetil	125-500 mg q12h		10-15 mg/kg q12h	
Cephalexin	250 mg-1 g q6h		6.25-25 mg/kg q6h	
Cephapirin		500 mg-2 g q4-6h		40-80 mg/kg/day, divided q4-6h
Cephradine	250 mg-1 g q6h or 500 mg-1 g q12h	500 mg-2 g q6h	6.25-25 mg/kg q6h or 12.5-50 mg/kg q12h	12.5-25 mg/kg q6h
Chloramphenicol[9]	12.5-25 mg/kg q6h	12.5-25 mg/kg[12] q6h	12.5-25 mg/kg q6h	12.5-25 mg/kg[12] q6h
Cidofovir		5 mg/kg once/wk × 2, then 5 mg/kg every other week		

‡But give usual dose after dialysis.
[12]Intravenous administration; dosage should be adjusted according to serum concentration.

Usual maximum dose/day	Dose	ADULT DOSAGE IN RENAL FAILURE FOR CREATININE CLEARANCE (ml/min) 80-50	50-10	<10	Extra dose after hemodialysis
4 g	500 mg	Change not required			yes
2 g	500 mg	q12-24h	q12-24h	q36h	yes
12 g	0.5-2 g	1-2 g q6h	1-2 g q8h	0.5-1 g q8-12h	yes
6 g	1 g	q8h	1 g q8-12h	1 g q24h	yes
600 mg	300 mg	No change	q24h	q24h	yes
6 g	2 g	q12h	1-2 g q24h	500 mg q24h	yes
400 mg	200-400 mg	q24h	q24h	200 mg q24h	no
2 g	0.5-2 g	0.5-1.5 g q24h	0.25-1 g q24-48h	0.25-1 g q3-5 days	no
12 g		Change not required			no
12 g	1-2 g	q4-8h	q6-12h	q12h	yes
6 g	1-3 g	q12h	q12-24h	q48h	yes
12 g	0.5-2g	1-2 g q8h	1-2 g q12h	0.5-1g q12-24h	yes
800 mg	200-400 mg	q12h	q24h	q24h	yes
1,000 mg	250-500 mg	No change	q24h	q24h	yes
6 g	0.5-2 g	q8-12h	1 g q12-24h	0.5 g q24-48h	yes
400 mg	400 mg	q24h	100-200 mg q24h	100 mg q24h	no‡
12 g	0.25-1.5 g	0.5-1.5 g q8h	0.25-1 g q12h	0.25-1 g q24-48h	yes
4 g		Change not required			no
9 g	0.75-1.5 g	q8h	q8-12h	q24h	yes
1,000 mg	250-500 mg	Change not required			yes
4 g	0.25-1 g	q6h	q8-12h	q12-48h	yes
12 g	0.5-2 g	q6h	q8h	q12h	yes
8 g	1-2 g	q6h	q8h	q12-72h	yes
4 g		Change not required			no*
	5 mg/kg	No change	1-2 mg/kg	0.5 mg/kg	no

Continued

Antimicrobial Drug Dosage[*]—cont'd

| | ADULTS | | CHILDREN | |
	Oral	Parenteral	Oral	Parenteral
Cinoxacin	250 mg q6h or 500 mg q12h			
Ciprofloxacin	250-750 mg q12h	200-400 mg q12h		
Clarithromycin	250-500 mg q12h		7.5 mg/kg q12h	
Clindamycin[9]	150-450 mg q6h	150-900 mg q6-8h	2-8 mg/kg q6-8h	2.5-10 mg/kg q6h
Cloxacillin	500 mg-1g q6h		12.5-25 mg/kg q6h	
Cycloserine[13]	250-500 mg q12h		5-10 mg/kg q12h	
Delavirdine	400 mg tid			
Dicloxacillin	125-500 mg		3.125-6.25 mg/kg	
Didanosine[14] (ddl)	≥60 kg:200 mg q12h <60 kg:125 mg q12h or 400 q24h	90-150 mg/m^2	q12h	
Dirithromycin	500 mg q24h			
Doxycycline	100 mg q12-24h	100 mg q12-24h	2.2 mg/kg[15] q12-24h	2.2 mg/kg[15] q12-24h
Efavirenz	600 mg q24h		200-400 mg q24h	
Enoxacin	200-400 mg q12h			
Erythromycin	250-500 mg q6h q6h	250 mg-1 g IV[16] q6h	7.5-12.5 mg/kg q6h q6h	3.75-12.5 mg/kg IV[16] q6h
Ethambutol[17]	15-25 mg/kg q24h		15-25 mg/kg q24h	
Ethionamide	250-500 mg q12h		7.5-10 mg/kg q12h	
Famciclovir	500 mg q8h[18]			
Fluconazole	50-400 mg q24h	100-400 mg q24h		
Flucytosine	12.5-37.5 mg/kg q6h		12.5-37.5 mg/kg q6h	
Foscarnet		60 mg/kg q8h or 90 mg/kg q12h[20]		

[13]Monitor concentrations, toxicity increases markedly above 30 µg/ml.
[14]Refers to chewable, dispersible tablets. For adults and children more than 1 year old, each dose should include two tablets to supply adequate buffer. Didanosine also available in powder for oral solution for adults: ≤60 kg: 250 mg q12h, <60 kg: 167 mg q12h. A pediatric powder formulation is also available.
[15]Not recommended for children less than 8 years old.
[16]By slow infusion to minimize thrombophlebitis
[17]Not recommended in children whose visual acuity cannot be monitored (<6 years old).

Usual maximum dose/day	Dose	ADULT DOSAGE IN RENAL FAILURE FOR CREATININE CLEARANCE (ml/min) 80-50	50-10	<10	Extra dose after hemodialysis
1 g	250-500 mg q8h	250 mg	250 mg q12-24h	250 mg q24h	no
2 g	250-750 mg	q12h q12-18h	250-500 mg q24h	250-500 mg	no*
1 g	250-500 mg	q12h	q24h	Unknown	Unknown
4.8 g		Change not required			no
4 g		Change not required			no
1 g	250 mg	No change q12-24h	250 mg q24-48h	250 mg	
1.2 g	400 mg	Change not required			no
4 g		Change not required			no
400 mg	125-200 mg	q12h	q12-24h	100 mg q24h	yes
500 mg		Change not required			no
200 mg	100 mg	q12-24h	q12-24h	q12-24h	no
600 mg	600 mg	Change not required			
800 mg	200-400 mg	q12h	q12h	q24h	no
4 g		Change not required			no
2.5 g	20 mg/kg	No change	q24-36h	q48h	
1 g	1 g	No change	No change q24h	500 mg	
1.5 g	500 mg	q12h	q24h	Not recommended	yes
400 mg	100-400 mg	q24h	q48h	≥q72h	yes
150 mg/kg	12.5-37.5 mg/kg	q6h	q12-24h	Not recommended[19]	yes
	60 mg/kg[20]	40-50 mg/kg q12h	50-60 mg/kg q24h	Not recommended	yes

[18]For herpes zoster. For first episode genital herpes, the dosage is 250 mg q8h. For genital herpes recurrence, it is 125 mg q12h. For suppression of genital herpes, it is 250 mg q12h.

[19]If treatment is essential, begin with 15-25 mg/kg q24h and adjust daily dose to maintain the plasma concentration between 50 and 75 µg/ml.

[20]For CMV, given over at least 1 hour for induction; for maintenance, 90-120 mg/kg daily over 2 hours. For HSV or VZV, 40 mg/kg q8h.

Continued

Antimicrobial Drug Dosage*—cont'd

	ADULTS		CHILDREN	
	Oral	Parenteral	Oral	Parenteral
Fosfomycin	3 g once			
Ganciclovir	1,000 mg q8h or 500 mg 6×	5 mg/kg[21]	q12h	5 mg/kg[21] q12h
Gatifloxacin	200-400 mg q24h	200-400 mg q24h		
Gentamicin		1-2.5 mg/kg q8h or 5-7 mg/kg q24h		1-2.5 mg/kg
Griseofulvin Microsize	500-1,000 mg q24h		11 mg/kg q24h	
Ultramicrosize	330-660 mg q24h		7.25 mg/kg q24h	
Imipenem		250 mg-1 g[22] q6-8h		15-25 mg/kg[22] q6h
Indinavir[9]	800 mg q8h		350 mg/m² q8h	
Isoniazid[9,24]	300 mg q24h		10-20 mg/kg q24h	
Itraconazole	100-200 mg q12-24h	200 mg q12h × 4, then 200 mg q24h	5 mg/kg q24h	
Kanamycin		5 mg/kg q8h or 7.5 mg/kg q12h		5 mg/kg/q8h or 7.5 mg/kg/q12h
Ketoconazole	200-400 mg q12-24h		3.3-6.6 mg/kg	q24h
Lamivudine	≥50 kg:150 mg q12h <50 kg: 2 mg/kg q12h		4 mg/kg q12h	
Levofloxacin	500 mg q24h	500 mg q24h		
Lomefloxacin	400 mg q24h			
Loracarbef	200-400 mg q12h		7.5-15 mg/kg	q12h
Meropenem		1-2 g q8h		20-40 mg/kg q8h
Methenamine hippurate[25]	1 g q12h		12.5-25 mg/kg q12h	
Methenamine mandelate[25]	1 g q6h		12.5-18.75 mg/kg q6h	
Metronidazole[9,26]	7.5 mg/kg q6h	7.5 mg/kg q6h	7.5 mg/kg q6h	7.5 mg/kg q6h

[21]For CMV induction, give IV at constant rate over 1 hour; for maintenance, 5 mg/kg 7 days/week or 6 mg/kg 5 days/week.
[22]Doses are for imipenem, which is combined with equal weight of cilastatin as Primaxin.
[23]Maximum dosage should be 4 g or 50 mg/kg, whichever is less.
[24]For prophylaxis of positive PPD in adults, 300 mg/d; in children, 10 mg/kg/d up to maximum of 300 mg.

Usual maximum dose/day	Dose	ADULT DOSAGE IN RENAL FAILURE FOR CREATININE CLEARANCE (ml/min)			Extra dose after hemodialysis
		80-50	50-10	<10	
3 g		Change not required			
10 mg/kg	5 mg/kg IV	2.5 mg/kg q12h	1.25-2.5 mg/kg q24h	1.25 mg/kg q24h	no*
	500 mg or 1,000 mg PO	500-1,000 mg q8h	500 mg once or q12h	500 mg 3×/week	no*
400 mg	400 mg	No change	400 mg once, then 200 mg q24h	400 mg once, then 200 mg q24h	no*
7 mg/kg	1.5 mg/kg	q8-12h	q12-24h	See footnote 2	yes
		Change not required			
		Change not required			
4 g[23]	250-500 mg	q6-8h	q8-12h Unknown	q12h	yes
300 mg	300 mg		Change not required		
400 mg			Change not required		
1.5 g	5-7.5 mg/kg	q24h	q24-72h	See footnote 2	yes
1 g			Change not required		no
300 mg	150 mg	q12h	150 mg once then 100-150 mg/d	50-150 mg once then 25-50 mg/d	no
500 mg	500 mg	No change	250 mg q24h	250 mg q48h	no
400 mg	400 mg	No change	400 mg once then 200 mg q24h	Unknown	no
800 mg	200-400 mg	q12h	q24h	q3-5 days	yes
6 g			0.5-1 g q12h	0.5 g q24h	
4 g	1 g	q12h	Not recommended		
4 g	1 g	q6h	Not recommended		
4 g	7.5 mg/kg		Change not required		no*

[25]Usually given with an acidifying agent

[26]Dosage for anaerobic bacterial infections. First dose should be 15 mg/kg loading dose. For antiparasitic dosages, see table beginning on page 104.

Continued

Antimicrobial Drug Dosage*—cont'd

	ADULTS		CHILDREN	
	Oral	*Parenteral*	*Oral*	*Parenteral*
Mezlocillin[9]		1.5-4 g q4-6h		50 mg/kg q4-6h
Miconazole[27]		600 mg-1.2 g q8h		6.6-13.3 mg/kg q8h
Moxifloxacin[9]	400 mg q24h			
Nafcillin	500 mg-1 g q6h	500 mg-1.5 g q4-6h	12.5-25 mg/kg q6h	25-50 mg/kg q6h
Nalidixic acid	1 g q6h		Not recommended	
Nelfinavir[9]	750 mg q8h		25-30 mg/kg q8h	
Netilmicin		1.5-3.25 mg/kg q12h or 1.3-2.2 mg/kg q8h		2.7-4 mg/kg q12h or 1.8-2.7 mg/kg q8h
Nevirapine	200 mg/d × 14, followed by 200 mg bid		120 mg/day × 14, followed by 120-200 mg/day q12h	
Nitrofurantoin	50-100 mg q6h	Not recommended	1.25-1.75 mg/kg q6h	Not recommended
Norfloxacin	400 mg q12h			
Ofloxacin	200-400 mg q12h	200-400 mg q12h		
Oseltamavir	75 mg q12h			
Oxacillin	500 mg-1 g q6h	500 mg-2 g q4-6h	12.5-25 mg/kg q6h	25-50 mg/kg q6h
Penicillin G[28]	250-500 mg q6h	1.2-24 million U/day, divided q2-12h[29]	6.25-12.5 mg/kg q6h	100,000-250,000 U/kg/day, divided q2-12h[29]
Penicillin V[28]	250-500 mg q6h		6.25-12.5 mg/kg	q6h
Piperacillin		3-4 g q4-6h		200-300 mg/kg/day, divided q4-6h
Piperacillin/ tazobactam		3 g q4-6h[31]		
Pyrazinamide	15-30 mg/kg q24h		15-30 mg/kg q24h	
Quinupristin/ dalfopristin		7.5 mg/kg q8-12h		5 mg/kg q24h
Rifabutin	150 mg q12h or 300 mg q24h		See footnote 32	
Rifampin[9,33]	600 mg/day	600 mg/day	10-20 mg/kg/day	10-20 mg/kg/day
Rifapentine	600 mg once or twice weekly		unknown	
Rimantadine[9]	100 mg once or q12h		5 mg/kg once	
Ritonavir[9]	600 mg q12h		400 mg/m² q12h	

[27]The manufacturer recommends an initial test dose of 200 mg.

[28]One mg is equal to 1,600 units.

[29]The interval between parenteral doses can be as short as 2 hours for initial intravenous treatment of meningococcemia, or as long as 12 hours between intramuscular doses of penicillin G procaine.

[30]Patients with severe renal insufficiency should be given no more than one third to one half the maximum daily dosage, i.e., instead of giving 24 million units per day, 10 million units could be given. Patients on lower doses usually tolerate full dosage even with severe renal insufficiency.

Usual maximum dose/day	Dose	ADULT DOSAGE IN RENAL FAILURE FOR CREATININE CLEARANCE (ml/min)			Extra dose after hemodialysis
		80-50	50-10	<10	
24 g	1.5-4 g	q4-6h	q6-8h	q8-12h	yes
3.6 g			Change not required		no
400 mg			Change not required		
12 g			Change not required		no
4 g	1 g	q6h	q6h	Not recommended	
2.5 g			Change not required		
6.5 mg/kg	1.3-2.2 mg/kg	q8-12h	q12-24h	q24-48h	yes
400 mg			Not known		
400 mg	50-100 mg	q6h	Not recommended		
800 mg	200-400 mg	q12h	q12-24h	q24h	no
800 mg	200-400 mg	q12h	q24h	half dose q24h	no
150 mg	75 mg	No change	q24h	Not recommended	
12 g			Change not required		no
24 million units			Change not required; see note 30		yes
4 g	250-500 mg		Change not required		yes
24 g	3-4 g	q4-6h	q6-12h	q12h	yes
18 g	2-3 g	No change	2 g q6h	2 g q8h	yes
2 g	2 g		Change not required		
None known			Change not required		
300 mg	300 mg		Change not required		no
600 mg			Change not required		no
600 mg			Unknown		

[31]Dosage based on piperacillin content. Piperacillin/tazobactam is supplied as 2 g piperacillin/250 mg tazobactam, 3 g piperacillin/375 mg tazobactam, and 4 g piperacillin/500 mg tazobactam.

[32]Safety has not been established but rifabutin, 5 mg/kg/day has been used in a limited number of children for treatment of *Mycobacterium avium* complex.

[33]For meningococcal carriers, dosage is 600 mg bid × 2 days for adults, 10 mg/kg q12h × 2 days for children more than 1 month old, and 5 mg/kg q12h × 2 days for infants less than 1 month old.

Continued

Antimicrobial Drug Dosage*—cont'd

	ADULTS		CHILDREN	
	Oral	*Parenteral*	*Oral*	*Parenteral*
Saquinavir[34]	1,200 mg q8h			
Sparfloxacin	400 mg day 1, then 200 mg days 2-10			
Spectinomycin		2 g once		40 mg/kg once
Stavudine[9]	≥60 kg: 40 mg q12h <60 kg: 30 mg q12h		>30 kg: 30 mg q12h <30 kg: 1 mg/kg q12h	
Streptomycin		500 mg-1 g q12h		10-15 mg/kg q12h
Sulfisoxazole	500 mg-1 g q6h	25 mg/kg q6h	150 mg/kg/day divided q4-6h	100 mg/kg/day divided q6-8h
Tetracyclines[15,35]	250-500 mg q6h		6.25-12.5 mg/kg q6h	
Ticarcillin		200-300 mg/kg/day, divided q4-6h		200-300 mg/kg/day, divided q4-6h
Ticarcillin/ clavulanic acid		3 g[36] q4-6h		200-300 mg/kg/day,[36] divided q4-6h
Tobramycin		1-2.5 mg/kg q8h or 5-7 mg/kg q24h		1-2.5 mg/kg q8h, or 5-7 mg/kg q24h
Trimethoprim	100 mg q12h or 200 mg q24h		2 mg/kg q12h	
Trimethoprim-sulfamethoxazole (TMP-SMX)	1 tablet[37] q6h or 2 tablets q12h[37]	4-5 mg/kg (TMP) q6-12h	4-5 mg/kg (TMP) q6h	4-5 mg/kg (TMP) q6-12h
Trovafloxacin	200 mg q24h	200-300 mg q24h		
Valacyclovir	1 g q8h[39]			
Vancomycin[40]	125-500 mg q6h[41]	1 g IV q12h	12.5 mg/kg q6h[41]	10 mg/kg IV q6h[42,43]
Zalcitabine (ddC)	0.375-0.75 mg q8h		0.005 to 0.01 mg/kg q8h	
Zanamivir	See footnote 44			
Zidovudine[9] (AZT)	200 mg q8h or 300 mg q12h		90-180 mg/m² q6-8h	

---

[34]Soft gelatin capsules.

[35]Tetracycline or oxytetracycline. The oral dose of demeclocycline for adults is 600 mg daily in two to four divided doses. The oral dose of minocycline for adults is 100 mg twice a day. The parenteral dose of minocycline is 100-200 mg/day, in one or two doses.

[36]Dosage based on ticarcillin component. A 3.1-g vial contains 3 g of ticarcillin and 0.1 g clavulanic acid; a 3.2-g vial contains 3 g of ticarcillin and 0.2 g clavulanic acid.

[37]Each tablet contains 80 mg trimethoprim and 400 mg sulfamethoxazole. Double-strength tablets are also available; the usual dosage of these is 1 tablet q12h. Suspension contains 40 mg trimethoprim and 200 mg sulfamethoxazole per 5 ml.

Usual maximum dose/day	Dose	ADULT DOSAGE IN RENAL FAILURE FOR CREATININE CLEARANCE (ml/min)			Extra dose after hemodialysis
		80-50	50-10	<10	
200 mg		Change not required			no
1200 mg		Change not required			no
3,600 mg	1200 mg	Change not required			
200 mg	200 mg	No change	q48h	q48h	
		No change	Not recommended		
80 mg	40 mg	q12h	20 mg q12-24h	Not recommended	
	30 mg	q12h	15 mg q12-24h		
2 g	0.5-1 g	q24h	q24-72h	q72-96h	yes
8 g	0.5-1 g	q6-8h	q8-12h	q12-24h	yes
2 g		Not recommended			
24-30 g	2-3 g	q4-6h	q6-8h	2 g q12h	yes
18 g	2-3.1 g	3.1 g q4h	2 g q4-8h	2 g q2h	yes
7 mg/kg	1-1.66 mg/kg	q8-12h	q12-24h	q24-48h	yes
200 mg	100 mg	q12h	q18-24h	Not recommended	
See footnote[38]	4-5 mg/kg (TMP)	q12h	q18h	Not recommended	yes
300 mg		Change not required			
3 g	1 g	q8h	1 g q12-24h	500 mg q24h	
2 g	1 g	q12-24h	q24h	See footnote 2	yes
2.25 mg	0.75 mg	No change	q12h	q24h	Unknown
		Change not required			
1.2 g	100 mg	No change			No change

[38]The usual maximum daily dose is 4 tablets orally or 1,200 mg trimethoprim with 6,000 mg sulfamethoxazole intravenously.

[39]For herpes zoster. For a first episode of genital herpes, the dosage is 1 g q12h. For recurrence of genital herpes, it is 500 mg q12h. For suppression of genital herpes, it is 1 g q24h.

[40]Vancomycin should be infused over a period of at least 60 minutes.

[41]Only for treatment of pseudomembranous colitis.

[42]Sixty mg/kg/day may be needed for staphylococcal CNS infections.

[43]Peak serum concentrations should be monitored.

[44]Inhalation, 10 mg q12h; intranasal, 16 mg q12h.

SAFETY OF ANTIMICROBIAL DRUGS IN PREGNANCY

Use of antimicrobial drugs during pregnancy is a frequent cause for concern. The table that follows summarizes the known prenatal risks of most antimicrobials, but the teratogenic potential of many agents remains unknown. The recommendations in the table are based on published data, the opinions of *Medical Letter* consultants, and on the importance of the drug and the availability of alternatives. Adverse effects not particularly related to pregnancy are not included here; they are summarized in the text beginning on p. 960. Serum levels of some renally excreted drugs (e.g., β-lactams, aminoglycosides) are decreased by 10% to 50% in late pregnancy. For serious infections, maximal recommended doses should be used and serum levels may need to be monitored (Korzeniowski, Infect Dis Clin North Am 1995;9:639).

Some Antimocrobial Agents in Pregnancy

Drug	Toxicity in pregnancy	Recommendation
Antibacterial		
Amikacin *(Amikin)*	Possible 8th-nerve toxicity in fetus	Caution*
Azithromycin *(Zithromax)*	None known	Caution*
Aztreonam *(Azactam)*	None known	Probably safe
Cephalosporins[1]	None known	Probably safe
Chloramphenicol (*Chloromycetin*, others)	Unknown—gray syndrome in newborn	Caution*, especially at term
Cinoxacin (*Cinobac*, others)	Arthropathy in immature animals	Contraindicated
Clarithromycin *(Biaxin)*	Teratogenic in animals	Contraindicated
Clindamycin (*Cleocin*, and others)	None known	Caution*
Dapsone	None known; carcinogenic in rats and mice; hemolytic reactions in neonates	Caution*, especially at term
Dirithromycin (*Dynabac* and others)	Retarded fetal development in rodents with high doses	Caution*
	Risk of cholestatic hepatitis appears to be increased in pregnant women	Contraindicated
Erythromycin (*Ery-Tab*, others)	None known	Probably safe but neonatal use has been associated with pyloric stenosis
Fosfomycin *(Monurol)*	Fetal toxicity in rabbits with maternally toxic doses	Caution*
Fluoroquinolones[2]	Arthropathy in immature animals	Contraindicated
Gentamicin (*Garamycin*, and others)	Possible 8th-nerve toxicity in fetus	Caution*
Imipenem-cilastatin *(Primaxin)*	Toxic in some pregnant animals	Caution*
Kanamycin (*Kantrex*, and others)	Possible 8th-nerve toxicity in fetus	Caution*
Methenamine mandelate (*Mandelamine*, and others)	Unknown	Probably safe

*Use only for strong clinical indication in absence of suitable alternative.

[1]Cefaclor (*Ceclor*, others), cefadroxil (*Duricef*, others), cefamandole *(Mandol)*, cefazolin (*Ancef*, others), cefepime *(Maxipime)*, cefdinir *(Omnicef)*, cefixime *(Suprax)*, cefonicid *(Monocid)*, cefoperazone *(Cefobid)*, cefotaxime *(Claforan)*, cefotetan *(Cefotan)*, cefoxitin *(Mefoxin)*, cefpodoxime *(Vantin)*, cefprozil *(Cefzil)*, ceftazidime *(Fortaz*, others), ceftibuten *(Cedax)*, ceftizoxime *(Cefizox)*, ceftriaxone *(Rocephin)*, cefuroxime (*Kefurox, Zinacef)*, cefuroxime axetil *(Ceftin)*, cephalexin (*Keflex*, others), cephapirin (*Cefadyl*, others), cephradine (*Velosef*, others), loracarbef *(Lorabid)*. Experience with newer agents is limited.

[2]Ciprofloxacin *(Cipro)*, enoxacin *(Penetrex)*, gatifloxacin *(Tequin)*, levofloxacin *(Levaquin)*, lomefloxacin *(Maxaquin)*, moxifloxacin *(Avelox)*, norfloxacin *(Noroxin)*, ofloxacin *(Floxin)*, sparfloxacin *(Xagam)*, trovafloxacin *(Trovan)*.

Some Antimocrobial Agents in Pregnancy—cont'd

Drug	Toxicity in pregnancy	Recommendation
Antibacterial—cont'd		
Metronidazole (*Flagyl*, and others)	None known – carcinogenic in rats and mice	Caution*
Nalidixic acid (*NegGram*, and others)	Arthropathy in immature animals; increased intracranial pressure in newborn	Contraindicated
Netilmicin (*Netromycin*)	Possible 8th-nerve toxicity in fetus	Caution*
Nitrofurantoin (*Macrodantin*, and others)	Hemolytic anemia in newborn	Caution*; contraindicated at term
Penicillins[3]	None known	Probably safe
Quinupristin/dalfopristin (*Synercid*)	Unknown	Caution*
Spectinomycin (*Trobicin*)	Unknown	Probably safe
Streptomycin	Possible 8th-nerve toxicity in fetus	Caution*
Sulfonamides	Hemolysis in newborn with G-6-PD deficiency; increased risk of kernicterus in newborn; teratogenic in some animal studies	Caution*; contraindicated at term
Tetracyclines[4]	Tooth discoloration and dysplasia, inhibition of bone growth in fetus; hepatic toxicity and azotemia with IV use in pregnant patients with decreased renal function or with overdosage	Contraindicated
Tobramycin (*Nebcin*, and others)	Possible 8th-nerve toxicity in fetus	Caution*
Trimethoprim (*Proloprim*, and others)	Folate antagonism; teratogenic in rats	Caution*
Trimethoprim-sulfamethoxazole (*Bactrim*, and others)	Same as sulfonamides and trimethoprim	Caution*; contraindicated at term
Vancomycin (*Vancocin*, and others)	Unknown—possible auditory and renal toxicity in fetus	Caution*
Antifungal		
Amphotericin B (*Fungizone*, and others)	None known	Caution*
Fluconazole (*Diflucan*)	Teratogenic	Contraindicated for high dose, caution for single dose
Flucytosine (*Ancobon*)	Teratogenic in rats	Contraindicated
Griseofulvin (*Fulvicin U/F*, and others)	Embryotoxic and teratogenic in animals; carcinogenic in rodents	Contraindicated
Itraconazole (*Sporanox*)	Teratogenic and embryotoxic in rats	Caution*
Ketoconazole (*Nizoral*)	Teratogenic and embryotoxic in rats	Caution*
Miconazole (*Monistat i.v.*)	None known	Caution*
Nystatin (*Mycostatin*, and others)	None reported	Probably safe
Antiparasitic		
Albendazole (*Albenza*)	Teratogenic and embryotoxic in animals	Caution*

[3]Amoxicillin (*Amoxil*, and others), amoxicillin/clavulanic acid (*Augmentin*), ampicillin (*Principen*, and others), ampicillin/sulbactam (*Unasyn*), carbenicillin indanyl (*Geocillin*), cloxacillin, dicloxacillin (*Dycill*, and others), methicillin, mezlocillin (*Mezlin*), nafcillin (*Nafcil*, and others), oxacillin, penicillin G, penicillin V, piperacillin (*Pipracil*), piperacillin/tazobactam (*Zosyn*), ticarcillin (*Ticar*), ticarcillin/clavulanic acid (*Timentin*). Experience with newer agents is limited.

[4]Doxycycline (*Vibramycin*, others), minocycline (*Minocin*, others), oxytetracycline (*Terramycin*), demeclocycline (*Declomycin*), tetracycline hydrochloride (*Sumycin*, others).

Continued

Some Antimocrobial Agents in Pregnancy—cont'd

Drug	Toxicity in pregnancy	Recommendation
Antiparasitic—cont'd		
Atovaquone (*Mepron*)	Maternal and fetal toxicity in animals	Caution*
Atovaquone/proguanil (*Malarone*)	Maternal and fetal toxicity in animals	Caution*
Chloroquine (*Aralen*, and others)	None known with doses recommended for malaria prophylaxis	Probably safe in low doses
Crotamiton (*Eurax*)	Unknown	Caution*
Diloxanide (*Furamide*)	Safety not established	Caution*
Furazolidone (*Furoxone*)	None known; carcinogenic in rodents; hemolysis with G-6-PD deficiency in newborn	Caution*; contraindicated at term
Hydroxychloroquine (*Plaquenil*)	None known with doses recommended for malaria prophylaxis	Probably safe in low doses
Lodoquinol (*Yodoxin*, and others)	Unknown	Caution*
Ivermectin (*Stromectol*)	Teratogenic in animals	Contraindicated
Lindane	Absorbed from the skin; potential CNS toxicity in fetus	Contraindicated
Malathion, topical (*Ovide*)	None known	Probably safe
Mebendazole (*Vermox*)	Teratogenic and embryotoxic in rats	Caution*
Mefloquine (*Lariam*)[5]	Teratogenic in animals	Caution*
Metronidazole (*Flagyl*, and others)	None known – carcinogenic in rats and mice	Caution*
Niclosamide (*Niclocide*)	Not absorbed; no known toxicity in fetus	Probably safe
Oxamniquine (*Vansil*)	Embryocidal in animals	Contraindicated
Paromomycin (*Humatin*)	Poorly absorbed; toxicity in fetus unknown	Probably safe
Pentamidine (*Pentam 300*, *NebuPent*, others)	Safety not established	Caution*
Permethrin (*Nix*, others)	Poorly absorbed; no known toxicity in fetus	Probably safe
Piperazine (*Antepar*, and others)	Unknown	Caution*
Praziquantel (*Biltricide*)	None known	Probably safe
Primaquine	Hemolysis in G-6-PD deficiency	Contraindicated
Pyrantel pamoate (*Antiminth*, others)	Absorbed in small amounts; no known toxicity in fetus	Probably safe
Pyrethrins and piperonyl butoxide (*RID*, others)	Poorly absorbed; no known toxicity in fetus	Probably safe
Pyrimethamine (*Daraprim*)	Teratogenic in animals	Caution*
Pyrimethamine-sulfadoxine (*Fansidar*)	Teratogenic in animals; increased risk of kernicterus in newborn	Caution*, especially at term
Quinacrine (*Atabrine*)	Safety not established	Caution*
Quinine	Large doses can cause abortion; auditory nerve hypoplasia, deafness in fetus; visual changes, limb anomalies, visceral defects also reported	Caution*
Suramin sodium (*Germanin*)	Teratogenic in mice	Caution*
Thiabendazole (*Mintezol*)	None known	Caution*
Antituberculosis		
Capreomycin (*Capastat*)	None known	Caution*
Cycloserine (*Seromycin*, others)	Unknown	Caution*

[5]See page 114, footnote 49 and 50.

Some Antimocrobial Agents in Pregnancy—cont'd

Drug	Toxicity in pregnancy	Recommendation
Antituberculosis—cont'd		
Ethambutol (Myambutol)	None known – teratogenic in animals	Caution*
Ethionamide (Trecator-SC)	Teratogenic in animals	Caution*
Isoniazid (Nydrazid, others)	Embryocidal in some animals	Probably safe
Pyrazinamide	Unknown	Caution*
Rifabutin (Mycobutin)	Unknown	Caution*
Rifampin (Rifadin, Rimactane)	Teratogenic in animals	Probably safe
Rifapentine (Priftin)	Teratogenic in animals	Caution*
Streptomycin	Possible 8th-nerve toxicity in fetus	Caution*
Antiviral		
Abacavir (Ziagen)	Teratogenic in animals	Caution*
Acyclovir (Zovirax, others)	None known	Caution*
Adefovir (Preveon)	Embryotoxic in mice	Caution*
Amantadine (Symmetrel, others)	Teratogenic and embryotoxic in rats	Contraindicated
Amprenavir (Agenerase)	Teratogenic in animals	Caution*
Cidofovir (Vistide)	Embryotoxic in rats and rabbits	Caution*
Delavirdine (Rescriptor)	Teratogenic in rats	Caution*
Didanosine (ddl; Videx)	None known	Caution*
Efavirenz (Sustiva)	Fetal abnormalities in monkeys	Contraindicated
Famciclovir (Famvir)	Animal toxicity	Contraindicated
Foscarnet (Foscavir)	Animal toxicity	Caution*
Ganciclovir (Cytovene; Vitrasert)	Teratogenic and embryotoxic in animals	Caution*
Indinavir (Crixivan)	None known	Caution*
Interferon-α (Intron A, others)	Large doses cause abortions in animals	Caution*
Lamivudine (3TC; Epivir)	Unknown	Caution*
Nelfinavir (Viracept)	No fetal toxicity in animals	Caution*
Nevirapine (Viramune)	Decrease in fetal weight in rats	Caution*
Oseltamivir (Tamiflu)	Some minor skeletal abnormalities in animals	Caution*
Ribavirin (Virazole)	Mutagenic, teratogenic, embryolethal in nearly all species, and possibly carcinogenic in animals	Contraindicated
Rimantadine (Flumadine)	Embryotoxic in rats	Contraindicated
Ritonavir (Norvir)	Animal toxicity	Caution*
Saquinavir (Invirase; Fortovase)	None known	Caution*
Stavudine (d4T; Zerit)	Animal toxicity with high doses	Caution*
Valacyclovir (Valtrex)	None known	Caution*
Vidarabine (Vira-A)	Teratogenic in rats and rabbits	Caution*
Zalcitabine (ddC; Hivid)	Teratogenic and embryotoxic in mice	Caution*
Zanamivir (Relenza)	None in animals	Caution*
Zidovudine (AZT; Retrovir)	Mutagenic in vitro	Indicated to prevent HIV infection of fetus

TRADE NAMES

abacavir—*Ziagen* (Glaxo Wellcome)

Abelcet (Liposome)—amphotericin B lipid complex

Actisite (Proctor & Gamble)—tetracycline HCl

*acyclovir—*Zovirax* (Glaxo Wellcome)

Aftate (Schering)—tolnaftate

Agenerase (Glaxo Wellcome)—amprenavir

*Also available generically.

Ala-Tet (Del-Ray)—tetracycline HCl

alatrofloxacin—*Trovan* (Pfizer)

Albamycin (Pharmacia & Upjohn)—novobiocin

albendazole—*Albenza* (SK Beecham)

Alferon N (Interferon Sciences)—interferon alfa-n3

*amantadine—*Symmetrel* (Du Pont), others

AmBisome (Fujisawa)—amphotericin B liposomal

amikacin—*Amikin* (Bristol-Myers Squibb)

Amikin (Bristol-Myers Squibb)—amikacin

*aminosalicylic acid—*Paser* (Jacobus)

*amoxicillin—*Amoxil* (SK Beecham), others

amoxicillin/clavulanic acid—*Augmentin* (SK Beecham)

Amoxil (SK Beecham)—amoxicillin

Amphotec (Sequus)—amphotericin B cholesteryl sulfate complex

*amphotericin B—*Fungizone* (Bristol-Myers Squibb), others

amphotericin B cholesteryl sulfate complex—*Amphotec* (Sequus)

amphotericin B lipid complex—*Abelcet* (Liposome)

amphotericin B liposomal—*AmBisome* (Fujisawa)

*ampicillin—*Principen* (Bristol-Myers Squibb), others

ampicillin/sulbactam—*Unasyn* (Pfizer)

amprenavir—*Agenerase* (Glaxo Wellcome)

Ancef (SK Beecham)—cefazolin

Ancobon (Roche)—flucytosine

Antiminth (Pfizer)—pyrantel pamoate

Aoracillin B (Vita Elixir)—penicillin V

Aralen (Sanofi)—chloroquine

†*Arsobal* (Aventis, France)—melarsoprol

artemether—*Artenam* (Arenco, Belgium)

atovaquone—*Mepron* (Glaxo Wellcome)

atovaquone/proguanil—*Malarone* (Glaxo Wellcome)

Augmentin (SK Beecham)—amoxicillin/clavulanic acid

Avelox (Bayer)—moxifloxacin

Azactam (Bristol-Myers Squibb)—aztreonam

AZT—see zidovudine

azithromycin—*Zithromax* (Pfizer)

aztreonam—*Azactam* (Bristol-Myers Squibb)

Bactrim (Roche)—trimethoprim-sulfamethoxazole

Beepen-VK (SK Beecham)—penicillin V

†benznidazole—*Rochagan* (Roche, Brazil)

Biaxin (Abbott)—clarithromycin

Bicillin LA (Wyeth-Ayerst)—penicillin G benzathine

Biltricide (Bayer)—praziquantel

Bio-cef (Intl Ethic Lab)—cephalexin

†bithionol—*Bitin* (Tanabe, Japan)

†*Bitin*—bithionol (Tanabe, Japan)

Brodspec (Truxton)—tetracycline HCl

butoconazole—*Femstat* (Bayer)

Capastat (Dura)—capreomycin

capreomycin—*Capastat* (Dura)

Ceclor (Lilly)—cefaclor

cefaclor—*Ceclor* (Lilly)

Cedax (Schering)—ceftibuten

*cefadroxil—*Duricef* (Bristol-Myers Squibb), others

Cefadyl (Bristol-Myers Squibb)—cephapirin

cefamandole—*Mandol* (Lilly)

*cefazolin—*Ancef* (SK Beecham), others

cefdinir—*Omnicef* (Parke-Davis)

cefepime—*Maxipime* (Bristol-Myers Squibb)

cefixime—*Suprax* (Lederle)

Cefizox (Fujisawa)—ceftizoxime

Cefobid (Pfizer)—cefoperazone

cefonicid—*Monocid* (SK Beecham)

cefoperazone—*Cefobid* (Pfizer)

Cefotan (Zeneca)—cefotetan

cefotaxime—*Claforan* (Aventis)

cefotetan—*Cefotan* (Zeneca)

cefoxitin—*Mefoxin* (Merck)

cefpodoxime—*Vantin* (Pharmacia & Upjohn)

cefprozil—*Cefzil* (Bristol-Myers Squibb)

ceftazidime—*Fortaz, Ceptaz* (Glaxo Wellcome), *Tazicef* (SK Beecham), *Tazidime* (Lilly)

ceftibuten—*Cedax* (Schering)

Ceftin (Glaxo Wellcome)—cefuroxime axetil

ceftizoxime—*Cefizox* (Fujisawa)

ceftriaxone—*Rocephin* (Roche)

cefuroxime—*Kefurox* (Lilly), *Zinacef* (Glaxo Wellcome)

cefuroxime axetil—*Ceftin* (Glaxo Wellcome)

Cefzil (Bristol-Myers Squibb)—cefprozil

*cephalexin—*Keflex* (Dista), others

cephapirin—*Cefadyl* (Bristol-Myers Squibb)

*cephradine—*Velosef* (Bristol-Myers Squibb), others

Ceptaz (Glaxo Wellcome)—ceftazidime

*chloramphenicol—*Chloromycetin* (Parke-Davis), others

Chloromycetin (Parke-Davis)—chloramphenicol

*chloroquine—*Aralen* (Sanofi), others

---

*Also available generically.
†Not commercially available in the United States.

*Also available generically.
†Not commercially available in the United States.

cidofovir—*Vistide* (Gilead)
Cinobac (Oclassen)—cinoxacin
*cinoxacin—*Cinobac* (Oclassen), others
Cipro (Bayer)—ciprofloxacin
ciprofloxacin—*Cipro* (Bayer)
Claforan (Aventis)—cefotaxime
clarithromycin—*Biaxin* (Abbott)
Cleocin (Pharmacia & Upjohn)—clindamycin
*clindamycin—*Cleocin* (Pharmacia & Upjohn), others
clofazimine—*Lamprene* (Novartis)
clotrimazole—*Mycelex* (Bayer)
*cloxacillin—generic
Cofatrim Fort (Ampharco)—trimethoprim-sulfamethoxazole
colistimethate—*Coly-Mycin* (Parke-Davis)
Coly-Mycin (Parke-Davis)—colistimethate
Combivir (Glaxo Wellcome)—lamivudine-zidovudine
Cotrim (Teva)—trimethoprim-sulfamethoxazole
crotamiton—*Eurax* (Westwood-Squibb)
Crixivan (Merck)—indinavir
†*Cryptaz* (Romark)—nitazoxanide
*cycloserine—*Seromycin* (Dura), others
Cytovene (Roche)—ganciclovir
ddC—see didanosine
ddI—see zalcitabine
*dapsone—generic (Jacobus)
Daraprim (Glaxo Wellcome)—pyrimethamine
Declomycin (Lederle)—demeclocycline
delavirdine—*Rescriptor* (Pharmacia & Upjohn)
demeclocycline—*Declomycin* (Lederle)
Denavir (SK Beecham)—penciclovir
*diclocacillin—*Dycill* (SK Beecham), others
didanosine—*Videx* (Bristol-Myers Squibb)
diethylcarbamazine—*Hetrazan* (Lederle)
Diflucan (Pfizer)—fluconazole
†diloxanide furoate—*Furamide* (Knoll, U.K.)
dirithromycin—*Dynabac* (Sanofi)
Doryx (Warner Chilcott)—doxycycline
*doxycycline—*Vibramycin* (Pfizer), others
Duricef (Bristol-Myers Squibb)—cefadroxil
Dycill (SK Beecham)—dicloxacillin
Dynabac (Sanofi)—dirithromycin
Dynapen (Bristol-Myers Squibb)—dicloxacillin
E.E.S. (Abbott)—erythromycin
efavirenz—*Sustiva* (DuPont)
†eflornithine—*Ornidyl* (Ilex Oncology)
Elimite (Allergan)—permethrin
Emtet-500 (EconoMed)—tetracycline HCl

E-Mycin (Knoll)—erythromycin
enoxacin—*Penetrex* (Aventis)
Epivir (Glaxo Wellcome) lamivudine
Ery-Tab (Abbott)—erythromycin
ERYC (Parke-Davis)—erythromycin
Erythrocin (Abbott)—erythromycin
*erythromycin—*Erythrocin* (Abbott), others
*erythromycin-sulfisoxazole—*Pediazole* (Ross/Abbott), others
Eryzole (Alra)—erythromycinsulfisoxazole
ethambutol—*Myambutol* (Lederle)
ethionamide—*Trecator-SC* (Wyeth-Ayerst)
Eurax (Westwood-Squibb)—crotamiton
Exelderm (Westwood-Squibb)—sulconazole
famciclovir—*Famvir* (SK Beecham)
Famvir (SK Beecham)—famciclovir
Fansidar (Roche)—pyrimethamine-sulfadoxine
†*Fasigyn* (Pfizer)—tinidazole
†*Fasinex* (Novartis Agribusiness)—triclabendazole
Femstat (Bayer)—butoconazole
Flagyl (Searle)—metronidazole
Floxin (Ortho-McNeill)—ofloxacin
fluconazole—*Diflucan* (Pfizer)
flucytosine—*Ancobon* (Roche)
Flumadine (Forest)—rimantadine
fomivirsen—*itravene* (Novartis)
Fortaz (Glaxo Wellcome)—ceftazidime
Fortovase (Roche)—saquinavir
foscarnet—*Foscavir* (Astra)
Foscavir (Astra)—foscarnet
fosfomycin—*Monurol* (Forest)
Fulvicin P/G (Schering)—griseofulvin
Fulvicin U/F (Schering)—griseofulvin
Fungizone (Bristol-Myers Squibb)—amphotericin B
Furacin (Roberts)—nitrofurazone
Furadantin (Dura)—nitrofurantoin
†*Furamide* (Knoll, U.K.)—diloxanide furoate
furazolidone—*Furoxone* (Roberts)
Furoxone (Roberts)—furazolidone
ganciclovir—*Cytovene* (Roche); *Vitrasert* (Chiron Vision)
Gantrisin (Roche)—sulfisoxazole
Garamycin (Schering)—gentamicin
gatifloxacin—*Tequin* (Bristol-Myers Squibb)
*gentamicin—*Garamycin* (Shering), others
†*Glucantime* (Aventis, France)—meglumine antimoniate
G-Mycin (Bolan)—gentamicin
Grifulvin V (Ortho)—griseofulvin

---

*Also available generically.
†Not commercially available in the United States.

Grisactin (Wyeth-Ayerst)—griseofulvin
*griseofulvin—*Fulvicin U/F* (Schering), others
Gris-PEG (Allergan)—griseofulvin
†*Halfan* (SK Beecham)—halofantrine
†halofantrine—*Halfan* (SK Beecham)
Hetrazan (Lederle)—diethylcarbamazine
Hiprex (Aventis)—methenamine hippurate
Hivid (Roche)—zalcitabine
Humatin (Parke-Davis)—paromomycin
hydroxychloroquine—*Plaquenil* (Sanofi)
Ilosone (Dista)—erythromycin estolate
imipenem-cilastatin—*Primaxin* (Merck)
indinavir—*Crixivan* (Merck)
Infergen (Amgen)—interferon alfacon-1
interferon alfa-2a—*Roferon-A* (Roche)
interferon alfa-2b—*Intron A* (Schering)
interferon alfa-n3—*Alferon N* (Interferon Sciences)
interferon alfacon-1—*Infergen* (Amgen)
Intron A (Schering)—interferon alfa-2b
Invirase (Roche)—saquinavir
*iodoquinol—*Yodoxin* (Glenwood), others
*isoniazid—*Nydrazid* (Bristol-Myers Squibb)
itraconazole—*Sporanox* (Janssen)
ivermectin—*Stromectol* (Merck)
*kanamycin—*Kantrex* (Bristol-Myers Squibb), others
Kantrex (Bristol-Myers Squibb)—kanamycin
Keflex (Dista)—cephalexin
Keftab (Dista)—cephalexin
Kefurox (Lilly)—cefuroxime
Kefzol (Lilly)—cefazolin
ketoconazole—*Nizoral* (Janssen)
lamivudine—*Epivir* (Glaxo Wellcome)
lamivudine-zidovudine—*Combivir* (Glaxo Wellcome)
†*Lampit* (Bayer, Germany)—nifurtimox
Lamprene (Novartis)—clofazimine
Lariam (Roche)—mefloquine
Ledercillin VK (Lederle)—penicillin V
levofloxacin—*Levaquin* (Ortho-McNeil)
Lincocin (Pharmacia & Upjohn)—lincomycin
*lincomycin—*Lincocin* (Pharmacia & Upjohn)
Lincorex (Hyrex)—lincomycin
†linezolid—*Zyvox* (Pharmacia & Upjohn)
lomefloxacin—*Maxaquin* (Searle)
Lorabid (Lilly)—loracarbef
loracarbef—*Lorabid* (Lilly)
Lyphocin (Lypho-Med)—vancomycin
Macrobid (Proctor & Gamble)—nitrofurantoin
Macrodantin (Proctor & Gamble)—nitrofurantoin

Malarone (Glaxo Wellcome)—atovaquone/proguanil
malathion—*Ovide* (Medicis)
Mandelamine (Warner Chilcott)—methenamine mandelate
Mandol (Lilly)—cefamandole
Marcillin (Marnel)—ampicillin
Maxaquin (Searle)—lomefloxacin
Maxipime (Bristol-Myers Squibb)—cefepime
mebendazole—*Vermox* (Janssen)
mefloquine—*Lariam* (Roche)
Mefoxin (Merck)—cefoxitin
†meglumine antimoniate—*lucantime* (Aventis, France)
†melarsoprol—*Arsobal* (Aventis, France)
meropenem—*Merrem* (Zeneca)
methenamine hippurate—*Hiprex* (Aventis), *Urex* (3M)
*methenamine mandelate—*Mandelamine* (Warner Chilcott), others
*metronidazole—*Flagyl* (Searle), others
Mezlin (Bayer)—mezlocillin
mezlocillin—*Mezlin* (Bayer)
*miconazole—*Monistat* (Ortho-McNeil), others
Minocin (Lederle)—minocycline
*minocycline—*Minocin* (Lederle), others
Mintezol (Merck)—thiabendazole
Monistat (Ortho-McNeil)—miconazole
Monodox (Oclassen)—doxycycline
Monurol (Forest)—fosfomycin
moxifloxacin—*Avelox* (Bayer)
Myambutol (Lederle)—ethambutol
Mycelex (Bayer)—clotrimazole
Mycobutin (Pharmacia & Upjohn)—rifabutin
Mycostatin (Bristol-Myers Squibb)—nystatin
My-E (Seneca)—erythromycin
nafcillin—*Unipen* (Wyeth-Ayerst)
*nalidixic acid—*NegGram* (Sanofi), others
Nallpen (Baxter)—nafcillin
Natacyn (Alcon)—natamycin
natamycin—*Natacyn* (Alcon)
Nebcin (Lilly)—tobramycin
NebuPent (Fujisawa)—pentamidine
NegGram (Sanofi)—nalidixic acid
nelfinavir—*Viracept* (Agouron)
*neomycin—many manufacturers
netilmicin—*Netromycin* (Schering)
Netromycin (Schering)—netilmicin
Neutrexin (US Bioscience)—trimetrexate
nevirapine—*Viramune* (Roxane)
†niclosamide—*Yomesan* (Bayer, Germany)
†nifurtimox—*Lampit* (Bayer, Germany)

---

*Also available generically.
†Not commercially available in the United States.

*Also available generically.
†Not commercially available in the United States.

Nilstat (Lederle)—nystatin

†nitazoxanide—*Cryptaz* (Romark)

*nitrofurantoin—*Macrodantin* (Proctor & Gamble), others

*nitrofurazone—*Furacin* (Roberts), others

Nix (Glaxo Wellcome)—permethrin

Nizoral (Janssen)—ketoconazole

norfloxacin—*Noroxin* (Merck)

Noroxin (Merck)—norfloxacin

Norvir (Abbott)—ritonavir

novobiocin—*Albamycin* (Pharmacia & Upjohn)

Nydrazid (Bristol-Myers Squibb)—isoniazid

*nystatin—*Mycostatin* (Bristol-Myers Squibb), others

Nystex (Savage)—nystatin

ofloxacin—*Floxin* (Ortho-McNeil)

Omnicef (Parke-Davis)—cefdinir

Omnipen (Wyeth-Ayerst)—ampicillin

†ornidazole—*iberal* (Hoffmann LaRoche, Switzerland)

†*Ornidyl* (Ilex Oncology)—eflornithine

oseltamivir—*Tamiflu* (Roche/Gilead)

Ovide (Medicis)—malathion

*oxacillin—generic

oxamniquine—*Vansil* (Pfizer)

oxytetracycline—*Terramycin* (Pfizer)

†*Paludrine* (Ayerst, Canada, ICI, U.K.)— proguanil

Panmycin (Pharmacia & Upjohn)—tetracycline HCl

paromomycin—*Humatin* (Parke-Davis)

Paser (Jacobus)—aminosalicylic acid

Pediazole (Ross/Abbott)—erythromycin-sulfisoxazole

penciclovir—*Denavir* (SK Beecham)

Penetrex (Aventis)—enoxacin

*penicillin G—many manufacturers

penicillin G benzathine—*Bicillin LA* (Wyeth-Ayerst), *Permapen* (Pfizer)

*penicillin G procaine—many manufacturers

*penicillin V—many manufacturers

Pentam 300 (Fujisawa)—pentamidine

*pentamidine isethionate—*Pentam 300* (Fujisawa), *NebuPent* (Fujisawa), others

†*Pentostam* (Glaxo Wellcome, U.K.)—sodium stibogluconate

Pen-V (Zenith Goldline)—penicillin V

Permapen (Pfizer)—penicillin G benzathine

*permethrin—*Elimite* (Allergan), *Nix* (Glaxo Wellcome)

piperacillin—*Pipracil* (Lederle)

piperacillin/tazobactam—*Zosyn* (Lederle)

Pipracil (Lederle)—piperacillin

Plaquenil (Sanofi)—hydroxychloroquine

*polymyxin B—generic

praziquantel—*Biltricide* (Bayer)

Priftin (Aventis)—rifapentine

primaquine phosphate (Sanofi)—generic

Primaxin (Merck)—imipenem-cilastatin sodium

Principen (Bristol-Myers Squibb)—ampicillin

†proguanil—*Paludrine* (Ayerst, Canada; ICI, U.K.)

Proloprim (Glaxo Wellcome)—trimethoprim

Pronto (Del)—pyrethrins with piperonyl butoxide

Protostat (Ortho-McNeil)—metronidazole

*pyrantel pamoate—*Antiminth* (Pfizer), others

*pyrazinamide—generic

*pyrethrins with piperonyl butoxide—*RID* (Pfizer), others

pyrimethamine—*Daraprim* (Glaxo Wellcome)

pyrimethamine-sulfadoxine—*Fansidar* (Roche)

*quinidine gluconate—many manufacturers

†quinine dihydrochloride

*quinine sulfate—many manufacturers

quinupristin–dalfopristin—*Synercid* (Aventis)

Rebetron (Schering)—ribavirin-interferon alfa-2b

Relenza (Glaxo Wellcome)—zanamivir

Rescriptor (Pharmacia & Upjohn)—delavirdine

Retrovir (Glaxo Wellcome)—zidovudine

ribavirin—*Virazole* (ICN)

ribavirin-interferon alpha-2b *Rebetron* (Schering)

RID (Pfizer)—pyrethrins with piperonyl butoxide

rifabutin—*Mycobutin* (Pharmacia & Upjohn)

Rifadin (Aventis)—rifampin

Rifamate (Aventis)—rifampinisoniazid

rifampin—*Rimactane* (Novartis), *Rifadin* (Aventis)

rifampin-isoniazid—*Rifamate* (Aventis)

rifapentine—*Priftin* (Aventis)

Rifater (Aventis)—rifampin, isoniazid and pyrazinamide

Rimactane (Novartis)—rifampin

rimantadine—*Flumadine* (Forest)

ritonavir—*Norvir* (Abbott)

Rocephin (Roche)—ceftriaxone

†*Rochagan* (Roche, Brazil)—benznidazole

Roferon-A (Roche)—interferon alfa-2a

†*Rovamycine* (Aventis)—spiramycin

saquinavir—*Fortovase; Invirase* (Roche)

Septra (Glaxo Wellcome)—trimethoprim-sulfamethoxazole

Seromycin (Lilly)—cycloserine

---

*Also available generically.

†Not commercially available in the United States.

†sodium stibogluconate—*Pentostam* (Glaxo Wellcome, U.K.)

Soxa (Vita Elixir)—sulfisoxazole

sparfloxacin—*Zagam* (Aventis)

spectinomycin—*Trobicin* (Pharmacia & Upjohn)

†spiramycin—*Rovamycine* (Aventis)

Sporanox (Janssen)—itraconazole

stavudine—*Zerit* (Bristol-Myers Squibb)

*streptomycin—generic

Stromectol (Merck)—ivermectin

sulconazole—*Exelderm* (Westwood-Squibb)

sulfatrim—trimethoprim-sulfamethoxazole

*sulfisoxazole—*Gantrisin* (Roche), others

Sumycin (Bristol-Myers Squibb)—tetracycline HCI

Suprax (Lederle)—cefixime

†suramin—(Bayer, Germany)

Suspen (Circle)—penicillin V

Sustiva (DuPont)—efavirenz

Symmetrel (Du Pont)—amantadine

Synercid (Aventis)—quinupristin-dalfopristin

Tamiflu (Roche/Gilead)—oseltamivir

TAO (Pfizer)—troleandomycin

Tazicef (SK Beecham)—ceftazidime

Tazidime (Lilly)—ceftazidime

Tequin (Bristol-Myers Squibb)—gatifloxacin

Terramycin (Pfizer)—oxytetracycline

Tetracap (Circle)—tetracycline HCI

Tetracon (Consolidated Midland)—tetracycline HCI

*tetracycline HCI—*Sumycin* (Bristol-Myers Squibb), others

thiabendazole—*Mintezol* (Merck)

†*Tiberal* (Hoffmann LaRoche, Switzerland)—ornidazole

Ticar (SK Beecham)—ticarcillin

ticarcillin—*Ticar* (SK Beecham)

ticarcillin/clavulanic acid—*Timentin* (SK Beecham)

†tinidazole—*Fasigyn* (Pfizer)

Timentin (SK Beecham)—ticarcillin/clavulanic acid

*tobramycin—*Nebcin* (Lilly), others

*tolnaftate—*Aftate* (Schering), others

Trecator-SC (Wyeth-Ayerst)—ethionamide

†triclabendazole—*Fasinex* (Novartis Agribusiness)

trifluridine—*Viroptic* (Glaxo Wellcome)

*trimethoprim—*Proloprim* (Glaxo Wellcome), others

*trimethoprim-sulfamethoxazole—*Bactrim* (Roche), *Septra* (Glaxo Wellcome), others

trimetrexate—*Neutrexin* (US Bioscience)

Trimox (Bristol-Myers Squibb)—amoxicillin

Trimpex (Roche)—trimethoprim

*trisulfapyrimidines—*Sultrin Triple Sulfa* (Ortho-McNeil), others

Trobicin (Pharmacia & Upjohn)—spectinomycin

troleandomycin—*TAO* (Pfizer)

trovafloxacin—*Trovan* (Pfizer)

Trovan (Pfizer)—trovafloxacin

Truxazole VK (Truxton)—sulfisoxazole

Truxcillin VK (Truxton)—penicillin V

Unasyn (Pfizer)—ampicillin/sulbactam

Unipen (Wyeth-Ayerst)—nafcillin

Urex (3M)—methenamine hippurate

valacyclovir—*Valtrex* (Glaxo Wellcome)

Valtrex (Glaxo Wellcome)—valacyclovir

Vancocin (Lilly)—vancomycin

Vancoled (Lederle)—vancomycin

*vancomycin—*Vancocin* (Lilly), others

Vansil (Pfizer)—oxamniquine

Vantin (Upjohn)—cefpodoxime

Veetids (Bristol-Myers Squibb)—penicillin V

Velosef (Bristol-Myers Squibb)—cephradine

Vermox (Janssen)—mebendazole

Vibramycin (Pfizer)—doxycycline

Vibra-Tabs (Pfizer)—doxycycline

vidarabine—*Vira-A* (Parke-Davis)

Videx (Bristol-Myers Squibb)—didanosine

Vira-A (Parke-Davis)—vidarabine

Virazole (ICN)—ribavirin

Viroptic (Glaxo Wellcome)—trifluridine

Vistide (Gilead)—cidofovir

Vitrasert (Chiron Vision)—ganciclovir

Vitravene (Novartis)—fomivirsen

Wesmycin (Wesley)—tetracycline HCI

Wycillin (Wyeth-Ayerst)—penicillin G

Wymox (Wyeth-Ayerst)—amoxicillin

Yodoxin (Glenwood)—iodoquinol

Yomesan (Bayer, Germany)—niclosamide

Zagam (Aventis)—parfloxacin

zalcitabine—*Hivid* (Roche)

zanamivir—*Relenza* (Glaxo Wellcome)

Zerit (Bristol-Myers Squibb)—stavudine

Ziagen (Glaxo Wellcome)—abacavir

zidovudine—*Retrovir* (Glaxo Wellcome)

zidovudine-lamivudine—*Combivir* (Glaxo Wellcome)

Zinacef (Glaxo Wellcome)—cefuroxime

Zithromax (Pfizer)—azithromycin

Zosyn (Lederle)—piperacillin/tazobactam

Zovirax (Glaxo Wellcome)—acyclovir

†*Zyvox* (Pharmacia & Upjohn)—linezolid

---

*Also available generically.
†Not commercially available in the United States.

*Also available generically.
†Not commercially available in the United States.

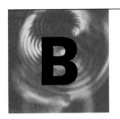

RECOMMENDED CHILDHOOD AND ADOLESCENT IMMUNIZATION SCHEDULE*

Each year, the Advisory Committee on Immunization Practices (ACIP) of the Centers for Disease Control and Prevention (CDC) reviews the recommended childhood and adolescent immunization schedule to ensure that it is current with changes in manufacturers' vaccine formulations and contains revised recommendations for the use of licensed vaccines, including those newly licensed. The recommended childhood immunization schedule for 2003 has remained the same in content and format since January 2002 (Figure B-1) (Centers for Disease Control and Prevention, 2002a). The recommendations and format have been approved by the ACIP, the American Academy of Family Physicians, and the American Academy of Pediatrics.

CATCH-UP CHILDHOOD AND ADOLESCENT IMMUNIZATION SCHEDULE

A new catch-up immunization schedule for children and adolescents who start late or who are >1 month behind is presented for the first time in 2003 (Tables B-1 and B-2). Minimum ages and minimum intervals between doses are provided for each of the routinely recommended childhood and adolescent vaccines. The schedule is divided into two age groups: children aged 4 months to 6 years and children/adolescents aged 7 to 18 years.

HEPATITIS B VACCINE

The schedule indicates a preference for administering the first dose of hepatitis B vaccine to all newborns soon after birth and before hospital discharge. Administering the first dose of

hepatitis B vaccine soon after birth should minimize the risk for infection caused by errors or delays in maternal hepatitis B surface antigen (HBsAg) testing or reporting, or by exposure to persons with chronic hepatitis B virus (HBV) infection in the household, and can increase the child's likelihood of completing the vaccine series. Only monovalent hepatitis B vaccine can be used for the birth dose. Either monovalent or combination vaccine can be used to complete the series. Four doses of hepatitis B vaccine can be administered to complete the series when a birth dose is given. In addition to receiving hepatitis B immune globulin (HBIG) and the hepatitis B vaccine series, infants born to HBsAg-positive mothers should be tested for HBsAg and antibody to HBsAg (anti-HBs) at age 9 to 15 months to identify those with chronic HBV infection or those who might require revaccination (Centers for Disease Control and Prevention, 1991).

INFLUENZA VACCINE

In addition to the recommendation to administer annual influenza vaccine to children at high risk, healthy children aged 6 to 23 months are encouraged to receive influenza vaccine when feasible. Children in this age group are at substantially increased risk for influenza-related hospitalizations (Centers for Disease Control and Prevention, 2002b).

INACTIVATED POLIOVIRUS VACCINE

The inactivated poliovirus (IPV) vaccine footnote has been removed from the Recommended Childhood and Adolescent Immunization Schedule, reflecting the cessation of the use of oral poliovirus (OPV) vaccine in the United States. An all-IPV schedule for routine childhood poliovirus vaccination has been recommended in the United States since January 1, 2000 (Centers

---

*Reprinted from Centers for Disease Control and Prevention: Recommended childhood and adolescent immunization schedule. MMWR January 31, 2003;52:Q1-Q4.

Recommended Childhood and Adolescent Immunization Schedule — United States, 2003

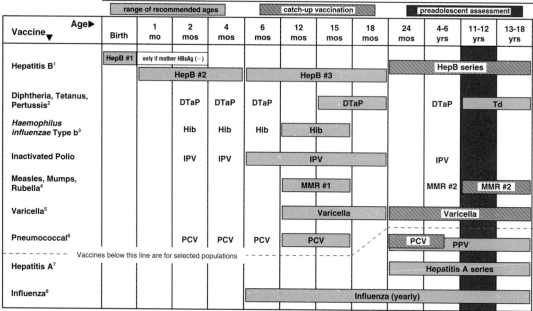

This schedule indicates the recommended ages for routine administration of currently licensed childhood vaccines, as of December 1, 2002, for children through age 18 years. Any dose not given at the recommended age should be given at any subsequent visit when indicated and feasible. ▨ Indicates age groups that warrant special effort to administer those vaccines not previously given. Additional vaccines may be licensed and recommended during the year. Licensed combination vaccines may be used whenever any components of the combination are indicated and the vaccine's other components are not contraindicated. Providers should consult the manufacturers' package inserts for detailed recommendations.

1. Hepatitis B vaccine (HepB). All infants should receive the first dose of hepatitis B vaccine soon after birth and before hospital discharge; the first dose may also be given by age 2 months if the infant's mother is HBsAg-negative. Only monovalent HepB can be used for the birth dose. Monovalent or combination vaccine containing HepB may be used to complete the series. Four doses of vaccine may be administered when a birth dose is given. The second dose should be given at least 4 weeks after the first dose, except for combination vaccines which cannot be administered before age 6 weeks. The third dose should be given at least 16 weeks after the first dose and at least 8 weeks after the second dose. The last dose in the vaccination series (third or fourth dose) should not be administered before age 6 months.

Infants born to HBsAg-positive mothers should receive HepB and 0.5 mL Hepatitis B Immune Globulin (HBIG) within 12 hours of birth at separate sites. The second dose is recommended at age 1-2 months. The last dose in the vaccination series should not be administered before age 6 months. These infants should be tested for HBsAg and anti-HBs at 9-15 months of age.

Infants born to mothers whose HBsAg status is unknown should receive the first dose of the HepB series within 12 hours of birth. Maternal blood should be drawn as soon as possible to determine the mother's HBsAg status; if the HBsAg test is positive, the infant should receive HBIG as soon as possible (no later than age 1 week). The second dose is recommended at age 1-2 months. The last dose in the vaccination series should not be administered before age 6 months.

2. Diphtheria and tetanus toxoids and acellular pertussis vaccine (DTaP). The fourth dose of DTaP may be administered as early as age 12 months, provided 6 months have elapsed since the third dose and the child is unlikely to return at age 15-18 months. **Tetanus and diphtheria toxoids (Td)** is recommended at age 11-12 years if at least 5 years have elapsed since the last dose of tetanus and diphtheria toxoid-containing vaccine. Subsequent routine Td boosters are recommended every 10 years.

3. *Haemophilus influenzae* type b (Hib) conjugate vaccine. Three Hib conjugate vaccines are licensed for infant use. If PRP-OMP (PedvaxHIB® or ComVax®[Merck]) is administered at ages 2 and 4 months, a dose at age 6 months is not required. DTaP/Hib combination products should not be used for primary immunization in infants at ages 2, 4 or 6 months, but can be used as boosters following any Hib vaccine.

4. Measles, mumps, and rubella vaccine (MMR). The second dose of MMR is recommended routinely at age 4-6 years but may be administered during any visit, provided at least 4 weeks have elapsed since the first dose and that both doses are administered beginning at or after age 12 months. Those who have not previously received the second dose should complete the schedule by the 11-12 year old visit.

5. Varicella vaccine. Varicella vaccine is recommended at any visit at or after age 12 months for susceptible children, i.e. those who lack a reliable history of chickenpox. Susceptible persons aged ≥13 years should receive two doses, given at least 4 weeks apart.

6. Pneumococcal vaccine. The heptavalent **pneumococcal conjugate vaccine (PCV)** is recommended for all children age 2-23 months. It is also recommended for certain children age 24-59 months. **Pneumococcal polysaccharide vaccine (PPV)** is recommended in addition to PCV for certain high-risk groups. See *MMWR* 2000;49(RR-9);1-38.

7. Hepatitis A vaccine. Hepatitis A vaccine is recommended for children and adolescents in selected states and regions, and for certain high-risk groups; consult your local public health authority. Children and adolescents in these states, regions, and high risk groups who have not been immunized against hepatitis A can begin the hepatitis A vaccination series during any visit. The two doses in the series should be administered at least 6 months apart. See *MMWR* 1999;48(RR-12);1-37.

8. Influenza vaccine. Influenza vaccine is recommended annually for children age 6 months with certain risk factors (including but not limited to asthma, cardiac disease, sickle cell disease, HIV, diabetes, and household members of persons in groups at high risk; see *MMWR* 2002;51(RR-3);1-31), and can be administered to all others wishing to obtain immunity. In addition, healthy children age 6-23 months are encouraged to receive influenza vaccine if feasible because children in this age group are at substantially increased risk for influenza-related hospitalizations. Children aged ≤12 years should receive vaccine in a dosage appropriate for their age (0.25 mL if age 6-35 months or 0.5 mL if aged 3 years). Children aged 8 years who are receiving influenza vaccine for the first time should receive two doses separated by at least 4 weeks.

For additional information about vaccines, including precautions and contraindications for immunization and vaccine shortages, please visit the National Immunization Program Website at www.cdc.gov/nip or call the National Immunization Information Hotline at 800-232-2522 (English) or 800-232-0233 (Spanish).

Approved by the Advisory Committee on Immunization Practices (www.cdc.gov/nip/acip), the American Academy of Pediatrics (www.aap.org), and the American Academy of Family Physicians (www.aafp.org).

Fig. B-1 Recommended childhood and adolescent immunization schedule—United States, 2003.

| TABLE B-1 | Catch-up Schedule for Children Ages 4 Months to 6 Years |

	MINIMUM INTERVAL BETWEEN DOSES			
Dose one (minimum age)	Dose one to dose two	Dose two to dose three	Dose three to dose four	Dose four to dose five
DTaP (6 weeks)	4 weeks	4 weeks	6 months	6 months[1]
IPV (6 weeks)	4 weeks	4 weeks	4 weeks[2]	
HepB[3] (birth)	4 weeks	8 weeks (and 16 weeks after first dose)		
MMR (12 months)	4 weeks[4]			
Varicella (12 months)				
Hib[5] (6 weeks)	4 weeks: if first dose given at age <12 months 8 weeks (as final dose): if first dose given at age 12 to 14 months No further doses needed: if first dose given at age ≥15 months	4 weeks[6]: if current age <12 months 8 weeks (as final dose)[6]: if current age ≥12 months and second dose given at age <15 months No further doses needed: if previous dose given at age ≥15 months	8 weeks (as final dose): this dose only necessary for children aged 12 months to 5 years who received 3 doses before age 12 months	
PCV[7] (6 weeks)	4 weeks: if first dose given at age <12 months and current age <24 months 8 weeks (as final dose): if first dose given at age ≥12 months or current age 24 to 59 months No further doses needed: for healthy children if first dose given at age ≥24 months	4 weeks: if current age <12 months 8 weeks (as final dose): if current age ≥12 months No further doses needed: for healthy children if previous dose given at age ≥24 months	8 weeks (as final dose): this dose only necessary for children aged 12 months to 5 years who received 3 doses before age 12 months	

[1]**Diphtheria and tetanus toxoids and acellular pertussis vaccine (DTaP):** The fifth dose is not necessary if the fourth dose was given after the fourth birthday.

[2]**Inactivated Polio (IPV):** For children who received an all-IPV or all-OPV series, a fourth dose is not necessary if third dose was given at age ≥4 years. If both OPV and IPV were given as part of a series, a total of 4 doses should be given, regardless of the child's current age.

[3]**Hepatitis B vaccine (HepB):** All children and adolescents who have not been vaccinated against hepatitis B should begin the hepatitis B vaccination series during any visit. Providers should make special efforts to immunize children who were born in areas of the world where hepatitis B virus infection is moderately or highly endemic.

[4]**Measles, mumps, and rubella vaccine (MMR):** The second dose of MMR is recommended routinely at age 4 to 6 years, but should be given earlier if desired.

[5]*Haemophilus influenzae* **type b (Hib):** Vaccine is not recommended generally for children aged ≥5 years.

[6]**Hib:** If current age is <12 months and the first 2 does were PRP-OMP (PedvaxHIB or ComVax [Merck]), the third (and final) dose should be given at age 12 to 15 months and at least 8 weeks after the second dose.

[7]**Pneumococcal conjugate vaccine (PCV):** Vaccine is not recommended generally for children aged ≥5 years.

Continued

TABLE B-2	Catch-up Schedule for Children Aged 7 to 18 Years—cont'd		
MINIMUM INTERVAL BETWEEN DOSES			
Dose one to dose two		*Dose two to dose three*	*Dose three to booster dose*
Td:	4 weeks	Td: 6 months	Td[1] 6 months: if first dose given at age <12 months and current age <11 years 5 years: if first dose given at age ≥12 months and third dose given at age <7 years and current age ≥11 years 10 years: if third dose given at age ≥7 years
IPV[2]:	4 weeks	IPV[2]: 4 weeks	IPV
HepB:	4 weeks	HepB: 8 weeks (and 16 weeks after first dose)	
MMR:	4 weeks		
Varicella[3]:	4 weeks		

[1]**Tetanus toxoids:** For children aged 7-10 years, the interval between the third and booster dose is determined by the age when the first dose was given. For adolescents aged 11-18 years, the interval is determined by the age when the third dose was given.

[2]**Inactivated Polio (IPV):** Vaccine is not recommended generally for persons aged ≥18 years.

[3]**Varicella:** Give 2-dose series to all susceptible adolescents aged ≥13 years.

for Disease Control and Prevention, 2001). All children should receive four doses of IPV at ages 2, 4, and 6 to 18 months and 4 to 6 years. For children who received an all-IPV or all-OPV series, a fourth dose is not necessary if the third dose was administered at age ≥4 years. If both OPV and IPV were administered as part of a series, a total of four doses should be administered regardless of the child's current age. These statements clarify the "Dose Three to Booster Dose" column in Table B-2 of the catch-up schedule. Routine poliovirus vaccination is not generally recommended for persons aged ≥18 years residing in the United States (Centers for Disease Control and Prevention, 1999).

VACCINE SUPPLY RECOMMENDATIONS

As a result of the vaccine supply shortage, deferral of some doses of pneumococcal conjugate vaccine (PCV) has been recommended (Centers for Disease Control and Prevention, 2000); health-care providers should record patients for whom vaccination has been deferred and should contact them once the supply has been restored. Supplies of tetanus and diphtheria toxoids (Td) vaccine; diphtheria and tetanus toxoids and acellular pertussis (DTaP) vaccine; measles, mumps, and rubella (MMR)

vaccine; and varicella vaccine in the United States have become sufficient to permit the resumption of the routine schedule for use as recommended by ACIP (Centers for Disease Control and Prevention, 2002c; Centers for Disease Control and Prevention, 2002d; Centers for Disease Control and Prevention, 2002e). The range of recommended ages for the Td vaccine has been extended to 18 years to emphasize that the vaccine can be administered during any visit if at least 5 years have elapsed since the last dose of tetanus and diphtheria toxoid—containing vaccine. Information about vaccine shortages is available from the CDC's National Immunization Program at http://www.cdc.gov/nip/news/shortages/default.htm.

VACCINE INFORMATION STATEMENTS

The National Childhood Vaccine Injury Act requires that all health-care providers give parents or patients copies of Vaccine Information Statements before administering each dose of the vaccines listed in the schedule. Additional information is available from state health departments and at http://www.cdc.gov/nip/publications/vis. Detailed recommendations for using vaccines are available from the manufacturers' package inserts, ACIP statements on specific vaccines, and the *2003 Red Book*

(American Academy of Pediatrics, 2003). ACIP statements for each recommended childhood vaccine can be viewed, downloaded, and printed from the CDC's National Immunization Program at http://www.cdc.gov/nip/publications/acip-list.htm; instructions on the use of the Vaccine Information Statements are available at http://www.cdc.gov/nip/publications/vis/vis-instructions.pdf.

REFERENCES

American Academy of Pediatrics. Active and passive immunization. In Pickering LK (ed). 2003 Red Book: Report of the Committee on Infectious Diseases, ed 26. Elk Grove Village, Ill: American Academy of Pediatrics, 2003.

Centers for Disease Control and Prevention. Hepatitis B virus: a comprehensive strategy for eliminating transmission in the United States through universal childhood vaccination: recommendations of the Advisory Committee on Immunization Practices (ACIP). MMWR Recomm Rep 1991;40.

Centers for Disease Control and Prevention. Recommendations of the Advisory Committee on Immunization Practices: revised recommendations for routine poliomyelitis vaccination. MMWR Morb Mortal Wkly Rep 1999; 48:590.

Centers for Disease Control and Prevention. Poliovirus prevention in the United States: updated recommendations of the Advisory Committee on Immunization Practices (ACIP). MMWR Recomm Rep 2000;49.

Centers for Disease Control and Prevention. Updated recommendations on the use of pneumococcal conjugate vaccine in a setting of vaccine shortage—Advisory Committee on Immunization Practices. MMWR Morb Mortal Wkly Rep 2001;50:1140-1142.

Centers for Disease Control and Prevention. Recommended childhood immunization schedule—United States, 2002. MMWR Morb Mortal Wkly Rep 2002a; 51: 31-33.

Centers for Disease Control and Prevention. Prevention and control of influenza: recommendations of the Advisory Committee on Immunization Practices (ACIP). MMWR Recomm Rep 2002b;51.

Centers for Disease Control and Prevention. Resumption of routine schedule for tetanus and diphtheria toxoids. MMWR Morb Mortal Wkly Rep 2002c;51:529-530.

Centers for Disease Control and Prevention. Resumption of routine schedule for diphtheria and tetanus toxoids and acellular pertussis vaccine and for measles, mumps, and rubella vaccine. MMWR Morb Mortal Wkly Rep 2002d;51:598-599.

Centers for Disease Control and Prevention. Resumption of routine schedule for varicella vaccine. MMWR Morb Mortal Wkly Rep 2002e;51:679.

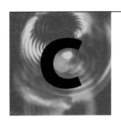

SEVERE ACUTE RESPIRATORY SYNDROME (SARS)

In late 2002, cases of a severe atypical pneumonia of unknown etiology were reported in Guangdong province of the People's Republic of China. Similar cases were subsequently detected in individuals in Hong Kong, Vietnam, and Canada during February and March of 2003, and the World Health Organization (WHO) issued a global alert for this illness, which was designated "severe acute respiratory syndrome" or SARS (WHO, 2003; MMWR, 2003). SARS was transmitted to household contacts and to healthcare workers who had cared for SARS patients, and the disease rapidly spread to over 25 countries and sickened thousands of individuals by April 2003. The global medical and scientific communities engaged in a truly cooperative effort that led with remarkable speed to progress in understanding and diagnosing this disease (Gerberding, 2003). It is hoped that this worldwide collaborative effort will lead in short order to strategies for prevention and treatment. Although the information in this chapter is current as of June 2003, progress is being made at record speed in this area and clearly much more will be known shortly. The Centers for Disease Control and Prevention (CDC) SARS website (http://www.cdc.gov/ncidod/sars/index.htm) is an excellent source for current information.

ETIOLOGY

In March 2003 a novel coronavirus was identified in association with cases of SARS (Peiris et al., 2003; Ksiazek et al., 2003; Drosten et al., 2003; Poutanen et al, 2003). The complete sequence of the SARS coronavirus (SARS-CoV) was determined (Rota et al., 2003; Marra et al., 2003), and initial characterization of the genome has been carried out (Rota et al, 2003). In addition, a paramyxovirus was isolated from several patients with SARS (Hassler et al., 2003) and the possible role of this virus in the development of

SARS has not yet been determined. Inoculation of monkeys with the SARS-associated coronavirus caused interstitial pneumonitis, and the virus could be isolated from the respiratory tract of the animals, proving that SARS-CoV causes SARS (Fouchier et al., 2003).

EPIDEMIOLOGY

SARS appears to spread primarily by close person-to-person contact. The incubation period is 2 to 10 days. Most cases of SARS thus far have been identified in individuals who cared for or lived with a patient, or had direct contact with infectious material from an infected person. It is also possible that certain individuals are "super spreaders" who transmit the virus widely before they can be identified and isolated.

CLINICAL MANIFESTATIONS

In general, SARS begins with a fever greater than 100.4° F (>38.0° C). Other symptoms may include headache, malaise, body aches, and mild respiratory symptoms. After 2 to 7 days, SARS patients may develop a dry cough and dyspnea. After 3 to 7 days, a lower respiratory phase begins with the onset of a dry, nonproductive cough or dyspnea, which might be accompanied by or progress to hypoxemia. The case-fatality rate among persons with illness meeting the current WHO case definition of SARS is thought to be between 4% and 50% and has not yet been adequately determined. Chest radiographs may be normal during the febrile prodrome; however, in a substantial proportion of patients the respiratory phase is characterized by focal interstitial infiltrates progressing to generalized, patchy, interstitial infiltrates. Some chest radiographs from patients in later stages of disease have shown areas of consolidation. At the peak of the respiratory illness, approximately 50% of patients have leukopenia and thrombocytopenia or low-normal platelet counts. Early in the respiratory phase, elevated creatine phosphokinase levels and hepatic transaminases (two to six times the upper limits of normal) have been noted (MMWR, 2003).

PATHOGENESIS

At the time of this writing (June 2003) the pathogenesis of SARS is still poorly understood. The infection results in an acute interstitial pneumonia, with the consequences described above, in some cases progressing to fatal lung disease (Nicholls et al., 2003). The immune response is not fully characterized and includes neutralizing antibodies with a possible cytotoxic lymphocyte (CTL) component. Virus can be shed in respiratory secretions, feces, and urine (Peiris et al., 2003; Drosten et al., 2003) and the duration of shedding has not yet been determined. It is not yet known whether persistent infection is established, and whether individuals are susceptible to reinfection. The possible contribution of immunopathology is not yet understood; however, in 10% of patients the interstitial pneumonitis is followed by progressive alveolar damage, and corticosteroids have been used in an attempt to decrease progression of this disease (Lee et al., 2003; Peiris et al., 2003; Chan-Yeung and Yu, 2003; Ksiazek et al., 2003).

DIAGNOSIS

Initial diagnostic testing for suspected SARS patients should include testing for viral respiratory pathogens in addition to SARS-CoV, notably influenza A and B and respiratory syncytial virus (RSV). Other studies should include a chest radiograph, pulse oximetry, blood cultures, and Gram's stain and culture of sputum. Clinicians should save available clinical specimens for additional testing until a specific diagnosis is made. Acute and convalescent (greater than 21 days after onset of symptoms) serum samples should be collected from each patient who meets the SARS case definition. At the time of this writing, paired sera and other clinical specimens can be forwarded through state and local health departments for testing at CDC. Specific instructions for collecting specimens from suspected SARS patients are available on the CDC web site listed above.

WHO/CDC CRITERIA

As of this writing, the WHO and CDC have established clinical, epidemiological, and laboratory criteria for the diagnosis of SARS. These are likely to be modified, but represent the state of understanding as of June 2003.

The clinical criteria for diagnosis are either mild or moderate respiratory illness with temperature of >100.4° F (>38° C), and one or more clinical findings of respiratory illness (e.g., cough, shortness of breath, difficulty breathing, or hypoxia). In the case of severe respiratory illness, the criteria include temperature of >100.4° F (>38° C), and one or more clinical findings of respiratory illness (e.g., cough, shortness of breath, difficulty breathing, or hypoxia), along with radiographic evidence of pneumonia, or respiratory distress syndrome, or autopsy findings consistent with pneumonia or respiratory distress syndrome without an identifiable cause. The epidemiologic criteria include travel (including transit in an airport) within 10 days of onset of symptoms to an area with current or previously documented or suspected community transmission of SARS, or close contact (within 10 days of onset of symptoms) with a person known or suspected to have SARS. The laboratory criteria for confirming the diagnosis include detection of antibody to SARS-CoV in specimens obtained during acute illness or more than 21 days after illness onset, detection of SARS-CoV RNA by RT-PCR confirmed by a second PCR assay (by using a second aliquot of the specimen and a different set of PCR primers), or isolation of SARS-CoV.

INFECTION CONTROL MEASURES

Rapid institution of rigorous infection control measures (Garner, 1996) has been critical in controlling the global and local spread of SARS. Patients with SARS pose a significant risk of transmission to close household contacts and healthcare personnel in close contact. Clinicians evaluating suspected cases should use standard precautions (hand hygiene) together with airborne (N-95 respirator) and contact (gowns and gloves) precautions, and refer to the updated infection control guidelines on the CDC website. At the time of writing, and until the mode of transmission has been better defined, eye protection also should be worn for all patient contact. For family members caring for a person with SARS, the CDC has developed interim infection control recommendations for patients with suspected SARS in the household, which will be updated regularly. These basic precautions should be followed for 10 days after respiratory symptoms and fever are gone. During that time, SARS patients should limit interactions outside the home (not go to work, school, or other public areas). The duration of time before or after onset of symptoms during which a patient with SARS can transmit the disease to others is unknown.

TRAVEL

Because of the rapid worldwide spread of SARS and the local geographic outbreaks, travel recommendations were rapidly developed. For individuals who must travel to an area with SARS, the CDC currently advises that travelers in an area with SARS wash their hands frequently and avoid close contact with large numbers of people as much as possible to minimize the possibility of infection. CDC does not currently recommend the routine use of masks or other personal protective equipment while in public areas (WHO, Wkly Epidemiol Rec, 2003).

TREATMENT AND PROPHYLAXIS

No specific treatment recommendations are yet available. There are currently no approved antiviral drugs that are effective against coronaviruses. Empiric therapy should include coverage for organisms associated with any community-acquired pneumonia of unclear etiology, including agents with activity against both typical and atypical respiratory pathogens. For the future, there are several steps in the coronavirus life cycle that could be targeted in order to develop antiviral strategies (Holmes and Enjuanes, 2003; Holmes, 2003; Anand et al., 2003). Coronavirus infection is initiated when the viral envelope spike protein binds to a cellular receptor, and this step, or the subsequent conformational change in the spike protein that results in fusion of the virus with the cell, could be targeted to prevent viral entry. Other targets may include the viral protease that cleaves the polyprotein encoded by the polymerase gene, the particular discontinuous RNA transcription carried out by this virus to replicate the RNA genome, virus assembly via the endocytic pathway, or the serine protease that may be required for cleavage activation of the spike glycoproteins. Passive immunization with convalescent serum, or administration of neutralizing antibodies against the coronavirus spike protein, are strategies that may be considered in an effort to prevent SARS in high-risk individuals (Holmes, 2003). Control of SARS in the future will likely await the development of vaccines. Live attenuated vaccines have been developed against coronaviruses of other animals and it is to be hoped that similar vaccines can be developed for SARS-CoV (Holmes, 2003).

REFERENCES

Anand K, Ziebuhr J, Wadhwani P, et al. Coronavirus main proteinase (3CLpro) structure: basis for design of anti-SARS drugs. Science. May 13, 2003.

Chan-Yeung M, Yu WC. Outbreak of severe acute respiratory syndrome in Hong Kong Special Administrative Region: case report. BMJ 2003;326:850-852.

Drosten C, Gunther S, Preiser W, et al. Identification of a novel coronavirus in patients with severe acute respiratory syndrome. N Engl J Med 2003;348(20):1967-1976; Epub 2003 Apr 10.

Fouchier RAM et al. Aetiology: Koch's postulates fulfilled for SARS virus. Nature 2003;423:240.

Garner JS and the Hospital Infection Control Practices Advisory Committee. Guideline for isolation precautions in hospitals. Part I. Evolution of isolation practices, Hospital Infection Control Practices Advisory Committee. Am J Infect Control 1996;24:24-52.

Gerberding JL. Faster. But fast enough? Responding to the epidemic of severe acute respiratory syndrome. N Engl J Med 2003;348(20):2030-2031, Epub 2003 Apr 02.

Hassler D, Schwarz TF, Braun R. [SARS: a new paramyxovirus or coronavirus?] Dtsch Med Wochenschr 2003; 128(15):786.

Holmes KV, Enjuanes L. Virology: the SARS coronavirus: a postgenomic era. Science 2003;300(5624):1377-1378.

Holmes KV. SARS coronavirus: a new challenge for prevention and therapy. J Clin Invest 2003;111:1605.

Ksiazek TG, Erdman D, Goldsmith CS, et al. A novel coronavirus associated with severe acute respiratory syndrome. N Engl J Med 2003;348(20):1953-1966.

Lee N, et al. A major outbreak of severe acute respiratory syndrome in Hong Kong. N Engl J Med 2003;348(20): 1986-1994. Epub 2003 Apr 07.

Marra MA, Jones SJ, Astell CR, et al. The Genome sequence of the SARS-associated coronavirus. Science 2003;300(5624):1399-1404.

MMWR Morb Mortal Wkly Rep. Preliminary clinical description of severe acute respiratory syndrome. 2003; 52:255-256.

Nicholls JM, Poon LL, Lee KC, et al. Lung pathology of fatal severe acute respiratory syndrome. Lancet 2003; 361(9371):1773-1778.

Peiris JS, Lai ST, Poon LL, et al. Coronavirus as a possible cause of severe acute respiratory syndrome. Lancet 2003;361(9366):1319-1325.

Poutanen SM, Low DE, Henry B, et al. Identification of severe acute respiratory syndrome in Canada. N Engl J Med 2003;348(20):1995-2005. Epub 2003 Mar 31.

Rota PA, Oberste MS, Monroe SS, et al. Characterization of a novel coronavirus associated with severe acute respiratory syndrome. Science 2003;300(5624):1394-1399.

WHO. Severe acute respiratory syndrome (SARS): multi-country outbreak. http://www.who.int/csr/don/2003_03-16/en/.

Wkly Epidemiol Rec. WHO recommended measures for persons undertaking international travel from areas affected by severe acute respiratory syndrome. Wkly Epidemiol Rec 2003;78:97-120.

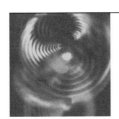

INDEX

A

Abacavir, 17
  adverse effects of, 960
  characteristics of, 952
  cost of, 950t
  dosage of, 974t-975t
Abdominal tuberculosis, 747-748
Abscess
  anorectal, 917-918
  appendiceal, 911
  brain, meningitis vs., 380
  intraabdominal, 903-906
  intracranial, 899-902
  peritonsillar, 657
  pilonidal, 893
  psoas, 915-917
  pyogenic liver, 911-913
  retroperitoneal, 914-915
  splenic, 913-914
  in urinary tract infection, 770
Abuse, sexual, 563-564
  bacterial vaginosis and, 598
  HIV infection and, 604
  human papillomavirus and, 601-602
  syphilis and, 588, 588t
  Trichomonas vaginalis and, 598t, 600
AC/HS test in toxoplasmosis, 717, 717t
AC/HSC, 727
Acanthamoeba keratitis, 175, 933t
Acellular vaccine, pertussis, 455-456
Acid-fastness of *Mycobacterium*, 732, 751-752
Acidosis
  cholera-related, 38-39
  in malaria, 347
Acoustic reflectometry, 421
Acquired immunodeficiency syndrome. *See also* Human immunodeficiency virus infection
  in adolescent, 9
  differential diagnosis of, 15-16
  epidemiology of, 6-9
  Epstein-Barr virus with, 153
  etiology of, 1-3
  laboratory diagnosis of, 5-6
  medical management of, 24-25
  pathogenesis of, 3-4
  pathology of, 4-5
  perinatal infection with, 7-8
  prognosis for, 25

Acquired immunodeficiency syndrome (*Continued*)
  prophylaxis for, 25-26
  toxoplasmosis in, treatment of, 723-724
  transfusion and coagulation factor acquired, 8-9
  treatment of, 16-22
Acrodermatitis, papular, 832-833
Actinobacillus, 102t
Actinomyces, bite wound and, 893
Actinomyces israelii, canaliculitis and, 163
Active hepatitis
  chronic, 822
  persistent, 822
  treatment of, 834-835
Active immunity
  to diphtheria toxin, 91
  to measles, 362
  to rubella, 535
Active immunization
  for mumps, 399-400
  varicella zoster and, 807-809
Acute endocarditis, 100-101
  clinical manifestations of, 104
  pathogenesis of, 101
Acute hepatitis, 830
Acute retinal necrosis, 178-179
Acyclovir
  adverse effects of, 960
  for cytomegalovirus prophylaxis, 64
  for herpes simplex virus infection, 268, 270-271, 271t, 273
  for herpesvirus 6, 284
  in immunocompromised host, 309
  for infectious mononucleosis, 152
  for neonatal sepsis, 554
  resistance to, 272
  for varicella zoster, 804-805
Adefovir
  characteristics of, 952-953
  for hepatitis, 836
Adenoid, enlarged, 424
Adenopathy in tuberculosis, 739f
Adenosine triphosphate in *Chlamydia trachomatis*, 589
Adenovirus
  enteric, 218, 218t
   epidemiology of, 220
  pneumonia caused by, 514
  urinary tract infection with, 770
Adenovirus keratitis, 175

Adhesin of *Staphylococcus*, 627-628
Adolescent
  Chlamydia trachomatis infection in, 590-592, 591t
   treatment of, 596
  gonococcal infection in, 568
  HIV infection in, 9
  human papillomavirus infection in, 603
  syphilis in, 586
  urinary tract infection in, 774, 780
Adverse drug effects, 960-972
Adverse reaction to hepatitis B vaccine, 846
Aedes mosquito, 74
Aeromonas infection
  clinical manifestations of, 211
  culture of, 215t
  epidemiology of, 207
  gastroenteritis caused by, 202
  pathology of, 9209
Agammaglobulinemia, 130
Age
  enterovirus and, 121
  Haemophilus influenzae type b and, 246-247
  hookworm and, 230
  Lyme disease and, 667
  rickettsialpox and, 681
  rubella and, 535-536
  tetanus and, 658
  tuberculosis and, 737
  urinary tract infection and, 778
Agglutinating antibody
  in tularemia, 673
  Vibrio cholerae and, 35
Agglutination
  in *Bordetella pertussis*, 444, 449
  Rocky Mountain spotted fever and, 680
  in toxoplasmosis, 714
Agglutinin in infectious mononucleosis, 149
AIDS. *See* Acquired immunodeficiency syndrome; Human immunodeficiency virus infection
AIDS-defining illness, 704-705
Airway obstruction
  in croup, 495
  tuberculosis causing, 736
Alanine aminotransferase
  in ehrlichiosis, 688